Abbreviations

Singular:

A.	=	Arteria
Lig.	=	Ligamentum
Ln.	=	Nodus lymphoideus
M.	=	Musculus
N.	=	Nervus
Proc.	=	Processus
R.	=	Ramus
V.	=	Vena
Var.	=	Variation

Plural:

Aa.	=	Arteriae
Ligg.	=	Ligamenta
Lnn.	=	Nodi lymphoidei
Mm.	=	Musculi
Nn.	=	Nervi
Procc.	=	Processus
Rr.	=	Rami
Vv.	=	Venae

Colour key

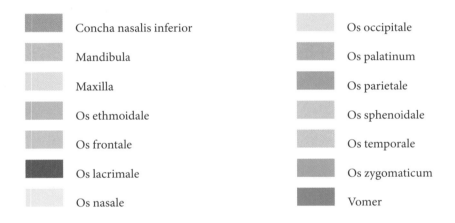

- Concha nasalis inferior
- Mandibula
- Maxilla
- Os ethmoidale
- Os frontale
- Os lacrimale
- Os nasale

- Os occipitale
- Os palatinum
- Os parietale
- Os sphenoidale
- Os temporale
- Os zygomaticum
- Vomer

For newborns, the following cranial bones are shown in the same colour:

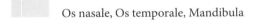

- Os nasale, Os temporale, Mandibula
- Maxilla, Os incisivum
- Os occipitale, Os palatinum

Edited by
J. Waschke, T.M. Böckers, F. Paulsen

Sobotta
ANATOMY TEXTBOOK

Edited by
Jens Waschke, Tobias M. Böckers, Friedrich Paulsen

Sobotta
ANATOMY TEXTBOOK
English edition with Latin nomenclature

First edition

With the assistance of:

Prof. Dr. Wolfgang Arnold, Witten
Prof. Dr. Ingo Bechmann, Leipzig
PD Dr. Anja Böckers, Ulm
Prof. Dr. Lars Bräuer, Erlangen
Prof. Dr. Faramarz Dehghani, Halle (Saale)
Prof. Dr. Thomas Deller, Frankfurt
Prof. Dr. Martin Gericke, Halle (Saale)
Prof. Dr. Bernhard Hirt, Tübingen

Dr. Martin Krüger, Leipzig
Dr. Daniela Kugelmann, Munich
Prof. Dr. Martin Scaal, Cologne
Prof. Dr. Dr. Michael J. Schmeißer, Magdeburg
Prof. Dr. Michael Scholz, Erlangen
PD Dr. Stephan Schwarzacher, Frankfurt
Prof. Dr. Volker Spindler, Basel
Prof. Dr. Andreas Vlachos, Freiburg

ELSEVIER

ELSEVIER

Hackerbrücke 6, 80335 Munich, Germany
Reply to books.cs.muc@elsevier.com

Original Publication:
Sobotta Anatomie – das Lehrbuch
© Elsevier GmbH, 2015.
All rights reserved.
ISBN 978-3-437-44080-9

This translation of Sobotta Anatomie – das Lehrbuch, 1st edition by Jens Waschke, Tobias M. Böckers and Friedrich Paulsen was undertaken by Elsevier GmbH.

ISBN 978-0-7020-6760-0
eISBN 978-0-7206-7617-4

All rights reserved
1st edition 2019
© Elsevier GmbH, Munich, Germany

Important note for the user
Medical knowledge is constantly evolving as a result of research and clinical experience. The editors and authors of this work have taken great care to ensure that the therapeutic information stated in this work (in particular with regard to therapeutic indications, dosages and adverse reactions) is fully up-to-date. This does not however mean that the users of this publication should refrain from consulting further written sources of information to check whether the details provided in such sources differ from those given in this publication, in order to responsibly prescribe a course of treatment. Protected trade names (trademarks) are usually marked as such (®). However, the lack of such identification does not automatically mean that the trade name is free.

The German National Library lists this publication in the German National Bibliography; detailed bibliographic data is available online at http://www.d-nb.de/.

19   20   21   22   23   5   4   3   2   1

For the copyright details of the images used, please see the picture credits.

In order not to disturb the flow of text, the grammatically masculine form has been used for patients and job titles. Of course this always refers to both women and men.

Content Strategist: Dr. Konstanze Knies, Susanne Szczepanek, Munich/Germany
Content Project Management: Martha Kürzl-Harrison, Munich/Germany
Translation: Lingo24 Ltd., Edinburgh/United Kingdom
Copyediting: Dr. rer med Steven Rand, Bissendorf/Germany; Marieke O'Connor, Oxford/United Kingdom
Proofreading: Carolyn Holleyman, Chorleywood/United Kingdom; Renate Hausdorf, Gräfelfing/Germany
Composed by: abavo GmbH, Buchloe/Germany; TNQ, Chennai/India
Printed and bound by: Drukarnia Dimograf Sp. z o. o., Bielsko-Biała/Poland
Cover Design: SpieszDesign, Neu-Ulm/Germany
Cover photo: Stephan Winkler, Munich/Germany

More information at **www.elsevier.com**

Preface

Anatomy is the study of the body's structure. The anatomical structure forms the morphological basis for functions. The combination of modern morphological methods with molecular biological, biochemical, biomechanical, bioinformatical and electrophysiological techniques have turned modern-day anatomy into functional, clinically orientated, structural research. Without the knowledge of anatomy, no functions can be deduced and without the knowledge of structure and function, no pathological changes can be understood.

- The question as to whether anything is still changing in anatomy often comes up, because we supposedly already know everything. This applies in particular to macroscopic anatomy and also to an anatomy textbook. So why do we need another anatomy textbook? In compiling this textbook, several issues were important to us:
- A textbook that works as closely as possible **in conjunction with an anatomy atlas** will facilitate learning. In doing so, we're continuing a tradition, since even the first issues of the Sobotta Atlas of Human Anatomy were accompanied by a manual. The fact that the textbook and atlas are put together by the same publisher, and that the editors of the atlas were also involved in the textbook, can only be an advantage. Within the field of neuroanatomy, we are very fortunate to have gathered numerous authors working as neuroanatomy researchers in the field of CNS, and who have thereby provided highly up-to-date and relevant content.
- The book is limited to **macroscopic anatomy** and related development (**embryology**) and refers to histological aspects only insofar as they are necessary for understanding macroscopic anatomy. This issue was important to us, since all students already have a book on histology and do not learn histology from an anatomy textbook.
- Most students do buy a separate book for **neuroanatomy**. The main reason for this is the fact that neuroanatomy is usually dealt with as a stand-alone course and in traditional anatomy textbooks is dealt with in different chapters. Usually, though, students cannot clearly understand the extent of the contents to be learned, nor where the details can be found in the book. In this textbook, neuroanatomy is displayed comprehensively and in its own section. Buying a stand-alone book on neuroanatomy is thereby no longer necessary.
- In the chapter 'Head' we have placed special emphasis on topics of interest to students of **dental medicine** and have displayed it in a clear and richly illustrated manner.
- Practical **case descriptions** show the relevance of anatomical knowledge to eventual clinical practice.
- The book intensively connects the macroscopic content **with functional and clinical aspects.** This means that students are not just learning about unalterable anatomy, but are also learning and transferring this knowledge within the context of their eventual profession as practical and clinically active doctors.
- Including suggestions on which skills are to be developed by studying the individual chapters, we consciously continue the current approaches of the new **National Competence Based Catalogues of Learning Objectives** for Undergraduate Medical Education (**NKLM**) and Dental Education (**NKLZ**).

Despite the new concept of this textbook, there is one thing it cannot do: it cannot do the learning for the students. Everyone must invest the time to learn. This textbook is designed to help facilitate learning through vivid representations of anatomical structures; we want to make you curious about your future career and present the contents in an exciting and interesting manner. It should be a welcome companion throughout all of your studies in human medicine, dentistry and molecular medicine.

We hope you enjoy the process.

Erlangen, Ulm, Munich, Summer of 2015
Friedrich Paulsen, Tobias M. Böckers and Jens Waschke

Acknowledgments

We would like to thank all our colleagues who contributed to the book as authors for the intense dedication, critical advice and great amount of time they have invested in the project.

As well as the authors, we would like to thank everyone at Elsevier who was involved in the planning process and release: we especially would like to thank Dr. Andrea Beilmann and Dr. Katja Weimann, who, with their many years of technical expertise took care of the book project as part of the Sobotta team. With their personal dedication they helped to guide it to its successful completion – the editors will miss the monthly telephone calls.

Our special thanks also to Martin Kortenhaus, who intensively edited all the chapters for the German edition, as well as our illustrators, who revised several images and created many new ones: Dr. Katja Dalkowski, Sonja Klebe, Jörg Mair and Stephan Winkler.

We would like to thank Sibylle Hartl for all aspects of production, Dr. Constance Spring and Dr Dorothea Hennessen for the overall coordination, as well as Alexandra Frntic and Elisa Imbery for the initial planning.

For the review and updating of chapter content we would very much like to thank Prof. Dr. Christopher Bohr (Department for Phoniatrics and Paediatric Audiology, University Clinic of Erlangen), Prof. (em.) Dr. Dr. h.c. Bodo Christ (Institute for Anatomy of the University of Freiburg), Prof. Dr. Christoph-Thomas Germer (Clinic and Polyclinic for General, Visceral, Vascular and Paediatric Surgery, University Clinic of Würzburg), Dr. Johannes Gottanka (Institute for Anatomy II, Friedrich-Alexander University of Nuremberg), Prof. Dr. Norbert Kleinsasser (University Clinic for Otolaryngology, Julius Maximilians University of Würzburg), Prof. Dr. Stephan Knipping (Clinic for ENT Medicine, Head & Neck Surgery, Städtisches Klinikum Dessau), Prof. Dr. Klaus Matzel (Coloproctology Department of Surgery, University of Erlangen), Prof. Dr. Felicitas Pröls (Institute for Anatomy II of the University of Cologne) and Dr. Nicolas Schlegel (Clinic and Polyclinic for General, Visceral, Vascular and Paediatric Surgery of the University Clinic of Würzburg). We are grateful to Dr. Gunther von Hagens (von Hagens Plastination, Guben) for allowing us to use the photographic documentation of plastinated palates, which form the basis for the illustrations in the chapter on the head/oral cavity and chewing apparatus, by Prof. Dr. Wolfgang Arnold. We are grateful to Dr. Stefanie Lescher and Prof. Dr. Joachim Berkefeldt (Neuroradiology, University Clinic of the Goethe University, Frankfurt) for the provision of neuroradiological images and helpful comments. We are grateful to Dr. Stephan Schwarzacher for his critical comments and critical review of chapter 13.9 Autonomic Nervous System. We are grateful to Dr. med. Tamas Sebesteny (Johannes Gutenberg University of Mainz, formerly: Goethe-University of Frankfurt) for creating excellent neuroanatomical specimens.

Erlangen, Ulm, Munich, Summer of 2015
Friedrich Paulsen, Tobias M. Böckers and Jens Waschke

List of editors and authors[1]

Editors

Prof. Dr. Jens Waschke
Ludwig Maximilians University of Munich
Institute of Anatomy – Department I
Pettenkoferstr. 11
80336 Munich

Prof. Dr. Tobias M. Böckers
University of Ulm
Institute of Anatomy and Cell Biology
Albert-Einstein-Allee 11
89081 Ulm

Prof. Dr. Friedrich Paulsen
Friedrich Alexander University
Erlangen-Nuremberg
Institute of Anatomy II
Universitätsstr. 19
91054 Erlangen

Authors

Prof. Dr. Wolfgang Arnold
University of Witten/Herdecke
Faculty of Dental, Mouth and Jaw Medicine
Alfred-Herrhausen-Str. 44
58455 Witten

PD Dr. Anja Böckers, MME
University of Ulm
Institute of Anatomy and Cell Biology
Albert-Einstein-Allee 11
89081 Ulm

Prof. Dr. Lars Bräuer
Friedrich Alexander University
of Nuremberg
Institute of Anatomy II
Universitätsstr. 19
91054 Erlangen

Prof. Dr. Faramarz Dehghani
Martin Luther University
of Halle-Wittenberg
Institute of Anatomy and Cell Biology
Große Steinstr. 52
06108 Halle (Saale)

Prof. Dr. Thomas Deller
Goethe University
Dr. Senckenbergische
Institute of Anatomy I
Clinical Neuroanatomy
Theodor-Stern-Kai 7
60590 Frankfurt

Dr. Martin Gericke
Leipzig University
Institute of Anatomy
Liebigstr. 13
04103 Leipzig

Prof. Dr. Bernhard Hirt
Eberhard Karls University of Tübingen
Institute of Anatomy
Sector of Macroscopic
and Clinical Anatomy
Elfriede-Aulhorn-Str. 8
72076 Tübingen

Dr. Martin Krüger
Leipzig University
Institute of Anatomy
Liebigstr. 13
04103 Leipzig

Dr. Daniela Kugelmann
Ludwig Maximilians University of Munich
Institute of Anatomy – Department I
Pettenkoferstr. 11
80336 Munich

Prof. Dr. Martin Scaal
University of Cologne
Institute of Anatomy II
Neuroanatomy and Macroscopic Anatomy
Joseph-Stelzmann-Str. 9
50931 Cologne

Dr. Dr. Michael J. Schmeißer
University of Ulm
Institute of Anatomy and Cell Biology
Albert-Einstein-Allee 11
89081 Ulm

Prof. Dr. Michael Scholz, MME
Friedrich Alexander University
of Erlangen-Nuremberg
Institute of Anatomy II
Universitätsstr. 19
91054 Erlangen

PD Dr. Stephan Schwarzacher
Goethe University
Dr. Senckenbergische Institute
of Anatomy I –
Clinical Neuroanatomy
Theodor-Stern-Kai 7
60590 Frankfurt

Prof. Dr. Volker Spindler
Ludwig Maximilians University of Munich
Institute of Anatomy – Department I
Pettenkoferstr. 11
80336 Munich

PD Dr. Andreas Vlachos
Goethe University
Dr. Senckenbergische
Institute of Anatomy I –
Clinical Neuroanatomy
Theodor-Stern-Kai 7
60590 Frankfurt

Contributors

Prof. Dr. Ingo Bechmann
Leipzig University
Institute of Anatomy
Liebigstr. 13
04103 Leipzig

---

[1] All editors and authors are located in Germany.

Picture credits

At the end of each caption for each image, a reference is given in square brackets to the relevant source for that image.

All charts and images not identified in this manner have been taken from the Sobotta Atlas of Human Anatomy, 23rd ed., Elsevier 2010, and previous editions, © Elsevier GmbH, Munich.

E347-09 Moore KL et al. The Developing Human. 9th ed. Saunders – Elsevier, 2011.

E402 Drake RL et al. Gray's Anatomy for Students. 1st ed. Churchill Livingstone – Elsevier, 2005.

E460 Drake RL et al. Gray's Atlas of Anatomy. 1st ed. Churchill Livingstone – Elsevier, 2008.

E581 Moore KL, Persaud TVN. The Developing Human. 7th ed. Saunders – Elsevier, 2003.

E838 Sharma R, Mitchell B. Embryology. 1st ed. Churchill Livingstone – Elsevier, 2005.

E943 Kanski YY. Clinical Ophthalmology. A Systematic Approach. 6th ed. Butterworth-Heinemann – Elsevier, 2007.

G210 Standring S. Gray's Anatomy. 40th ed. Churchill Livingstone – Elsevier, 2008.

G394 Schoenwolf G et al. Larsen's Human Embryology. 4th ed. Churchill Livingstone – Elsevier, 2008.

J787 Colourbox.com.

J787-023 Colourbox.com / Phovoir French Photolibrary.

J787-029 Colourbox.com / Pressmaster.

K340 Andreas Rumpf, Ottobrunn.

L106 Henriette Rintelen, Velbert

L126 Dr. Katja Dalkowski, Erlangen.

L127 Jörg Mair, Munich.

L141 Stefan Elsberger, Planegg.

L157 Susanne Adler, Lübeck.

L238 Sonja Klebe, Löhne.

L240 Horst Ruß, Munich.

L266 Stefan Winkler, Munich.

M375 Prof. Dr. Dr. Ulrich Welsch, Munich.

O541 Prof. Dr. Kurt Possinger, Medical Clinic and Outpatients' Clinic II specialising in Haematology and Oncology, Charité Mitte Campus, Berlin.

O932 Annegret Hegge, Osnabrück.

R234 Bruch HP, Trentz O. Berchtold Chirurgie. 6th ed. Urban & Fischer – Elsevier, 2008.

R235 Böcker W et al. Pathologie. 4th ed. Urban & Fischer – Elsevier, 2008.

R236 Classen M, Diehl V, Kochsiek K. Innere Medizin. 6th ed. Urban & Fischer, 2009.

R247 Deller T, Sebesteny T. Fotoatlas Neuroanatomie. 1st ed. Urban & Fischer – Elsevier, 2007.

R317 Trepel M. Neuroanatomie. 5th ed. Urban & Fischer – Elsevier, 2011.

S010-1-16 Benninghoff A. Anatomie, Vol. 1. 16th ed. Urban & Fischer, 2002.

S010-2-16 Benninghoff A. Anatomy, Vol. 2. 16th ed. Urban & Fischer – Elsevier, 2004.

S010-17 Benninghoff A, Drenckhahn D. Anatomie. Vol. 1. 17th ed. Urban & Fischer – Elsevier, 2008.

T719 Prof. Dr. Norbert Kleinsasser, ENT Clinic, University of Würzburg.

T785 Prof. Dr. Wolfgang Arnold, University Witten/Herdecke.

T786 Dr. Stefanie Lescher, Prof. Dr. Joachim Berkefeldt, Neuroradiology, University Clinic of the Goethe University, Frankfurt.

Table of contents

Table of contents

III INTERNAL ORGANS

IV HEAD AND THROAT

V NEUROANATOMY

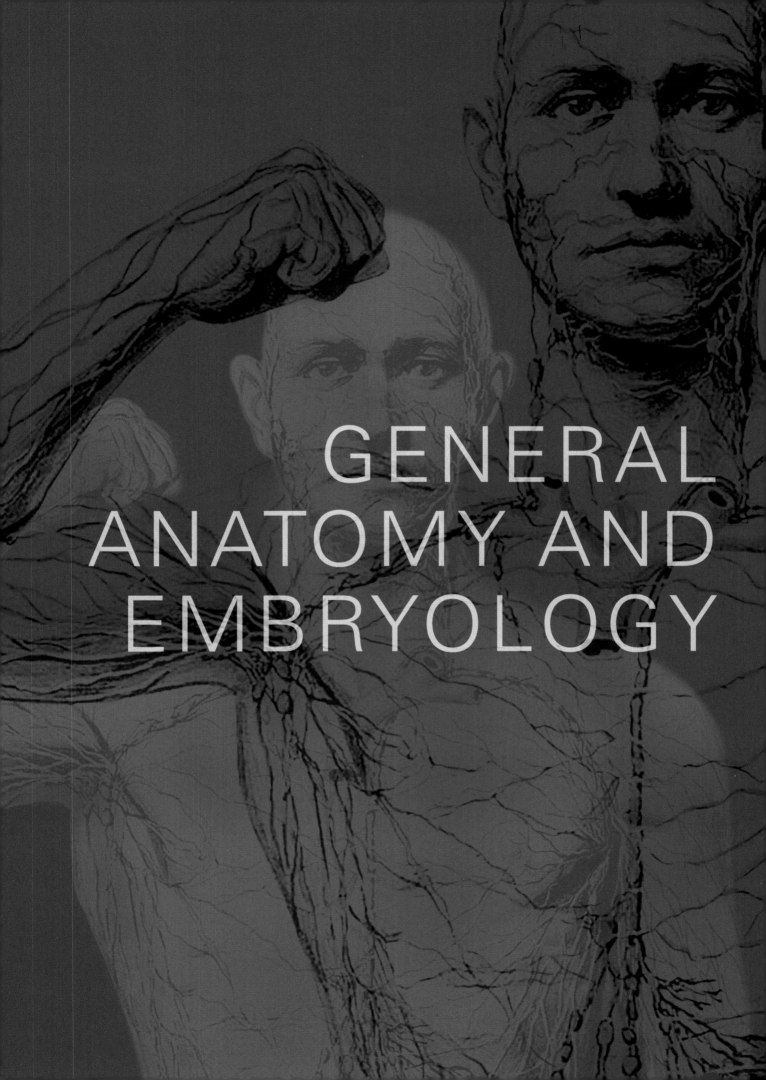

GENERAL ANATOMY AND EMBRYOLOGY

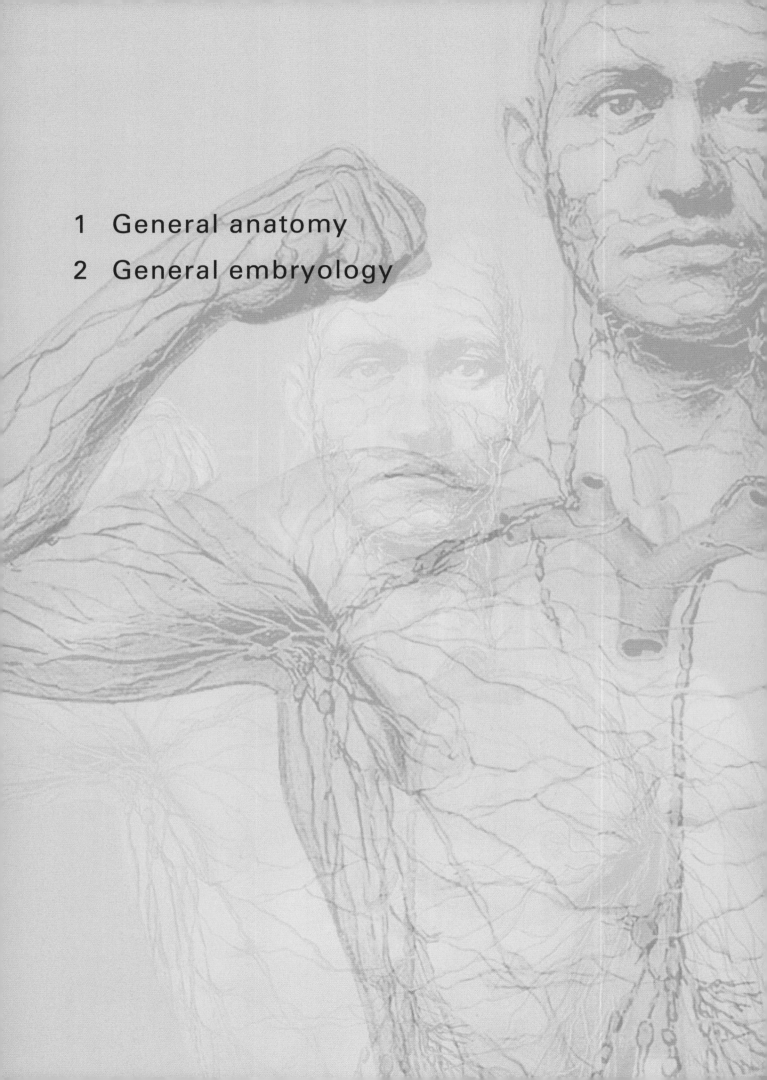

1 General anatomy

Friedrich Paulsen, Faramarz Dehghani

Gonarthrosis

Medical history

A 63-year-old patient has complained about increasing pain and restricted mobility of his left knee joint for several years. He had formerly practised a lot of sports. As a result, his menisci were lesioned twice. Painkillers no longer helped him, but caused increasingly stomach problems.

Initial examination

In the clinical examination it becomes apparent, among other things, that the left knee is slightly swollen and pressure on the medial joint space is painful. On mobilisation of the knee some friction noise (crepitus) can be felt and heard. The mobility is restricted. The knee can only be flexed up to approx. 80° and also cannot be fully stretched.

Further diagnostic

The radiological examination shows a significantly narrowed joint space, the bony tissue immediately below the cartilage is of higher density and there are small bone cysts. By appositional growth on the lateral side of the bone osteophytes (bony spurs) have been formed. The examination by the orthopaedist leads to the diagnosis of an advanced arthritis.

Treatment

Because of the relatively advanced pathology, the severely painful knee and its already restricted mobility, the orthopaedist advises the patient to undergo joint surface replacement. During the surgical procedure, the anterior region of the knee joint (Regio genus anterior) is opened by using a vertical incision of the skin and joint capsule. The direct view into the joint cavity confirms the diagnosis. The menisci are largely degenerated, the joint cartilage has almost completely disappeared, particularly on the medial side, and the underlying (subchondral) bone can already be seen. Also on the lateral side, two large lesions of the cartilage are visible. As the posterior surface of the patella looks macroscopically intact, the surgeons forego the replacement of the patellar cartilage. They perform a bicondylar surface replacement. In doing so, in contrast to the earlier frequently used total endoprosthesis of the knee joint, only the destroyed sliding surfaces of the joint are replaced, to sacrifice as little bone substance as possible. In addition, in the case of a bicondylar surface replacement, the replaced parts are not or only partially coupled to enable a more physiologic joint mobility.

Further development

Postoperatively the patient is already mobile on the 1st day. He receives special injections to prevent a thrombosis. A few days after the operation, the doctors detect that the lower leg is swollen. In this case, a lymphatic congestion (lymphoedema) had developed, which resolved within a few days by applying a lymphatic drainage. Twelve days after surgery, the suture staples were removed and the patient was discharged for the subsequent rehabilitative treatment. The subsequent rehabilitation is focused on an intense physical therapy for strengthening the muscles. The mobility was gradually increased and the coordination trained. Eight weeks later, the patient comes to the clinic for a follow-up examination. He has no more pain and can flex his knee now up to 95°. The scar is well healed, and he tells that he wants to attend dancing lessons in the near future.

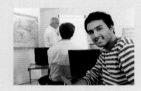

You may assist at your first operation as a trainee. The chief physician for orthopaedics is known for questioning his students on the patients, so you should prepare for the questions.

Question time in the surgery room!

<u>Hx:</u> 63-year-old patient (m), with increasing pain and restricted range of motion in his left knee for years; used to do a lot of sport → condition following a meniscus lesion. Improvement under pain medication ∅

CAVE: Stomach problems!

<u>CE:</u> Swelling left knee; range of motion: Flexion 80°, ∅ Fully consistent extension possible, crepitations, pain on pressure medial joint space

<u>DD.:</u> MRI/x-ray: joint gap narrowed, degenerated medial joint cartilage, densification of subchondral bone, bone cysts, osteophytes → **advanced gonarthrosis**

<u>TX:</u> bicondylar replacement of joint surfaces

After working through this chapter, you should be able to:
- classify the different parts of the human body and to define general anatomical terms
- categorise postnatal morphological changes, such as body proportions, body dimensions and sexual dimorphisms
- describe the structure of the skin and its appendages.
- understand the main features of the musculoskeletal system
- describe the various circulation systems
- define the structure of mucous membranes, glands and serous cavities
- categorise the nervous system clearly

Anatomy is derived of the Greek word *anatemnein* (cut open, dissect) and signifies **the art of dissecting.** It is a branch of morphology and deals with the structure of the healthy body (or in the broader sense of organisms) and is often referred to in conjunction with pathology and forensic medicine. However, pathology explores the emergence of structural changes in the body in the context of diseases, and forensic medicine (legal medicine) is concerned with the theory of development, diagnosis and assessment of legally relevant factors acting on the human body and deals with unexplained cases of death and injuries of victims.

1.1 Subdivisions

Anatomy is organised in various subdivisions:
- **Macroscopic anatomy:** describes the structures visible with the naked eye
- **Microscopic anatomy:** describes the structures that can be visualised by means of a light microscope or electron microscope
- **Molecular anatomy:** is linked to molecular biology, but pursues a morphological approach
- **Systematic anatomy:** groups the structures of the body into functionally related organ systems (e. g. the circulatory system)
- **Topographical anatomy:** describes the topographic relationship of individual structures according to their position to neighbouring structures
- **Functional anatomy:** describes the connections between structure and function
- **Descriptive anatomy:** pure description of the body architecture
- **Embryology:** describes all processes associated with the human development and therefore addresses the development of individual organisms (ontogenesis) (recent findings from early embryonic development show that interferences in this very sensitive [vulnerable] phase not only promote the emergence of well-known malformations, but are also responsible for numerous metabolic disorders in adulthood due to epigenetic modifications)
- **Comparative anatomy:** studies the body architecture of different animal species and compares it to that of humans; it allows an insight into the evolutionary history (phylogeny), which addresses the development of organs and organ functions in the course of evolution
- **Anatomy of living organisms:** uses anatomical knowledge on living organisms, e. g. when palpating bony points through the skin, feeling pulses, etc.; it serves as an intensive preparation for the future work with patients
- **Clinical anatomy:** connects the normal anatomy with diseases commonly encountered in the clinical practice; the clinical correlations originate in many different fields of medicine

Knowledge of human anatomy is fundamental for any practising doctor. The macroscopic anatomy plays a central role in the daily practical work on the patient. Apart from the (external) inspection of the body and the palpation (examination by touch) knowledge of the internal structures of the body plays a central role, e. g. for the evaluation of x-rays, CT and MRI scans, ultrasound and endoscopic findings, or in the context of operations, to be able to identify the relevant structures or to differentiate between 'sick' and 'healthy'. A standardised anatomical nomenclature used for the description is based on the Latin and Greek language. It consists of approx. 6 000 anatomical terms that are derived of about 600 linguistic (word) roots and have been summarised in the **Terminologia Anatomica,** an internationally valid nomenclature. In the teaching of anatomy, the dissection of a dead corpse has had a central role since ancient times. In modern times the dissection class is indispensable for medical students, because studying the anatomy of the real body can neither be replaced by anatomical models nor by images in an atlas. By dissections you get an idea of the shape, position and spatial relationships of the structures. The range of knowledge gained this way is supplemented by findings on the microscopic level of cells (cytology), tissues (histology) and organs (microscopic anatomy).

1.2 Architecture of the human body

1.2.1 Organisation

Topographical organisation
The human body is bilaterally symmetrical (➤ Fig. 1.1). It is divided topographically into:
- Head (Caput); represents the highest point of the upright body
- Neck (Collum)
- Trunk (Truncus)
- Chest (Thorax)
- Abdomen
- Pelvis
- Limbs (Membra)
- Upper limb (Membrum superius)
- Shoulder girdle
  - Clavicle (Clavicula)
  - Shoulder blade (Scapula)
  - Free upper limb
    - Upper arm (Brachium)
    - Forearm (Antebrachium)
    - Hand (Manus)
- Lower limb (Membrum inferius)
  - Pelvic girdle
  - Hip bone (Os coxae)
  - Sacrum (Os sacrum)
  - Free lower limb
    - Thigh (Femur)
    - Lower leg (Crus)
    - Foot (Pes)

Functional organisation
Dividing the body according to functions the following systems can be distinguished:
- Locomotor system (skeletal and muscular system)
- Respiratory system
- Circulatory system

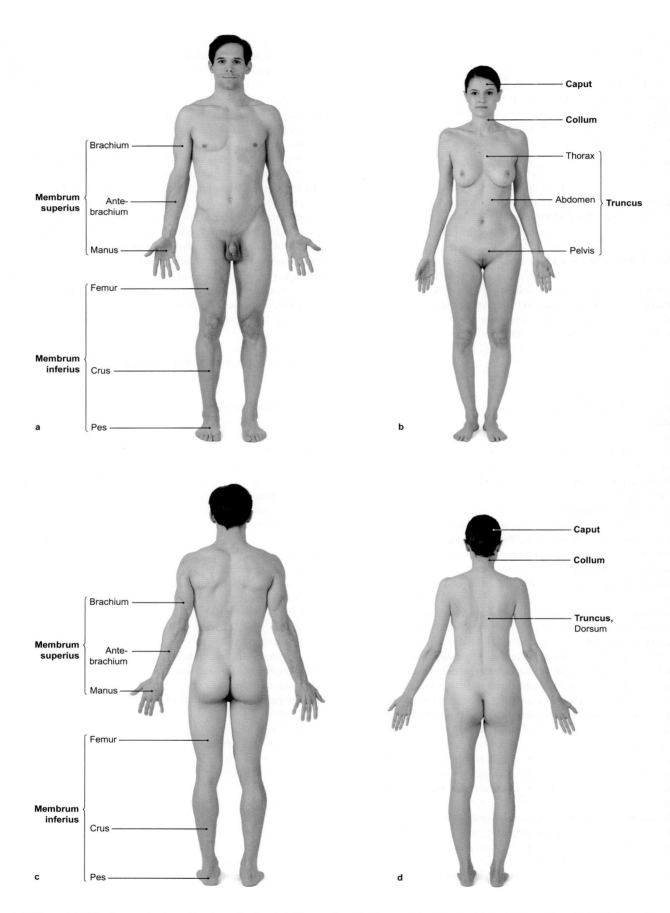

Fig. 1.1 Blueprint of the human body. a Man from the front. **b** Woman from the front. **c** Man from behind. **d** Woman from behind. [K340]

- Metabolic system
- Reproductive system
- Communication system
- Central control system

Bilateral symmetry and metamerism
The body is bilaterally symmetric (**bilateral symmetry**). Both halves of the body are laterally reversed and mirror each other on the right and the left side. The internal organs are an exception. **Metamerism** refers to the repetition or a series of similar elements (e. g. the ribs), which are arranged along an axis (vertebral column) (segmental or **metameric organisation**). Their origin lies in the development of somites (primary segments), which represent segmental units. The temporary occurrence of branchial arches (pharyngeal arches) is also known as **branchiometry**.

1.2.2 Body proportions

Age, sex, weight, body size and offspring (ethnic factors) affect the form and architecture of the body. The limbs, organs and regions of the body are connected to each other in a certain proportional manner at any age and grow at different speeds. These directly proportional relationships are most notable in infants and toddlers and also play the most important role in these age groups.

Developmental stages
In paediatrics, the postnatal period is divided into **developmental stages**:
- Neonatal period (the first 2 weeks of life)
- Infancy (up to the end of 1st year of life)
- Early childhood (up to the end of the 5th year of life)
- School age (up to the beginning of puberty)
- Puberty (maturation age, with variable duration)
- Adolescence (completion of the development and length growth of the skeletal system)

Since the middle of the 19th century there has been a general **acceleration** of development compared to previous generations, e. g. with respect to the growth or physical maturation processes. Improvements of life, sanitary and nutritional conditions as well as changes in the social environment are viewed as responsible for this.

External appearance
For the individual periods of life there are typical physical features, which shape the external appearance of an individual. Morphological differences are most marked as gender differences (**sexual dimorphism,** especially after sexual maturity). The skeletal system, the skeletal muscles, the distribution of the subcutaneous fatty tissue, the hair growth pattern and the body proportions contribute the largest part.

The genetically determined primary genitalia (testes or ovaries) which are responsible for the formation of gonads, are described as **primary sexual characteristics**. The **secondary sexual characteristics,** which develop during puberty, are mainly responsible for the external appearance. Their development is influenced by gonadotropins (hormones of the pituitary gland), which are responsible for the production of gender-specific gonadal hormones. The secondary sexual characteristics of *women* are:

- Mammary gland (mamma)
- Distribution pattern of the subcutaneous fat (more consistent, smoother outlines)
- Pubic hair pattern up to the Mons pubis
- Symmetrical (even) hairline
- Smaller body size
- Horizontally oval pelvis

The secondary sexual characteristics of *men* are:
- Pubic hair pattern up to the navel
- Beard growth
- Hair growth on the anterior thoracic and abdominal wall (varies greatly) as well as on the back and limbs
- Reduced hairline (receding hairline, partial baldness)
- Larger body size
- Narrower pelvis

Constitution refers to every person's physical and mental characteristics that are very individual in their interdependencies. According to Kretschmer, a distinction is made between 3 constitutional types:
- **Leptosome:** slim, slender body type, fragile limbs with light-weighted bones and thin muscles
- **Pyknic:** medium-sized, broad body type, having a tendency to become fat, rounded chest (below wider than above) and face, short neck; sedate, cosy, kind-hearted, sociable, serene temperament
- **Athletic:** muscular body type, broad shoulders and broad upper chest; in general serene temperament, outspoken, active

This classification is rejected by psychology today.

Body weight
For determining the normal weight and also the overweight and underweight of adults the body mass index (BMI, or Quetelet index) is used today. It is the quotient of body weight (in kg) and the square of the body size (in m). However, the age, gender and constitution must be taken into account in the evaluation. A BMI below 16 stands for severe underweight, 16–20 for underweight, 20–25 for normal weight, 30–40 for strong obesity and values over 40 for extreme obesity.

N O T E
Obesity (with a BMI above 30) per se is not an eating disorder: it is a disease, which can be caused by an eating disorder but not exclusively.

Skeletal age
In order to determine the skeletal age of *infants* and *toddlers* an x-ray image of the left hand is used. For assessing the skeletal age of *school children* the size and shape of the ossification centres in the knee joint region are evaluated. After *completion of the growth during puberty* the closure of the epiphyseal gaps is assessed.

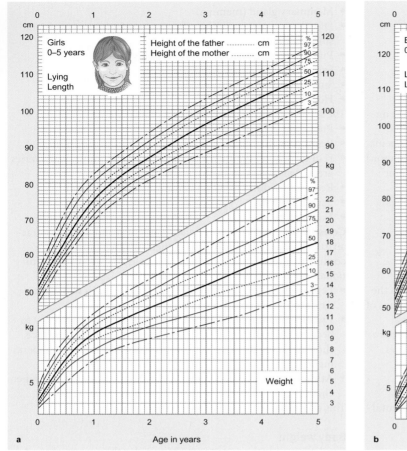

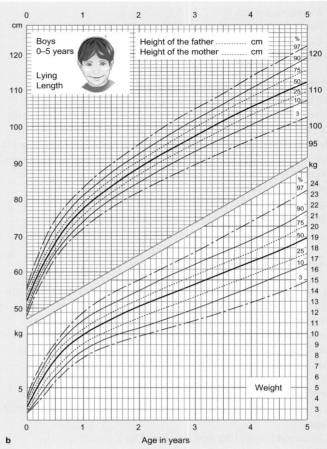

Fig. 1.2 Percentile growth curves. a Girls 0–5 years. **b** Boys 0–5 years. [L157]

For the assessment of a normal (standard) or deviating growth (variation) the measured body size, weight and cranial circumference of children are set in relation to their age and evaluated by using **percentile curves or tables** (➤ Fig. 1.2).

Body size

The body size or height is the length from the crown of the head to the soles of the feet. It is also referred to as the body length. The relative changes in the length of the body are shown in ➤ Fig. 1.3 compared with each other. Therefore, the head of an embryo at the end of the second month of pregnancy corresponds to the height of the rest of the body. The head of a newborn measures just a quarter, the head of a 6-year-old child a sixth and the head of an adult an eighth of the body length. The navel shifts from the lower abdomen (in an embryo) up to the waist during body growth.

1.2.3 Positional descriptions

Topographically, the body can be divided into regions (➤ Fig. 1.4). These regions are extremely useful to determine the exact position of the organs, to describe changes visible on the surface of the body or to document the process of surgical procedures (for regions of the head ➤ Fig. 9.11).

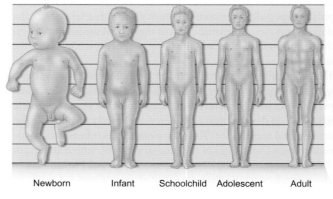

Fig. 1.3 Change of body proportions during growth. [L238]

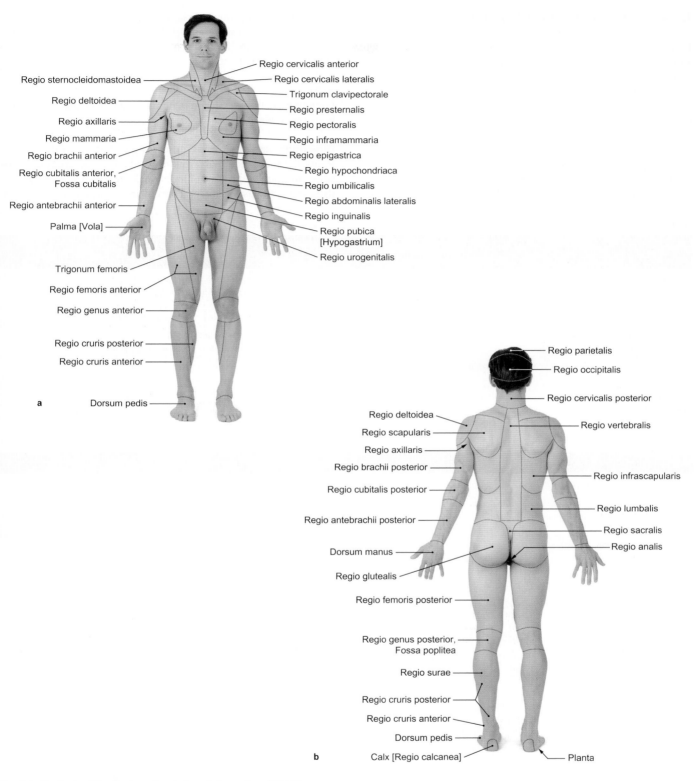

Regio cervicalis anterior
Regio sternocleidomastoidea
Regio cervicalis lateralis
Trigonum clavipectorale
Regio deltoidea
Regio presternalis
Regio axillaris
Regio pectoralis
Regio mammaria
Regio inframammaria
Regio brachii anterior
Regio epigastrica
Regio cubitalis anterior,
Fossa cubitalis
Regio hypochondriaca
Regio umbilicalis
Regio antebrachii anterior
Regio abdominalis lateralis
Regio inguinalis
Palma [Vola]
Regio pubica
[Hypogastrium]
Regio urogenitalis
Trigonum femoris
Regio femoris anterior
Regio genus anterior
Regio cruris posterior
Regio cruris anterior

a Dorsum pedis

Regio parietalis
Regio occipitalis
Regio cervicalis posterior
Regio deltoidea
Regio vertebralis
Regio scapularis
Regio axillaris
Regio brachii posterior
Regio infrascapularis
Regio cubitalis posterior
Regio antebrachii posterior
Regio lumbalis
Regio sacralis
Dorsum manus
Regio analis
Regio glutealis
Regio femoris posterior
Regio genus posterior,
Fossa poplitea
Regio surae
Regio cruris posterior
Regio cruris anterior
Dorsum pedis
b Calx [Regio calcanea]
Planta

Fig. 1.4 Regions of the body. a Front view. **b** Rear view. [K340]

1.2.4 General anatomical descriptions

In medicine the positional and directional terms are transferred to a three-dimensional coordinate system with 3 axes and planes perpendicular to each other. This corresponds to a person standing upright, with the head facing forward, the arms hanging at the sides, the palms facing forward and the feet next to each other **(anatomical position)**.

Planes
The cardinal planes of the body are the frontal, the transverse, the sagittal, and the median planes (> Table 1.1, > Fig. 1.5). These cardinal planes can be shifted arbitrarily to all parallel levels with

the exception of the median plane. In radiographic imaging techniques (computed tomography, CT and magnetic resonance imaging, MRI) the three cardinal anatomical planes are defined as layers with their own nomenclature.

Axes
Longitudinal, transverse and sagittal axes are the main axes of the body (> Table 1.2).

Directional and positional terms for parts of the body
Positional and directional terms are used for the description of position, location and course of individual structures. Sometimes these terms are also an integral part of anatomical names. Position-

Table 1.1 Cardinal planes.

Plane	Corresponding radiological sectional planes	Description
Frontal plane (coronal plane) (> Fig. 1.5)	Coronal plane	• Movement plane visible in the front view of humans • Any plane that divides the body into front and back, and runs parallel to the forehead • Movements in this plane take place from left to right or from top to bottom
Transverse plane (axial plane, horizontal plane, transaxial plane) (> Fig. 1.5)	Axial layer	• Any plane perpendicular to the longitudinal axis • Therefore each horizontal plane when standing upright
Sagittal plane (> Fig. 1.5)	Sagittal layer	• Any plane crossing the body from front to back • Runs parallel to the midsagittal plane
Median (or midsagittal) plane (> Fig. 1.5)	Sagittal layer	• Sagittal plane passing from front to back through the centre of the body and dividing it into two equal halves

Table 1.2 Cardinal axes.

Axis	Description
Longitudinal axis (vertical axis) (> Fig. 1.5)	Longitudinal axis passing through the body from top to bottom (or vice versa)
Transverse axis (horizontal axis) (> Fig. 1.5)	Crossing the body from the left to the right half (or vice versa)
Sagittal axis (ventrodorsal axis) (> Fig. 1.5)	Penetrates the body in the direction of the arrow from front to back (or vice versa)

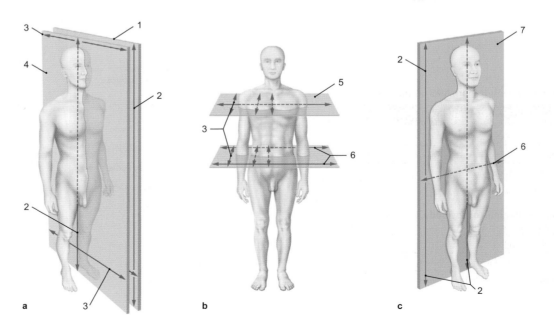

1 Sagittal plane
2 Longitudinal axis
3 Sagittal axis
4 Median sagittal plane
5 Transversal plane
6 Transverse axis
7 Frontal plane

Fig. 1.5 Planes and axes. a Sagittal plane (Planum sagittale), through which sagittal and longitudinal axes pass. **b** Transverse plane = horizontal plane (Planum transversale), through which transverse and sagittal axes pass. **c** Frontal plane = coronal plane (Planum frontale), through which longitudinal and transverse axes pass. [L127]

Table 1.3 Directional and positional terms for the body parts.

Term	Meaning
Cranial or superior	Towards the head
Caudal or inferior	Towards the tail bone (sacrum)
Anterior or ventral	Towards the front or abdomen
Posterior or dorsal	Towards the back
Lateral	Towards the side, away from the midline
Medial	Centred, in the middle or towards the midline
Median or medianus	Within the median plane
Intermediate	Lying in between
Central	Towards the interior of the body
Peripheral	Towards the surface of the body
Profunda	Lying deep inside
Superficial	Lying close to or on the surface
External	Outside
Internal	Inside
Apical	Directed or related to the tip
Basal	Directed towards the base
Dexter	Right
Sinister	Left
Proximal	Towards the trunk or torso
Distal	Towards the end of the limbs
Ulnar	Towards the ulna
Radial	Towards the radius
Tibial	Towards the tibia
Fibular	Towards the fibula
Volar or palmar	Towards the palm of hand
Plantar	Towards the sole of the foot
Dorsal	(Extremities) towards the back (dorsum) of hand or foot
Frontal	Towards the front
Rostral	Towards the mouth or tip of nose (literally: towards the beak; used only for head-related terms)

al terms are independent of the actual position of the body. The positional descriptions always refer to the anatomical position. The key terms are summarised in ➤ Table 1.3 and partially represented in ➤ Fig. 1.5. In ➤ Fig. 1.6 and ➤ Table 1.4 the orientation lines on the body are also summarised.

Terms of movement

In order to describe changes of position and location of individual parts of the body in relation to the biomechanical movements occurring in their joints, defined terms are used (➤ Table 1.5, ➤ Fig. 1.7). These terms are not always clearly differentiated, as the joints allow different degrees of freedom or range of motion, so that their movements depend on the type of joint involved, and thus combinations are possible. The movement terms differ according to the specific body region.

Range of motion

The **range** or **freedom of motion** in a joint is the maximum excursion from its neutral position: when standing upright, the arms hanging loosely down at the sides of the body, the thumbs facing forward, the elbow and knee joints not completely extended but minimally flexed (➤ Fig. 1.8). This **neutral ('zero') position** corresponds to the anatomical position with the exception that the thumbs are pointing forward. The freedom of motion can be limited by bony and soft tissue structures (joint inhibition):

- **Bone-guided inhibition:** If two bones touch in a certain joint position, the movement may not be continued, e. g. the extension in the elbow joint when the Olecranon clicks into the Fossa olecrani.
- **Ligament-guided inhibition:** In this case the joint movement comes to a standstill by a tense or stretched ligament, e. g. the retroversion in the hip joint induced by extension of the Lig. iliofemorale.
- **Soft tissue or mass-guided inhibition:** If soft tissues oppose each other in a certain joint position, the movement may not be continued, e. g. when the bending in the elbow joint is restricted by overdeveloped muscles of the arm and forearm.
- **Muscle-guided inhibition:** The arrangement of muscles can be the limiting factor, e. g. in a maximum flexed position of the wrist it is not possible to close the fist (➤ Chap. 1.4.4, active and passive insufficiency).

Table 1.4 Orientation lines on the body.

Line	Legend
Linea mediana anterior	Front midline that divides the body in 2 symmetrical halves
Linea sternalis	Parallel to the Linea mediana anterior at the lateral margin of the breastbone (sternum)
Linea parasternalis	Parallel to the Linea mediana anterior, just between Linea sternalis and Linea medioclavicularis
Linea medioclavicularis	Parallel to the Linea mediana anterior, right through the centre of the clavicle
Linea axillaris anterior	Parallel to the Linea mediana anterior, just through the anterior border of the axilla
Linea axillaris posterior	Parallel to the Linea mediana posterior, just through the posterior border of the axilla
Linea scapularis	Parallel to the Linea mediana posterior, just through the lower angle (Angulus inferior) of the shoulder blade (scapula)
Linea paravertebralis	Parallel to the Linea mediana posterior at the lateral margin of the spine
Linea mediana posterior	Posterior midline that divides the body in 2 symmetrical halves

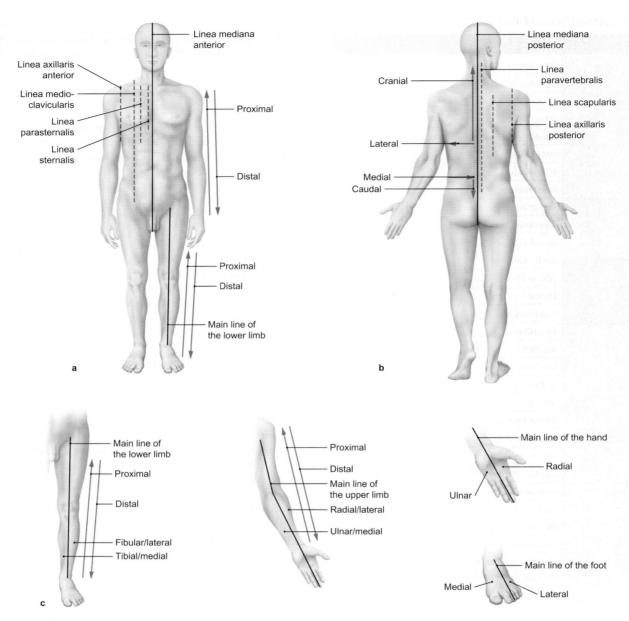

Fig. 1.6 Orientation lines, directional and positional terms. [L127]

Table 1.5 Anatomical terms of movement.

Region	Term	Movement
Extremities	Extension	Elongation
	Flexion	Bending
	Abduction	Pulling away from the body
	Adduction	Pulling towards the body
	Elevation	Raising of the arm/shoulder above the horizontal plane
	Depression	Lowering the arm/shoulder from above the horizontal plane
	Inner rotation	Inward rotation
	Outer rotation	Outward rotation
	Pronation	Rotation movement of hand/foot with hand turned inwards or sole of foot turned outwards
	Supination	Rotation movement of hand/foot with palm of hand turned outwards or sole of foot turned inwards
	Radial abduction	Swivelling hand/fingers towards the radius
	Ulnar abduction	Swivelling hand/fingers towards the ulna
	Palmar flexion/Volar flexion	Bending palm of hand towards back of arm
	Plantar flexion	Bending sole of the foot towards back of leg
	Dorsiflexion	Extending hand/foot towards the back of arm/leg
	Opposition	Comparison of thumb vs. little finger
	Reposition	Repositioning of the thumb next to the index finger
	Inversion	Lifting the inner side of the foot using the talocalcaneonavicular joint
	Eversion	Lifting the outside of the foot using the talocalcaneonavicular joint
Spine	Rotation	Rotation of the spine in the longitudinal axis
	Lateral flexion	Lateral tilt
	Inclination (flexion)	Forward tilt
	Reclination (extension)	Backward tilt
Pelvis	Flexion (anterior/ventral rotation)	Pelvic tilt towards the front
	Extension (dorsal rotation)	Pelvic lying towards the back
Temporomandibular joint	Abduction	Opening the jaw
	Adduction	Closing the jaw
	Protrusion/protraction	Pushing the lower jaw forward
	Retrusion/retraction	Pulling the lower jaw back
	Occlusion	Interlocking the upper and lower jaw teeth
	Mediotrusion	Ventral-medial translation of the lower jaw on one side
	Laterotrusion	Dorsal-lateral translation of the lower jaw on one side

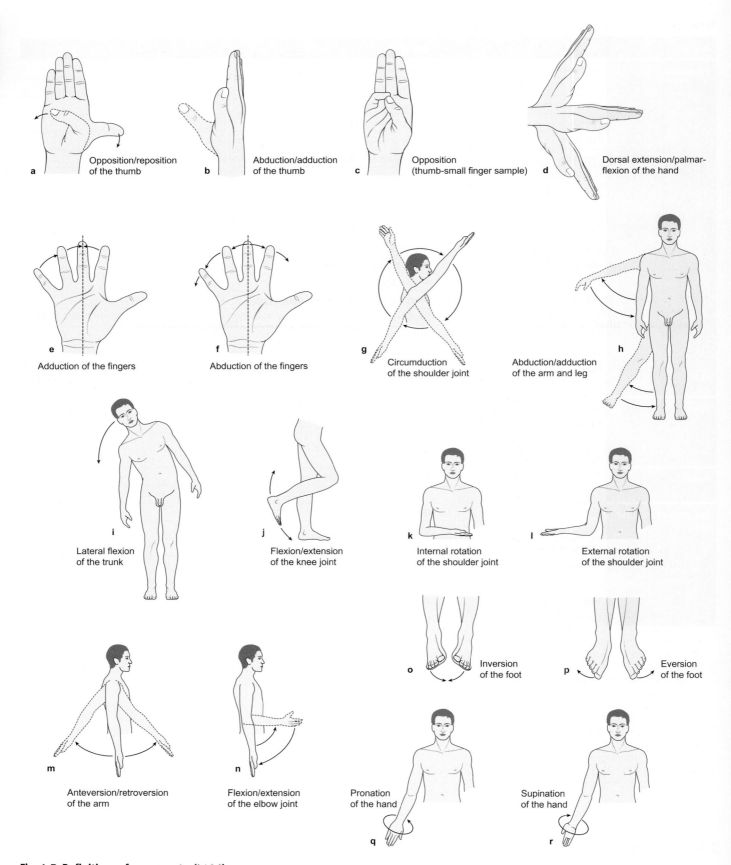

Fig. 1.7 Definitions of movements. [L126]

a Opposition/reposition of the thumb

b Abduction/adduction of the thumb

c Opposition (thumb-small finger sample)

d Dorsal extension/palmarflexion of the hand

e Adduction of the fingers

f Abduction of the fingers

g Circumduction of the shoulder joint

h Abduction/adduction of the arm and leg

i Lateral flexion of the trunk

j Flexion/extension of the knee joint

k Internal rotation of the shoulder joint

l External rotation of the shoulder joint

m Anteversion/retroversion of the arm

n Flexion/extension of the elbow joint

o Inversion of the foot

p Eversion of the foot

q Pronation of the hand

r Supination of the hand

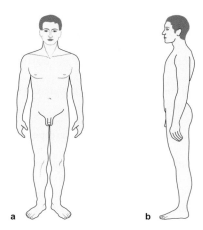

Fig. 1.8 Neutral position. a Front view. **b** Lateral view.

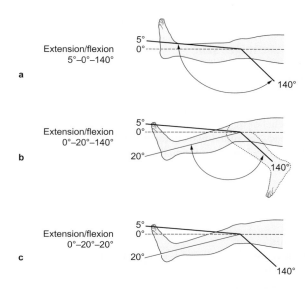

Fig. 1.9 Documentation of the range of motion of joints.
a Normal range of motion of the knee joint. **b** Extension of the knee is not possible. **c** Complete stiffening of the knee.

NOTE
In order to describe the range of motion of a joint and to make the measurements comprehensible for follow-up examiners, one uses the **neutral-zero method** (➤ Fig. 1.8).

Clinical remarks

The **neutral-zero method** is a standardised orthopaedic evaluation and documentation system for describing the mobility of joints. Starting from the neutral or 'zero' position (➤ Fig. 1.8) the achievable range of motion around a specific axis is measured and defined as degrees of angle. First the range of motion leading away from the body is determined, followed by the range of motion leading back towards the body (➤ Fig. 1.9). Thus, the mobility can be clearly defined and documented in findings and medical documents. All restrictions of the mobility are determined and assessed by comparison with standard values. They can serve as a basis for expert opinions. For example, the **normal range of motion** of the knee joint is 5° extension and 140° flexion. The straight extended or minimally flexed knee is the neutral or 'zero' position of the joint. However, the neutral or 'zero' position of the foot is at right angles to the lower leg. From this position, a maximum of 20° extension and 40° flexion is possible. Therefore the normal range of motion in the knee joint is defined as 5°–0°–140° (extending the knee, passing the 'zero' position and bending the knee, ➤ Fig. 1.9a); for the foot it is defined as 20°–0°–40° (dorsal extension, passing the 'zero' position, and plantar flexion).
Restrictions of joint mobility can be reproduced exactly by the neutral 'zero' method. If, for example, there is a **flexion contracture in the knee joint** of 0°–20°–140° (➤ Fig. 1.9b), the knee cannot be extended or pass the 'zero' position, it remains in a 20° flexed position at the maximum range of extension, but can be further bent up to 140°. In the case of a **complete knee stiffening** of 0°–20°–20° (➤ Fig. 1.9c) neither extension nor bending of the knee is possible, and the 'zero' position is not achieved.

1.3 Skin and skin appendages

The skin covering the body has with 1.5–2 m² the largest extension or surface area of all organs of the body. It has a total weight between 3 and 4 kg (and together with the subcutaneous fat up to 16 kg). The thickness of the skin varies between 1 and 2 mm depending on the body region. It has the following **functions:**

- Protection (as a mechanical, thermal, chemical or immunological barrier)
- Registration of pressure, touch, vibration, pain, temperature
- Energy storage
- Heat insulation

NOTE
Condition and appearance of the skin and skin appendages significantly influence the social acceptance and the subjective impression of a person. For the medical professionals they provide information about age, life style, health, general condition and mood of a person.

Clinical remarks

For a grading of **burns** by the body surface affected, the **Neuner rule** is applied, which allows a prognostic estimation of the burnt skin surface:
- Adults:
  - Arms and head 9 % respectively
  - Chest/abdomen, back and legs 18 % respectively
  - Palm of hands including fingers and genital region 1 % respectively
- Children up to 5 years:
  - Arms 9.5 %
  - Chest/abdomen, back 16 % respectively
  - Legs 17 %
  - Head 12 % (age-dependent)
If more than 20 % of the skin surface is burnt, it is a severe burn. From 40 % on the probability is extremely high that the patient dies. From 5 % in children and 10 % in adults there is a risk of shock. Inpatient treatment in a hospital is nearly always indicated, and should be reserved for specialised centres for patients with burns, in order to treat the patient in the best way possible.

1.3.1 Skin types and skin layers

Meshed and ridged skin

A distinction is made due to the morphological structure between meshed and ridged skin. **Meshed skin** has glands and hairs and makes up the largest part of the body surface area. It has a variable thickness in different regions of the body. **Ridged skin** forms the surface relief of the palms and soles and is – being genetically determined – an individual characteristic of each person (fingerprint). This enables an individual identification.

Skin layers

The **skin (Cutis)** consists of epidermis, dermis and subcutis (➤ Fig. 1.10).

Epidermis

The **epidermis (Epithelium)** is the surface of the skin and has characteristic layers:

- Stratum corneum
- Stratum lucidum (only ridged skin)
- Stratum granulosum
- Stratum spinosum
- Stratum basale

It is a multi-layer (or stratified) squamous epithelium without blood vessels, containing numerous sensory receptors in the form of free nerve endings (mechanical, temperature and/or pain perception) and MERKEL cells (pressure sensation). In addition, there are melanocytes and dendritic cells (immune cells, LANGERHANS cells).

Dermis

The layer below the epidermis is the **dermis (or Corium)**, is a layer of connective tissue with a superficial capillary plexus (Plexus superficialis) on the border between the epidermis and dermis and a deep vascular plexus (Plexus profundus) on the border between dermis and underlying subcutis. These vascular plexuses not only play a role in the blood circulation, but also in the heat regulation. The dermis has two layers:

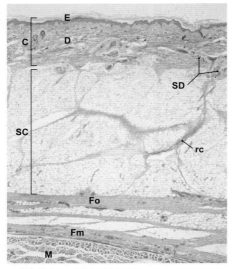

Fig. 1.10 Layers of the skin (integument). C = Cutis, E = Epidermis, D = Dermis, SC = Subcutis, Fo = Surface fascia, Fm = Muscle fascia, M = Muscle, rc = Retinaculum cutis, SD = Eccrine sweat glands; H&E staining, magnification x22. [S010–2–16]

- Stratum papillare: papillae of collagenous and elastic connective tissue link (indent) the dermis with the epidermis. In each papilla a capillary of the Plexus superficialis runs to the tip.
- Stratum reticulare: tense collagenous and elastic connective tissue

The dermis is well vascularised and innervated. It houses various specialised receptors:

- MERKEL cells for pressure sensation
- MEISSNER tactile corpuscles for touch (especially Stratum papillare)
- RUFFINI corpuscles for stretching sensation (especially Stratum reticulare)
- VATER-PACINI corpuscles for vibration sensation
- Free nerve endings for mechanical, thermal and/or pain perception

Furthermore there are nerves, lymphatic vessels, immune cells, melanotropin-producing cells (UV protection), sweat glands, hair follicles, sebaceous glands and smooth muscle cells in the dermis. Epidermis and dermis are linked via the papillae of the Stratum papillare. Below this follows the Stratum reticulare of the dermis. The latter is mainly responsible for the elasticity of the skin.

Clinical remarks

The epidermis and the Stratum papillare of the dermis (dermo-epidermal transition zone) are interlocked by various proteins and other structures. If one or more of these proteins or adhesive structures is missing (e. g. genetically) or undergoes destruction (e. g. mechanically), **bubbles** (Bullae) may occur, and in rare cases there may be a large-scale detachment of the epidermis. There are also conditions such as the **bullous pemphigoid,** in which antibodies are formed against components of the adhesive structures (auto-antibodies). In the case of **pemphigus** the antibodies disturb the adhesion of the cells within the epidermis.

Subcutis

Below the dermis lies the subcutis, consisting of loose connective tissue and adipose tissue (subcutaneous fat tissue).

Clinical remarks

The main orientation of the collagen fibres in the Stratum reticulare of the dermis determines the so-called **cleavage lines** of the skin, which play an important role for correct incisions in surgery. If incisions are opposing these cleavage lines, this leads to increased scarring and the formation of non-physiological wrinkles in later life.

1.3.2 Skin appendages

The skin appendages (or organs) include, apart from hair and nails, numerous large and small sweat glands, sebaceous glands and the mammary glands (lacteal glands, Mammae).

Hair

Hair (Pili) are viewed as remnants which once served as heat insulation. In the evolutionary development this function became obsolete and has receded. Today, hair contributes substantially to the external appearance of a person and plays a major role in social acceptance and aesthetic perceptions. Furthermore hair serves as a protective shield against UV light and heat, as well as conveying tactile sensations.

Hair is the product of keratinisation, which begins in **matrix cells** at the bottom of invaginations in the epidermis (➤ Fig. 1.11). The cells derived of the matrix cells differentiate to become horny cells which form the hair shaft.

Basic types

Postnatally, a distinction is made between two basic types of hair:

- **Vellus hair (fluffy hair):** are soft and short hairs, with hair follicles (see below) in the epidermis. The thin and nearly colourless vellus hairs have no medulla (see below) and correspond to the foetal *lanugo hair*. It covers the largest part of the body in children and women.
- **Terminal hair (long hair):** is strong and long, with hair follicles extending into the subcutis. The thick and coloured (pigmented) terminal hairs have shafts with medulla, and occur in various

forms, such as scalp hair, eyelashes, eyebrows, pubic hair, axillary hair and beard hair, which usually differ considerably in the various ethnic groups. Terminal hair is classified as short (eyelashes, eyebrows) and long hairs (all other). Its structure depends on genetic factors and gender.

Hair follicles

Hairs begin to develop in depressions (invaginations) of the columnar epithelium, which extend to the dermis or the subcutis. These **hair follicles** are nourished by blood vessels and consist of a **hair bulb** and a **hair papilla**. Here the hair growth begins. Each hair follicle is associated with a sebaceous gland (**pilo-sebaceous gland unit**) and a smooth muscle (**M. arrector pili**). The latter can straighten the hair by indenting the epidermis (*goose bumps*). In the hair, a distinction is made between (➤ Fig. 1.11):

- **Hair shaft:** completely keratinised with an epithelial hair root sheath
- **Hair bulb:** the distended epithelial part where the hair begins to grow, and which contains matrix cells capable of cell division
- **Hair papilla:** a cell-rich connective tissue extension of the dermis, indenting from below into the hair bulb
- **Hair funnel:** opening of the hair follicle to the skin surface; the duct of the associated sebaceous gland ends here
- **Epithelial root sheath:** divided into the inner and the outer root sheath
  - Inner root sheath: with the following layers from inside to outside
    - Cuticle (of sheath)
    - HUXLEY's layer
    - HENLE's layer
  - Outer root sheath: consists of several layers of bright, non-keratinised cells that only become horny in the area of the hair funnel and pass here to the epidermis of the skin

Genetic factors and the pigment content (melanin) of the hair are responsible for a person's characteristic hair colour. Once the production of melanin ceases, the hair appears grey or white.

Nails

On the upper side of the fingers and toes, there are approximately 0.5 mm thick nails. Each **nail (Unguis)** is a convex, translucent keratin plate (body of nail), which protects the finger tips and supports the grasping function (➤ Fig. 1.12). The nail structures are:

- **Body of nail** (Corpus unguis)
- **Nail wall** (Vallum unguis): on both sides of the body of nail
- **Nail fold:** skin fold, which rises above the nail wall
- **Cuticle of nail** (Eponychium, Cuticula): epithelium of the nail wall, lying dorsally on the body of nail.

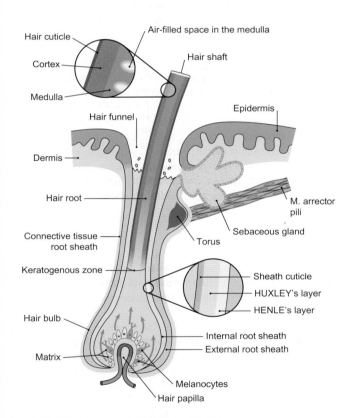

Fig. 1.11 Structure of a hair follicle. [L141]

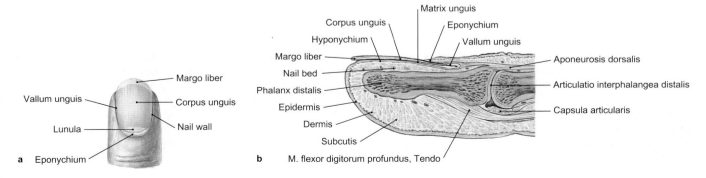

Fig. 1.12 Structure of a nail (distal phalanx, Phalanx distalis). **a** View from above. **b** Sagittal section.

- **Hyponychium:** epithelium, covered by the body of nail
- **Nail matrix** (Matrix unguis): epithelium proximal of the hyponychium, from which the body of nail emerges
- **Nail bed:** connective tissue below the nail matrix, which is firmly fused with the periosteum of the distal phalanx
- **Lunule of nail:** crescent-shaped whitish part of the Matrix unguis, from which the body of nail emerges; the Lunula is visible through the nail

---

Clinical remarks

Some people have **white spots** under their nails. This signifies, that the nail is insufficiently fixed on the nail bed. Changes in light reflection at these points cause the nail to appear milky-white (similar to the lunule). Possible reasons for this are impacts against the nail, medication or various diseases. A lack of biotin (vitamin H) is a common cause for **brittle nails,** because biotin is required for the production of keratin, the main component of the body of nail.

Numerous systemic diseases are associated with nail disorders. Psoriasis, for example, causes the formation of **pitted nails, oil-drop signs, crumbly nails** or **nail dystrophy. Onychomycoses** (fungal colonisation/mycosis of the nails) are a common cause for consulting a dermatologist (skin specialist). The treatment is often lengthy.

Skin glands

Sweat glands

Sweat glands (Glandulae sudoriferae) occur as small and large sweat glands.

- **Small sweat glands** are distributed over the entire body surface. The density varies from 50/cm^2 (on the back) to 300/cm^2 (in the palms). The excretory ducts open onto cutaneous ridges or raised points of the epidermis. Functionally, they provide a regulation of the body's temperature: With increased secretion of sweat, this hypotonic fluid evaporates and heat is removed from the body (evaporative cooling). Generally, in 12 hours approximately 250 ml of sweat is secreted. If the ambient temperature is elevated, this amount may increase many times over. Bacteria that colonise the skin physiologically, change the composition of the sweat and add a characteristic odour.
- **Large sweat glands** (scent glands) only occur regionally, e. g. in the armpit, around the nipples, in the eyelids, in the external acoustic meatus, in the perigenital and perianal regions. They only become fully functional in puberty and influence – by bacterial modification of the secretion – the individual body odour of a person.

Sebaceous glands

Sebaceous glands mostly occur in association with hair (pilo-sebaceous gland unit, see above). However, there are also regions of the body, where sebaceous glands occur independently of hair, e. g. in the eyelids (MEIBOMIAN glands), in the external acoustic meatus, on the nipples, lips and in the genital region. Sebaceous glands produce an oily discharge, which greases hair and skin, or for example covers the tear film and protects it from evaporation.

Mammary gland

The mammary gland is described in ➤ Chap. 3.1.2 together with the chest or thoracic wall.

1.4 Musculoskeletal system

The musculoskeletal system consists of passive (bone, cartilage, ligaments and joints) and active (muscles and tendons) elements.

1.4.1 Cartilage

Cartilage like bone belongs to the supportive tissues of the body. It is only briefly mentioned here for further understanding. Cartilage consists of cartilaginous cells (chondrocytes) and the extracellular matrix (ECM), with proteoglycans and collagen fibrils as key components. Cartilage has a high elasticity on pressure. This is based on its solid consistency, which helps to only slightly change its form under pressure and to return it back to its old form when the pressure subsides. Due to the composition, a distinction is made between three different types of cartilage:

- **Hyaline cartilage:** This most common type of cartilage (joint cartilage, respiratory tract, nose tip, nasal septum, larynx, trachea, bronchi, ribs, epiphyses, primordial bones before ossification) consists of cartilaginous cell (chondrocyte) clusters and ECM. The collagen fibres are not visible in histological sections (they are masked).
- **Elastic cartilage:** structured similar to hyaline cartilage, it contains additionally a larger quantity of elastic fibres in the ECM and has smaller chondrocytes. It occurs in the auricle, in the external acoustic meatus, in the pharyngo-tympanic tube, the epiglottis, as the small laryngeal cartilage and in the smallest bronchi.
- **Fibrous cartilage:** In this type of cartilage the cells are separate, and the collagen fibres are not masked, so they are visible in histological sections (hence the name). Fibrous cartilage occurs in the intervertebral discs, the pubic symphysis, articulardiscs, menisci, in chondrotendinous insertions, sliding tendons, and in the temporomandibular joint.

1.4.2 Bones

The bones (Ossa) form the bony skeleton of the body. The adult skeleton is made up of nearly 200 single bones, which are connected by joints.

Bone is not a dead, but a living tissue that is very well supplied with blood. In 10 % of bones there is a constant remodelling of bone even after completed growth. If osteogenesis and osteoclasis take place at different sites, this will change the form (shape) of the bone *(modelling);* if both processes take place at the same site, the form does not change *(remodelling).* With a constant loading of bones, osteogenesis and osteoclasis will be balanced. Only when one process outweighs the other, does the bony structure begin to change: if osteogenesis predominates, this leads to a greater density of bones (osteosclerosis); if more bone is degenerated (by osteoclasis) than newly formed, one speaks of osteolysis or osteoporosis. These processes can be localised or generalised.

Bone consists of organic substances (mainly type I collagen, and bone cells [osteocytes, osteoblasts, osteoclasts]) and inorganic matrix (containing salts such as calcium phosphate, magnesium phosphate and calcium carbonate as well as calcium, potassium and sodium compounds with chlorine and fluorine). 99 % of the body's calcium reserves are bound in the bone. This is equivalent to 1–1.5 kg calcium in the human body. Only 1 % is not bound in bone, but is found elsewhere, e. g. in the blood or muscles. Organic substances and inorganic matrices form a composite, its mechanical properties depend on the ratio of the individual components. Osteogenesis *(bone formation)* and osteoclasis *(bone resorption)* are influenced by various factors such as mechanical load, hormones, growth factors, matrix molecules and cytokines.

Functions of bone are:
- **Support** (the entire skeletal system)
- **Protection** (skull and vertebral canal)
- **Calcium reservoir** (the entire skeletal system)
- **Blood formation** (the entire skeletal system, age-dependent)

Clinical remarks

In the case of inactivity or immobilisation (e. g. by a plaster cast), lack of gravity (astronauts), and diseases such as osteoporosis or spreading of malignant tumour cells in bone (bone metastases) the **bone mass is reduced,** and the stability of the bone is at risk. The goal of treatment is to balance this disequilibrium in favour of a regeneration (osteogenesis) or preservation of bone mass by means of an early initiated therapy with exercises or drugs. The functional early mobilisation after injury and operations through physical therapy is therefore of very great importance.

Classification of bones

The bones are divided into different types, based on their structure and their appearance (➤ Table 1.6, ➤ Fig. 1.13).

Table 1.6 Classification of bones.

Description	Example	Explanation
Long bones (Ossa longa)	Femur, Humerus	• Have a shaft (Corpus) and ends (Extremitates) • The medullary cavity (Cavitas medullaris) is in the shaft
Flat bones (Ossa plana)	Os parietale, Scapula	Consist of 2 compact lamellae with integrated cancellous bone in between
Short bones (Ossa brevia)	Carpal bones, tarsal bone	Have no medullary cavity, but a core of cancellous bone
Irregular bones (Ossa irregularia)	Vertebrae	Bones that do not fit into the above categories
Air-filled bones (Ossa pneumatica)	Maxilla, Os ethmoidale	Bones with one or more air-filled spaces and lined with mucosa
Sesamoid bones (Ossa sesamoidea)	Patella, Os pisiforme	Bones embedded in tendons
Accessory bones (Ossa accessoria)	Os trigonum	Accessory bones that do not occur regularly

Functional adaptation

Construction principle/architecture

The shape of bones is genetically determined; in contrast their structure depends considerably on the type and amount of mechanical stresses acting upon them. In this respect, bones are formed according to an **economic construction principle**: with a minimum of material, a maximum of strength is achieved (minimum-maximum principle). The tube (of long bones) is the optimal architectural element for a body that is subject to bending: being hollow inside and flexible in all directions (high peripheral tensions, inside = 0 = neutral fibre = no tension). The **light weight construction** is particularly evident when one considers the weight relations: the bones account for only 10 % of body weight, the muscles over 40 %.

Bones have an outer layer of compact or cortical bone (**Substantia compacta or corticalis**) consisting of osteons and lamellae, and an inner light weight construction due to trabeculae (**Substantia spongiosa, cancellous or spongy bone trabeculae**) with interposed spaces, filled with bone marrow or medulla (➤ Fig. 1.14). The plate-like structure of flat bones allows the distinction between an outer and an inner cortical layer with spongy bone in between. On the flat cranial bones, the outer layer of the Substantia compacta is referred to as **Lamina externa** and the inner layer as **Lamina interna.** The Substantia spongiosa is referred to as **diploe.** The hollow spaces of pneumatised (air-filled) bones are lined with mucous membrane. This construction, which is only found in the cranial region, is a useful means of minimising the weight.

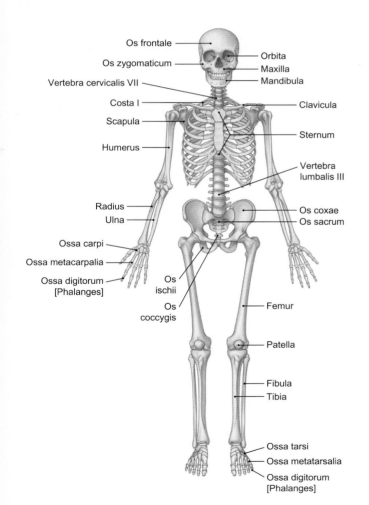

Os frontale
Os zygomaticum
Vertebra cervicalis VII
Costa I
Scapula
Humerus
Radius
Ulna
Ossa carpi
Ossa metacarpalia
Ossa digitorum [Phalanges]
Os ischii
Os coccygis

Orbita
Maxilla
Mandibula
Clavicula
Sternum
Vertebra lumbalis III
Os coxae
Os sacrum
Femur
Patella
Fibula
Tibia
Ossa tarsi
Ossa metatarsalia
Ossa digitorum [Phalanges]

Fig. 1.13 Skeleton. Ventral view. [E460]

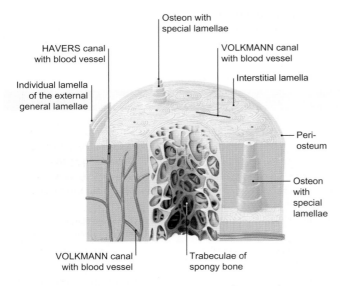

Fig. 1.14 Structure of a bone with compact and spongy bone.

Adaptation

The compact bone is reinforced in areas exposed to higher compressive loads by external forces (**quantitative adaptation**). Thus, for example, the cortical bone of the femur is reinforced on the medial side of the thigh (thickened cortical bone, Linea aspera), because it is exposed to a large bending stress here in the frontal plane (➤ Fig. 1.15a). The spongy bone trabeculae are aligned according to the compressive and tensile forces acting on the bone in this area, e. g. pressure trabeculae = pressure trajectories, tension trabeculae = tension trajectories (**qualitative adaptation**) (➤ Fig. 1.15b). Pressure trabeculae run like compression trajectories, and tension trabeculae like stretching trajectories.

In unloaded areas of the bone (so-called **neutral fibres**), no cancellous or spongy bone exists, e. g. in the long bones.

Clinical remarks

The femoral neck angle (angle between the neck and shaft of the femur; also **CCD angle = Centrum-Collum-Diaphyseal angle;** ➤ Chap. 5.3.1) of adults measures normally approximately 126° in the frontal plane. If the angle is below 120°, one speaks of a coxa vara. In this case more tension trabeculae are formed in the bone to counteract the high load by tensile stresses in the femoral neck. However, these adaptive processes are possible only up to a certain extent. If the load on the femoral neck in coxa vara exceeds the adaptive capacities of the bone, a femoral neck fracture can occur. In the case of coxa vara a fracture can be caused by considerably lower forces than in the case of a normal femoral neck angle (coxa norma).

Architecture of a long bone

Regardless of their absolute length long bones are divided into a shaft (**diaphysis**) with normally 2 ends (**epiphysis proximalis and epiphysis distalis**) (➤ Fig. 1.16). These epiphyses are covered by articular cartilage on their ends; between epiphysis and diaphysis lies the cartilaginous growth zone (epiphyseal gap) during the time of length growth. After completion of the bone growth, you can still see the former growth zone in sections through the bone (Linea epiphysialis). The **metaphysis** is directly linked to the growth zone or Linea epiphysialis. It represents the zone of the bone formation (osteogenesis) emerging in the course of growth. Other bony protrusions or prominences are referred to as **apophyses**. They are formed by the insertions of tendons and ligaments and have their own ossification centres during development. Areas where the bone surface is not smooth but rough, are referred to as roughness or tu-

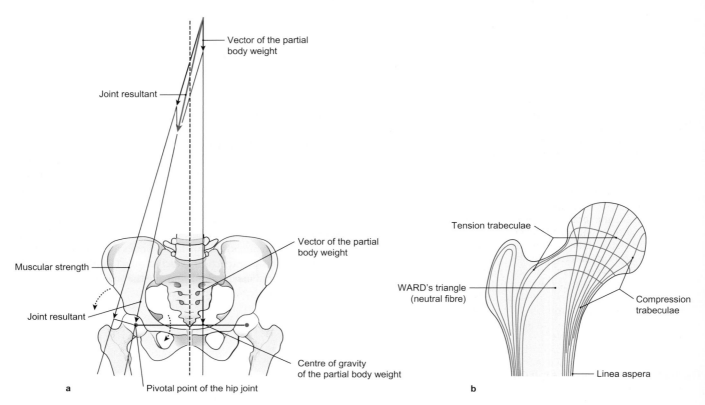

Fig. 1.15 Functional adaptation of bones exemplified by the femur. **a** Vectors of forces in the medial and lateral cortical tissues of the femoral head and neck. **b** Course of the corresponding trajectories.

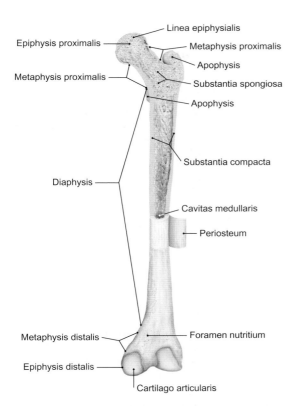

Linea epiphysialis
Epiphysis proximalis
Metaphysis proximalis
Apophysis
Metaphysis proximalis
Substantia spongiosa
Apophysis
Substantia compacta
Diaphysis
Cavitas medullaris
Periosteum
Metaphysis distalis
Foramen nutritium
Epiphysis distalis
Cartilago articularis

Fig. 1.16 Structure of a long bone (Os longum) exemplified by the femur. Dorsal view.

berosity *(Tuberositas)*. Furthermore there are osseous combs or ridges *(Cristae)*, lips *(Labiae)* or rough lines *(Lineae)*. All these different types of roughness serve as a connection with muscles and ligaments. Depending on its use the thickness of bone and the ratio of compact and spongy bone will be adapted (see above). The medullary cavity (Cavitas medullaris) is filled with bone marrow that also extends between the spongy bone trabeculae.

Clinical remarks

If the load on a bone exceeds its strength, a **fracture** may occur. This results in 2 or more bone fragments, which can be shifted (dislocation). Apart from pain, the typical clinical signs of a fracture include abnormal mobility, grinding sounds with movement (crepitation), axial misalignment, and an initial stupor (lack of muscular activity). The diagnosis is confirmed by an x-ray image. For the healing of a fracture it should be ideally immobilised without any stress or movement. This involves a fixation of the fragments until the bone can be completely fused, and for the recovery of long bones it is necessary to restore the medullary cavity, e. g. by a plaster cast, screws, or plates. If the fracture gap is small (< 5 mm) and not irritated, a **primary fracture healing** is possible without formation of callus. However, this succeeds almost only after surgical osteosynthesis with screws and plates, when the fracture ends have been optimally adapted. The **secondary fracture healing** occurs after the formation of callus which is then gradually ossified and becomes functional.

In the adult organism there is red marrow (Medulla ossium rubra) in the epiphyses and yellow **bone marrow** (Medulla ossium flava) in the diaphyses. Red marrow fulfils the task of blood formation (haematopoiesis); yellow bone marrow consists mainly of adipose and connective tissues. Under abnormal (pathological) conditions (e. g. massive blood loss), the yellow bone marrow in the diaphyses can be replaced by red

marrow within a short time. The diagnosis of diseases, e. g. of the haematopoietic system (leukaemia) can then be confirmed with a bone marrow biopsy of the spongy bone (punch biopsy) of the iliac crest or of the sternum (sternal biopsy– conducted only rarely today).

Bone development (osteogenesis)

The development of bones begins with cartilaginous or fibrous precursor cells (condensed mesenchyme, blastema). The processes of **desmal** (fibrous, direct) and **endochondral** (cartilaginous, indirect) bone formation **(osteogenesis),** the structure of immature **(woven bone, fibrous bone, primary bone)** and mature bones **(lamellar bone, secondary bone)** as well as the processes in the growth zones of bones are dealt with in detail in histology textbooks. Bone formation (osteogenesis) does not, however, take place in all parts of the skeleton at the same time. It starts as early as in the 2nd embryonic month at the clavicle (Clavicula) and ends around the 20th year of life with the closure of the epiphyseal gaps of certain long bones. During this development, due to an endochondral ossification in the epiphyses and apophyses secondary **ossification centres** occur. They are usually formed in a limited period of time and in a typical sequence for each skeletal element. The skeletal age can be determined by comparing at which time the ossification centres emerge and the ossification pattern of the bones (➤ Fig. 1.17). A distinction is made between primary ossification centres, which emerge during the foetal period in the area of the diaphyses **(diaphyseal ossification)** and secondary ossification centres, which develop partly in the 2nd half of the foetal period and partly in the first years of life within the cartilaginous epiphyses and apophyses **(epiphyseal and apophyseal ossification).** With the closure of the epiphyseal gaps (synostosis, see below) the length growth is completed. Thereafter, isolated ossification centres are no longer visible in X-ray images.

Clinical remarks

In orthopaedics the **determination of the skeletal age** and of a potential 'growth reserve' plays an important role for the treatment planning and the outcome of orthopaedic disorders and malformations in childhood.

Periosteum and endosteum

With the exception of joint surfaces or direct insertions of tendons, all other parts of bones are covered with **periosteum**. The periosteum consists of an outer fibrous layer *(Stratum fibrosum)* and an inner nourishing regenerative layer *(Stratum osteogenicum)*. The collagen fibres of the Stratum fibrosum run in a longitudinal direction. The off-branching collagen fibres are *SHARPEY fibres* which course through the vascularised and densely innervated Stratum osteogenicum to the compact bone, and firmly anchor the periosteum to the bone. The periosteum is very well innervated and supplied with blood. Inside, the spongy bone (cancellous bone trabeculae) is covered by a single epithelial layer, the **endosteum.** The blood supply of the bone and the bone marrow is provided by larger vessels, which penetrate the bone via osseous channels **(Vasa nutritia).** They are visible as holes in the bones of a skeleton.

NOTE

Due to the good innervation of the periosteum, impacts against bones are always extremely painful (kick against the shin). The regeneration of a bone fracture begins in the periosteum and endosteum.

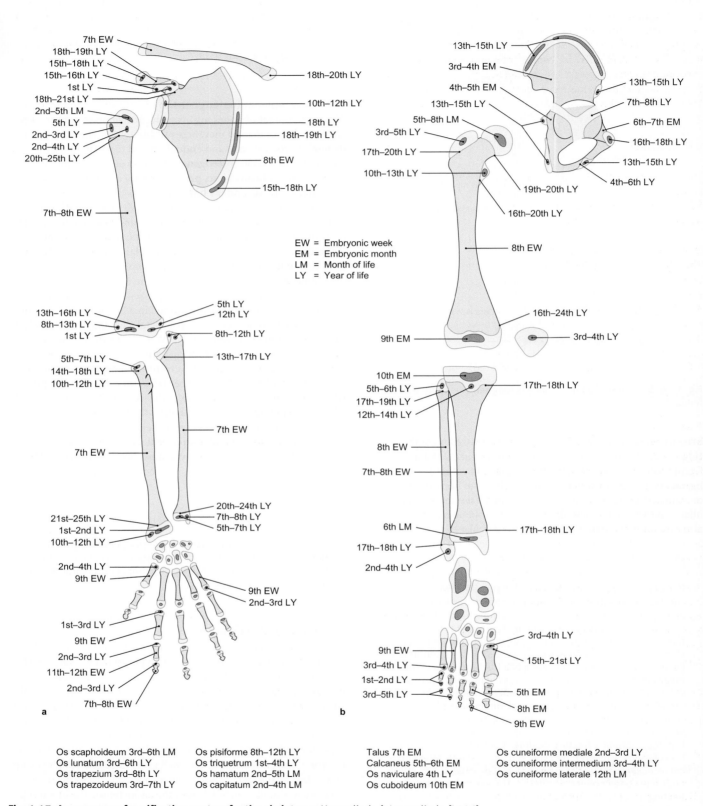

EW = Embryonic week
EM = Embryonic month
LM = Month of life
LY = Year of life

Os scaphoideum 3rd–6th LM
Os lunatum 3rd–6th LY
Os trapezium 3rd–8th LY
Os trapezoideum 3rd–7th LY

Os pisiforme 8th–12th LY
Os triquetrum 1st–4th LY
Os hamatum 2nd–5th LM
Os capitatum 2nd–4th LM

Talus 7th EM
Calcaneus 5th–6th EM
Os naviculare 4th LY
Os cuboideum 10th EM

Os cuneiforme mediale 2nd–3rd LY
Os cuneiforme intermedium 3rd–4th LY
Os cuneiforme laterale 12th LM

Fig. 1.17 Appearance of ossification centres for the skeleton. a Upper limb. **b** Lower limb. [L126]

Blood supply

For the continuous remodelling processes in bone, haematopoiesis in the bone marrow and calcium homoeostasis, a good blood supply is needed. For this reason, there are afferent and efferent blood vessels (**Vasa nutritia**), which enter and leave the bone via corresponding passageways (**Foramina nutritia**). The compact bone of the long bones has a specific vascular system, consisting of HAVERS and VOLKMANN canals.

1.4.3 Joints

Joints are flexible connections (junctures) between cartilaginous and/or bony skeletal elements. They allow movements and a transfer of forces without reaching critical values of load in the bones, which could lead to a fracture.

Joint connections (junctures)

The adjacent bones of the skeletal system can be connected continuously or articulate intermittently, and therefore two types of joints exist:
- 'false' joints (**synarthroses,** as continuous connections)
- 'true' joints (**diarthroses,** as discontinuous connections)

'False' joints are immobile articulations characterised by filling tissue between the skeletal elements; there is no joint space; they are referred to as symphysis, junctures, syndesmosis or synchondrosis. In contrast, true joints have a joint space between the articulating skeletal elements.

False joints

Synarthroses (➤ Table 1.7, ➤ Fig. 1.18) differ according to the type of filling tissue which can consist of connective tissue, cartilage or bone. Normally synarthroses allow only a low-grade to moderate mobility (connective or cartilaginous tissue) or no movement at all (bony tissue) between the skeletal elements. The freedom of movement also depends on the type and amount of the filling tissue, which in turn develops in the sense of a functional adaptation depending on the mechanical stresses to which the synarthrosis is exposed. In this way syndesmoses are loaded by traction; in synchondroses, depending on the type of loading, hyaline cartilage (compressive stress) or fibrous cartilage (shear stress) may occur. One example is the pubic symphysis (➤ Fig. 1.19). It is reinforced above and below by 2 ligaments (Ligg. pubica superius and inferius), which absorb traction forces; the hyaline cartilage in the gap of the pubic symphysis absorbs compressive forces and the fibrous cartilage absorbs shear stresses.

Syndesmosis [ligamentous juncture, Junctura fibrosa]

The adjacent bones of ligamentous articulations or junctures are connected by:

- Collagen tissue fibres – e. g. Membrana interossea radioulnaris
- Elastic tissue fibres – e. g. Ligg. flava between adjacent vertebral arches

Syndesmoses include the Membrana interossea cruris, and the Syndesmosis tibiofibularis as well as the cranial sutures and fontanelles. The **cranial sutures** are bridged by connective tissue, that has developed from embryonic tissue and that shortly after birth, has covered even larger areas between the developing cranial bones in the form of fontanelles (➤ Chap. 9.1.3). According to the form of sutures, a distinction is made between:

- **Sutura serrata** (serrate suture): a toothed connection, very solid (e. g. Sutura lambdoidea)
- **Sutura squamosa** (squamous suture): a scale-like bevelled bone surface (e. g. Squama ossis temporalis or Os parietale)
- **Sutura plana** (plane suture): with almost even, smooth and parallel bone edges (e. g. Sutura palatina mediana)
- **Schindylesis** ('tongue and groove' suture): a bony crest sunken into a slit-like deepening (e. g. the vomer in the Os sphenoidale)
- **Gomphosis** (pouring in): as the dental root 'plugged' in the alveolar bone

Synchondrosis [cartilaginous articulation or juncture, Junctura cartilaginea]

The adjacent bones of a synchondrosis are connected by hyaline cartilage. These junctures include the costal cartilage between ribs and sternum, the epiphyses (growth zones) and also the Synchondrosis sphenooccipitalis of the skull. A **symphysis** (fused) like the Symphysis pubica represents a special form. Fibrous cartilage occurs here as well as in the intervertebral discs (Disci intervertebrales).

Synostosis [osseous juncture or union, Junctura ossea]

Two bones are secondarily fused by bony tissue, e. g. the Os sacrum and hip bones.

Clinical remarks

If two bones of an existing joint become fused, e. g. after a joint infection or due to immobilisation, this is defined as **ankylosis.**

True joints

Characteristic features of diarthroses are (➤ Fig. 1.20):
- articulating skeletal elements
- a joint space
- joint surfaces (Facies articulares) covered with cartilage
- a joint cavity (Cavitas articularis)
- a surrounding joint capsule (Capsula articularis)
- ligaments reinforcing the joint capsule
- and muscles that move and stabilise the joint

Table 1.7 Synarthroses.

Synarthrosis	Synonym	Filling tissue	Description	Examples
Ligamentous articulation (➤ Fig. 1.18a)	Syndesmosis, Junctura fibrosa	Connective tissue (collagen, elastic fibres)	2 bones are connected by connective tissue	• Membrana interossea cruris, Syndesmosis tibiofibularis, (cranial) fontanelles • Special form: gomphosis (attachment of a tooth in the alveolar part of the jaws)
Cartilaginous articulation (➤ Fig. 1.18b)	Synchondrosis, Junctura cartilaginea	Cartilage (hyaline cartilage, fibrous cartilage)	2 bones are connected by cartilage	Epiphyseal gaps, rib cartilage, Symphysis pubica
Osseous union (➤ Fig. 1.18c)	Synostosis, Junctura ossea	Bones	2 bones are secondarily fused by bony tissue	Os sacrum, Os coxae, ossified epiphyseal gaps after completed growth, individual cranial sutures

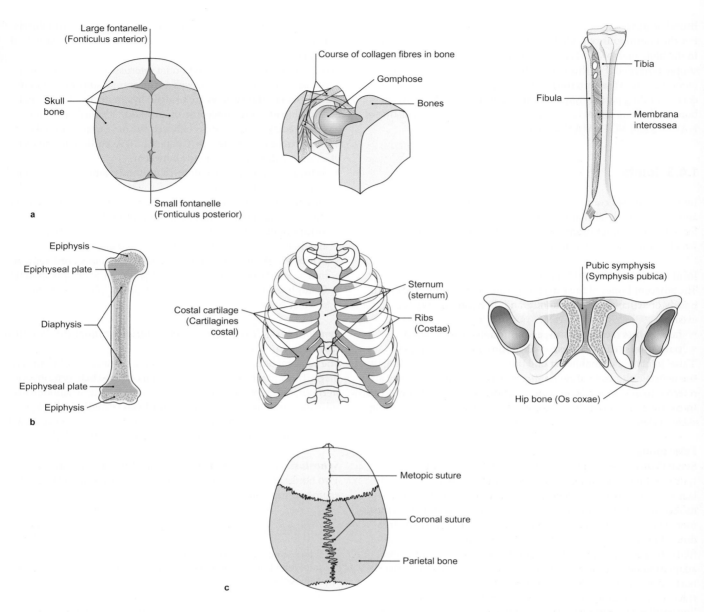

Fig. 1.18 Synarthrosis. a Ligamentous articulation [syndesmosis]. **b** Cartilaginous articulation [synchondrosis]. **c** Osseous union [synostosis]. [L126]

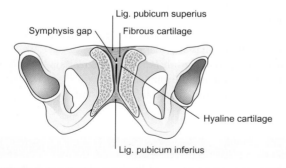

Fig. 1.19 Functional adaptation via connective and supporting tissues exemplified by the pubic symphysis (symphysis pubica). [L126]

These structures form a functional unit. Joints, which have very limited mobility due to a tense joint capsule are called **amphiarthroses** or fixed joints (e. g. Articulatio sacroiliaca, numerous carpal joints of hand and foot).

Joint development

The primordial limbs (➤ Chap. 4.2) consist of a mesenchymal blastema, which originates from the parietal mesoderm of the body wall (somatopleura). Within the mesenchyme, cell consolidations (precartilage blastema) occur, from which preformed cartilaginous skeletal elements develop. At the future locations of joints, an intensive cell consolidation takes place. Thereby joints can develop in two ways:

- **Carve out (carve out joints):** In this most common type, splitting within a preformed skeletal element occurs, e. g. hip joint, knee joint.
- **Apposition (apposition joints):** In this case two preformed skeletal elements grow towards each other. In the area of their first contact initially a bursa develops which is later transformed into a joint cavity. In addition, there are articular discs (see below), e. g. in the temporomandibular joint, the sternoclavicular joint or the posterior joint of pelvic girdle (sacroiliac joint).

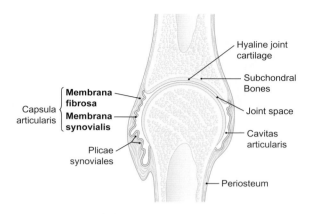

Fig. 1.20 Synovial or 'true' joint (Junctura synovialis, articulation, diarthrosis). The muscles moving the joint and the ligaments enhancing the joint capsule are not shown here.

In the development of carve out joints the following processes occur:
- Within the blastema and under the influence of hox genes cell consolidations are organised, from which **precartilage** is differentiated (precursor of the later joint cartilage) with a cell-poor homogeneous intermediate zone (**inter-zone,** becoming the later joint space).
- Due to the synchronised developmental processes, the characteristic shape of the precartilaginous preformed skeletal elements can be seen as early as the *6th embryonic week.*
- In the *8th embryonic week* a cracking (joint space or line) and the formation of the **joint cavity** occur in the inter-zone. The peripheral areas of the inter-zone differentiate into the **joint capsule,** and the inner layer of the capsule starts producing the synovial fluid. The precartilage immediately adjacent to the joint space differentiates further into the hyaline **joint cartilage.**
- The processes are completed in the middle of the *3rd embryonic month.* Since then any further increase in size is achieved by interstitial and appositional growth. However, the nutrition of the cartilage by diffusion from the differentiated perichondrium and from the synovia of the joint cavity will soon become insufficient, therefore in the *13th embryonic week* **blood vessels** emerge in the hyaline cartilage. Only areas close to the perichondrium and the joint space remain avascular. The regular growth of joint bodies therefore also depends greatly on the blood supply. However, this blood supply is not linked to the genetically determined beginning of the endochondral osteogenesis.

Intra-articular structures such as menisci, ligaments, joint lips and articular discs (see below) all originate from the blastema of the inter-zone. In contrast to diarthroses, in **synarthroses** the gap formation in the inter-zone is omitted. Here, the filling tissue of the corresponding synarthrosis (connective tissue or cartilage) differentiates from the cells of the inter-zone.

Clinical remarks

In the case of disruptions or disturbances of joint development, fusions of skeletal elements can occur **(synostoses, Coalition),** which appear most commonly in the hand and foot skeleton.

Types of joint
Joints (Juncturae synoviales, articulation, diarthroses) typically have a significant range of motion and can be classified according to:

- Number of movement axes (according to the body axes) or degrees of freedom:
  - uni-axial
  - biaxial
  - multiaxial
- Number of articulating skeletal elements:
  - Simple joints (Articulationes simplices): 2 bones articulate with each other (e. g. hip joint)
  - Composite joints (Articulationes compositae): several bones articulate with each other (e. g. elbow joint, knee joint)
- Form and shape of the joint surfaces (➤ Fig. 1.21):
  - **Cylindrical or roll-like joints** (Articulatio cylindrica):
    - **Hinge joint** (Ginglymus): uni-axial joint, which allows flexion and extension (e. g. Articulatio talocruralis, ➤ Fig. 1.21a)
    - **Pivot joint** (Articulatio conoidea): uni-axial joint, which allows rotational movements (e. g. Articulatio radioulnaris proximalis, ➤ Fig. 1.21b); the pivot rotates as a joint head in a concave joint cavity
    - **Wheel-like or trochoid joint** (Articulatio trochoidea): uni-axial joint, which allows rotational movements (e. g. Articulatio atlantoaxialis mediana, ➤ Fig. 1.21c); the concave joint cavity turns around a fixed pivot
  - **Condyloid or ellipsoid joint** (Articulatio ovoidea, Articulatio ellipsoidea): biaxial joint which allows flexion, extension, abduction, adduction and slight rotatory movements (e. g. proximal wrist, ➤ Fig. 1.21d)
  - **Saddle joint** (Articulatio sellaris): biaxial joint, which allows flexion, extension, abduction, adduction and slight rotatory movements (e. g. carpometacarpal joint of the thumb, ➤ Fig. 1.21e)
  - **Ball-and-socket joint** (Articulatio spheroidea): joint with 3 axes, which allows flexion and extension, abduction and adduction, internal and external rotation as well as rotatory movements (e. g. shoulder joint, ➤ Fig. 1.21f)
  - **Plane or flat joint** (Articulatio plana): joint which allows simple gliding movements in different directions (e. g. vertebral joints, ➤ Fig. 1.21g)

A special form are **condylar joints** (Articulationes bicondylares). They have similar curved surfaces like ellipsoid and cylindrical joints. Their main characteristics are biconvex bony prominences (condyles), which articulate with concave joint surfaces. These biaxial joints allow rotational, shifting (translational) and rolling movements (e. g. temporomandibular joint, Articulatio femorotibialis).

NOTE

Uni-axial joints have one axis of movement, and the orientation of this axis is responsible for the type of movement. They have therefore only one degree of freedom. The movement in biaxial joints occurs around two axes perpendicular to each other, which intersect in the centre of the joint. The mobility of the joint bodies (articulating bones) in biaxial joints is therefore greater than in uni-axial and lesser than in three-axial joints.

Structure of joints
A characteristic feature of diarthroses is a synovial joint space **(Cavitas articularis).** With the help of the lubricating synovial fluid the articulating bones can move against each other.

General structure
Despite the different types of joints some basic structural characteristics can be distinguished:

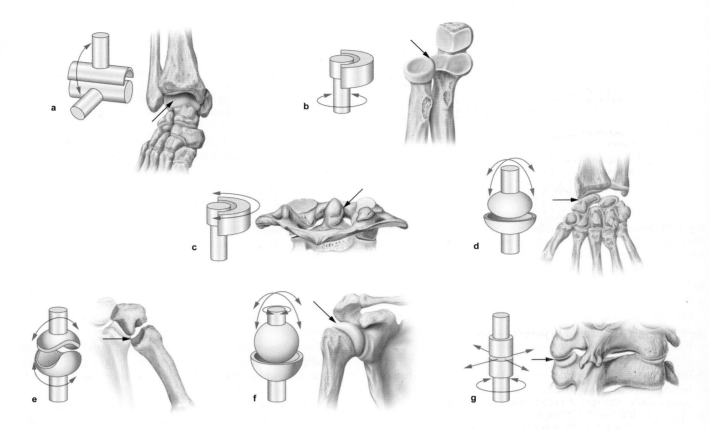

Fig. 1.21 Types of joints (Juncturis synovialis). **a** Hinge joint. **b** Conoid pivot joint. **c** Trochoid pivot joint. **d** Condyloid joint. **e** Saddle joint. **f** Ball-and-socket joint. **g** Plane joint. [L127]

- **Caput articulare** (joint head)
- **Fossa articularis** (joint socket)
- **Coating of hyaline cartilage** (on joint head and joint socket)

N O T E

Exceptions to the rule of a hyaline cartilage covering can be found in the temporomandibular joint and the sternoclavicular joint. They are covered by fibrous cartilage.

Joint cartilage

The articulating bone ends (joint surfaces, Facies articulares) of synovial joints are covered with **hyaline cartilage** of varying thickness according to their exposure to biomechanical stresses (or loads). For example, the patella has a particularly thick joint cartilage (up to 7 mm), in the sacroiliac joint the cartilage on the joint surface of the sacrum is much thicker (4 mm) than on the joint surface of the ilium (1 mm); the thickness of the joint cartilage in the hip joint is 2–4 mm, and in the finger joints only 1–2 mm. Healthy joint cartilage appears whitish and is devoid of a perichondrium and blood vessels. So it has to be supplied via diffusion and convection by blood vessels in the synovia of the joint space and the subchondral bone. Joint cartilage is structured according to its exposure to biomechanical stresses: the collagen fibrils in the joint cartilage (specific type II collagen) run in a corresponding direction; the cartilaginous cells (chondrocytes), which form the collagen fibrils as well as the basic substance (glycosaminoglycans and proteoglycans, particularly the water-binding aggrecan), have a distinct morphology in different areas of the joint cartilage. For

this reason, joint cartilage can be divided into different zones (➤ Fig. 1.22a):

- The superficial **zone of tangential fibres** (zone I) is directly adjacent to the joint space. The chondrocytes are spindle-shaped, and the orientation of the collagen fibres is parallel to the surface. Due to the composition of the extracellular matrix, the retention of water in this zone is particularly high.
- In the **transition zone** (zone II) the collagen fibrils run obliquely to the surface of the cartilage and cross the collagen fibrils of the opposite direction at right angles. The chondrocytes are arranged in so-called isogenic groups (clusters of several cells).
- The **radiate zone** (zone III) is the widest layer, here the collagen fibrils converge radially to the underlying layers. The chondrocytes are arranged in small columnar groups. The caudal border forms a limiting line ('tide mark') between the non-mineralised cartilage and the underlying mineralised cartilage.
- The **zone of mineralised cartilage** (zone IV) consists of calcified cartilage, which is the connection to the underlying subchondral bone and transfers the biomechanical forces onto the bone.

Functionally, the joint cartilage serves as a smooth surface which reduces the friction between the articulating bones. This enables an equal distribution of pressure onto the subchondral bone. The various zones of joint cartilage adapt and balance the different elasticity modules of the tissues and prevent an overloading of the structures. When exposed to compressive forces, the cartilage conveys water towards the joint space and reabsorbs it when the pressure subsides (convection). The joint surfaces can reversibly deform to a certain degree.

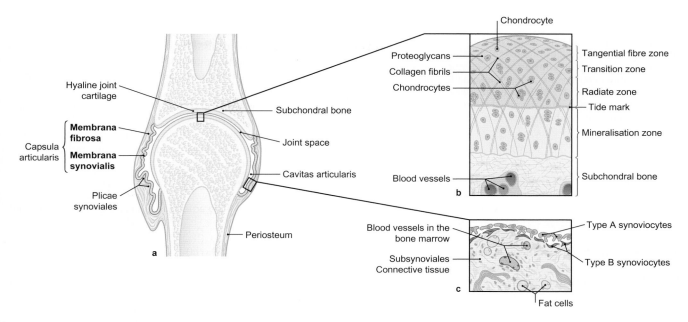

Fig. 1.22 General structure of a joint. a General structure. **b** Joint cartilage. **c** Joint capsule. [L126]

Joint capsule
The joint cavity of synovial joints is completely surrounded by a joint capsule (Capsula articularis) (➤ Fig. 1.22b) that seals the joint cavity airtight. The joint capsule consists of the following structures:
• **Membrana fibrosa:** this outer fibrous layer contains mainly type I collagen and only a few elastic fibres; in many joints it is reinforced additionally by ligaments; it continues peripherally into the periosteum of the bone.
• **Membrana synovialis:** the inner lining of the joint capsule and thus the layer directly adjacent to the joint space, is the cell-rich synovial membrane which is further divided into:

– The **innermost synovial layer or Tunica intima** (consists of 2 cell populations):
– *Type A synoviocytes,* have many vacuoles and are capable of phagocytosis, take up waste products of the cartilage cell metabolism, lie superficial to the joint cavity
– *Type B synoviocytes,* are fibroblast-like, rich in endoplasmic reticulum and produce the lubricating synovial fluid, lie below the type-a synovialocytes.
– **Subsynovial tissue,** containing fibroblasts, fat cells (adipocytes), macrophages, mastocytes, pain receptors and mechanoreceptors, as well as large quantities of blood vessels and lymphatic vessels)
The surface area of the synovia is enlarged by synovial folds and villi, and can easily follow joint movements.

Synovia
The highly viscous **synovia or synovial fluid ('lubricant' of the joint)** is a clear, slightly yellowish fluid consisting of proteohyaluronate and a transudate of blood, that is similar to the blood serum. Normally, there is only a small amount of synovia in a joint (e. g. in the knee joint only 3–6 ml).
The synovial fluid produced by type B synoviocytes in the Tunica intima has a pH value of 7.3–7.7 and consists of hyaluronic acid (2–3 mg/ml), proteins (10–30 mg/ml), glucose (0.5–0.7 mg/ml), water and desquamated cells.
Its **functions** are:
• **Nutrition** of the joint cartilage and of parts of the intra-articular structures
• **Lubrication** (friction-free gliding of the joint surfaces)
• **Shock absorption** (by an even distribution of the compressive forces)

Joint loading

The joint cartilage is loaded under physiological conditions by axial pressure, as the transfer of forces from a joint surface to the other is perpendicular to the cartilage surface. Forces that act on the joint are:

- **Partial body weight** (e. g. with unilateral loaded hip joint, the weight of the torso, neck, head and upper limbs)
- **Muscular and ligamentous forces** (e. g. with unilateral loaded hip joint exerted by the iliotibial tract and the muscles acting on it, as the M. tensor fasciae latae, M. gluteus maximus, M. vastus lateralis)

The partial body weight is reduced by the action of antagonistic muscles and ligaments. The result is the actual **load of the joint** ($\succ$ Fig. 1.15), which is referred to as the **joint resultant (R)** and can be represented as the sum of vectors of gravitational (partial body weight), muscular and ligamentous forces. It passes in accordance with the laws of balance through the respective fulcrum of the joint ($\succ$ Fig. 1.15). With movements in the joint, size, direction and position of the joint resultant will change.

The actual pressure on the cartilage (intra-articular pressure and surface contact) depends not only on the joint resultant (joint load) but also on the size of the surface exposed to the force. The smaller the surface is, the greater the pressure is: the small area of a stiletto heel will leave pits in a new wooden floor, whereas the larger area of the flat sole does not.

Auxiliary or accessory structures

In several joints there are auxiliary or accessory intra-articular structures that are essential for the biomechanical function and the range of motion of joints:

- **Interposed discs**
  - Disci articulares
  - Menisci articulares
- **Joint lips** (Labra articularia)

In addition, **bursae** (Bursae synoviales) occur, which form elastic pads or cushions and enable the sliding of tendons and muscles against bone, as well as **ligaments** (Ligamenta) which reinforce the capsule, guide or inhibit movements.

Intra-articular discs

They can compensate for uneven areas (incongruence) of the articulating joint surfaces and are exposed to compressive forces. They can be complete discs (Disci, like a full moon) or partial discs (Menisci, crescent-shaped moon).

- **Disci articulares** consist of dense connective tissue and fibrous cartilage. They fill the joint cavity completely and are often attached to the joint capsule (e. g. Discus articularis of the temporomandibular joint).
- **Menisci articulares** also consist of dense connective tissue and fibrous tissue. They look crescent-like seen from above, and wedge-shaped in profile, and they cover the margins or the periphery of the joint surfaces (medial meniscus, and lateral meniscus of the knee joint).

NOTE

In contrast to menisci the articular discs completely cover the joint surface.

Joint lips (Labra articularia)

These structures are composed of connective tissue and fibrous cartilage, and they serve to enlarge the sockets of joints. In the human body, **joint lips (Labra)** are found in the shoulder joint (Labrum glenoidale) and in the hip joint (Labrum acetabuli). They are anchored in the bony ring (Limbus) of the respective joint socket.

Bursae

A **bursa (Bursa synovialis)** is, in principle, structured like a joint capsule. You can imagine it as a fluid-filled cushion. It is surrounded by a layer of connective tissue (Membrana fibrosa) and inside there is a synovial membrane (Membrana synovialis), which produces the fluid in the lumen of the bursa. The composition of the fluid is almost identical with the synovial fluid in joints. The elastic bursae allow the sliding of tendons and muscles on bones and tendons. They can communicate with the joint cavity (e. g. Bursa subscapularis in the shoulder joint) or occur as independent bursa (e. g. Bursa prepatellaris).

Ligaments

Ligaments (Ligamenta) consist of tight collagenous tissue. The fibres are usually arranged in parallel. Ligaments can be flat or string-like and form a connection of mobile skeletal elements. In addition to the tight ligaments of the locomotor system (e. g. the Lig. cruciatum anterius or anterior cruciate ligament in the knee joint) there are thin, delicate connections between structures within body cavities (e. g. the Lig. hepatoduodenale, a ligament between liver and duodenum). The ligaments of the locomotor system occur as **intra-articular ligaments** (e. g. Lig. cruciatum anterius) within joints or as **extra-articular ligaments** outside the joints (e. g. the Lig. collaterale fibulare, the lateral or outer collateral ligament of the knee joint). If ligaments are integrated into the joint capsule, one speaks of **intracapsular ligaments** as opposed to extracapsular ligaments, which are separated from the joint capsule by loose connective tissue.

Extracapsular ligaments are divided according to their function in:
- **Reinforcing ligaments** of the joint capsule, e. g. the Lig. pubofemorale at the hip joint
- **Guiding ligaments,** for the guidance of joint movements, e. g. the Lig. anulare radii at the elbow joint
- **Inhibiting or restricting ligaments,** which limit joint movements, e. g. the Lig. iliofemorale at the hip joint

Ligaments usually do not have just one, but several functions (of the three mentioned above).

1.4.4 General considerations on muscles

There are three different types of muscular tissue:
- Striated skeletal muscles
- Cardiac muscle
- Smooth muscles

The **striated skeletal muscles** represent the active locomotor system. The skeletal muscles comprise approximately 300 muscles including their tendons and muscle-specific connective tissue. Skeletal muscles exist, apart from the axial system, in the tongue, pharynx, larynx, in parts of the oesophagus and in the anal region. Each skeletal muscle consists of a varying number of *muscle fibres,* which are their smallest distinct structural units.

Skeletal muscles actively move the bones of joints. Additional **functions of muscles** can be:
- Stabilisation of joints (postural securing)
- Tension banding (reduction of bending stress of long bones)
- Energy storage when stretched (attenuation in the joint with dynamic activity)

Clinical remarks

After strong, unusual loads (mostly in sports) the muscle tissue can become disrupted. This is called a **tear of muscle fibres** or in the case of a severe damage as **muscle rupture** (depending on the extent of muscle damage). The muscles of the thigh or lower leg are most often affected. It is differentiated from muscle **strain** in which no macroscopic structural changes with destruction of muscle cells and bleeding can be recognised.

Muscle ache is a pain that occurs after physical exertion, especially after high stress of certain muscle parts. It is usually only first detectable hours after the respective activity. It used to be attributed to an acidification of the respective muscle by lactic acid (lactate) but this has been refuted. This is caused by small microtears in the muscle fibrils with a subsequent inflammatory reaction.

Structure of skeletal muscle

Skeletal muscle can be differentiated into:
- **Belly of a muscle** (venter musculi): shaped differently
- **Tendon** (tendo musculi): transmits the muscle tension directly or indirectly to the skeletal or connective tissue elements:
  - **Origin (Origo):** original tendon, close to torso (proximal) attachment point
  - **Attachment (Insertio):** attachment tendon, far from torso (distal) attachment point
  - **Fixation point:** attachment site on an immovable skeletal element
  - **Mobile point:** attachment site on a movable skeletal element

NOTE

Muscle origin and muscle attachment are arbitrarily determined. They must not be confused with the Punctum fixum and the Punctum mobile.

It is not necessarily always the case that the Punctum fixum and muscular origin match, because Punctum fixum and Punctum mobile can also change depending on the movement. Muscles on the back of the thigh (ischiocrural muscles) can, for example, on contraction cause either knee joint flexion (Punctum fixum and muscle origin match) or in the case of a distal Punctum fixum support a backward tilt of the pelvis in the hip joint.

Types of muscle

There are several ways to grade muscles:
- **Arrangement of muscle fibres:**
  - parallel course of muscle fibres (to pulling direction of the tendon); extensive movements are possible with little force
  - pinnate, i.e. an oblique course of muscle fibres in a certain acute angle (pinnate angle) to long, wide tendons, high muscle strength
- **Number of heads:** 1, 2 or more heads
- **Differences according to joint involvement:** depending on whether a muscle is involved in movements in 1 or 2 joints or has no relationship to a joint, a distinction can be made between:
  - single joint muscles
  - double joint muscles
  - mimicry muscles (no joint involvement)
- **Shape:** according to their form muscles are divided into (➤ Fig. 1.23):
  - single-headed, parallel fibre muscles (M. fusiformis)
  - two-headed parallel fibre muscles (M. biceps)

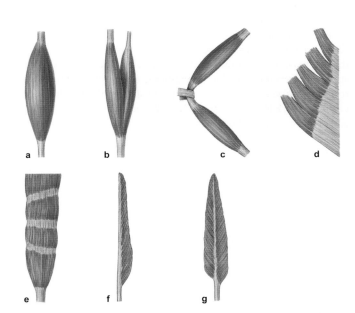

Fig. 1.23 Types of muscles. a Single-headed muscle with parallel fibres. **b** Two-headed muscle with parallel fibres. **c** Two-bellied muscle with parallel fibres. **d** Multi-headed flat muscle. **e** Multi-bellied muscle with tendinous intersections. **f** Unipennate muscle. **g** Multipennate muscle.

- two-lobed, parallel fibre muscles (M. biventer)
- multilobed, flat muscles (M. planus)
- multilobed muscles divided by intermediate tendon (M. intersectus)
- semipennate muscles (M. semipennatus)
- multipennate muscles (M. pennatus)

Tendon

Tendons are constructed of dense parallel fibrous connective tissue and have special facilities at the muscle-tendon transition, as well as in the area of the attachment zones to the skeleton. They are extremely tear-resistant, elastic and can be plastically deformed. At the same time, however, they can only be slightly stretched (5–10 %). They have the function to transfer the force created in the contraction of a muscle to the skeletal elements. The transfer of the force takes place mainly at the muscle-tendon transition. The shape of the tendons differs from muscle to muscle. Some tendons are so short that they cannot be seen macroscopically (fleshy attachment), while others are extremely thin and flat, so that they are referred to as aponeuroses.

Types

From a structural and functional point of view, a distinction is made between tension tendons and sliding tendons:

- **Tension tendons** are located in the main direction of the muscle and are exclusively used in tensile stress. They have the typical tendon structure.
- **Sliding or pressure tendons** change their course direction by pulling around a bone or a connective tissue structure. The bone/connective tissue structure is used as a pivot point (hypomochlion). On the side facing the bone/connective tissue structure, strain is placed on the tendon under pressure and slides at this point. Fibrous tissue at the deflection point is stored in the tendon.

Muscle-tendon transition

The **myotendinous zone** is the connection between the muscle fibre and the collagen fibres of the origin and attachment areas. It is characterised by an extensive surface enlargement (factor 10) of the cytoplasmic membrane at the muscle fibre end. In the area of surface enlargement the basal membrane of the muscle fibre is surrounded by a microfibre network (thin collagen fibres). The fibrils of the network interlace internally with microfibres of the tendon and create a fixed anchorage.

Tendon attachment zones

Tendon attachment zones are present to adapt the different elasticity modules of connective tissue, cartilage and bone to each other, to avoid detachment or tearing of the tendons in the attachment area. You can imagine this as a spring embedded in the insertion area. According to the structure and the position, a distinction is made between 2 types of tendon attachment zones (➤ Fig. 1.24):

- **Chondral apophyseal attachment zones:** They occur in all muscles, which insert in areas of previous cartilaginous apophyses and also in some other muscles (e. g. the tendons of the masticatory muscles on the skull skeleton). It is characteristic that fibrous cartilage is embedded at the insertion site, of which the layer directly covering the bone is mineralised. In the area of insertion the periosteum is missing and the collagen fibres penetrate into the bone.
- **Periosteal diaphyseal attachment zones:** They are typical for the diaphyses of the long bones. The collagen fibres of the planar tendons radiate into the periosteum and anchor the tendon into the cortical bone. In this way, the force is transmitted over a very large area. In some cases the collagen fibres penetrate directly into the bone. At this point, the periosteum is missing. Periosteal diaphyseal attachments are characterised by roughness (tuberosities) to the bone.

Clinical remarks

Overloading of chondreal apophyseal tendon attachment zones can lead to degenerative changes with pain in the area of the attachment zone (e. g. **tennis elbow**). In periosteal diaphyseal tendon attachment zones, increased bone formation with pain sometimes occurs (e. g. in the area of the Achilles tendon insertion at the heel bone as **calcaneal spur** or in the insertion area of the quadriceps femoris muscle to the patella as **patellar tip syndrome**).

Auxiliary equipment for muscles and tendons

All muscles and tendons need additional structures to varying degrees, to

- adapt to the environment
- to protect against mechanical damage
- to prevent friction losses and to reduce
- power loss.

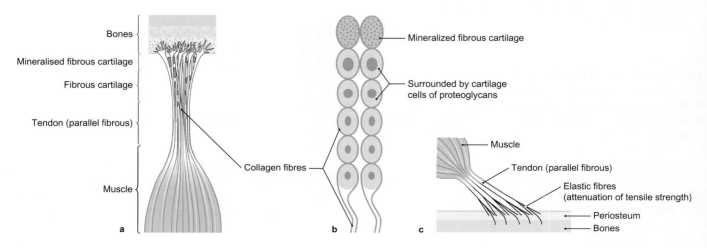

Fig. 1.24 Structure of tendinous insertions or attachment zones. a Chondroapophyseal attachment zone. **b** Schematic drawing of a chondroapophyseal attachment zone with chondrocytes, proteoglycans and collagen fibres. **c** Periosteal-diaphyseal attachment zone. [L126]

Additional structures are:
- **Fascia** (connective tissue sheath)
- **Retinacula** (connective tissue retaining ligaments)
- **Tendon sheaths**
- **Bursa**
- **Sesamoid bones**

Fascia

The fascias, which are also known as muscular facias are sheaths made of collagen connective tissue which surround individual muscles, several muscles (muscle groups) and tendons like a sheath or a stocking. Fascias can be considered as an outer layer of the musculature. The fascias allow the muscle to contract almost invisibly without the surrounding tissue also contracting.
A distinction is made between:
- **Single fascia:** enveloping a muscle
- **Group fascias:** encasement of several muscles of a muscle group (but each individual muscle of the muscle group has its own individual fascia)
- **Body fascia:** originate from the general body fascia (superficial fascia) and cover the underlying muscles (which are already inserted into individual and group fascias)

N O T E

Group fascias form the interosseous membrane or the intermuscular septum (also a fascia) **osteofibrous channels,** especially in the area of the lower leg of the lower extremities, together with the periosteum of the adjacent bones in which single muscle groups lie. They are referred to as **fascial compartments.** Each muscle group is supplied by independent blood and lymph vessels.
The importance of fascias for the body is greater than generally assumed. Consequently fascias led a shadowy scientific existence. Only in the last few years have they increasingly become the goal of scientific focus. Because they are innervated, pain can also be transmitted through them. Paramedically, there are now trends towards 'fascial fitness'.

--- Clinical remarks ---

Injuries of the blood vessels for individual muscular compartments in the context of major trauma (e. g. traffic accident) may cause a collection of effluent blood in the respective muscle compartment (osteofibrous canal) and compression of the (muscle) tissue. This is referred to as **compartment syndrome** (compartment = muscle group). If the osteofibrous canal is not relieved (opened) as soon as possible, the muscle tissue can be irreversibly damaged.

Retinacula

Retinacula are connective tissue retaining ligaments for tissue layers or organs. In the extremities they ensure e. g. on the hand or foot joints that the tendons do not become detached from the bones in muscle contraction. You can look at it as a belt that keeps them in their typical position.

Tendon sheaths

A tendon sheath (**Vagina tendinis**) encloses a tendon everywhere where it runs directly on the bone or is deflected (hypomochlion). It protects the tendon and enables improved gliding. Tendon

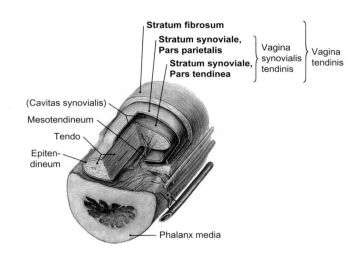

Fig. 1.25 Structure of a tendon sheath.

sheaths are comparable in their design to joint capsules (➤ Fig. 1.25). The **inner tendon sheath sheet (Stratum synoviale, Pars tendinea)** is fused with the tendon, the **outer tendon sheath sheet (Stratum synoviale, Pars parietale)** with the fibrous layer of the tendon sheath. In the gliding space (**Cavitas synovialis**) a fluid comparable to synovial fluid is emitted. Small blood vessels guarantee the nourishment of the tendon via small ligaments of the mesotendon (Vincula brevia and longa) into the tendon.

--- Clinical remarks ---

Overuse can lead to painful **tenosynovitis (inflammation of the tendon sheath)** that is particularly common on hands and feet. A **tenosynovitis stenosans** (stenosing tenosynovitis) is characteristic of overuse of hand flexor muscles. It is especially common in activities with a stereotypic movement, e. g. tradespeople, athletes, piano players or frequent long-term work on a computer keyboard (is sometimes recognised as an occupational disease). The overload leads to minor injuries in the tendon, which the body attempts to repair with an inflammatory reaction. The associated swelling of the tendon constricts the tendon sheath (Tenosynovitis stenosans) and leads to the formation of tendon nodules, which for every finger flexion has to pass through small circular ligaments (ring ligaments, Ligg. annularia, affixing the tendon sheaths on the bone) and can be trapped there. This secondarily gives rise to the **phenomenon of 'trigger finger'**.

Bursa

The pressure elastic bursae facilitate the sliding of tendons and muscles over bones and tendons (➤ Chap. 1.4.3).

Sesamoid bone

Sesamoid bones (Ossa sesamoidea) are bones which are stored in tendons and functionally protect the tendon
- against too much friction or
- extend the lever arm and thus save muscle strength.
They emerge in the sense of a functional fit of tissue in the area of pressure tendons. Examples are the kneecap (Patella) or the pisiform bone (Os pisiforme) of the wrist.

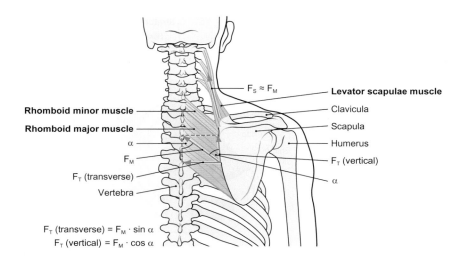

F_S ≈ F_M
Levator scapulae muscle
Rhomboid minor muscle
Clavicula
Rhomboid major muscle
Scapula
α
Humerus
F_M
F_T (vertical)
F_T (transverse)
α
Vertebra

$F_T \text{ (transverse)} = F_M \cdot \sin \alpha$
$F_T \text{ (vertical)} = F_M \cdot \cos \alpha$

Fig. 1.26 Muscle work. Transfer of muscle force on tendon force depending on the orientation of muscle fibres in relation to the tendons.

General muscle mechanisms
Muscle activation and coordination
The central nervous system coordinates movements by sending pulses along the peripheral nerves to muscles. As a rule, several muscles will be addressed at the same time, which support a certain movement in the same direction (**synergists**) or their counteracting (**antagonists**). An activation of the synergists is paired with inhibition of antagonists. Physiologically the nerve impulses constantly reach the muscles and ensure that some of the muscle fibres are in the contraction state. Consequently, tension is built up, which is designated as **basic tone (resting tone)**.

The visible contraction of a muscle commences only when an initial resistance against the tone of the antagonists is overcome. Initially only the tension condition increases in the muscle, without shortening of the muscle fibres (**isometric contraction**). Only then does a shortening of the muscle fibres (**isotonic contraction**) occur at the same level of tension that leads to visible movement.

Muscle work
Lifting force/lifting height
The work of a muscle depends on
* its power development (lifting force) and
* the extent of its reduction (lifting height)

and can be calculated using the simple formula: work = force (F) × distance. The force is referred to as a lifting force, the path as a lifting height.
* **Lifting force:** It depends on the physiological cross-section (total cross-section) and from the pennate angle (the angle through which the muscle fibres insert in the tendon, see above).
* **Lifting height:** It depends on the length of the muscle fibres and on the pennate angle.

There is a direct proportional relationship between muscle force and physiological cross-section of the muscle (lifting force of a muscle relative to the cross-section of all muscle fibres positioned perpendicular to the direction of fibres): if the tendon of the muscle runs parallel to its tension direction (e. g. M. levator scapulae, ➤ Fig. 1.26), the complete momentum generated (*absolute muscle force)* is transferred to the tendon. Thereby, the muscle force (F_M) and the tendon force (F_T) are nearly identical. If the muscle fibres are at an angle to the tension direction of the tendon (e. g. Mm. rhomboidei major and minor, ➤ Fig. 1.26), only a part of their contraction force is transferred to the tendon. Thereby the vertical tendon force (F_T [vertical]) compared to the muscle force (F_M) is reduced by the factor cos α and the transverse tendon force (F_T [transversal]) is reduced by the factor sin α.

Muscle cross-section
A distinction is made on the muscle between an
* **Anatomical cross-section** (is perpendicular to the main line in the thickest part of the muscle) and a
* **Physiological cross-section** (is identical with the cross-sectional area of all muscle fibres and therefore a measure of the absolute contraction force of all muscle fibres).

Anatomical and physiological cross-sections only rarely match (only in the case of parallel fibrous and spindle-shaped muscles).

Lever arm and muscle activity
For understanding the muscle work it is also necessary to include the distance of the insertion point of the tendon from the joint pivot point in the considerations. In simple terms the necessary power can be estimated with lever principles and the extent of the movement can be determined. As with a lever,
* **Load arm** (body section to be moved),
* **Force arm** (muscles acting on the joint with their tendons) and
* **Pivot point** (at the joint)

can be defined on the skeleton. The amount of force a muscle can transfer to a joint depends on the length of the respective **lever** (vertical distance of the vector force of the muscle to the rotational axis of the joint = force arm) (➤ Fig. 1.27). The length of the lever varies depending on the joint position and is known as **virtual lever arm**. The torque of a muscle is calculated according to the simple formula: Torque = Force (F) × virtual lever arm.

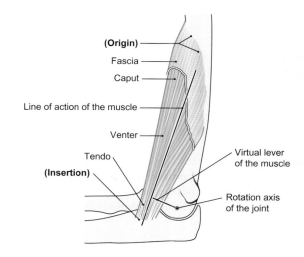

(Origin)
Fascia
Caput
Line of action of the muscle
Venter
Tendo
Virtual lever of the muscle
(Insertion)
Rotation axis of the joint

Fig. 1.27 Basic structure of a skeletal muscle.

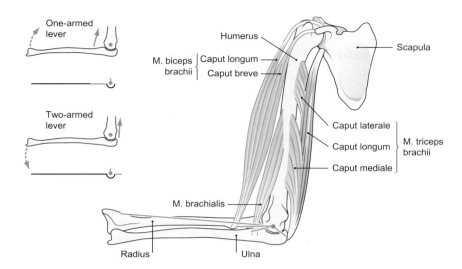

Fig. 1.28 Lever arm and muscle action. [L126]

For skeletal components to be moved around a rotational axis of a joint, a muscle must, as described, use an anatomical (= existing) lever arm to generate torque. The length of the lever arm depends on the distance between the muscle attachment and the centre of rotation of the joint. Thus, e.g. the **M. brachioradialis** has a long and the **M. brachialis** a short anatomical lever arm, when the arm is moved towards the torso (➤ Fig. 1.28). If a muscle engages a single arm lever, the skeletal element is moved in the tension direction of the muscle (e. g. M. brachioradialis, M. biceps brachii, M. brachialis, ➤ Fig. 1.28). In the case of two-arm levers, the muscular attachment point is moved in the tension direction of the muscle and the main part of the skeletal element is shifted in the opposite direction (e. g. M. triceps brachii, ➤ Fig. 1.28, see ➤ Fig. 1.27).

Work and performance
The product achieved from lifting height and lifting force is the **mechanical work** of a muscle and is measured in *joules*. The **work** a muscle performs per unit time is measured in *watts*.

Active and passive insufficiency
If a muscle is already fully reduced but the joint function has not yet reached the final position that would be possible via the maximum contraction of the muscle, one speaks of **active insufficiency.** Therefore, e. g. the knee joint cannot be bent above 125° (in neutral zero position in the hip joint). Only when there is additional flexion in the hip joint can 140° be achieved.
Passive insufficiency is when a muscle is prevented from achieving an active joint position due to its limited stretching (the muscle could shorten further but this is prevented by its antagonists). Therefore, e. g. in a flexed wrist the fist cannot be closed.

1.5 Circulation systems

Warmth, gases, nutrients, metabolic end products, hormones, among other things, and immune cells must be distributed in the body. To ensure this, the body has different circulation systems:
• Body circulation
• Pulmonary circulation
• Portal vein circulation
• Prenatal (or fetal) circulation
• Lymphatic circulation

1.5.1 Body and pulmonary circulation

Blood
Blood is the most important means of transport for gases, active substances, nutrients, waste materials and warmth. It is a liquid tissue. In the adult, the blood volume is between 4 and 6 l. Approximately 44 % are solid components (cells). The most frequent type of cell is the *erythrocyte* (red blood cells), used for gas transport (O_2 and CO_2). In second place are the thrombocytes, which act within the framework of blood coagulation (platelets). *Leukocytes* (white blood cells) describe a heterogeneous group of 5 different types of nucleated cells in the blood, which undertake all functions within the framework of the immune system (3 groups of granulocytes, monocytes and lymphocytes). They use the blood only as a means of transport and are all capable of actively leaving the vascular system and thus leave the blood through amoeboid movement to actively arrive at their deployment site in the surrounding tissue.

Blood vessel system
Blood is transported in a tube system made of blood vessels. The motor for the continuous blood flow is the heart which is divided into a left and a right ventricle. The left ventricle serves the body circulation, which supplies the individual organs with blood and the right ventricle drives the pulmonary circulation for deposition of CO_2 and the intake of O_2 (➤ Fig. 1.29).

Circulation
The **heart** is a muscular hollow organ. For each heart contraction approximately 70 ml of blood are pumped from the heart ventricles into each artery. For the left ventricle this is the main artery (aorta) and for the right ventricle the pulmonary trunk from which the left and right pulmonary arteries emerge. The permanent branching of the main vessels creates increasingly smaller **arteries** and finally, **arterioles** accomplish the transition into a capillary network, in which material and gas exchange takes place. The return transport of the blood from the capillary network is carried out via **venules**

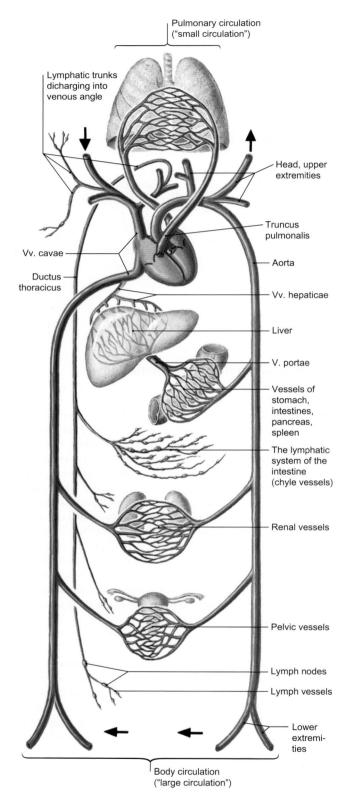

Pulmonary circulation
("small circulation")

Lymphatic trunks
dicharging into
venous angle

Head, upper
extremities

Truncus
pulmonalis

Vv. cavae

Aorta

Ductus
thoracicus

Vv. hepaticae

Liver

V. portae

Vessels of
stomach,
intestines,
pancreas,
spleen

The lymphatic
system of the
intestine
(chyle vessels)

Renal vessels

Pelvic vessels

Lymph nodes

Lymph vessels

Lower
extremi-
ties

Body circulation
("large circulation")

Fig. 1.29 Systemic and pulmonary circulation.

and then continuously larger **veins,** which transport the blood from the body circulation via the upper (Vena cava superior) and lower vena cava (Vena cava inferior) into the right atrium and from the pulmonary circulation via the pulmonary veins into the left atrium. Finally, the blood from the atria goes back into the respective ventricle (from the left atrium into the left ventricle and from

the right atrium into the right ventricle) and the circulation cycle starts again. Arterioles, capillary system and venules are jointly referred to as **terminal vessels.** Together they form the main cross-sectional area of the vascular system. In the region of the terminal vessels in which the exchange of substances and fluid volume shifts occur, more fluid leaves the vessel bed than is reabsorbed so that only approximately 98 % of the fluid volume sent by the heart into the body and pulmonary circulations is returned to the venous system. The missing 2 % is drained via the lymph circulation and thus takes a short cut just before the heart back into the venous arm of the bloodstream and thus back into the blood circulation.

High-pressure and low-pressure systems
According to the blood pressure, the circulation system is differentiated into the high-pressure system (left heart chamber and arteries) and low-pressure system (capillaries, veins, right heart, lung circulation and left atrium). In the high-pressure system the blood pressure (RR = after RIVA-ROCCI) under physiological conditions is between 60 and 130 mmHg (millimeters of mercury) and in the low-pressure system the blood pressure at the heart level is between 9 and 12 mmHg.

Vasa publica and Vasa privata
Some organs, e. g. the lungs or liver, have 2 independently functioning vessel systems:
- **Vasa publica:** these vessels have a function for the whole body circulation (in the lungs they are responsible for gas exchange – Aa. and Vv. pulmonales).
- **Vasa privata:** these vessels are responsible for the specific organ blood flow (in the lungs they serve the blood supply to the lung tissue – bronchial arteries).

In the case of other organs (e. g. renal arteries) the arteries have a dual function and operate simultaneously as Vasa publica and Vasa privata.

Heart
The heart is the muscular pump for blood circulation. It conducts rhythmically coordinated muscle contractions. The muscles consist of specialised heart muscle cells. The muscle contractions create pressure in the chambers of the heart, which is guided in one direction (from the atria into the ventricles and from the ventricles into the arteries) by the opening and closing of cardiac valves between the atria and the chambers of the heart and between the chambers of the heart and the connected arteries (aorta, pulmonary trunk). The heart contraction is called **systole;** the relaxation phase is called **diastole.**

Heart wall
The heart wall consists of three layers:
- **Endocardium:** endothelium (coated inner layer) and connective tissue
- **Myocardium:** Cardiac muscle and connective tissue
- **Epicardium:** Connective tissue and mesothelium (specialised outer layer)

The heart is located in a heart sac (**pericardium).** There is a capillary gap between the epicardium and the pericardium (serous cavity, ➤ Chap. 1.6.3).

Heart valve
Each heart ventricle has 2 openings (ostia) in which the heart valves (➤ Table 1.8) are located – one to the corresponding atrium and the other to the corresponding artery. The valves between the

atria and ventricles are referred to as **atrioventricular valves**. They are named according to their structure as *sail valves* (on the left **mitral valve,** consisting of 2 sails on the right the **tricuspid valve,** consisting of 3 sails). The valves to the arteries (aorta, pulmonary trunk) are *pocket flaps* (on the left the **aortic valve** with 3 pockets and on the right the **pulmonary valve** with 3 pockets). All 4 ostia for the valves are located on a common level **(valve level),** in which the connective tissue of the heart skeleton is also located, which serves as a fixation point for the cardiac muscle.

The heart valves open and close depending on the prevalent pressure gradient (➤ Table 1.9). In the case of closure of the heart valves the free edges of the sail and pocket flaps are close to each other. In contrast to the pocket flaps, the sail flaps have a holding apparatus of **papillary muscles (Mm. papillares),** which are attached via **tendon cords (Chordae tendineae)** to the free underside of the sails and prevent penetration. In contrast, the pocket flaps work as non-return valves.

Arteries and veins

The blood vessel system occurs macroscopically as a tubular network of arteries and veins, which is distributed throughout the body (➤ Fig. 1.30). The naming of the blood vessels depends on the direction of the blood flow in relation to the heart. Arteries transport blood from the heart to the periphery of the body or the lungs (➤ Fig. 1.30a) and veins transport blood from the periphery of the body or the lungs back to the heart (➤ Fig. 1.30b).

Table 1.8 Heart valves.

Valve type	Name	Number of cusps or leaflets	Position
Atrioventricular valves	Mitral valve (Valva atrioventricularis sinistra)	2	Between left atrium and left ventricle
	Tricuspid valve (Valva atrioventricularis dextra)	3	Between right atrium and right ventricle
Semilunar valves	Aortic valve (Valva aortae)	3	Between left ventricle and aorta
	Pulmonary valve (Valva trunci pulmonalis)	3	Between right ventricle and Truncus pulmonalis

Table 1.9 Cardiac action.

Cardiac action	Phase	Heart valves, AV-valves	Semilunar valves
Systole	Contraction phase of the ventricular myocardium	Closed	Closed
	Ejection phase of the ventricular myocardium	Closed	Open
Diastole	Relaxation phase of the ventricular myocardium	Closed	Closed
	Filling phase (relaxed ventricular myocardium)	Open	Closed

Structure

In this respect, arteries and veins principally have the same structure. The wall of the larger vessels consists from the inside to the outside of three layers:

- **Tunica intima** (intima, inner layer): this flat endothelial cell layer is separated from the internal elastic membrane by a basal membrane. The former is substantially stronger in arteries than in veins.
- **Tunica media** (media, middle layer): a layer of coats of smooth muscle cells, which in the case of arteries are of the elastic type (see below) containing strong networks of elastic fibres. The smooth muscle cells regulate the vessel cross-section by contraction and thus the resistance to flow. This is joined on the outside to an external elastic membrane.
- **Tunica adventitia** (Adventitia, Tunica externa, outer layer): it contains collagenic connective tissue, which incorporates and anchors the blood vessel in the surroundings. Nerves, and in the case of vessels with a large diameter, blood vessels run here for the blood supply of the vessel (Vasa vasorum).

> **N O T E**
> Arteries typically have roughly the same circumference as veins. Their wall is, however, significantly thicker and the lumen is consequently smaller.

The wall of arterioles, capillaries and venules shows an alternative structure. Here we refer to textbooks on histology and to textbooks on physiology with respect to the pressure conditions in the individual vessels, vessel number, vessel diameter, vessel motility (vasomotor), vascular resistance and cross-sectional area.

Some vessels have special facilities within the vascular system (e. g. the liver sinusoids). Here, too, we refer to textbooks on histology. In some regions of the body or organs, the capillary bed can be circumvented. Here, arteries and veins are directly linked with each other **(arteriovenous anastomoses).** These play a large role e. g. in the skin for thermal regulation.

Arteries

Due to their histological structure a distinction is made between:

- **Arteries of the elastic type:** in these arteries (e. g. aorta, arteries near the heart) the elastic wall structure is used to store a part of the energy occurring during systole in the form of passive wall distension for a short time and then release it again when returning to the starting position (windkessel function). This ensures that the discontinuous blood flow initially resulting due to the heart contraction is converted into a more continuous blood flow.
- **Arteries of the muscular type** (most arteries, e. g. brachial artery, femoral artery).
- **Contractile arteries:** these specialised arteries have an irregularly grouped longitudinal muscle layer. The intima bulges into the vessel lumen and on contraction is able to reduce or stop the blood flow to the downstream areas. They occur, e. g. in the genital organs (e. g. cavernous body of the penis).

There is a gradual transition between the arteries of the elastic and those of the muscular type. The arteries of the muscular type become increasingly smaller in the body periphery, form an increasing number of branches and eventually reach the capillary bed via

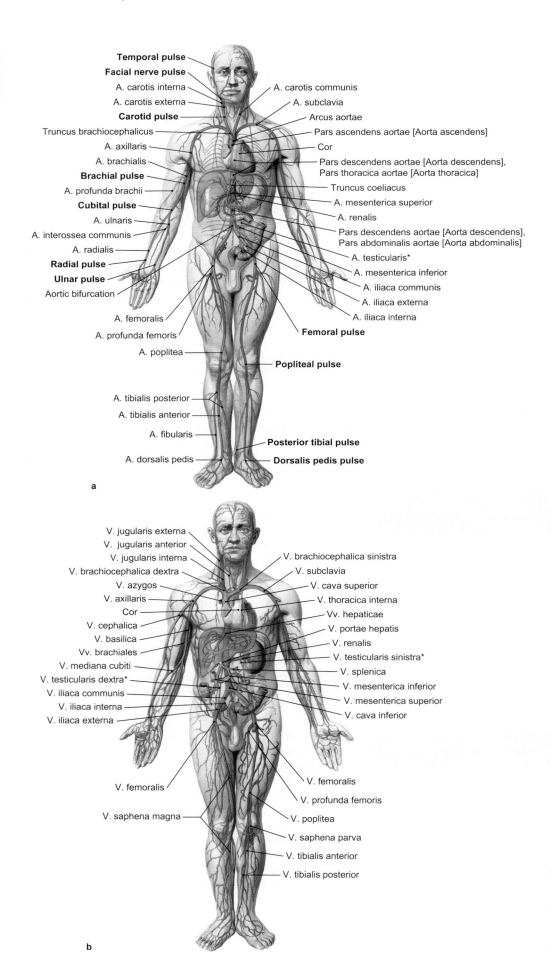

Temporal pulse
Facial nerve pulse
A. carotis interna
A. carotis externa
Carotid pulse
Truncus brachiocephalicus
A. axillaris
A. brachialis
Brachial pulse
A. profunda brachii
Cubital pulse
A. ulnaris
A. interossea communis
A. radialis
Radial pulse
Ulnar pulse
Aortic bifurcation
A. femoralis
A. profunda femoris
A. poplitea
A. tibialis posterior
A. tibialis anterior
A. fibularis
A. dorsalis pedis

A. carotis communis
A. subclavia
Arcus aortae
Pars ascendens aortae [Aorta ascendens]
Cor
Pars descendens aortae [Aorta descendens],
Pars thoracica aortae [Aorta thoracica]
Truncus coeliacus
A. mesenterica superior
A. renalis
Pars descendens aortae [Aorta descendens],
Pars abdominalis aortae [Aorta abdominalis]
A. testicularis*
A. mesenterica inferior
A. iliaca communis
A. iliaca externa
A. iliaca interna
Femoral pulse
Popliteal pulse
Posterior tibial pulse
Dorsalis pedis pulse

a

V. jugularis externa
V. jugularis anterior
V. jugularis interna
V. brachiocephalica dextra
V. azygos
V. axillaris
Cor
V. cephalica
V. basilica
Vv. brachiales
V. mediana cubiti
V. testicularis dextra*
V. iliaca communis
V. iliaca interna
V. iliaca externa
V. femoralis
V. saphena magna

V. brachiocephalica sinistra
V. subclavia
V. cava superior
V. thoracica interna
Vv. hepaticae
V. portae hepatis
V. renalis
V. testicularis sinistra*
V. splenica
V. mesenterica inferior
V. mesenterica superior
V. cava inferior
V. femoralis
V. profunda femoris
V. poplitea
V. saphena parva
V. tibialis anterior
V. tibialis posterior

b

Fig. 1.30 Arteries and veins of the systemic circulation. **a** Arteries; * in women: A. ovarica. **b** Veins; deep veins are shown on the left arm and the left side of the head, superficial veins on the right arm and the right side of the head.

arterioles (smallest arteries). The wall structure of the arterioles makes a significant contribution to the maintenance of blood pressure. They constitute in their entirety approximately half of the peripheral resistance.

> **N O T E**
>
> In many parts of the body, large and medium-sized arteries run near the body surface. Here, the delayed heart contraction can be palpated as a **pulse** (➤ Fig. 1.30a) by gently pressing the artery against a harder underlying structure (e. g. bone). The palpable pulse most distal and thus farthest from the heart is the pulse of the **dorsalis pedis artery** on the arch of the foot. Palpation of the pulse provides numerous indications, e. g. on the frequency of the heartbeat, on possible circulation differences in the upper and lower extremities or, more generally, on the state of the blood circulation in a body section.

Veins

Veins transport blood from the periphery of the body and the lungs back to the heart. Their wall is easily expandable and provides a reservoir function. The veins of the systemic circulation transport deoxygenated blood and those of the lung circulation transport oxygenated blood. Most veins are concomitant to arteries, i.e. they run parallel to corresponding arteries (**accompanying veins**). Overall, the course of veins is much more versatile than that of arteries and can show great individual variation. However, the large vein stems occur regularly in all people. Veins together with capillaries and venules belong to the low pressure system of the blood circulation (see above). Since in an upright position most veins have to transport the blood to the heart against gravity, the larger veins of the extremities and the lower neck region have **venous valves** (➤ Fig. 1.31), which support the venous return flow. They ensure that the blood flow is only possible in the direction of the heart. Venous valves are opposing bag-shaped projections of the intima (intima duplicators). They open in the case of blood flow towards the heart and when the blood flow returns due to the pressure conditions, blood flows into the pockets and closes them. Most of the body sections have a superficial venous system in the subcutaneous fat tissue and a deep venous system, running mostly parallel to the arteries. Both **venous systems** are interconnected via short veins but the venous blood only flows in a superficial to deep direction, as venous valves stipulate the flow direction in the connecting veins.

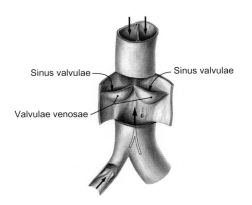

Sinus valvulae — — Sinus valvulae

Valvulae venosae —

Fig. 1.31 Venous valves.

> **N O T E**
>
> The **venous return flow to the heart** is guaranteed by:
> - Venous valves (responsible for the directional return flow)
> - The arterial pulse running through the arteries, which compresses the walls of the accompanying veins (arteriovenous coupling)
> - Contraction of the surrounding muscles (muscle pump), which also leads to compression of the walls of the veins
> - Suction effect of the heart (only near the heart)
> - Pressure differences in the chest (during inhalation and exhalation)

> **Clinical remarks**
>
> Defects of the venous valves in the connecting veins between the superficial and the deep venous system of the lower extremities lead to the formation of **varicose veins (varices),** which can be distinguished on the leg from the outside as greatly expanded and tortuously running vessels under the skin.

Some veins have a specialised structure:
- **Capacitance veins:** These are venous sections with very thin media, while at the same time having a large cross-section. They can store large volumes of blood, are usually downstream of contractile arteries and play a role for cavernous bodies (e. g. in the nasal mucosa/nasal conchae or the efferent tear ducts).
- **Jugular veins:** Just like contractile arteries they have (see above) irregularly grouped longitudinal muscle bundles in the media. They are often downstream of capacitance veins but also occur independently (e. g. in the adrenal medulla). In the case of muscle contraction the blood flow is reduced or stopped, so that the blood in the upstream vessel sections is staunched.

1.5.2 Portal vein circulation

The portal vein circulation (➤ Fig. 1.32) holds a special position within the systemic circulation. It is used to supply nutrients to the liver for further metabolism by the shortest routes via the gastrointestinal tract. For this purpose, the blood of the unpaired abdominal organs (stomach, gut, pancreas, spleen) is not directly fed to the body through veins, but is taken from the capillary system to an interim switched venous system, draining the blood into the portal vein, which leads directly into the liver. After this blood has flowed through the liver (and the nutrients have been metabolised), it enters the inferior vena cava and thus back into the body circulation.

> **Clinical remarks**
>
> In the context of various diseases (e. g. alcohol abuse), cirrhosis of the liver can develop. The normal blood flow from the portal vein into the liver is disrupted and blood backs up into the portal vein and the veins upstream of the portal vein. The **portal vein pressure is increased.** The body tries to compensate for the increased pressure via bypass circuits. In doing so, the blood is drained via **portacaval anastomoses** (connection routes between portal vein and the superior and inferior vena cavae) past the liver. However, the veins in the anastomotic region are inadequate for the increased blood flow and are widened in a varicose manner. These **varicose veins** (extended, tortuously running veins) can arise:

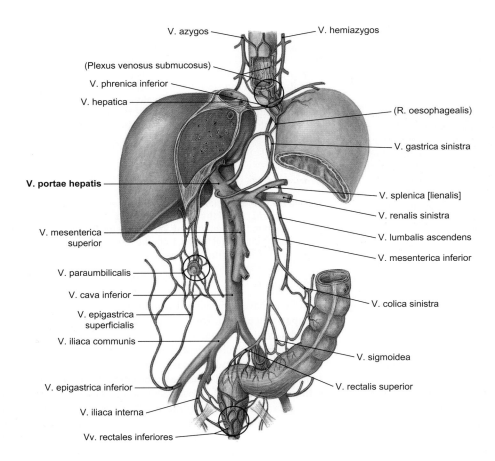

V. azygos — — V. hemiazygos

(Plexus venosus submucosus)

V. phrenica inferior

V. hepatica

— (R. oesophagealis)

— V. gastrica sinistra

V. portae hepatis

— V. splenica [lienalis]

— V. renalis sinistra

— V. lumbalis ascendens

— V. mesenterica inferior

V. mesenterica superior

V. paraumbilicalis

V. cava inferior

— V. colica sinistra

V. epigastrica superficialis

V. iliaca communis

— V. sigmoidea

V. epigastrica inferior

— V. rectalis superior

V. iliaca interna

Vv. rectales inferiores

Fig. 1.32 Portal vein circulation.

- at the transition from the stomach to the esophagus (submucosal esophageal varices can be easily damaged during food intake and lead to life-threatening bleeding).
- In the veins around the navel (paraumbilical veins), whereby the image of a so-called caput medusae (Medusa's head- from Greek mythology) emerges.
- In the anal canal.

Table 1.10 Structures of the prenatal circulation.

Shunt	Prenatal	Postnatal
Between right and left atrium	Foramen ovale	Fossa ovalis in the atrial septum
Between pulmonary trunk and aortic arch	Ductus arteriosus (BOTALLI)	Lig. arteriosum
Between portal vein and inferior vena cava	Ductus venosus (ARANTII)	Lig. venosum

1.5.3 Prenatal circulation

The prenatal circulation is different from the circulation after birth (➤ Fig. 1.33). Before birth, nutrients and oxygen are taken up via the umbilical cord through the placenta and metabolic products are delivered in a reverse way. The lungs of the unborn child are not yet ventilated and there is still no gas exchange. The pulmonary circulation is therefore almost entirely disconnected from the body; the blood is routed past the lungs via short circuits (➤ Table 1.10). The majority of the blood flows through a connecting opening in the atrial septum (**Foramen ovale**) directly from the right into the left atrium and therefore circumvents the lungs. A further part is taken from the pulmonary trunk, which joins the right ventricle, via a connecting shunt (**Ductus arteriosus**) into the aortic arch and also circumvents the lungs. Since the liver is not yet fully matured, the blood is transported for the most part via another short circuit (**Ductus venosus**) from the umbilical vein directly into the inferior vena cava. Immediately after birth the foramen ovale closes and the ductus arteriosus (BOTALLI) and the ductus venosus (ARANTII) obliterate. Now the blood flows through the pulmonary circulation and through the liver.

Clinical remarks

If the foramen ovale closes only partially or not at all a **left-to-right shunt** is formed after birth when the blood flows in the reverse direction. These shunts are among the most common congenital heart defects.

1.5.4 Lymphatic circulation

The lymphatic circulation is in addition to the systemic circulation a system of tubes (lymph vessels) that transports lymph. It begins blind with lymph vessels in the interstices, which absorb approximately 2 % of the fluid emitted by the capillary system of the blood circulation, and lead through the lymph vessel system and the venous arm of the blood circulation again before entering the superior vena cava. Lymph nodes are integrated into the lymphatic circulation, which have to be traversed by the draining lymphatic fluid (lymph). They are used for immune defence.

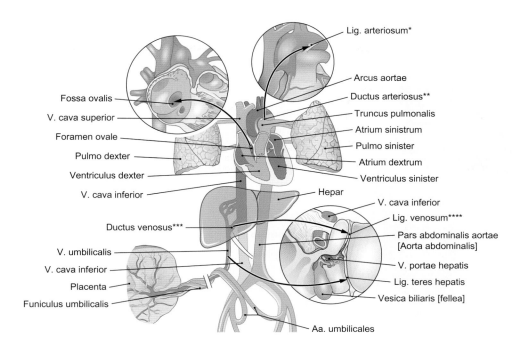

Fig. 1.33 Prenatal cardiovascular system;
* Ligament BOTALLI,
** Ductus arteriosus BOTALLI,
*** Ductus venosus ARANTII,
**** Ligament ARANTII.

Labels (left): Fossa ovalis, V. cava superior, Foramen ovale, Pulmo dexter, Ventriculus dexter, V. cava inferior, Ductus venosus***, V. umbilicalis, V. cava inferior, Placenta, Funiculus umbilicalis, Aa. umbilicales

Labels (top/right): Lig. arteriosum*, Arcus aortae, Ductus arteriosus**, Truncus pulmonalis, Atrium sinistrum, Pulmo sinister, Atrium dextrum, Ventriculus sinister, Hepar, V. cava inferior, Lig. venosum****, Pars abdominalis aortae [Aorta abdominalis], V. portae hepatis, Lig. teres hepatis, Vesica biliaris [fellea]

Lymph vessel system

The lymph vessel system is a system comparable to the blood vessel system from vessels that are coupled together (see below).

Functions

Functions of the lymph vessel system are:
- **Liquid transport:** transport of a part of the liquid overflowed from the capillaries into the interstices (including substances dissolved in it) as *lymph* back into the venous arm of the systemic circulation
- **Fat transport:** transport of fats resorbed in the gut as *chyle* and transferred to the venous arm of the systemic circulation
- **Immune defence** by interpositioned lymph nodes

Chyle (milk juice) is the fat-rich milky lymph coming from the gut (the resorbed dietary fat is transported in the form of chylomicrons not in the blood but in the lymph in contrast to carbohydrates and amino acids).

Structure

The lymph vessel system starts with **lymph capillaries** (Vasa lymphocapillaria), which form networks similar to the blood capillaries in interstitial tissue of most organs (exception: central nervous system, cartilage, bone marrow). The lymph capillaries are blind incipient tubes, which are anchored in the surrounding tissue so that they are opened by the tension from the connective tissue or pressure from the interstitial fluid. From the capillary system the vessels enlarge on a continuous basis. These are joined to:
- **Lymph collectors** (collection vessels)
- **Lymph vessels:** Vasa lymphatica, transport vessels, and intermediary lymphoid organs, which are responsible for the filtration of a body region *(regional lymph nodes)* or receive the lymph of various other lymph nodes *(collection lymph nodes)*
- **Lymphatic trunks** (Trunci lymphatici, ➤ Table 1.11)
- Large lymphatic trunks (they lead the lymph into the venous blood vessel system of the systemic circulation; at the confluence of the lymph vessel trunks from the lower body [lumbar trunk] into the thoracic duct this is expanded to the *Cisterna chyli*)

The major part of the lymph is drained by the **Ductus thoracicus** into the left venous angle (between the Vv. jugularis interna sinistra and subclavia sinistra, ➤ Fig. 1.34). In contrast, the lymph of the right upper quadrant of the body drains via the **Ductus lymphaticus dexter** into the right venous angle (between the Vv. jugularis interna dextra and subclavia dextra) (➤ Fig. 1.34).

To enable a directional lymph flow to the feeder centres above the heart into the venous vascular system, lymph collectors and lymph vessels have pocket flaps (**lymph vessel valves**); the structure is basically the same as the venous valves. The **wall of the lymph vessels** consists, like the wall of the veins, of:
- an endothelial cell layer (Intima)
- a muscular layer (Media)
- a surrounding adventitia (Externa)

However, the media is much thinner than in the veins. The lymph is transported within the vascular system by both muscle contraction of the media and as in the veins through the arterial pulse wave, the muscle pump of the skeletal muscles and the suction effect of the thorax when breathing (➤ Chap. 1.5.1).

Lymph nodes

In the human body there are up to 1000 lymph nodes, which are incorporated in the lymph vessel system. Within the lymph node there is a compartmentalization into cortex and medulla. Every

Table 1.11 Large lymphatic trunks.

Lymphatic trunk	Localisation	Drainage area
Truncus jugularis	Cranial neck region	Head
Truncus subclavius	Lateral neck region	Arm, chest (or thoracic) wall, back
Truncus bronchomediastinalis	Mediastinum	Thoracic organs
Trunci intestinales	Radix mesenterii (root of the mesentery)	Gut
Truncus lumbalis	Lumbar region	Abdominal wall, buttocks, pelvis, leg

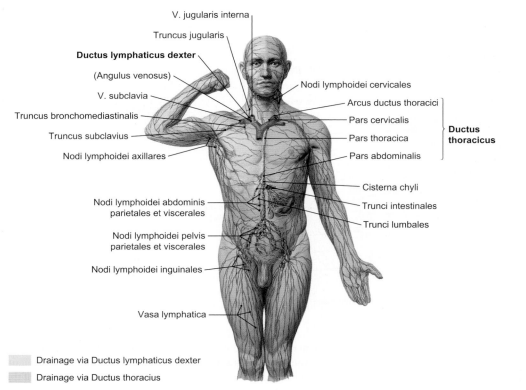

V. jugularis interna

Truncus jugularis

Ductus lymphaticus dexter

(Angulus venosus)

V. subclavia

Truncus bronchomediastinalis

Truncus subclavius

Nodi lymphoidei axillares

Nodi lymphoidei abdominis
parietales et viscerales

Nodi lymphoidei pelvis
parietales et viscerales

Nodi lymphoidei inguinales

Vasa lymphatica

Nodi lymphoidei cervicales

Arcus ductus thoracici

Pars cervicalis

Pars thoracica

Pars abdominalis

**Ductus
thoracicus**

Cisterna chyli

Trunci intestinales

Trunci lumbales

Drainage via Ductus lymphaticus dexter

Drainage via Ductus thoracius

Fig. 1.34 Overview of the lymphatic system.

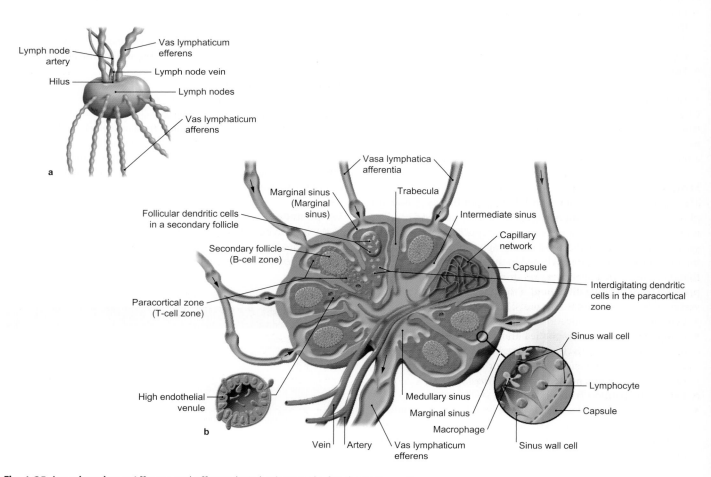

Lymph node
artery

Hilus

Vas lymphaticum
efferens

Lymph node vein

Lymph nodes

Vas lymphaticum
afferens

a

Follicular dendritic cells
in a secondary follicle

Secondary follicle
(B-cell zone)

Paracortical zone
(T-cell zone)

High endothelial
venule

Vasa lymphatica
afferentia

Marginal sinus
(Marginal
sinus)

Trabecula

Intermediate sinus

Capillary
network

Capsule

Interdigitating dendritic
cells in the paracortical
zone

Sinus wall cell

Lymphocyte

Capsule

Medullary sinus

Marginal sinus

Macrophage

Sinus wall cell

Vein   Artery   Vas lymphaticum
efferens

b

Fig. 1.35 Lymph nodes. a Afferent and efferent lymphatic vessels. **b** Schematic section.

lymph node has numerous afferent and few efferent but large lumen lymph vessels (➤ Fig. 1.35):

- The afferent **Vasa lymphatica afferentia** lead the lymph via border sinuses and intermediary sinuses to medullary sinuses, via which the lymph is routed to the efferent vessels. Between the sinuses there is organised lymphatic tissue.
- The **Vasa lymphatica efferentia** leave the lymph nodes at the hilus of the lymph node. Supplying blood vessels also enter and exit from here (➤ Fig. 1.35).

The lymph nodes come in various shapes (mostly lens or bean-shaped with a diameter of roughly 5–20 mm).

Up to the confluence into the venous blood vessel system, the lymph flows mostly through several serially arranged lymph nodes. Lymph nodes belong functionally together with the spleen, tonsils ('almonds') and lymphoid tissue of the intestines and the rest of the mucous membranes to the **secondary lymphatic organs,** which are opposed to the primary lymphatic organs (bone marrow, thymus) and all of which serve the immune defence system.

Clinical remarks

The **examination of lymph nodes** is part of every detailed physical examination of a patient in the palpable regions of the throat area, axilla (armpit) and groin.
Lymph node enlargements can be a first indication of inflammation processes (lymphadenitis) or malignant diseases (metastasis of a malignant tumor [lymphogenic tumour metastasis] or of a generalised disease of the lymphatic system, e. g. HODGKIN's disease.
Congestion within the lymph vessels, e. g. in the case of certain diseases or after separation of lymph vessels in the context of operations may cause a **lymphodoema**. The interstitial tissue is hardened (indured) and the fluid collection in the tissue cannot be pressed away as in normal tissue oedema. After surgery, a manual lymphatic drainage therapy is often conducted.

1.6 Mucous membranes, glands, serous cavities

The inner surfaces of the body (e. g. respiratory tract, digestive tract, urogenital tract and also ocular surfaces, efferent lacrimal system and middle ear with adjacent spaces) are covered by **mucous membranes**, which undertake organ-specific functions such as secretion and/or resorption except for a barrier function against micro-organisms.

There are also **glands,** which are functionally linked to the mucous membranes or independently undertake functions in the body. Glands are cell associations that produce a secretion, which they release as exocrine glands through a duct system to the mucosal surface or that they secrete into the blood as hormones (endocrine glands).

Serous cavities are recesses in the body, which serve the relocation of highly movable organs (lungs, heart, bowels). They are not associated with the external surroundings (with the exception of the peritoneal cavity of women) and are lined by a thin serous coat (serosa).

1.6.1 Mucous membranes

Depending on function the structure of the mucous membranes is very different. Nevertheless, a distinction can be made between a basic, uniform and three-layer blueprints. This consists of

- **Lamina epithelialis mucosae:** specialised epithelium, that functions as protection, secretion and/or resorption
- **Lamina propria mucosae:** contains blood and lymph capillaries and serves the transport of substances and the immune defence system
- **Lamina muscularis mucosae** (only present in the gut): smooth muscles, which serve the motility of the mucous membrane

Under the mucous membrane there is a **Tela submucosa** (submucosal connective tissue) joined with with blood and lymph vessels.

1.6.2 Glands

Exocrine glands

Exocrine glands drains the secretions via a duct system to the surface anatomy (skin, mucous membranes). Exocrine glands are e. g. sweat glands, sebaceous glands, scent glands, salivary glands, lacrimal glands, pancreatic glands, liver. The excretory duct system begins with an end piece, in which the glandular cells excrete the produced secretions. The excretory duct system often shows specializations, which further modify the extravasated secretions (e. g. salinity, viscosity). Exocrine glands are derivatives of epithelium and enter at the site on the epithelium, from which their development took their source (exoepithelial glands). Some glands are formed as single cells (e. g. cup cell) or in the form of multiple cells, small intraepithelial units, known as endoepithelial glands.

Endocrine glands

Endocrine glands have no independent duct system. The secretion-forming (hormone-forming) cells are covered directly from a blood vessel network into which the hormones are directly fed. Hormones are neurotransmitters that act via special receptors on target tissue (e. g. the thyroid stimulating hormone (TSH) produced in the pituitary gland only works on thyroid cells).

1.6.3 Serous cavities

Serous cavities of the body are:

- **Cavitas pleuralis** (pleural cavity)
- **Cavitas pericardialis** (pericardial cavity)
- **Cavitas peritonealis** (peritoneal cavity)
- **Tunica vaginalis testis** (testicular sheath; it is a separation from the peritoneal cavity)

Serous cavities are capillary spaces, which are filled with a thin layer of protein-rich liquids. The specialised epithelium (Serosa, Tunica serosa, mesothelium) creates a moist smooth surface, which reduces the friction caused by the movement of the organs to a minimum and keeps the organs together (capillary adhesion, comparable to two glass panels bonded together with fluid).

The joint cavities (➤ Chap. 1.4.3), the covering of the tendinous sheaths and bursae (➤ Chap. 1.4.4) are similar to the structure of serous cavities.

Parietal and visceral sheet

You can imagine a serous cavity as a closed bag. One side is the interior of the bag and is referred to as the parietal sheet (Serosa parietalis). The other side covers the respective organ and is referred to as a visceral sheet (Serosa visceralis) (➤ Table 1.12).

Table 1.12 Names/nomenclature of the serous membranes.

Organ	Parietal layer	Visceral layer
Lungs	Parietal pleura	Visceral pleura
Heart	Pericardium	Epicardium
Stomach, intestines	Parietal peritoneum	Viscera peritoneum
Testis	Periorchium	Epiorchium

Clinical remarks

Serous cavities can expand under pathological conditions to air or liquid-filled spaces. Thus, an injury to the lungs may cause a drawing in of air into the gap with collapsing of the lungs **(pneumothorax)** or, under certain conditions this can lead to an overflow of fluid from the blood into the respective cavity **(pleural effusion, pericardial effusion, ascites),** which is then gradually filled with this liquid.
Adhesions of the two sheets after inflammation can severely inhibit normal organ function, e. g. in the peritoneal cavity it is referred to as adhesions.

The serosa consists of three layers:
- Serosal epithelium (mesothelium)
- Lamina propria (serosa connective tissue with blood and lymph vessels)
- Subserosal tela (subserous layer)

Functionally its purpose is to guarantee the formation of a transudate (thin liquid film) for the reduction of friction between the parietal and visceral sheets, as well as for absorption of excess generated liquid to a uniform thin liquid film.

Mesenteries

As described above parietal and visceral serosa form a closed bag. The envelope area of both sheets from the wall of the body cavity on the respective organ include the supply route (blood and lymph vessels and nerve fibres) and the suspension device from connective tissue. It is a serosa duplication and is depicted in the broader sense (generic term) as **mesentery (mesentery or meso)**. Examples are:
- Mesogastrium (gastric mesentery)
- Mesentery (small bowel mesentery, in the narrower sense)
- Mesocolon (large bowel mesentery)
- Mesohepaticum (liver mesentery)
- Mesovarium (ovarian mesentery)
- Mesosalpinx (mesentery of fallopian tubes)
- Mesometrium (uterine mesentery)

The attachment of the meso on the body cavity is often referred to as **radix** (e. g. the Radix mesenterii.) Functionally, the mesenteries are therefore responsible for supplying blood and lymph vessels, innervation, the storage of excretory ducts (e. g. bile ducts) as well as the fixation of the organs involved in the form of retaining bands (ligaments), e. g. as:
- **Broad ligament of the uterus** (womb, uterus)
- **Gastrocolic ligament** (ligament between stomach and large intestine)
- **Hepatoduodenal ligament** (ligament between liver and duodenum)

The firmness of these 'ligaments' is much lower than the ligaments in the musculoskeletal system. Smaller peritoneal duplicatures are referred to as folds **(Plicae)** (e. g. caecal fold, recto-uterine fold). The special form of peritoneal skin duplication is the large network (greater omentum) that has no holding function, but a defence function through the accumulation of immune defence cells.

Location of the abdominal and pelvic organs

The position of organs in the abdomen and pelvic cavity is defined as follows:
- **Intraperitoneal:** the organ is connected via a meso with the peritoneal wall and/or neighbouring organs (e. g. stomach, spleen).
- **Retroperitoneal:** the organ lies 'behind' the parietal peritoneum, its other wall surfaces are surrounded by retroperitoneal connective tissue (e. g. kidneys).
- **Secondary retroperitoneal:** the organ has been shifted during development from a former intraperitoneal position onto the wall of the peritoneal cavity, so that on the wall side the visceral peritoneum and parietal peritoneum are adhered to each other (e. g. parts of the duodenum, colon, pancreas).
- **Extraperitoneal:** the organ has no relation to the peritoneal cavity and is surrounded by connective tissue (e. g. prostate gland).

1.7 Nervous system

The nervous system serves to
- Receive stimuli,
- Transfer stimuli,
- Stimulus processing and
- Stimulus response
and forms the basis of
- Emotions
- Memory and
- Thought processes.

The nervous system (➤ Fig. 1.36) is divided into:
- **Central nervous system (CNS):** consisting of the brain (encephalon) and spinal cord (Medulla spinalis)
- **Peripheral nervous system (PNS):** consisting of spinal nerves (including the cervical plexus, brachial plexus, lumbosacral plexus) and cranial nerves (Nn. craniales)

The nervous system controls the activity of muscles and viscera, is used to communicate with the environment and the interior of the body (inner environment) and fulfils complex functions, such as storage of experience (memory), development of ideas (thinking) as well as emotions and is used for rapid adjustment of the whole organism to changes in the outside world and the interior of the body. A distinction is made between:
- **Autonomic nervous system** (vegetative, visceral nervous system) for control of visceral activity, mostly involuntary (➤ Fig. 1.37); consisting of:
  - **Sympathetic nervous system:** mobilization of the body in the event of activity and in emergency situations, antagonist of the parasympathetic nervous system. The nerve cells are located in the lateral horn of the thoracolumbar segment of the spinal cord. It also includes the adrenal medulla.
  - **Parasympathetic nervous system:** food intake and processing as well as sexual arousal, antagonist of the sympathetic nervous system. The neurons are located in the brain stem and the sacral medulla.

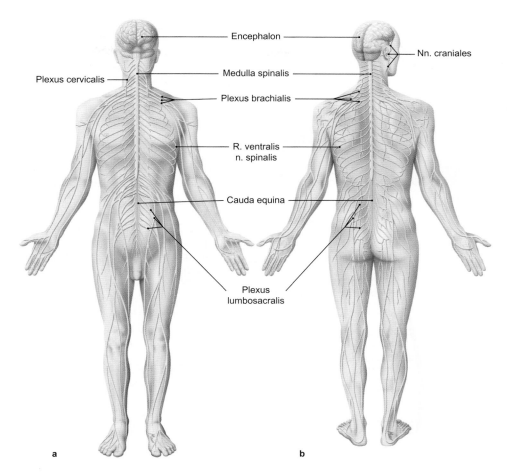

Fig. 1.36 **Structure of the nervous system. a** Ventral view. **b** Dorsal view.

- **Enteral nervous system (intestinal nervous system):** regulation of intestinal activity, is under the influence of the sympathetic and parasympathetic nervous systems.
- **Somatic nervous system** (innervation of skeletal muscles, voluntary perception of sensory input, communication with the environment)

Both systems are closely interlaced and interact with each other. Besides the nervous system, the endocrine system also participates in the regulation of the total organism.

Clinical remarks

1.7.1 Disorders of peripheral nerves
Various diseases (e. g. diabetes mellitus, lack of vitamin B, intoxication with heavy metals and drugs, impaired blood circulation and excessive alcohol consumption) can cause disorders of the peripheral nerves. In this respect, deficits and/or overexcitation of nerve cells (neurons) are possible. If many nerves are affected at the same time, this is referred to as **polyneuropathy.**

1.7.2 Disorders of the autonomic nervous system
Disorders of the autonomic nervous system play a role in almost all medical disciplines. They can occur as independent diseases (e. g. inherited **autonomic neuropathy**), as a result of other diseases (e. g. autonomic neuropathy in diabetes mellitus or PARKINSON's DISEASE) or as a response to external influences or other disorders (e. g. **autonomic dysregulation** in the case of stress, severe pain or psychiatric disorders). Depending on the region of the autonomic nervous system affected, disorders of the circulatory system, digestion, sexual function or other functions can be predominant.

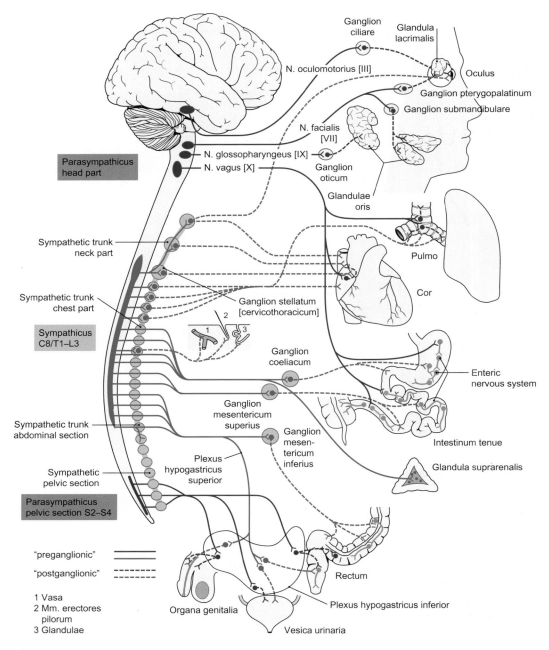

Fig. 1.37 **Autonomic nervous system**.

2 General embryology

Martin Scaal

Gastroschisis

History

A 24-year-old female student confirms her pregnancy with a rapid test. She goes with her boyfriend to the gynaecologist at the beginning of the 9th week of pregnancy. The ultrasound findings are inconspicuous. In a follow-up visit to the gynaecologist at the beginning of the 5th month of pregnancy, ultrasound findings show normal growth of the foetus, but determine an irregular convolute on the foetal abdominal wall.

Further diagnostics and diagnosis

From the detailed ultrasound it can be seen that intestinal loops emerge through an opening in the abdominal wall to the right of the navel and protrude into the amniotic cavity. The diagnosis is gastroschisis. Gastroschisis occurs in approximately 4.5 out of 10,000 births; however, the embryological reason for gastroschisis is unclear.

Further procedure

Through close regular monitoring using fine ultrasound, the development of the abdominal wall and the condition of the protruding intestinal segments are kept under observation. If the opening becomes smaller (with the risk of incarceration of the intestinal loops) or the intestinal wall is damaged by the amniotic fluid, an immediate caesarean section is indicated. Immediately after birth damaged intestinal segments can be surgically removed, the intestinal loops transferred into the abdominal cavity, and the abdominal wall closed. Postoperatively, the child is temporarily fed parenterally until the intestines have regenerated. Regular controls are carried out to exclude an ileus (bowel occlusion). The long-term prognosis of the child is very good.

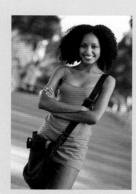

The 24-year-old student is a girlfriend of yours. Immediately after the gynecologist gave the diagnosis, she was so nervous that she stopped listening to the doctor. Therefore, she asks you to explain again exactly how the treatment will work. In addition, she would like to know how good the prognosis of the disease is.
You make notes so that you do not forget:

A friend in need ...

TX: Sectio caesarea in the 34th-36th week of pregnancy with prior induction of the lung maturation, postpartum gastric outlet probe, parenteral nutrition via infusion, antibiotic prophylaxis, elimination of torsion in the gut, humidity and sterile packaging of the leaked abdominal viscera in a plastic bag, no mask ventilation, operation: primary abdominal wall closure in the event of a large defect a) suturing of a patch or b) provisional closure using a silicone bag ("silo bag"), from which the viscera will be reduced little by little so that the bag continues to shrink

Prognosis: 90% chance of survival, volvulus with intestinal necrosis as possible complication → resection: short bowel syndrome

2.1 Introduction

Human life begins with the fusion of two germ cells from the parents, a paternal spermatozoan and a maternal ovum, to create a genetically new cellular individual, the **zygote.** The zygote contains in its genome all the genetic information which autonomously controls the subsequent development to become an adult human. This development includes not only cell proliferation, but also the formation of different cell types and their arrangement into anatomical structures. The basis for the differentiation of cells into specific cell types is **differential gene expression.** Although each cell of an organism contains all the genes of the individual genome, in each cell only certain genes are selectively expressed and so only a certain set of proteins are synthesised. The determination of an embryonic cell for a specific developmental outcome is called **determination** (syn.: specification), their conversion into a particular type of cell is called **differentiation.** Crucial to both steps are molecular signals, which are either formed by the cell itself (cellautonomous) or originate from cells in the environment **(induction).** Inductive interactions between cells also play an important role in the subsequent developmental stages. Similar differentiated cells are arranged into cell groups and tissues **(histogenesis).** The cell groups and tissues are arranged as specific anatomical forms **(morphogenesis)** and the forms in turn, together with other tissue groups and make up to superordinate anatomical structures with a specific spatial alignment, corresponding to the specific patterns of human anatomy **(pattern formation).**
This is simply illustrated using the example of the development of the humerus: from a cell population in the central mesenchyme of the position of the extremities (determination), cartilage cells emerge (differentiation). The resulting hyaline cartilage (histogenesis) is arranged in the form of a tubular bone with epiphyses and diaphyses (morphogenesis), which lies between the shoulder blade position and the position of the forearm bones (pattern formation). Thus, in embryogenesis all organ systems of the body exist in a functional cluster, which corresponds to the human blueprint.
In the ensuing **foetal period** this leads to coordinated growth and to functional maturation of organ systems until birth. Postnatal development through childhood, puberty, adults and senium are also part of the developmental process of humans, which begins with the zygote and finally ends in death.
This chapter entitled 'General embryology', describes early human development from insemination to the formation of the basic blueprint of the body (basic body form). Special embryology (development of the organ systems) is dealt with in the respective chapters.

N O T E
Embryonic development is regulated by developmental genes, which specify the initially naive cells of the early embryo to form different cell types, and which orchestrate the arrangement of the diverse cell types into tissues, organs and the entire anatomical bauplan of the body.

2.2 Fertilisation

2.2.1 Translocation and capacitation

Insemination, the fusion of female and male germ cells for formation of the zygote, usually takes place in the ampulla of the fallopian tube (uterine tube, oviduct). Both the ovum and the spermatozoa have to get there from the gonads **(translocation):**
- In ovulation (➤ Fig. 2.1) the ovum leaves **(oocyte),** their ovary wrapped in the **Zona pellucida** and in the **Corona radiata,** and enters the **fimbrial funnel** of the fallopian tube. This is assisted by sweeping movements of the fimbria, which during ovulation lay close to the ovary. The resulting flow of the liquid in the tubes, assisted by peristaltic contractions of the fallopian tubes, transports the ovum slowly into the ampulla.
- The **spermatozoa,** as the cellular part of the semen, are deposited by ejaculation into the vaginal vault (Fornix vaginae). By beating the tails of the cilia, the spermatozoa actively pass through the mucus barrier of the uterine cervix, which is passable due to the effect of oestrogen, into the uterine lumen and from there move largely passively by contractions of the uterus into the fallopian tube. Here the spermatozoa undergo a maturation process under the influence of the tube epithelium called **capacitation.** This process changes the protein configuration and the electrophysiological characteristics of the cell membrane at the sperm head. The spermatozoa are only capable of fertilisation at this point. When they are in the vicinity of the ovum, the capacitated spermatozoa greatly increase their beating action and reach the oocyte by following a temperature gradient **(thermotaxis;** the temperature in the ampulla is slightly higher than in the proximal oviduct) and the concentration gradient of the molecules secreted by the oocyte **(chemotaxis,** including progesterone). Although more than 200 million spermatozoa are

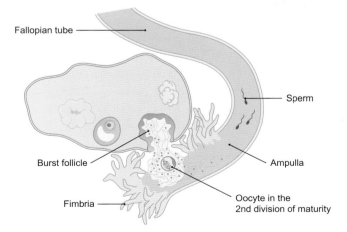

Fallopian tube

Sperm

Ampulla

Burst follicle

Oocyte in the 2nd division of maturity

Fimbria

Fig. 2.1 Ovulation. The ovum is expelled from the GRAAF's follicle and escapes via the fimbrial funnel into the ampullary part of the fallopian tube, where it comes into contact with capacitated spermatozoa. [L126]

ejaculated into the vagina, only approximately 200 reach the ovum.

The translocation of spermatozoa can take between 30 minutes up to several days. It is not necessarily the fastest spermatozoon that fertilises the ovum because for capacitation to take place, a sufficiently long contact with the tube epithelium is required.

Clinical remarks

Birth control (contraception) can be achieved by restricting the translocation of spermatozoa (condom, vaginal diaphragm, intrauterine device) or by preventing ovulation (hormonal contraceptives, 'the pill') or implantation (interception, emergency postcoital contraception).

NOTE

The fertilisation of the ovum by the spermatozoon typically occurs in the ampulla of the uterine tube.

2.2.2 Acrosome reaction and fusion of the germ cells

The oocyte progresses into the fallopian tube surrounded by a loose circle of follicular cells (**Corona radiata**) and a dense sheath of glycoproteins (**Zona pellucida**). Both layers must be penetrated by the spermatozoon that has reached the ovum, in order to reach the actual oocyte (➤ Fig. 2.2). Receptor proteins in the cell membrane of the head of the spermatozoon, which has been prepared by capacitation, bind to the glycoproteins of the Zona pellucida (zona proteins, ZP). As a result, the **acrosome reaction** is initiated, whereby the vesicle membrane of the acrosome, a vesicle filled with proteases on the tip of the sperm head, fuses with the superficial cell membrane of the spermatozoon, so releasing the contents of the acrosome. As a result of protease digestion, a channel is created in the Zona pellucida through which the sperm can penetrate into the ovum. The sperm head is located at a tangent to the cell membrane of the oocyte, and the cell membrane of the sperm head then fuses with that of the oocyte.

Triggered by the fusion, the ovum protects itself against multiple fertilisation (polyspermy) by releasing enzymes from vesicles under its cell membrane (**cortical granules**) by exocytosis into the Zona pellucida, which modifies the sperm receptors of the zona proteins in such a way as to prevent attachment of a spermatozoon (**zona reaction**). The fusion of the spermatozoon with the oocyte also leads to **activation of the ovum**, which is accompanied by an oscillating increase in Ca^{2+} concentration in the cytoplasm and is a prerequisite for the subsequent steps in fertilisation.

Clinical remarks

In **extracorporeal fertilisation (in vitro fertilisation, IVF)** the oocytes are removed transvaginally by puncture of the ovary which has previously been hormonally stimulated and mixed in a nutrient solution with spermatozoa which have been capacitated by preincubation in a special medium. After successful fertilisation up to 3 embryos in the 4-8 cell stage are introduced into the uterus (embryo transfer). The Zona pellucida can be removed mechanically or using a laser before embryo transfer to facilitate implantation. In the case of insufficient sperm motility, a single spermatozoon can be selectively injected into an ovum in vitro. **Intracytoplasmic sperm injection (ICSI)**.
During **preimplantation genetic diagnostics (PGD)** individual embryo blastomeres are removed before the embryo transfer and are examined at a molecular genetic level for the presence of any gene defects. Due to the totipotency of early blastomeres, this sampling does not generally adversely affect the development of the embryo; however, trophoblast cells are increasingly being used for PGD at the blastocyst stage (blastocyst biopsy). After selection, only healthy embryos are introduced into the uterus and the other embryos are discarded. This is why PGD is ethically and legally controversial.

2.2.3 Fusion of genetic material

At the time of fertilisation the ovulated oocyte is at the **metaphase of the 2nd division of maturity.** Only when both germ cells fuse will the 2nd division of maturity be continued and finalised. In doing so, another polar body is emitted, and the nucleus of the oocyte is pres-

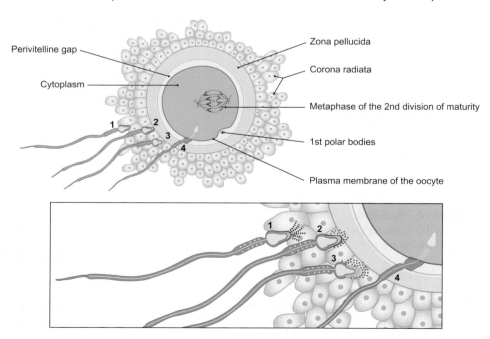

Perivitelline gap

Cytoplasm

Zona pellucida

Corona radiata

Metaphase of the 2nd division of maturity

1st polar bodies

Plasma membrane of the oocyte

Fig. 2.2   Acrosome reaction and fusion of the germ cells. Spermatozoa penetrate through the Corona radiata with secreted enzymes (1) and lie with their heads on the Zona pellucida (2). The acrosomal proteases are released by the acrosome reaction, and they penetrate the Zona pellucida (3), so that the spermatozoa can advance into the oocyte. By the fusion of the cell membranes of both germ cells, the nucleus and also parts of the middle and the tail of the spermatozoa succeed in entering the cytoplasm of the oocyte (4). [E347-09]

ent in the haploid state. It is now described as a **female pronucleus** (➤ Fig. 2.3a). Apart from the nucleus, parts of the neck and the tail of the spermatozoon penetrate into the oocyte, but are rapidly broken down. The compressed core of the spermatozoon loosens after fusion and becomes the **male pronucleus.** Both pronuclei replicate their DNA, together with their own centrosomes forming asters (star-shaped arrangements of microtubules) and come nearer to each other (➤ Fig. 2.3b, c). With the fusion of both pronuclei both nuclear envelopes collapse; the chromosomes are arranged on a common spindle apparatus and are rapidly distributed to both daughter nuclei of the **zygote,** without forming an actual zygote core with a common nuclear envelope (➤ Fig. 2.3d, ➤ Fig. 2.4). In

humans the zygote is only a transient division stage. After fertilisation of the ovum, the 2-cell stage of the genetically new embryo immediately follows (➤ Fig. 2.4c). The gender of the embryo is determined by the spermatozoon: if the fused spermatozoon carries a Y chromosome, the gene located on it **SRY** ('sex-determining region of Y') ensures the formation of the male phenotype.

NOTE

In fertilisation, the cell membranes of oocyte and spermatozoon fuse, so the haploid nucleus of spermatozoon enters the oocyte as a male pronucleus, and male and female pronuclei jointly form the cell nucleus of the zygote.

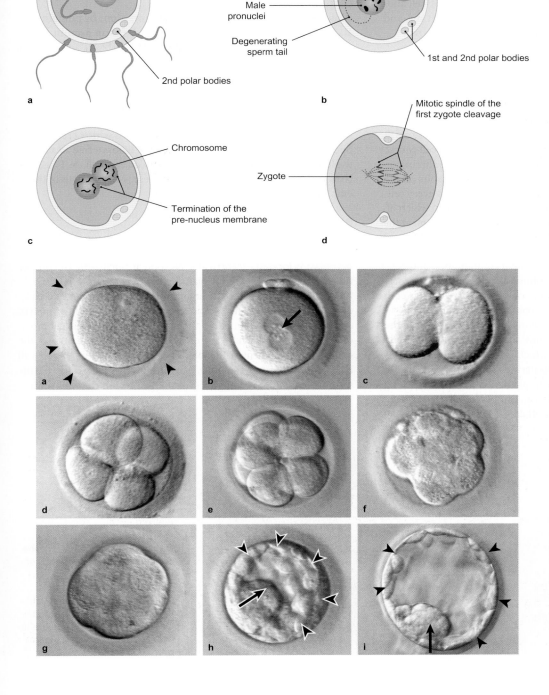

Fig. 2.3 Formation of the zygote.
a After a spermatozoon has penetrated into the ovum, further ingress by other spermatozoa is prevented by the zonal reaction and the 2nd meiosis of the oocyte is completed.
b The tail and mitochondria of the spermatozoon degenerate, and the nucleus increases in size to the male pronucleus.
c Male and female pronuclei approach and merge by dissolution of the nuclear membranes to become a zygote. **d** The chromosomes of both pronuclei are immediately aligned to the division spindle and the zygote initiates the first cleavage division. [E347-09]

Fig. 2.4 Cleavage, compaction and blastocysts. Illustrations of human embryos in vitro.
a Oocyte shortly before fertilisation. Arrows = Zona pellucida.
b Zygote with fused, male and female pronuclei (= arrow).
c First cleavage for 2-cell stage.
d 4-cell stage. **e** 8-cell stage. The blastomeres are still rounded.
f Morula stage at the beginning of compaction. The cells are compacted together and form a epithelium-like outer cell layer.
g Morula after compaction.
h Early blastocyst still within the Zona pellucida, with blastocoel between the outer shell of the trophoblast and the inner embryoblast. **i** Blastocyst after leaving the Zona pellucida. Arrowhead = trophoblast, arrow = embryoblast. [G394]

2.3 Preimplantation development

2.3.1 Cleavage and compaction

Cleavage positions
After fertilisation multiple mitotic divisions occur in the zygote while still in the Zona pellucida, which separate the cytoplasm of the oocytes into several daughter cells **(blastomeres)** (cleavage positions). The cleavage positions occur relatively slowly at intervals of several hours, with staggered division levels. This means that the first division of zygote cleavage occurs meridionally, whereas the second cleavage division runs around its equator and that the cadence of division rhythm is individual in each daughter cell; therefore an odd number of blastomeres can also be present (➤ Fig. 2.4). During the first two division steps, the proteins which are required for cell maintenance and mitotic cell division, i.e. **maternal genes,** are synthesised by the mRNA of the oocyte, and are released for translation by activation of the ovum. Between the 4-cell and 8-cell stages the **zygotic genes** are activated for the first time, and from now on the embryo takes over the expression of its own genes, independently of the mother.

Compaction
After the 8-cell stage and the 3rd division (➤ Fig. 2.4) another decisive event takes place: while the blastomeres so far approximately resemble round balls that are loosely joined together, the outer cells closely join together in an epithelium-like lattice. They close off the internal cells from the outside world by forming cell to cell contact between them (e.g. via the cell adhesion molecule E-cadherin) and tight junctions **(compaction,** ➤ Fig. 2.4f). Up to this point all the cells of the young embryo are **totipotent,** meaning that every cell has the potential to form a complete embryo on its own, which often happens in the case of identical twins. With compaction at the 16-cell stage **(morula stage,** ➤ Fig. 2.4f, g) now the **first differentiation** of cells takes place as the outer cells become differentiated from inner cells in terms of shape, protein configuration and developmental outcome. While the **trophoblast cells** and the chorion of the placenta develop from the outer cells, the embryo itself is entirely made up of the inner cells **(embryoblast** or internal cell mass). After the 64-cell stage, there is no more cell exchange between the two cell populations. Up to this point, the entire development takes place within the Zona pellucida, which migrates through the fallopian tube to the uterus during this period. The Zona pellucida protects the embryo from premature implantation in the mucosa of the fallopian tube, which would lead to an ectopic (tubal) pregnancy and is life-threatening for both, mother and embryo.

Clinical remarks

In the case of **ectopic pregnancies** implantation occurs outside the uterus. Over 90 % of these occur in the fallopian tube (tubal pregnancy) which can lead to the rupture of the fallopian tube and a life-threatening haemorrhage in the mother. The reason for this is often adhesions to the mucous membranes of the tube.
If after fertilisation the zygote passes through the fimbrian funnel back into the abdominal cavity, the embryo can implant in various locations within the peritoneum. Usually, it leads to intra-abdominal bleeding and miscarriage, but in exceptional cases it can lead to abdominal cavity pregnancies carried to full term and delivered by caesarean section.

2.3.2 Blastocysts and implantation

Cavitation
After compaction the trophoblast cells deliver ions by pumping Na^+ into the interior of the morula, which draws an osmotic wake of water behind it and the space between trophoblasts and embryoblasts is widened into a fluid-filled cavity (cavitation).

Hatching
At the fifth day, the embryo which has now reached the lumen of the uterus, leaves the narrowing Zona pellucida (➤ Fig. 2.4i, ➤ Fig. 2.5). The trophoblasts secrete proteases which create an opening in the Zona pellucida allowing the embryo free access to the lumen of the uterus, like hatching from an eggshell, ➤ Fig. 2.5a). Now not only cell division occurs, but there is also growth of the embryo.

Blastocysts and implantation
Due to fluid retention, the embryo now has the shape of a blister (blastocyst, ➤ Fig. 2.5, ➤ Fig. 2.6) and on its inner wall the embryoblast is located excentrically. As soon as the blastocyst comes into contact with the uterine wall, generally in the fundus of the uterus, it is attached with the embryonic pole to the maternal endometrial cells and to the abundantly suffused extracellular matrix. After successful attachment of the blastocyst the trophoblast produces proteases, which locally digest the extracellular matrix of the endometrium and enable the blastocyst to sink into the uterus wall **(implantation,** syn.: nidation). Approximately 10 days after fertilisation, the embryo is completely enveloped by the endometrium.

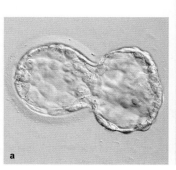

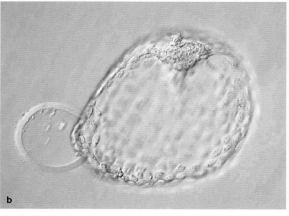

Fig. 2.5 Blastocyst leaving the Zona pellucida. Illustrations of human embryos in vitro.
a Hatching of the blastocyst from the Zona pellucida (left).
b Blastocyst leaving the Zona pellucida; the empty zona pellucida is to the left of the blastocyst. [G210]

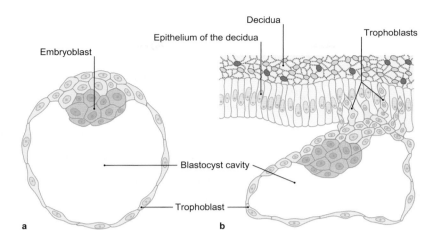

Decidua

Epithelium of the decidua

Trophoblasts

Embryoblast

Blastocyst cavity

Trophoblast

a   b

Fig. 2.6 Blastocyst and incipient implantation.
a Free blastocyst. **b** The blastocyst attaches with the embryonic pole to the uterine mucosa; the trophoblast begins to penetrate into the maternal tissue. [L126]

2.4 Gastrulation

2.4.1 Two-leaved germinal disc

While the trophoblast of the implanted blastocyst develops into parts of the placenta to serve nutrition of the embryo, the **embryoblast** undergoes further differentiation of cells (➤ Fig. 2.7). Embryoblast cells which express the transcription factor Nanog are arranged on the side facing the trophoblast, whereas those which do not express Nanog, but the transcription factor Gata6 form a layer adjacent to the blastocyst cavity. Both layers appear as round discs. This creates the **two-leaved germinal disc,** in which the embryoblast is divided into 2 epithelioid leaves – the **epiblast** (Nanog-positive) and the **hypoblast** (Gata6-positive). Simultaneously, the first of the 3 **body axes** of the embryo is defined, as the epiblast lies on the future dorsal side and the hypoblast lies on the ventral side. The hypoblast cells proliferate and grow around the lumen of the blastocyst cavity, where they are now referred to as extra-embryonic entoderm and form the epithelium of the **primary yolk sac** emerging from the blastocyte cavity. (➤ Fig. 2.7b).

In the epiblast, a thin cell sheet is secreted along the trophoblast shell that is increasingly detached by confluent splits from the underlying epiblast cells. This thin cell sheet, which is also referred to as **amnioblast,** is the precursor of the later amniotic epithelium and, together with the remaining epiblast, encloses a fluid-filled cavity, the **amniotic sac** (➤ Fig. 2.7a). All that remains as material of the embryo are the residual epiblast, which can therefore also be referred to as embryonic epiblasts. Before the start of gastrulation the embryo enclosed by trophoblast is made up of the two-leaved germinal disc with the epiblast and hypoblast, and ventrally and dorsally a fluid-filled cavity is present (**the two-vesicle stage**): dorsally from the amniotic cavity covered by amnioblast, ventrally the yolk sac coated in extra-embryonic entoderm emerging from the hypoblast .

2.4.2 Creation of the germinal layers

Before gastrulation, the embryo is present as a flat disc made of morphologically uniform epithelioid cells, the embryonic epiblast. From now onwards, the aim of **gastrulation** is to form the basic blueprint of the body from the epiblast, consisting of an outer shell (ectoderm) a lining of the inner surface, i.e. the intestinal tube (entoderm), and the tissue lying between it (mesoderm).

On the edge of the epiblast disc there is a protrusion, caused by the apicobasal elevation of the highly prismatic cells, which increasingly extends in a stripe-like fashion towards the middle of the germinal disc (**primitive streak**). This shows a nodular thickening there (**primitive node,** HENSEN's node, ➤ Fig. 2.8). The extension of the primitive streak is achieved by intercalating of the cells along the longitudinal axis of the primitive streak (convergent extension). The position and cell movements of the primitive streak are controlled by inductive signals from the underlying hypoblast. The primitive node is located on the upper pole of the primitive streak. Thus, even at this early stage, all other **body axes** are ultimately determined by the dorsoventral body axis, in particular the craniocaudal longitudinal axis, and also the left-right axis. On both sides of the primitive streak, the epiblast cells release E-cadherin-mediated cell to cell contacts, expand into the intercellular spaces by synthesising hyaluronan, and move in the direction of the primitive streak. The cells migrate into the primitive streak through a groove along the central line of the strip called the **primitive groove,** at a depth, i.e. ventrally.

The first cells arriving there penetrate from a medial direction between the hypoblast cells and completely displace them laterally into the wall of the yolk sac. Now the migrating cells form the ventral floor of the embryo and are the progenitor cells of the **entoderm.** The epiblast cells migrating somewhat later through the primitive groove spread out driven laterally and cranially by repulsive signals (e.g. secreted fibroblast growth factor, FGF) into the primitive streak. They form a loose mesenchymal cell association between the epiblast and newly-formed entoderm and together they form the **mesoderm.** This means that the location of the migration through the primitive streak is crucial to the future position of the mesoderm cells:

- The most cranially positioned migrating cells, i.e. through the primitive node, penetrate between the entoderm cells and migrate cranially where they initially form the **head process** and, as

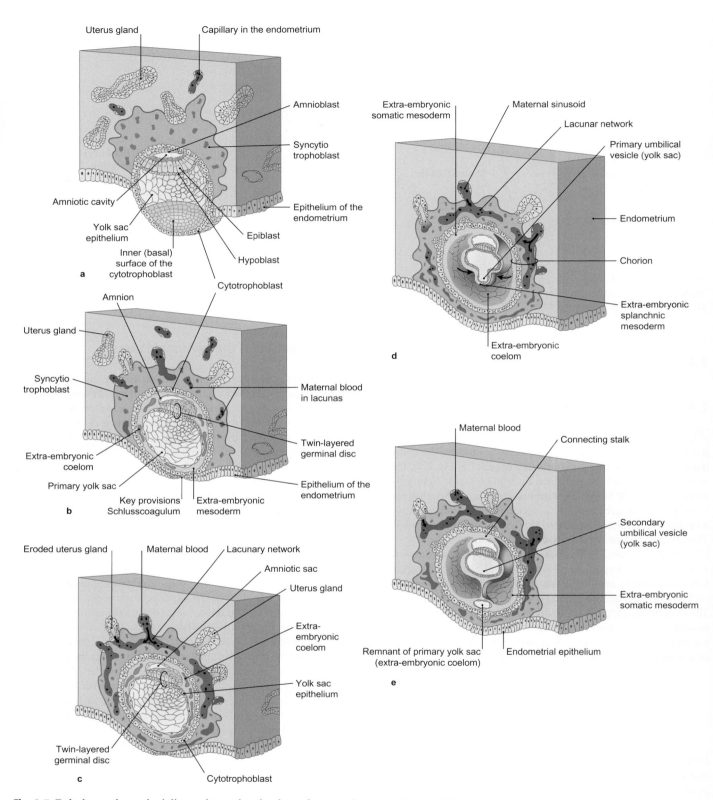

Fig. 2.7 Twin-layered germinal disc and complete implantation. a In the embryoblast epiblast, hypoblast and amnioblast have separated. The amniotic sac is formed between the epiblast and the amnioblast. In the trophoblast, the cells adjacent to the endometrium join together into multinuclear giant cell, syncytiotrophoblast. **b** The yolk sac epithelium developing from the hypoblast (syn.: extra-embryonic entoderm) has fully surrounded the blastocyst cavity formation, now referred to as the primary yolk sac. The extra-embryonic mesoderm grows in between the cytotrophoblast and the primary yolk sac. The syncytiotrophoblast arrodes the first endometrial vessels and the blood flows into the trophoblastic lacunae. **c** The cavities in the extra-embryonic mesoderm merge together with the extra-embryonic coelom. The trophoblastic lacunae coalesce into a coherent network, through which the mother's blood flows. **d** The extra-embryonic coelom flows into a contiguous cavity (chorionic cavity) that separates the yolk sac from the trophoblast. Thus the extra-embryonic mesoderm is divided into a visceral and a parietal sheet. The primary yolk sac becomes increasingly constricted. **e** The chorionic cavity surrounds the entire nucleus, which only comes into contact with the trophoblast via the connecting stalk. The proximal part of the constricted primary yolk sac forms the secondary yolk sac, the distal part becomes the rudimentary exocoelomic cyst. [E347-09]

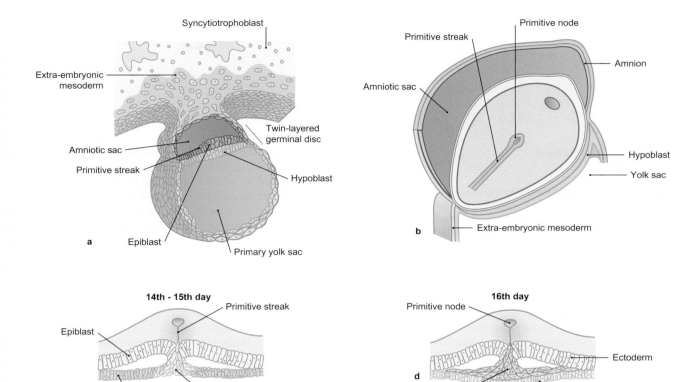

Fig. 2.8 Gastrulation. a At the start of gastrulation the primitive streak is formed in the epiblast. **b** Epiblast cells migrate deeper through the primitive groove which runs along the primitive streak and propagate on all sides beneath the epiblast. **c** The first cells migrating through the primitive groove laterally displace the hypoblast and form the epithelial entoderm. **d** The subsequent cells remain as mesenchymal cells and form the middle germ layer (mesoderm) separating the remaining epiblast cells, which are now known as ectoderm and entoderm. [L126]

gastrulation progresses, the **Chorda dorsalis** or **notochord** as the embryonic central axis.

- The cells migrating caudally to the primitive node through the cranial section of the primitive streak form the mesoderm lateral to the central axis, the **paraxial mesoderm.**
- The cells migrate increasingly caudally to correspondingly form the **intermediate mesoderm** and finally form the **lateral mesoderm** (side plate mesoderm, ➤ Fig. 2.9).

The cells of the epiblast that do not migrate deep through the primitive streak but after the completion of gastrulation remain in the former epiblasts, now form another germinal layer to be the dorsal surface epithelium called the **ectoderm.** As a result of gas-

trulation, the epiblast of the two-leaved germinal disc become the **three germ-layered embryo** which is still present as a flat germinal disc but which together with the ectoderm, mesoderm and entoderm already shows the principal structure of the vertebrate body; its body axes are defined in all three spatial planes.

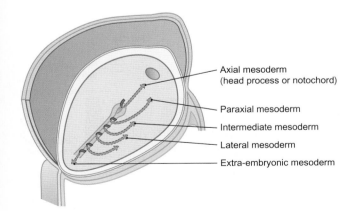

Fig. 2.9 Migration of mesoderm sections through the primitive streak. The more cranially the mesoderm progenitor cells migrate through the primitive streak or the primitive node, the further medially the mesoderm sections are formed. [L126]

Clinical remarks

Identical (monozygotic) twins are caused by the division of cells of a single germ cell at various stages of development. The most common is the division of blastomeres during cleavage, and more rarely by the division of the embryoblast in the blastocyst. In very rare cases, the separation occurs only during gastrulation, with 2 primitive streaks being created. Where incomplete separation of the two primitive streaks occurs, both twins remain partially conjoined (**'Siamese twins'**).

NOTE

During gastrulation three germ layers arise from the epiblast, the ectoderm, mesoderm and entoderm, and axes of the body are established.

2.5 Development of the ectoderm

2.5.1 Induction of the neuroectoderm

The cells of the epiblast, which during gastrulation do not migrate deep in the primitive streak but remain in the layer of the former

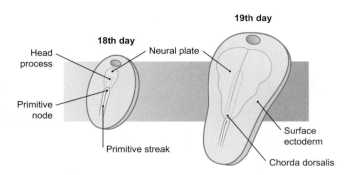

Fig. 2.10 Formation of neural plate. The thickened neural plate is formed from neuroectoderm under the influence of the head extension or the chordamesoderm migrating through the primitive node. In the brain area the neural plate is wide, whereas in the spinal cord area it is narrow. [L126]

epiblast, are referred to as **ectoderm**. Initially the ectoderm is a flat, slightly oval epithelial disc. With progressive gastrulation, in the medial third of the ectoderm there is an elevation of the multilayered epithelium, which stretches in a craniocaudal direction from the prechordal plate up to the primitive node, and viewed from the dorsal side displays an almost pear-shaped outline (➤ Fig. 2.10). This thickened ectoderm section (**neural plate**) provides the material for the nervous system (**neuroectoderm**), while the surrounding ectodermal epithelium forms the future **superficial ectoderm**.

The formation of the neural plate is based on **induction** by the underlying axial mesoderm. The primitive node and the mesoderm sections emerging from the primitive node, the head process and the notochord, function as a so-called **organiser**. They secrete signal molecules which induce the formation of the neural plate in the ectoderm above it (e.g. fibroblast growth factor 8, FGF8) and also inhibit the development of ectoderm cells into superficial ectoderm ('bone morphogenetic protein antagonists', BMPs, such as chordin). BMP seems to be a key molecule in the first differentiation of the ectoderm: if the BMP signal pathway is active, superficial ectoderm is formed and if it is inhibited (by the axial mesoderm) neuroectoderm is formed.

At the end of the 3rd week, the neural plate approximately resembles the outline of a violin with a broad section at the head in which the structure of the forebrain and midbrain are already prominent and a narrow, elongated section in the area of what will become the hindbrain and spinal cord (➤ Fig. 2.10).

2.5.2 Neurulation

Shortly after the formation of the neural plate, its lateral edges, together with the lateral superficial ectoderm begin to bulge dorsally (**neural bulge**), while at the same time, a longitudinal furrow is formed along the midline of the neural plate (**neural groove**) (➤ Fig. 2.11).

At this point, the neural plate in the area of neural groove comes temporarily into contact with the underlying notochord, whereby a hinge is simultaneously formed, dorsally raising the neural folds up to the median sagittal axis just like the compressed pages of a book (➤ Fig. 2.12).

The driving force for this is the apical constriction of the cells in the neural groove induced by the **chorda dorsalis** which take on a wedge shape and the strong growth of the ectoderm sited laterally to the neural plate, which together with the underlying mesoderm, displaces the neural bulge dorsally and medially. At the end of this process, the neural bulges touch both sides dorsally at the midline, firstly in the head and throat transition area and then progressing like a zip cranially and caudally (➤ Fig. 2.11c, ➤ Fig. 2.12d). This leads to the division of different parts of the neural bulges: the lateral portions of both neural bulges fuse at the furthest dorsal section and connect the superficial ectoderm on both sides by a full epithelial coat, from which the **epidermis** of the skin results. The respective medial components of both neural bulges join together with the neural tube below the superficial ectoderm **neural tube** from which the brain and spinal cord arise (➤ Fig. 2.11c, d ➤ Fig. 2.12e, f). At the end of neurulation the cranially and caudally progressing neural tube terminus remains as an open connection to the amniotic cavity (**anterior or posterior neuropore**), which only closes later on. The posterior neuropore is located at the level of the sacral medulla and the caudally positioned subsequent sacral and coccygeal segments of the spinal cord are formed by a fundamentally different mechanism (**secondary neurulation**). From the mesenchyme of the tail bud, which as a derivative of the primitive streak provides the building material for the coccyx area in the 4th week, a solid cord of neural tissue initially develops, which receives a lumen (**cavitation**) by detachment of the cell contacts inside it and soon connects to the caudal end of the neural tube formed by (primary) neurulation.

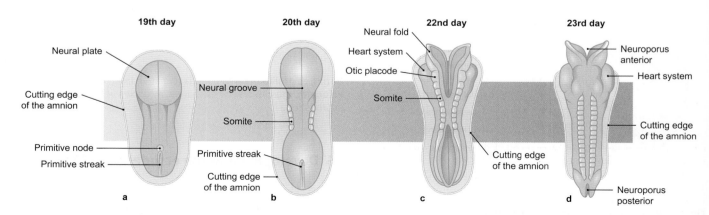

Fig. 2.11 Neurulation. a, b The neural plate bulges on both sides of the centre line in the form of dorsal neural folds and forms the neural groove. **c** At the start of the 3rd week, the neural folds fuse like a zip and form the neural tube. **d** Via Neuroporus anterior and posterior, the neural tube remains fused for some time with the amniotic cavity. [L126]

NOTE

In neurulation, the neural plate folds into 2 neural bulges that close dorsally in the median line to the neural tube.

2.5.3 Neural crest

Between the superficial ectoderm and the neural plate, i.e. directly ventral to the fusing neural bulges, a 3rd cell population becomes arranged, the **neural crest cells** (➤ Fig. 2.12f). The neural crest cells leave the ectodermal epithelial association (epithelial-mesenchyme transition, EMT) and as **mesenchymal progenitor cells** migrate to various points in the embryonic body. Emerging from them are various derivatives, such as the neurons of the peripheral nervous system, chromaffin cells of the adrenal gland and skin melanocytes **(truncal neural crest)**, and in the head area the skeleton and connective tissue **(head neural crest)**. The neural crest cells are guided on their migration to the sometimes distant target areas by the nature of the extracellular matrix and controlled by attraction and repulsion of molecular gradients **(chemotaxis)**. In the truncal neural crest 3 cell flows can be distinguished (➤ Fig. 2.13):
- under the superficial ectoderm laterally (melanocyte precursor)
- in each cranial half of the somites (progenitors of spinal ganglion cells)
- ventrally between the neural tube and somites (progenitors of sympathetic ganglion cells, ganglion cells of the intramural plexus of the viscera and the adrenal medulla).

Only after arrival at the destination do the cells differentiate according to their location; however, the determination probably already occurs in the course of migration created by environmental signals (specification of cell outcomes by induction).

Clinical remarks

Congenital bowel disease **(congenital megacolon, HIRSCHSPRUNG's disease)** is based on a defect of the migration behaviour of neural crest cells that form the intramural ganglia of the enteral nervous system of the large intestine. These

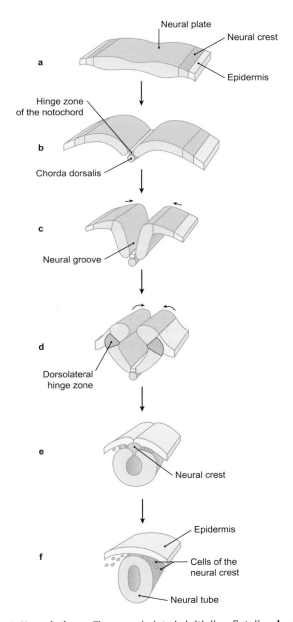

Fig. 2.12 Neurulation. a The neural plate is initially a flat disc. **b, c** It then increasingly develops along a hinge zone in contact with the chorda dorsalis to neural folds. **d, e** Due to the growth of the surface ectoderm, the neural folds are pressed in a medial direction along a dorsolateral hinge zone **(d)** and finally fuse in the midline into a closed neural tube **(e). f** Thereby the neuroectoderm is separated from the surface ectoderm and the neural crest cells migrate from the neuroectodermal epithelium. [L126]

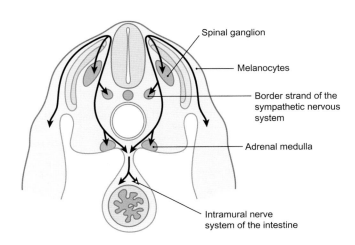

Fig. 2.13 Migration routes of neural crest cells in the trunk. The neural crest cells migrate at the time of neural tube closure from the neural folds to their target areas. The main routes are the subectodermal mesenchymal dorsal to the somites (melanocyte precursors), through the cranial half of the sclerotome (spinal ganglion precursor) and ventrally between somites and neural tube (precursor of chromaffin cells of the adrenal gland and the intestinal ganglia). [L126]

neural crest cells chemotactically follow the molecular attractant glial cell line-derived neurotrophic factor (GDNF), which they recognise through the RET membrane receptor. In the case of defects in either the expression of the GDNF ligand or the RET receptor, the innervation of the affected intestinal segments is omitted. Due to the resulting lack of peristalsis the contents of the intestines oral to the diseased intestinal portion accumulate and must therefore be surgically removed.

NOTE

Neural crest cells originate from the ectodermal neural bulges and migrate to the end of the neural tube as mesenchymal progenitor cells in very different target areas of the body, where they are differentiated as different cell types.

2.6 Development of the mesoderm

2.6.1 Axial mesoderm

The epiblast cells, which during gastrulation penetrate through the **primitive node,** i.e. the most cranial section of the primitive streak into the middle germ layer, remain in the midline of the embryo and migrate cranially as **axial mesoderm** past the primitive node. In doing so they temporarily penetrate the newly formed entoderm of the midline, displacing it laterally. At this stage, the axial mesoderm is referred to as the **chordal process** (syn.: chordal plate, head process). The chordal process subsequently dissolves as a solid strand from the entoderm dorsally, and the entoderm cells coalesce again in the midline and form the pharyngeal entoderm of the future (prospective) foregut (> Fig. 2.14). Thus the rod-shaped **chorda dorsalis** is formed from epitheloid mesoderm cells.
Only the most cranial part of the axial mesoderm remains mesenchymal as part of the **prechordal mesoderm** (head mesoderm) and in the course of further development forms the extraocular muscles. In the further process of gastrulation, the primitive node shifts increasingly in a caudal direction, while continuously emitting mesoderm cells in a cranial direction. The notochord is equal-

ly extended caudally in the 'fairway' of the primitive node (> Fig. 2.8, > Fig. 2.9). At the same time, the primitive streak is gradually shortened, while the germinal disc grows in total, becomes longer and in the cranial section the structures of the head are already formed. Finally, at the caudal aspect of the embryo, only the **tail bud** remains as the rudiment of the primitive streak where gastrulation continues to take place in a modified form until the formation of the mesoderm of the embryo is completed towards the end of the *4th week*.

NOTE

The notochord forms an embryonic axis organ. It is made up of mesoderm cells from the primitive node and plays an important role as a signal centre in the development of the nervous system and the somites. In the course of the formation of the vertebral column, the cells of the chorda presumably enter the nucleus pulposus of the intervertebral discs.

2.6.2 Paraxial mesoderm

Somitogenesis
The mesoderm cells, which in the course of gastrulation movements come to rest on both sides immediately lateral to the midline, form the **paraxial mesoderm.** They originate from cells that migrate caudally of the primitive node through the cranial primitive streak. Presumably cells of the caudal portion of the primitive node also succeed in entering the paraxial mesoderm. The paraxial mesoderm is initially created as solid mesenchyme strips bilateral to the notochord and is referred to as presomitic mesoderm (syn.: **segment plate**). The cells at the cranial end of the segment plate undergo a mesenchyme epithelial transition (MET) and are arranged into epithelial balls (**somites**) enclosing within it a central lumen filled with some mesenchymal cells (**somitocoel**). This process progresses as a result of rhythmic motion of a caudally progressing gastrulation every 4–5 hours, so that the segment plates are continuously segmented as they are extended caudally, in a craniocaudal direction by the formation of somites (**somitogenesis** > Fig. 2.15).

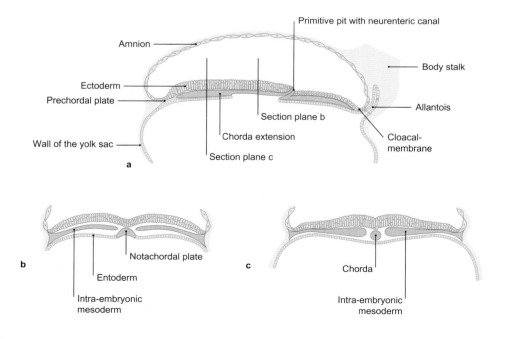

Amnion
Primitive pit with neurenteric canal
Body stalk
Ectoderm
Prechordal plate
Section plane b
Allantois
Wall of the yolk sac
Chorda extension
Cloacal-membrane
Section plane c
a

Notochordal plate
b
Entoderm
Intra-embryonic mesoderm

c
Chorda
Intra-embryonic mesoderm

Fig. 2.14 Development of the axial mesoderm. a Longitudinal section through an embryo in the middle of the 3rd week. The mesodermal cells migrating through the primitive nodes travel cranially in the midline and form the chordal process and then the prechordal mesoderm and the chorda dorsalis. **b** The chordal process displaces the entoderm temporarily into the midline. **c** Later the chordal process splits from the entoderm, coming to rest between the entoderm and the neural tube and forms the chorda dorsalis. [L126]

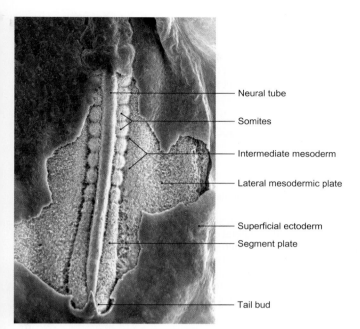

Neural tube

Somites

Intermediate mesoderm

Lateral mesodermic plate

Superficial ectoderm

Segment plate

Tail bud

Fig. 2.15 Somitogenesis. Scanning electron microscopy image of somitogenesis in a bird embryo. The paraxial mesoderm migrating during gastrulation on both sides of the neural tube through the cranial primitive streak forms a mesenchymal stripe (segment plate), which continuously produces somites at the cranial end by drawing in of segment limits. In the course of development the segment plate is extended by continuation of gastrulation in the tail bud, so that during somitogenesis the embryo continuously grows in a caudal direction. [G394]

The somitogenesis of both halves of the body occurs in a strictly synchronous manner and is temporally regulated by the oscillating expression of genes, e.g. of the notch signalling pathway, syn.: 'segmentation clock'). Somitogenesis begins on the *20th day of development* at the level of the auditory placodes, and comes to a stop after the creation of the coccygeal segments in the *5th week*. This creates the foundation for the segmental blueprint of the trunk: 5 occipital, 7 cervical, 12 thoracic, 5 lumbar, 5 sacral and 8–10 coccygeal pairs of somites develop, whereby the most recently formed coccygeal somites partially degenerate again. The **segmental identity** of somites, i.e. their region-specific properties, e.g. as cervical segments, will be conferred on them by a different expression of various **Hox genes,** in each segment, which encode transcription factors with homeobox DNA-binding domains (segment-specific 'Hox code').

The paraxial mesoderm positioned cranially to the auditory placode (**paraxial head mesoderm**) does not undergo any segmentation and, together with the prechordal mesoderm provides the building material for parts of the muscles and connective tissue of the head.

N O T E

Somites are segmental portions of the paraxial mesoderm, from which the skeletal muscles of the body and the axial skeleton originate.

Somite maturation: sclerotome

Only a few hours after their formation, the ventral side of the epithelial somites dissolves into a loose mesenchymal cell bond (**epithelial-mesenchyme transition,** EMT, ➤ Fig. 2.16). The reason for this is the signal protein formed in the notochord and the basal plate of the tube called sonic hedgehog (Shh), which reaches the ventral so-

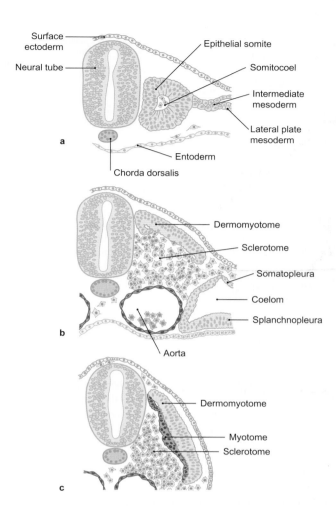

Surface ectoderm

Neural tube

Epithelial somite

Somitocoel

Intermediate mesoderm

Lateral plate mesoderm

a

Entoderm

Chorda dorsalis

Dermomyotome

Sclerotome

Somatopleura

Coelom

Splanchnopleura

b

Aorta

Dermomyotome

Myotome

Sclerotome

c

Fig. 2.16 Somite maturation. a Transverse section through an embryo at the level of a newly formed somite. The somite is a hollow epithelial ball, whose somitocoel contains mesenchyme. **b** After a few hours the ventral half of the somite becomes mesenchymal and forms the sclerotome. The dorsal half forms an epithelial sheet, the dermomyotome. **c** From the dermomyotome, cells migrate ventrally and form a 3rd compartment, the myotome, containing embryonic muscle cells. [L126]

mites by diffusion and induces EMT. These mesenchymal cells form the building material of the body skeleton and are therefore referred to as **sclerotome** (Gr.: 'skleros', hard). Accordingly, the sclerotome cells migrate in an amoeba-like way (➤ Fig. 2.17)

• in a ventromedial direction around the notochord to form the vertebral body,
• in a dorsomedial direction around the neural tube to form the vertebral arches and
• in the lateral abdominal wall to form the ribs.

The dura mater of the vertebral canal also originates from the sclerotome. Within a segment the cranial and caudal halves of the sclerotome have different properties. Due to the expression of the repellent effects of the signal molecule ephrin in the caudal half of the sclerotome, neural crest cells and motor neurons migrate from the spinal cord only into the cranial half of the respective sclerotome, in order to form the **spinal nerves**. The segmental organisation of the peripheral nervous system therefore emerges secondarily as a result of the segmentation of the paraxial mesoderm.

Somite maturation: dermomyotome and myotome

The epithelial cells of the dorsal half of the somites remaining outside the effect of Shh, form a nearly rectangular sheet under the

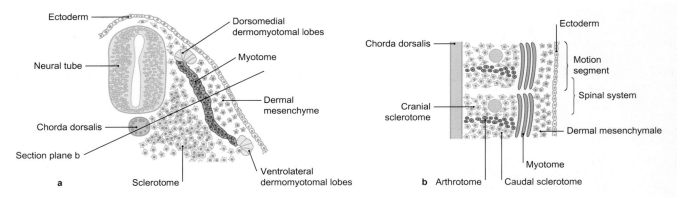

Fig. 2.17 Somite differentiation. a Transverse section through a mature somite. The sclerotomal mesenchyme (yellow) encloses the chorda dorsalis and the neural tube as an annex to the vertebral body and vertebral arch and forms a lateral offshoot as the annex of the ribs. Dorsolaterally, the sclerotome is limited by the myotomal annex of the back muscles. On one side the epithelial dermomyotome develops into myotome cells and on the other side into dermal connective tissue progenitor cells. The dermomyotomal epithelium only survives at the dermomyotomal lips and provides further annex material for both cell lines. **b** Oblique horizontal section through **a.** In the cranial section, neural crest cells form spinal ganglia. Between the cranial and caudal halves of the somite lie the cells of the arthrotome, from which the vertebral joints develop. They mark the future border between two vertebrae. A mobile segment consists at this stage of two adjacent vertebral systems, the intermediate joint system and the myotomal muscle fibres of a somite. [L126]

influence of signals from the superficial ectoderm (especially secreted glycoproteins of the Wnt family, otherwise called 'Wint') and the cover plate of the neural tube. This sheet is made up of highly prismatic epithelial cells called the **dermomyotome** . This designation gives the impression that the cells of the dermomyotome form the building material of dermal connective tissue and skeletal muscles. Following successful EMT, migrating dermomyotomal cells take several steps ventrally between the dermomyotome and the sclerotome, and there form a third somite compartment, called the **myotome**. The myotome consists of primordial, single mononuclear muscle fibres which extend in a craniocaudal direction from segment border to segment border and form the

site of the segmentally organised **trunk musculature** (➤ Fig. 2.17, ➤ Fig. 2.18). The specification of the dermomyotomal progenitor cells to skeletal muscles is in turn induced by Wnt signals that are formed in the cover plate of the neural tube and the superficial ectoderm. The Wnt signals induce the expression of muscle-specific regulator genes in the dermomyotome cells, such as the transcription factor **MyoD,** which determine the fate of their development as muscle cells and initiate the muscle-specific differentiation of cells. From the medial (**epaxial**) section of the myotome the autochthonous back muscles develop, while from the lateral (**hypaxial**) section the intercostal muscles and the muscles of the abdominal wall develop. The segmental arrangement of myotome fibres

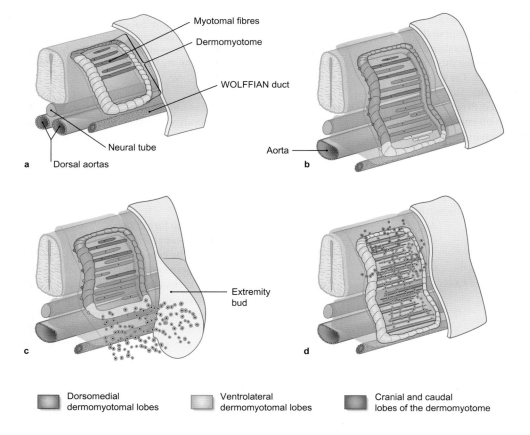

Fig. 2.18 Myotome formation. a The first myotome cells formed are taken from the dorsomedial lip of the dermomyotome and form the epaxial myotome fibres from which the autochthonous muscles later arise. **b** Then the ventrolateral lip of the dermomyotome forms hypaxial myotome fibres, from which the ventrolateral abdominal wall muscles are formed. In addition, the cranial and caudal edges of the dermomyotome and later on also the central dermomyotome contribute myotome fibres. **c** At the level of the extremity system no hypaxial myotomes are formed. The hypaxial dermomyotome cells migrate as muscle progenitor cells into the extremity system. **d** After the dissolution of the central dermomyotome, the cells migrate into both the myotome and the subectodermal mesenchyme where they form the dermis and subcutis. [G210]

remains unchanged in the deep layers of the back muscles and in the intercostal muscles and in the cross-segmental systems of the trunk muscles it is only shown in the innervation. In the area of the **extremity position** no hypaxial myotome is formed, instead the cells of the lateral (hypaxial) dermomyotome migrate into the extremity buds as a precursor of the muscles of the extremities a (➤ Fig. 2.21).

Dermomyotomal cells that do not form muscles, migrate dorsally under the superficial ectoderm and form the **dermis** and subcutis of the back (➤ Fig. 2.17, ➤ Fig. 2.18). These cells are often referred to according to their developmental outcome as **dermatomes** but within the dermomyotome cannot be morphologically distinguished. Only the dermis of the back is derived from somites, the dermis of the ventral trunk wall and the extremities derive from the side plate mesoderm and that of the head originates from the neural crest of the head.

N O T E

Origin of the musculoskeletal system: the autochthonous musculature arises from the epaxial myotomes, the thoracic and abdominal wall musculature arise from the hypaxial myotomes and the extremity muscles arise from muscle progenitor cells, which migrate from the lateral dermomyotomes to the extremity site. The skeletal muscle in the region of the pharyngeal arches is derived from the lateral dermomyotomes of the occipital somites and the unsegmented paraxial head mesoderm.

Development of the movement segment

The derivatives of a single somite form a so-called **movement segment,** i.e. the adjacent halves of two neighbouring vertebrae and the joints, muscles and ligaments lying between them (➤ Fig. 2.17b). The vertebral joints and intervertebral discs arise from the somitocoel cells located at the centre of the somite (**arthrotome**), with the border between two vertebrae running through the middle of the somites. A single vertebral body is conversely formed from the cranial and caudal halves of the sclerotome of two neighbouring somites. Therefore, the macroscopically visible segmentation of the spine is offset towards the **primary segmentation** of the embryo by the somites in one half of a segment (**resegmentation**).

Clinical remarks

Errors in the regulation of Hox gene expression in the paraxial mesoderm can lead to shifts in the segment identity of individual vertebrae **(homeotic transformation).** Examples include **cervical ribs,** for which topographically cervical vertebrae have a thoracic identity, or **atlas assimilation,** where the topographically highest cervical vertebra has an occipital identity and becomes part of the occiput. Particularly clinically relevant is the sacralisation of the lumbar vertebral vein. It leads to the extension of the birth canal (assimilation canal pelvis or 'long pelvis') and can be an indication for birth by caesarean section.

N O T E

A cervical vertebra arises from the sclerotomes of each of two adjacent halves of somites.

2.6.3 Intermediate mesoderm

The paraxial mesoderm is associated with the lateral mesoderm by a narrow strip of mesenchymal cells, referred to as **intermediate mesoderm** and contains the building material of the embryonic kidneys (➤ Fig. 2.16, ➤ Fig. 2.19). At the level of the occipital somites, the intermediate mesoderm appears to be absent. In the area of cervical segments, at the start of the *4th week* an initially solid thread from the mesenchyme is dorsolaterally affiliated, which rapidly becomes an epithelial tube channel (**prerenal duct**). It is extended in a caudal direction in the course of the caudally progressing growth of the embryo in approximately the same way as the segmentation front of the paraxial mesoderm. This growth is ensured by the proliferation of a blastema at the caudal tip of the duct. As a result, the intermediate mesoderm is divided into:

- the epithelial prenephric and **mesonephric duct** (ductus mesonephricus, WOLFFIAN duct), which reaches as far as the cloaca caudally, and
- the ventromedially adjacent mesenchyme, which depending on the developmental stage of the kidneys (pronephros and mesonephros) is referred to as pronephrogenic or mesonephrogenic mesenchyme.

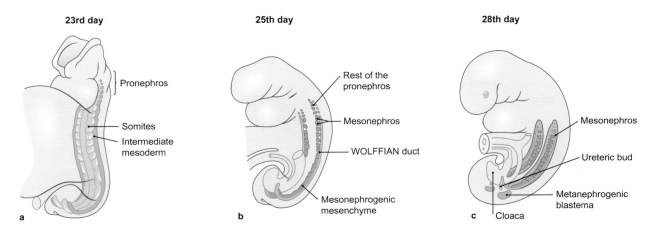

23rd day

Pronephros
Somites
Intermediate mesoderm

25th day

Rest of the pronephros
Mesonephros
WOLFFIAN duct
Mesonephrogenic mesenchyme

28th day

Mesonephros
Ureteric bud
Metanephrogenic blastema
Cloaca

a   b   c

Fig. 2.19 Development of the intermediate mesoderm. Embryo drawn to demonstrate the intermediate mesoderm, shown transparently.
a The intermediate mesoderm lies laterally to the somite and on day 23 is made up of pronephrogenic and mesonephrogenic mesenchyme.
b The distant cranially lying pronephros degenerates after inducing the formation of the WOLFFIAN duct. The mesonephros begins to form urinary corpuscles. **c** Before the junction of the WOLFFIAN duct into the cloaca, the ureteric bud grows together into the metanephric mesenchyme and forms the definitive kidney (metanephros). [L126]

While the pronephros remains without any function and degenerates, the WOLFFIAN duct and mesonephrogenic mesenchyme form the functioning embryonic **mesonephros** by mutual induction. As development continues, the ureteric bud branches off from the caudal portion of the WOLFFIAN duct; in males the cranial portion of the WOLFFIAN duct becomes the seminal duct (Vas deferens, ➤ Fig. 2.19).

> **NOTE**
> The kidneys as well as the urinary and seminal tracts arise from the intermediate mesoderm.

2.6.4 Lateral mesoderm

Coelom
Laterally to the intermediate mesoderm there extends over the entire length of the trunk a wide, unsegmented tissue stripe **(lateral mesoderm)**, which in the early embryo changes laterally into the extra-embryonic mesoderm and thus constitutes the lateral margin of the germinal disc. The lateral mesoderm (syn.: **side plate mesoderm**) is divided into two superimposed epithelial plates, which are separated by a slit-shaped cavity **(coelom)**:

- The posterior plate is referred to as the somatic (syn.: parietal) side plate mesoderm (➤ Fig. 2.16). Together with the overlying superficial ectoderm, it forms the outer wall of the coelom (**somatopleure).**
- The plate located ventrally to the coelom is called the visceral side plate mesoderm and together with the underlying entoderm forms the inner wall of the coelomic cavity (**splanchnopleure,** ➤ Fig. 2.20).

The coelomic cavity opens laterally in the germinal disc stage into the **extra-embryonic coelom** (syn.: chorionic cavity). After the ventral closure of the embryo resulting from the lateral cleavage (➤ Chap. 2.8.2), the lateral mesoderm fuses ventromedially to the ventral trunk wall, with the exception of the umbilical cord. The coelom joins onto the embryonic **abdominal cavity.**

The mesodermal cell layer of the somatopleure and splanchnopleure directly adjacent to the coelomic cavity remains epithelial and covers the abdominal cavity as parietal and visceral **serosa.** The deeper lying cells of both mesodermal layers become mesenchymal (EMT) and form the **somatic mesenchyme** between the serosa and the ectoderm and the **visceral mesenchyme** located between the serosa and the entoderm (➤ Fig. 2.21).

> **NOTE**
> The intra-embryonic coelom is the primary abdominal cavity and separates the side plate mesoderm into a parietal and a visceral sheet. From the coelom, the body cavities (peritoneal cavity, pleural cavity, pericardial cavity) develop.

Somatopleure
From the mesenchyme of the somatopleure during further development, the connective tissue of the ventrolateral trunk wall and extremities arise, including the dermis and subcutis of the skin; however, thoracic and abdominal wall muscles and the ribs come from somites. Streams of migrating cells from the lateral sclerotome penetrate the mesenchymal matrix of the **thoracic somatopleure** in a segmental arrangement and form the ribs. Therefore, the ribs in developmental terms are extensions of the spine. In the trunk the only skeletal element is the **sternum** from the mesenchyme of the somatopleure. It is produced by chondral ossification from 2 bilateral systems **(sternal borders),** which fuse with the ventral closure of the embryo.

The thoracic hypaxial myotomes push forward between the segmental rib sites by the consecutive recruitment of muscle progenitor cells from the hypaxial dermomyotomes ventrolaterally, and form the intercostal muscles. In the abdominal area where no ribs are formed, the hypaxial myotomes, having lost their morphologically recognisable segmentation, grow into the somatopleure and form the abdominal wall muscles. Aponeuroses and connective tissue of the thoracic and abdominal wall muscles arise from the side plate mesoderm.

The **limb systems** arise from a local bulging of the somatopleure due to the strong proliferation of the somatic mesenchyme (➤ Fig. 2.21, ➤ Chap. 2.10). This creates the connective tissue and the **skeleton of the extremities** from the somatic side plate mesenchyme. The skeletal muscles of the extremities arise in turn from the somites. Unlike the trunk muscles, they do not originate from the myotomes, but they arise from highly mobile **myogenic progenitor cells**, which are disassociated from the hypaxial dermomyotomes of the somites at the level of the extremity systems, and migrate into the mesenchymal matrix of the extremity buds, where they are differentiated into muscle fibres (➤ Fig. 2.21).

> **NOTE**
> The ventrolateral body wall and the extremities arise from the somatopleure, with the exception of the muscles, which originate from the somites.

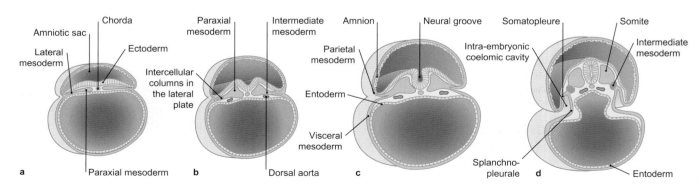

Fig. 2.20 Development of the lateral mesoderm. a The lateral mesoderm or lateral plate mesoderm lies at the edge of the germinal disc laterally to the paraxial and intermediate mesoderm. **b** The coelom is formed by the formation of fissures in the lateral mesoderm. **c** The dorsal portion of the lateral plate mesoderm and the ectoderm (somatopleure) lying above it are merged into the wall of the amniotic cavity. The ventral portion of the side plate mesoderm and the underlying entoderm (splanchnopleure) are included in the wall of the yolk sac. **d** The coelom is located between the somatopleure and the splanchnopleure. [L126]

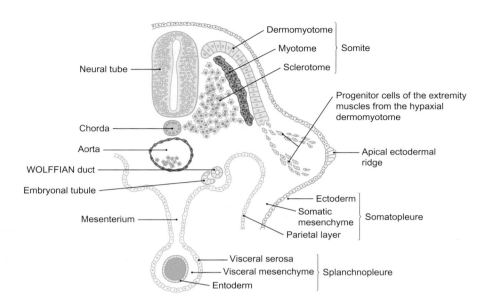

Fig. 2.21 Mesoderm development. Semi-schematic cross-section through an embryo towards the end of the 4th week. The somatopleure forms the ventrolateral abdominal wall and the splanchnopleure forms the wall of the gut and the mesentery. The extremity annex occurs as a thickening of the somatopleure and is colonised by myogenic progenitor cells from the somites, which are arranged ventrally and dorsally as a premuscle mass. [L126]

Splanchnopleure

The splanchnopleure envelops the entodermal intestinal tube and its appendages after the ventral closure of the abdominal wall (➤ Fig. 2.21). It forms the **visceral serosa** and the underlying subperitoneal, subpleural and subpericardial connective tissue as well as the connective tissue and the **smooth muscles** of the gastrointestinal tract and the lungs. In the most cranial section of the lateral mesoderm, the site material of the myocardium (**cardioembryonic plate**) forms in the splanchnopleure which, after fusion of the paired heart system is surrounded by the most cranial section of the coelom as the pericardial cavity.

> **N O T E**
> The splanchnopleure gives rise to the mesodermal wall of the gastrointestinal tract and the heart.

2.7 Development of the entoderm

The **entoderm** is initially present as a flat, epithelial layer of the ventral surface of the three-leaved germinal disc. The embryo forms the roof of the **yolk sac** with quasi 'open abdomen'. As part of the formation of the definitive body shape by cleavage movements of the embryo (➤ Chap. 2.8), the entoderm is ventromedially drilled in and attaches to the ventrally closed **intestinal tube** (➤ Fig. 2.21). The connection to the yolk sac remains only at the navel in the form of the **vitelline duct** (Ductus omphaloentericus, Ductus vitellinus). The intestinal section in the area of the vitelline duct is referred to as the **midgut**, sections located further towards the mouth are defined as the **foregut**; and the sections located aborally thereof are designated as the **hindgut** (➤ Fig. 2.22). The embryonic intestinal tube remains closed at its cranial and caudal end:

- The **buccopharyngeal membrane** arises from the mesoderm-free prechordal plate and closes the entodermal foregut opposite the ectoderm-lined stomatodeum.
- The **cloacal membrane** opens into the hindgut opposite the ectoderm-lined proctodeum.

After the repositioning of the development-linked umbilical hernia towards the end of the *3rd month* the vitelline duct obliterates but can persist in the adult ileum in approximately 3% of cases as **MECKEL's diverticulum**.

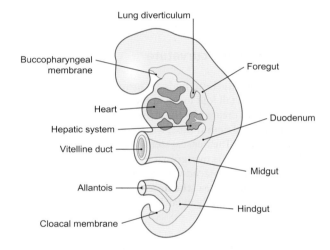

Fig. 2.22 Development of the entoderm. Embryo towards the end of the 4th week. The vitelline duct divides the intestines into the foregut, midgut and hindgut. The oral and anal openings of the gut are initially closed (buccopharyngeal membrane or cloacal membrane). [L126]

The wall of the gastrointestinal tract and the organs annexed to the intestines, including the lungs, are formed from the entodermal epithelium of the intestinal tube by inductive interaction with the surrounding mesenchyme of the **splanchnopleure** (and the neural crest in the pharyngeal gut).

> **N O T E**
> The epithelial lining of the intestinal tube and its annex organs develop from the embryonic entoderm. Conversely, the smooth muscles and connective tissue of the gastrointestinal tract are derived from the splanchnopleure.

2.8 Folding movements of the embryo

Until the start of the *4th week*, the embryo is a flat **germinal disc,** which has stretched from an initial round plate into a longitudinally oval plate. Along the primitive streak, the germ layers of ectoderm, mesoderm and entoderm are formed as part of gastrulation. Dorsally above the embryo is the **amniotic cavity,** the base of which is formed from superficial ectoderm. Ventrally beneath the embryo is the **secondary yolk sac,** the roof of which is formed by the entoderm. The germ layers and the coelom merge laterally and seamlessly into the **extra-embryonic tissue.** The embryonic ectoderm merges into the amniotic epithelium, the somatic lateral mesoderm merges into the extra-embryonic mesoderm of the chorionic cavity, the visceral lateral mesoderm merges into the extra-embryonic mesoderm of the yolk sac, and the entoderm merges into the yolk sac epithelium. The embryonic coelom is openly connected laterally to the **chorionic cavity.** The three-dimensional shape of the embryo, in which the body wall encloses the abdominal cavity and the intestinal tube, only emerges in the course of the 4th week by **folding movements** of the germinal disc in the sagittal and transverse planes. In this way the embryo develops a blueprint typical of vertebrates **(basic body form).** The extra-embryonic parts of the embryo then form the foetal parts of the placenta, and the embryo only remains linked to this via the umbilical cord.

> NOTE
> The three-dimensional shape of the embryo occurs in the course of the 4th week by craniocaudal and lateral cleavage movements.

2.8.1 Craniocaudal curvature

In the sagittal plane the head folds are formed at the cranial end of the embryo and the tail fold forms at the caudal end:
- The **head fold** is created by the strong growth of the brain system in the cranial neural tube, which bulges in a cranial and ventral direction. The heart system positioned in front of the head of the embryo is overgrown by the head structures pressing cranially and displaced ventrally and caudally in relation to the head and throat area **(the descent of the heart).** The yolk sac is narrowed cranially in such a way that the **vitelline duct**

(Ductus omphaloentericus) comes to rest caudally to the heart (➤ Fig. 2.23).
- The **tail bud** is raised at the caudal end of the embryo from the amnion, and curves together with the hindgut ventrally. The **allantois** comes to rest in the area of what will later become the umbilical cord, caudal of the vitelline duct. The resulting blind ending section of the gut arising from the tail fold **(tail gut),** caudal to the cloaca, is then obliterated.

2.8.2 Lateral folding up

As a result of the strong growth in the course of the *4th week,* the germinal disc bulges to form a cap lying over the yolk sac, which is narrowing at the same time to become the vitelline duct (➤ Fig. 2.24). As a consequence as well as the craniocaudal curvature, there is **lateral folding; somatopleure** and **splanchnopleure** (➤ Chap. 2.6.4) bend ventromedially, while the paraxial mesoderm and the axillary organs (notochord and neural tube) retain their dorsal location. The somatopleure and splanchnopleure finally fuse in a zip-like fashion in the ventral centre line; only in the area of the navel does the embryo remain ventrally open to the yolk sac. On the outside the **amnion,** which is attached to the ectoderm, unfolds together with the somatopleure of the embryo and lies over the thus formed umbilical cord as an epithelial cover. Therefore, the embryo is covered on all sides by the amniotic cavity, and the ectoderm of the amniotic fluid flows round it.

On the ventral side, the **entoderm** curves together with the splanchnopleure ventromedially and attaches in the ventral centre line to the **foregut.** As a result, the left and right embryonic coelom cavities also connect to the shared **abdominal cavity,** and the connection between the embryonic coelom and the chorionic cavity, which exists up to this point, is closed.

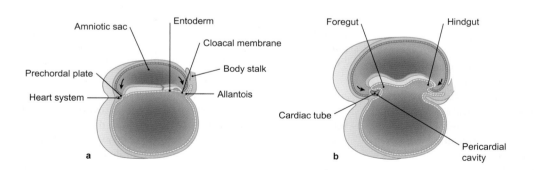

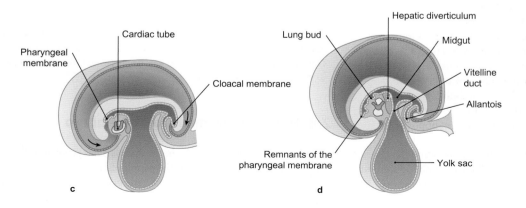

Fig. 2.23 Craniocaudal curvature; longitudinal sections. **a** An 18-day-old embryo in the germinal disc stage. **b** A 20-day-old embryo during neurulation. Heart system and tail bud rotate ventrally. **c** A 21-day-old embryo. As a result of the descent of the heart and the formation of the hind gut, the yolk sac becomes increasingly constricted. **d** A 30-day-old embryo. The intestinal tube has closed and only remains in contact with the yolk sac via the vitelline duct. [L126]

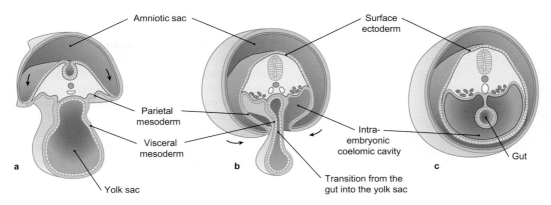

Amniotic sac

Surface ectoderm

Parietal mesoderm

Visceral mesoderm

Intra-embryonic coelomic cavity

Gut

Transition from the gut into the yolk sac

a   b   c

Yolk sac

Fig. 2.24 Lateral folding; cross-sections. **a** A 21-day-old embryo. Somatopleure and amnion grow together ventrolaterally. **b** A 22-day-old embryo. The yolk sac becomes increasingly constricted. **c** A 30-day-old embryo. The splanchnopleure together with the entoderm has closed to become the intestinal tube. The somatopleure together with the ectoderm has closed onto the ventral wall of the trunk and the amnion completely envelops the embryo. Between the somatopleure and the splanchnopleure the coelom which is now closed becomes the embryonic abdominal cavity. [L126]

Clinical remarks

If as part of the lateral folding, the ventromedial closure of the abdominal wall remains incomplete, the coelom remains open towards the amniotic cavity and intestinal loops can freely protrude into the abdomen (**gastroschisis**), or in the thorax the heart can protrude freely in the amniotic cavity (**Ectopia cordis**).

2.9 Extra-embryonic tissue

Only some of the cells of the early embryo become part of the actual embryo (➤ Chap. 2.3.1). Other cells develop into **extra-embryonic structures,** whose function is to supply the embryo with nutrients and oxygen and the creation of a favourable intrauterine environment. Finally, the extra-embryonic tissues largely go into the **placenta** and at birth are expelled as the afterbirth.

2.9.1 Trophoblast

As early as the first week the embryoblast and trophoblast separate in the blastocyst (➤ Chap. 2.3.1). At implantation, the trophoblast fully penetrates into the **endometrium** of the uterus and as such is the contact with the maternal tissues. At the edge of the endometrium, the trophoblast cells fuse into a single giant cell with multiple nuclei (**syncytium),** which surrounds the embryo like a shell. In the course of further growth, the cells of the highly proliferating cellular trophoblasts are in constant fusion (**cytotrophoblast**) with the external **syncytiotrophoblast,** thus growing and penetrating further into the uterus wall. Within the syncytiotrophoblasts, membrane-covered, extracytoplasmic vacuoles (**trophoblastic lacunae**) are formed, which increasingly fuse and form an intracellular, fluid-filled system of channels. Where syncytiotrophoblast come into contact with maternal blood vessels, their vessel walls dissolve and the maternal blood flows into the trophoblastic lacunae. Thus the syncytiotrophoblast is switched towards the end of the *2nd week* between the arterial and venous leg of the endometrial vessels, and the incipient **uteroplacental circulation** enables the supply of the growing embryo by the maternal blood.

2.9.2 Chorionic cavity and yolk sac

In the middle of the *2nd week* the embryo still displays the basic form of the blastocyst despite the differentiation processes in the embryoblast and trophoblast; however, the **blastocoel** will be referred to thereafter as the **primary yolk sac**. This is covered on the inside by the hypoblast cells displaced laterally during gastrulation (➤ Chap. 2.4) (**primary yolk sack epithelium,** syn.: HEUSER's membrane). Between the cytotrophoblast and primary yolk sac epithelium migrates as a loose aggregation into the cells of the **extra-embryonic mesoderm**. While trophoblast and extra-embryonic mesoderm display strong growth, the primary yolk sac lags behind in terms of growth and becomes detached from the cytotrophoblasts. This creates **lacunae** in the growing extra-embryonic mesoderm, which continue to coalesce and finally form a large, continuous cavity between the primary yolk sac and the trophoblast (**chorionic cavity,** syn.: extra-embryonic coelom, ➤ Fig. 2.25). The extra-embryonic mesoderm covers the chorionic cavity externally at the border to the cytotrophoblast (**parietal extra-embryonic mesoderm**) as well as inside at the border to the yolk sac (**visceral extra-embryonic mesoderm**). In the primary yolk sac, however, there is annular constriction and detachment of the distal part of the yolk sac, which loses its connection to the embryo (**exocoelomic cyst**) and finally perishes (➤ Fig. 2.25). The proximal part of the yolk sac is lined by a succeeding population of hypoblast cells and now forms the **secondary** (syn.: definitive) **yolk sac.** This means that the wall of the secondary yolk sac consists of an inner epithelial layer formed from hypoblast (extra-embryonic entoderm) and an outer layer of visceral extra-embryonic mesoderm, demarcating the yolk sac from the chorionic cavity. Later blood cells (haematopoiesis) and original germ cells arise from the visceral extra-embryonic mesoderm of the yolk sac. The outer wall of the embryo, which is made up of parietal extra-embryonic mesoderm and the trophoblast, is named the **chorion**. The majority of the **foetal placenta** arise later from the chorion.

> **NOTE**
> Although the embryo of mammals and of humans has no yolk, a yolk sac is formed as with the embryos of egg-laying vertebrates. The yolk sac is phylogenetically preserved, because the original germ cells and blood cells arise from the wall of the yolk sac, making it also essential for mammalian embryos.

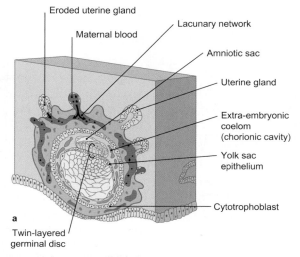

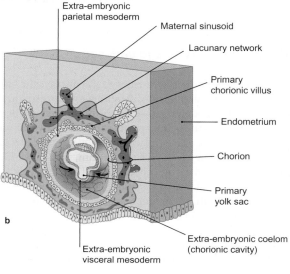

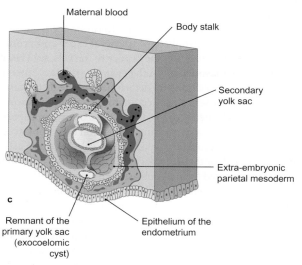

Fig. 2.25 Early development of extra-embryonic tissue.
a A 12-day-old embryo. The syncytiotrophoblast taps into vessels of the maternal endometrium so that the maternal blood flows freely into the trophoblast lacunae. Due to the formation of fissures the chorionic cavity forms in the extra-embryonic mesoderm. **b** A 13-day-old embryo. As a result of the confluence of the chorionic fissures, the chorionic cavity becomes a cohesive cavity. The primary yolk sac is constricted annularly. **c** A 14-day-old embryo. The rest of the primary yolk sac is cut off as the exocoelomic cyst; the secondary yolk sac is coated with entoderm cells. [E347-09]

2.9.3 Amnion

The **amniotic epithelium** exists from the beginning of the *2nd week* as a separation of the dorsal epiblast and envelopes the **amniotic cavity** lying initially dorsal to the germinal disc. It merges on the border into the surface ectoderm of the germinal disc and is therefore referred to as **extra-embryonic ectoderm**. In the course of embryonic folding movements in the *3rd week* (➤ Chap. 2.8), the amniotic cavity completely envelopes the entire embryo up to the body stalk. Together with the yolk sac, the amniotic epithelium facing the chorionic cavity is covered with **visceral extra-embryonic mesoderm**. In the course of the *2nd month* , the embryo and the amnion surrounding it grow stronger than both enveloping chorionic cavities so that at the end of the *3rd month* the lumen of the chorionic cavity is entirely displaced by the amnion and, together with the chorion, the amnion forms the wall of the **amniotic sac** (➤ Fig. 2.26).

Phylogenetically, the amnion should be understood as an adaptation to **life on land**. It enables embryonic development within the egg in dry environments, in the form of a liquid-filled amniotic cavity, which encloses the embryo similar to an aquarium, and protects it from drying out. In the secondary development transposed within the moist environment of the uterus of mammals and humans this feature again becomes less important. Due to their development in the amniotic cavity, reptiles, birds and mammals are grouped together as **amniotes**.

> **Clinical remarks**
>
> The amniotic fluid is formed from the amniotic epithelium, drunk by the foetus, partly reabsorbed by the foetal intestines and passed through the placenta into the maternal blood, partly excreted through the foetal kidneys and urine back into the amniotic sac. If this balance is disturbed, too little (**oligohydramnios,** risk of malformations due to compression) or too much (**polyhydramnios,** risk of rupture of the membrane) amniotic fluid may be present. This can be treated by amniotic infusion or amniotic puncture.
>
> In cases of a suspected foetal **genetic abnormality**, as part of the prenatal diagnosis, the amniotic cavity can be punctured through the abdominal wall, uterine wall, chorion and amnion. The paediatric cells floating in the amniotic fluid can be removed at minimum risk to the foetus and genetically tested (**amniocentesis).**

> **N O T E**
>
> The amnion completely envelops the foetus and in the foetal period forms the amniotic sac and the foetal portion of the placenta together with the chorion.

2.9.4 Allantois

From the ventral wall of the **hind gut** an entodermal diverticulum called the **allantois,** is pulled into the extra-embryonic mesoderm of the body stalk. Here it seems to play a role in the development of the umbilical vessels. The important function of the allantois for other amniotes is the storage of nitrogen metabolites (embryonic bladder); this is irrelevant in mammals and humans due to the excretory function of the placenta. The allantois becomes narrower as it continues in its developmental process into a duct (**urachus),** which is obliterated postnatally to **the Lig. umbiliacale medianum.** The bladder is at the junction of the allantois into the entodermal cloaca.

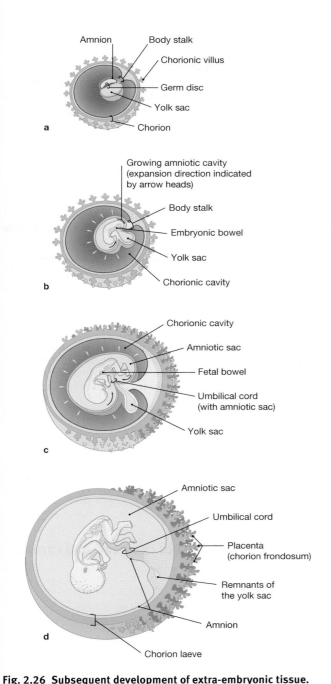

Fig. 2.26 Subsequent development of extra-embryonic tissue.
a 3rd week: the amnion covers the dorsal surface of the embryo, the chorionic cavity between the embryo and the trophoblast is relatively large. **b** 4th week: in the course of the unfolding movements, the amnion envelopes the entire embryo except the umbilical cord. **c** The amnion grows strongly, while the lumen of the chorionic cavity and yolk sac become relatively smaller. **d** The amnion has fully displaced the chorionic cavity and now forms the amniotic sac. The yolk sac recedes back to the rudimentary stage. [E347-09]

2.10 Early development of the extremities

2.10.1 Formation of the extremity buds

In the *4th week* laterally protruding arch-shaped bulges (**extremity buds**) form in the **somatopleure**, bilaterally at the level of the lower cervical and the lower lumbosacral somites. The extremity buds are made up of a highly proliferating **mesenchymal nucleus** made from

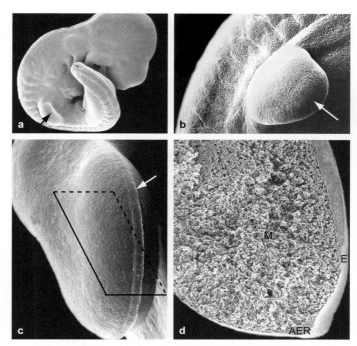

Fig. 2.27 Extremity buds; scanning electron microscopy images. **a** A 26-day-old embryo. The arm system (arrow) is already recognisable, the leg system first appears later on day 28. **b** A 29-day-old embryo with well-demarcated arm bud (arrow). It is located in the side plate mesoderm lateral to the segmental somites. **c** A 32-day-old embryo, lateral view of an extremity bud. The apical ectodermal ridge (AER, arrow) pulls as an ectodermal sickle-shaped thickening in an antero-posterior direction over the tip of the extremity bud. The rectangle indicates the sectional plane in d. **d** Longitudinal section through a limb bud; E = ectoderm, M = mesenchyme. In the area of apical ecto-dermal ridge (AER) the ectoderm is thickened. [G394]

somatic side plate mesoderm and an **epithelial sheath** made from ec-toderm (➤ Fig. 2.27). The strong growth of the extremity buds comes from the action of growth factors of the **FGF family** (fibroblast growth factor). The expression of FGF10 in the mesenchyme of the extremity buds induces the expression of FGF8 in the distal ecto-derm, which maintains the expression of FGF10 in the mesenchyme and so, by mutual **induction** (positive feedback loop), interacts with the continued proliferation of the mesenchyme of the extremities.

2.10.2 Pattern formation in the extremities positions

The position of the basic blueprint of the extremities (pattern for-mation) along the three spatial axes is largely determined by 3 sig-nal centres.
A decisive factor for the **creation of the longitudinal axis (proxi-modistal pattern formation)** of the limbs are signals from the distal ectoderm of the extremities bud. These cells become increasingly highly prismatic and form a crescent moon-shaped (**apical ectoder-mal ridge, AER),** which runs crescent-shaped from the posterior to the anterior edge over the tip of the extremities bud (➤ Fig. 2.21, ➤ Fig. 2.27, ➤ Fig. 2.28). The cells of the AER continually secrete FGF8 (➤ Chap. 2.10.1) and by doing so not only control the length of growth of the limb, but also the successive creation of the shoul-der, upper arm, forearm and hand, with the proximal structures cre-ated earlier and the distal structures created later. Apparently, the mesenchymal cells form more distal structures, the longer and stron-ger they are exposed to the FGF signals from the AER.
Anteroposterior pattern formation, i.e. the arrangement of ana-tomical structures in the radioulnar or tibiofibular axis, is based on

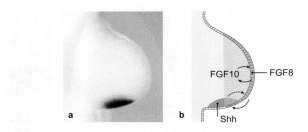

Fig. 2.28 Induction processes in the development of the extremities.
a Proof of the expression of sonic hedgehog (Shh) in the zone of polarising activity (ZPA) by in situ hybridisation. [G394] **b** Simplified presentation of induction processes in the extremities bud. FGF8 from the AER induces the expression of FGF10 in the extremity mesenchyme and this in turn, maintains the expression of FGF8 (positive feedback loop). In addition, the Shh in the ZPA indirectly maintains the expression of FGF8 in the AER and vice versa. As a result, the proximodistal pattern formation via FGF and the anteroposterior pattern formation via Shh are coupled together. [L126]

the activity of the signal molecule sonic hedgehog (Shh). The Shh is expressed in a mesenchymal area on the posterior edge of the extremities mesenchyme (**zone of polarising activity, ZPA,** ➤ Fig. 2.28). Based on the ZPA, the expression of Shh, which is in turn activated by FGF from the AER, forms a concentration gradient by diffusion in the extracellular fluid space of the extremities mesenchyme along the anteroposterior axis. The Shh acts as a **morphogen**: a high concentration of Shh and long-lasting exposure of the cells in the posterior mesenchyme conveys ulnar positional information, a low concentration of Shh in the anterior mesenchyme conveys radial positional information.

As with the regionalisation of the paraxial mesoderm (➤ Chap. 2.6.2), **Hox genes** play an important role in the specification of the cells along both the proximodistal and anteroposterior axes (➤ Fig. 2.29). Thus, for example, the skeleton of the forearm (zeugopod) is specified by a combined expression of Hox11, in addition to Hox9 and Hox10 (hox code).

The **dorsoventral pattern formation** of the extremities is controlled by the interaction of multiple genes in ectoderm and mesenchyme; a key role is played by a secreted signal molecule (**Wnt7a**), which is expressed exclusively in the dorsal ectoderm and at the beginning of a signal cascade seems to control the different development of flexor and extensor sides of the extremities.

N O T E
The proximodistal pattern formation of the extremities is controlled by signals from the apical ectodermal ridge (AER) and the anteroposterior pattern formation of the extremities is controlled by signals from the zone of polarising activity (ZPA).

2.10.3 Origin of the skeleton and the muscles of the extremities

The precursor extremity mesenchyme from the **somatopleure** of the lateral mesoderm provides the building material for connective and supporting tissues of the limb. Here the mesenchyme is consolidated, dependent on the above-mentioned pattern formation processes to become **chondrogenic zones,** from which the later parts of the skeleton arise.

The musculature of the extremities, on the other hand, is not derived from the somatopleure but is formed from the progenitor cells (**myoblasts**) from the **hypaxial dermomyotomes** of the somites, which migrate into the connective tissue matrix of the extremities systems and are arranged as ventral and dorsal **premuscle masses** on the future flexor and extensor sides of the extremities (➤ Fig. 2.21). The splitting and positioning of the **anatomical muscles** arising from the premuscle masses is probably controlled by signals from the local connective tissue.

Clinical remarks

Disorders of the complex regulation of pattern formation of the extremities can lead to a variety of congenital malformations, e.g. **polydactylism** as a result of a mutation of Shh regulator sequences and **brachydactylism** as a result of a mutation in the gene for an FGF receptor.

N O T E
The skeleton of the extremities develops locally in the extremity buds and originates from the mesenchyme of the somatopleure. The musculature migrates into the extremity buds and derives from the somites.

2.11 Early development of the head and throat area

2.11.1 Pharyngeal arches

In the body wall of the head-throat area the **pharyngeal arches** are formed in the *4th week* in cranio caudal sequence, (pharyngeal arches, branchial or gill arches). Phylogenetically these go back to the gill arches of fish and, in their basic arrangement recall the gill apparatus of sharks. Between the **pharyngeal grooves** depressed into the surface ectoderm and in the entodermal gut wall of everted **pharyngeal pouches** the pharyngeal arches protrude as mesen-

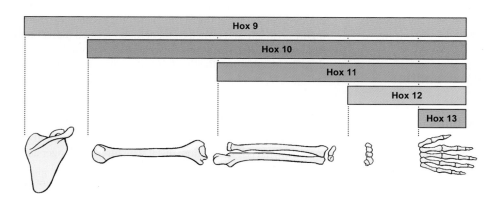

Fig. 2.29 Hox genes determine the identity of the arm skeleton. The pattern formation of the extremities skeleton, such as hand, wrist, forearm, upper arm and shoulder blade is determined by different combinations of expression of hox genes (here hox 9-13). [G394]

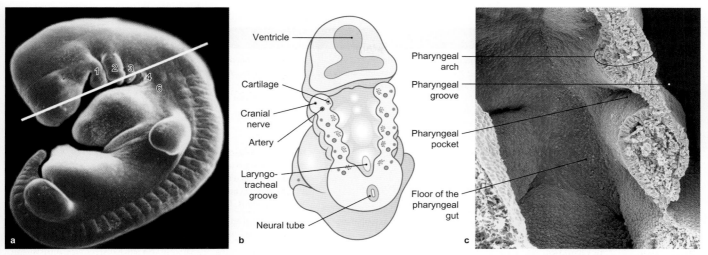

Fig. 2.30 Pharyngeal arches. a Scanning electron microscopy image of the embryo at the beginning of the 5th week. The numbers 1–4 and 6 identify the individual pharyngeal arches; the line shows the section direction in b. **b** Frontal section through the pharyngeal arch region, dorsal view. Each pharyngeal arch has a skeletal element, an artery and a cranial nerve branch. **c** Scanning electron microscopy image of a pharyngeal arch by frontal section as in b. Each pharyngeal arch is covered on the inside by entodermal epithelium and on the outside by ectodermal epithelium and is filled with mesenchyme. a und c: [G394]; b: [L126]

chymal ridges (➤ Fig. 2.30). Unlike fish gills the pharyngeal grooves and pouches, which are equivalent to gill slits, are not continuous, instead they are closed at one end. In humans, only 5 of the original 6 pharyngeal arches are formed. They are designated from cranial to caudal as arches 1 (**mandibular arch**), 2 (**hyoid arch**), 3, 4 and 6 (➤ Table 2.1). From comparative anatomy we know that the 5th arch is absent in humans. Again, equivalent to fish gills each arch contains a **skeletal element,** an **artery** as a branch of the ventral aorta and a characteristic **cranial nerve** (➤ Fig. 2.30). The mesenchyme, from which the skeleton and connective tissue of the pharyngeal arch originates, comes from

the **cranial neural crest. Skeletal musculature** also migrates into the mesenchyme of the pharangeal arches. It comes from both the dermomyotomes of the **occipital somites** (and form the muscles of the larynx and tongue) as well as from the unsegmented cranially located **paraxial cranial mesoderm** (forms the head muscles). Thus, each pharyngeal arch is covered laterally by ectoderm and medially by entoderm and contains the derivative of neural crest mesenchyme and a skeletal element arising from it. There is a cranial nerve branch, an aortic arch and skeletal muscle migrated from the paraxial mesoderm (➤ Fig. 2.30, ➤ Fig. 2.31, ➤ Fig. 2.32, ➤ Fig. 2.33, ➤ Fig. 2.34).

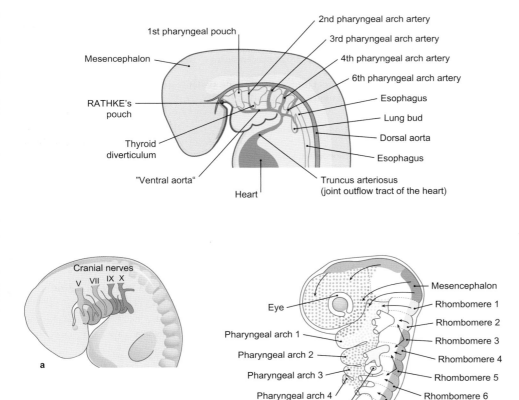

Fig. 2.31 Pharyngeal arch arteries. The pharyngeal arch arteries run in the same way as the gill arteries of fish, from the ventral aorta through the pharyngeal arches to the dorsal aorta. [E347-09]

Fig. 2.32 Innervation of the pharyngeal arches and origin of the neural crest cells. a The pharyngeal arches are supplied by the cranial nerves, trigeminal nerve [V], facial nerve [VII], glossopharyngeal nerve [IX] and vagus nerve [X] **b** The pharyngeal arch mesenchyme of the respective arches originates from the head neural crest of different sections of the embryonic brain (rhombomeres). The neural crest cells migrate into the pharyngeal arches depending on the segment. [E347-09]

Table 2.1 Pharyngeal arches.

Pharyngeal arch	Skeletal element	Nerve	Muscles	Artery
1 (Mandibular arch)	• From maxillary cartilage (quadratus): Incus, Ala major ossis sphenoidalis • From MECKEL's cartilage: Malleus, Lig. sphenomandibulare • By desmal ossification: Os maxillare, Os zygomaticum, Os temporale pars squamosa, Mandibula	N. trigeminus [V], N. mandibularis [V/3], N. maxillaris [V/2]	From paraxial head mesoderm: masticatory muscles, M. digastricus ventor anterior, M. tensor veli palatini, M. tensor tympani	(A. maxillaris)
2 (Hyoid arch)	From REICHERT's cartilage: Stapes, Proc. styloideus, Lig. stylohyoideum, Cornu minus and upper part of the hyoid bone	N. facialis [VII]	From paraxial head mesoderm: mimic facial muscles including M. buccinator and Mm. auriculares, M. digastricus venter posterior, M. stylohyoideus, M. stapedius	(A. stapedia)
3	Cornu majus and lower part of the hyoid bone	N. glossopharyngeus [IX]	From paraxial head mesoderm: M. stylopharyngeus	Parts of the A. carotis communis and A. carotis interna
4	Laryngeal skeleton	N. vagus [X], N. laryngeus superior	From occipital somites: M. cricothyroideus, M. levator veli palatini, M. constrictor pharyngis	• 4th left aortic arch: Arcus Aortae • 4th right aortic arch: Truncus brachiocephalicus
6	Laryngeal skeleton	N. vagus [X], N. laryngeus inferior	From occipital somites: inner laryngeal muscles	A. pulmonalis

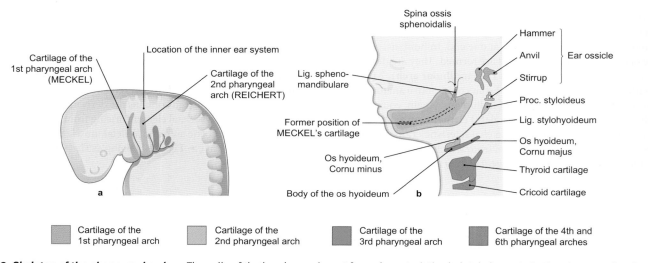

Fig. 2.33 Skeleton of the pharyngeal arches. The cells of the head neural crest form characteristic skeletal elements in the pharyngeal arches; from these, in the course of further development, different bones and ligaments arise. [E347-09]

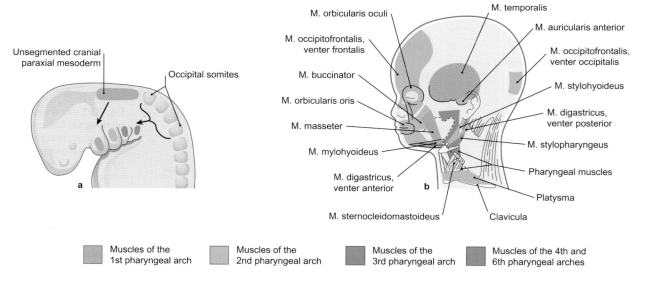

Fig. 2.34 Muscles of the pharyngeal arch. a The skeletal muscles of the pharyngeal arches develop from the cranial paraxial mesoderm, both from the unsegmented cranial mesoderm as well as from the occipital somites. **b** From here the myogenic cells migrate into the pharyngeal arch mesenchyme and differentiate into individual muscle groups that are innervated by the cranial nerves according to their origin. [E347-09]

Mandibular arch

The **1st pharyngeal arch (mandibular arch,** ➤ Table 2.1) arises at the beginning of the *4th week* as the first of the pharyngeal arches. It is arched like a brace and consists of two branches, a cranial **maxillary ridge** and the caudally connecting **mandibular ridge.** Between them is the **stomatodeum;** ➤ Fig. 2.37. However, some authors consider the maxillary ridge to be a separate formation of the mesenchyme of the head cranial to the 1st pharyngeal arch. The mesenchyme of the mandibular arch is derived from neural crest cells of the mesencephalon and segments **(rhombomeres) 1 and 2** of the hind brain. A cartilage element **(Quadratum)** is formed in the maxillary ridge, which by chondral ossification later becomes

the hammer **(malleus)** of the middle ear, and in the mandibular ridge **MECKEL's cartilage,** becomes the anvil **(incus)** of the middle ear. The bones of the definitive upper and lower jaw are created by **desmal ossification** from the neural crest mesenchyme. The main nerve is the N. trigeminus with the **N. maxillaris[V/2]** and the **N. mandibularis [v3],** supplying the immigrated musculature in the mandibular arch (e.g. masticatory and palate muscles). The 1st **aortic arch** passing through the mandibular arch probably remains partially unchanged as the maxillary artery.

Hyoid arch

Approximately 2 days after the mandibular arch the hyoid arch is formed as the **2nd pharyngeal arch** (➤ Table 2.1). Its mesenchyme is mainly derived from **rhombomere 4** and forms **REICHERT's cartilage,** from which the stirrup **(stapes)** of the middle ear, the **styloid process** and parts of the **hyoid bone** arise. The main nerve is the N. facialis [VII] which innervates the muscles of the middle

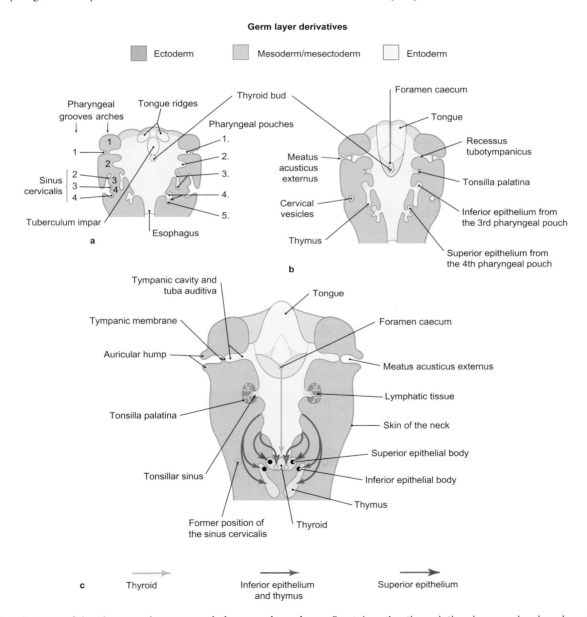

Fig. 2.35 Development of the pharyngeal grooves and pharyngeal pouches. a Frontal section through the pharyngeal arch region of a 5-week-old embryo. The 2nd pharyngeal arch grows in a caudal direction and covers the 3rd and 4th pharyngeal grooves, so that the cervical sinus is temporarily made from them. **b** Only the first pharyngeal groove survives as the external acoustic meatus. From the first pharyngeal pouch, the tubotympanic recess forms as a precursor of the tympanic cavity and the entodermal neck organs develop from the 2nd–4th pharyngeal pouches. **c** Derivatives of pharyngeal pouches and their caudal displacement. [E347-09]

ear and throat formed by the muscle cells of the 2nd pharyngeal arch (stapedius muscle, stylohyoid muscle and posterior digastric muscle) and the **mimetic muscles** probably migrating from the 2nd pharyngeal arch in the subcutis of the head and neck. Whether remnants of the 2nd aortic arch, which passes through the hyoid arch, remain in the arteries of the middle ear (e.g. A. stapedia), is contentious.

3rd pharyngeal arch

Pharyngeal arches 3–6 do not have individual names. The **3rd pharyngeal arch** (➤ Table 2.1) is mainly formed from neural crest cells of **rhombomere 6**, which, together with the hyoid arch, forms the **Os hyoideum.** It is innervated by the **N. glossopharyngeus [IX]** and contains the myoblasts (muscle progenitor cells) of the stylopharyngeus muscle. The **3rd aortic arch** enters the A. carotis communis and the proximal portion of the A. carotis interna.

4th and 6th pharyngeal arch

The caudal pharyngeal arches form (➤ Table 2.1) only at the start of the *5th week* and are morphologically less clearly defined than the first 3 arches; they show only vague grooves. They contain neural crest cells from the most caudal sections of the hindbrain at the transition to the neural tube and form the cartilage skeleton of the larynx. Together, they are innervated by the **N. vagus [X]** and accordingly assigned to the muscles of the larynx and throat of the 4th and 6th pharyngeal arches. The **4th aortic arch** takes on the definitive aortic function, even if it is asymmetric, and forms the aortic arch on the left and the innominate artery on the right. The **6th aortic arch** becomes on both sides the A. pulmonalis.

2.11.2 Pharyngeal grooves and pharyngeal pouches

Pharyngeal grooves and **pharyngeal pouches** delimit the pharyngeal arches from each other superficially or towards the pharynx. Only the **1st pharyngeal groove** remains, and develops into the **external ear canal,** which is only separated by the tympanic membrane from the **1st pharyngeal pouch;** from the pharynx, the tympanic cavity of the **middle ear** and the Tuba auditiva arise. Hence the eardrum is covered up to the ear canal by ectodermal epithelium, and up to the tympanic cavity it is covered by entodermal epithelium. All other pharyngeal grooves disappear because the 2nd pharyngeal arch grows caudally over to close pharyngeal grooves 2–4. By the inductive interaction of the entodermal epithelium with the mesenchyme of the pharyngeal arches, the pharyngeal pouches 2–4 develop into the lymphatic and endocrine appending organs of the pharynx. Thus,

- from the **2nd pharyngeal pouch** the **Tonsilla palatina** emerges,
- from the **3rd pharyngeal pouch** the **Glandula parathyroidea inferior** and part of the thymus and
- from the **4th pharyngeal pouch,** the **Glandula parathyroidea superior**

are formed. The existence of a **5th pharyngeal pouch** as a protrusion from the 4th pharyngeal pouch, from which the **ultimobranchial body** (C-cells of the thyroid gland) arises, is still a matter of contention (➤ Fig. 2.35).

2.11.3 Development of the tongue and thyroid gland

At the ventral floor of the pharynx, where the pharyngeal arches come together bilaterally in the median line, at the end of the *4th week* unpaired, entoderm-covered (at the junction to the stomodeum, also ectoderm covered) mesenchyme ridges protrude (➤ Fig. 2.36). In the mandibular arch area, this is the **Tuberculum impar,** which is flanked on both sides by the paired **lateral lingual swellings.** Caudal from here follows the **Copula,** in the area of the hyoid arch, in the area of arches 3 and 4 of the **hypobranchial eminence** and immediately prior to the inlet of the larynx of the epiglottal eminence. The lateral tongue swellings of the mandibular arch strongly proliferate and overgrow the Tuberculum impar, and in doing so they fuse in the midline and form the anterior two thirds of the dorsum of tongue, with its mucous membrane coming from the **ectoderm.** The Copula of the 2nd pharyngeal arch is overgrown by the hypobranchial eminence forming the rear third of the back of the dorsum of the tongue, the mucosa of which is at least partially derived from the **entoderm.** The rearmost part of the tongue at the junction to the oropharynx comes from part of the

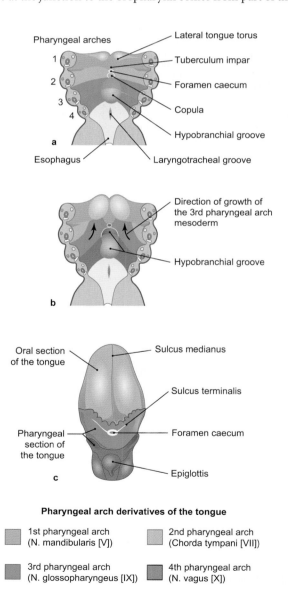

Pharyngeal arch derivatives of the tongue

▢ 1st pharyngeal arch (N. mandibularis [V])	▢ 2nd pharyngeal arch (Chorda tympani [VII])
▢ 3rd pharyngeal arch (N. glossopharyngeus [IX])	▢ 4th pharyngeal arch (N. vagus [X])

Fig. 2.36 Development of the tongue. View of the floor of the pharynx in frontal section. **a, b** Development of the tongue structures during the 4th–6th weeks. **c** Adult tongue. [E347-09]

epiglottal eminence and has entodermal mucous membrane. The muscles of the tongue arise from migrating myoblasts of the occipital **somites.** The heterogeneous origin of the tongue from various pharyngeal arches and the paraxial mesoderm is the reason for its complex innervation.

The **Foramen caecum** is depressed between the Tuberculum impar and the Copula in the floor of the pharynx. At its base, a solid entodermal epithelium bud grows ventrally and caudally to the mesenchyme of the neck **(Ductus thyroglossus),** which soon loses its connection to the tongue system, and at the end of the *7th week* as an isolated, twin-lobed entodermal island approaches the entodermal tracheal tube, where it is already developing laterally in the *12th week* as a functional **thyroid gland.**

NOTE

The tongue is formed in the base of the pharynx as part of the pharyngeal arches 1–6 and myoblasts of the occipital somites.

2.11.4 Facial development

The face develops, starting at the end of the *4th week,* from **5 facial eminences,** the paired **maxillary and mandibular swellings** of the 1st pharyngeal arch and the unpaired **frontal process,** which covers the forebrain (➤ Fig. 2.37). The frontal process consists of mesenchyme originating from the cranial neural crest from the midbrain and forebrain, and, like the facial eminences of the mandibular arch, is covered with **ectoderm.** The facial eminences demarcate the ectodermal **stomodeum,** which is then sealed off by the **buccopharyn-**

geal membrane from the foregut. On the border of the two maxillary bulges, the ectoderm of the frontal process thickens to form paired **olfactory placodes.** In the middle of each of these, the ectoderm sinks to form **olfactory pits,** from which the olfactory area of the nose is formed. The ectoderm bulges in a horseshoe shape around the olfactory pits with the underlying mesenchyme forming the **medial and lateral nasal bulge.** Both nasal bulges grow much larger, increasingly overgrowing the olfactory pits. The **nasolacrimal groove** sinks between the lateral nasal bulge and the maxillary bulge from which the Ductus nasolacrimalis will later arise. Together with the maxillary bulges and the eyes positioned to the sides of the frontal process, the nasal bulges on both sides are increasingly shifted medially. At the end of the *7th week* the medial nose bulges on both sides fuse together in the midline into the **nasal bridge,** nasal septum and philtrum (➤ Fig. 2.37). The lateral nasal bulge forms the lateral nasal wall and the **nostrils.** The nasolacrimal groove is overgrown by the lateral nasal bulge and the maxillary bulge, so that both fuse together. In the meantime, the **eyes** migrate from their original lateral position towards the front, taking up their final position on both sides of the nose. The mandibular bulges on both sides, positioned caudally to the stomodeum, are medially joined forming the arch-shaped **lower jaw system.**

NOTE

The face is essentially created in a paired fashion and develops from the left and right maxillary and nasal bulges, which migrate from lateral to medial, fusing together with the unpaired forehead bulge in the midline. The mandibular bulges, which form the lower jaw, are joined medially from the beginning.

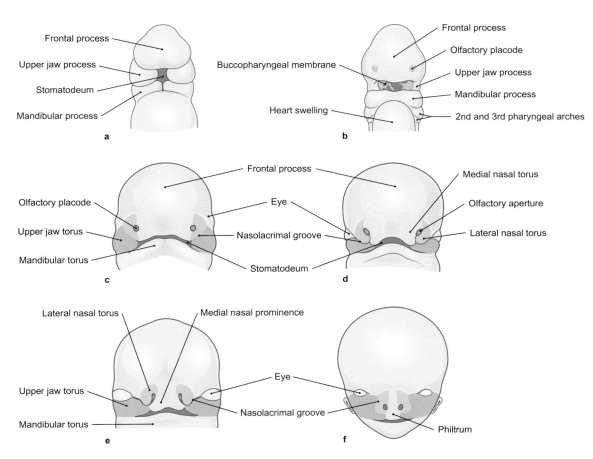

Fig. 2.37 Facial development. The face develops from the unpaired forehead projection and the paired maxillary and nasal ridges by shifting the structures medially, where they finally fuse. [L126]
a 3.5 weeks. **b** 4 weeks. **c** 5 weeks. **d** 6 weeks. **e** 7 weeks. **f** 10 weeks.

2.11.5 Development of the oral and nasal cavities

Nasal and maxillary bulges do not only fuse on the surface, but also in the depths of the stomodeum (> Fig. 2.38). The buccopharyngeal membrane is torn down at the end of the *3rd week* and connects the ectodermal **oral cavity** with the entodermal foregut. From the **maxillary processes** in the roof of the mouth the developing **palatal plates** from both sides grow initially downwards to the floor of the mouth, then rise balcony-like in a medial direction and finally join together at the end of the *7th week* in the midline. Therefore, together with the **intermaxillary segment (primary palate)** arising from the medial nasal bulges, the **secondary palate** is formed, separating the mouth from the nasal cavity. The paired **primary nasal cavities** originate from the tubular **olfactory pits** growing far into the mesenchyme of the frontal process. Its floor is formed from the **intermaxillary segment** and later from the thin **bucconasal membrane** (syn.: oronasal membrane). After rupturing at the end of the *6th week*, the two primary nasal cavities open via the **primitive choanae** into the oral cavity. As a result of the fusion of the palate plates and the formation of the secondary palate, the internal nostrils shift via the **definitive choanae** into the nasopharynx. Within the resulting **definitive nasal cavity**, which arises in the rear section of the oral cavity, the **nasal septum** grows arising from the medial nasal prominences with the palate, completely separating both halves of the nose from each other. The **paranasal sinuses** occur postnatally as sacculations of the nasal cavity.

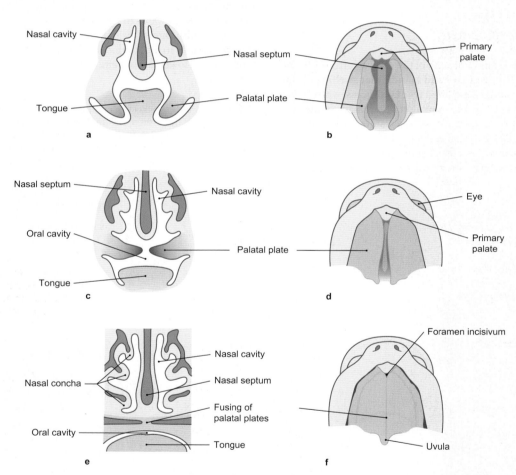

Fig. 2.38 Development of oral and nasal cavities. The primary oral cavity is divided by the medial fusion of the palatal plates of the maxillary ridges into the oral cavity and the nasal cavity. [L126]
a, b 6.5 weeks. **c, d** 7.5 weeks. **e, f** 10 weeks.

MUSCULO-SKELETAL SYSTEM

3 Torso

3.1 Ventral torso wall

Martin Gericke, Martin Krüger (with contribution from Ingo Bechmann)

3.1.1 General structure

The ventral trunk wall ranges from the Clavicula and the Insisura jugularis notch of the breastbone up to the iliac crests, the ligaments and the upper edge of the Symphysis pubica. It comprises the lateral and anterior chest wall, as well as the lateral and anterior abdominal wall. The costal arch forms the border between the thoracic and abdominal wall. The border to the dorsal torso wall constitutes the rear axillary line (Linea axillaris posterior, see below).

Orientation lines

For everyday clinical application, it is practical to use a uniform and unambiguous nomenclature to describe locations on the skin, for the precise identification of puncture and auscultation sites, or surgical access routes. The course of the ribs or the intercostal

spaces (ICS) are used as horizontal orientation lines, and vertical orientation lines are also used, so that certain points can be described, similar to a coordinate system (➤ Table 1.4, ➤ Fig. 1.6).

Palpable bone points

Palpable bone points on the ventral trunk wall are:
- Claviculae
- Insisura jungularis sterni
- Acromioclavicular joint (shoulder joint)
- Sternum with Angulus sterni (LUDOVICI, transition between the Manubrium sterni and Corpus sterni; serves as orientation for counting the ribs)
- Proc. xiphoideus
- Ribs (exception: Ist rib)
- Costal arch
- Crista iliaca, Spina iliaca anterior superior, Tuberculum pubicum, Symphysis pubica

> **NOTE**
> To reliably determine the height of the ribs and the intercostal spaces (ICS), one begins at the **Angulus sterni,** which corresponds to the attachment of the 2nd rib. The Ist rib is not palpable under the Clavicula, so that one palpates downwards from the Angulus sterni.

In the transition area to the neck, the clavicle and the Incisura jugularis of the Manubrium sterni are cranially easily palpable. Below the collar bones, the **M. pectoralis major** can be well defined. Between the **M. pectoralis major** and the **M. deltoideus,** lies the **Fossa infraclavicularis** (MOHRENHEIM'S fossa, ➤ Chap. 4.10.1), in the depths of which the neurovascular bundle runs to the arm. In the case of lean bodied people, the coracoid process of the shoulder blade can be felt at its **lateral margin** of the **Proc. coracoideus.** This can be facilitated by abducting and adducting the arm at the same time; however, palpation of the Proc. coracoideus does not often succeed due to the body's constitution. Laterally the muscle serrations of the **M. serratus anterior** can be recognized, especially in an abducted arm which intrudes into the upper serrations of the **M. obliquus externus abdominis** with its lower serrations. This zigzag line is referred to as **GERDY's line.** The transition to the epigastrium is marked by the easily palpable costal arch and the **Proc. xiphoideus.**

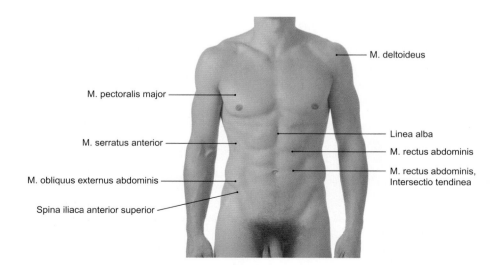

M. deltoideus

M. pectoralis major

M. serratus anterior

M. obliquus externus abdominis

Spina iliaca anterior superior

Linea alba

M. rectus abdominis

M. rectus abdominis, Intersectio tendinea

Fig. 3.1 Surface relief of the thoracic and abdominal wall of a young man.

Surface relief

The construction of the anterior torso wall (➤ Fig. 3.1) shows significant individual differences. Apart from the gender and age-specific shape of the thorax and the pelvis as well as the size and shape of the mammary glands, it is essentially dependent on the expression of the subcutaneous and intra-abdominal fat tissue and the muscles.

In the case of muscular people of normal weight it is easy to recognize the **M. pectoralis major** (in women mostly covered by the breasts). It also stands out in a well-trained 'six-pack' on the abdominal wall (**M. rectus abdominis** with Intersectiones tendineae and Linea alba). Laterally, the **M. obliquus externus abdominis** can be seen, the muscle-aponeurosis transition of which is particularly elevated, slightly above the Spina iliaca anterior superior as muscle covering. Its muscle serrations interfere with the muscle serrations of the **M. serratus anterior** in the area of the lateral rib arch. The superficial veins often shimmer through the abdominal skin.

3.1.2 Thoracic wall

Clinical case

Pneumothorax

Case study

A 23-year-old man presents in the emergency department of the university clinic. While presenting his case to the on-call doctor he reports the sudden occurrence of chest pains, which are accompanied by substantial shortage of breath during stress. The pain first started 2 hours ago at rest when he was standing in the shower. The patient does not complain of any other disorders, such as diarrhoea, nausea or dizziness. There are also no pre-existing conditions. The patient has also not undertaken any long distance car or air travel recently, which would indicate a risk factor for a pulmonary embolism. The medical history also shows an 'appendectomy' at the age of 9 years. The patient does not smoke and does not take any medications.

Initial examination

The patient is 188 cm tall and of slim build. He weighs 72 kg. The vital parameters (blood pressure, heart rate, oxygen saturation, body temperature) are initially within normal range. On auscultation there is an attenuated respiratory sound above the right lung.

Further diagnostics

The subsequent chest x-ray confirms that the suspected diagnosis of a spontaneous pneumothorax is confirmed.

Therapy and follow-up

Due to the increasing shortness of breath and the deteriorating vital signs, the doctor decides to conduct a thoracic drainage in the emergency department (BÜLAU drainage). During the inpatient stay the patient recovers quickly and can be discharged from hospital 7 days later.

Clinical symptoms

A pneumothorax is a condition where air has entered the pleural space, which would normally not be found there. In cases of pneumothorax the air from the outside enters the pleural space due to a defect in the chest wall and the Pleura parietalis or from the inside by a defect of the Pleura visceralis and leads to the cancellation of the negative pressure in the pleural space. The normally existing adhesion between the pleural sheets is annulled and the lung retracts toward the hilus due to its elastic properties. If this occurs with no identified cause or injury from the outside, it is called an idiopathic spontaneous pneumothorax. Typically, it occurs in tall, slim built males and patients with otherwise healthy lungs (gender balance men to women around 3 : 1). The cause is often malformed lung tissue in the form of so-called bullae in the tips of the lungs, which are spontaneously ruptured. The incidence of idiopathic spontaneous pneumothorax is given as 4 per 100,000. Small sized pneumothorax (tips or coating pneumothorax) can be treated conservatively. In the case of attenuated breathing sounds, severe shortness of breath or a change in vital parameters (hypotension, a drop in oxygen saturation) the placement of a thorax drainage is indicated. This should be done in the case of a life-threatening tension pneumothorax even at the scene of the accident and should not be postponed until arrival in hospital or even until after the x-ray diagnostics.

The chest wall is differentiated into four layers:
- Superficial: skin, subcutaneous fat and mammary glands
- Ventral muscles of the shoulder girdle and the upper limbs
- Sternum, ribs and intercostal muscles
- Inner layers: Fascia endothoracica and Pleura parietalis

Superficial layer
Skin

On the sternum the skin is relatively tightly connected with the Membrana sterni but otherwise it can be easily relocated. In women and children there is often lanugo on the breast skin; in men this is often stronger terminal hair. If it is less well-developed, there is often stronger and longer terminal hair around the areolae.

Subcutaneous tissue, Tela subcutanea

In the area of the mammary glands the subcutaneous fat is well-pronounced, otherwise less distinctly pronounced. Starting from the throat area the **Platysma** radiates as a mimetic skin muscle via the clavicle into the subcutis. In the area of the sternum phylogenetic residues of this skin muscle can sometimes remain, which then can be referred to as **M. sternalis**.

Vascular, lymphatic and nervous systems
Arteries

The arterial supply of the skin (➤ Fig. 3.12, ➤ Fig. 3.13, ➤ Fig. 3.2) is ensured through
- Rr. perforantes of the **A. thoracica interna**
- Rr. cutanei laterales of the **Aa. intercostales posteriores**
- **A. thoracica lateralis** (branch of the A. axillaris)
- **A. thoracodorsalis**

Veins

The venous drainage (➤ Fig. 3.14, ➤ Fig. 3.2, ➤ Fig. 3.15) takes place via:
- Accompanying veins of the abovenamed arteries
- the **V. thoracoepigastrica,** which in turn leads into the V. axillaris

Cutaneous nerves

The chest area is sensitively innervated (➤ Fig. 3.2) by
- cranial: **Nn. supraclaviculares (C3–C4)** from the Plexus cervicalis
- caudal: segmentally from the **intercostal nerves,** of which the **Rr. cutanei laterales** in the midaxillary line perforate the fascia

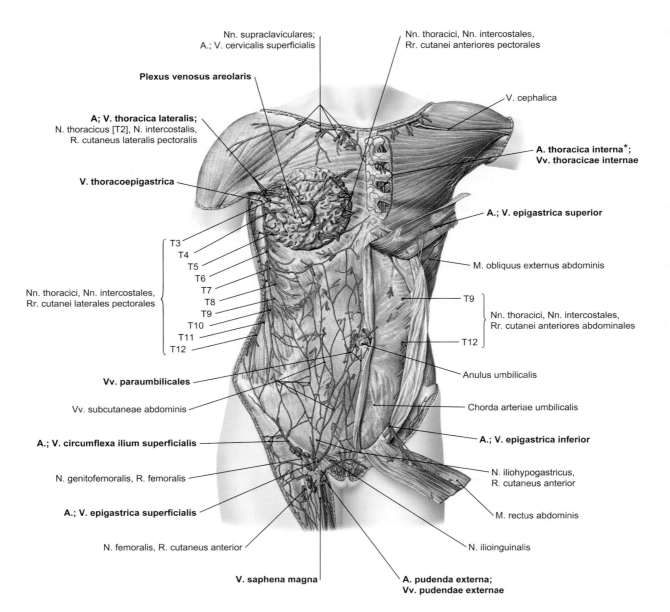

Fig. 3.2 Epifascial and deep vessels and nerves of the abdominal wall in the female. Ventral view; * clinically also A. mammaria interna.

- medial: **Rr. cutanei anteriores,** which extend from parasternal to lateral in the area above the M. pectoralis major

Mammary gland
Development
As early as the *4th developmental week* a thickening of the ectoderm stands out on the lateral abdominal wall, the **ventral epidermal ridges** . It develops during the *5th week* to a **milk line,** whereby it results in the sprouting of 6 strands in the underlying mesenchyme. In animals, the milk line extends at regular intervals from the axillary region to the groin and differentiates further; in humans it recedes back to the **4th pair of glands** at the level of the IIIrd–Vth ribs. Originating from the milk line, in humans a lenticular protrusion is formed, which sinks like a cone into the underlying mesenchyme. Several epithelial cones sprout from this epithelial bulb, from which the **Sinus and Ductus lactiferi** later emerge. The blunt ends of the epithelial cones branch out later and form the subsequent lobar structure. Under the influence of sex hormones, the epithelial structures are channelled in the *7th–8th month* and form a lumen. The milk ducts drain into the skin on a gland field, which at the time of birth is still at the level of the body surface and only later, sometimes only after puberty, forms the nipple. The apocrine **Glandulae areolares** of the areolae occur in the *5th–6th foetal month*.

Location, structure and function
The mammary gland (breast, ➤ Fig. 3.3) is formed in both sexes and is regarded as a **secondary sexual characteristic.** Its functional status and its macroscopic and microscopic structure are subject to hormone-related, distinctive sex and age differences. The fully formed mammary gland of a woman of childbearing age ranges craniocaudally from around the IInd or IIIrd to VIth rib, as well as in the horizontal expansion of the parasternal line to the front axillary line and often towers over a craniolateral offshoot (Proc. axillaris) up into the armpit. As **Lobus axillaris** it can transcend the lower margin of the M. pectoralis major. The main part of the glandular body is movably connected with the Fascia pectoralis superficialis and the Lobus axillaris with the fascia of the M. serratus anterior. Both breasts are separated in the area of the sternum by the **mammary sinus (Sinus mammarum).**

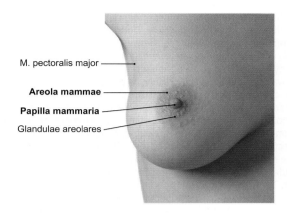

Fig. 3.3 Breast (Mamma). Ventral view.

On the usually much darker pigmented **Areola (Areola mammae)** the tapered **nipple (Papilla mammae)** rises into which 12–15 milk ducts flow (➤ Fig. 3.3). The position is usually projected in men onto the **4th intercostal space (ICS).** The situation is much more variable in women. In both sexes, it also depends on the nutritional status and the condition of the connective tissue, which changes in particular due to age. The projection onto the chest wall can be significantly shifted due to this.

The **Areola mammae** is surrounded by a ring of 10–15 small elevations, which are formed by larger packages of apocrine scent glands (Glandulae areolares). Together with sebaceous and eccrine sweat glands, the secretions during breastfeeding create an airtight closure between the oral cavity of the infant and the nipple of the mother, which is important for the suckling process, ensuring that the child does not constantly inspire additional air. Due to the complex arrangement of smooth muscle fibres in the area of the nipple and areola, the nipple can become erect, partly due to tactile stimuli and as such becomes 'tangible' for the infant.

The glandular body of each breast is structured by strong connective tissue septa into **15–24 glandular lobes**, each of which has a separate excretory duct (**Ductus lactifer**) (➤ Fig. 3.4). Each Ductus lactifer extends from the outlet in the area of the Papilla mammae to the Sinus lactifer. By merging several ducts the number of openings does not always correspond to the number of glandular lobes. The individual glandular lobes in turn are structured into smaller lobes, from which the excretory ducts flow into the respective Ductus lactifer.

The support of the glandular body is guaranteed by connective tissue strands (**Ligg. suspensoria mammaria, COOPER ligaments**) which extend from the skin to the Fascia pectoralis superficialis (➤ Fig. 3.4). The spaces between this connective tissue framework are filled with adipose tissue.

In the case of pregnancy, the glandular bodies are supplied with a much greater amount of blood. It increases under hormonal influence and thus displaces the interlobular connective tissue. The milk secretion takes place after birth essentially by the influence of **prolactin,** which is formed in the anterior lobes of the pituitary gland. The milk supply is ensured by oxytocin from the posterior lobe of the pituitary gland, which leads to contraction of myoepithelial cells. Breast milk is an emulsion of fat droplets in an aqueous sugar and electrolyte-containing protein solution. In the first few days after birth the breast gland secretes the **first milk (Colostrum),** which is characterised by an extremely high content of immunoglobulins that guarantees the infant 'nest protection' and protection against infections.

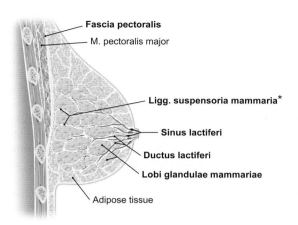

Fig. 3.4 Breast (Mamma). Sagittal section; * clinically also COOPER ligaments.

Clinical remarks

In rare cases the nipples **(athelia)** or breasts **(amastia, breast aplasia)** are missing on one or both sides. Also excess nipples **(polythelia)** or breasts **(polymastia)** along the entire milk line are possible. This is usually hereditary and can also affect men. The rudimentary mammary tissue does not usually develop further in men after birth. Particularly in the context of hormonal disorders, men can nevertheless grow breasts **(gynaecomastia)** . This is more common in puberty and should not regarded as pathological at this point in time.

Too large breasts **(mammary hypertrophy)** not only disturbs the affected women cosmetically, but is often also associated with shoulder and back pain.

Through the transfer of maternal hormones from breast-feeding mothers, the mammary glands of infants of both sexes can secrete the first milk (Colostrum) (used to be more commonly known as 'witches' milk').

Vascular, lymphatic and nervous systems

Arteries

The **arterial blood supply** (➤ Fig. 3.5, ➤ Fig. 3.2) occurs from

- **Rr. mammarii mediales** (via Rr. perforantes from Aa. intercostales anteriores) of the A. thoracica interna
- **Rr. mammarii laterales** of the (via Rr. cutanei laterales) from Aa. intercostales posteriores
- **Rr. mammarii laterales** of the A. thoracica lateralis.

Veins

The venous drainage takes place via two venous networks (➤ Fig. 3.5, ➤ Fig. 3.2):

- A superficial vein network with the **Plexus venosus areolaris** drains into the V. thoracica lateralis and further into the V. axillaris.
- A deep vein network drains via the anterior intercostal veins into the V. thoracica interna to the V. brachiocephalica.

N O T E

During pregnancy and breast feeding the superficial veins can be elevated due to increased circulation through the surface of the skin.

Lymph vessels

The lymph vessels have a great practical clinical significance due to the high prevalence of breast cancer. In the same way as for the veins, the lymph drainage is divided into a superficial and a deep network. The latter is located in the glandular body and is connected to the superficial network. There are 3 main lymph drainage passages (➤ Fig. 3.5):

- **Axillary drainage:** this passage is the most important (about three quarters of the lymph of the breasts). The lymph of the lateral parts is drained via the **Nodi lymphoidei paramammarii** and **Nodi lymphoidei axillares pectorales** to paraclavicular and cervical lymph nodes.
- **Interpectoral drainage:** the lymph of the rear parts of the glandular body are drained between the Mm. pectoralis major and minor via the **Nodi lymphoidei interpectorales** to the Nodi lymphoidei axillares apicales.
- **Parasternal drainage:** the lymph of the medial parts of the breast is drained via the **Nodi lymphoidei parasternales** cranially to the deep cervical lymph nodes and/or into the Truncus jugularis.

Nerves

The sensory innervation takes place via **Rr. cutanei anteriores** and **laterales** of the intercostal nerves, which mainly originate from segments **T2–6**.

Clinical remarks

Breast cancer (➤ Fig. 3.6) is the most common malignant tumour disease in women between 35 and 55 years old in Germany. In rare cases men can also be affected. Overall, breast cancer is the main cause of cancer-related deaths after lung cancer and bowel cancer in women. In about 60% of all cases the upper outer quadrant of the breast is affected (➤ Fig. 3.7). Breast carcinoma originates mostly from the epithelium of the Ductus lactiferi (ductal carcinoma) and metastasizes into the axillary lymph nodes, less often into the parasternal (retrosternal) lymph nodes.

In the context of breast cancer screening, breast cancer should be detected as early as possible. During inspection, attention should be paid to differences between both breasts, contraction of the skin and other superficial changes. The glandular body is inspected by palpation for calluses or nodes and the movability in the glandular body, as well as assessment across the chest wall. For this purpose, the chest is divided into 4 quadrants, which meet in the mamilla and must be carefully palpated within the framework of the screening examination. It is important to ensure that the submamillary region is not neglected, which is often referred to clinically as a '5th quadrant'. The regional lymph nodes are also palpated. They are divided under clinical topographic and oncosurgical aspects into **3 levels**. The M. pectoralis minor acts as a border (➤ Fig. 3.5):

- **Level I:** lateral to the M. pectoralis minor (Nodi lymphoidei axillares humerales [laterales], Nodi lymphoidei axillares subscapulares, Nodi lymphoidei axillares pectorales, Nodi lymphoidei paramammarii)
- **Level II:** below or above the M. pectoralis minor (Nodi lymphoidei axillares centrales, Nodi lymphoidei interpectorales)
- **Level III:** medial of the M. pectoralis minor (Nodi lymphoidei axillares apicales).

Lymph drainage takes place from level I to level II and from there to the Nodi lymphoidei axillares apicales in level III. From here the lymph passes into the Truncus subclavius. The parasternal drainage passages on both sides are interconnected. They drain into mediastinal and intercostal drainage passages that are clinically relevant for metastases in the lungs, pleura and mediastinum.

The **sentinel lymph nodes** are understood as the first lymph node situated in the lymph drainage area of a malignant tumor. In most cases it is therefore the first metastatic lymph node to be colonised. The number of affected lymph nodes in the three levels is directly related to the survival rate in breast cancer. Metastases on the contralateral side are possible via the connected parasternal lymph nodes.

Lymph node metastases within the Nodi lymphoidei axillares pectorales **(SORGIUS group)** may cause irritation of the **N. intercostobrachialis** resulting in radiating pain in the affected arm. This can even be the first indication of breast cancer.

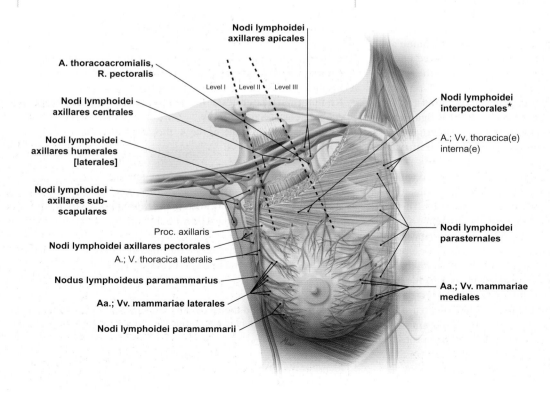

Fig. 3.5 Blood supply and mammary gland lymph drainage;
* clinically also ROTTER nodes.

Nodi lymphoidei axillares apicales

A. thoracoacromialis, R. pectoralis

Level I Level II Level III

Nodi lymphoidei axillares centrales

Nodi lymphoidei axillares humerales [laterales]

Nodi lymphoidei axillares subscapulares

Proc. axillaris

Nodi lymphoidei axillares pectorales

A.; V. thoracica lateralis

Nodus lymphoideus paramammarius

Aa.; Vv. mammariae laterales

Nodi lymphoidei paramammarii

Nodi lymphoidei interpectorales*

A.; Vv. thoracica(e) interna(e)

Nodi lymphoidei parasternales

Aa.; Vv. mammariae mediales

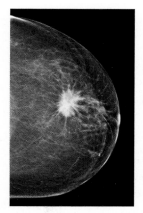

Fig. 3.6 Mammography of malignant breast cancer. [O541]

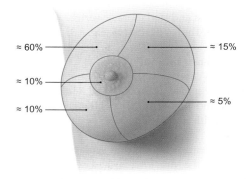

≈ 60%
≈ 15%
≈ 10%
≈ 10%
≈ 5%

Fig. 3.7 Frequency of occurrence of breast cancer in relation to the localisation in percent.

Ventral muscles of the shoulder girdle and the upper extremity

These include the Mm. subclavius, pectoralis major , pectoral minor and serratus anterior. These so-called immigrated muscles are discussed in ➤ Chap. 4.3.4.

Thoracic wall muscles

Note: to be able to understand the location and function of the thoracic wall muscles, it is helpful to first read the section 'Bony thorax'. This is discussed in ➤ Chap. 3.3.4.
The **autochthonous muscles** of the rib cage include the **intercostal muscles**, the **M. subcostalis** and the **M. transversus thoracis**. In evolution the **Mm. serrati posteriores** have the same origin; however, during ontogenesis they have shifted dorsally over the autochthonous muscles of the back. Also the parts of the **Mm. levatores**

costarum innervated by the Rr. ventrales of the intercostal nerves originate from these ventral positions.

Intercostal muscles

The intercostal muscles (Mm. intercostales, ➤ Table 3.1) are taken from the ventral attachments of myomas and keep their metamere (segmental) arrangement in ontogenesis. According to location and course of the intercostal muscles, a distinction is made between (➤ Fig. 3.8, ➤ Fig. 3.9, ➤ Fig. 3.10):
• **Mm. intercostales externi**
• **Mm. intercostales interni**
• **Mm. intercostales intimi**
The Mm. intercostales externi (exterior) are inspiration muscles (inspiration), the Mm. intercostales interni (middle) and intimi (interior) are expiration muscles (expiration).

Mm. intercostales externi

The Mm. intercostales externi (➤ Fig. 3.8, ➤ Fig. 3.10, ➤ Table 3.1) correspond with the course of the M. obliquus externus abdominis. Hence, they run from the upper posterior to lower anterior. Therefore, they extend from the **Tubercula costarum** to the transition of the **cartilage bone border of the ribs.** Their origin each lies on the Crista costae. From here, each muscle runs to the respective next lower rib. The Mm. intercostales externi pass between the rib cartilage in a connective tissue tendon plate (**Membrana intercostalis externa**). The Mm. intercostales externi are covered by the **Fascia thoracica externa** between the ribs.

Mm. intercostales interni

The Mm. intercostales interni (➤ Fig. 3.8, ➤ Fig. 3.10, ➤ Table 3.1) run analogue to the M. obliquus internus abdominis and cross the Mm. intercostales externi vertically. They extend dorsally from the **Angulus costae** ventrally to the sternum. They extend obliquely in a cranioventral direction from the top edges of the inner surface of each rib to insert into the next higher rib. The Mm. intercostales interni pass from the Angulus costae medially into the **Membrana intercostalis interna**. Between the rib cartilages, they are referred to as **Mm. intercartilaginei**. Between the ribs, the Mm. intercostales are covered on the inside of the chest, apart from by their own muscle fascia (Fascia thoracica interna) by the **Fascia endothoracica**.

Mm. intercostales intimi

The intercostales intimi muscles (➤ Table 3.1) are an inconstant separation of the Mm. intercostales interni and thus have the same course as they do, and together include the intercostal vessels and nerves. In many textbooks the Mm. intercostales intimi are not viewed as independent muscles, but counted as Mm. intercostales

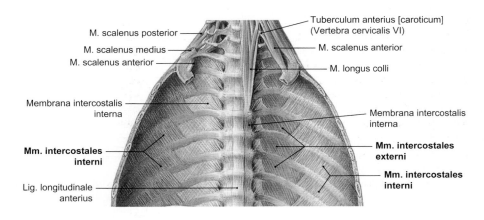

M. scalenus posterior
M. scalenus medius
M. scalenus anterior
Membrana intercostalis interna
Mm. intercostales interni
Lig. longitudinale anterius

Tuberculum anterius [caroticum] (Vertebra cervicalis VI)
M. scalenus anterior
M. longus colli
Membrana intercostalis interna
Mm. intercostales externi
Mm. intercostales interni

Fig. 3.8 Posterior wall of the thorax (Cavea thoracis). Ventral view.

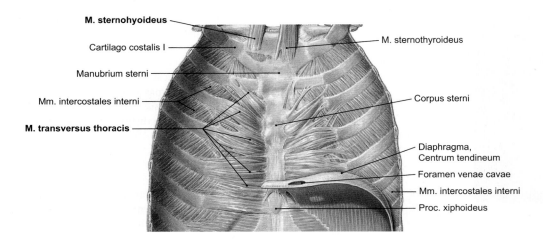

M. sternohyoideus

Cartilago costalis I

Manubrium sterni

Mm. intercostales interni

M. transversus thoracis

M. sternothyroideus

Corpus sterni

Diaphragma, Centrum tendineum

Foramen venae cavae

Mm. intercostales interni

Proc. xiphoideus

Fig. 3.9 Anterior wall of the thorax (Cavea thoracis). Dorsal view.

interni. As part of the Mm. intercostales interni, the Mm. intercostales intimi are covered on the inside of the chest by the Fascia endothoracica (see below).

Mm. subcostales
The Mm. subcostales are referred to as the lower rib muscles (➤ Table 3.1) and have the same fibre course as the Mm. intercostales interni; however, they skip at least one segment, so that muscular connections to adjacent intercostal space (ICS) are created. They vary in number and frequency.

M. transversus thoracis
The M. transversus thoracis (➤ Fig. 3.9, ➤ Table 3.1) is located on the inside of the chest. It originates from the sides of the sternum and from the Proc. xiphoideus and is attached to the rib cartilage of the IInd–VIth ribs. The muscle fibres run horizontally or in a slightly ascending course.

M. serratus posterior superior
The very thin muscle is covered by the M. rhomboideus and runs on both sides of the Procc. spinosi of the VIth and VIIth cervical

vertebrae and the Ist and IInd thoracic vertebra obliquely caudally and laterally to the IInd–Vth ribs (➤ Fig. 3.33, ➤ Table 3.1).

M. serratus posterior inferior
The thin muscle is covered by the M. latissimus and runs on both sides of the Procc. spinosi of the XIth and XIIth thoracic vertebrae and the Ist and IInd lumbar vertebra obliquely caudally and laterally to the IXth –XIIth ribs (➤ Fig. 3.33, ➤ Table 3.1).

Function of the ventral thoracic musculature
The contraction of the Mm. intercostales externi and intercartilaginei leads to **elevation of the ribs.** This increases the volume of the thorax. These are sometimes referred to as inspiration muscles or inspirators because they enable **inspiration.** The Mm. intercostales interni and M. transversus thoracis act as **rib lowerers;** they are supported by the Mm. intercostales intimi and the Mm. subcostales. As a result, these muscles effect the **expiration.**

Inner layers of the chest wall
Fascia endothoracica
The **Fascia endothoracica** is a layer of connective tissue, which covers the inside of the thorax (➤ Fig. 3.10). It therefore represents

Table 3.1 Thoracic wall muscles.

Innervation	Origin	Attachment	Function
Mm. intercostales externi			
Nn. intercostales	Crista costae	Next deeper rib	Rib lifter, inspiration
Mm. intercostales interni			
Nn. intercostales	Inner surface of the upper rib edge	Sulcus costae	Rib sinker, expiration
Mm. intercostales intimi			
Nn. intercostales	Inner surface of the upper rib edge	Sulcus costae (inside)	Rib sinker, expiration
Mm. subcostales			
Nn. intercostales	Inner surface of the upper rib edge	Sulcus costae (inside)	Rib sinker, expiration
M. transversus thoracis			
Nn. intercostales (T2–6)	Sternum	Costal cartilage (II–VI)	Rib sinker, expiration
M. serratus posterior superior			
Cranial Nn. intercostales	Procc. spinosi of the VIth and VIIth cervical vertebrae and the Ist and IInd thoracic vertebrae	IInd–Vth rib each lateral to the Angulus costae	Rib lifter, inspiration
M. serratus posterior inferior			
Caudal Nn. intercostales	Procc. spinosi of the XIth and XIIth thoracic vertebrae and the Ist and IInd lumbar vertebrae	Caudal edge of the IXth–XIIth rib	Lowers the IXth to XIIth rib, as an antagonist of the diaphragm and also active on forced inspiration

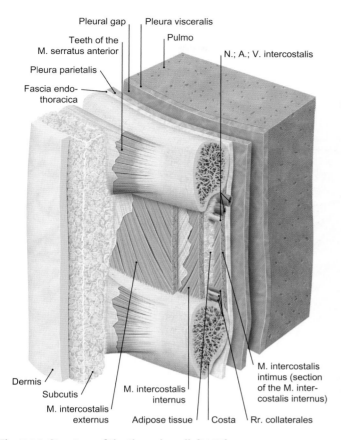

Fig. 3.10 **Structure of the thoracic wall.** [L127]

Labels (from image):
- Pleural gap
- Teeth of the M. serratus anterior
- Pleura parietalis
- Fascia endo-thoracica
- Pleura visceralis
- Pulmo
- N.; A.; V. intercostalis
- Dermis
- Subcutis
- M. intercostalis externus
- M. intercostalis internus
- Adipose tissue
- Costa
- M. intercostalis intimus (section of the M. inter-costalis internus)
- Rr. collaterales

pleura costalis), the vertebral body, the sternum and the upper diaphragmic surface (**Pleura diaphragmatica**) as well as the area of the mediastinum as **Pleura mediastinalis** (➤ Fig. 3.10). It consists of one layer of squamous epithelium.

Vascular, lymphatic and nervous systems of the chest wall

The vessels and nerves of the thoracic wall are arranged segmentally analogue to the intercostal muscles and the skeleton. They run as Aa. and Vv. intercostales posteriores and Rr. ventrales of the spinal nerves (intercostal nerves) to the anterior axillary line in the Sulcus costae. The vein lies above and the accompanying nerve below the artery (➤ Fig. 3.11).

Arteries

The **Aa. intercostales posteriores** (1 and 2) of the two top ICS are branches of the **A. intercostalis suprema,** which originate from the Truncus costocervicalis from the A. subclavia. The Aa. intercostales posteriores of the ICS 3–11, as well as the **Aa. subcostales** are direct branches from the **Aorta thoracica** (➤ Fig. 3.12). As it is located slightly left of the spine, the respective right intercostal arteries are longer. They extend in front of the spine, but behind the oesophagus and behind the V. azygos, as well as the right sympathetic trunk to the respective Sulcus costae. The left-sided Aa. intercostales posteriores run behind the V. hemiazygos accessoria and the V. hemiazygos to the ICS.

Approximately at the height of the rib heads, the arteries emit one **R. dorsalis**, from which the **R. spinalis** for the supply of the spinal cord, the spinal meninges and the spinal nerve emerge. After formation of branches to supply the autochthonous back muscles, the R. dorsalis divides into a **R. cutaneus medialis** and a **R. cutaneus lateralis** (➤ Fig. 3.13, ➤ Fig. 3.65). The main trunk courses further to the lower edge of the respective rib ventrally and emits in its course a **R. collateralis (R. supracostalis)** to the upper edge of the respective lower rib and a **R. cutaneus lateralis** to the skin (➤ Fig. 3.13). Ventrally, the top 6 ICS are supplied by the **A. thoracica interna** (➤ Fig. 3.13) and the lower ICS by the **A. musculophrenica**. These usually emit 2 **Aa. (Rr.) intercostales anteriores** per ICR, which anastomise with the respective Aa. intercostales posteriores and the Rr. collaterales.

The A. thoracica interna runs as a branch of the A. subclavia on both sides of the sternum caudally. In the area of the **Trigonum sternocostale** of the diaphragm it emits the A. musculophrenica (➤ Fig. 3.12).

the connective tissue contact between the thorax inner wall in the form of the costal periosteum and internal thoracic fascia covering the Mm. intercostales interni/intimi on one side and the Pleura parietalis on the other side. The Fascia endothoracica is strongly formed, especially in the area of the pleural dome and is referred to as SIBSON's **fascia (Membrana suprapleuralis, cervicothoracic diaphagm).** The stability of the pleural dome is also improved by connective tissue threads from the Ist rib (**Lig. costopleurale**) and fibres of the Fascia prevertebralis (**Lig. pleurovertebrale**).

Pleura parietalis

The parietal pleura (rib lining) covers the inside of the thorax in the area of the cervical pleura (Cupula pleurae), the ribs (rib lining,

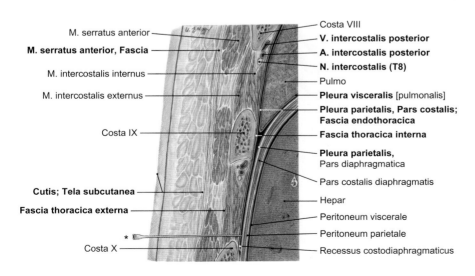

Labels (from image):
- M. serratus anterior
- **M. serratus anterior, Fascia**
- M. intercostalis internus
- M. intercostalis externus
- Costa IX
- **Cutis; Tela subcutanea**
- **Fascia thoracica externa**
- Costa X
- Costa VIII
- **V. intercostalis posterior**
- **A. intercostalis posterior**
- **N. intercostalis (T8)**
- Pulmo
- **Pleura visceralis [pulmonalis]**
- **Pleura parietalis, Pars costalis; Fascia endothoracica**
- **Fascia thoracica interna**
- **Pleura parietalis,** Pars diaphragmatica
- Pars costalis diaphragmatis
- Hepar
- Peritoneum viscerale
- Peritoneum parietale
- Recessus costodiaphragmaticus

Fig. 3.11 **Intercostal space in cross-section;** * Position of the needle during thoracentesis

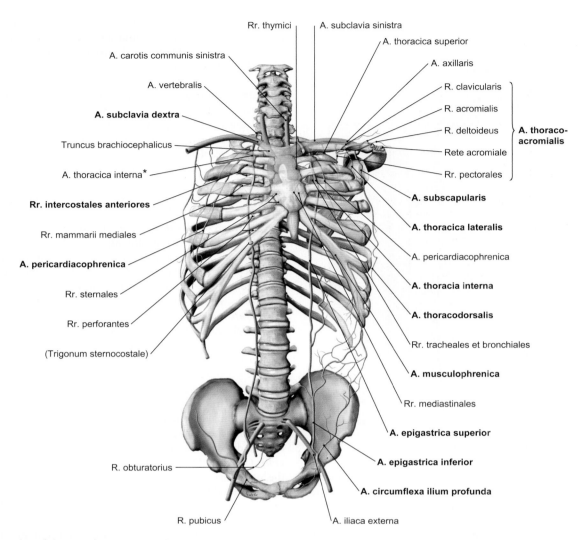

Rr. thymici
A. subclavia sinistra
A. thoracica superior
A. carotis communis sinistra
A. axillaris
A. vertebralis
R. clavicularis
A. subclavia dextra
R. acromialis
R. deltoideus
A. thoraco-
acromialis
Truncus brachiocephalicus
Rete acromiale
A. thoracica interna*
Rr. pectorales
Rr. intercostales anteriores
A. subscapularis
Rr. mammarii mediales
A. thoracica lateralis
A. pericardiacophrenica
A. pericardiacophrenica
A. thoracia interna
Rr. sternales
A. thoracodorsalis
Rr. perforantes
Rr. tracheales et bronchiales
(Trigonum sternocostale)
A. musculophrenica
Rr. mediastinales
A. epigastrica superior
A. epigastrica inferior
R. obturatorius
A. circumflexa ilium profunda
R. pubicus
A. iliaca externa

Fig. 3.12 Arteries of the anterior torso wall; * clinically also A. mammaria interna.

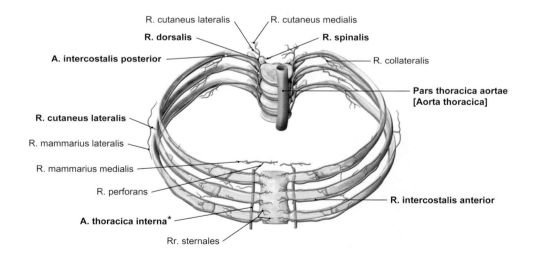

R. cutaneus lateralis
R. cutaneus medialis
R. dorsalis
R. spinalis
A. intercostalis posterior
R. collateralis
**Pars thoracica aortae
[Aorta thoracica]**
R. cutaneus lateralis
R. mammarius lateralis
R. mammarius medialis
R. perforans
R. intercostalis anterior
A. thoracica interna*
Rr. sternales

**Fig. 3.13 Course and exit points
of the intercostal arteries in the
intercostal space;** * clinically
also A. mammaria interna.

Clinical remarks

An **aortic coarctation** (Coarctatio aorta) is a narrowing of the aorta in the area of the aortic arch, which is considered as a vascular malformation. Due to the constriction bypass circulations are formed in order to maintain blood supply to parts of the trunk wall and lower extremities (➤ Fig. 6.11):

- **Horizontal bypass circulation:** between the Aa. thoracicae internae and Aorta thoracica via Rr. intercostales anteriores and Aa. intercostales posteriores to supply the thoracic and abdominal organs (➤ Fig. 3.13). The intercostal arteries expand and lead to rib usures.
- **Vertical bypass circulation:** to supply the trunk wall and the lower extremities between Aa. subclaviae and Aa. iliacae externae via Aa. thoracicae internae, epigastricae superiores and epigastricae inferiores (within the rectus sheath, see below) as well as in the area of the abdominal wall over the Aa. musculophrenicae, epigastricae inferiores and circumflexae ilium profundae (➤ Fig. 3.12).

For the operative revascularization of the heart (bypass operation) in the case of severe **coronary stenosis** (coronary artery narrowing), the A. thoracica interna is primarily used, except for the superficial V. saphena magna (of the leg).

Veins

The venous drainage takes place via veins, which run together with the respective arteries. The **Vv. intercostales anteriores** flow ventral-ly into the **V. thoracica interna** (➤ Fig. 3.14, ➤ Fig. 3.15) and dorsally into the **Vv. azygos and hemiazygos and hemiazygos accessoria** (➤ Fig. 3.16). In doing so, they form venous anastomoses between both drains. The **V. intercostalis suprema** flows from the first intercostal space into the V. vertebralis or V. brachiocephalica. The **Vv. intercostales posteriores** of the 2nd and 3rd ICS unite on both sides to the **V. intercostalis superior,** which flows into the V. azygos on the right(➤ Fig. 3.16) and into the V. brachiocephalica on the left.

Clinical remarks

Thrombosis, masses or the growth of tumours can lead to inflow congestion of the Vv. cavae superior and inferior or the Vv. iliacae communes. As a result, the following bypass circulations can form between the V. cava superior and V. cava inferior **(cavocaval anastomoses,** ➤ Fig. 3.14):

- between the V. iliaca externa and V. cava superior via V. epigastrica inferior, V. epigastrica superior, V. thoracica interna and V. brachiocephalica
- between the V. femoralis and V. cava superior via V. circumflexa ilium superficialis/epigastrica superficialis, V. thoracoepigastrica, V. axillaris and V. brachiocephalica
- between the V. iliaca interna and V. cava superior via Plexus venosus sacralis, Plexus venosi vertebrales externi and interni, Vv. azygos and hemiazygos
- between the Vv. lumbales and V. cava superior via Vv. lumbales ascendentes, Vv. azygos and hemiazygos.

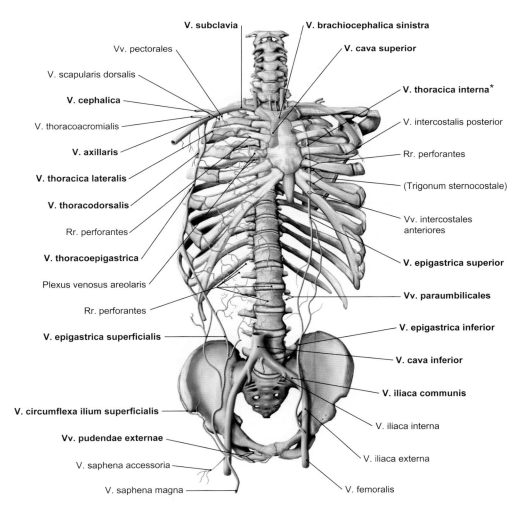

Fig. 3.14 Veins of the anterior torso wall; * clinically also V. mammaria interna.

Cavocaval anastomoses are differentiated from portocaval anastomoses. The latter are circumventions of the liver between the portal vein and upper/lower vena cava (➤ Chap. 7.3.11).

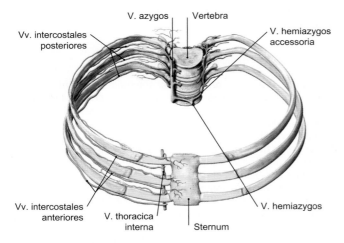

Fig. 3.15 Course and exit points of the intercostal veins in the intercostal space. [L266]

Lymph vessels

The lymph vessels of the Pleura parietalis and intercostal muscles run dorsally to the **Nodi lymphoidei intercostales** in the area of the Angulus costae and drain from here into the **Ductus thoracicus** . The ventral parts of the deep chest wall layers drain into the **Nodi lymphoidei parasternales,** which are located along the A. and V. thoracica interna. From there, the lymph moves cranially via the **Nodi lymphoidei cervicales profundi** in the **Truncus jugularis** and left into the Ductus thoracicus.

Innervation

The ventral trunk wall is innervated segmentally from the **Rr. ventrales** of the thoracic spinal nerves and thus from the **intercostal nerves.** Cranially, the **Nn. supraclaviculares** from the Plexus cervicalis are involved in the sensory innervation in the area of the clavicle . In the course of the intercostal nerves the sensitive **Rr. cutanei laterales** exit at around the height of the middle axillary line. In the segments T1–3 they branch to the **Nn. intercostobrachiales** which sensitively innervate the skin of the medial upper arm. The segments T4–6 emit **Rr. mammarii laterales** to the mammary glands. In the area of the first 6 ICS the **Rr. cutanei anteriores** of the intercostal nerves pass parasternally through the fascia and innervate the skin in the ventral area. From here the **Rr. mammarii mediales** pass from the segments T3–6 to the mammary glands.

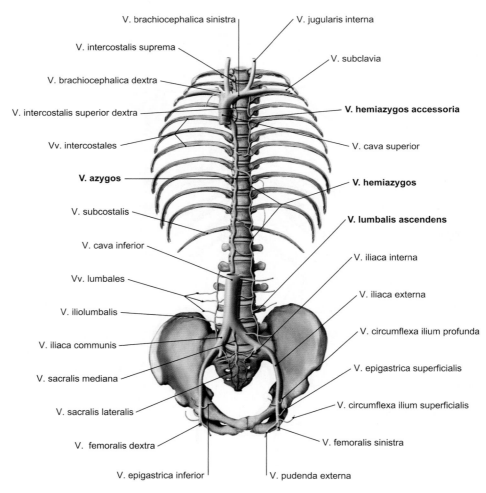

Fig. 3.16 Azygos system.

Clinical remarks

The intercostal spaces are of high practical clinical relevance. For various reasons, there may be an accumulation of fluid in the pleural space between the chest wall and lung surface. If a **thoracentesis** has to be conducted to remove liquid, the positional relationships of the vascular, lymphatic and nervous systems on the lower edge of the ribs are important. The punctures are performed so that the puncture needle is inserted into the thorax directly above the upper edge of the rib to minimise the risk of vascular injuries (➤ Fig. 3.11). This procedure involves penetration of the following structures with the puncture needle in the order from outside to inside (➤ Fig. 3.10):

- Cutis/Subcutis
- Fascia musculi serrati
- M. serratus anterior
- Fascia thoracica externa
- M. intercostalis externus
- M. intercostalis internus/intimus
- Fascia thoracica interna
- Fascia endothoracica
- Parietal pleura

A longer-term accumulation of fluid or air in the pleural space often requires **pleural drainage**, which is usually created in the 4th–5th ICS in the front or middle axillary line (➤ Fig. 6.49). It is conducted for serothorax (serous effusion), haemothorax (blood effusion), pyothorax (bacterial putrid effusion) or haematopneumothorax (blood and air after trauma) mostly as a BÜLAU drainage. This corresponds to the puncture in the 'triangle of safety', i.e. between the lateral margin of the M. pectoralis major and the anterior margin of the M. latissimus dorsi at the height of the nipples. Pleural tapping or drainage below the 6th ICS is avoided due to the risk of injuries to the liver or spleen. In the case of pneumothorax a MONALDI drainage is usually conducted through the 2nd ICS in the midclavicular line. The MONALDI drainage differs from the BÜLAU drainage by a smaller lumen.

3.1.3 Diaphragm

The dome-shaped **diaphragm (Diaphragma)** separates the thoracic cavity from the abdominal cavity. It shows characteristic passageways for the oesophagus, blood and lymph vessels and nerves. The diaphragm is also the most important inspiration muscle.

Development

The development is based on 4 structures:

- Septum transversum
- Plicae pleuroperitoneales
- Periesophageal connective tissue
- Mesodermal ridges growing on the side of the body wall

The **Septum transversum** forms a mesenchymal plate between the heart and liver. The largest part of the Centrum tendineum emerges from the septum. The **Plicae pleuroperitoneales** close the coelomic canals (pleuroperitoneal canals). In doing so, they grow from lateral and dorsal to the septum transversum and join together with the septum and with the mesenchyme surrounding the oesophagus (**perioesophageal connective tissue**). Tissue projections of the parietal **mesoderm** seal the diaphragm borders and attach it to the body wall. The developmental process does not occur in the chest, but in the neck area. Therefore, the diaphragm is innervated

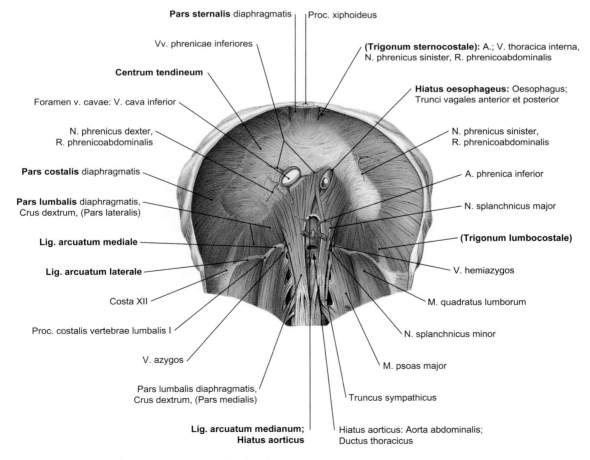

Fig. 3.17 Diaphragm (Diaphragma) and posterior abdominal wall.

mainly from the cervical segments C3–C5. The nerve fibres of the 3 segments together form the **N. phrenicus**. With the descent of the heart and growth in length, the diaphragm shifts up to the inferior thoracic aperture and the N. phrenicus on both sides extends in length (30 cm in adults); however, the intercostal nerves are also involved in the innervation.

Structure

The diaphragm (➤ Fig. 3.17) consists of a muscular (**Pars muscularis**) and a fibrous part (**Centrum tendineum**), which serves the diaphragm muscles as an attachment due to its central position. The sinewy muscle origins include the whole lower thoracic aperture of the lumbar spine via the ribs to the sternum. The muscle origins are divided accordingly into **Pars lumbalis, Pars costalis** and **Pars sternalis.**

Pars lumbalis

The muscle-packed **pars lumbalis** originates on both sides of the ventral side of the spine, so that a differentiation can be made between the right (**Crus dextrum**) and left crus of the diaphragm (**Crus sinistrum**). Both diaphragm legs are muscle strands:

- **Crus dextrum:** it is longer and wider than the Crus sinistrum and originates in the lumbar bodies I–IV, as well as the intervening Disci intervertebrales.
- **Crus sinistrum:** it is shorter and narrower than the Crus dextrum and fixed to the lumbar bodies I and II, as well as the corresponding intervertebral discs.

Depending on the school of teaching, both crura are divided into 2 (Crus mediale and Crus laterale) or 3 sections (Pars lateralis, Pars intermedia and Pars medialis). Here, the division is into three sections. The Pars medialis of the Crus dextrum forms a loop around the oesophagus (**Hiatus oesophageus**). and is connected to the Pars medialis of the Crus sinistrum on the midline via a connective tissue arch (**Lig. arcuatum medianum, aortic arcade**). The aorta (**Hiatus aorticus**) and the Ductus thoracicus run behind the arch, but in front of the spine.

Further laterally the Pars intermedia of the Crus dextrum forms a 2nd tendinous arch, which extends beyond the M. psoas (**psoas arcade**) and is referred to as **Lig. arcuatum mediale**. On the left side, the Lig. arcuatum mediale of the Pars medialis and the Pars intermedia is formed. The tendon arches are on the sides of the Ist and IInd lumbar vertebrae and fixed laterally at the Proc. transversus of the Ist lumbar vertebra.

Even further laterally the Partes laterales of the Crus dextrum and the Crus sinistrum each bridge the M. quadratus lumborum (**quadratus arcade**) as the **Lig. arcuatum laterale** . The arch is medial both at the Proc. transversus of the Ist lumbar vertebra and fixed laterally to the XIIth rib.

The Ligg. arcuata mediale and laterale are also called HALLER'S arches.

> NOTE
>
> The Pars lumbalis diaphragmatis is divided into:
> - Crus dextrum (Pars lateralis, Pars intermedia, Pars medialis)
> - Crus sinistrum (Pars lateralis, Pars intermedia, Pars medialis)

Pars costalis

The greater Pars costalis originates on the right and left of the costal arch and of the cartilaginous parts of the VIIth–XIIth ribs and extends to the Centrum tendineum.

Pars sternalis

The Pars sternalis originates on the rear surface of the Proc. xiphoideus of the breastbone and with smaller parts from the rear lamina of the rectus sheath and extends to the Centrum tendineum.

Centrum tendineum

The Centrum tendineum (➤ Fig. 3.17) forms the joint attachment tendon of the muscular parts of the diaphragm. To the right of the centre line it is limited by the **Foramen venae cavae,** through which the V. cava inferior passes. Projected into the respiratory central position, the Centrum tendineum is approximately at the height of the border between the Corpus and Proc. xiphoideus of the sternum. The Centrum tendineum is fused on the thoracic side with the pericardium and on the abdominal side it is fused with the Area nuda of the liver.

Topographical relationships of the diaphragm

Above the liver the right diaphragmatic dome is approximately 1–2 cm higher than the left, whereby in meteorism (excessive gas deposits in the gut, distension) the left diaphragmatic dome can approach the height of the right one. At maximum expiration the right pleural dome projects to the upper edge of the IVth rib and at the height of the VIIIth thoracic vertebrae. In inspiration position the right diaphragmatic dome is in contrast at the height of the VIth rib and XIth thoracic vertebrae. On the left the pleural dome is situated both for inspiration and expiration positions, by half or one ICS and half a vertebra lower than on the right side. The diaphragm is higher when lying than when standing.

Diaphragm openings and penetrating structures

Numerous structures penetrate or move around the diaphragm (➤ Fig. 3.17):

- The **Trigonum sternocostale** is located at the transition between Pars sternalis and Pars costalis. The **A. epigastrica superior** runs ventral in front of the fibrous triangle as a terminal branch of the A. thoracica interna and its accompanying veins and with lymph vessels.

Note: The Trigonum sternocostale is referred to clinically and also in many anatomy textbooks as the 'LARREY cleft'; however, this term should not be used, as when LARREY described his work on pericardial puncture he did not puncture caudally (i.e. from the peritoneal cavity) through the Trigonum sternocostale but penetrated the diaphragm left and cranially with a scalpel after a puncture between the costal arch and Proc. xiphoideus. The usual teaching opinion that the A. thoracica interna penetrates through this triangle and passes into the A. epigastrica superior is also not entirely correct since the vessels run ventrally of the Trigonum sternocostale.

- At the transition of the Pars costalis and Pars lumbalis there is usually a muscle-free triangle (**Trigonum lumbocostale, BOCHDALEK triangle**) which is sealed by connective tissue and serous membranes.
- The **Nn. splanchnici major and minor** run on both sides through the diaphragm crus (usually between the Pars medialis and Pars intermedia of the respective Crus dextrum or sinistrum).
- The **V. azygos** (not always, see below) and the **V. hemiazygos** pass through the right or left diaphragm crus (between Pars medialis and Pars intermedia).
- The **oesophagus** penetrates into the oesophageal hiatus slightly left above the Hiatus aorticus at the height of the Xth thoracic vertebra through the Pars medialis of the Crus dextrum. With it

run the **Trunci vagales anterior and posterior,** the **Rr. oesopha-geales** of the A. and V. gastrica sinistra as well as lymph vessels.
- The **aorta** runs behind the tendinous arch (Lig. arcuatum medi-anum, aortic arcade) of the Partes mediales of the Crus dextrum and Crus sinistrum and in front of the XIIth thoracic vertebra a little to the left of the centre line (Hiatus aorticus). The **Ductus thoracicus** and sometimes the **V. azygos.** also penetrate through the Hiatus aorticus.
- The **Foramen venae cavae** lies in the Centrum tendineum ap-proximately at the height of the transition from the VIIIth to the IXth thoracic vertebrae slightly to the right of the spine. The V. cava inferior penetrates through the foramen from the abdominal cavity into the chest. The Foramen venae cavae is also used by the **N. phrenicus dexter** for passage.
- The **N. phrenicus sinister** penetrates the Pars costalis on the left-hand side or enters through the Hiatus oesophageus.
- The **sympathetic trunks** run on both sides behind the Lig. ar-cuatum mediale.

Other small vessels and nerves, e. g. for the diaphragm muscles or branches of some intercostal nerves also penetrate at certain places through the diaphragm.

N O T E

The **diaphragm** (Daphragma) is the main breathing muscle, without which adequate breathing is not possible. It separates the thoracic cavity from the abdominal cavity and is penetrated by many struc-tures, such as the oesophagus and V. cava inferior.

─ Clinical remarks ─────────────────

Diaphragmatic hernia (Hernia diaphragmatica) can be con-genital or acquired. In both cases, abdominal viscera pass over into the thoracic cavity. If the shifted organs are covered by peritoneum (hernial sac), one speaks of true hernias:
- Congenital diaphragmatic hernias (BOCHDALEK hernias) are usually gaps in the diaphragm through which abdominal or-gans (stomach, intestines, liver, spleen) pass into the thorax and can impair lung growth and breathing after birth. In ad-dition to life-threatening dyspnea in a newborn child, cardi-ac symptoms may also occur due to suppression of the heart. Congenital diaphragmatic hernias are more likely to be on the left than on the right side, usually have no hernial sac and are often in the Trigonum sternocostale (MORGAGNI hernia) or lumbocostale (BOCHDALEK hernia).
- Acquired diaphragmatic hernias are usually hiatal hernias or paraesophageal hiatal hernias. In a hiatal hernia part of the stomach also passes through the slit-shaped Hiatus oesophageus (➤ Fig. 3.18). If the cardia of the stomach is pulled up through the diaphragm into the chest, it is called an axial hiatal hernia (➤ Fig. 3.18). There are also mixed forms. In severe cases, the majority of the stomach can slide into the chest (thoracic stomach, 'upside-down stomach').

A **flattening of the pleural dome** in the x-ray image can indi-cate a reduced retraction force of the lungs, e. g. in the case of an emphysema or pneumothorax. During pregnancy or in the case of fluid accumulation in the abdominal cavity (ascites) there can be a **shift of the diaphragm borders** in a cranial di-rection.

Vascular, lymphatic and nervous systems
Arteries
The diaphragm is supplied at its upper and lower side with blood:
- from the thoracic cavity side:
  - **Aa. musculophrenicae** (branches of the A. thoracica interna)

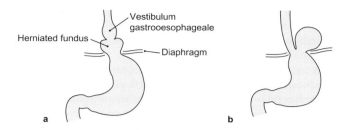

Fig. 3.18 Acquired diaphragmatic hernias (scheme). **a** Axial hiatal hernia. **b** Paraesophageal hiatal hernia. [L141]

  - **Aa. pericardiacophrenicae** (branches of the A. thoracica in-terna)
  - **Aa. phrenicae superiores** (branches of the Aorta thoracica).
- From the abdominal cavity side:
  - **Aa. phrenicae inferiores** (branches of the Aorta abdominalis).

Veins
The venous drainage occurs via:
- **Vv. phrenicae superiores** into the V. azygos and the V. hemiazy-gos
- **Vv. phrenicae inferiores** into the V. cava inferior.

Lymph vessels
The lymph drainage takes place within the muscles via its own lymph ducts to the lymph ducts of the pleura and peritoneum.

Innervation
The motor and sensory innervation for the most part is effected by the **Nn. phrenici** from the segments **C3–C5** of the Plexus cervica-lis. The Nn. phrenici run left and right over the front of the M. sca-lenus anterior and pass through the upper thoracic aperture into the chest. Here they stretch between Pleura mediastinalis and peri-cardium through the thoracic cavity to the diaphragm surface. In their course they sensitively innervate the Pleura mediastinalis, the Pleura diaphragmatica and the pericardium. On the right, the N. phrenicus penetrates through the Foramen venae cavae in the Cen-trum tendineum; on the left, it usually passes alone near the Cen-trum tendineum through the Pars costalis diaphragmatis. Both Nn. phrenici branch out below the diaphragm and motor innervate the muscles and sensory the Peritoneum parietale on the diaphragm. In addition, the adjacent intercostal nerves are involved and the **N. subclavius** as the so-called *accessory phrenic nerve* can be involved in the innervation.

N O T E

The diaphragm innervation is carried out via the N. phrenicus. It in-nervates
- by motor nerves
  - diaphragm muscles
- by sensory nerves
  - Pleura mediastinalis
  - Pleura diaphragmatica
  - Pericardium
  - Peritoneum parietale on the diaphragm

─ Clinical remarks ─────────────────

Damage to the N. phrenicus causes paralysis of the muscles on the affected side with an elevated diaphragm (Relaxatio diaphragmatica).

Diaphragm function, respiratory mechanics and accessory breathing muscles

Respiration and the breathing muscles are also described in ➤ Chap. 6.5.4.

Based on the relaxed breathing position, contraction of the **Mm. intercostales externi,** the **Mm. intercartilaginei, Mm. scaleni** and the **diaphragm** results in **inspiration:** The ribs are raised, the diaphragm is flattened out and the thoracic volume is increased. The external forces that act on the chest and also the elastic restorative forces of the chest and the lungs are therefore overcome. The further the ribs are lifted, the greater the resistance and the more power is required. In doing so, the thorax in the upper section expands more in the longitudinal diameter (**sternocostal breathing type**) and stretches more in the lower section in the diameter (flank breathing). The enlargement in the caudal section leads to the expansion of the diaphragm, thereby enabling a mechanically favourable starting position for diaphragm contraction (**costodiaphragmatic breathing type**). The interplay of extension of the inferior thoracic aperture and contraction-related flattening of the diaphragm expands the **Recessus costodiaphragmaticus** on both sides. Under physiological conditions both types of breathing are normally combined. Under resting conditions the inspiration is dominated by contraction of the Mm. scaleni, which slightly raise the Ist and IInd ribs. Through the tone of the intercostal muscles the rest of the ribs are raised slightly so that the chest is mainly expanded from below by diaphragm contraction. The Mm. intercostales externi and intercartilaginei are only activated for increased inspiration. In addition to the abovementioned muscles that act on inspiration, the following muscles can be activated in forced inspiration due to physical stress or during illnesses (e. g. bronchial asthma) (**accessory breathing muscles**). The burden of the weight of the shoulder girdle on the thorax can be reduced by the **Mm. rhomboidei, levatores scapulae** and **trapezii.** As the force of the shoulder girdle acts in an expirational manner on the chest, less force has to be applied on inspiration due to the elevation of the shoulder girdle. By supporting the arms on the thighs, as can frequently be observed in athletes following a competitive event, the **Mm. pectorales majores, minores** and **serrati anteriores** are also able to lift the ribs and expand the chest. In this way they also have an inspirational effect (by reversal of punctum fixum and punctum mobile by resting the arms).

On **expiration** the **elastic restorative forces** of the lungs and the thorax as well as gravity have the effect that the chest springs back to its initial position, as soon as the inspiratory muscles become fatigued. Only when breathing is continued via the breathing resting position, does contraction of the **Mm. intercostales interni** and the **M. transversus thoracis** cause a further sinking of the ribs. A crucial role for forced expiration is also played by the **abdominal muscles** (➤ Chap. 3.1.4). Their contraction lowers the thorax further, narrows the lower thoracic aperture and increases the intra-abdominal pressure, causing the abdominal organs and the diaphragm to be pushed upwards at the expense of the intrathoracic volume. Therefore the abdominal muscles are the most important auxiliary muscles for expiration. When the arms are at rest, the **M. latissimus dorsi** also supports expiration by lowering the ribs.

3.1.4 Abdominal wall

Clinical case

Indirect inguinal hernia

Case study

An 84-year-old retired man in poor general state of health visits a general practitioner for a second opinion. The patient has suffered severe weight loss (approx. 8 kg) and a significant loss of power within 1 year. He also reports cramp-like abdominal pains after each food intake, which have the effect that he hardly eats anything at all. Today, in particular, he feels particularly unwell and has not yet eaten anything. He sometimes also suffers from severe diarrhoea. His family doctor treated it from the onset of the complaints with the suspected diagnosis 'heartburn'. The prescribed tablets to reduce gastric acid production had not helped him. A gastroscopy 3 months ago has shown no pathological findings. Previous conditions reported by the patient include 2 operations (1945 shrapnel injury; 1991 inguinal hernia left) and a well-adjusted high blood pressure (current measurement RR 125/80). Until a few months ago, he had independently managed a large plot of land and looked after his wife who recently received a 'new hip'.

Initial examination

During physical examination a dry tongue and persisting skin folds give an indication of severe exsiccosis. Blood pressure, heart rate and auscultation findings are normal. The pulse is easily palpable on both sides and the indicative neurological examination is without pathological findings. When the doctor asks the patient to take off his clothes for a rectal examination, the old man asks whether this is really necessary. His old family doctor had always spared him that procedure. The doctor tells him that many ulcers in bowel cancer may be easily detected in the early stages with the finger or through blood on the glove. One should also regularly check the prostate at his age. The patient then reluctantly agrees to the manual palpation examination. The investigation, however, remains without pathological findings, except for an enlarged prostate gland which is in keeping with the age of the patient. During the inspection of the patient's inguinal region, the doctor notices a clearly visible swelling on the right side. The more detailed examination consolidates the suspicion that this is a hernia. The hernial sac cannot be manually shifted back into the abdominal cavity. On an ausculatory level bowel sounds are perceptible in the patient's scrotum, indicating that there are intestinal components here. The doctor explains to the patient that intestinal components are trapped in his abdominal wall. This is obstructing the transport of the food mass at this point and could explain his symptoms. In the worst case, this could lead to an intestinal infarct caused by clamping of the blood supply to the intestine. Due to the alarming findings, the doctor immediately refers the patient to the local hospital.

Further diagnostics

In the subsequent x-ray of the abdomen the level of fluid in the small intestines is noticeable, which indicates a partial or complete closure of the intestinal passage (subileus or ileus) due to the inguinal hernia.

Therapy and follow-up

The senior surgical consultant conducts emergency surgery 3 hours later in which he confirms an indirect inguinal hernia. He can move the section of the small intestine back without having to resect it.

During the morning visit the next day the patient thanks the doctor for his rapid assistance and asks when he can finally get back home to support his wife.

Clinical picture

The inguinal canal is the most common localisation (approx. 80%) of abdominal wall hernias. A distinction is made between indirect and direct inguinal hernias depending on the hernial ring. Indirect inguinal hernias are the most common abdominal wall hernias in adulthood (approximately two thirds of all hernias) and occur particularly in men. The hernial sac continues via the inguinal canal through the outer inguinal ring into the scrotum or to the labia majora. Direct inguinal hernias (about one third of all hernias) make a direct course through the abdominal wall, by penetrating the abdominal wall in the Fossa inguinalis medialis.

The abdominal wall surrounds the abdominal cavity (**peritoneal cavity, cavitas peritonealis**) and the organs of the abdominal cavity (Cavitas abdominalis) in the **extraperitoneal space (Spatium extraperitoneale)**. It is cranial to the chest, dorsal to the spine and caudal to the pelvis. It is primarily formed from 4 flat abdominal muscles and their tendon plates (aponeuroses), which extend between the chest and pelvis. Together, they form the abdominal wall and the lateral parts are also referred to as the flanks. The abdomen wall runs continuously into the pelvic wall. It can be divided into three layers:

- Superficial layer
  - Skin and subcutaneous tissue
  - General body fascia (Fascia abdominis superficialis)
- Middle layer
  - Front, side and back abdominal muscles with aponeuroses
- Deep layer
  - Inner abdominal wall fascia (Fascia abdominis interna)
  - Subserosal connective tissue (Tela subserosa)
  - Parietale peritoneum (Peritoneum parietale)

Superficial layer
Cutis

The cutis is elastic and approximately 2 mm thick. The gender-specific pubic hair (pubes) in men usually extends up to the navel and in the case of women ends above the mons pubis. The collagen fibrils of skin have a certain alignment (LANGER'S lines), which need to be taken into account during surgery to avoid extensive scars.

Clinical remarks

Skin overstretching of the abdominal wall or thighs, e.g. in the case of obesity or during pregnancy, can evoke stripe-like tears (stretch marks) in the dermis and visible striae distensae.

Subcutis

In the **Tela subcutanea** there is gender-specific storage of fat depending on the nutritional status. The subcutaneous adipose tissue is missing in the umbilical area.

The **subcutis** is a layer of connective tissue particularly below the umbilicus, which consists of connective tissue membranes and is stored in the adipose tissue. It is referred to as the **Stratum membranosum (CAMPER's fascia)**. The connective tissue contains large quantities of elastic fibres and is fused with the outer ring of the rectus sheath (see below). Fibre bundles of CAMPER's fascia extend to the penis root as the Lig. fundiforme (**Lig. fundiforme penis**) or to the clitoris (**Lig. fundiforme clitoridis**).

Superficial fascia

The superficial fascia (**Fascia abdominis superficialis, SCARPA's fascia**) is fused with the M. obliquus externus abdominis and its aponeurosis. Fibres of the fascia join together with fibres of the M. obliquus externus abdominis aponeurosis and form the **Lig. suspensorium penis** on the upper side of the penis and at the top of the clitoris the **Lig. suspensorium clitoridis.** They connect these with the lower edge of the symphysis pubica.

The Fascia abdominis superficialis passes cranially continuously to the superficial chest wall fascia (Fascia pectoralis) and to the Fascia axillaris; caudally it continues under the Lig. inguinale in the fascia of the thigh (Fascia lata) and dorsal in the back fascia (Fascia thoracolumbalis).

Vascular, lymphatic and nervous systems of the superficial layer
Arteries

The arterial blood supply takes place partially segmentally; in some cases the supply deviates from this (➤ Fig. 3.12, ➤ Fig. 3.2):

- Segmentally
  - **Rr. cutanei laterales** of the Aa. intercostales posteriores (VIIth to XIth) reach the skin at the edge of the M. obliquus externus abdominis
- Not segmentally
  - Branches of the Aa. epigastricae superior and inferior to the skin
  - **A. epigastrica superficialis**
  - **A. circumflexa ilium superficialis**
  - **Aa. pudendae externae superficialis et profunda**

Veins

The veins in the subcutis of the abdominal wall form a network which drains into the

- **V. thoracoepigastrica** (in the upper section) and into the
- **V. epigastrica superficialis** (in the lower section).

The V. thoracoepigastrica leads the blood into the V. axillaris. The V. epigastrica superficialis drains the blood to the vein cross (Hiatus saphenus). The V circumflexa ilium superficialis and the Vv. pudendae externae merge here. The **Vv. paraumbilicales** are connected with the Vv. thoracoepigastrica et epigastrica superficialis and also drain through the abdominal wall to the V. portae hepatis (➤ Chap. 7.8.3). Segmentally arranged, the main veins accompanying the arteries carry blood to the Vv. intercostales posteriores and Vv. epigastricae superior et inferior.

Lymph vessels

Regional lymph nodes of the cutis and subcutis (➤ Fig. 3.19, ➤ Fig. 3.5) are:

- Above the navel:
  - **Nodi lymphoidei pectorales**
  - **Nodi lymphoidei intercostales**
  - **Nodi lymphoidei parasternales**
- Below the navel:
  - **Nodi lymphoidei inguinales superficiales** (Tractus horizontalis: Nodi lymphoidei superomediales and nodi lymphoidei superolaterales)

Innervation

The innervation of the abdominal wall takes place segmentally (➤ Fig. 3.2). The contributing main nerves are branches of the

- Nn. intercostales VI–XI
- N. subcostalis
- N. iliohypogastricus
- N. ilioinguinalis

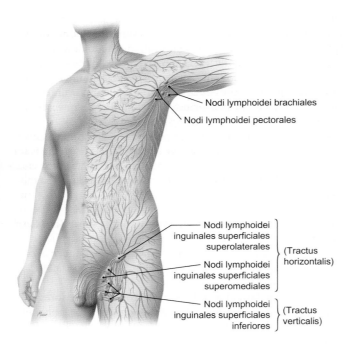

Nodi lymphoidei brachiales

Nodi lymphoidei pectorales

Nodi lymphoidei
inguinales superficiales
superolaterales } (Tractus
horizontalis)

Nodi lymphoidei
inguinales superficiales
superomediales

Nodi lymphoidei
inguinales superficiales
inferiores } (Tractus
verticalis)

Fig. 3.19 Superficial lymph vessels and regional lymph nodes of the anterior torso wall.

Rr. cutanei anteriores mediales of the intercostal nerves reach the skin beside the linea alba; the corresponding **Rr. cutanei anteriores laterales** reach the subcutis in the area of origin of the M. obliquus externus abdominis.

The **R. medialis** of the **N. iliohypogastricus** arrives at the surface anatomy a little above the Anulus inguinalis superficialis and innervates the skin around the annulus and the mons pubis. The terminal branch of the **N. ilioinguinalis** leaves the Canalis inguinalis to innervate the skin above and medial of the Anulus inguinalis superficialis and the mons pubis. In addition, its branches innervate parts of the Labia majora as **Rr. labiales anteriores** and as **Rr. scrotales anteriores** the front of the scrotum.

Middle layer

The middle layer of the abdominal wall includes the front and lateral abdominal muscles and their aponeuroses and a group of deeper abdominal muscles. According to their location, the muscles are divided into:

- Front (straight) abdominal muscles
- Lateral (angled) abdominal muscles
- Rear (deep) abdominal muscles

The muscles of the abdominal wall (**Mm. abdominis**) form together with their aponeuroses and suffused fascia the actual abdominal wall, which covers the area between the chest wall and pelvic ring. Innervation, attachment, origin and function of the muscles are summarised in ➤ Table 3.2. The fascia, which cover the muscles outside (Fascia abdominis superficialis) and inside (Fascia transversalis), belong to the superficial or deep layer of the abdominal wall.

Development

The abdominal muscles emerge from the ventral dermomyotome, which divides in the 5th week into a larger ventral group of mesenchymal cells (hypomere) and a smaller dorsal group (epimere). The epimere becomes the indigenous back muscles. Apart from the Mm. scaleni, the prevertebral neck muscles, the infrahyoid muscles, the Mm. intercostales, the Mm. subcostales and the M. trans-

versus thoracis, 3 muscle layers are differentiated from the hypomere in the abdominal area:

- M. obliquus externus abdominis
- M. obliquus internus abdominis
- M. transversus abdominis

The following also emerge from the hypomere:

- M. rectus abdominis
- M. quadratus lumborum
- Pelvic floor muscles and closing muscles of the urethra and anus.

Front (straight) abdominal muscles
M. rectus abdominis

The paired M. rectus abdominis has a straight fibre trend, which is displaced by 90° with the fibres of the M. transversus abdominis (➤ Fig. 3.20, ➤ Fig. 3.22). It lies paramedially from the pubic bone to the thorax and is embedded in a fibre canal (rectus sheath, see below), which is formed by the aponeuroses of the oblique abdominal muscles. The M. rectus abdominis muscle has 4–5 muscle bellies, which are impressive when there is a low level of subcutaneous adipose tissue and well-trained muscles in the form of a 'six-pack'. The muscle parts do not comply with the segmental myotomes and are separated by 3–4, rarely by 5 **Intersectiones tendineae**. The inter-sections are individually arranged at different heights and often also vary between the two sides. They are fused with the frontal lamina (Lamina anterior) of the rectus sheath. On the back the branches of the intercostal nerves (T7–12) and supplying blood vessels (Aa./Vv. epigastricae superior et inferior) can reach the muscle. The muscle is of great significance for the torso flexion and plays a role together with the oblique abdominal muscles in abdominal pressing and forced expiration.

M. pyramidalis

The M. pyramidalis is a small triangular-shaped muscle between the aponeuroses of the oblique abdominal muscles or behind the front lamina of the rectus sheath (➤ Fig. 3.20). It spans the Linea alba. It is missing in 10–25% of people.

Lateral (angled) abdominal muscles

Lateral abdominal muscles (Mm. obliquus externus abdominis, M. obliquus internus abdominis, M. transversus abdominis) overlap each other in 3 layers. The fibres of these muscles run differently. They cover a large area, but are relatively thin. In the area of the midclavicular line, the muscles pass into their aponeuroses, from which the rectus sheath of the right and left side are formed and which interweave into the midline to the Linea alba (see below).

M. obliquus externus abdominis

The M. obliquus externus abdominis is the most superficial and largest of the lateral abdominal muscles (➤ Fig. 3.20, ➤ Table 3.2). The muscle has a serrated shape, with the attachments of the M. serratus anterior alternating origin line that extends up to the Vth rib. In the case of trained persons the line is clearly visible on the side of the thorax (GERDY's line). The course of the muscle fibres of the M. obliquus externus abdominis continues over the line on the M. serratus anterior to cranial. Caudally, on the opposite side (via an imaginary line through the two rectus sheaths), the muscle fibre course continues to the M. obliquus internus abdominis of the opposite side and thus forms a slanted muscle loop. This explains the strong force effect of the M. obliquus externus abdominis in torso diffraction, torso rotation and when throwing (M. serratus anterior in continuation on the shoulder girdle). The caudal limit of the aponeurosis of the M. obliquus externus abdominis is formed by the inguinal ligament (Lig. inguinale). The aponeurosis has a gap for the outflow of the inguinal canal (outer inguinal ring, Anulus inguinalis superficialis) and is involved in the development of the front lamina of the rectus sheath.

M. obliquus internus abdominis

The M. obliquus internus abdominis lies between the M. transversus abdominis and M. obliquus externus abdominis (➤ Fig. 3.20, ➤ Fig. 3.21, ➤ Table 3.2). Its muscle fibres radiate from the Spina iliaca anterior superior in a fan shape and insert into the Linea alba and the bottom edge of the rib arch. The fibre course continues here in the Mm. intercostales interni. Thus, the muscle fibres run obliquely above the pelvic comb and thus perpendicular to the M. obliquus externus abdominis. At the height of the Spina iliaca anterior superior the muscle fibre course is horizontal and below it downwards. The descending fibres overlie the spermatic cord and at the same time form the roof of the inguinal canal. Caudal muscle fibres accompany the spermatic cord as the M. cremaster (Funiculus spermaticus, see below). The internus aponeurosis branches above the Linea arcuata (➤ Fig. 3.25) in 2 parts: the front portion combines with the aponeurosis of the M. obliquus externus abdominis to the front lamina of the rectus sheath; the rear portion combines with the aponeurosis of the M. transversus abdominis to the rear lamina of the rectus sheath (see below). Below the Linea arcuata both parts extend to the front lamina of the rectus sheath.

M. transversus abdominis

The M. transversus abdominis is the deepest of the lateral abdominal muscles (➤ Fig. 3.22, ➤ Table 3.2). Its fibres run approximately

horizontally and pass laterally from the M. rectus abdominis into a crescent-shaped line (**Linea semilunaris, SPIEGHEL line**) into its aponeurosis. Lower muscle fibres emerging from the inguinal ligament pass over the inguinal canal (➤ Fig. 3.26). The aponeurosis combines above the Linea arcuata (➤ Fig. 3.30) with the posterior part of the aponeurosis of the M. obliquus internus abdominis to the rear lamina of the rectus sheath. The part emerging below the Linea arcuata from the inguinal ligament of the aponeurosis is fused with the M. obliquus internus abdominis (M. complexus) and runs ventrally to strengthen the front face of the rectus sheath. Some fibres are usually involved in the formation of the M. cremaster. As the **Falx inguinalis** is the radiating part of the attachment tendon of the M. transversus abdominis it is referred to as the Tuberculum pubicum. The fibres previously run in an arch shape on the border to the rectus sheath downwards (transversus sinew arch, transversus sinew arcade, Tendo conjunctivus) and laterally limit the Trigonum inguinale (HESSELBACH's triangle, see below).

Rear (deep) abdominal muscles

Dorsally, the abdominal wall is formed by 2 pairs of muscles, which lie ventrally of the deep lamina of the Fascia thoracodorsalis and of the original area of the M. transversus abdominis:

- **M. psoas major**
- **M. quadratus lumborum**

Both muscles form the base of the Fossa lumbalis, a muscular niche, which extends between the lumbar spine, XIIth rib and iliac crest.

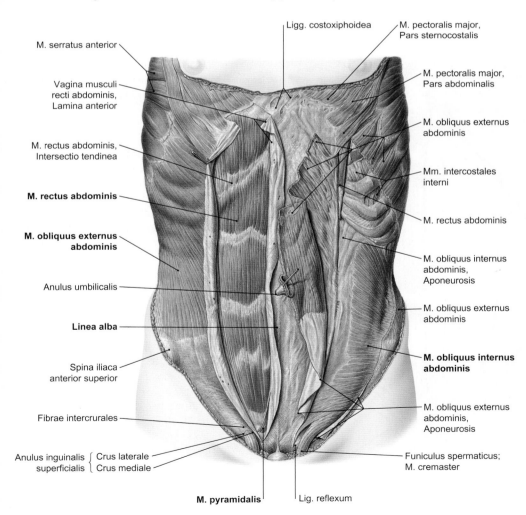

M. serratus anterior

Vagina musculi recti abdominis, Lamina anterior

M. rectus abdominis, Intersectio tendinea

M. rectus abdominis

M. obliquus externus abdominis

Anulus umbilicalis

Linea alba

Spina iliaca anterior superior

Fibrae intercrurales

Anulus inguinalis superficialis { Crus laterale / Crus mediale

M. pyramidalis

Lig. reflexum

Ligg. costoxiphoidea

M. pectoralis major, Pars sternocostalis

M. pectoralis major, Pars abdominalis

M. obliquus externus abdominis

Mm. intercostales interni

M. rectus abdominis

M. obliquus internus abdominis, Aponeurosis

M. obliquus externus abdominis

M. obliquus internus abdominis

M. obliquus externus abdominis, Aponeurosis

Funiculus spermaticus; M. cremaster

Fig. 3.20 Superficial and middle layer of the abdominal muscles, Mm. abdominis. Ventral view.

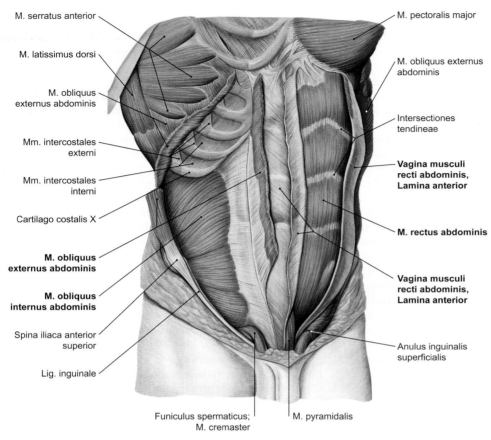

M. serratus anterior

M. latissimus dorsi

M. obliquus externus abdominis

Mm. intercostales externi

Mm. intercostales interni

Cartilago costalis X

M. obliquus externus abdominis

M. obliquus internus abdominis

Spina iliaca anterior superior

Lig. inguinale

M. pectoralis major

M. obliquus externus abdominis

Intersectiones tendineae

Vagina musculi recti abdominis, Lamina anterior

M. rectus abdominis

Vagina musculi recti abdominis, Lamina anterior

Anulus inguinalis superficialis

Funiculus spermaticus; M. cremaster

M. pyramidalis

Fig. 3.21 Middle layer of the abdominal muscles, Mm. abdominis. Ventral view.

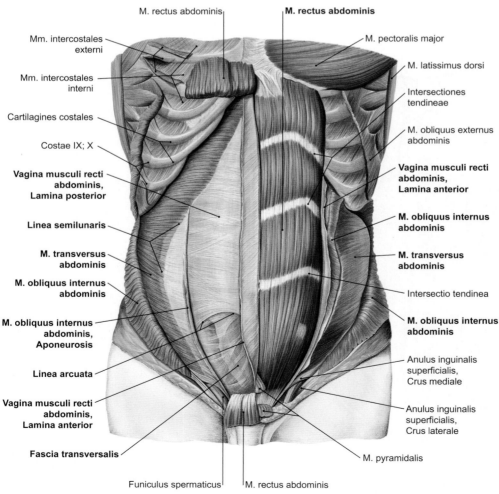

M. rectus abdominis

M. rectus abdominis

Mm. intercostales externi

Mm. intercostales interni

Cartilagines costales

Costae IX; X

Vagina musculi recti abdominis, Lamina posterior

Linea semilunaris

M. transversus abdominis

M. obliquus internus abdominis

M. obliquus internus abdominis, Aponeurosis

Linea arcuata

Vagina musculi recti abdominis, Lamina anterior

Fascia transversalis

Funiculus spermaticus

M. rectus abdominis

M. pectoralis major

M. latissimus dorsi

Intersectiones tendineae

M. obliquus externus abdominis

Vagina musculi recti abdominis, Lamina anterior

M. obliquus internus abdominis

M. transversus abdominis

Intersectio tendinea

M. obliquus internus abdominis

Anulus inguinalis superficialis, Crus mediale

Anulus inguinalis superficialis, Crus laterale

M. pyramidalis

Fig. 3.22 Deep layer of the abdominal muscles, Mm. abdominis. Ventral view.

Table 3.2 Abdominal muscles.

Innervation	Origin	Attachment	Function
Anterior muscles of the abdominal wall			
M. rectus abdominis			
Nn. intercostales, N. subcostalis, N. iliohypogastricus	• Outer surface of the Vth–VIIth rib • Proc. xiphoideus • Ligg. costoxiphoideus	• Os pubis • Symphysis pubica	Pull the thorax against the pelvis, abdominal pressing, abdominal breathing (expiration)
M. pyramidalis			
N. subcostalis, N. iliohypogastricus	Os pubis (ventral to the M. rectus abdominis)	Linea alba	Tensing of the Linea alba
Lateral muscles of the abdominal wall			
M. obliquus externus abdominis			
Nn. intercostales, N. subcostalis	Vth–XIIth ribs (outer surface)	• Iliac crest • Lig. inguinale (complete) • Os pubis • Linea alba	• Unilateral contraction: thoracic rotation (synergistically with M. obliquus internus of the contralateral side), lateral flexion (synergistically with M. internus externus on the ipsilateral side) • Bilateral contraction: pulls the thorax against the pelvis, abdominal pressing, abdominal breathing (expiration)
M. obliquus internus abdominis			
Nn. intercostales, N. subcostalis, N. iliohypogastricus, N. ilioinguinalis	• Fascia thoracolumbalis • Crista iliaca • Spinor iliaca anterior superior • Lig. inguinale (only lateral)	• IXth–XIIth ribs (lower edge) • Linea alba	• Unilateral contraction: thoracic rotation (synergistically with M. obliquus externus on the contralateral side), lateral flexion (synergistically with M. obliquus externus on the ipsilateral side) • Bilateral contraction: pulls the thorax against the pelvis, abdominal pressing, abdominal breathing (expiration) • M. cremaster: elevation of the testes
M. transversus abdominis			
Nn. intercostales, N. subcostalis, N. iliohypogastricus, N. ilioinguinalis, N. genitofemoralis	• VIIth–XIIth ribs (inner surface) • Fascia thoracolumbalis • Crista iliaca • Lig. inguinale (only lateral)	• Linea alba • Os pubis	• Unilateral contraction: torso rotation • Bilateral contraction: abdominal press, abdominal breathing (expiration) • M. cremaster: elevation of the testes
Posterior (deep) muscles of the abdominal wall			
M. quadratus lumborum			
N. subcostalis, Rr. musculares of the Plexus lumborum	• Crista iliaca • Lig. iliolumbale	• XIIth rib • Proc. costales of the lumbar vertebral body	Lateral flexion of the torso, lowering of the ribs (expiration)
M. psoas major			
Rr. musculares of the Plexus lumborum	Ist–IVth lumbar vertebras (Corpus and Proc. costalis)	Trochanter minor (together with M. iliacus)	• Unilateral contraction: sideways inclination of the torso, flexion of the hips • Bilateral contraction: elevation of the torso
M. psoas minor (inconstant)			
Rr. musculares of the Plexus lumborum	• XIIth thoracic vertebral body • Ist lumbar body	• Fascia of the M. iliopsoas • Arcus iliopectineus	• Unilateral contraction: sideways inclination of the torso • Bilateral contraction: elevation of the torso

Psoas major

The M. psoas major belongs functionally to the hip muscles and is discussed there (➤ Chap. 5.3.4). Its fascia forms a closed funnel-shaped box together with the fascia of the M. iliacus (Fascia iliopsoas), which extends from the diaphragm and from the Os ilium up to the trochanter minor. The Psoas fascia is part of the Fascia lumbalis and has cranial connections to the fascia on the diaphragm, where it is involved in the formation of the Lig. arcuatum mediale (psoas arcade, internal HALLER's arches).

M. quadratus lumborum

The M. quadratus lumborum is located adjacent to the vertebral column on the deep lamina (Lamina profunda) of the Fascia thoracolumbalis (➤ Fig. 3.23, ➤ Table 3.2). It consists of a front and a rear portion. The front part is covered by the Fascia musculi quadrati lumborum, which represents a continuation of the Fascia transversalis (see below). Medially it passes into the fascia of the M. psoas major. Cranially, the quadratus fascia is strengthened to a tendinous arch, which extends from the Proc. costalis of the Ist lumbar vertebra to the top of the XIIth rib and forms the Lig. arcuatum laterale (quadratus arcade, outer HALLER's arches).

A contraction of the muscle lowers the XIIth rib. In addition the muscle stabilises the XIIth rib during the contraction of the diaphragm and is therefore also important for inspiration. The muscle shows a large number of muscle spindles. This indicates a fine regulated muscle tension from spinal reflexes, as it is often found in support motor functions.

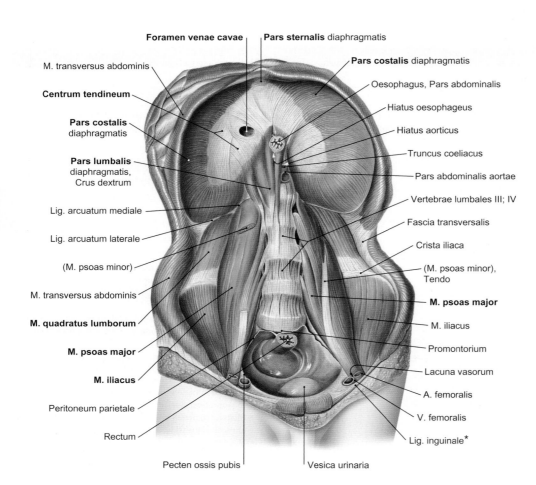

Foramen venae cavae | Pars sternalis diaphragmatis

M. transversus abdominis

Centrum tendineum

Pars costalis diaphragmatis

Pars lumbalis diaphragmatis, Crus dextrum

Lig. arcuatum mediale

Lig. arcuatum laterale

(M. psoas minor)

M. transversus abdominis

M. quadratus lumborum

M. psoas major

M. iliacus

Peritoneum parietale

Rectum

Pecten ossis pubis

Pars costalis diaphragmatis

Oesophagus, Pars abdominalis

Hiatus oesophageus

Hiatus aorticus

Truncus coeliacus

Pars abdominalis aortae

Vertebrae lumbales III; IV

Fascia transversalis

Crista iliaca

(M. psoas minor), Tendo

M. psoas major

M. iliacus

Promontorium

Lacuna vasorum

A. femoralis

V. femoralis

Lig. inguinale*

Vesica urinaria

Fig. 3.23 Diaphragm (Diaphragma) and abdominal muscles (Mm. abdominis). Ventral view. * FALLOPIAN ligament or POUPART's ligament

Functions of the abdominal muscles

Functionally the lateral abdominal muscles form through their opposite fibre course via the midline belt-shaped muscle loops in 4 levels around the abdominal cavity and brace it. The muscle loops are of functional importance in the selective contraction of different muscles parts in the *lateral flexion* or the *forward bending of the torso* (ventral flexion). They also play a major role in *torso rotation* (torsion) and therefore when throwing. Simultaneous contraction of all abdominal muscles leads to an intra-abdominal pressure increase *(abdominal pressing),* which has different functions depending on whether the glottis is opened or closed:

- In the case of a **closed glottis** the abdominal pressing supports micturition and/or defaecation (after surgical removal of the larynx patients can no longer retain air in the lungs by arbitrarily closing the glottis and have to manually close the artificially produced exit of their trachea in the throat area [tracheostoma] during abdominal pressing). The abdominal pressing is also essential during parturition and to support contractions during the expulsion phase.
- In the case of an **open glottis** the abdominal pressing can help to expel inspired air and thus to increase the volume of a vocal sound. In addition, the simultaneous contraction of all abdominal muscles when the glottis is open causes the diaphragm to bulge into the thorax, the lungs become compressed and as such exhalation is accelerated (forced expiration).

Vascular, lymphatic and nervous systems of the middle layer
Arteries

- The arteries have a segmental arrangement and run along the side of the abdominal wall ventrally. The **Aa. intercostales VI–XI** leave the corresponding ICS at the rib arch and pass between the Mm. obliquus internus abdominis et transversus abdominis forward below to the rectus sheath (➤ Fig. 3.2). On their way they emit branches to the M. obliquus externus abdominis. The terminal branches pass through the aponeuroses of the abdominal muscles to the side into the rectus sheath and supply the M. rectus abdominis. Here they anastomose with the Aa. epigastricae superiores et inferiores.
- The **A. epigastrica superior** is the continuation of the A. thoracica interna. They are usually connected within the rectus sheath on the back or side of the M. rectus abdominis with the A. epigastrica inferior.
- The **A. epigastrica inferior** exits from the A. iliaca externa shortly before it enters the Lacuna vasorum and runs on the Lig. interfoveolare (see below) in a cranial direction to the rectus sheath. On the rear surface of the abdominal wall it emits, together with its associated vein, the Plica umbilicalis lateralis (epigastrica). After entering the rectus sheath it runs on the back of the M. rectus abdominis further cranially and connects with the A. epigastrica superior approximately at the height of the centre of the rectus sheath. In its course the following emerge from the A. epigastrica inferior:
  - **A. cremasterica** (in men): it supplies the M. cremaster.
  - **A. ligamenti teretis uteri** (in women): it supplies the Lig. teres uteri.

– **R. pubicus:** it extends to the pubic bone.
– **R. obturatorius:** it normally forms an anastomosis with the R. pubicus of the A. obturatoria.
• Another branch for blood supply to the abdominal wall musculature in the lower section (➤ Fig. 3.41) is the **A. circumflexa ilium profunda**. It extends with a **R. ascendens** between the M. obliquus internus and the M. transversus abdominis and connects here with the Aa. lumbales, of the A. iliolumbalis and the A. epigastrica inferior.

> **Clinical remarks**
>
> A **Corona mortis** (lat. wreath of death) is an ectopic origin of the A. obturatoria from the A. epigastrica inferior. In this case, a powerful R. obturatorius of the A. epigastrica inferior replaces the unformed A. obturatoria. This common vessel variation (up to 30%) used to frequently lead to fatal bleeding in surgery on the groin (predominantly in leg hernias).

Veins
The abovementioned arteries are accompanied by ordered veins running segmentally (**Vv. intercostales VI–XI, Vv. epigastrica superior, Vv. epigastrica inferior**) (➤ Fig. 3.2, ➤ Fig. 3.14). The Vv. epigastricae superiores drain into the Vv. thoracicae internae; the Vv. epigastricae inferiores pass into the v. iliaca externa.

Lymph vessels
The lymph of the middle and deep layers of the lateral abdominal wall drain into the

– **Nodi lymphoidei iliaci communes**
– **Nodi lymphoidei lumbales**.
The lymph of the abdominal wall flows into lymph vessels that accompany the Vasa epigastrica and which drain into the
– **Nodi lymphoidei epigastrici inferiores**
– **Nodi lymphoidei parasternales**.

Innervation
The innervation of the middle layer of the abdominal wall takes place via (➤ Fig. 3.24):
• **Nn. intercostales V–XI:** they run together with the intercostal vessels between the M. obliquus internus abdominis and m. transversus abdominis. Their branches innervate the lateral abdominal muscles and after penetration of the rectus sheath the M. rectus abdominis.
• **N. subcostalis:** it runs like the Nn. intercostales V–XI and innervates the lateral abdominal muscles and the M. rectus abdominis. It is also involved in the innervation of the M. quadratus lumborum and the M. pyramidalis.
• **N. iliohypogastricus:** the muscle branch of the N. iliohypogastricus extends between the M. obliquus internus abdominis and M. transversus abdominis, which it also innervates, medially and also innervates the M. rectus abdominis and the M. pyramidalis.
• **N. ilioinguinalis:** it extends on the top inside edge of the Os ilium between M. obliquus internus abdominis and M. transversus abdominis while emitting muscle branches medially. At the level of the Spina iliaca anterior superior it penetrates the M. obliquus internus abdominis and runs parallel to the Lig. inguinale caudally covered by the external aponeuroses. In men, the nerve

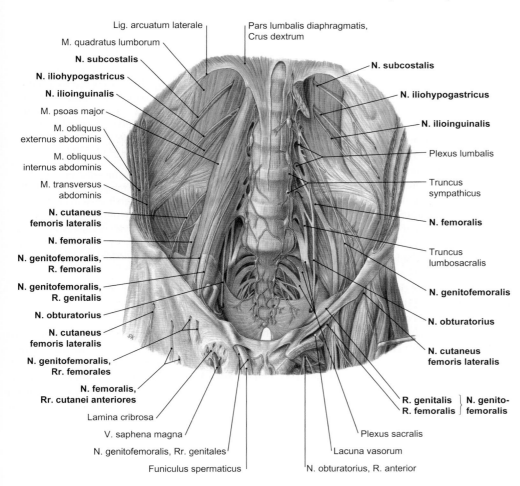

Fig. 3.24 Nerve branches for innervation of abdominal wall muscles. Ventral view.

joins the Funiculus spermaticus, in women it runs with the Lig. teres uteri. In the area of the Anulus inguinalis superficialis it leaves the inguinal canal and divides into its terminal branches (Nn. scrotales anteriores or Nn. labiales anteriores).

- **N. genitofemoralis:** its R. genitalis extends over the Fossa inguinalis lateralis to the inguinal canal. Shortly before entering, it emits muscle branches to the M. transversus abdominis and innervates the M. cremaster in the inguinal canal (see below).

NOTE

Rapid stroking of the abdominal skin of the relaxed patient, lying on his/her back with a pointed object (tip of the reflex hammer, rods and back of the fingernail) from lateral to medial triggers the **abdominal skin reflex** of the equilateral abdominal muscles. This belongs to the physiological foreign reflexes. An examination is conducted on both sides below the ribs, at the height of the navel and above the groin. Absence can provide important clinical evidence (e.g. on a pyramid tract lesion).

Clinical remarks

The Nn. ilioinguinalis and iliohypogastricus from the Plexus lumbalis break through the M. transversus abdominis dorsal to the kidneys and then run ventrally between the M. transversus abdominis and M. obliquus internus abdominis. **Damage to the nerves** during dorsal surgical access to the retroperitoneal space (e.g. kidneys, adrenal glands) can cause postoperative pain in the groin area or lead to an abdominal wall weakness on the affected side.
For the treatment of pain or in the context of inguinal hernia surgery, the N. ilioinguinalis medial of the Spina iliaca anterior superior can be blocked using infiltration anaesthesia. Because of its close proximity, the N. iliohypogastricus it often simultaneously blocked.

Rectus sheath
The paired **rectus sheath (Vagina musculi recti abdominis)** is a connective tissue guide tube, in which the M. rectus abdominis and the M. pyramidalis are located. It is formed by the lateral abdominal muscles and the abdominal wall fascia (➤ Fig. 3.20, ➤ Fig. 3.21, ➤ Fig. 3.22). The tube consists of a **front (Lamina anterior)** and a **rear lamina (Lamina posterior).** Slightly below the navel (**Linea arcuata,** Linea semicircularis, DOUGLAS' line, it is sometimes not a clear line but a transition zone, Zona arcuata) the structure changes (➤ Fig. 3.22). Above the Linea arcuata, the Lamina anterior of the rectus sheath is formed from the aponeurosis of the M. obliquus externus abdominis and the front lamina of the aponeurosis of the M. obliquus internus abdominis; below the Linea/Zona arcuata the rear lamina of the internus aponeuroses and the transversus aponeuroses are involved in the formation of the Lamina anterior of the rectus sheath (➤ Table 3.3, ➤ Fig. 3.25). The Lamina posterior above the Linea/Zona arcuata consists of the rear lamina of the aponeurosis of the M. obliquus internus abdominis, M. transversus abdominis, Fascia transversalis and Peritoneum parietale; below the Linea/Zona arcuata only the Fascia transversalis and the Peritoneum parietale are involved (➤ Table 3.3, ➤ Fig. 3.25). The medial edge of the rectus sheath is formed by the **Linea alba** (see below); the lateral edge, which represents the transition zone of the lateral abdominal muscles in their aponeuroses, is the **Linea semilunaris** (➤ Fig. 3.22). The transversus fascia between Linea arcuata and lateral edge of the rectus sheath is referred to clinically as SPIEGHEL fascia.

Table 3.3 Structure of the rectus sheath.

Above Linea/Zona arcuata	Below Linea/Zona arcuata
Lamina anterior	
Aponeurosis of the M. obliquus externus abdominis	Aponeurosis of the M. obliquus externus abdominis
Anterior lamina of the aponeurosis of the M. obliquus internus abdominis	Anterior lamina of the aponeurosis of the M. obliquus internus abdominis
	Posterior lamina of the aponeurosis of the M. obliquus internus abdominis
	Aponeurosis of the M. transversus abdominis
Lamina posterior	
Posterior lamina of the aponeurosis of the M. obliquus internus abdominis	
Aponeurosis of the M. transversus abdominis	
Fascia transversalis	Fascia transversalis
Parietal peritoneum	Parietal peritoneum

Clinical remarks

The area of the abdominal wall is frequently the site of formation of **hernias.** They are characterised by:
- A **hernial sac** (bulge of the Peritoneum parietale)
- A **hernial ring** or hernial canal (preformed or acquired gap in the abdominal wall)
- A **hernial content** (e. g. intestinal components, internal organs)

The hernial sac pushes through the hernial ring or hernial canal to the outside and can contain hernial contents. Approximately 10% of all hernias are scar hernias following surgery or via the abdominal wall. The incisions are often quite large to attain good access and optimal visibility into the abdominal cavity and to be able to display the contents. The most common incision is the central craniocaudal incision from the Proc. xiphoideus up to the Symphysis pubica in the area of the Linea alba. It enables large-scale access to the entire abdominal cavity contents with exploratory laparotomy; however, laparotomy has receded into the background in favour of a far less invasive laparoscopy. In **laparoscopy** the abdominal wall is only cut in a few points to be in a position to inspect the stomach contents by means of optics that are introduced through small abdominal wall cuts. Using inserted instruments it is now possible, e.g. to remove the gall bladder (cholecystectomy) or the appendix. The patient can also be discharged much earlier, and the rate of complications (e.g. developing a post-operative incisional hernia) is significantly lower.
Rarely a **SPIGELIAN hernia** can occur between the lateral margin of the Linea arcuata and Linea semilunaris.

Linea alba
The interdependence of the tight connective tissue of all aponeuroses of the flat stomach muscles of both sides in the median plane forms the **Linea alba.** It is 1–3 cm wide and runs from the Proc. xiphoideus up to the Symphysis pubica, where it enters via the triangular Adminiculum lineae albae (Lig. triangulare) at the Lig. pubicum superius. It is slightly wider only around the navel, where it is interrupted by the umbilical port. It is significantly narrower below the navel.

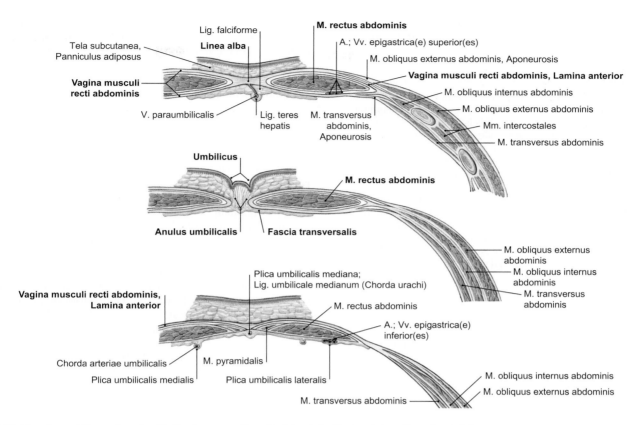

Fig. 3.25 Structure of the rectus sheath, Vagina musculi recti abdominis. Horizontal section; Caudal view.

Clinical remarks

A **Diastasis recti abdominis** is the separation of the two Mm. recti abdominis by more than 2 cm in the area of the Linea alba. It can be either congenital or acquired and occurs more often in women and above the Linea arcuata than below:

- Causes of acquired Diastasis recti abdominis are pregnancy and birth (in particular multiple births, strong pressing), obesity and chronic constipation. With increasing enlargement of the Diastasis recti, the abdominal muscles become increasingly insufficient and it also predisposes to abdominal wall hernias (see below).
- The physiological Diastasis recti abdominis in a normal pregnancy (from the 5th month of pregnancy), which occurs in nearly every pregnant woman and gradually regresses after birth, should be differentiated from those pathological forms of Diastasis recti that do not recede. Regression exercises can be beneficial here.

The abdominal wall in abdominal cavity operations can be opened along the Linea alba without causing any major bleeding **(median laparotomy).**

Umbilicus

Structure of the abdominal wall

Around the **navel (Umbilicus)** in adults, there is a special structure around the abdominal wall: the outer skin is fused above the **umbilical papilla (Papilla umbilicalis,** an opening in the Linea alba) with the Fascia umbilicalis (a consolidation of the Fascia transversalis) directly with the Peritoneum parietale. At this point, since the subcutaneous adipose tissue is missing, there is an **umbilical recess.** The umbilical recess is surrounded by circularly running connective tissue fibres of the Linea alba, which form the easily palpable **navel ring (Anulus umbilicalis).**

Development

Between the *3rd and 4th week,* the entodermal germinal layer bulges inwards and forms the central gut (precursor of the small intestines). Initially, the connection between the midgut and yolk sac is still large, but increasingly becomes a narrow tube (yolk sac stalk **Ductus vitellinus, Ductus omphaloentericus,** body stalk). The attachment point of the amnion is reduced around the Ductus vitellinus at the ventral embryo surface to a narrow oval area (umbilical ring) and also the connection between the intra-embryonic and extra-embryonic coelom will soon be only a narrow connection, which circularly surrounds the yolk sac stalk. The navel and the umbilical cord (contains extra-embryonic coelom = navel coelom, yolk corridor, system for navel vessels and allantoin) have evolved. In the first instance, the amnion supplies the epithelial surface of the umbilical cord. Due to its good blood supply via the A. mesenterica superior, the midgut grows relatively quickly in the abdominal cavity. The maturing liver and mesonephros are already there. The space is not sufficient and the midgut deviates depending on the path of least resistance into the navel coelom (the evolving umbilical cord). A **developmental umbilical hernia** occurs (the term physiological umbilical hernia is inaccurate and should not be used for this purpose). This process takes place in the *6th-10th week.* In doing so, the gut is not only displaced to the umbilical cord, but it also rotates through 90° counter-clockwise around the A. mesenterica superior. At the end of the 10th week the gut can be brought back, because in the meantime the abdominal cavity has become sufficiently large. The extra-embryonic coelom and the yolk sac obliterate completely. During the foetal period the strong **Aa. umbilicales** and the **V. umbilicalis** run through the navel. Both arteries are fused to the navel ring here; the V. umbilicalis is, in contrast, only loosely connected with the navel ring. After birth, and separation of the umbilical cord, rapid obliteration and accretion take place; the remnants of the severed umbilical vessels form a firm closure of the navel together with the navel ring and the skin.

Clinical remarks

If the gut does not completely shift back into the abdominal cavity at the end of the 10th week, this results in an **omphalocele** (congenital omphalocele). This is an inhibition malformation with an incidence of 1:5000. The abdominal wall lies outside a bladder surrounded by an amnion, which contains bowel loops, mesentery and branches of the A. mesenterica superior (internal organs such as the liver or spleen are rarely included).

In contrast to an omphalocele a **congenital umbilical hernia** is covered by skin. The hernial ring is the not yet formed umbilical papilla. **Acquired umbilical hernias** occur in adults due to the separation of the connective tissue from the umbilical papilla in pronounced hyperextension of the abdominal wall (pregnancy, obesity). The hernial ring is, in this case, the navel ring.

Deep layer

The deep layer comprises the inner lining of the abdominal wall. It involves:

- Fascia transversalis
- Peritoneum parietale

Fascia transversalis

The Fascia transversalis is not only a rough muscle fascia on the inner surface of the muscle part of the M. transversalis but also covers all muscles and structures that limit the abdominal wall. Therefore, we speak of the **Fascia abdominis interna.** Dorsally, the Mm. quadratus lumborum et psoas major are covered by the Fascia transversalis. In addition, it extends over the lumbar spine and participates ventrally in the establishment of the rectus sheath. Here it is fused above the Linea arcuata with the aponeurosis of the M. transversus abdominis; below it the transversus aponeuroses and Fascia transversalis are separate. The transversus aponeuroses connects below the Linea arcuata with the aponeuroses of M. obliquus internus abdominis and M. obliquus externus abdominis and run in front of the M. rectus abdominis. The Fascia transversalis runs further caudally and, together with the Peritoneum parietale forms the rear lamina of the rectus sheath in this area. Around the navel the Fascia transversalis is reinforced to the Fascia umbilicalis. Cranially, the Fascia transversalis continues into the Fascia diaphragmatica; caudally, it is secured to the Lig. inguinale and passes into the Fascia iliaca. At the inner inguinal ring (see below) the Fascia transversalis bulges into the inguinal canal and runs as the Fascia spermatica interna enveloping the spermatic cord to the testes.

Peritoneum parietale

The peritoneum is a serous skin, which ensures the smooth sliding of the organs in the abdominal cavity. It is divided into a visceral lamina (**Peritoneum viscerale**), which covers the abdominal organs, and a parietal lamina (**Peritoneum parietale**), which covers the front and side abdominal cavity wall. It is divided from the Fascia transversalis by a **Tela subserosa**, which is developed to a differing degree depending on the region. Above the navel (especially Linea alba) and around the navel the Tela subserosa is so thin that the Peritoneum parietale and Fascia transversalis are connected almost immoveably.

Vascular, lymphatic and nervous systems of the deep layer

Vessel supply lymph drainage and innervation correspond to the middle layer of the abdominal wall.

Inguinal region

The groin (inguinal region, Regio inguinalis) includes the transitional area between the abdominal wall and thigh. This includes not only the inguinal ligament (Lig. inguinale), but also the osteofibrous canal lying beneath the inguinal ligament, which is separated by a connective tissue separation of the inguinal ligament (**Arcus iliopectineus**) into a medial access site for vessels (**Lacuna vasorum**) and a lateral access site for muscles (**Lacuna musculorum**).

Inguinal ligament

The **inguinal ligament (Lig. inguinale)** is made of firm collagenous connective tissue and spans between the Spina iliaca anterior superior and Tuberculum pubicum (➤ Fig. 3.26, also ➤ Chap. 5.10.1, ➤ Fig. 5.71). It forms the floor of the inguinal canal (see below). Covering skin and inguinal ligament are fused mainly by tight Retinacula cutis; subcutaneous fat tissue is extensively lacking, so that the Lig. inguinale is easily palpable. The Lig. inguinale is not a ligament in the true sense, but a fusion of different fibrous structures:

- Lower section of the aponeurose of the M. obliquus externus abdominis
- Lower section of the fused aponeuroses of the M. obliquus internus abdominis and M. transversus abdominis
- Fascia transversalis (medial)
- Fascia iliopsoas (lateral)
- Fascia lata (caudal)

At the medial margin of the inguinal ligament a small part of the fibres from the inferior margin of the inguinal ligament extends in a downward curve to the Os pubis. This fibre content, the **Lig. lacunare** (➤ Fig. 5.71), medially limits the Lacuna vasorum. The fixing of the Lig. lacunare on Pecten ossis pubis is referred to as the Llig. pectineum. The abovementioned **Arcus iliopectineus** is a curved connective tissue structure and part of the Fascia iliaca. It spans between the Lig. inguinale and Eminentia iliopubica and demarcates the Lacuna musculorum from the Lacuna vasorum (➤ Chap. 5.10.1, ➤ Fig. 5.71 for penetrating structures).

Inguinal canal

The **inguinal canal (Canalis inguinalis)** is approx. 4–5 cm long and penetrates through the abdominal wall at an oblique angle from the top externally to the bottom internally. In men, the spermatic cord runs through the inguinal canal; in women the Lig. teres uteri together with lymph vessels passes from the tube angle on both sides of the Labia majora via the inguinal canal. The structures penetrating the canal normally fill the canal completely and are usually connected with it via loose connective tissue. **Entry and exit points** for the inguinal canal are:

- **Internal inguinal ring (Anulus inguinalis profundus):** it is visible as a deepening on the inside of the abdominal wall, in the Fossa inguinalis lateralis (see below). Its medial border is strengthened by the Lig. interfoveolare (sickle-shaped reinforcement of the Fascia transversalis) and by the muscle fibres of the M. transversus abdominis (M. interfoveolaris). More muscle fibres of the M. transversus abdominis also wind around the inner inguinal ring, which is referred to as the transversus loop.
- **Outer inguinal ring (Anulus inguinalis superficialis):** it enters through the aponeurosis of the M. obliquus externus abdominis. At this point, the aponeurosis forms 2 connective tissue legs

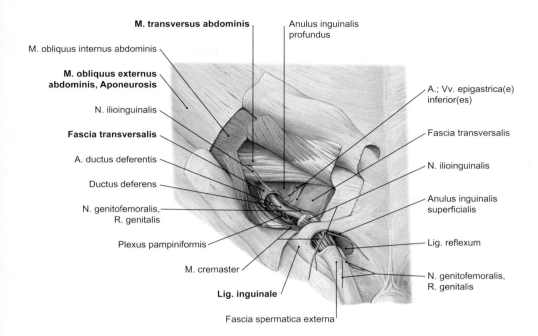

Fig. 3.26 **Walls and contents of the inguinal canal (Canalis inguinalis), right.** Ventral view. [S010-17]

(Crus mediale and Crus laterale), which are held together at the top with other connective tissue fibres of the M. obliquus externus abdominis (Fibrae intercrurales). Below the legs are held together by a trench-type tendon plate (Lig. reflexum).

The **walls of the inguinal canal** are formed (➤ Fig. 3.26):

- **Above:** under the edge of the M. obliquus internus abdominis and M. transversus abdominis and its fused aponeuroses; the roof is laterally structured from muscle fibres, medially from connective tissue
- **Bottom:** Lig. inguinale and medial Lig. reflexum
- **Front:** aponeurosis of the M. obliquus externus abdominis with Fibrae intercrurales
- **Rear:** Fascia transversalis, subserous connective tissue and Peritoneum parietale, reinforced by the Lig. interfoveolare with the M. interfoveolaris; hence, a muscle-free triangle is formed when viewed from the inside (Trigonum inguinale, HESSELBACH's triangle)

Development

Spermatogenesis requires a lower temperature than the average body temperature of approximately 37 °C. Therefore, the testes shift during the foetal period outside the abdominal cavity. For this purpose, the testes migrate along the lower Gubernaculum testis under the Peritoneum parietale at the side of the body wall into the scrotum downwards and partially take the abdominal wall layers with them (➤ Fig. 3.27). The Peritoneum parietale forms a pouch in the inguinal canal (Proc. vaginalis peritonei), reaching down to the scrotum and ending above the testes. With the exception of a remnant in the testis region (Tunica vaginalis testis), the Proc. vaginalis peritonei obliterates shortly after birth.

Clinical remarks

Disorders of Descensus testis are frequent (approximately 3% of all newborns). The testicles can lie in the abdominal cavity or in the inguinal canal (testicular retention, cryptorchidism, ectopic testis) and fertility problems and an increased risk of malignant degeneration may occur. The Descensus testis into the scrotum is a sign of foetal maturity at birth.

Covering of the spermatic cord and the scrotum

The spermatic cord (Funiculus spermaticus) and testicles (testis) lie in a pouch of the abdominal wall which extends into the scrotum caused by the descensus testis. The spermatic cord and scrotum are therefore constructed in the same way as the abdominal wall. In this process the following structures become separated (➤ Fig. 3.28):

- **Fascia spermatica externa:** this is a continuation of the lower portion of the aponeurosis of the M. obliquus externus abdominis on the Funiculus spermaticus.
- **Fascia cremasterica with M. cremaster:** the M. cremaster with its fascia forms a separation of the lower portion of the M.

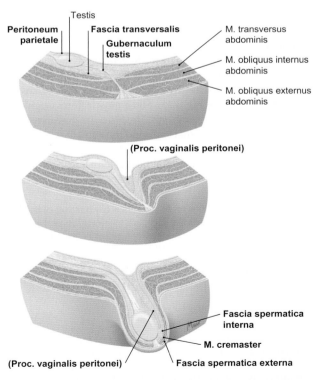

Fig. 3.27 **Descensus testis from the 7th week (postconception) until delivery.**

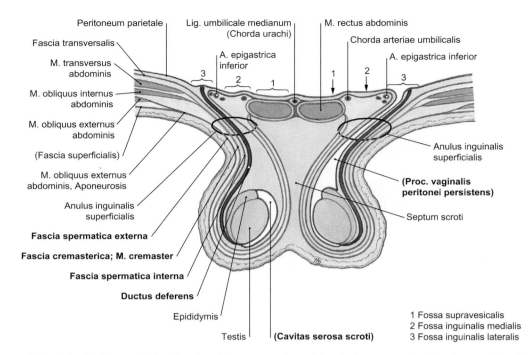

Peritoneum parietale
Fascia transversalis
M. transversus abdominis
M. obliquus internus abdominis
M. obliquus externus abdominis
(Fascia superficialis)
M. obliquus externus abdominis, Aponeurosis
Anulus inguinalis superficialis
Fascia spermatica externa
Fascia cremasterica; M. cremaster
Fascia spermatica interna
Ductus deferens
Epididymis
Testis
(Cavitas serosa scroti)

Lig. umbilicale medianum (Chorda urachi)
A. epigastrica inferior
M. rectus abdominis
Chorda arteriae umbilicalis
A. epigastrica inferior
Anulus inguinalis superficialis
(Proc. vaginalis peritonei persistens)
Septum scroti

1 Fossa supravesicalis
2 Fossa inguinalis medialis
3 Fossa inguinalis lateralis

Fig. 3.28 Structure of the abdominal wall and the sheaths of the spermatic cord (Funiculus spermaticus) and testes (Testis). Schematic presentation. [L240]

obliquus internus abdominis. Often lower muscle fibres of the m. transversus abdominis also participate in this.

- **Fascia spermatica interna:** this continues the Fascia transversalis and envelopes the Funiculus spermaticus.
- **Vestigium processus vaginalis:** this relates to a Proc. vaginalis peritonei, which is obliterated with the exception of a remnant in the testicular region (Tunica vaginalis testis with Lamina parietalis = Periorchium and Lamina visceralis = Epiorchium).

The content of the Funiculus spermaticus, the structure of the Tunica dartos, the blood supply, the lymph drainage and the innervation of the testes and the scrotum are outlined in ➤ Chap. 8.5.

M. cremaster

The M. cremaster is innervated by the R. genitalis of the N. genitofemoralis and emerges from the lower fibres of the M. obliquus internus abdominis and usually from fibres of the M. transversus abdominis (➤ Fig. 3.21, ➤ Fig. 3.26). Some muscle fibres originate at the front lamina of the rectus sheath. The fibres are positioned in men as single muscle fibres that surround the Funiculus spermaticus between the Fascia spermatica externa and Fascia spermatica interna to the scrotum. In women they join the Lig. teres uteri.

NOTE

Stroking of the inside of the thigh triggers a contraction of the M. cremaster **(cremasteric reflex)**. This causes elevation of the testicles on the same lamina. The cremasteric reflex is one of the physiological extrinsic reflex actions. Afferent fibres run in the R. femoralis of the N. genitofemoralis and the efferent fibres in the R. genitalis of the N. genitofemoralis.

Clinical remarks

The inguinal canal is a predilection site for hernias **(Inguinal hernias)**. A distinction is made between indirect and direct inguinal hernias depending on the hernial ring:

- **Indirect inguinal hernias (canal hernias)** are the most common abdominal wall hernias in adulthood (approximately

two thirds of all hernias) and occur primarily in men. During this process, the hernial sac in the Fossa inguinalis lateralis passes through the Anulus inguinalis profundus into the inguinal canal or completely through the inguinal canal up into the scrotum or the Labia majora (➤ Fig. 3.29). The hernial ring is identical to the inner inguinal ring and lies lateral to the Vasa epigastrica inferiora. Since these vessels in the surgical site are easy to identify, they are referred to as lateral inguinal hernias (Herniae inguinales laterales). Indirect hernias can also occur innately. In this case the Proc. vaginalis testis is not closed, but persists (Proc. vaginalis peritonei persistens ➤ Fig. 3.28). There is an open connection between the abdominal cavity and Cavitas serosa scroti, through which the hernia content can advance into the scrotum. In general, however, indirect hernias are acquired.

- **Direct inguinal hernia** (about one third of all hernias) penetrate through the muscle-free trigonum inguinale (HESSELBACH's triangle, ➤ Fig. 3.31) into the Fossa inguinalis medialis which is a weak spot, because the abdominal wall here only consists of the Fascia transversalis and Peritoneum parietale. Because the hernial ring lies medial of the Vasa epigastrica inferiora, one also talks about medial inguinal hernias (Herniae inguinales mediales, ➤ Fig. 3.29).

Side hernias (approx. 10% of all hernias) are more frequent in women. The hernial ring is in contrast to inguinal hernias beneath the Lig. inguinale either in the Lacuna vasorum (more frequently) or the Lacuna musculorum (less frequently).

NOTE

Preferred points for **abdominal wall hernias** are in the inguinal canal (80%), the side channel (10%), the navel (5%), the Linea alba (5%), the Linea semilunaris, the Canalis obturatorius and the Trigonum lumbale (the latter 3 together under 1%). In the case of inguinal hernias, a distinction is made between direct and indirect inguinal hernias. Indirect inguinal hernias are the most common abdominal wall hernias in adulthood (approximately two thirds of all hernias) and are more common in men. The hernial sac follows the course of the inguinal canal. Direct inguinal hernia (about one third of all hernias) break through the abdominal wall directly into the Fossa inguinalis medialis, i.e. not through the inner inguinal ring.

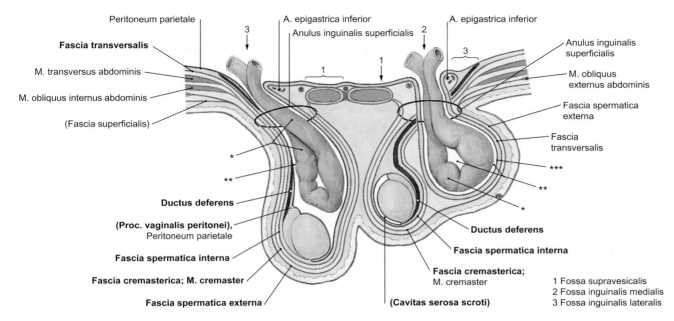

Fig. 3.29 Hernias, schematic presentation. Left image: lateral, indirect hernia; right image: medial, direct hernia; [L240]
* Intestinal loop in the hernial sac, ** peritoneal space, *** newly formed peritoneal hernia sac. [L240]

Inner outline of the abdominal wall

The abdominal wall has on its inside a distinctive inner outline of folds and recesses, all of which are covered by the Peritoneum parietale (➤ Fig. 3.30, ➤ Fig. 3.31). Behind the symphysis the bladder body (Corpus vesicae) protrudes. When moderately filled it has a transversus furrow (Plica vesicalis transversa). In addition, the following folds can be defined on the inside of the abdominal wall:

- **Plica umbilicalis mediana** (unpaired): this runs from the vertex of the bladder to the navel and contains the Lig. umbilicale medianum, which has emerged from the obliteration of the former urachus, which runs from the bladder to the navel (original urinary passage).
- **Plica umbilicalis medialis** (paired): this runs from the lateral bladder wall to the navel and contains the Lig. umbilicale later-

ale, which emerged from the obliteration of the former A. umbilicalis. In some cases, the A. umbilicalis can still be preserved.

- **Plica umbilicalis lateralis** (paired): this arises from the course of the Vasa epigastric inferiora, coming from the Vasa iliaca externa and passing to the back wall of the rectus sheath, and thus has no connection to the navel. In the lower section of the Plica umbilicalis lateralis, the Fascia transversalis is reinforced by the **Lig. interfoveolare (HESSELBACH's ligament)** (➤ Fig. 3.30, ➤ Fig. 3.31) and by the M. interfoveolaris. Both structures are divisions of the M. transversus abdominis and limit the muscle-free triangle (Trigonum inguinale, HESSELBACH's triangle) (➤ Fig. 3.30, ➤ Fig. 3.31).

Between the folds and lateral to the Plica umbilicalis lateralis the following recesses can be defined (➤ Fig. 3.30):

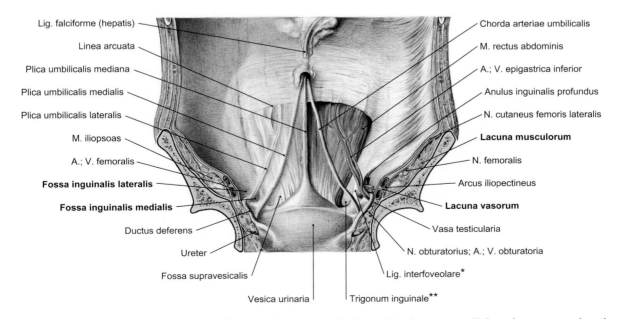

Fig. 3.30 Anterior abdominal wall. View from the inside; The Peritoneum parietale and Fascia transversalis have been removed on the right side of the body; * HESSELBACH's ligament, ** HESSELBACH's triangle.

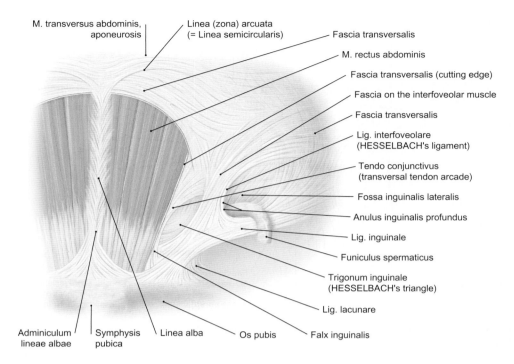

Fig. 3.31 Anterior abdominal wall. View from the inside; right side; Peritoneum parietale and Fascia transversalis have been partially removed; presentation of HESSELBACH's ligament and HESSELBACH's triangle. [L127]

- **Fossa supravesicalis** (paired): it is located between the Plica umbilicalis mediana and Plica umbilicalis medialis.
- **Fossa inguinalis medialis** (pair, medial inguinal recess): It is located between the Plica umbilicalis medialis and Plica umbilicalis lateralis in the area of the muscle-free triangle (HESSELBACH's triangle) (➤ Fig. 3.30, ➤ Fig. 3.31).
- **Fossa inguinalis lateralis** (pair, lateral inguinal recess): It is located laterally to the Plica umbilicalis lateralis. The inner inguinal ring (Anulus inguinalis profundus) lies within it. In addition, the structures involved in the development of the spermatic cord run together below the Peritoneum parietale. At the Anulus inguinalis profundus the Fascia transversalis lowers into the inguinal canal and becomes the Fascia spermatica interna.

In addition to the 5 lower abdominal wall folds an upper fold on the inner abdominal wall extends from the navel to the liver. It contains the **Lig. teres hepatis,** which represents the obliterated V. umbilicalis (➤ Fig. 3.30).

Clinical remarks

The technique formerly commonly practiced for **inguinal hernia surgery** (SHOULDICE's technique) doubling of the Fascia transversalis fascia in the HESSELBACH's triangle for reinforcement of the rear wall of the inguinal canal is now almost a thing of the past. It has been replaced by minimally invasive techniques such as the TEPP (total extraperitoneal patch plastic) or the TAPP procedure (transabdominal preperitoneal hernioplasty). As part of the TEPP an endoscopy (in contrast to TAPP) is conducted on the abdominal wall through 2–3 incisions. Within the framework of the operation a thin plastic mesh is laid between the layers of the abdominal wall (behind the M. transversus and under the Peritoneum parietale). The advantage of this surgical procedure is the immediate ability to sustain pressure, which generally makes it possible to do even intense sport within 1 week. Surgery is open, the LICHTENSTEIN's operation is generally used in which a mesh is also inserted. Due to the good results and the excellent compatibility of the meshes, these are used substantially today in operative inguinal hernia surgery.

3.2 Dorsal torso wall
Friedrich Paulsen, Jens Waschke

3.2.1 General structure

Depending on fitness, the back outline is basically formed by the back muscles on the surface, the M. trapezius, Mm. rhomboidei, M. latissimus dorsi and M. teres major. The expansion of the back area ranges from the Linea nuchalis superior at the Os occipitale to the Os coccygis along the spine and laterally to the dorsally visible part of the thoracic and abdominal wall.

Surface anatomy
Lines and palpable bone points are used for guidance and for height localisation.

Orientation lines
Vertically running orientation lines on the dorsal abdominal wall are (➤ Fig. 1.6):
- Linea mediana posterior (via the spinous processes)
- Linea paravertebralis (via the vertebral transverse processes)
- Linea scapularis (through the Angulus inferior of the Scapula with relaxed hanging arms)

Palpable bone points
Palpable bone points on the dorsal abdominal wall are:
- Spina scapulae (lies on both sides just under the skin, and can be traced laterally to the acromion); a horizontal line between the two spinae scapulae is at the height of the spinous process of the IIIrd thoracic vertebra
- Angulus superior scapulae (moves when the arms are moved)
- Margo medialis scapulae (moves when the arms are moved)
- Angulus inferior scapulae (moves when the arms are moved)
- Vertebra prominens (spinous process of the VIIth cervical vertebra)
- Ribs

- Crista iliaca
- Spina iliaca posterior superior
- Tuber ischiadicum
- Os sacrum
- Procc. spinosi

Surface relief

The skin on the back has a rough corium and is therefore relatively thick. In the Regio vertebralis the surface outline is defined by the back groove and the laterally lying autochthonous back muscles (> Chap. 3.2.2). The Fascia thoracolumbalis lies lumbarly above the autochthonous back muscles (> Chap. 3.2.2). The superficial back muscles define the outline laterally up to the neck area, as already mentioned above. Where the Regio vertebralis passes into the Regio sacralis, the sacral triangle is formed in men and the MICHAELIS rhomboid (Venus rhomboid) in women. The sacral triangle and Venus rhomboid are created from palpable bone points lying directly under the skin without underlying muscles or subcutaneous fatty tissue. The points resemble groove-like indentations.

Sacral triangle

The sacral triangle (> Fig. 3.32) is formed by:
- The two Spinae iliacae posteriores superiores
- the start of the Crena ani (vertical gap between the buttocks, anal groove)

MICHAELIS' rhomboid

The MICHAELIS' rhomboid (> Fig. 3.32) is formed by:
- The dimple-shaped indentation of skin above the spinous process of the IVth or Vth lumbar vertebra
- The two Spinae iliacae posteriores superiores

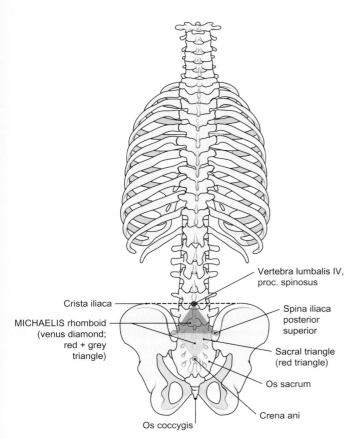

Fig. 3.32 Tactile and visible bone points of the MICHAELIS rhomboid and the sacral triangle. Dorsal view. [L126]

Crista iliaca

MICHAELIS rhomboid (venus diamond; red + grey triangle)

Vertebra lumbalis IV, proc. spinosus

Spina iliaca posterior superior

Sacral triangle (red triangle)

Os sacrum

Crena ani

Os coccygis

- The start of the Crena ani

Spinal regions

The neck section of the spinal region is referred to as the neck region (Regio cervicalis posterior, Regio colli, Regio nuchae) (> Fig. 1.4b). The muscles of this area are discussed in > Chap. 3.2.2, blood supply and topographic aspects in > Chap. 10. Other regions of the dorsal abdominal wall are the Regiones vertebralis, scapularis, infrascapularis, lumbalis, sacralis et glutealis (> Fig. 1.4b). There are 2 weak points in the Regio lumbalis (> Fig. 3.33):
- The **upper lumbar triangle** (Trigonum lumbale superius, GRYNFELT triangle, Trigonum lumbale fibrosum, spatium tendineum lumbale) has the following limits:
  - Cranial: the XIIth rib
  - Lateral: M. obliquus internus abdominis
  - Medial: autochthonous back muscles
  - Base: original aponeurosis of the M. transversus abdominis
  - Coverage: M. serratus posterior inferior, M. latissimus dorsi
- The **lower lumbar triangle** (Trigonum lumbale inferius, PETIT triangle) has the following limits:
  - Medial: edge of the M. latissimus dorsi
  - Lateral: rear edge of the M. obliquus externus abdominis
  - Caudal: Crista iliaca
  - Base: original aponeurosis of the M. transversus abdominis and Fascia transversalis with Peritoneum parietale

3.2.2 Back muscles

Overview

All muscles on the dorsal side of the torso are referred to as **back muscles** (Mm. dorsi). This also includes the muscles of the throat area, which topographically lie in the Regio cervicalis posterior and thus at the neck, but due to their course systematically correspond with the back muscles.

The back muscles form 2 layers that differ developmentally and functionally:
- The **deep back muscles** are already created on the dorsal side of the torso. Therefore they are referred to as primary or autochthonous (= local) back muscles (Mm. dorsi proprii). They are innervated by the R. posterior of the spinal nerves, are used for the correction and extension of the torso and are functionally collectively known as 'M. erector spinae'.
- In contrast, the **superficial back muscles** develop not at the back but on the ventral torso wall, the arm position or arise from the material for the formation of the soft tissues of the head and only

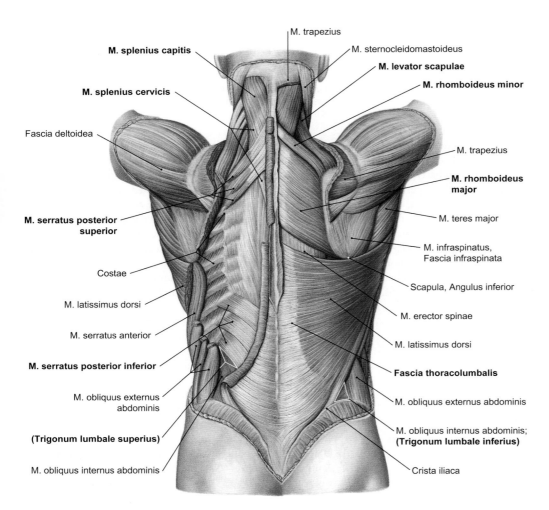

M. splenius capitis

M. trapezius

M. sternocleidomastoideus

M. levator scapulae

M. splenius cervicis

M. rhomboideus minor

Fascia deltoidea

M. trapezius

M. rhomboideus major

M. serratus posterior superior

M. teres major

M. infraspinatus, Fascia infraspinata

Costae

Scapula, Angulus inferior

M. latissimus dorsi

M. erector spinae

M. serratus anterior

M. latissimus dorsi

M. serratus posterior inferior

Fascia thoracolumbalis

M. obliquus externus abdominis

M. obliquus externus abdominis

(Trigonum lumbale superius)

M. obliquus internus abdominis; **(Trigonum lumbale inferius)**

M. obliquus internus abdominis

Crista iliaca

Fig. 3.33 Deep layer of the torso arm and torso shoulder girdle muscles. Dorsal view. The M. trapezius has been removed on the right side of the body, the Mm. rhomboidei and the M. latissimus dorsi from the left side of the body.

shift to the back during the development as secondary back muscles. They are innervated according to their original territory from the R. anterior of the spinal nerves, from the Plexus brachialis or the N. accessorius [XI]. Most superficial back muscles are used mainly for the upper extremities and are therefore functional parts of the shoulder and shoulder girdle muscles.

> **NOTE**
> The back muscles are divided into two layers:
> - The **primary (= autochthonous) back muscles** lie deep and are innervated by the R. posterior of the spinal nerves. They are used for the correction and extension of the torso (M. erector spinae).
> - The **secondary (= immigrant) back muscles** lie superficially and are innervated by the Rr. anterior of the spinal nerves, from the Plexus brachialis or the cranial nerves. They are used for the movement of the upper extremity and the ribs.

Both the deep and the superficial back muscles can be divided into systems that are useful for understanding the function of individual muscle groups.

Autochthonous (deep) back muscles

The deep back muscles are referred to collectively as **M. erector spinae** (M. erector trunci). The M. erector spinae extends from the pelvis to the occiput (➤ Fig. 3.34, ➤ Fig. 3.35) and fills the trench formed by the skeleton formed between the spinous processes and the ribs or the rib equivalents. It can be structurally and functionally divided into a **medial and a lateral tract** which lie in their own fascial tubes. The tracts are separated by an envelope system of taut connective tissue, from the **Fascia thoracolumbalis,** to the superficial back muscles. A further distinction is made in systems. The description of the systems essentially relays the course of muscles, from which the function (see below) can be derived from the individual muscle groups (➤ Fig. 3.34). The abdominal muscles and the M. erector spinae together act as a functional unit (bow-string-arch principle).

Medial tract

The medial tract (➤ Table 3.4) is located near the mid-axis, deep and the muscles act via short lever arms. It consists of two systems (➤ Fig. 3.34):
- **spinal system** (M. spinalis and Mm. interspinales, ➤ Fig. 3.35, ➤ Fig. 3.36, ➤ Fig. 3.37, ➤ Fig. 3.39)
- **transversospinal system** (M. semispinalis, Mm. multifidi, Mm. rotatores, ➤ Fig. 3.35, ➤ Fig. 3.36, ➤ Fig. 3.39)

The deep neck muscles assume a special position (Mm. suboccipitales) (see below).

In the area of the head joints, the medial tract of the M. erector spinae has been reshaped during evolution to ensure as free and closely controlled movement of the head as possible. Here, four pairs of muscles are differentiated that are referred to collectively as **deep neck muscles** or dorsal muscles of the short head joint muscles (Mm. suboccipitales) (➤ Fig. 3.37, ➤ Fig. 3.38, ➤ Table 3.5):
- **M. rectus capitis posterior major**
- **M. rectus capitis posterior minor**
- **M. obliquus capitis superior**
- **M. obliquus capitis inferior**

Tract	Straight system		Oblique system	Tract

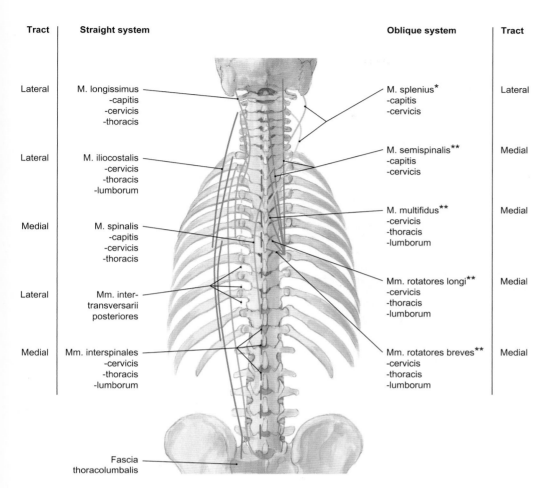

Tract	Straight system	Oblique system	Tract
Lateral	M. longissimus -capitis -cervicis -thoracis	M. splenius* -capitis -cervicis	Lateral
Lateral	M. iliocostalis -cervicis -thoracis -lumborum	M. semispinalis** -capitis -cervicis	Medial
Medial	M. spinalis -capitis -cervicis -thoracis	M. multifidus** -cervicis -thoracis -lumborum	Medial
Lateral	Mm. inter-transversarii posteriores	Mm. rotatores longi** -cervicis -thoracis -lumborum	Medial
Medial	Mm. interspinales -cervicis -thoracis -lumborum	Mm. rotatores breves** -cervicis -thoracis -lumborum	Medial
	Fascia thoracolumbalis		

Fig. 3.34 Autochthonous (deep) back muscles; orientation scheme of the muscle groups;
* Spinotransversal,
** Transversospinal.

Table 3.4 Autochthonous muscles of the back, medial tract.

Innervation	Origin	Attachment	Function
Spinal system			
Mm. interspinales (lumborum, thoracis [inconstant], cervicis)			
Rr. posteriores of the Nn. spinales	Procc. spinosi in the median level	Procc. spinosi in the median level	Support for the extension, stabilization and fine tuning of the motion segments
M. spinalis (thoracis, cervicis, capitis [inconstant])			
Rr. posteriores of the Nn. spinales	Procc. spinosi lateral to the median plane	Procc. spinosi lateral to the median plane, superior nuchal line	• Unilaterally active: support of the lateral inclination of the spine • Bilaterally active: extension of the spine
Transversospinal system			
Mm. rotatores breves et longi (lumborum [inconstant], thoracis, cervicis [inconstant]), pull to the next or skip a segment			
Rr. posteriores of the Nn. spinales	Procc. mamillares of the lumbar spine, Procc. transversi of the thoracic and cervical vertebrae	Procc. spinosi of the next highest (breve) or second highest (longi) vertebra	• Unilaterally active: low lateral inclination and rotation to the contralateral side • Bilaterally active: low extension, stabilisation of the mobile segments
Mm. multifidi (lumborum [particularly strong], thoracis, cervicis), skip 2–3 segments			
Rr. posteriores of the Nn. spinales	Facies dorsalis of the Os sacrum, Crista iliaca, Procc. mamillares of the lumbar vertebrae, Procc. transversi of the thoracic vertebrae, Procc. articulares of the cervical vertebrae	Procc. spinosi	• Unilaterally active: rotation of the vertebral column to the contralateral side and support of lateral inclination • Bilaterally active: extension and tension as well as stabilisation of the spinal column
M. semispinalis (thoracis, cervicis, capitis), skip 4–7 segments			
Rr. posteriores of the Nn. spinales	• Procc. transversi of the thoracic spine and cervical spine • M. semispinalis capitis superimposes the other sections	Procc. spinosi, Linea nuchalis superior	• Unilaterally active: rotating the head, the cervical spine and thoracic spine to the contralateral side, lateral inclination of the head, cervical spine and thoracic spine to the ipsilateral side • Bilaterally active: extension of the head and spine, tension and stabilisation of the cervical spine and thoracic spine

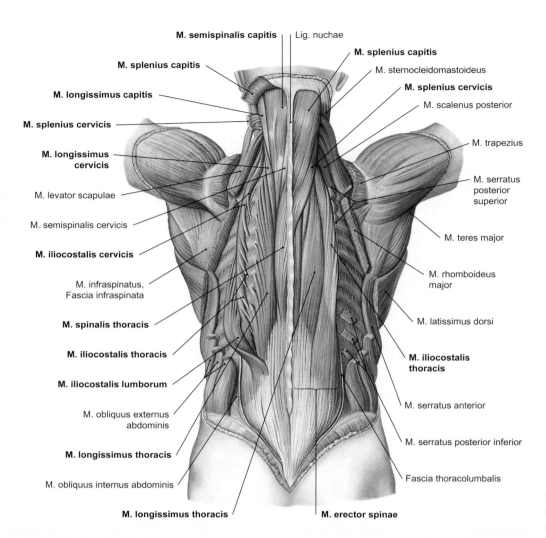

M. semispinalis capitis | Lig. nuchae
M. splenius capitis
M. longissimus capitis
M. splenius cervicis
M. longissimus cervicis
M. levator scapulae
M. semispinalis cervicis
M. iliocostalis cervicis
M. infraspinatus, Fascia infraspinata
M. spinalis thoracis
M. iliocostalis thoracis
M. iliocostalis lumborum
M. obliquus externus abdominis
M. longissimus thoracis
M. obliquus internus abdominis
M. longissimus thoracis
M. erector spinae

M. splenius capitis
M. sternocleidomastoideus
M. splenius cervicis
M. scalenus posterior
M. trapezius
M. serratus posterior superior
M. teres major
M. rhomboideus major
M. latissimus dorsi
M. iliocostalis thoracis
M. serratus anterior
M. serratus posterior inferior
Fascia thoracolumbalis

Fig. 3.35 Autochthonous back muscles; superficial layer. Dorsal view.

M. rectus capitis posterior major, M. obliquus capitis superior and M. obliquus capitis inferior form the deep neck triangle (Vertebralis triangle).

Apart from the deep neck muscles that form the dorsal group of Mm. suboccipitales, 2 more muscle pairs belong to the short head joint muscles (Mm. suboccipitales, ➤ Chap. 10.2.2, ➤ Tab. 10.8, ➤ Fig. 10.8):

- **M. rectus capitis anterior**
- **M. rectus capitis lateralis** (➤ Fig. 3.37)

They form the ventral group. All 6 muscle pairs together make up their insertion of the Axis, Atlas and Os occipitale. In contrast to the dorsal group the ventral group is innervated by Rr. anteriores of the spinal nerves. Together with the dorsal group they influence the fine tuning of the head in the atlantooccipital joints. Apart from the deep neck muscles, however, further muscles of the M. erector spinae and parts of the shoulder girdle muscles are involved in the movement of the head.

Lateral tract

The lateral tract not only lies lateral to the medial tract, but also partially overlaps it. The muscles are aligned laterocranially and the individual muscles are much longer in relation to the muscles of the medial tract (longer lever arms). The lateral tract can be divided into 4 muscle systems (➤ Table 3.6, ➤ Fig. 3.34, ➤ Fig. 3.35, ➤ Fig. 3.36, ➤ Fig. 3.37, ➤ Fig. 3.38):

- **Sacrospinal system** (M. longissimus, M. iliocostalis)
- **Spinotransversal system** (M. splenius)

- **Intertransversal system** (Mm. intertransversarii)
- **Mm. levatores costarum**

Functions

The autochthonous back muscles, apart from the passive musculoskeletal system (bone, discs, joints, ligaments), are of vital importance for the **movement and the posture of the spine, of the torso and the head** as active components of a standing and walking person (➤ Fig. 3.46):

- Straightening of the torso (M. erector spinae)
- Stretching (both sides) and lateral flexion (one-sided) of the torso
- Rotation of the torso
- Proprioception: location of body position in the room (especially Mm. suboccipitales)

The participation of the individual muscle systems can be deduced from their course:

- Bilateral contraction always causes stretching
- Straight median muscles (spinal system) can only stretch
- Straight lateral muscles (intertransversal system) can only lean to the side
- Oblique muscles are used for rotation:
  - Muscles, which run laterally, rotate in the same direction (spinotransversal system)
  - Muscles that run medially, rotate in the opposite direction (transversospinal system).

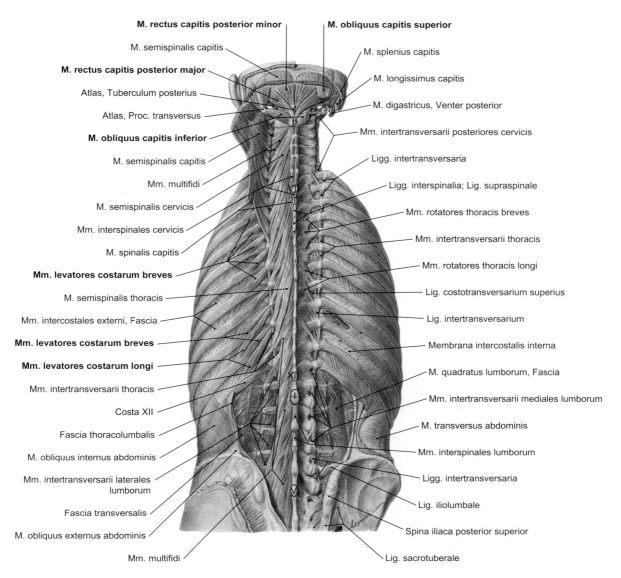

M. rectus capitis posterior minor

M. semispinalis capitis

M. rectus capitis posterior major

Atlas, Tuberculum posterius

Atlas, Proc. transversus

M. obliquus capitis inferior

M. semispinalis capitis

Mm. multifidi

M. semispinalis cervicis

Mm. interspinales cervicis

M. spinalis capitis

Mm. levatores costarum breves

M. semispinalis thoracis

Mm. intercostales externi, Fascia

Mm. levatores costarum breves

Mm. levatores costarum longi

Mm. intertransversarii thoracis

Costa XII

Fascia thoracolumbalis

M. obliquus internus abdominis

Mm. intertransversarii laterales lumborum

Fascia transversalis

M. obliquus externus abdominis

Mm. multifidi

M. obliquus capitis superior

M. splenius capitis

M. longissimus capitis

M. digastricus, Venter posterior

Mm. intertransversarii posteriores cervicis

Ligg. intertransversaria

Ligg. interspinalia; Lig. supraspinale

Mm. rotatores thoracis breves

Mm. intertransversarii thoracis

Mm. rotatores thoracis longi

Lig. costotransversarium superius

Lig. intertransversarium

Membrana intercostalis interna

M. quadratus lumborum, Fascia

Mm. intertransversarii mediales lumborum

M. transversus abdominis

Mm. interspinales lumborum

Ligg. intertransversaria

Lig. iliolumbale

Spina iliaca posterior superior

Lig. sacrotuberale

Fig. 3.36 Autochthonous back muscles, deep layer, and neck muscles (Mm. suboccipitales). Dorsal view.

Table 3.5 Deep neck muscles, dorsal group of short cranial joint muscles (M. suboccipitales).

Innervation	Origin	Attachment	Function
M. rectus capitis posterior major			
R. posterior of the 1st spinal nerve (N. suboccipitalis)	Proc. spinosus of the Axis	Middle third of the Linea nuchalis inferior	• Unilaterally active: rotates and tilts the head slightly to the ipsilateral side, fine tuning of the head in the atlantooccipital joint • Bilaterally active: slight extension of the cranial joints
M. rectus capitis posterior minor			
R. posterior of the 1st spinal nerve (N. suboccipitalis)	Tuberculum posterius of the Arcus posterior of the Atlas	Medial below the Linea nuchalis inferior	• Unilaterally active: rotates and tilts the head to the ipsilateral side, fine tuning of the head in the atlantooccipital joint • Bilaterally active: extension of the cranial joints
M. obliquus capitis superior			
R. posterior of the 1st spinal nerve (N. suboccipitalis)	Proc. transversus of the Atlas	Lateral third of the Linea nuchalis inferior	• Unilaterally active: tilts the head to the ipsilateral side, fine tuning of the head in the cranial joints • Bilaterally active: extension of the cranial joints
M. obliquus capitis inferior			
R. posterior of the 1st spinal nerve (N. suboccipitalis)	Proc. spinosus of the Axis	Proc. transversus of the Atlas	• Unilaterally active: rotates and tilts the head to the ipsilateral side, fine tuning of the head in the cranial joints • Bilaterally active: extension of the cranial joints

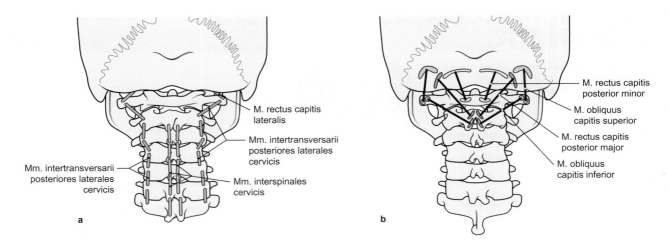

Fig. 3.37 Short neck and head joint muscles. a Short neck muscles. **b** Short head joint muscles (Mm. suboccipitales). [L126]

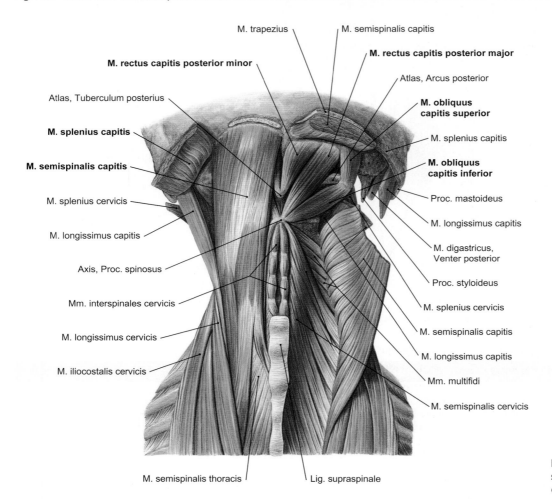

Fig. 3.38 Neck muscles (Mm. suboccipitales) and back muscles (Mm. dorsi). Dorsal view.

Due to their cross-section the **M. longissimus** , the **M. iliocostalis** and the **M. spinalis** are particularly responsible for straightening the torso and are therefore also strictly speaking referred to by *Terminologia Anatomica* as M. erector spinae. The short muscles (**Mm. interspinales and inter-transversarii, Mm. rotatores, Mm. levatores costarum**) are used primarily for stabilisation of the individual movement segments of the spinal column.
The exact courses are only important for muscles that lead to the head:

- **Mm. suboccipitales**
- **M. spinalis** and **m. semispinalis capitis**

- **M. longissimus capitis**
- **M. splenius capitis**

These muscles sometimes have contrary functions, except for the extension on unilateral contraction! The Mm. suboccipitales are responsible for fine tuning of head movements because they perceive proprioceptive functions due to the large number of muscle spindles and also mostly only skip one vertebral segment (exception: M. rectus capitis posterior major).

Table 3.6 Autochthonous muscles of the back, lateral tract.

Innervation	Origin	Attachment	Function
Sacrospinal system			
M. iliocostalis (lumborum, thoracis, cervicis)			
Rr. posteriores of the Nn. spinales	Facies dorsalis of the Os sacrum, Crista iliaca, Crista sacralis lateralis, Procc. spinosi of the lumbar vertebrae, Lamina superficialis of the Fascia thoracolumbalis, medial from the Angulus costae of the IIIrd–XIIth ribs	Procc. costales of the upper lumbar spine, Angulus costae of the Ist–XIIth ribs, Tubercula posteriora of the IIIrd–VIth cervical vertebrae	• Unilaterally active: lateral flexion and rotation of the vertebral column to the ipsilateral side • Bilaterally active: extension and tension of the spinal column, expiration (by lowering the ribs)
M. longissimus (thoracis, cervicis, capitis)			
Rr. posteriores of the Nn. spinales	Facies dorsalis of the Os sacrum, Crista sacralis lateralis, Crista iliaca, Lamina superficialis of the Fascia thoracolumbalis, Procc. spinosi of the lumbar vertebrae, Procc. transversi and Procc. articulares of the thoracic and cervical vertebrae	Procc. transversi of the thoracic and cervical vertebrae, Angulus costae, Tubercula posteriora of the IInd–VIIth cervical vertebrae, Proc. mastoideus	• Unilaterally active: lateral flexion and rotation of the head and spine to the ipsilateral side • Bilaterally active: extension of cervical spine and head, spinal tension
Intertransversal system, Mm. intertransversarii (lumborum, cervicis)			
Rr. posteriores (and anteriores) of the Nn. spinales	Tuberculum posterius of the Procc. transversi of the Ist to IVth cervical vertebrae, Procc. accessorii of the Ist–IVth lumbar vertebra	Tuberculum posterius of the Procc. transversi of the IInd–Vth cervical vertebrae, Procc. accessorii and Procc. mamillares of the IInd–Vth lumbar vertebrae	• Unilaterally active: support of lateral flexion • Bilaterally active: low extension
Spinotransversal system, M. splenius (cervicis, capitis)			
Rr. posteriores (and anteriores) of the Nn. spinales	Procc. spinosi of the IIIrd–VIIth cervical vertebrae and the Ist–IVth thoracic vertebrae	Proc. mastoideus and lateral portion of the Linea nuchalis superior, Procc. transversi of the Ist-IIIrd cervical vertebrae	• Unilaterally active: lateral flexion and rotation of the cervical spine and head to the ipsilateral side, tension of the cervical spine • Bilaterally active: extension of cervical spine and head
Mm. levatores costarum			
Rr. posteriores (and anteriores) of the Nn. spinales	Procc. transversi of the thoracic vertebrae	Next lower (breve) and second lowest (longi) rib (lateral from Angulus costae)	• Unilaterally active: rotation of the vertebral column to the contralateral side and lateral flexion to the ipsilateral side • Bilaterally active: extension of the spine and elevation of the ribs (inspiration)

Fascia thoracolumbalis

The Fascia thoracolumbalis consists of 2 sheets (➤ Fig. 3.39, ➤ Fig. 3.40):
- **Superficial lamina (Lamina superficialis):** originates at the rear of the sacrum and the spinous processes of the spine
- **Deep lamina (Lamina profunda):** connects the Crista iliaca via the Procc. costales of the lumbar vertebra with the XIIth rib; the coarse section between the ribs process of the Ist lumbar vertebra and XIIth rib is referred to as lumbocostal ligament.

The Fascia thoracolumbalis together with the spinal column forms an **osteofibrous canal,** in which the autochthonous muscles are embedded (➤ Fig. 3.39, ➤ Fig. 3.40). The Fascia thoracolumbalis is also the origin for the following abdominal muscles, secondary back muscles and hip muscles:
- Superficial lamina:
  - M. latissimus dorsi
  - M. serratus posterior inferior
  - M. gluteus maximus
- Deep lamina:
  - M. obliquus internus abdominis
  - M. transversus abdominis

This enables the thoracolumbar fascia to interact with these muscle groups in the movement of the torso and extremities.

┌─ Clinical remarks ─

In the case of pathologically increased tone (spasticity) in the muscles, that lead to the head, a **muscular twisted neck** (Torticollis spasmodicus) may occur with rotation of the head. This is treated, among other things, by interrupting synaptic transmission to the muscular end plate with an injection of botulinum toxin. Primarily the two strongest and most superficial muscles (M. splenius capitis and M. semispinalis capitis) come into question; however, since they rotate the head to opposite sides and the M. splenius is also very thin, it must be ensured according to the symptoms that only one of the two muscles is affected.
The muscular twisted neck belongs to the group of **myogeloses** (muscle tension). This consists of circumscribed palpable,

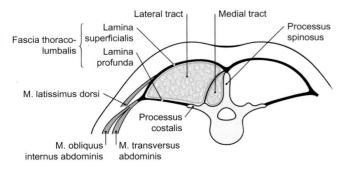

Fig. 3.39 Fascia thoracolumbalis and autochthonous back muscles; scheme. [L126]

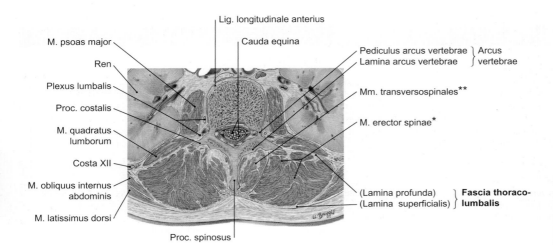

Fig. 3.40 Autochthonous back muscles and Fascia thoracolumbalis. Transversal section at the level of the IInd lumbar vertebra; caudal view; * lateral tract, ** medial tract.

mostly pressure pain thickenings of a muscle with contractile muscle bundles, such as nodes or swellings, which are common in chronic pain conditions of the back.

Superficial muscles of the back

The superficial back muscles are used for the movement of the arms and the ribs. According to their course, they can be divided into three systems:

- Spinohumeral system: M. latissimus dorsi
- Spinoscapular system: M. trapezius, Mm. rhomboidei, M. levator scapulae
- Spinocostal system: Mm. serrati posteriores superior et inferior

Course and function of the muscles are explained in more detail in the upper extremities (➤ Chap. 4.3.4) or have already been discussed for the ventral torso wall (spinocostal system) (➤ Chap. 3.1.2, ➤ Table 3.1, ➤ Fig. 3.33).

3.2.3 Vascular, lymphatic and nervous systems of the dorsal torso wall

Arteries

The dorsal torso wall is supplied with blood, to a large extent directly from the aorta but also from branches of the Aa. subclavia et axillaris (throat area) as well as the Aa. iliacae externa et femoralis via anastomoses with the ventral torso wall arteries. The blood supply to the neck muscles is discussed in ➤ Chap. 10.4.

Branches of the Aorta thoracica

The branches of the Aorta thoracica (Pars thoracica aortae) show the typical segmental classification (therefore also referred to as chest segment arteries) and supply the intercostal muscles, the upper part of the stomach muscles, the skin at the side and back chest wall and join the blood supply of the mammary gland (➤ Fig. 3.13). From the Aorta thoracica, the paired **Aa. intercostales posteriores** emerge. The 3rd–11th arteries originate directly from the thoracic aorta and the 1st and 2nd arteries from the **A. intercostalis suprema** of the Truncus costocervicalis of the A. subclavia. The intercostal arteries course in the respective ICS on the bottom edge of the rib in the Sulcus costalis. The 12th chest segment artery still runs under the XIIth rib, but no longer in an ICS. It is therefore called the **A. subcostalis**. Branches of the intercostal arteries are respectively (➤ Fig. 3.13):

- **Posterior branch:** supplies the back muscles but also the skin, the vertebrae and the spinal canal with spinal cord and spinal cord membranes. It leads to the Rr. spinales and is divided into the R. cutaneus medialis and the R. cutaneus lateralis.
- **Collateral branch:** supplies the intercostal muscles and together with the Aa. intercostales it is anastomosed with the Aa. intercostales anteriores (see below).
- **Lateral cutaneous branch:** supplies the skin in the area of the axillary line and divides into an anterior and posterior branch. The anterior branches of the Rr. cutanei laterales of the Aa. intercostales posteriores II–IV supply the mammary glands as the Rr. mammarii laterales.

Branches of the Aorta abdominalis

The branches of the Aorta abdominalis supply the back muscles and the skin of the back with blood, partially the lower portion of the abdominal muscles and are involved in the blood supply of the vertebral canal in the lumbar region and the diaphragm (➤ Fig. 3.41). Central branches are 4 paired Aa. **lumbales,** which leave the aorta on their rear wall and pass to the abdominal wall at the level of the I–IV lumbar vertebrae behind the M. psoas and the M. quadratus lumborum. Here they pass between the M. obliquus internus abdominis and the M. transversus abdominis and anastomoses with the Aa. intercostales posteriores, A. epigastrica inferior, A. iliolumbalis and the A. circumflexa ilium profunda. From each A. lumbalis originates a

- **Posterior branch:** this supplies, analogue to the posterior branch, the Aorta thoracica (see above), the back muscles, also the skin, the vertebra and the spinal canal with Cauda equina and spinal cord membranes. The Rr. spinales arises from it and divides into the main branches R. cutaneus medialis and the R. cutaneus lateralis.

At the level of the diaphragm the paired **A. phrenica inferior** arises on the anterior side of the aorta at the height of the aortic hiatus. It branches off on the underside of the diaphragm and anastomoses with the lower intercostal arteries and visceral arteries.

Veins

The venous drainage of the dorsal torso wall is divided into 3 systems as in the ventral torso wall:

- Epifascial venous system
- Subfascial venous system
- Venous system of the spine

The course of the veins can be extremely variable, particularly in the epifascial and subfascial venous systems.

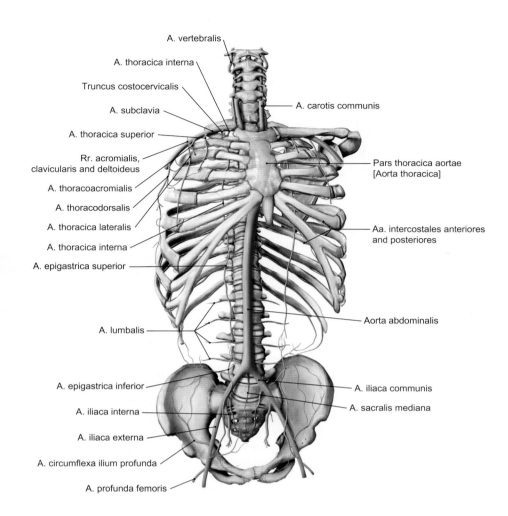

A. vertebralis
A. thoracica interna
Truncus costocervicalis
A. subclavia
A. thoracica superior
Rr. acromialis, clavicularis and deltoideus
A. thoracoacromialis
A. thoracodorsalis
A. thoracica lateralis
A. thoracica interna
A. epigastrica superior
A. lumbalis
A. epigastrica inferior
A. iliaca interna
A. iliaca externa
A. circumflexa ilium profunda
A. profunda femoris

A. carotis communis
Pars thoracica aortae [Aorta thoracica]
Aa. intercostales anteriores and posteriores
Aorta abdominalis
A. iliaca communis
A. sacralis mediana

Fig. 3.41 Arteries of the torso wall. Anterior view. [L266]

Epifascial venous system

The epifascial veins lie in the subcutis and form a densely ramified network on the dorsal torso wall. The lumen diameter varies considerably from person to person, and in contrast with the ventral torso wall, where there are larger vein stems with their own terminology, there is no terminology for these veins at the dorsal torso wall.

Subfascial venous system

The subfascial venous system is similar to the arteries, which are accompanied by these veins; however, there are exceptions on the dorsal torso wall. The azygos system (➤ Fig. 3.16) is here, consisting of the V. azygos, V. hemiazygos and the V. hemiazygos accessoria. The following belong to the subfascial venous system of the dorsal torso wall:

- **Vv. intercostales posteriores:** They receive blood from the intercostal muscles and the overlying skin of the dorsal torso wall and from the back muscles (R. dorsalis) and the vertebral canal (R. intervertebralis, R. spinalis). The upper intercostal veins (II–III) drain to the right via the V. intercostalis superior dextra into the V. azygos and to the left via the left superior intercostal vein into the V. left innominate vein. The lower intercostal veins (IV–XI) drain to the right into the V. azygos, left into the V. hemiazygos and the V. hemiazygos accessoria.
- **Vv. lumbales** (I–IV): they drain the blood of the posterior abdominal wall into the Vilumbalis ascendens and from there into the V. iliaca communis. The 3rd and 4th lumbar veins usually flow directly into the V. cava inferior.
- **V. azygos:** this leads the blood up into the V. cava superior and down into the V. cava inferior.

- **V. hemiazygos:** drains into the A. subclavior azygos, V. cava inferior, V. illiaca communis and V. illiaca externor.
- **V. hemiazygos accessoria:** Supplies blood to the V. azygos and the A. subclavior.

Venous system of the spine

The veins of the spine are referred to in their entirety as **Vv. columnae vertebralis**. They can be divided into an outer and inner venous network (➤ Fig. 3.65). They are discussed in ➤ Chap. 3.3.2.

Lymph vessels

Epifascial lymph vessels above the navel drain into the axillary lymph nodes (**Nodi lymphoidei axillares**); epifascial lymph vessels below this drain into the superficial inguinal lymph nodes (**Nodi lymphoidei inguinales superficiales**), Nodi lymphoidei superomedialis and superolateralis of the superficial inguinal Lymph nodes.

Subfascial lymph vessels on the inside of the dorsal torso wall drain into the **Nodi lymphoidei intercostalis** lying paravertebrally, which also take up the lymph of the Pleura parietalis in this area. With the Aorta abdominalis there is also a lymph discharge to the **Nodi lymphoidei lumbales** and along the A. iliaca externa to the **Nodi lymphoidei iliaci externi**.

Innervation

The dorsal torso wall is innervated segmentally from the branches of the **thoracic and lumbar spinal nerves** (➤ Fig. 3.42).
The Rr. **posteriores of the Nn. spinales thoracici and lumbales** each divide into a **R. mediales** and a **R. laterales** (➤ Fig. 3.43).

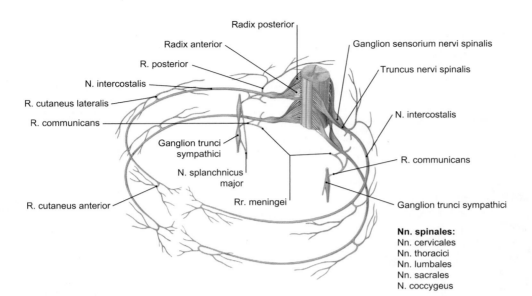

Nn. spinales:
Nn. cervicales
Nn. thoracici
Nn. lumbales
Nn. sacrales
N. coccygeus

Fig. 3.42 Construction principle of spinal nerve (N. spinalis) and spinal cord segment, exemplified by two thoracic nerves (Nn. thoracici). Anterior oblique view.

They innervate the autochthonous back muscles and the overlying skin. The lateral cutaneous branches are well developed in the lower back and, depending on the location are referred to as Rr. cutanei posteriores or Nn. clunium superiores.

The **Rr. anteriores (ventrales) of the Nn. spinales thoracici (intercostales)** are the intercostal nerves (they are shown here completely because of their origin in the area of the dorsal torso wall, although they innervate the ventral torso wall). They innervate the intercostal and abdominal muscles and the Mm. serrati posteriores superior et inferior. Their sensitive branches are used for the innervation of the Pleura parietalis and Peritoneum parietale:

- N. intercostalis I is part of the brachial plexus.
- Nn. intercostales II–VI run in the ICS up to the sternum.
- Nn. intercostales VII–XI run partly in the ICS, then leave and run almost near to the midline. In the process they cross the attachment area of the diaphragm and run between the M. obliquus internus abdominis and the M. transversus abdominis up to the rectus sheath, enter this and innervate the M. rectus abdominis.
- The 12th intercostal nerve runs under the XIIth rib and is called the **N. subcostalis**. It has the same course as the Nn. intercostalis

VII–XI and is involved in the innervation of the M. rectus abdomini.

In the axillary line each intercostal nerve emits a **R. cutaneus lateralis** and in the front sternal line a **R. cutaneus anterior** to the skin. Depending on the region to be innervated, the branches are called:

- Rr. cutanei laterales pectorales
- Rr. cutanei anteriores pectorales
- Rr. mammarii laterales
- Rr. mammarii mediales
- Rr. cutanei lateralis abdominis
- Rr. cutanei antierores abdominis

The Rr. cutanei laterales of the (1st, 2nd and 3rd) intercostal nerve extend as the **N. or Nn. intercostobrachiales** on the medial side of the arm and combine here with the N. cutaneus brachii medialis (➤ Chap. 4.6.1).

The Rr. cutanei anteriores of the 1st (and 2nd) Intercostal nerves are missing. The skin is innervated here by the Nn. supraclaviculares from the Plexus cervicalis.

> **Clinical remarks**
>
> Due to the segmental sensory innervation of the skin of the torso wall, nipples (T5), navel (T10) and the inguinal region (L1) are used as reference points for **height localisation.** Pain in the chest wall can be projected into the arm via the **Nn. intercostobrachiales** (e.g. when mammary carcinoma metastases are present in the axillary lymph nodes that grow into the nerves).

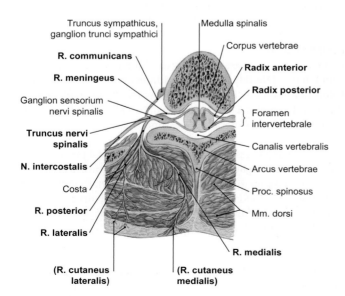

Fig. 3.43 Spinal nerve (N. spinalis) in the thoracic region. Caudal view.

3.3 Spine, spinal cord and thorax
Bernhard Hirt, Friedrich Paulsen

The vertebral column (Columna vertebralis), together with the axial skeleton, is located at the back of the torso and is thus eccentric, carrying the weight of the head, the upper extremities, the torso and the thoracic and abdominal viscera and transferring it to the pelvic girdle. The chest wall skeleton is connected by a joint system with the spine. The special structure of the free (presacral) spine with generally 24 individually moving vertebrae and 23 intervertebral discs (Disci intervertebrales) as well as the ligaments of the spine provide excellent power transfer during free movement. The weight is transferred caudally via the sacrum (Os sacrum), which is integrated into the pelvic girdle to which the coccyx (Os coccygis) is connected. The spinal cord is located in the vertebral canal (Canalis vertebralis); the spinal nerve branches enter and exit via the intervertebral foramina (Foramina intervertebralia). The dorsal root ganglia are also found here.

3.3.1 Embryology

Development of the axis organs and somites

On the *16th day of development* the Chorda dorsalis as a rod-shaped structure in the median plane of the middle germ layer (mesoderm). It is located in the axial plane as a support rod and releases inductive messengers, which cause the paraxial mesoderm (➤ Chap. 2.6.2) to differentiate (see below). Parallel to this, the neural tube is formed. The notochord and neural tube are referred to as the axis organs. The close relationship between the spine and the spinal cord is thus already created. Through consolidation of the paraxial mesoderm in the following period (up to the *5th week*) 42–44 pairs of somites are created (syn.: original segments), which are positioned beside the axis organ like a string of pearls. This structure of the mesoderm in somites is the basis of the segmental structure of the body (metamerism).

Differentiation of somites

The cells of the somites differentiate sequentially into sclerotomes, myotomes and dermatomes. Vertebrae, parts of the intervertebral discs and the ligaments develop from the **sclerotomes**. For this purpose, the somite cells migrate medially to the Chorda dorsalis and to the neural tube. The vertebral bodies differentiate in the cranial and caudal halves of two neighbouring somites. Thus, the vertebral body positions are located between the somites and the positions of the intervertebral discs each lie in the middle of the somites. The vertebral arch positions arise from two neighbouring paraxial somite parts lying beside the Chorda dorsalis.

The initially centrally located Chorda dorsalis in the vertebral system becomes degenerated. As a relic of the notochord the only thing remaining is the gelatinous core of the intervertebral discs (Nucleus pulposus).

The initially organised 42–44 somite pairs are distributed in the course of development.

- The cranial 4½ somites evolve to parts of the occipital bone.
- The coccyx evolves from 3–5 vertebral positions.
- The caudal 5–7 somites regress.

From the *6th embryonic week* the cartilaginous reconstruction of mesenchymal precursor tissue occurs based on cartilage centres in the area of the vertebral body and the arch roots. Ossification (**endochondral ossification**) begins in the *4th foetal month* with the formation of bone cores in the vertebral bodies and the vertebral arches. In neonates the vertebral bodies are usually already ossified.

Clinical remarks

Vertebral malformations can be associated with pathological vertebral body shapes:
- The fusion of 2 or more vertebral bodies in the context of development leads to a dysontogenetic **block vertebra.** Vertebral fusion occurs on the cervical spine, e.g. in the case of KLIPPEL–FEIL's syndrome (congenital cervical vertebrae synostosis) with characteristic shoulder blade elevation and deep hairline.

- In the case of **wedge-shaped vertebrae** (hemivertebrae) the front surface of the vertebral body is lower than the rear surface. This occurs when two cartilage centres appear instead of just one. Wedge-shaped vertebrae change the spinal form (kyphosisation) and the spinal static.
- In adults if two vertebrae fuse under degeneration of the intervertebral disc, **block vertebrae** are created.

If single or multiple **vertebral arches** do not fuse together, the result is a divided, dorsally open spine **(Spina bifida):**
- In the simplest form, the fissure formation lies under the skin and is not externally visible (Spina bifida occulta).
- If the neural folds are also open to the outside, it is called rachischisis (Spina bifida aperta).
- If the spinal cord is also affected, this can be associated with paralysis in the affected area and below.

SCHEUERMANN's disease (Scheuermann's disease, adolescent kyphosis, juvenile kyphosis, osteochondritis deformans juvenilis dorsi) is an etiologically unclear (probably inherited) spinal disease (probably giving rise to disorders in the ring apophyses/growth zones) that form in children and adolescents aged between 11 and 17 years. Boys are much more likely to be affected. In this case, the front part of the vertebral body (especially on the lower thoracic spine) is decreased, the top and base plates are irregularly outlined, SCHMORL's cartilage nodes can be found on the end and base plates and the vertebral body is extended on the ventral side. Those affected suffer from back pain, stooping, movement restrictions and overloading of adjacent spinal sections. Physiotherapy, sport and a spinal support (by orthoses) are used for treatment.

3.3.2 Spine

The spine accounts for two fifths of the size of a human. A quarter of the vertebral column length is attributable to the intervertebral discs (Disci intervertebrales).

Structure and form

Sections

The vertebral column (Columna vertebralis, ➤ Fig. 3.44) is divided into 5 sections. The sections differ in the number of vertebrae, and in the rotation and tilting of the vertebrae in relation to each other. The 24 presacral vertebrae are divided into
- 7 cervical vertebrae **(Vertebrae cervicales),**
- 12 thoracic vertebrae **(Vertebrae thoracicae)** and
- 5 lumbar vertebrae **(Vertebrae lumbales).**

The following are immovable
- 5 synostotically fused vertebrae called the sacrum **(Os sacrum)** and the
- coccyx consisting of 3–5 fused vertebrae **(Os coccygis).**

The boundary between the lumbar spine and the sacrum is the **Promontorium.**

NOTE

In 5–6 % of the population there is a transition vertebra in form of a **sacralisation.** In the process, lumbar vertebra V is fused with the sacrum and there are only 23 presacral vertebrae. A sacralisation is very often associated with the cervical ribs. There is also a predisposition for a slipped disc in the segment lying above.

Another form of a transition vertebra is **lumbalisation,** which is slightly less common than the sacralisation. In the process, the sacral vertebra I is not fused with the rest of the sacrum to a bone, but remains as a free vertebra. In this case there are 25 presacral vertebrae.

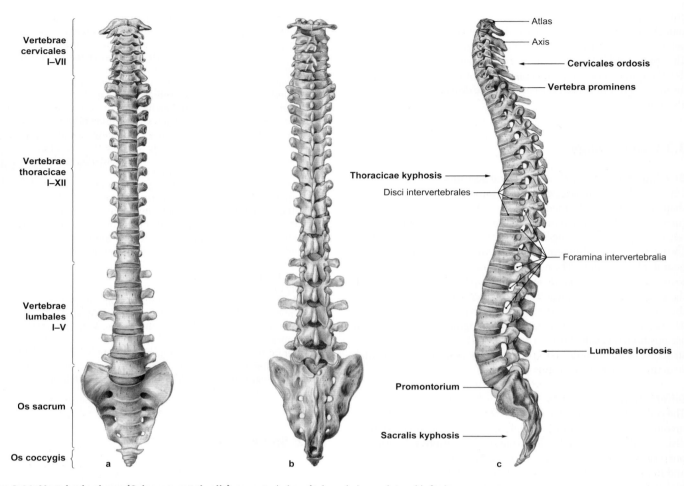

Atlas
Axis
Cervicales ordosis
Vertebra prominens

Vertebrae cervicales I–VII

Vertebrae thoracicae I–XII

Thoracicae kyphosis
Disci intervertebrales

Foramina intervertebralia

Vertebrae lumbales I–V

Lumbales lordosis

Os sacrum

Promontorium

Sacralis kyphosis

Os coccygis

a   b   c

Fig. 3.44 Vertebral column (Columna vertebralis). a ventral view. **b** dorsal view. **c** lateral left view.

Curvatures

The spine has physiological curvatures in the sagittal plane (➤ Fig. 3.44), which give it its double-S-shape. These are not yet in existence in neonates. Only a flat kyphotic curve in the thoracic spine, and in the sacrum and coccyx are dominant. The curvature in the throat and lumbar regions are formed with the burden on the spine through raising the head, sitting and standing upright in the 1st year of life and beyond. The cervical and lumbar spine are ventrally bent and convex which is referred to as **lordosis** (cervical lordosis, lumbar lordosis), the thoracic spine and Os sacrum/Oscoccygis are bent ventrally and concave, which is referred to as **kyphosis** (thoracic kyphosis, sacral kyphosis). The curvature of the spine in adults is not exactly transferable to the various sections of the spine; therefore, cervical lordosis refers to the cervical vertebrae I–VI and thoracic kyphosis to the VI cervical to IX thoracic vertebrae and lumbar lordosis from the IX thoracic to the V lumbar vertebra.

Clinical remarks

Excessive curvature of the spine in the frontal plane is referred to as **scoliosis** and is always pathological. This growth deformity of the spine results in a fixed lateral curvature. In the thoracic spine a scoliosis in conjunction with a fixed twisting (torsion) of individual vertebrae and rib-vertebrae joints (rotation of axial organs) also leads to a deformity of the rib cage with hump formation (Gibbus), which can no longer be compensated on a muscular level. This often has an impact on the pulmonary and circulatory function. Scoliosis has been a well-known orthopaedic condition since ancient times but its treat-

ment remains difficult even today; however, almost everyone has a minimal level of scoliosis, because most people's legs differ slightly in length. Degenerative or inflammatory changes, developmental disorders or compression fractures of the spine may result in a hyperkyphosis of the upper thoracic spine and the formation of a round back.

Vertebrae and their connections
Basic form of a vertebra

Each free presacral vertebra, ➤ Fig. 3.45) consists of:
- Vertebral body (Corpus vertebrae)
- Vertebral arch (Arcus vertebrae)
- Vertebral arch processes (Procc. arcus vertebrae)

The exception is in the first two cervical vertebra (Atlas and Axis). All other vertebrae of the freely movable spine are structured in this way, but show characteristic shape and position variations in their structure in the various sections of the spine.

Vertebral bodies

The vertebral body (➤ Fig. 3.45) has cranially and caudally a transverse oriented surface (**Facies intervertebralis**), which is surrounded in a circular form by a border rim (**Epiphysis anularis**). The border rim is made of dense bone in the same way as the side wall of the vertebral body. The central area is also made up of compact bone but only a thin layer, so that it directly connects with the underlying cancellous bone of the vertebral body. The vertebral body surface is covered by hyaline cartilage; cranially it is referred to as a cover plate and caudally as a ground or base plate. The top

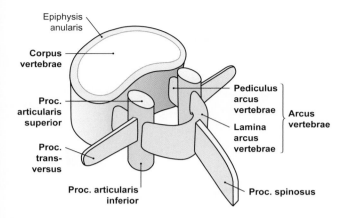

Epiphysis anularis
Corpus vertebrae
Proc. articularis superior
Proc. trans- versus
Proc. articularis inferior
Pediculus arcus vertebrae
Lamina arcus vertebrae
Arcus vertebrae
Proc. spinosus

Fig. 3.45 Structural elements of a vertebra, schematic. Posterior oblique view. [L126]

and bottom plates are solidly connected with the adjacent intervertebral disc (disc, Discus intervertebralis, see below).

Clinical remarks

In Germany approximately 6 million adults suffer from **osteoporosis** (bone loss) and 80% are women. Osteoporosis is a systemic disease of aging of the skeleton, which changes the cancellous bone architecture and makes the bones susceptible to fractures. It is characterised by a decrease in bone mass, whereby less bone is formed than degraded. In particular, very spongiose constructed skeletal elements, such as the vertebral body are affected, as the conversion rate in ancellous bone (approximately 28%) is significantly higher than in compact bone (approx. 4%). Risk factors for osteoporosis are family history, white skin colour, age, oestrogen deficiency, vitamin D deficiency, low calcium intake, smoking, excessive alcohol intake and an inactive life style. The most common cause is oestrogen deficiency after menopause (as with men in old age). In this process the bone loss increases as oestrogen inhibits the osteoclast activity. A lack of oestrogen means that too many osteoclasts are created and live for too long. In the vertebral bodies, particularly the cancellous bone trabeculae, there is thinning and consequently microfractures. Vertical cancellous bone trabeculae heal together again via secondary fracture healing (via callus), because the fracture ends adjoin each other. Horizontal fracture ends are pressed apart by the forces acting on the vertebral bodies and can no longer grow together. They are degraded. At some point, the vertebra can no longer withstand the physical stress acting on it and collapses (sinter down). This can occur completely or only affect the front or rear part, so that deformation of the axial skeleton (with reduction in body height) and deficits can be the result. New drugs against osteoporosis intervene in the bone metabolism, e.g. antibodies against the membrane component protein RANKL on osteoblasts or against the osteocyte protein sclerostin. The previously conducted postmenopausal oestrogen treatment has been abandoned due to adverse side effects (e.g. a significantly increased risk of breast cancer).

Vertebral arches

The vertebral arches (**Arcus vertebrae,** ➤ Fig. 3.45) are located dorsally on the vertebrae and on both sides consists of 2 units:
• Pedicle of the vertebral arch (**Pediculus arcus vertebrae**)
• Lamina of the vertebral arch (**Lamina arcus vertebrae**)
The vertebral arch plates of both sides meet in the spinal process (**Proc. spinosus**) and thus form the vertebral foramen (**Foramen**

vertebrale). The vertebral foramen of all vertebrae form in their entirety the vertebral canal (**Canalis vertebralis**), which contains the marginal ligaments, the spinal cord and the spinal meninges.

Vertebral arch processes

Between the pedicle and the arch plate (lamina) a laterally facing vertebral arch process is located on both sides (**transverse process, Proc. transversus**). On each side one articular process protrudes up and down, respectively, (**Procc. articulares superior et inferior**) for flexible connection with the above and underlying vertebrae or bones. The pedicle is constricted at the top and bottom in the lateral view (Incisurae vertebrales superiores et inferiores). Through the corresponding upper and lower constrictions of the pediculi of adjacent vertebrae, the vertebral arch foramina are created (**Foramina intervertebralia**), which enter and exit through the spinal nerve roots and contain the portions of the spinal ganglia.

Clinical remarks

Clinicians often use the short forms lamina and pedicle. The term lateral mass, which is frequently used for all vertebrae, for the region of the joint and transverse process between the arch root and the arch plate is incorrect. The lateral masses are exclusively structures of the first cervical vertebrae (Atlas, see below).

In spinal surgery the removal of the vertebral arch plate plays a significant role (**laminectomy,** e.g. in the operative treatment of a disc prolapse, see below). Screws that are introduced into the vertebral arch root to stabilise the spine, are called pedicle screws.

A **spondylolysis** is a lateral cleft in the vertebral arch that leads to the separation of the inferior articular process from the rear part of the arch and of the spinal process from the rest of the vertebral parts. They can occur as a congenital defect or as acquired stress fracture of the lamina. The bony separation of the isthmus (➤ Fig. 3.60) can cause vertebral slippage (**spondylolisthesis**). The latter is an instability of the spine, in which the upper portion of the spine slides forward with the slipped vertebra over the underlying vertebral body. In most cases, spondylolisthesis is an incidental finding but it can be accompanied by nerve and spinal cord involvement up to failure symptoms.

Mobile segments of the spinal column

The term **mobile segment** refers to two neighbouring vertebrae with their connections and the ligamentous and muscular structures. The entire vertebral column is therefore made up of various mobile segments. The range of movement within a mobile segment is not particularly large. The sum of all mobile segments leads to an extraordinarily large range of movement of the vertebral column (➤ Fig. 3.46) in the various movements.

N O T E

The intervertebral discs act as connections between the vertebrae (Disci intervertebrales) and the vertebral arch joints (Articulationes zygapophyseales).

Intervertebral discs

The spine has 23 **intervertebral discs (Disci intervertebrales),** located between the vertebral bodies (➤ Fig. 3.47) and in healthy adults they account for approximately one quarter of the total length of the spine. Skull and atlas as well as atlas and axis (the first two cervical vertebrae) are linked by true joints (diarthroses). There are no intervertebral discs here. The intervertebral discs connect the top and base plates of adjacent vertebral bodies and are tightly connected

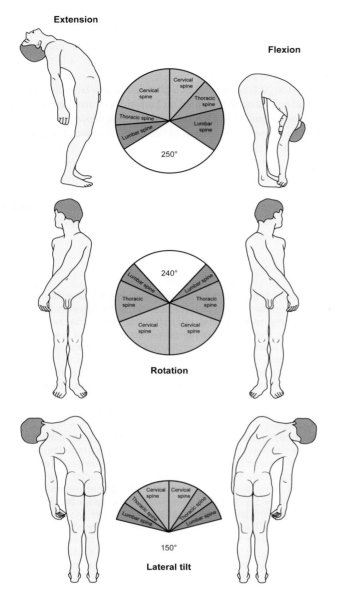

Fig. 3.46 Range of movement of the spinal sections (equivalent to neutral-null method). [L126]

with these by collagen fibres. The thickness of the intervertebral discs increases from cranial to caudal corresponding to the mechanical load. The height of each individual intervertebral disc is subject to a daily time fluctuation due to pressure-dependent fluid volume disturbances in the extracellular spaces (this means that in the morning after sleep one can be 2.5 cm taller than in the evening).

Structure

A Discus intervertebralis (➤ Fig. 3.47) consists of an outer fibrous ring (Anulus fibrosus) and an inner jelly-like core (Nucleus pulposus). The **Anulus fibrosus** is further divided into an external zone, an internal zone and a transition zone.

- **External zone:** consists of dense connective tissue arranged in lamellae made of collagen fibrils which run in opposition, in the form of a herringbone pattern (rhombic lattice scissors grid, Venetian scissors) (in particular type I collagen), which is anchored to the bony edge of the vertebral body. Between the collagen fibrils there are large quantities of proteoglycans (approximately 66%), which form a functional unit with the collagen fibrils. There are also numerous elastic fibres.

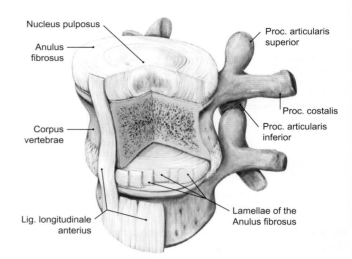

Fig. 3.47 Structure of the Disci intervertebrales. Anterior oblique view. [L266]

- **Internal zone:** consists of wider lamellae made of fibrous cartilage (type I and type II collagen), which are also arranged in the shape of a herringbone pattern.
- **Transition zone:** the inner zone passes into the Nucleus pulposus without any clear demarcation and as a transition zone consists of loose connective tissue.

The **Nucleus pulposus** borders cranially and caudally with the cartilage plates of the vertebral body and laterally on the Anulus fibrosus. It consists primarily of an extracellular matrix with a high proportion of proteoglycans and a correspondingly high water-binding capacity.

Function

The water-binding capacity of the Nucleus pulposus leads to a uniform source pressure, which is aligned against the base and top plates of two adjacent vertebrae and is released laterally (axial pressure load). In this way the fibres of the Anulus fibrosus are always kept under tension. The Nucleus pulposus acts like a centrally-loaded water cushion, which distributes the physical pressure evenly on the top and base plates of the vertebral body. The grid-like interwoven fibres of the Anulus fibrosus hold the Nucleus pulposus in position and make it impossible for the vertebrae to shift against each other when the intervertebral disc is intact. The fibres of the Anulus fibrosus, convert eccentrically acting pressure and shear forces on the Nucleus pulposus into tensile forces on the marginal edge of the vertebral body.

Nutrition

The outer zone of the Anulus fibrosus is supplied with vessels in the case of healthy and young intervertebral discs, but this ceases with age. The other zones are avascular. The tissue of the intervertebral discs is bradytrophic, has a low metabolic activity and can hardly regenerate. Nutrition is carried out using convection of nutrients from the blood vessels of the vertebral body and the peripheral zone of the Anulus fibrosus. Convection is expedited by the fluid displacement that take place throughout the day.

NOTE

In old age a large part of the proteoglycans of the intervertebral discs is lost. The reasons for this have not been conclusively established. As a result, the water retention capacity in the Anulus fibrosus decreases by 20%. This can be compensated by muscle training. If this compensation is missing, degenerative changes occur that can lead to complaints.

With age, the water-binding capacity of the Anulus fibrosus and Nucleus pulposus continuously decreases. Small tears appear in the Anulus fibrosus **(chondrosis)**. This can be detected radiologically by a reduction in height and functionally by an instability with increased mobility in the motion segment. The height of the disc is reduced and its mechanical buffer function diminished. This results in the top and base plates of the vertebral body being stressed to a greater level, which can be expressed radiologically as sclerotisation (increased radiation density, osteochondrosis). In addition, spondylophytes (bony marginal spikes) can form on the vertebral bodies.

If this type of predamaged intervertebral disc is overstressed, the Anulus fibrosus can rupture and the jelly-like centre can penetrate at different points through the now discontinuous Anulus fibrosus (so-called slipped disc):

- Most common is a **laterodorsal prolapse** (➤ Fig. 3.48), which restricts the intervertebral foramen and compresses the spinal nerve root of the corresponding segment. The result is a so-called spinal radicular syndrome with back pain (lumbago), possibly referred pain in the arms (brachialgia) or legs (ischialgia) and sensory disturbances or muscle paresis in the innervation area of the affected spinal nerve; however, a prolapse can also be asymptomatic. Due to the high complication rate there is a strict indication for surgery.
- A **mediodorsal disc prolapse** can also compress the spinal cord at a corresponding height (➤ Fig. 3.48). This situation is an emergency, because the spinal cord has to be rapidly relieved.

Degeneratively linked slipped discs are most common in the lumbar and cervical spine. The segments S1, L5 and L4 are most often affected. The slipped discs arise in the cervical spine after rupture of the intervertebral discs, which lie in the uncovertebral joints (see below).

Vertebral arch joints

The vertebrae are connected on both sides under each other via vertebral arch joints (Articulationes zygapophysiales). Dorsal of the vertebral bodies and intervertebral discs, the upper articular process **(Proc. articularis superius)** of a vertebra forms a true joint (diarthrosis) with the corresponding inferior articular process **(Proc. articularis inferius)** of the overlying vertebra. The shape, size and position of the joint facets **(Facies articulares superior et inferior)** are regionally different and are distinctive structural features of the individual spinal sections (➤ Fig. 3.49).

Within a mobile segment the two vertebral arch joints absorb pressure forces in this way and have an important kinematic function in the movement control of the individual regions of the spine. The function of this is closely linked to the spatial position of the articular surfaces.

> **N O T E**
>
> The Articulationes zygapophysiales are often referred to as **facet joints** due to the shape and position of the joint facets in the various sections of the spine.

An irritation (mostly chronic) of the facet joints (Articulationes zygapophyseales) leads to pain, which is referred to as facet syndrome or **facet joint syndrome**. It is the most common cause of back pain, which in turn is the most common reason to seek medical consultation in Germany. The cause of the pain is degenerative changes (osteoarthritis, spondyloarthrosis) in one or in most cases in several adjacent facet joints. The lumbar spine is most often affected because here the stress of the body weight coupled with high mobility is at a high level. Obesity is an additional important factor. Characteristically, there is pain at the height of the affected joints or somewhat below them radiating to the legs. Within the framework of the joint changes the nerves innervated in the joints are also stimulated (facet joint nerves), which are branches of the corresponding spinal nerve roots. The symptoms correspond to a root stimulus symptom (radiculopathy), but without the sensation disorders typical for a radicular syndrome. These are sometimes referred to as pseudoradicular pain.

Ligaments of the vertebral column

The spine has strong ligaments. The ligaments extend between the spinal vertebrae or over larger sections. A distinction is made between vertebral body ligaments and vertebral arch ligaments.

Vertebral body ligaments

The vertebral bodies are connected ventrally and dorsally via a longitudinal ligament:

- Lig. longitudinale anterius
- Lig. longitudinale posterius

The **Lig. longitudinale anterius** (➤ Fig. 3.50, ➤ Fig. 3.51) extends from the anterior atlas arch to the Os sacrum and ends there as the Lig. sacrococcygeum. The ventral superficial fibre components of the ligament extend over several vertebral bodies; the dorsal, deep fibre components connect the bony edges between two adjacent vertebrae. A connection to the intervertebral discs does not exist. The ligament becomes broader from cranial to caudal.

The **Lig. longitudinale posterius** (➤ Fig. 3.50, ➤ Fig. 3.51) extends from the Os occipitale to the Os sacrum, limits the vertebral canal at the front and lies on the back of the vertebral body. Overall, it is narrower than the Lig. longitudinale anterius and ends as deep Lig. sacrococcygeum posterius profundum in the sacral canal. The fibres, which run at the front, each spread over the intervertebral discs and are fused with them.

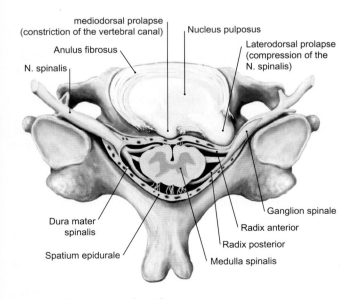

mediodorsal prolapse
(constriction of the vertebral canal)
Nucleus pulposus
Anulus fibrosus
Laterodorsal prolapse
(compression of the
N. spinalis)
N. spinalis
Ganglion spinale
Dura mater
spinalis
Radix anterior
Radix posterior
Spatium epidurale
Medulla spinalis

Fig. 3.48 Disc prolapse. [L266]

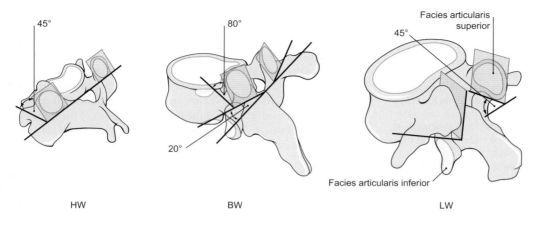

Fig. 3.49 Position of the vertebral arch joints at the cervical, thoracic and lumbar vertebrae. [L126]

HW   BW   LW

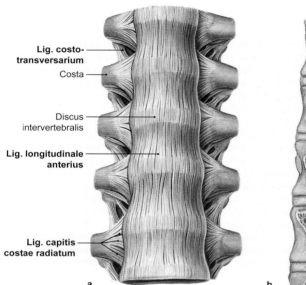

Lig. costo-transversarium
Costa
Discus intervertebralis
Lig. longitudinale anterius
Lig. capitis costae radiatum

a

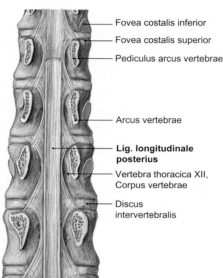

Fovea costalis inferior
Fovea costalis superior
Pediculus arcus vertebrae
Arcus vertebrae
Lig. longitudinale posterius
Vertebra thoracica XII, Corpus vertebrae
Discus intervertebralis

b

Fig. 3.50 Ligmaments of the spine. a Lig. longitudinale anterius (using the example of the lower thoracic spine). **b** Lig. longitudinale posterius (using the example of the lower thoracic and upper lumbar spine).

Clinical remarks

In the case of **BECHTEREW's DISEASE (Spondylitis anky-losans),** a genetically caused painful, inflammatory rheumatic disease, there is increasing ossification of all ligament structures, particularly of the spine. In the early stages, often only the sacroiliac joints are affected. Later, the spine is like a fixed rod and the back has the appearance of being 'smoothly ironed', the chest wall excursions are significantly reduced with reduced respiratory capacity. The occiput wall distance when standing is significantly increased.

Vertebral arch ligaments

The vertebral arches are also very well secured by ligaments (➤ Fig. 3.51). These include:

- **Lig. flava:** They join the Laminae arcus vertebrale and form the posterior limit of the Foramina intervertebralior and the lateral and posterior limitation of the vertebral canal. The Ligg. flava have a very high proportion of elastic fibres (hence the yellow colour) and help the autochthonous back muscles (see below) when holding the spine straight. In the process they act against a front-facing force.
- **Ligg. interspinalia:** They join adjacent spinal processes (Procc. spinosi) and are closely connected to the tendons of the autochthonous back muscles. At the tip of the spinal processes they

pass into the Lig. supraspinale. They limit ventral flexion and also the sliding movement of the vertebrae.
- **Lig. supraspinale:** the ligament consists of long fibres and connects the tips of multiple Proc. spinosi. Cranially, it passes into the Lig. nuchae. It limits the ventral flexion of the spine.
- **Lig. nuchae:** The Lig. nuchae is a sagittally situated, thin, rough plate of connective tissue between the Protuberantior occipitalis externa and the Proc. spinosus of the VIIth cervical vertebra (Vertebra prominens, see below). It is fused in the area of the neck groove with the general body fascia.
- **Ligg. intertransversaria:** The ligaments connect adjacent Procc. transversi of the thoracic spine and Proc. accessori of the lumbar spine and limit lateral flexion and rotation.

Characteristics of the individual regions of the spine

According to the regional differences in the movement of the spinal sections, there is a difference between the form of the vertebral bodies, of the spinal processes, the transverses process and the joint processes.

Based on these characteristics, individual vertebrae can be assigned to the respective spinal section. The specific structure of the individual mobile segments lead to differences of mobility in the individual spinal regions. These are measured according to the neutral-null method.

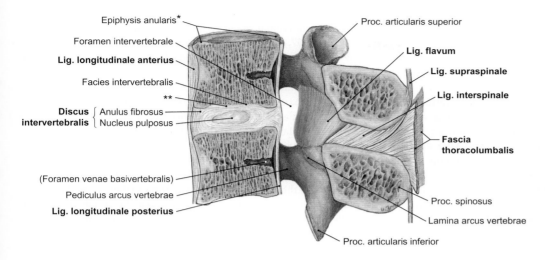

Fig. 3.51 Lumbar mobile segment with ligaments of the spine. Median section; left view.
* also: marginal ridge,
** hyaline cartilaginous covering on the base plate

NOTE

The objectification of movement restrictions can be performed via the Fingertip-to-Floor (FTF) test and function tests according to OTT (thoracic spine) and SCHOBER (lumbar spine).

- The **FTF** measures the distance between the finger tips and the floor when bent forwards with straight legs. A young person should always reach the floor (finger floor distance = 0).
- In the **test according to SCHOBER** (➤ Fig. 3.52) a mark is made on the skin at the spinal process of S1 and 10 cm cranial of this point. At maximum flexion (forward flexion) the markings typically deviate 5 cm apart, in the retroflexion the distance is reduced by 1–2 cm.
- In the **test according to OTT** (➤ Fig. 3.52) a mark is made on the skin above the Proc. spinosus process of the VIIth cervical vertebra (Vertebra prominens) and a further 30 cm caudal of this point. At the maximum flexion markings typically deviate 3–4 cm apart.

The mobility of the spine is e.g. in the case of ankylosing spondylitis (BECHTEREW's disease) limited.

Craniocervical junction

The Os occipitale and the first two cervical vertebra (atlas and axis) are connected to one another via a total of 5 joints and facilitate the freedom of movement of the head in 3 axes. In principle, the mobile segments differ in their morphological structure from those of the lower sections.

Os occipitale

The unpaired occipital bone (Os occipitale) consists of 3 units (Pars basilaris, Partes laterales and Squamor occipitalis, ➤ Fig. 9.10).

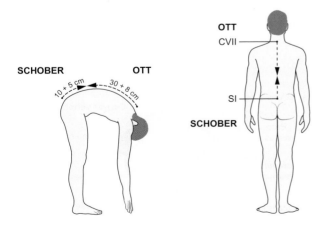

Fig. 3.52 **Objective assessment of movement restrictions** of the lumbar spine (method according to SCHOBER) and the thoracic spine (OTT sign).

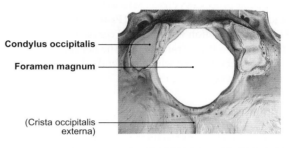

Fig. 3.53 **Section with the Os occipitale and the condyles for the upper cranial joint.** The condyles of the skull are located at the front lateral to the Foramen magnum.

The convex and slightly rostrally converging joint surfaces for articulation with the first cervical vertebra (Condyli occipitales skull conyles, skull condyles) are located at the side of the Foramen magnum in the two Partes laterales ossis occipitalis (➤ Fig. 3.53). Both hinge ligaments (Lig. alaria) begin rostromedial of the Condyli occipitales. In the median the Faciculus Longitudinalis inserts at the anterior margin of the Foramen magnum, the superior longitudinal bundle and the widely spread Membrana tectoria (➤ Fig. 3.56).

Atlas

The atlas (Ist cervical vertebra, ➤ Fig. 3.54) has no vertebral body, instead an anterior atlas arch (**Arcus anterior atlantis**) connects two lateral masses (**Massae laterales**), on which the upper and lower joint surfaces (Facies articulares superior et inferior) for articulation with the skull condyles and the axis can be found (IInd cervical vertebra), as well as the transverse process with the **Foramen transversarium** for the passage of the A. vertebralis. At the front the anterior atlas arch has a **Tuberculum anterius**. The posterior atlas arch (**Arcus posterior atlantis**) has a trench for the A. vertebralis (Sulcus arteriae vertebralis) and a posterior tubercle (**Tuberculum posterius**). A spinous process is missing.

Clinical remarks

Especially in motor vehicle accidents, there may be isolated **fractures of the atlas arches** which is now happening less frequently due to the improved protective devices in cars (air bags). They have to be differentiated from atlas variants (e.g. Canalis arteriae vertebralis) or malformations (e.g. fusion of atlas and occipital bone = atlas assimilation) as well as frequently occurring cleft formations in the region of the vertebral arch.

Axis

The axis (IInd cervical vertebra, ➤ Fig. 3.55) has a vertebral body which has a massive tooth-shaped projection, the **Dens axis**. From an evolutionary perspective the Dens axis is the former vertebral body of the Atlas. From the top of the dens axis (**Apex dentis**) the **Lig. apicis dentis** originates (➤ Fig. 3.56) and from the lateral areas the **Ligg. alaria** arise laterally and wing-shaped. On the ventral side there is a joint surface at the Dens axis (Facies articularis anterior) for articulation with the anterior vertebral arch of the Atlas, on the dorsal side there is an area (Facies articularis posterior) by which **Lig. transversum atlantis** holds the Dens axis in position. The axis has a vertebral arch, which laterally supports the connection from the vertebral body on the lower edge of the dens axis of 2 upper articular processes (**Procc. articulares superiores**) to the atlas and below 2 articular processes (**Procc. articulares inferiores**) for the articulation with the IIIrd cervical vertebra. In addition, the axis has a **Proc. transversus**. The **Foramen transversarium** for the vertebral artery, which is slightly slanted from lower inside to upper outside, lies in this.

Clinical remarks

In road accidents, **dens fractures** can occur or a **fracture of the arch root (Hangman's fracture)** with the risk of cervical cord compression. These fractures are very difficult to diagnose and can occur even in young children.

Cranial joints

A differentiation is made between 2 cranial joints (➤ Fig. 3.56, ➤ Fig. 3.57, ➤ Fig. 3.58):
- Upper cranial joint (Articulatio atlantooccipitalis): connects the skull with the atlas
- Lower cranial joint (Articulatio atlantoaxialis): connects the atlas and axis and is divided into the following:
  - Articulatio antlantoaxialis mediana (unpaired)
  - Articulatio antlantoaxilialis lateralis (paired)

All of these joints are true joints (diarthroses) without intervertebral discs.

In the **Articulatio atlantooccipitalis** the Condyli occipitales articulate with the Facies articulares superiores atlantis (➤ Fig. 3.57). The upper articular surfaces of the atlas can be designed individually and intervariably and also have biconvex joint surfaces. The joint capsule is wide (➤ Fig. 3.56b) and reinforced on both sides by a lateral ligament (**Lig. atlantooccipitale laterale**).

In the **Articulatio atlantooccipitalis** the atlas and the axis are connected via 3 individual joints:
- The **Articulatio atlantoaxialis mediana** has 2 joint surfaces for the Dens axis. In the anterior joint chamber the Facies articularis anterior of the Dens axis articulates with the Fovea dentis of the anterior atlas arch (➤ Fig. 3.58). In the posterior joint chamber the Facies articularis posterior of the Dens axis articulates with the **Lig. transversum atlantis** (➤ Fig. 3.58), which originates on both sides at the Massae laterales atlantis and crosses over the root and the main body of the Dens axis.
- The **Articulatio atlantoaxialis lateralis** are made up of joint connections between the Facies articularis inferior atlantis caudal of the Massa lateralis atlantis and the Facies articularis superior axis on both sides (➤ Fig. 3.56, ➤ Fig. 3.57). Both joint surfaces are convex and thus incongruent.

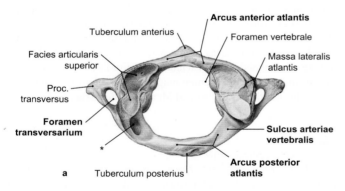
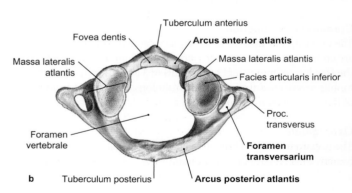

Fig. 3.54 I. Cervical vertebra, atlas. a cranial view. **b** caudal view. * variant: Canalis arteriae vertebralis

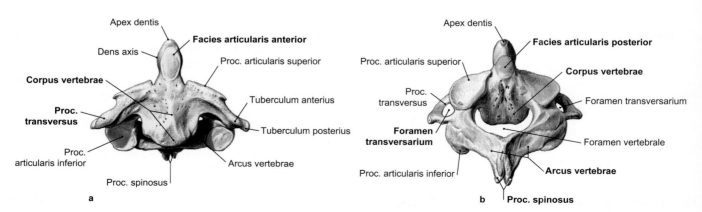

Fig. 3.55 II. Cervical vertebrae, axis. a ventral view. **b** dorsal view.

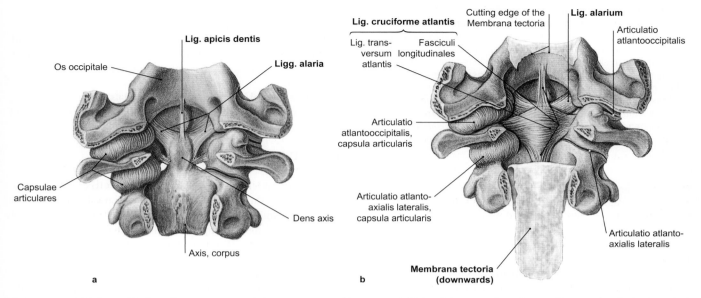

Fig. 3.56 Cranial joints with deep ligaments. Dorsal view. **a** Upper and lower cranial joint, joint capsules, Lig. cruciforme atlantis. **b** Ligg. alaria and Lig. apicis dentis.

Ligaments

The stability of the craniocervical junction is ensured by an elaborate ligament back-up, which still allows maximum freedom of movement. A multi-layer structure of the ligament structures prevents dislocation of the vertebral bodies, ensuring the integrity of the vertebral canal with the structures important for the vital functions of the Medulla oblongata and the cervical cord:

- **Membrane atlantooccipitalis anterior** (➤ Fig. 3.57, ➤ Fig. 3.58): This passes as a continuation of the Lig. longitudinale anterius extending from the anterior atlas arch to the underside of the occipital bone in front of the Foramen magnum and inhibits extension of the head.
- **Membranor atlantooccipitalis posterior** (➤ Fig. 3.58): This moves from the posterior atlas arch to the dorsal margin of the Foramen magnum and inhibits flexion of the head.
- **Membrana tectoria** (➤ Fig. 3.56b, ➤ Fig. 3.58): This continues the Lig. longitudinale posterior and runs from the posterior edge of the axis body to the anterior edge of the foramen magnum and to the Clivus. It limits the forward tilt of the head.
- **Lig. cruciforme atlantis** (➤ Fig. 3.56b, ➤ Fig. 3.58): The ligament consists of several units that cross in their fibre direction. The **Lig. transversum atlantis** extends between the two Massae laterales of the atlas, runs behind the Facies articularis posterior of the dens axis and as such holds the Dens axis in position at

the anterior Atlas arch. In the area of the joint surface, the ligament is made of fibrous tissue. A **Fasciculus longitudinalis superior** runs in the vertical direction from the front edge of the Foramen magnum to the Lig. transversum atlantis; a **Fasciculus longitudinalis inferior** comes from the rear surface of the axis body and radiates caudally into the Lig. transversum atlantis. The Lig. cruciforme atlantis inhibits the forward inclination of the head with both units.

- **Ligg. alaria** (➤ Fig. 3.56a): The wing ligaments extend to the side from the Dens axis to the medial edge of the Foramen magnum and limit the rotation in the Articulatio atlantoaxialis mediana as well as the forward inclination of the head.
- **Lig. apicis dentis** (➤ Fig. 3.56a, ➤ Fig. 3.58): Extends from the Apex dentis to the anterior edge of the foramen magnum and inhibits forward inclination of the head.

Clinical remarks

In the case of a **cervical fracture** the Lig. transversum atlantis or the Lig. cruciforme atlantis tear. The Dens axis tilts dorsally into the vertebral canal and presses on the Medulla oblongata, in which the respiratory and circulatory centres are located, and on the spinal cord. This results in immediate death.

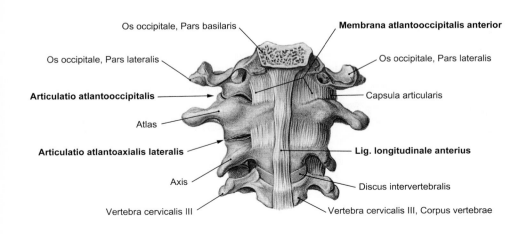

Fig. 3.57 Cranial joints with ligaments and upper cervical spine.

Occasionally, a missing or incomplete formation of the Dens axis may cause an **atlantoaxial subluxation**. Injury to the ligaments of the cranial joints can cause **atlantoaxial instability**. Such injuries are often overlooked in clinical practice, as the patient reactively shows increased muscle tension (protection spasm). Symptoms of such atlantoaxial instabilities are often intermittent circulatory disorders of the vertebral arteries, the A. carotis interna and the V. jugularis with a dazed feeling, dizziness, visual disturbances (Mouches volantes = seeing stars), headache and nausea.

N O T E
The cranial joints are at the height of the oropharynx. When the mouth is open and a finger is inserted as far as the pharyngeal wall, this lies at the height of the atlantoaxial joint.

Mechanisms
Together, the two cranial joints act like a ball joint, which enables all-round movements of the head; however, the overall extent of

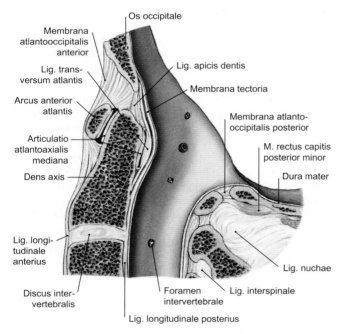

Fig. 3.58 **Cervico-occipital transition region** with intermediate atlantoaxial joint and ligamentous apparatus. Median sagittal section, left view.

mobility results from the interaction with the other mobile segments in the cervical spine.

The **upper cranial joint** is a ellipsoid joint, which enables the nodding movements of the head around a transversal axis of a total of 20–35°. Around a sagittal axis, minor side movements of 10–15° are possible.

The **lower cranial joint** is a hinge joint and its vertical axis runs through the Dens axis. It allows rotational movements of a total of 35–55° and a small nodding movement.

IIIrd–VIIth cervical vertebrae
Characteristics
One can only refer to characteristic cervical vertebrae (**Vertebrae cervicales**) for the IIIrd–VIIth cervical vertebrae, because only these 5 are similarly structured (➤ Fig. 3.59). The overall relatively small vertebrae have an approximately rectangular shape. Special features of the cervical vertebrae are:

* The margins of the cervical vertebrae each have an upturned process with sagittal alignment (**Proc. uncinatus;** syn.: Uncus corporis). When viewed from the front it looks as if the lateral edges of the vertebral body cover plates are bent upwards (➤ Fig. 3.59a).
* The transverse process consists of a posterior part (**Tuberculum posterius**), the actual transverse process and a front portion (**Tuberculum anterius**), which corresponds to the rib rudiment (➤ Fig. 3.59b). The transversus process has a lateral-directed deepening for the course of spinal nerve branches (**Sulcus nervi spinalis**) and the IIIrd–VIth cervical vertebrae usually have a **Foramen transversarium** for the passage of the A. vertebralis.
* The articular processes are flat and incline approximately 45° to the rear (➤ Fig. 3.59b).
* The spinal process of the vertebral bodies III–VI are short and bifurcated (bipartite, ➤ Fig. 3.59b).
* The Tuberculum anterius of the VIth cervical vertebra is palpable from ventral (Tuberculum caroticum).
* The interspinous process of the VIIth cervical vertebra is long and well palpable (Vertebra prominens) from the outside.

Uncovertebral joints
Around the *10th year of life,* at the upper spine (IIIrd–VIth cervical vertebrae) there is a physiological fissure formation in the lateral portions of the Disci intervertebralis. This creates new joint-like connective tissue structures, which are referred to as uncovertebral joints (**Hemiarthroses uncovertebrales, VON LUSCHKA's joints**) (➤ Fig. 3.60). The cleft formation often continues to the Nucleus pulposus, so that the intervertebral disc is virtually halved horizon-

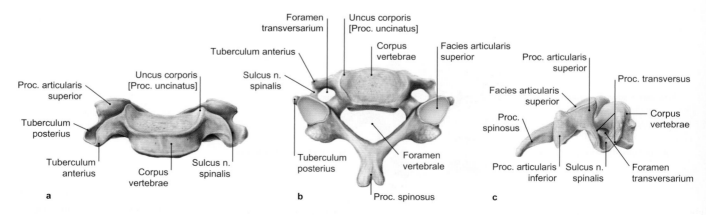

Fig. 3.59 **Cervical vertebra. a** Ventral view. **b** Dorsal view. **c** Right lateral view. [L266]

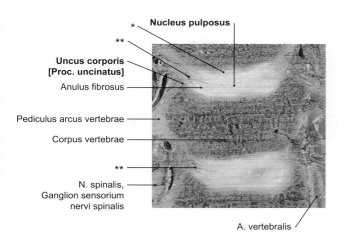

Fig. 3.60 Uncovertebral joints; * hyaline cartilaginous coverages of the end plates; ** so-called uncovertebral cleft.

tally. This creates structure loosening, which is compensated by the strong ligaments. On the lower cervical spine the uncovertebral joints are usually only weakly developed.

It is discussed that these joints allow ventral and dorsal movements, while lateral movements are restricted; however, the function has not been conclusively clarified.

Mechanisms

In the cervical spine below the cranial joints, anteflexion and dorsal flexion as well as lateral flexion and rotational movements to a certain extent are possible. Overall, the cervical spine is very flexible (➤ Fig. 3.46).

Thoracic vertebrae
Characteristics

The vertebral bodies of the thoracic spine (**Vertebrae thoracicae,** ➤ Fig. 3.61) are dorsally indented, so that the base and top plates have a heart shape. They are lower ventrally than dorsally and thus enable thoracic kyphosis. As a special feature, the Ist–IXth thoracic vertebral body dorsolaterally have cranial and caudal joint surfaces (**Foveae costales superior et inferior**). An Fovea costalis inferior always forms a common joint cavity with a Fovea costalis superior facet of the underlying vertebra for a rib head (**Articulatio capitis costae,** rib head joint, ➤ Chapter 3.3.4). The Xth and XIth thoracic vertebral body only have a Fovea costalis. In the case of the XIIth thoracic vertebral body, the Fovea costalis posterior lies centrally on the vertebral body. The transverse processes are inclined towards dorsolateral and the Ist–Xth vertebral bodies have joint surfaces (Foveae costales processus transversi) for connection to the costotransverse joints (**Articulationes costotransversariae,** ➤ Chapter 3.3.4). The upper articular processes (**Procc. articulares superiores**) are directed dorsally and the lower (**Procc. artic-**

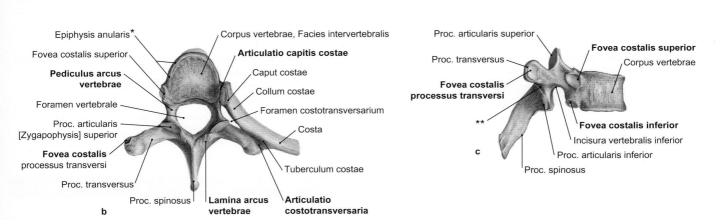

Fig. 3.61 Thoracic vertebra. a Ventral view; * marginal ridge. **b** Dorsal view. **c** Right lateral view; ** region of the vertebral arch between the superior and inferior joint extension (so-called isthmus = interarticular portion).

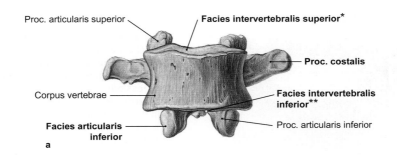

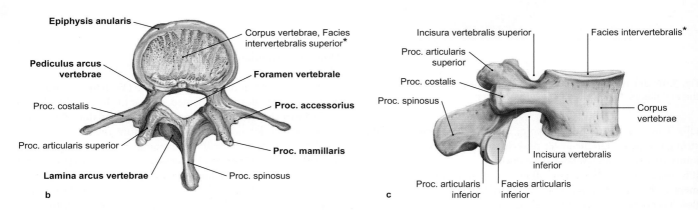

Fig. 3.62 Lumbar vertebra. a Ventral view. **b** Dorsal view; * cover plate, ** base plate. **c** Right lateral view. [L266]

ulares inferiores) ventrally. The joint surfaces are located approximately in the frontal plane (➤ Fig. 3.49). The spinous processes are long and aligned caudally. They overlap like roof tiles and protect the Canalis vertebralis (➤ Fig. 3.44c).

Mechanisms
The vertebrae are connected to the chest wall. In spite of the larger number of vertebrae, the thoracic spine is less mobile than the other sections of the spine. Slight ventral flexion and dorsal flexion movements and lateral flexion and rotational motions are possible (➤ Fig. 3.46).

Lumbar vertebrae
Characteristics
The vertebral bodies of the lumbar spine (**Vertebrae lumbales,** ➤ Fig. 3.62) are large; the transverse diameter is larger than the sagittal, the base and top plates are ventrally retracted into a kidney shape. They are higher ventrally than dorsally and thus enable lumbar lordosis. The long and laterally oriented processes are referred to as **Proc. costalis** (rib process). The actual transverse processes lie as rudiments at the base of the Procc. costales and are called **Procc. accessorii.** The articular processes are aligned dorsally. The **Proc. articularis superior** dorsally bears a hump (**Proc. mamillaris).** With the exception of the lumbar vertebral vein the joint surfaces are aligned in the sagittal plane (➤ Fig. 3.49). The spinous processes are almost straight and aligned dorsally.

> **NOTE**
> In clinical terms both the Procc. costales as well as the Procc. accessorii of the lumbar vertebrae are often summarised as **Procc. transversi** in the analogy to the other spinal sections.

Mechanisms
The sagittal position of the joint surfaces of the Articulationes zygapophyseales in the upper 4 mobile segments of the lumbar spine en-

ables extension and flexion and brakes rotational movements. Due to the condylar position of the joint processes, the rotary motion takes place between the lumbar vertebral vein and the sacrum. A lateral flexion is extensively possible in the lumbar spine (➤ Fig. 3.46).

Sacrum
The **sacrum (Os sacrum;** ➤ Fig. 3.63) is composed of 5 sacral vertebrae that in adolescence are still connected via cartilage and later fuse synostotically; however, in later life disc tissue can still be found between the synostotically connected former vertebral bodies. The sacrum is connected to the two hip bones (Ossa coxae) via the Articulationes sacroiliacae and shows significant gender differences (➤ Table 3.7). The base (**Basis ossis sacri)** is connected via a large intervertebral disc to the lumbar vertebral vein. The front edge of the sacrum base bulges ventrally into the lumbosacral transition and into the pelvis (**Promontorium**). On the front surface (**Facies pelvica)** the original borders of the sacral vertebrae can be recognised as **Lineae transversae** (➤ Fig. 3.63a). The **Foramina intervertebralia** has merged to bony channels, which have 4 openings at the front (**Foramina sacralia anteriora)** for the ventral spinal nerve branches. Dorsally, (**Facies dorsalis)** multiple longitudinally running strips are present (➤ Fig. 3.63b):
- **Crista sacralis mediana** (unpaired): they are located in the area of the former spinous process.
- **Crista sacralis medialis** (paired): located in the area of the former articular process.
- **Crista sacralis lateralis** (paired): located in the area of the former transverse process.

Table 3.7 Gender differences of the sacrum (Os sacrum).

Form	Women	Men
Length	Shorter	Longer
Expression	Wider	Narrower
Curvature	Weaker	Stronger

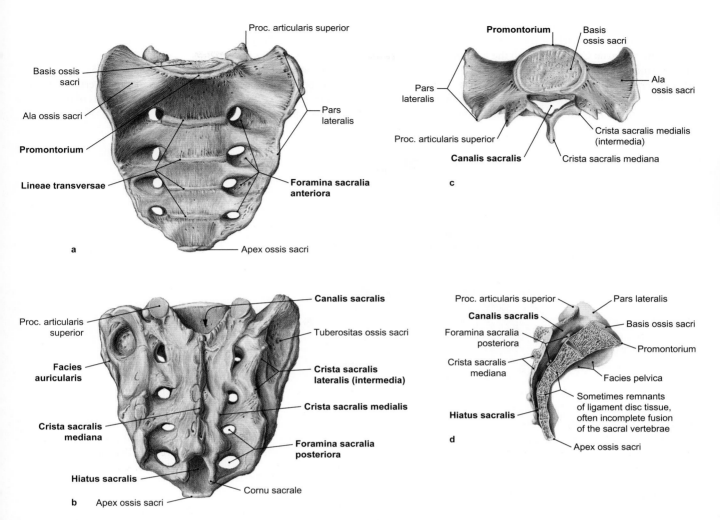

Fig. 3.63 Sacrum, Os sacrum. a Ventral view. **b** Dorsal view. **c** View from above. **d** Mediosagittal section.

Caudally to the Crista sacralis mediana is the access to the sacral canal (**Canalis sacralis**), in form of the **Hiatus sacralis**. The **Foramina sacralia posteriora** are the exit points of the dorsal spinal nerve branches. The region at the side of the rear openings is referred to as the **Pars lateralis**. On their lateral surface are the **Facies auricularis** which are the joint surfaces for articulation and the **Tuberositas ossis sacri** for fibrous connection with the Os ilium of the hip bone (sacroiliac joint, Articulatio iliosacralis, ➤ Chap. 5.2.3).

Coccyx

The **coccyx** (**Os coccygis**; ➤ Fig. 3.64) is normally constructed of 3–5 rudimentary vertebrae. Only the two coccygeal horns (**Cornua coccygea**) of the Ist coccygeal vertebra as rudiments of the upper articular process enable the origin as vertebrae to be recognised. The Cornua coccygea can articulate with rudiments of the left and right lower articular processes of the sacral vertebral vein (**Articulatio sacrococcygea**). The coccyx is otherwise connected by carti-

lage to the sacrum. In younger people there can also be an intervertebral disc.

Vascular, lymphatic and nervous systems
Arteries
Cervical spine
The mobile segments of the cervical spine are supplied with blood via the branches of the **A. carotis externa** (A. occipitalis) and the **A. subclavia** (A. vertebralis, A. cervicalis profunda from the Truncus costocervicalis, A. transversa colli from the Truncus thyrocervicalis).

The **A. vertebralis** arises on the rear wall of the A. subclavia. It is divided into 4 sections:

- **Pars prevertebralis:** Course on the M. longus colli to the Foramen transversarium of VIth cervical vertebra (approx. 90% of cases). Also a shorter distance to the VIIth cervical vertebra (approximately 2% of cases; then the VIIth cervical vertebra also has Fo-

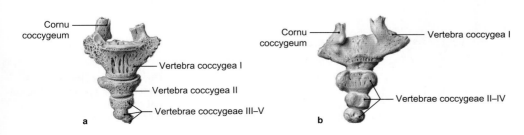

**Fig. 3.64 Coccyx, Os coccygis.
a** Ventral view. **b** Dorsal view.

ramina transversaria) or a longer distance with entry into the Vth, IVth or IIIrd cervical vertebrae is possible (➤ Fig. 10.14).

- **Pars transversaria:** Course through the Foramina transversaria, accompanied by the Plexus venosus of the V. vertebralis and the Plexus vertebralis (sympathetic nerve network around the A. vertebralis). From the Pars transversaria segmental branches emit through the Foramina intervertebralia into the vertebral

canal, and supply the meninges (**Rr. spinales**) and the spinal cord (**Rr. radiculares**). **Rr. musculares** run to the deep neck muscles.

- **Pars atlantica, Pars intracranialis:** Chap. 11.1.5.

In the posterior cranial fossa the right and left A. vertebralis connect to the A. basilaris on the clivus. Further details of the A. vertebralis are presented in Chap. 11.1.5.

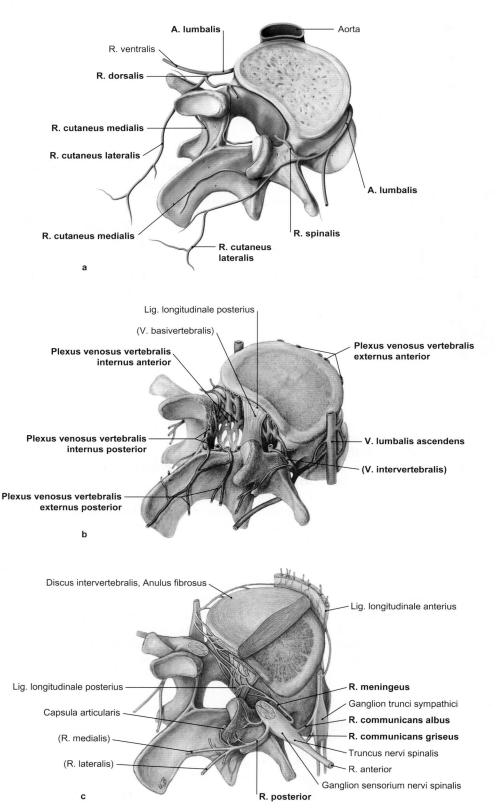

Fig. 3.65 Vascular, lymphatic and nervous systems of the spinal canal. Right oblique view. **a** Arteries [L266]. **b** Veins. **c** Nerves.

Thoracic and lumbar vertebral column

A strictly segmental arterial supply is at the height of the thoracic and lumbar spine. Eleven paired **Aa. intercostales posteriores,** the paired **A. subcostalis** and 4 paired **Aa. lumbales** exit as segmental branches from the Aorta thoracica or the Aorta abdominalis to supply the adjacent vertebrae with blood (➤ Fig. 3.13).
The arteries each emit a **R. dorsalis** from which a **R. spinalis** passes through the Foramen intervertebrale of the corresponding mobile segment and enters the vertebral canal (➤ Fig. 3.65a). The segmental spinal arteries anastomose at different heights in the vertebral canal via ascending and descending branches. The posterior artery branches each reach the arch plates (laminae) and the spinosus processes from the inside. The terminal branches of the Rr. posteriores are the **Rr. cutanei mediales** and **Rr. cutanei laterales,** which run parallel with the dorsal spinal nerve branches of the same name, supply blood to the posterior bony structures from the outside and their end branches penetrate the dorsal back muscles and supply the skin.

Sacrum and coccyx

The supply of the sacrum takes place via the **A. sacralis mediana** running along the ventral side from the abdominal aorta (➤ Fig. 3.41) and via the lateral sacral arteries (**Aa. sacrales laterales**) from the A. iliaca interna. The lateral sacral arteries emit **Rr. spinales** into the Foramina sacralia pelvina and reach the coccyx as terminal branches.

Veins

The venous drainage from the spine and the spinal cord takes place via venous networks (➤ Fig. 3.65b). The veins are valveless and have connections to the veins in the skull and the azygos system. They can be divided into an outer and inner venous network:
- **Outer venous system:**
  - The **Plexus venosus vertebralis externus anterior** is to the side and in front of the vertebral body and includes veins that come from the lateral surface of the vertebral body and the neighbouring ligaments.
  - The **Plexus venosus vertebralis externus posterior** is to the side and behind the arch roots and the spinous processes. It takes up the blood from these, the neighbouring ligaments, the autochthonous back muscles and the skin on the back.
- **Inner venous system:**
  - The **Plexus venosus vertebralis internus anterior** is located on the rear of the vertebral body in the vertebral canal laterally to the Lig. longitudinale posterius and take blood from the vertebral bodies, which is supplied from the Vv. basivertebrales (a horizontally running vein network in the cancellous bone of the vertebral body). It also drains blood from the spinal cord (Vv. spinales anteriores).
  - The **Plexus venosus vertebralis internus posterior** is located on the inside of the vertebral arches and drains the blood from the vertebral arches and the neighbouring ligaments, as well as from the spinal cord (Vv. spinales posteriores).

The outer and inner venous systems are connected with abundant anastomoses. In the craniocervical junction there is a link between extracranial and intracranial veins. In the throat area the venous plexuses drain into the V. vertebralis and the V. cervicalis profunda.

On the thoracic and lumbar spine the vein networks drain via the Vv. intercostales posteriores or Vv. lumbales into the azygos system (Vv. azygos, hemiazygos et hemiazygos accessoria, ➤ Fig. 3.16) and via the vein networks of the pelvis into the V. iliaca interna.

Innervation of the vertebral arch joints

The innervation of the joint capsule of the vertebral arch joints takes place from the Rr. mediales of the Rr. posteriores of the spinal nerves (➤ Fig. 3.65c).

3.3.3 Spinal cord site

Spinal canal

The vertebral canal (also spinal canal; **Canalis vertebralis**) extends from the Foramen magnum of the Os occipitale to the Hiatus sacralis of the sacrum. It follows the curvature of the spine in the presacral area and at the height of sacrum is referred to as the sacral canal.
In the **presacral, free part** of the spine, the vertebral canal is limited ventrally by the vertebral bodies, the intervertebral discs and the posteriorly attached Lig. longitudinale posterius (➤ Fig. 3.51). Laterally and dorsally it is limited by the vertebral arches and the connecting Ligg. flava and the Lig. interspinale. The intvertebral formina (Foramina intervertebralia) lie laterally between the individual vertebrae.
The **caudal section** of the vertebral canal is the sacral canal (**Canalis sacralis**, ➤ Fig. 3.63), which is bordered on all sides by bone and is covered with offshoots of the Lig. longitudinale posterius. It ends at variable heights in the Hiatus sacralis. The Foramina sacralia anteriora connect the sacral canal with the pelvic space and the Foramina sacralia dorsalia with the sacral region.

Clinical remarks

A narrowing of the vertebral canal is referred to as a **spinal canal stenosis.** The cause is often bony projections (spondylophytes) of the vertebral body or the intervertebral joints, which emerge during degenerative changes of the spine. The patients report radicularly radiating pain of the affected segments. The pain often increases when walking. In this case it is known as a **claudicatio spinalis.**

Spinal meninges
Hard spinal meninges

The hard meninges (**Dura mater encephali**) passes into the hard spinal meninges at the Foramen magnum (**Dura mater spinalis**). At the craniocervical junction the Dura mater spinalis is firmly connected via the periosteum to the bony wall of the foramen magnum and of the vertebral canal. Below the axis, there are only a few connections between the Dura mater spinalis and the vertebral arches (➤ Fig. 3.66a). Lateral bulges of the Dura mater spinalis extend into the Foramina intervertebralia. The dural sac usually ends caudally at the height of the IInd sacral vertebrae and from there goes over into the thin offshoots of the Filum terminale (also ➤ Chap. 12.6.2).

Soft spinal meninges

The two soft meninges (**Leptomeninx encephali,** consisting of the Arachnoidea mater encephali and Pia mater encephali) continuously pass into the soft spinal meninges, (**Leptomeninx spinalis**). The outer lamina of the **Arachnoidea mater spinalis** attaches to the inner surface of the Dura mater spinalis (➤ Fig. 3.66b). The

129

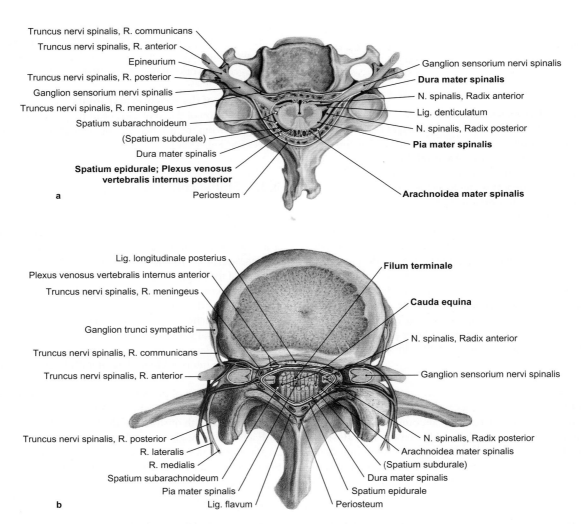

Fig. 3.66 **Content of the spinal canal (Canalis vertebralis);** cranial view. **a** Cross-section at the height of the cervical vertebral vein. **b** Cross-section at the height of the IIIrd lumbar vertebra.

subarachnoid space is between the Arachnoid mater spinalis and Pia mater spinalis (**Spatium subarachnoideum**), which shows continuity with the intracranial subarachnoid space and contains the Liquor cerebrospinalis.

The **Pia mater spinalis** is firmly attached to the spinal cord and the spinal nerve roots (➤ Fig. 3.66). The spinal cord and the spinal nerve roots, the spinal ganglion and the Truncus nervi spinalis are surrounded by Liquor cerebrospinalis. The subarachnoid space is traversed by thin trabeculae of the Arachnoidea spinalis. The **Lig. denticulatum** extends laterally as a loose connective tissue plate through the subarachnoid space into the Foramina intervertebralia (➤ Fig. 3.67a). There it separates and stabilises the two spinal nerve roots.

Extensions of the subarachnoid space are referred to as **cisterns**:

- At the craniocervical junction there is a posterior extension of the subarachnoid space due to the attachment of the Dura mater spinalis on the wall of the vertebral canal (**Cisterna rebello-medullaris,** ➤ Chap. 11.4.4).
- Caudally to the spinal cord are the spinal nerve roots (**Cauda equina**) in the cerebrospinal fluid-filled subarachnoid space (➤ Fig. 3.67b). This area is also referred to as the **Cisterna lumbalis.**

Clinical remarks

Through a **puncture of the subarachnoid space** Liquor cerebrospinalis can be removed for research purposes, or medication can be administered in the fluid space. In most cases, the Cisterna lumbalis (in the area of the Cauda equina) is punctured for this (lumbar puncture). It lies caudally to the spinal cord below the IInd lumbar vertebra, usually between the spinous processes L3/L4 or L4/L5 and has the advantage that the spinal nerve roots in the subarachnoid space can avoid the puncture needle and injury to the spinal cord can be excluded. The puncture needle is inserted through the Ligg. supraspinale et interspinale, the epidural space, the Dura mater, and the Arachnoidea until the needle enters the subarachnoid space. Alternatively, a suboccipital puncture is also possible, in which the Cisterna cerebellomedullaris is punctured at the craniocervical junction (more often in children).

Spinal cord

The **spinal cord (Medulla spinalis)** lies protected, surrounded by the spinal cord meninges within the vertebral canal (➤ Fig. 3.66a). It does not fill the vertebral canal completely, so that the dural sac lies in the loose connective tissue of the epidural space. The caudal end of the spinal cord is referred to as the **Conus medullaris** (also ➤ Chap. 12.6.2). The growth in length of the spinal cord lags behind compared to the length growth of the axial skeleton. In neo-

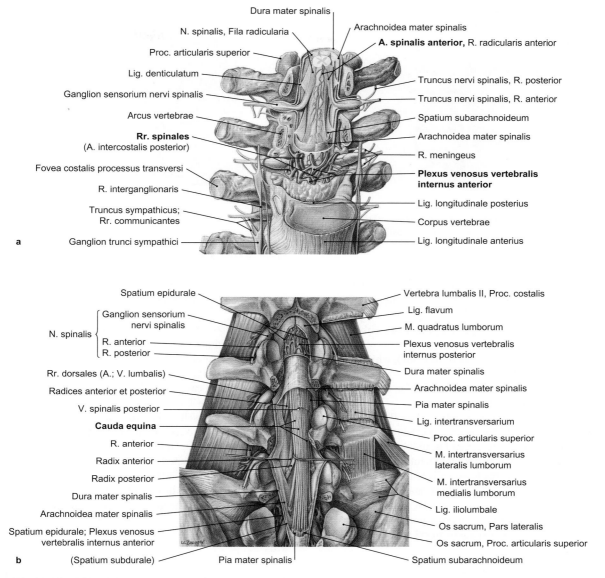

Fig. 3.67 Opened spinal canal. a Thoracic spine with spinal cord (Medulla spinalis) and sympathetic trunk (Truncus sympathicus); ventral view. **b** Lumbar spine with Cauda equina; dorsal view.

nates the spinal cord ends at the height of the IIIrd lumbar vertebra, in adults it is usually between the Ist and IInd lumbar vertebrae.

In the area of the entry and exit points of the spinal nerve roots for the extremities, the spinal cord is thickened:

- **Intumescentia cervicalis:** between the IIIrd cervical vertebra and the IIIrd thoracic vertebra with the spinal nerve roots for the Plexus cervicalis and the Plexus brachialis
- **Intumescentia lumbosacralis:** between the Xth thoracic vertebra and the Ist lumbar vertebra with the spinal nerve roots for the Plexus lumbosacralis

Spinal nerve roots
Lateral to the spinal cord, the entry and exit points of the spinal nerve roots are located (**Radices anteriores et posteriores,** ➤ Fig. 3.66, ➤ Fig. 3.67). Because the spinal cord grows more slowly than the axial skeleton, the spinal nerve roots run in the subarachnoid space at the height of the cervical spine almost horizontally to the intervertebral foramina, while they steeply extend caudally at the height of the lumbar spine. The spinal nerve roots of the lumbar

and sacral spinal cord, which partially run over a long distance caudally to the Conus medullaris in the subarachnoid space, are amalgamated as the **Cauda equina** (horse tail). The almost vertical course of the caudal spinal nerve roots changes direction when it enters into the horizontally aligned intervertebral foramina (➤ Fig. 3.67).

Intervertebral foramina
Bony and ligamentary borders
The **intervertebral foramina (Foramina intervertebralia)** are formed in the presacral section of the spine by contractions (**Incisurae vertebrales inferior et superior**), which are created between adjacent vertebrae dorsal to the vertebral bodies and the intervertebral disc and ventral of the vertebral arch joints in the area of the Pediculi arcus vertebrae (➤ Fig. 3.51). Since the Foramina intervertebralia are formed by 2 articulated interconnected vertebrae, the diameter of the Foramina changes during movement in the respective motion segment. At the lumbar spine, the foramina intervertebralia are limited dorsally by the Ligg. flava (➤ Fig. 3.51, ➤ Fig. 3.68).

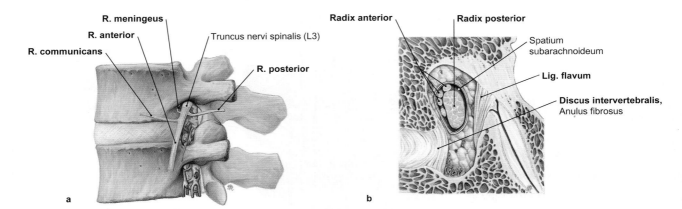

Fig. 3.68 Foramen intervertebrale using the example of the lumbar spine; left view. **a** Content of the Foramen intervertebrale. **b** Sagittal section at the height of the Foramen intervertebrale. [S010-17]

Contents

The intervertebral foramina are each 7–10 mm deep and can therefore be considered as connecting canals between the vertebral canal and the paravertebral region. Each Foramen intervertebrale contains:

- the posterior spinal nerve root (**Radix posterior**) with the spinal ganglion (Ganglion spinale)
- the anterior spinal nerve root (**Radix anterior**), which usually consists of several bundles
- the retrograde **R. meningeus** for the innervation of the meninges
- the **R. spinalis** of the segment artery
- **Connecting veins** for connection between the Plexus venosus vertebralis internus and Plexus venosus vertebralis externus.

The Radix posterior, Radix anterior and R. meningeus are located as parts of the spinal segment in the subarachnoid space and are sheathed by hard meninges. The R. spinalis of the segment artery and the connecting veins lie in the epidural space of the Foramen intervertebrale, embedded in loose connective tissue. Outside of the Foramen intervertebrale is the merging point of the spinal roots to the spinal nerve stem (**Truncus nervi spinalis**).

Clinical remarks

An osteophyte formation in arthrosis of the vertebral arch joints **(Osteochondrosis vertebralis)** or the uncovertebral joints (on the cervical spine) can constrict the Foramina intervertebralia and as such damage the spinal nerve roots or the spinal nerve stem. Patients complain in most cases of radiating radicular pain or even muscle paresis depending on the spinal cord segment affected.

3.3.4 Thorax

Bony thorax and joints

The chest (**Cavea thoracis, thorax**, ➤ Fig. 3.69) is formed from:

- 12 thoracic vertebrae (Vertebrae thoracicae I–XII)
- 12 pairs of ribs (Costae I–XII)
- Breastbone (Sternum)

The **rib pairs I–X** are connected via the rib cartilage and the rib-sternal joints with the sternum. Dorsally the ribs articulate with the thoracic spine via rib-vertebral joints. In each case 2 ribs border an intercostal space (**Spatium intercostale**) with intercostal muscles and vascular, lymphatic and nervous systems. The 10th and 11th ICS are already part of the abdominal wall. The chest en-

closes the thoracic cavity (**Cavitas thoracis**). Functionally the chest forms a stable protective enclosure for vital organs, such as the heart and lungs; it is the attachment point for many muscles (including the diaphragm) and enables breathing through the movable ribs.

The upper chest opening (**Apertura thoracis superior**) is limited by the first thoracic vertebra, both first ribs and the Manubrium sterni. The lower chest opening (**Apertura thoracis inferior**) is significantly greater than the upper. It is limited by the XIIth thoracic vertebra, in each case by the XIIth ribs, the cartilaginous ends of the Xth and XIth ribs and the cartilaginous costal arch (Angulus infrasternalis) as well as the Proc. xiphoideus of the sternum.

The shape of the thorax goes through age and gender-specific changes and also displays individual differences. In newborns the thorax is still bell-shaped and the ribs are almost horizontally aligned. Therefore, an infant breathes far more abdominally. With the growth in length, the course of the ribs becomes more crescent-shaped. This is the mechanical prerequisite for more efficient thoracic breathing.

Ribs

Normally there are 12 rib pairs (**Costae**). Most of the ribs in young adults are formed from a larger bony and a smaller cartilaginous portion. A differentiation is made depending on whether the ribs have contact to the sternum or to the cartilaginous costal arch or have no contact with the sternum or rib arch (➤ Fig. 3.70):

- **True ribs** (**Costale verae**, ribs I–VII), their rib cartilage is directly connected and articulated to the sternum
- **False ribs** (**Costal spuriae**, ribs VIII–XII), they are not directly connected with the sternum
- **Free ribs** (**Costae fluctuantes**, ribs XI and XII, variably also the Xth rib), they end free between the pectoral muscles

The VIIIth and IXth ribs, as well as the Xth rib, are involved in the development of the rib arch (Arcus costae) in approximately one third of the cases. In doing so, the cartilaginous parts accumulate from below on the next higher rib.

Basic structure of the ribs

The bony part of the rib (**Os costae**) is articulated in contact with the vertebrae and continues forward as cartilage (**Cartilago costalis**). On the Os costae, a distinction is made between (➤ Fig. 3.71):

- Rib head (**Caput costae**): articulates with the thoracic vertebral bodies
- Rib neck (**Collum costae**): connects to the rib head
- Rib tubercle (**Tuberculum costae**): articulates with the Proc. transversus of the vertebral body

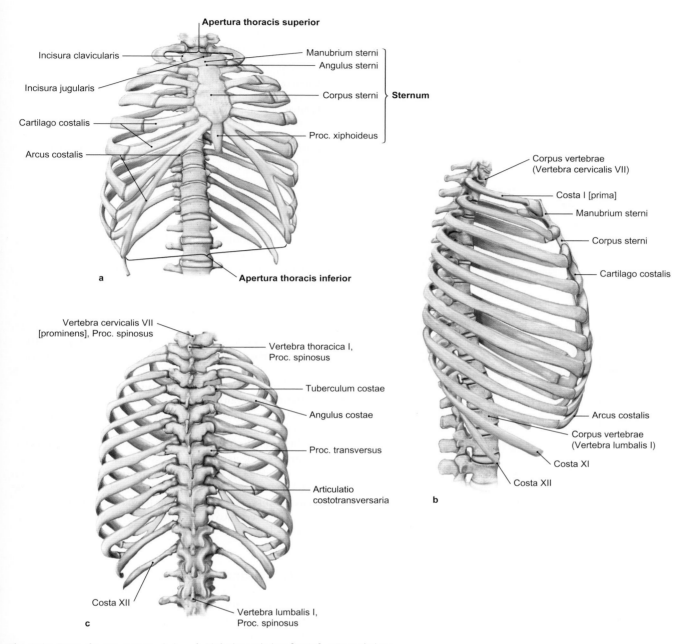

Apertura thoracis superior

Incisura clavicularis

Incisura jugularis

Cartilago costalis

Arcus costalis

Manubrium sterni

Angulus sterni

Corpus sterni ⟩ **Sternum**

Proc. xiphoideus

Apertura thoracis inferior

a

Corpus vertebrae
(Vertebra cervicalis VII)

Costa I [prima]

Manubrium sterni

Corpus sterni

Cartilago costalis

Arcus costalis

Corpus vertebrae
(Vertebra lumbalis I)

Costa XI

Costa XII

b

Vertebra cervicalis VII
[prominens], Proc. spinosus

Vertebra thoracica I,
Proc. spinosus

Tuberculum costae

Angulus costae

Proc. transversus

Articulatio
costotransversaria

Costa XII

Vertebra lumbalis I,
Proc. spinosus

c

Fig. 3.69 Bony thorax. a Ventral view. **b** Right lateral view [L266]. **c** Dorsal view.

- Rib angle (**Angulus costae**): connects with the Tuberculum costae
- Rib body (**Corpus costae**): continues to the front into the rib cartilage

From the IVth rib, the cartilaginous portions of the ribs become longer, form an arch and pull cranially ascending in the direction of the sternum. The bony parts, particularly the rib body, display 3 different curvatures:

- **Surface curvature:** outer surface is bent downwards and to the outside
- **Edge curvature:** the rib head is higher compared to the ventral rib ends by 2 vertebrae
- **Rib torsion:** the ribs are twisted around their longitudinal axis

All curvatures are strongly formed particularly in the upper ribs (exception Ist rib) and thus regionally different. This has an impact on the respiratory mechanics (see below).

Individual differences

The IIIrd–Xth ribs are the typical ribs. The Ist, IInd, XIth and XIIth ribs deviate from the typical rib structure (➤ Fig. 3.70, ➤ Fig. 3.71).

- **Costae III–X:** they have the typical rib form with wedge-shaped **Caput costae,** which each bear 2 joint facets (Facies articulares capitis costae). The **Tuberculum costae** has a joint surface (Facies articularis tuberculi costae). The intercostal vessels and nerves (V., A. and N. intercostalis) are positioned on the **Sulcus costae.** The Corpus costae exhibits a cavity for contact with the rib cartilage at the ventral end.
- **Costa I:** is flattened, shorter, wider and more strongly bent than the rest of the ribs. The **Sulcus arteriae subclaviae** and the **Sulcus venae subclaviae** (for the vessels of the same name) run along the surface. In addition, the attachment zones for the Mm. scaleni anterioris (Tuberculum musculi scaleni anterioris) and medius can be recognised. Their head only has one joint facet

133

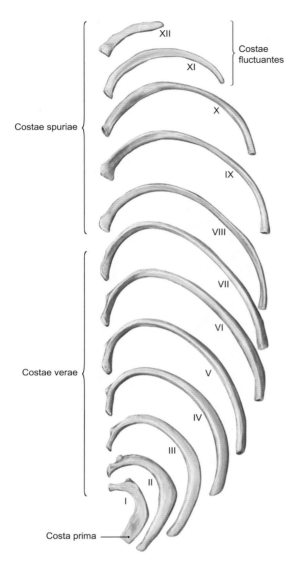

Costae fluctuantes

Costae spuriae

Costae verae

XII
XI
X
IX
VIII
VII
VI
V
IV
III
II
I

Costa prima

Fig. 3.70 Bony part of the ribs I–XII left side, superior view. [L266]

and it is more strongly curved (surface curvature). Edge curvature and rib torsion are missing.

- **Costa II:** the Sulcus costae is only indicated. There is also a **Tuberositas musculi serrati anterioris** for the origin of the M. serratus anterior. The IInd ribs have 2 joint facets like the IIIrd–Xth ribs.
- **Costae XI and XII:** they do not have a Tuberculum costae and no Sulcus costae. They do not have contact with the costal arch; their front end is pointed. They have only one joint surface on their head.

Clinical remarks

Ribs anomalies often occur in the population (approximately 6%):

- **Cervical ribs** (approx. 1 % of the population): the rib system at the VIIth cervical vertebra is enlarged. The additional ribs can be unilateral or bilateral but only the Proc. transversus can also be enlarged in isolation. If the additional ribs are in contact with the sternum (either via connective tissue or even bones), the lower roots of the brachial plexus can be compressed, which leads to sensory disorders and motor deficits in the innervation area of the spinal nerves C8 and T1.

- **Two-headed ribs:** two ribs are partially fused.
- **Fork ribs:** the rib forks in the front portion into 2 ends.
- **Rib notching:** asures are extensions of the intercostal arteries, which run in the Sulcus costae, in the case of aortic coarctation and the resulting pressure on the bone are referred to as rib erosion. The vessels then usually run in an extremely tortuous shape.
- **Lumbar ribs** (approx. 7–8 % of the population): these are additional ribs that are similar to the XIth and XIIth ribs and begin at the Ist or IInd lumbar vertebral body. They can have a topographic relationship to the kidneys and cause pain here.

Rib-vertebral joints

Caput and Tuberculum costae articulate with the thoracic vertebrae in the **Articulationes costovertebrales** (true joints). In doing so, the rib head articulates in the Articulationes capitis costae; the rib tubercles in the Articulationes costotransversariae:

- **Articulatio capitis costae:** The Ist, XIth and XIIth ribs articulate with the corresponding thoracic vertebral bodies via an articular facet. The IInd–Xth ribs articulate in contrast with the higher, as well as the corresponding thoracic vertebral body (➤ Fig. 3.72). The resulting 2 joints are separated by a ligament (**Lig. capitis costae intraarticulare,** ➤ Fig. 3.72b), which runs from the intervertebral disc to the centre of the rib head. The joint capsule is reinforced by the circular **Lig. capitis costae radiatum.**
- **Articulatio costotransversaria:** The rib tubercles of the Ist–Xth ribs articulate with the Procc. transversi of the corresponding vertebra (➤ Fig. 3.72, ➤ Fig. 3.73). The joint capsules are reinforced by strong ligaments. Dorsally, the **Lig. costotransversarium laterale** connects the Proc. transversus and Angulus costae and ventrally the **Lig. costotransversarium** is stretched between Proc. transversus and Collum or Caput costae (➤ Fig. 3.73). The **Lig. costotransversarium superius** from the rib neck reaches the Proc. transversus of the next highest vertebra and suspends the ribs (➤ Fig. 3.73).

Sternum

The **breastbone (Sternum)** in adults, is a composite flat bone consisting of 3 pieces (➤ Fig. 3.74). It consists of:

- **Handle (Manubrium sterni):** articulates with the Claviculae and the Ist and IInd pair of ribs and has a cranial indentation (**Incisura jugularis**).
- **Body of the sternum (Corpus sterni):** articulates with the rib pairs II–VII.
- **Xiphoid process (Proc. xiphoideus):** can be created with cartilage or bone.

The 3 bones are interconnected via synchondroses. The Manubrium is slightly tilted in the sagittal plane against the Corpus in a craniodorsal direction and forming the **Angulus sterni (LUDOVICI).** In more than 30% of cases, a gap filled with synovial fluid occurs between the Manubrium and Corpus sterni. In this case, one speaks of a **Symphysis manubriosternalis.** The cartilage adhesion between Corpus sterni and Proc. xiphoideus consists of fibrous cartilage (**Symphysis xiphosternalis**). With increasing age (from the *40th year of life*) the 3 sections fuse mostly by bone with each other. The sternum articulates with the collar bones (**Articulationes sternoclaviculares**) and the rib pairs and I–VII (**Articulationes sternocostales,** see below).

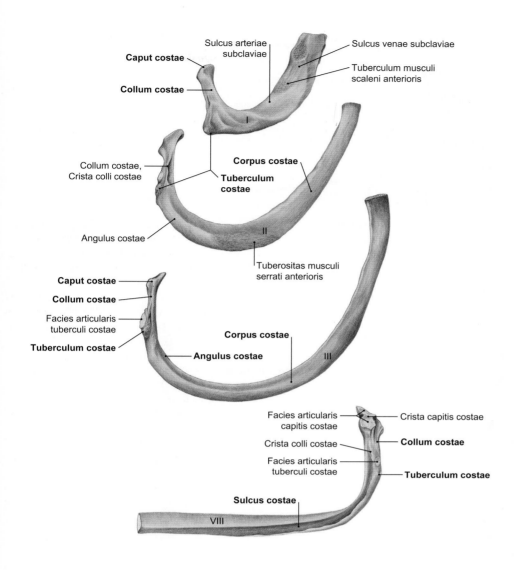

Caput costae
Sulcus arteriae subclaviae
Sulcus venae subclaviae
Collum costae
Tuberculum musculi scaleni anterioris
I

Collum costae, Crista colli costae
Corpus costae
Tuberculum costae
Angulus costae
II
Tuberositas musculi serrati anterioris

Caput costae
Collum costae
Facies articularis tuberculi costae
Tuberculum costae
Corpus costae
Angulus costae
III

Facies articularis capitis costae
Crista capitis costae
Crista colli costae
Collum costae
Facies articularis tuberculi costae
Tuberculum costae
Sulcus costae
VIII

Fig. 3.71 Ribs, Costae; Ist–IIIrd ribs (cranial view) and VIIIth rib (caudal view).

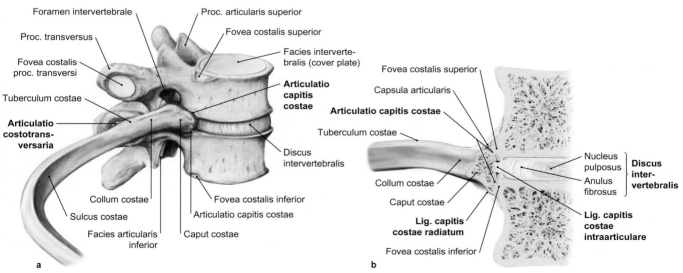

Foramen intervertebrale
Proc. transversus
Fovea costalis proc. transversi
Tuberculum costae
Articulatio costotransversaria
Collum costae
Sulcus costae
Facies articularis inferior
Proc. articularis superior
Fovea costalis superior
Facies intervertebralis (cover plate)
Articulatio capitis costae
Discus intervertebralis
Fovea costalis inferior
Articulatio capitis costae
Caput costae

Fovea costalis superior
Capsula articularis
Articulatio capitis costae
Tuberculum costae
Collum costae
Caput costae
Lig. capitis costae radiatum
Fovea costalis inferior
Nucleus pulposus
Anulus fibrosus
Discus intervertebralis
Lig. capitis costae intraarticulare

a
b

Fig. 3.72 Costovertebral joints (Articulationes costovertebrales). a Costovertebral joints at the height of the VIIth and VIIIth thoracic vertebrae; right lateral view. **b** Rib head joint (Articulatio capitis costae), right lateral view. [L266]

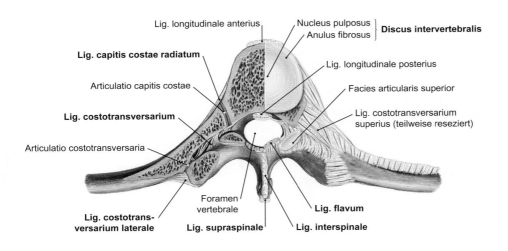

Fig. 3.73 Ligaments of the costovertebral joints (Articulationes costovertebrales).

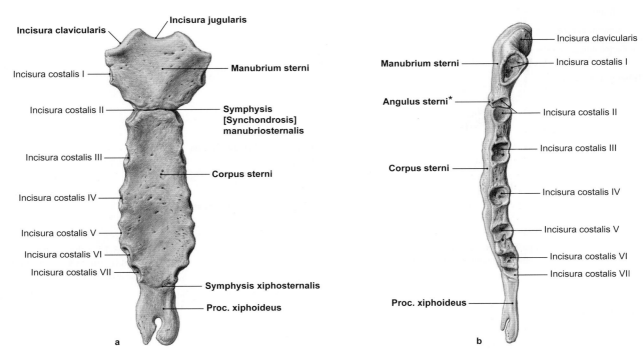

Fig. 3.74 Sternum. a Ventral view. **b** Lateral view from the left side. * LUDOVICI

Clinical remarks

For the assessment of bone marrow cells (bone marrow smear) the bone is punctured, typically at the iliac crest. A **sternal puncture** is also possible; however, it is only very rarely carried out today. For this purpose, one uses a strong biopsy needle with Arretier plate and punctures under local anaesthesia in the median line of the Corpus sterni between the attachments of the IInd and IIIrd ribs. Punctures should not be made in the vicinity of the costosternal connections (occurrence of the synchondroses), and the lower two thirds of the Corpus sterni (there can be a Fissura sterni congenita caused by the paired bone system of the sternum) are also obsolete, because the puncture needle could easily enter the heart or the lungs (pleura).

Sternoclavicular joint

Sternoclavicular joint (**Articulatio sternoclavicularis**) is a functional ball and socket joint with three degrees of freedom. The Facies articularis sternalis articulates with the Incisura clavicularis sterni. Due to the incongruity of the articular surface, the joint has a fibre cartilaginous Discus articularis, which divides the joint into two chambers (dithalamic joint). The shape of the joint enables multiaxial movements and extremely different stresses in various joint positions, which are of importance for the shoulder girdle (➤ Chapter 4.3). The joint capsule is strengthened by:
- Lig. sternoclaviculare anterius
- Lig. sternoclaviculare posterius
- Lig. interclaviculare
- Lig. costoclaviculare

The joint is also discussed in the context of the upper extremities (➤ Chap. 4.3.2).

Rib-sternal joints

The Ist rib and often also the VIth and VIIth ribs are connected to the sternum with their cartilaginous component as synchondroses (**Articulationes costochondrales**). In rare cases true joints (diarthroses, **sternocostal joints**) can occur, such as between the IInd and Vth ribs (➤ Fig. 3.75). Each of the Incisura costalis sterni articulates with the ventral end of the rib cartilage.

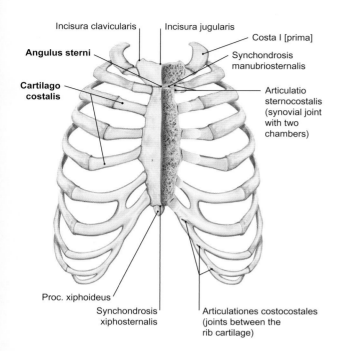

Fig. 3.75 Articulationes sternocostales. Ventral view. [L266]

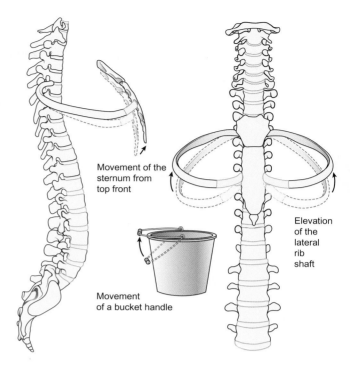

Fig. 3.76 Movement of the thoracic wall. [L126]

The 2nd sternocostal joint regularly has a **Lig. sternocostale intraarticulare**. The joint capsules of the rib-sternum joints are reinforced by the **Ligg. sternocostalia radiata**. At the front the ligaments connect to the Membrana sterni externa and at the back to the Membrana sterni interna. The ligaments radiate caudally as **Ligg. costoxiphoidea** to the xiphoid process. The cartilage connections on the rib arch are referred to as **Articulationes interchondrales**. Joint clefts can sometimes occur here.

In the course of life the rib cartilage ossifies fully up to old age.

> **N O T E**
>
> In the case of a cardiac arrest a **cardiac massage** is performed as a life-saving measure. In this case, there are often rib fractures in the ossified rib cartilage even when correctly executed. These are normal and do not pose further far-reaching risks for the patient. Cardiac massage should therefore be continued even after one or more rib fractures.

Thorax mechanisms

A key feature of the bony and cartilaginous chest wall are movements that serve to alter the chest volume, and to enable transport of air in and out of the lungs. The central elements are the **Articulationes costovertebrales** (Articulationes capitis costae radiatae and Articulationes costotransversariae form a functional unit) and the **Articulationes sternocostales**. They therefore serve the respiratory mechanisms. In the context of breathing, the thoracic skeleton (➤ Fig. 3.76):

- moves the sternum to the upper front. The movement comes about when the front end of the ribs are lower than the rear. In this process, the angle between Manubrium and Corpus sterni slightly flattens. The movement changes the extent of the thorax in an anteroposterior direction.
- elevates the lateral rib shafts (lifting for inspiration, lowering for expiration). This results in changes in the lateral and anteroposterior directions. The ribs move laterally like a bucket handle. The middle portions of the rib shafts are even lower than the ends of the two ribs at different heights.

The elastic rib cartilages are also significantly involved in the positional changes of the ribs. With the ossification of the rib cartilage in old age, thoracic mobility is restricted and the respiratory width decreases.

The muscles responsible for the movements of the thorax are discussed in ➤ Chap. 3.1.2.

4 Upper extremity

Volker Spindler, Jens Waschke

Humeral shaft fracture

Case study

A 33-year-old man is brought into hospital in an ambulance. Whilst cycling he was clipped by an overtaking lorry and fell onto his right arm and upper body. As a matter of routine, the patient is sent into the trauma room of A & E and examined in detail after the A & E doctor has removed the vacuum splint.

Findings

The patient is conscious and fully orientated. He has severe pain, especially in the right upper arm. Heart rate (90/min), respiratory rate (30/min) and blood pressure (140/100 mm Hg) are all slightly increased. The A & E doctor reports an approximately 6 × 8 cm sized wound on the right upper arm with visible bone fragments in the wound bed. Due to the possibility of an operation, the attached compresses are initially not removed. During manual examination of the remaining bony skeleton no abnormal mobility or grinding noises (crepitations) are triggered. Neurological examination shows a limply drooping right hand that the patient can raise only minimally against gravity. In addition, there is a noticeable numbness on the radial side of right forearm and back of the hand, especially between thumb and forefinger. The blood flow of the right hand is not restricted. Apart from multiple grazing and bruising on the face, the right upper body and both hands, the rest of the physical examination yields nothing remarkable.

Diagnostics

A computer tomography (CT) of the whole body, as conducted routinely in the trauma room, shows a comminuted fracture of the right humerus in the area of the shaft. Otherwise, no other fractures or organ damage are noticeable.

Diagnosis

Comminuted fracture of the right humeral shaft with damage to the N. radialis.

Treatment

Due to the complex fracture with an obvious nerve lesion, an operation is indicated. After exposing the fracture area, the N. radialis is examined. A few small splinters of bone which have penetrated into the nerve are removed. Also, a larger bone fragment that was compressing the nerve is repositioned. The fracture is extensively repositioned and stabilised with a plate whilst preserving the N. radialis.

Further developments

On the day after the procedure physiotherapy is started. Full mobility of the shoulder and elbow is achieved again after a few weeks; however, it is many more weeks before the patient can extend his wrist again and no further sensory disorders are detectable.

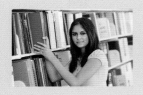

You were present during your practical year while the patient was in the emergency department. Everything went quite quickly and on leaving, the senior consultant gives you 2 bullet points to think about...

Rep safe and unsafe fracture signs
Safe fracture signs: bone rub (Crepitatio), open fracture (visible bone fragments), abnormal mobility, axle deformity of the bone
Unsafe fracture signs: pain, swelling, haematoma, Increased warmth, movement restrictions
Rep peripheral paralysis
(traumat.) nerve paralysis → those muscles supplied by the nerve are no longer innervated → function failure
Wrist drop: paralysis of radial nerve: back of the hand can no longer be raised → falls down = drop hand

4.1 Overview

Dissection of the extremities necessitates much time and effort in the dissection process until in particular the complicated areas, such as the axilla (Fossa axillaris) and the hand with their entire vascular, lymphatic and nervous systems, are laid bare. As always during preparation, the individual structures can only be presented carefully and completely with good theoretical knowledge.

In a **clinical setting** the anatomy of the passive (bone, joints with ligaments) and active (muscles) musculoskeletal system of the limbs are of great significance for the specialties of orthopaedics, emergency surgery and radiology, since injuries and degenerative changes to arms and legs are frequent. In addition, peripheral neuroanatomy (branches of the spinal nerves) is particularly important for diagnostics in neurology and general medicine. Since in neurology, e.g. in the case of spastic tonus escalation, individual muscles are also increasingly being treated by injection of botulinum toxin, the exact topography of individual muscles has also become increasingly relevant in addition to their function. Also, in anaesthesia, targeted nerve plexuses and individual nerves are anaesthetised locally. Knowledge of the blood vessels is particularly relevant in the case of circulation disorders and thromboses (internal medicine, vascular surgery) and lymph vessels with their individual lymph node stations for tumour diagnosis in various fields, such as dermatology and gynaecology (breast cancer with the possibility of metastases in axillary lymph nodes).

Through its distinctive movement possibilities, the **upper extremity** of a person is adapted to its functions as a gripping organ and an important instrument of interaction with the environment. It is divided into the shoulder girdle (Cingulum pectorale) and the arm as a free-swinging part. The arm is divided into upper arm (Brachium), forearm (Antebrachium) and hand (Manus) (➤ Fig. 4.1). The longitudinal axis of the upper arm and forearm bones laterally form the arm exterior angle of 170°. The rotational axis of the upper arm in the shoulder joint corresponds to the line connecting the humeral head and elbow joint. It is extended as a diagonal axis of the forearm from the proximal to the distal joint between the forearm (radioulnar joints). Turning/rotational movement (pronation/supination) of the forearm takes place around this axis.

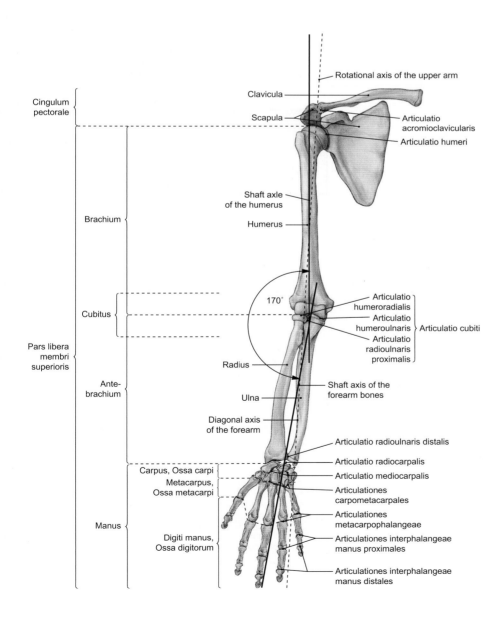

Fig. 4.1 Skeleton of the upper extremity, Membrum superius, right. Ventral view.

4.2 Development of upper and lower extremities

4.2.1 Course

The limbs develop in the *4th week*. A fin-like arm bud forms on the 26th–27th day and therefore 2 days earlier than the leg bud. The extremity systems at this point in time consist of a core of connective tissue (mesenchymal), which is derived from the mesodermal somatopleura, and of an encasing surface ectoderm which later forms the epidermal layer of the skin (➤ Fig. 4.2).

The extremity buds can be distinguished in different sections into a division of arm and leg systems in the *5th–6th week*. From the 6th week the finger rays separate from each other through pro-

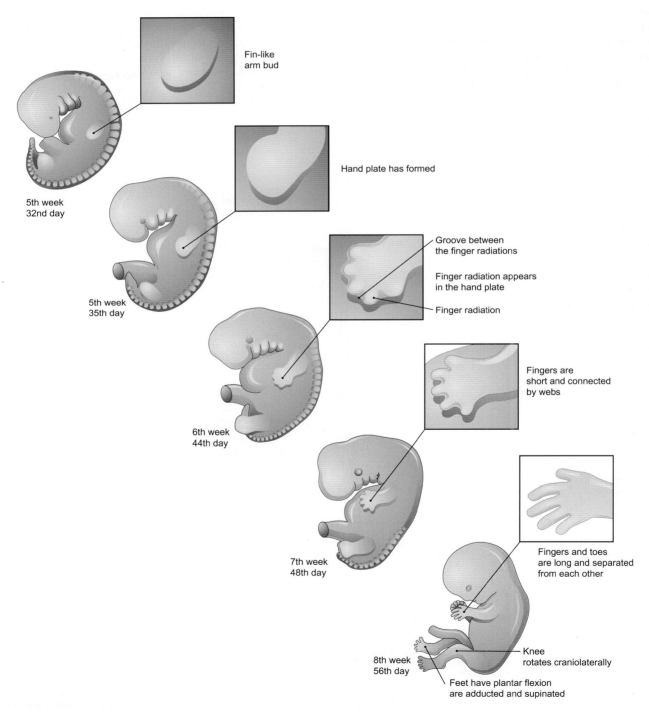

Fin-like
arm bud

Hand plate has formed

Groove between
the finger radiations

Finger radiation appears
in the hand plate

Finger radiation

Fingers are
short and connected
by webs

Fingers and toes
are long and separated
from each other

Knee
rotates craniolaterally

Feet have plantar flexion
are adducted and supinated

5th week
32nd day

5th week
35th day

6th week
44th day

7th week
48th day

8th week
56th day

Fig. 4.2 Embryonic limb development (5th–8th week). [E581]

grammed cell death (apoptosis) in the interlying tissue. By the *end of the 8th week* the fingers and toes are completely separated. In the *8th week* there is a rotation of the extremities systems (➤ Fig. 4.2): the arm system revolves 90°, so that the elbow is aligned caudally. The flexor muscles then lie ventrally and the extensor muscles dorsally. The leg system also rotates by almost 90° but in the opposite direction, so that the knee points in a craniolateral direction. This means that with the leg the extensor muscles of the upper and lower leg lie ventrally, but the flexor muscles lie dorsally. Furthermore, in the *8th week* the foot is initially plantarflected, adducted and supinated. By the *11th week,* however, this foot position is normally reversed.

4.2.2 Bones

The mesenchyme of the arm bud is consolidated and forms a cartilaginous skeleton as the precursors of later bones in the *4th–6th week on the arm* and in the *6th–8th week on the leg* (➤ Fig. 4.3). This process advances from proximal to distal. In this cartilaginous skeleton bone cores form *from the 7th week* which initiate ossification and thus the conversion of the cartilaginous skeleton into bone tissue (**chondral ossification**). Ossification progresses according to a specific pattern:

- By the *12th week* bone cores can be found in all bones of the *upper extremity* apart from the wrist (➤ Fig. 4.4a). The bone cores of the wrist first emerge postnatally between the *1st and 8th year of age.* An exception is the Clavicula, which is the first bone *(7th week)* to form, emerges without a cartilaginous skeleton and thus directly from the mesenchyme (**desmal ossification**).
- In the *lower extremity* ossification develops a little later (➤ Fig. 4.4b). In the thigh and leg bones the first bone cores emerge roughly in the *8th embryonic week,* but they only first emerge in the toes between the *9th week* and the *9th month.* The tarsal bones *(1st–4th year of life)* and the pelvic girdle (partly up to the *20th year of life*) ossify postnatally.

The **epiphyseal plates** join between the *14th and 25th years* and in most bones up to the *21st year of life.* The growth length of the extremities is thereby terminated.

Joints (diarthroses) between the individual bones are present from the start of the foetal period (from the *9th week*).

4.2.3 Muscular system

The muscle cells of the limbs differentiate into the limb buds (➤ Fig. 4.5a and b). The ectoderm at the distal edge of the limb buds (ectodermal marginal ridge) forms growth factors, which attract precursors of muscle cells from the somites of the mesoderm into the torso region. By the *6th week the precursor cells in the limb systems form* the ventral and dorsal **muscle masses,** from which the flexor and extensor muscles later develop. Since the limb muscles develop out of precursor cells from the ventral (hypaxial) muscle system of somites, the muscles of the limbs are all later innervated by the anterior branches of the spinal nerves. The **motor nerve fibres** grow in the *5th week* into the limb systems. The muscle fibres for the arms then develop from the muscle systems of segments C5–T1, which form the anterior branches of the spinal

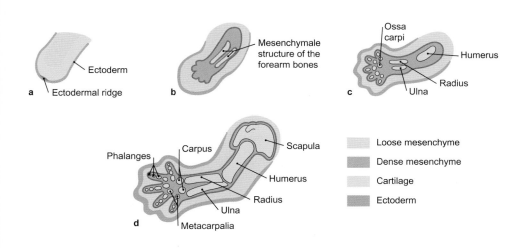

Ectoderm
Ectodermal ridge
a

Mesenchymale structure of the forearm bones
b

Ossa carpi
Humerus
Radius
Ulna
c

Phalanges
Carpus
Scapula
Humerus
Radius
Ulna
Metacarpalia
d

Loose mesenchyme
Dense mesenchyme
Cartilage
Ectoderm

Fig. 4.3 Development of cartilaginous primary stages of the arm skeleton. a 28th day, **b** 44th day, **c** 48th day and **d** 56th day of development. [E581]

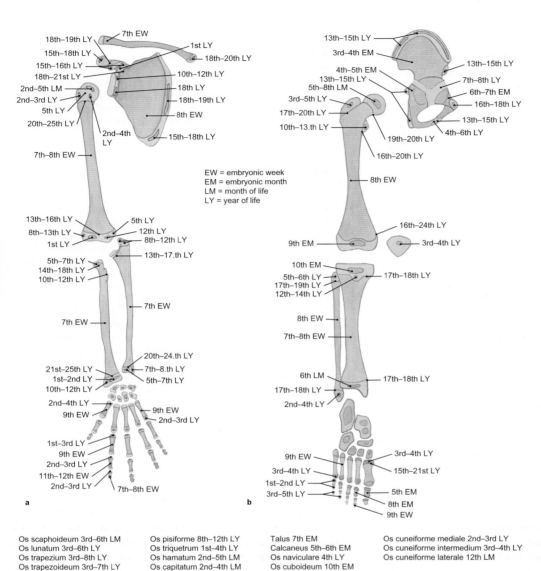

EW = embryonic week
EM = embryonic month
LM = month of life
LY = year of life

Fig. 4.4 Ossification of the skeleton, location of the ossification centres and chronological sequence of ossification centre development. a Upper extremity. **b** Lower extremity.

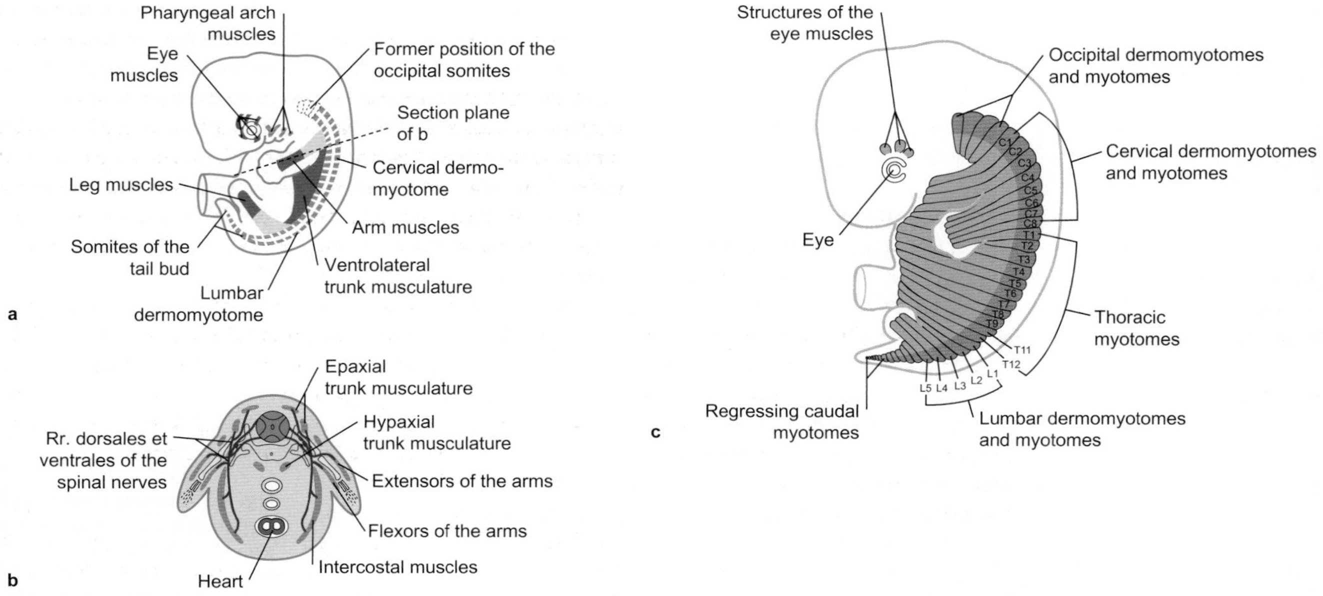

Os scaphoideum 3rd–6th LM	Os pisiforme 8th–12th LY
Os lunatum 3rd–6th LY	Os triquetrum 1st–4th LY
Os trapezium 3rd–8th LY	Os hamatum 2nd–5th LM
Os trapezoideum 3rd–7th LY	Os capitatum 2nd–4th LM

Talus 7th EM	Os cuneiforme mediale 2nd–3rd LY
Calcaneus 5th–6th EM	Os cuneiforme intermedium 3rd–4th LY
Os naviculare 4th LY	Os cuneiforme laterale 12th LM
Os cuboideum 10th EM	

Fig. 4.5 Development of the musculature in the 6th week. a, c Schematic diagram. **b** Cross-section. [E347-09]

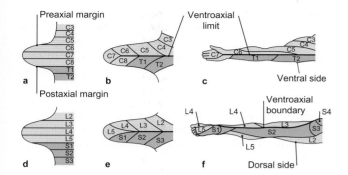

Fig. 4.6 Development of dermatomes. a–c Upper extremity. [E581] **d–f** Lower extremity. Arrangement of the dermatomes at the beginning (a and d) and end of the 5th week (b and e) as well as in adults (c and f). The ventroaxial boundary marks the area in which there is hardly any overlapping of the innervation areas. [E581]

nerves of the Plexus brachialis from their spinal cord segments (> Fig. 4.5c). The muscle precursor cells for the legs originate from segments L2–S3, the motoneurons of which are correspondingly merged in the Plexus lumbosacralis.

4.2.4 Nerves

The **sensory nerve fibres** grow out along the motor fibres and initially reach segmentally arranged skin areas (> Fig. 4.6a and b). Due to the growing out of the limbs, the arrangement of the cutaneous areas, which are innervated by a spinal cord segment also changes. (**dermatomes = radicular fields**). In contrast to the torso, where dermatomes are arranged in a belt shape, dermatomes in the limbs initially proceed almost longitudinally and later during development in an increasingly oblique direction (> Fig. 4.6). Arms and legs exhibit a ventroaxial border in which the individual sensory innervated areas hardly overlap.

4.2.5 Blood vessels

The blood vessels of the limb systems originate from the dorsal intersegmental arteries (> section 6.1.3). Firstly, an **axial artery** forms in the median plane, from which later on branches grow out at the distal end. In the arm the axial artery forms the **A. brachialis,** but remains on the forearm behind the growth of the limb system and later forms the **A. interossea communis** with its branches. The **A. mediana,** emerges distally from the axial artery, which, however, is only temporarily formed and later becomes reduced to the A. comitans nervi mediani. Then the **A. ulnaris** and **A. radialis** form as the main vessels of the forearm and maintain connection to the digital arteries.

The axial artery in the leg is called the **A. ischiadica** because it accompanies the N. ischiadicus. It regresses at the thigh and is later replaced by the newly growing **A. femoralis.** Emerging from it in the lower leg are the **A. tibialis anterior** and the **A. tibialis posterior.**

Clinical remarks

Remnants of the axial arteries can remain as variants. The **A. mediana** can, e.g. as a variant as a strong vessel on the forearm still be connected to the palmar arches. What can be particularly relevant is a **superficial A. brachialis** (present in 8%

of cases), which can remain if the distal portion of the A. brachialis is not replaced by a more deeply coursing segment. This superficial A. brachialis then courses subcutaneously through the elbow and in the case of accidental puncture during blood collection or administration of medication can lead to spurting bleeding or incorrect arterial injection. Therefore, before puncture there should always be a manual palpation to test whether the respective vessel in the elbow still actually has a pulse and can thus be seen as an artery.

4.3 Shoulder girdle

Skills

After working through this chapter, you should be able to:
• explain on a skeleton the bony structures of the shoulder girdle and its joints together with the range of movement
• explain the course of the ligaments of the shoulder girdle as well as all muscles with origin, attachment and function, and show these on a skeleton or specimen.

4.3.1 Bones of the shoulder girdle

The bones of the shoulder girdle are:
• Clavicle (Clavicula)
• Shoulder blade (Scapula)

Clavicula

The Clavicula joins the sternum with the shoulder blade and is well palpable nearly horizontally. It has a thickened medial end, **Extremitas sternalis,** and a flattened lateral end, **Extremitas acromialis,** > Fig. 4.7). Because of 2 bends the Clavicula is curved and slightly S-shaped, so that ventrally the lateral half is concave and the medial half is convex. Dorsally located underneath at the lateral bend is the **Tuberculum conoideum** as a small apophysis. From here, the **Linea trapezoidea** extends laterally. Both parts of the Lig. coracoclaviculare are fastened to these structures. Also on the underside of the lateral third is a depression, the **Sulcus musculi subclavii,** in which the M. subclavius lies against the bone. The Clavicula originates predominantly by membrane ossification and in the *7th week* is the first osseous skeletal element of an embryo.

Clinical remarks

Because of the exposed position of the Clavicula and its S-shape that e. g. cannot withstand axial loads arising from falls onto an outstretched arm, **fractures** are frequent. In a typical fracture in the middle third of the Clavicula the lateral part is dragged downwards by the weight of the arm, but the medial part, on the other hand, is dragged upwards by the pull of the M. sternocleidomastoideus.

Shoulder blade (Scapula)

The Scapula is a triangular, mostly flat bone with an anterior surface facing the thorax (**Facies costalis**) and a posterior surface (**Facies posterior**) (> Fig. 4.8a). Corresponding to the triangle shape, a distinction is made between 3 sides (**Margo lateralis, medialis and superior**) and 3 angles (**Anguli lateralis, inferior and superior**).

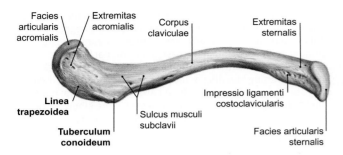

Fig. 4.7 Clavicle, Clavicula, right. Caudal view.

A short neck piece, the **Collum scapulae,** forms an appendage which protrudes in the lateral angle, into which the **Cavitas glenoidalis** is sunken. It forms the joint socket for the head of the humerus. There are 2 small elevations on its upper and lower edges, the **Tubercula supraglenoidale and infraglenoidale** as the origins for the Caput longum of the M. biceps brachii and the M. triceps brachii, respectively (➤ Fig. 4.8). At the Margo superior of the Scapula the **coracoid process (Proc. coracoideus)** bends forwards. Medial to the Proc. coracoideus, the superior border is indented by the **Incisura scapulae,** which is bridged by a ligament (Lig. transversum scapulae superius). Spine of the Scapula (**Spina scapulae**) is elevated from the Facies posterior and articulates with the Clavicula with its end section, the acromion. From the base of the Spina scapulae there is a ligament connection (Lig. transversum scapulae inferius) to the neck of the shoulder blade.

On the Scapula there are 3 recesses:
- **Fossa subscapularis,** Ventral; origin of the M. subscapularis
- **Fossa supraspinata,** dorsal to and above the Spina scapulae; origin of the M. supraspinatus
- **Fossa infraspinata,** dorsal below the Spina scapulae; origin of the M. infraspinatus

4.3.2 Joints and ligament connections of the shoulder girdle

A distinction is made between 2 joints on the shoulder girdle:
- Medial clavicular joint (**Articulatio sternoclavicularis**)
- Lateral clavicular joint (**Articulatio acromioclavicularis**)

Medial clavicular joint

The Articulatio sternoclavicularis is the only truly articulated connection between the upper extremity and the torso (➤ Fig. 4.9). The **joint surfaces** of the Extremitas sternalis of the Clavicula and the Incisura clavicularis of the Manubrium sterni are both slightly saddle-shaped but functionally they are ball joints. A **Discus articularis** divides the joint almost completely. Because of the very strong ligaments, luxation of the joint is extremely rare.

The following **ligaments** secure the medial clavicular joint:
- **Ligg. sternoclavicularia anterius and posterius** on the front and back of the joint
- **Lig. interclaviculare,** which connect both clavicles with each other along the top of the breastbone
- **Lig. costoclaviculare,** which stretches from the cartilage of the first rib to the medial end of the Clavicula.

Also, the **M. subclavius,** which stretches from the first rib to the Clavicula, supports the fixation of the Clavicula to the thorax and thus acts as an active ligament.

Lateral clavicular joint

The lateral clavicular joint (Articulatio acromioclavicularis) is a plane joint and connects the lateral end of the Clavicula with the acromion of the Scapula (➤ Fig. 4.10). It is stabilised by 3 **ligaments:**
- **Lig. acromioclaviculare,** which constitutes a reinforcement of the joint capsule
- **Lig. trapezoideum** from the Linea trapezoidea of the Clavicula to the Proc. coracoideus
- **Lig. conoideum** from the Tuberculum conoideum of the Clavicula to the Proc. coracoideus.

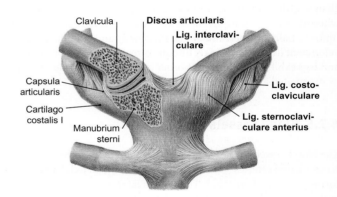

Fig. 4.9 Medial clavicular joint, Articulatio sternoclavicularis, Ventral view.

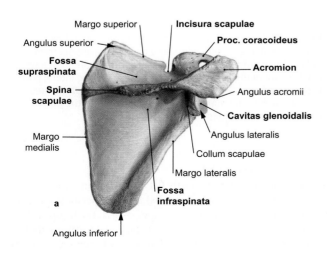

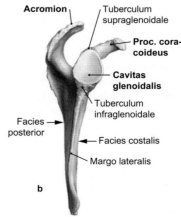

Fig. 4.8 Shoulder blade, Scapula, right. a Dorsal view. **b** Lateral view.

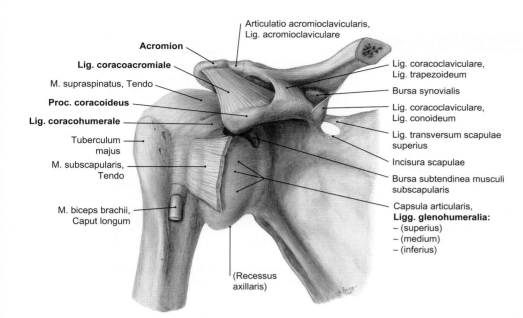

Acromion

Lig. coracoacromiale

M. supraspinatus, Tendo

Proc. coracoideus

Lig. coracohumerale

Tuberculum majus

M. subscapularis, Tendo

M. biceps brachii, Caput longum

Articulatio acromioclavicularis, Lig. acromioclaviculare

Lig. coracoclaviculare, Lig. trapezoideum

Bursa synovialis

Lig. coracoclaviculare, Lig. conoideum

Lig. transversum scapulae superius

Incisura scapulae

Bursa subtendinea musculi subscapularis

Capsula articularis, Ligg. glenohumeralia:
– (superius)
– (medium)
– (inferius)

(Recessus axillaris)

Fig. 4.10 Lateral clavicular joint, right. Ventral view.

The Ligg. trapezoideum (lateral) and conoideum (medial) are merged into the **Ligg. trapezoideum (lateral) and conoideum (medial)**. Three other ligament connections have no direct relation to the clavicular joints:

- The **Lig. coracoacromiale** connects the Proc. coracoideus and Acromion and together with them forms the so-called roof of the shoulder.
- The **Lig. transversum scapulae superius** bridges the Incisura scapulae.
- The **Lig. transversum scapulae inferius** is only inconsistently formed and is located directly below the lateral end of the Spina scapulae.

Clinical remarks

In contrast to injuries to the medial clavicular joint, trauma to the Articulatio acromioclavicularis (clinical: **dropped shoulder**) is common. Typically they arise through a fall onto the shoulder with an outstretched arm, often through sports accidents. A distinction is made according to TOSSY, between 3 levels of severity:
- TOSSY I: strain or partial rupture of the Lig. acromioclaviculare (1 ligament affected)

- TOSSY II: additional partial rupture of the Lig. coracoclaviculare (2 ligaments affected)
- TOSSY III: complete tear of the Lig. acromioclaviculare and the Lig. coracoclaviculare (all 3 ligaments torn)
Especially in the case of TOSSY III the lateral end of the Clavicula is higher than the Acromion. The clear step formation can be pushed back into the normal position ('**piano key phenomenon**', ➤ Fig. 4.11).
Clinically, a classification by ROCKWOOD based on that by TOSSY is now primarily used, as this is more suitable for whether an operation is indicated.

4.3.3 Shoulder girdle mechanics

The **Clavicula** can be dislocated in the sternoclavicular joint around the sagittal and longitudinal axes (➤ Fig. 4.12, ➤ Table 4.1). Thereby the Clavicula moves in the form of a cone with the tip in the sternoclavicular joint and the base in the acromioclavicular joint ('circles of the shoulder'). In addition, due to the relatively weakly developed saddle form of the articular surfaces of the sternoclavicular joint, light rotational movements of the Clavicula

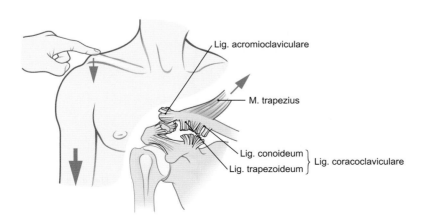

Lig. acromioclaviculare

M. trapezius

Lig. conoideum
Lig. trapezoideum } Lig. coracoclaviculare

Fig. 4.11 Piano key phenomenon in the case of avulsion of the Lig. acromioclaviculare and Lig. coracoclaviculare.

147

Table 4.1 Range of movement in the shoulder girdle.

Movement	Range of movement
Elevation/depression	40°–0°–10°
Protraction/retraction	25°–0°–25°

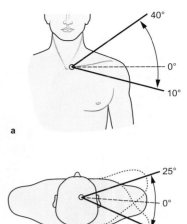

around its longitudinal axis are possible. Functionally, the clavicular joints act together as *ball joints*.

During movements in the clavicular joints the **Scapula** is by necessity always moved as well. In the process it slides extensively with its anterior side on the thorax. In addition, the Scapula also rotates around a sagittal axis. Thus, the Angulus inferior can be rotated approximately 30° medially and approximately 60° laterally. This rotation capability is essential for abduction of the arm in the shoulder joint beyond 90°, which is designated as **elevation**.

> **NOTE**
>
> The Scapula can be moved extensively against the torso:
> • Shifting movements to **ventral** (e.g. enclosing the contralateral upper arm with the hand) and to **dorsal** (e.g. tying an apron)
> • Shift movement to **cranial** (e.g. shrugging the shoulders) and to **caudal**
> • Rotation around a **sagittal** axis (e.g. in arm elevation)

4.3.4 Shoulder girdle muscles

Shoulder girdle muscles are designated according to their function as muscles, which have their origin at the torso skeleton and skull and their attachment to the Scapula or Clavicula (➤ Fig. 4.13, ➤ Fig. 4.14). Accordingly, they move only these two bones. A special situation here is the ability to deploy some of these muscles as auxiliary respiratory muscles for **respiratory support**. In the case of a fixed shoulder girdle (e.g. propping up on a handrail) they induce elevation of the rib cage and inspiration.

The **ventral muscles** of the shoulder girdle (➤ Fig. 4.13, ➤ Table 4.2) include:
• M. serratus anterior
• M. pectoralis minor
• M. subclavius

The ventral group originates on the anterior side of the thoracic cage of the ribs.

Fig. 4.12 Range of movement in the shoulder girdle. a Elevation/depression. **b** Protraction/retraction.

The **dorsal muscles** of this group (➤ Fig. 4.14, ➤ Table 4.3) are
• M. trapezius
• M. levator scapulae
• M. rhomboideus major
• M. rhomboideus minor

The dorsal group lies superficially on the back; however, the muscles did not develop in the area of the torso, but in the arm system. They are also not innervated by the Rr. posteriores of the spinal nerves, like true back muscles are. Therefore, these muscles are also referred to as **migrated (secondary) back muscles.**

The Clavicula and Scapula are moved by the shoulder girdle muscles as a unit against the abdominal wall. Functionally **4 muscle slings** are differentiated, which mediate the shift and rotational movements of the Scapula on the thoracic wall (➤ Fig. 4.15).
• **longitudinal sling:** M. levator scapulae and Pars ascendens of the M. trapezius
• **transverse sling:** Pars transversa of the trapezius, Pars superior and pars divergens of the M. serratus anterior
• **upper oblique sling:** Pars descendens of the M. trapezius, M. pectoralis minor
• **inferior oblique sling:** Mm. rhomboidei and Pars convergens of the M. serratus anterior

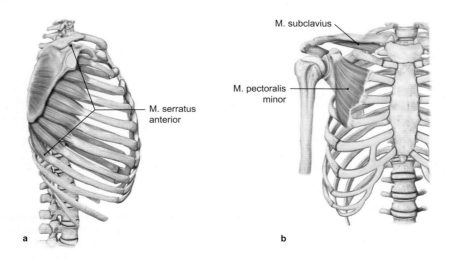

Fig. 4.13 Ventral shoulder girdle muscles. a M. serratus anterior. **b** M. pectoralis minor and M. subclavius.

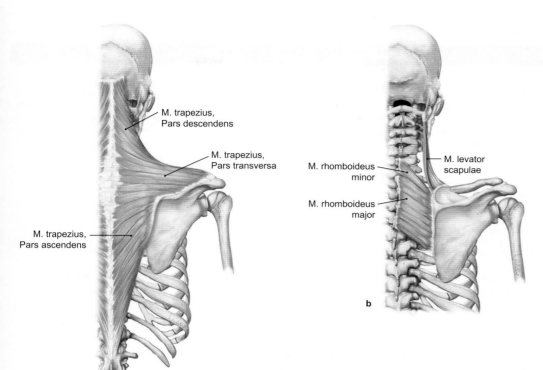

Fig. 4.14 Dorsal shoulder girdle muscles. a M. trapezius. **b** M. levator scapulae and Mm. rhomboidei.

The 2 muscles of a sling act as antagonists and thus move the Scapula in opposing directions. If both muscles of a sling contract the Scapula is pressed onto the thorax. Here the transverse sling is the most important. During rotation of the Scapula in a lateral direction (movement of the Cavitas glenoidalis cranially) the M. serratus anterior and the Partes descendens and ascendens of the M. trapezius work together.

in a wing shape **(Scapula alata).** This is particularly visible when propped up by a wall or in bed. Failure of the M. subclavius and M. pectoralis minor are functionally insignificant.

> ### Clinical remarks
>
> In **the event of failure of the M. serratus anterior** patients are particularly impaired, as arm elevation is not possible. It is also noticeable that the medial border of the Scapula projects

> ### Clinical remarks
>
> In the event of **failure of the M. trapezius** and also the **Mm. rhomboidei** the medial border of the Scapula is elevated and in the case of a **lesion of the M. levator scapulae** the shoulder is slightly lowered. Since during elevation the M. trapezius is also involved in rotation of the Scapula, this is restricted and the Cavitas glenoidalis is directed downwards.

Table 4.2 Ventral shoulder girdle muscles.

Innervation	Origin	Attachment	Function
M. pectoralis minor			
Nn. pectorales medialis and lateralis	(II) III–V ribs near the bone cartilage margin	Tip of the Proc. coracoideus	*Shoulder girdle:* lower *Thorax:* raises the upper ribs (inspiration: auxiliary breathing muscle)
M. subclavius			
N. subclavius	Cartilage bone margin of I rib	Lateral third of the Clavicula	*Shoulder girdle:* stabilises the sternoclavicular joint, protects Vasa subclavia; the fascia of the M. subclavius is firmly fused with the adventitia of the V. subclavia and thereby holds it open.
M. serratus anterior			
N. thoracicus longus	I–IX rib	Medial on the Scapula • Pars superior: Angulus superior • Pars divergens: Margo medialis • Pars convergens: Angulus inferior	*Shoulder girdle:* pulls the Scapula ventro-laterally, together with the Mm. rhomboidei presses the Scapula onto the thorax • Pars superior: lifts the Scapula • Pars divergens: lowers the Scapula • Pars convergens: lowers the Scapula and turns its lower angle outwards for elevation of the arm above the horizontal plane together with the M. trapezius *Thorax:* raises the ribs (inspiration) whilst the Scapula is fixed

Table 4.3 Dorsal shoulder girdle muscles.

Innervation	Origin	Attachment	Function
M. trapezius			
N. accessorius [XI] and branches of the Plexus cervicalis	• At the Os occipitale between the Linea nuchalis suprema and Linea nuchalis superior • Procc. spinosi of the cervical and thoracic vertebrae	• Pars descendens: acromial third of the Clavicula • Pars transversa: Acromion • Pars ascendens: Spina scapulae	• Pars descendens: prevents lowering of the shoulder girdle and the arm (e.g. when carrying suitcases), lifts the Scapula and turns its lower angle outwardly for elevation of the arm, with fixed shoulders rotates the head to the contralateral side, stretches the cervical spine in bilateral innervation • Pars transversa: pulls the Scapula downwards • Pars ascendens: lowers the Scapula and turns it downwards
M. levator scapulae			
Dorsal scapular nerve, (direct branches of the Plexus cervicalis)	Tubercula posteriora of the Procc. transversi of I–IV cervical vertebrae	Angulus superior of the Scapula	*Shoulder girdle:* lifts the Scapula
M. rhomboideus minor and major			
N. dorsalis scapulae	Proc. spinosus of the VI. and VII. cervical vertebrae (minor) and the 4 upper thoracic vertebrae (major)	Margo medialis of the cranial (minor) and caudal (major) Scapula of the Spina scapulae	Pulls the Scapula medially and cranially, together with the M. serratus anterior fixes the Scapula to the torso

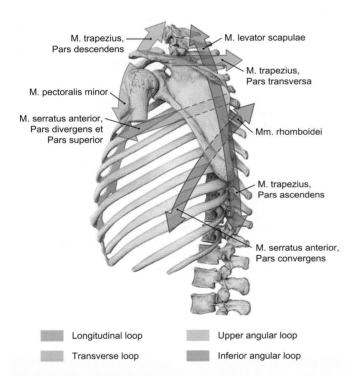

M. trapezius, Pars descendens

M. levator scapulae

M. trapezius, Pars transversa

M. pectoralis minor

M. serratus anterior, Pars divergens et Pars superior

Mm. rhomboidei

M. trapezius, Pars ascendens

M. serratus anterior, Pars convergens

Longitudinal loop

Upper angular loop

Transverse loop

Inferior angular loop

Fig. 4.15 Muscle slings for moving the Scapula.

4.4 Upper arm

Skills

After working through this chapter, you should be able to:
• explain the bony structures of the humerus as well as the development and range of movement of the shoulder joint
• demonstrate the ligaments of the shoulder joint and explain their significance for the mobility of the shoulder joint
• know all shoulder muscles with origin, attachment and function and show them on a specimen
• demonstrate the interplay of shoulder girdle and shoulder joint for the mobility of the upper extremity

4.4.1 Humerus

At the proximal end of the humerus (Humerus) a distinction is made between an anatomical and a clinical neck section: the **Collum anatomicum** separates the Caput humeri from the laterally located **Tuberculum majus** and the ventrally directed **Tuberculum minus** (➤ Fig. 4.16a). Both tubercles are separated by the **Sulcus intertubercularis** and taper out distally as the Crista tuberculi majoris and minoris. At the **Collum chirurgicum** distal to the two tubercula, fractures of the humerus are common.

The **Tuberositas deltoidea** for the attachment of the M. deltoideus is located on the shaft (**Corpus humeri**) . The **Sulcus nervi radialis** serves the N. radialis on the posterior side as a guiding furrow (➤ Fig. 4.16b) in which it can be damaged in the case of humeral shaft fractures .

The distal end of the humerus, is formed by the **Condylus humeri** (➤ Fig. 4.16c). This carries both joint plates of the elbow joint, **the Trochlea humeri** medial/ulnar and **the Capitulum humeri** lateral/radial. Above the two joint plates are 2 indentations that come into contact with the two forearm bones during flexion. The Fossa coronoidea for the corresponding extension of the Ulna is medial and the Fossa radialis is lateral. Dorsally the Fossa olecrani impedes extending movement through contact with the olecranon of the Ulna. Proximal to the Condylus the **Epicondyli medialis and lateralis** are elevated as apophyses, which taper out upwards on both sides as the Cristae supraepicondylares medialis and lateralis. On the dorsal side of the Epicondylus medialis is the Sulcus nervi ulnaris (➤ Fig. 4.16b), in which the N. ulnaris is palpably located under the skin. If it is compressed against the bone here, painful paraesthesia ensues (*'funny bone'*).

4.4.2 Shoulder joint

In the shoulder joint (**Articulatio humeri**) the almost spherical humeral head articulates with the Cavitas glenoidalis of the Scapula. The surface of the Cavitas glenoidalis is, however, much smaller than that of the humeral head. A loose connective tissue joint lip (Labrum glenoidale) therefore enlarges the joint plate. The shoulder joint is the *ball joint* with the largest range of movement in the human body.

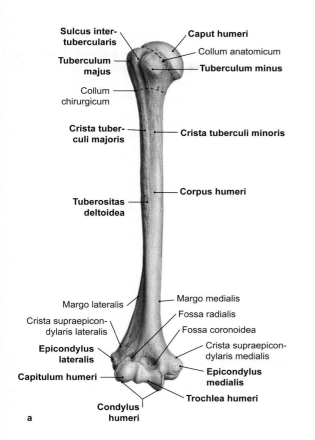

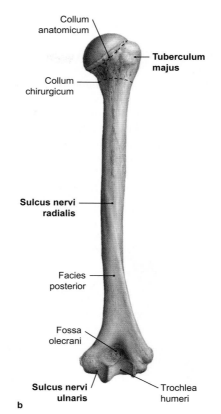

Fig. 4.16 Humerus, right.
a Ventral view. **b** Dorsal view.

The wide **joint capsule** originates at the Labrum glenoidale and extends to the Collum anatomicum of the humerus. When the arm hangs down, it has a reserve fold caudally ('Recessus axillaris', ➤ Fig. 4.10). The following **ligaments** reinforce the joint capsule (➤ Fig. 4.10, ➤ Fig. 4.17):

- **Lig. coracohumerale** (cranially) from the base of the Proc. coracoideus to the joint capsule
- **Ligg. glenohumeralia superius, medius and inferius** (ventrally), from the Collum scapulae to the joint capsule

In addition, the end tendons of the 4 muscles of the **rotator cuff** radiate into the joint capsule and reinforce and tense them (➤ Fig. 4.17):

- **M. supraspinatus** (cranial)
- **M. infraspinatus** (dorsal above)

- **M. teres minor** (dorsal below)
- **M. subscapularis** (ventral)

As a special feature the original tendon of the Caput longum of the **M. biceps brachii** runs through the joint cavity and attaches to the humerus in the Sulcus intertubercularis (➤ Fig. 4.10).

Cranially, the shoulder joint is delineated by the **'shoulder roof'**. This is formed by the Acromion and Proc. coracoideus of the Scapula, which are connected by the Lig. coracoacromiale. Below the shoulder roof there are larger **bursae:**

- The **Bursa subacromialis** on the attachment tendon of the M. supraspinatus (➤ Fig. 4.17) connects mostly laterally with the **Bursa subdeltoidea**. The two bursae are also referred to as 'subacromial accessory joints', as they ensure low friction gliding of the head of the humerus under the shoulder roof.
- The **Bursa subcoracoidea** under the Proc. coracoideus often connects with the **Bursa subtendinea musculi subscapularis** under the tendon attachment of the M. subscapularis and communicates with the joint cavity.

Clinical remarks

The wide joint capsule can become 'sticky' during longer **immobilisation of the shoulder joint,** especially in the area of the so-called Recessus axillaris. Therefore, in the case of operations in the area of the shoulder joint attempts should be made to facilitate movement of the shoulder joint as early as possible.

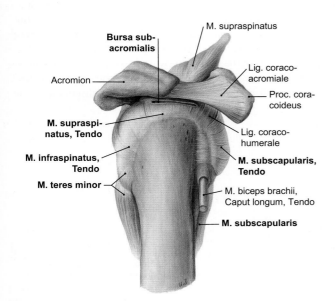

Fig. 4.17 Shoulder joint, right. Lateral view.

4.4.3 Shoulder joint mechanics

The shoulder joint is the joint with the largest range of movement of the human body. It is a ball joint with **mobility potential** around 3 axes:

- *Anteversion* and *retroversion* around a transverse axis: movement of the arm to the front or back
- *Abduction* and *adduction* around a sagittal axis: movement of the arm towards and away from the torso
- *External rotation* and *internal rotation* around an axis along the humeral shaft: rotation of the arm outwards or inwards.

The large range of movement in the shoulder joint is due to the fact that the stability of the joint is accomplished less by bone inhibition and ligament guidance, but mainly by muscles. In addition, during shoulder movement the shoulder girdle is usually also moved. This noticeably increases the range of movement of the upper extremity compared to movements in the shoulder joint alone (➤ Table 4.4, ➤ Fig. 4.18).

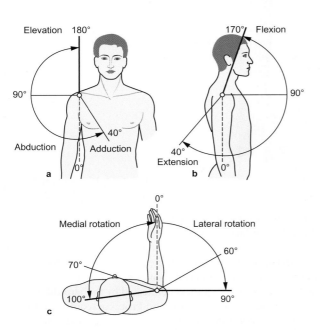

Fig. 4.18 Range of movement in the shoulder joint involving the shoulder girdle (thick line) as well as in the shoulder joint alone (thin line).

Table 4.4 Range of movement in the shoulder joint with and without the involvement of the shoulder girdle.

Movement	Shoulder joint	Shoulder joint and shoulder girdle
Abduction/adduction	90° – 0° – 40°	180° – 0° – 40°
Anteversion/retroversion	90° – 0° – 40°	170° – 0° – 40°
External rotation/internal rotation	60° – 0° – 70°	90° – 0° – 100°

Abduction beyond 90° is designated as **elevation**. This movement can only be carried out in combination with a rotation of the Scapula, as the shoulder roof impedes further abduction in the shoulder joint; however, rotational movements of the Scapula begin long before reaching the maximum abduction in the shoulder joint of 90°.

Clinical remarks

Due to weak ligament protection and bone guidance **luxations of the shoulder joint** are very common. The most common luxation is ventral and caudal under the Proc. coracoideus (Luxatio subcoracoidea). A patient with such a first luxation usually suffers from severe pain. The shoulder curvature is reduced and the affected arm appears longer in a lateral comparison (➤ Fig. 4.19). For repositioning, the ARLT method is often used (➤ Fig. 4.19). In this case the patient sits down and places the arm over the back of a padded chair that serves as an abutment. With a bent elbow joint, the doctor pulls along the axis of the humerus until the head of the humerus 'jumps' back into the plate under light internal rotation.

4.4.4 Shoulder muscles

Shoulder muscles refer to the muscles that move the shoulder joint and have an attachment in the upper arm. The muscles are divided according to their location into **3 groups**:

- **Ventral group:**
  - M. pectoralis major
  - M. coracobrachialis
- **Lateral group:**
  - M. deltoideus
  - M. supraspinatus
- **Dorsal group:**
  - M. infraspinatus
  - M. teres minor
  - M. teres major
  - M. subscapularis
  - M. latissimus dorsi

Ventral group

The large, fan-shaped **M. pectoralis major** (➤ Fig. 4.20, ➤ Table 4.5) is located very superficially and is thus responsible for the expression of the chest wall relief. Its fibres cross each other laterally, so that those of the Pars clavicularis join distally to the Crista tuberculi majoris of the Humerus, which, in contrast, proximally forms the Pars sternoclavicularis and thereby the anterior axillary fold. In an elevation movement the muscle fibres disentangle. The

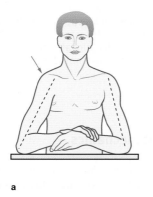

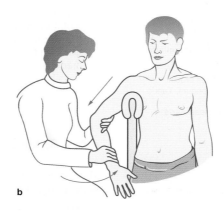

Fig. 4.19 Luxation of the shoulder joint. a Reduction of the shoulder bulge to the right in Luxatio subacromialis. **b** Repositioning manoeuvre following the METHOD OF ARLT.

Table 4.5 Ventral shoulder muscles.

Innervation	Origin	Attachment	Function
M. pectoralis major			
Nn. pectorales medialis and lateralis	• Pars clavicularis: sternal half of the Clavicula • Pars sternocostalis: Manubrium und Corpus sterni, cartilage of the II–VII ribs • Pars abdominalis: anterior lamina of the rectus sheath	Crista tuberculi majoris of the humerus	*Shoulder joint:* adduction *(most important muscle)*, internal rotation, anteversion *(most important muscle)*, retroversion from anteversion position *Thorax:* with fixed shoulder girdle lifts the sternum and ribs (inspiration: auxiliary breathing muscles)
M. coracobrachialis			
➤ See Chap. 4.5.5			

M. pectoralis major is the most important muscle for adduction and anteversion. In the case of propped up arms, it is an important auxiliary respiratory muscle.

The **M. coracobrachialis** performs the same functions as the M. pectoralis major. Corresponding to its location and innervation, however, it is usually numbered amongst the upper arm muscles (➤ Chap. 4.5.5). From the group of upper arm muscles the **M. biceps brachii** and the **M. triceps brachii** also impact (only the Caput longum) on the shoulder joint. Corresponding to their lever arms, however, they are only minimally involved in the corresponding joint excursions but together with the M. deltoideus and the M. coracobrachialis they primarily assist the stabilisation of the humeral head in the socket.

Clinical remarks

In the case of **failure of the M. pectoralis major** anteversion and adduction are severely impaired; therefore, the arms cannot be crossed in front of the body! The anterior axillary fold can wear away through atrophy of the muscle.

Lateral group

The **M. deltoideus** is a massive, complexly built muscle in the form of a triangle standing on its apex (➤ Fig. 4.21a, ➤ Table 4.6). In this way it gives the shoulder its contour. It can be involved in all movements depending on the position of the shoulder joint. With its **Pars acromialis** it is the most important muscle for abduction. The **Pars clavicularis** is situated in front of the transverse and rotational axes, thus this part can be anteverted and rotated inwards. For the **Pars spinalis** the reverse is true; it is located dorsally of the two axes and thus causes retroversion and external rotation. Both parts ad-

duct in a neutral position because at this juncture they are located below the sagittal axis of the shoulder joint. In the case of greater abduction (> 60°) of the arm, however, they end up above this axis and therefore support the Pars acromialis in further abduction. This means that the **supraspinatus** also functions synergistically (➤ Fig. 4.21b, ➤ Table 4.6) and its attachment tendon is separated by the Bursa subdeltoidea of the M. deltoideus. It is most important at the start of an abduction movement ('ignition function' of the M. supraspinatus).

Clinical remarks

In **the event of failure of the M. deltoideus** the arm can practically no longer be abducted because the M. supraspinatus is too weak to hold the arm. In the case of a longer lasting le-

---

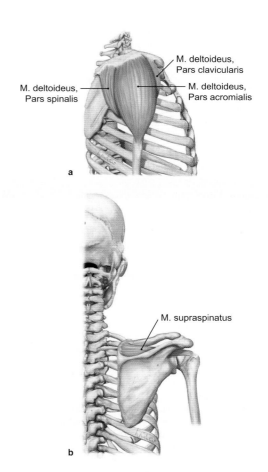

a

b

Fig. 4.21 Lateral shoulder muscles. a M. deltoideus, lateral view. **b** M. supraspinatus, dorsal view.

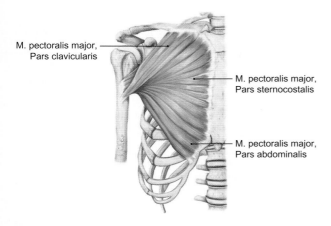

Fig. 4.20 Ventral shoulder muscles – M. pectoralis major, right. Ventral view.

sion, atrophy of the shoulder is visible. Also in the case of a **M. supraspinatus lesion** abduction is limited as the 'ignition function' is missing.

The attachment tendon of the **M. supraspinatus** runs below the shoulder roof in the 'subacromial space'. Due to the local spatial restriction the tendon is, e. g. in the case of chronic inflammation of the bursa, very vulnerable and ruptures (supraspinatus or shoulder impingement syndrome) commonly ensue.

Dorsal group

The **M. infraspinatus** is the most important lateral rotator in the shoulder joint, and is supported in this by the **M. teres minor** (➤ Fig. 4.22a, ➤ Table 4.7). Both muscles originate from the Scapula and run dorsally to the Humerus to the Tuberculum majus. The most important medial rotator is the **M. subscapularis** (➤ Fig. 4.22b, ➤ Table 4.7), which is the only muscle to originate from the ventral side of the Scapula. It stretches ventrally from the Humerus to the Tuberculum minus.

The largest muscle of the human body with respect to surface area is the **M. latissimus dorsi,** which covers the posterior side of the trunk in the lower thoracic and lumbar regions and in forming the rear posterior axillary fold stretches to the humerus (➤ Fig. 4.22c,

➤ Table 4.7). The muscle is important for retroversion from an anteversion position (thrust movement). Here, it acts synergistically with the M. pectoralis major, which is why both muscles are very well-defined in swimmers or high bar gymnasts. Since the M. latissimus dorsi lies over the rib cage, it can support exhalation as an auxiliary expiration respiratory muscle, e. g. during coughing. The **M. teres major** (➤ Fig. 4.22a, ➤ Table 4.7) supports the M. latissimus dorsi in movement against resistance.

Clinical remarks

In **the event of failure of the M. infraspinatus** the external rotation is severely affected. If, however, the **M. subscapularis** is not innervated, the internal rotation is considerably limited, so that the arms cannot be brought behind the back. Despite its size **failure of the M. latissimus dorsi** is in contrast functionally relatively insignificant. In the examination, however, it becomes obvious that the arms cannot be crossed behind the back ('apron grip') and the rear axillary fold is smoothed out. This muscle can be well utilized for reconstruction of the female breast, e.g. after resection for breast cancer. For this purpose, a part of the muscle in the area of origin is detached and moved ventrally. Failure of the Mm. teres major and minor is functionally insignificant.

Table 4.6 Lateral shoulder muscles.

Innervation	Origin	Attachment	Function
M. deltoideus			
N. axillaris	• Pars clavicularis: acromial third of the Clavicula • Pars acromialis: Acromion • Pars spinalis: Spina scapulae	Tuberositas deltoidea	*Shoulder joint:* abduction *(most important muscle)* • Pars clavicularis: adduction (from approx. 60° increasingly abduction), medial rotation, anteversion • Pars acromialis: abduction up to the horizontal plane • Pars spinalis: adduction (from approx. 60° onwards increasingly abduction), lateral rotation, retroversion
M. supraspinatus			
N. suprascapularis	Fossa supraspinata, Fascia supraspinata	Upper facet of the Tuberculum majus, joint capsule	*Shoulder joint:* abduction up to the horizontal plane, low lateral rotation; strengthening of the joint capsule *(rotator cuff)*

Table 4.7 Dorsal shoulder muscles.

Innervation	Origin	Attachment	Function
M. infraspinatus			
N. suprascapularis	Fossa infraspinata, Fascia infraspinata	Middle facet of the Tuberculum majus, joint capsule	*Shoulder joint:* lateral rotation *(most important muscle);* strengthening of the joint capsule *(rotator cuff)*
M. teres minor			
N. axillaris	Middle third of the Margo lateralis	Lower facet of the Tuberculum majus, joint capsule	*Shoulder joint:* external rotation, adduction; strengthening of the joint capsule *(rotator cuff)*
M. teres major			
N. thoracodorsalis	Angulus inferior	Crista tuberculi minoris	*Shoulder joint:* medial rotation, adduction, retroversion
M. subscapularis			
Nn. subscapulares	Fossa subscapularis	Tuberculum minus, joint capsule	*Shoulder joint:* medial rotation *(most important muscle);* strengthening of the joint capsule *(rotator cuff)*
M. latissimus dorsi			
N. thoracodorsalis	• Procc. spinosi of the 6 lower thoracic vertebrae and of the lumbar vertebrae • Fascia thoracolumbalis • Facies dorsalis of the Os sacrum • Labium externum of the Crista iliaca • IX–XII ribs • Frequently Angulus inferior of the Scapula	Crista tuberculi minoris	*Shoulder joint:* adduction, medial rotation, retroversion *(most important muscle)*

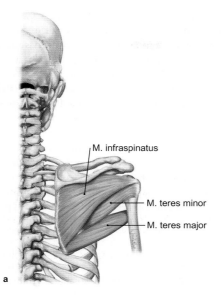

M. infraspinatus

M. teres minor

M. teres major

a

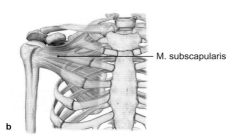

M. subscapularis

b

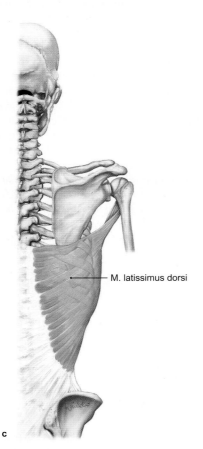

M. latissimus dorsi

c

In addition, the upper arm muscles **M. biceps brachii**, the **M. coracobrachialis** and the **M. triceps brachii** also participate in movements in the shoulder joint.

The following muscles are involved in the respective movements (most important muscle in bold type):

Abduction:
- **M. deltoideus**
- M. supraspinatus
- M. infraspinatus (cranial part)
- M. biceps brachii (Caput longum)

Adduction:
- **M. pectoralis major**
- Mm. teres major and minor
- M. latissimus dorsi
- M. deltoideus (Pars spinalis and Pars clavicularis)
- M. triceps brachii (Caput longum)
- M. biceps brachii (Caput breve)
- M. coracobrachialis
- M. infraspinatus (caudal part)

Anteversion:
- **M. pectoralis major**
- M. deltoideus (Pars clavicularis)
- M. biceps brachii
- M. coracobrachialis

Retroversion:
- **M. latissimus dorsi**
- M. deltoideus (Pars spinalis)
- M. teres major
- M. triceps brachii (Caput longum)

Lateral rotation:
- **M. infraspinatus**
- M. teres minor
- M. deltoideus (Pars spinalis)

Medial rotation:
- **M. subscapularis**
- M. pectoralis major
- M. latissimus dorsi
- M. teres major
- M. deltoideus (Pars clavicularis)
- M. coracobrachialis

4.5 Forearm and hand

Skills

After working through this chapter, you should be able to:
- explain the bony structures of the forearm and hand, as well as the structure and function of all joints on a specimen
- know the course of the ligaments of the elbow joint and the basics of the ligaments of the hand joints
- know the origin, attachment, function and innervation of all muscles and to show this on a specimen
- explain the functions of the M. biceps brachii depending on the position of the elbow joint as well as explain its interaction with the M. brachialis
- know the importance of tendon sheaths and retinacula for the function of muscles and to explain the functional relationship between the short finger muscles and the dorsal aponeurosis

Fig. 4.22 Dorsal shoulder muscles. a M. infraspinatus, M. teres major and M. teres minor, dorsal view. **b** M. subscapularis, ventral view. **c** M. latissimus dorsi, dorsal view.

4.5.1 Bones of the forearm

The forearm is formed by two bones:
- Radius
- Ulna

The radius and ulna are articulated by 2 **joints** (the Articulatio radioulnaris proximalis and Articulatio radioulnaris distalis) as well as by a rigid syndesmosis, the Membrana interossea antebrachii (➤ Fig. 4.23).

The **Caput radii** is located proximally and has 2 joint plates, the Fovea articularis (cranial) and the Circumferentia articularis (lateral) that are involved in the structure of the elbow joint.

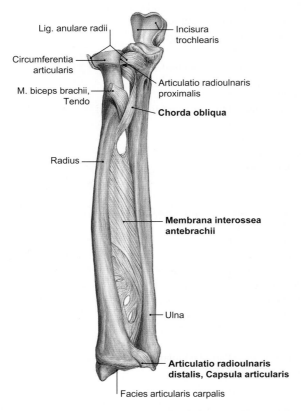

Fig. 4.23 labels:
- Lig. anulare radii
- Incisura trochlearis
- Circumferentia articularis
- M. biceps brachii, Tendo
- Articulatio radioulnaris proximalis
- **Chorda obliqua**
- Radius
- **Membrana interossea antebrachii**
- Ulna
- **Articulatio radioulnaris distalis, Capsula articularis**
- Facies articularis carpalis

Fig. 4.23 Bone and bone connections of the forearm, right. Ventral view.

The **diaphysis** of the radius is connected with the Caput radii via the radial neck (**Collum radii**) and is triangular in cross-section, so that 3 borders arise (**Margines anterior, interosseus and posterior**). Ventral is the **Tuberositas radii,** which serves as an attachment for the M. biceps brachii.

The **distal radial epiphysis** carries the stylus process (**Proc. styloideus radii**) and an articular surface for the distal radioulnar joint, the Incisura ulnaris.

Proximally on the dorsal side, the ulna has a prominent apophysis, the **olecranon** (elbow). Ventral to the apophysis is the **Proc. coronoideus,** where there are also two joint surfaces, the Incisura trochlearis and the Incisura radialis.

As for the radius, for the **diaphysis** a differentiation is made between 3 borders (**Margines anterior, interosseus and posterior**). Ventral is the **Tuberositas ulnae** for the attachment of the M. brachialis.

The **Caput ulnae** is located distally and with the Circumferentia articularis supports the ulnar part of the joint surface for the distal radioulnar joint as well as the **Proc. styloideus ulnae.**

> **N O T E**
> The radius and ulna each have a slim head and a thickened end. In the case of the radius the head is located proximally (at the elbow joint), whereas it is distal in the case of the ulna (in the direction of the wrist).

4.5.2 Elbow joint

The elbow joint (**Articulatio cubiti**) is a composite joint, which is formed by the humerus, radius and ulna (➤ Fig. 4.24). It is further divided into 3 joints:
- **Articulatio humeroulnaris**
- **Articulatio humeroradialis**
- **Articulatio radioulnaris proximalis**

All 3 parts of the joint are surrounded by a common joint capsule. In their entirety, the partial joints act as a *hinge-pivot joint.*

The **Articulatio humeroulnaris** is a pure *hinge joint,* in which the trochlea of the humerus articulates with the Incisura trochlearis of the ulna. Here the bone guidance is very well-defined by the trochlea, which is shaped like a horizontal hourglass.

In the **Articulatio humeroradialis** the Capitulum humeri and the Fovea articularis of the Caput radiale move against each other. From the shape of the articular surfaces this joint is a *ball joint;*

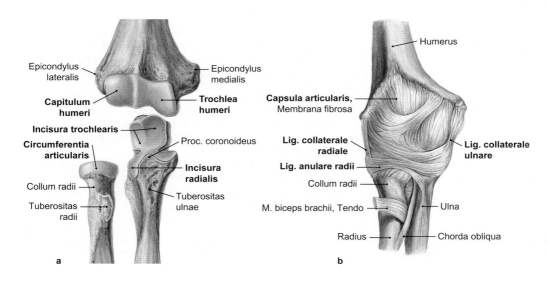

Fig. 4.24 a labels:
- Epicondylus lateralis
- Epicondylus medialis
- **Capitulum humeri**
- **Trochlea humeri**
- **Incisura trochlearis**
- Proc. coronoideus
- **Circumferentia articularis**
- **Incisura radialis**
- Collum radii
- Tuberositas ulnae
- Tuberositas radii

Fig. 4.24 b labels:
- Humerus
- **Capsula articularis,** Membrana fibrosa
- **Lig. collaterale radiale**
- **Lig. collaterale ulnare**
- **Lig. anulare radii**
- Collum radii
- M. biceps brachii, Tendo
- Ulna
- Radius
- Chorda obliqua

Fig. 4.24 Elbow joint (Articulatio cubiti), right. Ventral view. **a** Joint surfaces of the elbow joint. **b** Ligaments of the elbow joint.

however, coupling of the radius to the ulna by an annular ligament (**Lig. anulare radii**) and to the Membrana interossea antebrachii prevents abduction and adduction movements.

The **Articulatio radioulnaris proximalis** is a *pivot joint*. The joint head is formed by the hoop-shaped Circumferentia articularis which encompasses the Caput radii. This moves against the Incisura radialis ulnae and the Lig. anulare radii. The annular ligament is fixed to the front edge of the Incisura radialis ulnae and winds around the Circumferentia articularis in order to reinsert at the posterior edge of the Incisura radialis.

The **joint capsule** encloses all 3 joint surfaces and extends from the humerus somewhat distally of the Epicondyli to about 1 cm distal of the Lig. anulare radii. The elbow joint is further stabilised by 2 strong ligaments that reinforce the joint capsule laterally and medially (➤ Fig. 4.24b):

- **Lig. collaterale ulnare:** runs from the Epicondylus medialis of the humerus and extends in a triangular shape ventrally to the Proc. coroideus and dorsally to the olecranon
- **Lig. collaterale radiale:** runs from the Epicondylus lateralis of the humerus with 2 parts into the Lig. anulare radii and thus inserts at the anterior and posterior edges of the Incisura radialis ulnae

4.5.3 Joint connections between the forearm bones

Turning/rotational movements of the forearm (pronation and supination) are carried out in both joints together. The axis is thus the diagonal axis of the forearm, which connects the two radioulnar joints to each other:

- **Articulatio radioulnaris proximalis** (part of the elbow joint, ➤ Chap. 4.5.2)
- **Articulatio radioulnaris distalis**

The **distal radioulnar joint** is formed by the Incisura ulnaris radii and the Circumferentia articularis ulnae. This is a pivot joint with a movement axis.

The **Membrana interossea antebrachii** spans between the two Margines interosseae of the radius and ulna and forms a *syndesmosis* (➤ Fig. 4.23). It is important for stabilising rotational movements of the forearm. It also serves as a muscle origin and in the process separates the flexor muscles of the forearm from the extensor muscles. Proximally the Membrana interossea antebrachii has an entry point for the A./V. interossea posterior and a hollow to create space for the Tuberositas radii in pronation and supination movements. Located there with the **Chorda obliqua** is a ligament tension directed against the fibre course of the Membrana interossea.

4.5.4 Elbow joint and distal radioulnar joint mechanics

In the elbow joint **flexion** and **extension movements** are carried out around the transverse axis. In addition, in conjunction with the distal radioulnar joint **rotational movements** occur around an axis, which runs diagonally through the forearm from the radial to the ulnar head, and is referred to as **pronation** and **supination** (➤ Fig. 4.25, ➤ Table 4.8; also ➤ Fig. 4.39).

A clear extension is not possible because it is prevented by the bone constraint of the olecranon in the Fossa olecrani of the humerus prevents. The flexion, however, is not limited by bony structures, but by the soft tissue constraint of the upper arm muscles. Rotational movements of the forearm can be carried out in isolation only when the elbow is flexed and the upper arm is laid flat, otherwise movements in the shoulder joint also occur. In **supination**

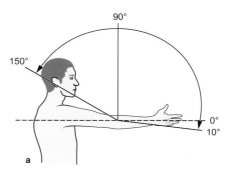

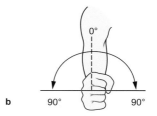

Fig. 4.25 Range of movement of the elbow joint. a Lateral view. **b** Ventral view.

Table 4.8 Range of movement of the elbow joint:

Movement	Range of movement
Extension/flexion	10°–0°–150°
Supination/pronation	90°–0°–90°

(thumbs to lateral, the palm pointing upwards) the radius and ulna are parallel (➤ Fig. 4.39b). In **pronation** (thumb pointing medially, the palm pointing downwards), both bones cross each other(➤ Fig. 4.39a). Thus, in rotational movements the radius circles around the ulna, guided in the process by the Lig. anulare radiai and the Membrana interossea.

4.5.5 Muscles

The most important muscles for movement in the elbow joint are located on the upper arm. Besides flexion and extension, they are also significantly involved in supination movements. A distinction is made between 3 ventral and 2 dorsal muscles (➤ Fig. 4.26b, ➤ Table 4.9):

Ventral group:
- M. biceps brachii
- M. brachialis
- M. coracobrachialis

Dorsal group:
- M. triceps brachii
- M. anconeus

Ventral group

The **M. biceps brachii** is superficial and thus determines the relief of the ventral upper arm (➤ Fig. 4.26). The original tendon of the **Caput longum** originates at the Tuberculum supraglenoidale of the Scapula within the joint capsule of the shoulder joint. It runs through the joint cavity and leaves the capsule space in the Sulcus intertubercularis. In this way, the tendon is involved in stabilisation of the shoulder joint. The **Caput breve** originates at the Proc. coracoideus. In addition to its attachment to the Tuberositas radii, the

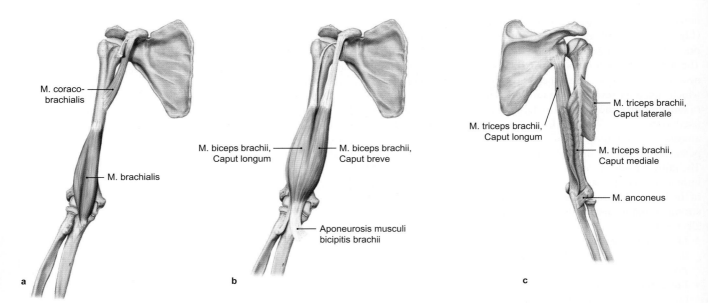

Fig. 4.26 Upper arm muscles, right. a M. brachialis and M. coracobrachialis, ventral view. **b** M. biceps brachii, ventral view. **c** M. triceps brachii and M. anconeus, dorsal view.

Table 4.9 Ventral upper arm muscles.

Innervation	Origin	Attachment	Function
M. biceps brachii[1]			
N. musculocutaneus	• Caput longum: Tuberculum supraglenoidale • Caput breve: tip of the Proc. coracoideus	Tuberositas radii, Fascia antebrachii	*Shoulder joint:* anteversion, medial rotation, abduction (Caput longum), adduction (Caput breve) *elbow joint:* flexion *(most important muscle),* supination *(most important muscle of the flexed elbow)*
M. brachialis			
N. musculocutaneus	Facies anterior of the humerus (lower half)	Tuberositas ulnae	*Elbow joint:* flexion, tenses joint capsule
M. coracobrachialis[2]			
N. musculocutaneus	Proc. coracoideus	Medial to the middle of the Humerus	*Shoulder joint:* medial rotation, adduction, anteversion

[1] The tendon of the Caput longum runs freely through the shoulder joint.
[2] The muscle is normally penetrated by the N. musculocutaneus.

M. biceps brachii runs into the Aponeurosis musculi bicipitis brachii, which is integrated into the superficial muscle fascia of the forearm, the Fascia antebrachii. The M. biceps brachii is the *strongest flexor in the elbow joint* and is also involved in movements of the shoulder joint. It is also the *most important supinator of the flexed elbow joint.* The muscle is particularly effective from the pronation position since its tendon winds around the radius, bolstered by the Bursa bicipitoradialis. In contraction, the tendon curls up similarly to a yo-yo (➤ Fig. 4.27). In the case of an extended arm, however, the tension axis of the M. biceps brachii runs parallel to the pronation/supination axis so that it can exert no force.

The **M. brachialis** is located under the M. biceps brachii (➤ Fig. 4.26a). It is a classical example of a flexor muscle because with its short lever it can carry out a large flexion movement with little contraction. In this way, it brings the M. biceps brachii into a more favourable position, so that it can aid flexion better. Thus, both muscles act synergistically (➤ Fig. 4.28).

Due to its position and innervation the **M. coracobrachialis** is also counted among the upper arm muscles (➤ Fig. 4.26a); however, it does not move the elbow joint, but only the shoulder joint. Because its muscle belly is normally (in approx. 90% of cases) penetrated by the N. musculocutaneus, it is an important orientation mark for the Plexus brachialis.

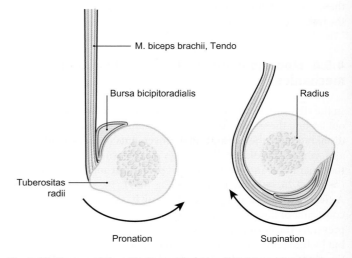

Fig. 4.27 Course of the attachment tendon of M. biceps brachii in relation to the radius during pronation (left) and supination (right). [L126]

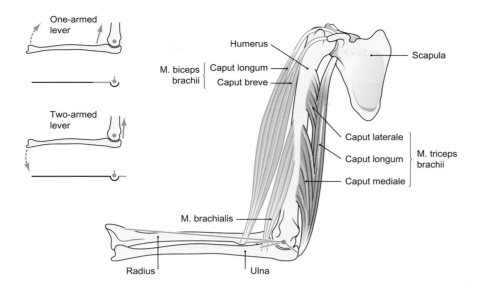

Fig. 4.28 Synergism of upper arm flexors.

In the event of a **failure of the M. biceps brachii** and the **M. brachialis,** mostly caused by a lesion of the N. musculocutaneus, flexion of the elbow is significantly impaired. Minimal bending, however, is still possible since the impaired flexors of the forearm (innervation by N. medianus) and also the radial muscle group of the forearm (innervation by N. radialis) can bend. If the M. biceps brachii is affected, supination of the flexed elbow is restricted and the biceps tendon reflex (triggered by a blow to the attachment tendon above the Tuberositas radii) is eliminated. A failure of the M. coracobrachialis, on the other hand, is relatively insignificant.

In the case of **lesions of the M. triceps brachii,** extending the elbow is impossible and the triceps tendon reflex (triggered by a blow to the attachment tendon above the olecranon) cannot be triggered.

The **M. biceps brachii** is the **marker muscle** for spinal cord segment **C6,** and the **M. triceps brachii** for **segment C7,** because both muscles are predominantly supplied by the respective segments. This plays an important role in in the diagnosis of herniated discs in the area of the cervical spine since in these cases, only one of the two muscles fails and not the remaining muscles supplied by the same nerve.

Dorsal group

The **M. triceps brachii** is the most important extensor in the elbow region (➤ Fig. 4.26c, ➤ Table 4.10). The Caput mediale and Caput laterale only have an effect on the elbow joint; the Caput longum is additionally involved in retroversion and adduction in the shoulder joint and separates the lateral and medial shoulder gaps from each other.

The **M. anconeus** is functionally insignificant and is to be seen rather as a distal separation of the M. triceps brachii (➤ Fig. 4.26c).

4.5.6 Structure and bones of the hand

The hand (**Manus**) is divided into three sections (➤ Fig. 4.29):

- Wrist (**Carpus**)
- Middle hand (**Metacarpus**)
- Fingers (**Digiti manus**)

The digits and the bones of the metacarpus are numbered I–V from radial to ulnar. The first digit is the thumb (Pollex); the second digit is the index finger (Index); the third digit the middle finger (Digitus medius); the fourth digit the ring finger (Digitus anularis); and the fifth digit the little finger (Digitus minimus).

The 8 carpal bones are arranged in 2 rows of 4 bones each (➤ Fig. 4.29).

Proximal row (from radial to ulnar):

- Scaphoid bone (**Os scaphoideum**)
- Semilunar bone (**Os lunatum**)
- Triquetral bone (**Os triquetrum**)
- Pisiform bone (**Os pisiforme**)

Distal row (from radial to ulnar):

- Greater multangular bone (**Os trapezium**)
- Lesser multangular bone (**Os trapezoideum**)
- Capitate bone (**Os capitatum**)
- Hamate bone **Os hamatum**)

Table 4.10 Dorsal muscles of upper arm.

Innervation	Origin	Attachment	Function
M. triceps brachii			
N. radialis	• Caput longum: Tuberculum infraglenoidale • Caput mediale: Facies posterior to the medial humerus and distal to the Sulcus nervi radialis • Caput laterale: Facies posterior of the lateral humerus proximal to the Sulcus nervi radialis	Olecranon	_Shoulder joint:_ adduction, retroversion (Caput longum) _Elbow joint:_ extension (_most important muscle_)
M. anconeus[1]			
N. radialis	Epicondylus lateralis humeri	Facies posterior of the ulna, Olecranon	_Elbow joint:_ extension

[1] The muscle lies on the lateral part of the Caput mediale of the M. triceps brachii.

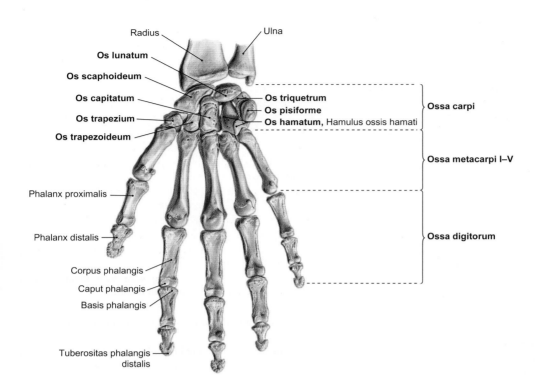

Radius — Ulna
Os lunatum
Os scaphoideum
Os capitatum — Os triquetrum
— Os pisiforme
Os trapezium — Os hamatum, Hamulus ossis hamati
Os trapezoideum

Ossa carpi

Ossa metacarpi I–V

Phalanx proximalis

Phalanx distalis

Ossa digitorum

Corpus phalangis
Caput phalangis
Basis phalangis

Tuberositas phalangis
distalis

Fig. 4.29 Hand skeleton, right. Palmar view.

NOTE

Surprisingly, the relatively senseless mneumonic 'Some Lovers Try Positions That They Can't Handle' can, nevertheless, be quite helpful in learning the sequence of the individual carpal bones and is therefore well known to any medical student.

The carpal bones form the base of the **carpal tunnel (Canalis carpi).** On both the Os scaphoideum and the Os trapezium a palmar tubercle is formed (Tubercula ossis scaphoidei and trapezii). These form the radial wall of the carpal tunnel 'Eminentia carpi radialis'. The ulnar wall is formed by the Os pisiforme together with a prominence of the hamate bone (Hamulus ossis hamati) 'Eminentia carpi ulnaris'. In this way a groove is formed, referred to as the Sulcus carpi. As a roof, the Retinaculum musculorum flexorum closes the groove to the carpal tunnel, through which the tendons of the long finger flexors and also the N. medianus pass. The **pisiform bone** is also embedded in the tendon of the M. flexor carpi ulnaris and is thus functionally a sesamoid bone.

The 5 metacarpals form the bones of the **middle hand.** In each case, a distinction is made between basis, corpus and caput. As an anomaly the Os metacarpal III has a Proc. styloideus.

Even in the **fingers** there are differences. Whereas the thumb consists of 2 bones (**Phalanges proximalis and distalis),** in the other 4 digits there are three bones (**Phalanges proximalis, media and distalis).** Just like on the metacarpal bones, here there is also a differentiation between basis, corpus and caput.

NOTE

All bones of the metacarpus and of the digits are divided into basis, corpus and caput. The thumb skeleton consists only of 2 bones.

4.5.7 Joints of the hand

A differentiation is made between the following joints or **joint groups** on the hand:
- Proximal wrist joint (**Articulatio radiocarpalis**) between the radius and proximal row of carpal bones
- Distal wrist joint (**Articulatio mediocarpalis**) between the proximal and distal rows of carpal bones
- **Articulationes intercarpales** between individual carpal bones
- **Articulationes carpometacarpales** between the distal row of carpal bones and the Ossa metacarpi
- **Articulationes intermetacarpales** between the Ossa metacarpi
- Metacarpophalangeal joints (**Articulationes metacarpophalangeae**) between the Ossa metacarpi and Phalanges proximales
- **Articulationes interphalangeae manus** between the bones of the digits

Accordingly, the **ligaments of the joints** of the hand are divided into different groups:
- Ligaments between forearm and wrist
- Ligaments between the carpal bones
- Ligaments between carpal bones and metacarpus
- Ligaments between the metacarpal bones
- Ligaments between metacarpal bones and proximal phalanges of the digits
- Ligaments between the phalanges

NOTE

Wrist joints in the proper sense of the word refer to the Articulatio radiocarpalis and the Articulatio mediocarpalis, because they ensure the movement of the hand opposite the forearm.
Clinically, abbreviations for the **finger joints** are often used:
MCP = metacarpophalangeal joint (finger basis joint)
PIP = proximal interphalangeal joint (finger middle joint)
DIP = distal interphalangeal joint (finger end joint)

Proximal and distal wrist joints

The proximal wrist (**Articulatio radiocarpalis**) is a *condyloid joint* (➤ Fig. 4.30). The proximal articular surface is formed by the Facies articularis carpalis of the radius as well as by a Discus articularis distal of the Caput ulnae. The distal articular surface is created by 3 of the 4 bones of the proximal row of carpal bones. In this way the Os scaphoideum and Os lunatum articulate directly with the radius; in contrast, the Os triquetrum articulates with the Discus articularis.

These 3 bones in turn form the proximal articular surfaces of the distal wrist joint (**Articulatio mediocarpalis**) and articulate here with all 4 bones of the distal row of carpal bones. Due to the transverse intersection of wave-shaped articular surfaces, the distal wrist joint is an *interlocking hinge joint;* however, functionally it works together with the proximal wrist joint in the sense of a condyloid joint. The Os pisiform is not involved in the formation of the wrist and, therefore, is actually not even a carpal bone.

> **N O T E**
>
> In the case of a palmar flexed hand, 2 grooves of skin on the intersection from forearm to hand are usually noticeable. The proximal flexor groove (**'Restricta'**) projects approximately onto the proximal wrist joint, the distal flexor groove (**'Rascetta'**) roughly onto the distal wrist joint.

Ligaments between forearm and carpal bones (➤ Fig. 4.31):
The following 2 ligaments inhibit **ulnar abduction** of the hand:
- **Lig. collaterale carpi radiale:** strong ligament between Proc. styloideus radii and Os scaphoideum.
- **Ligg. radiocarpale palmare:** on palmar side runs diagonally from the radius to the centrally located carpal bones located near the ulna. The distal contractions inhibit ulnar abduction and the proximal parts inhibit adial abduction.

The following 3 ligaments inhibit **radial abduction** of the hand:
- **Lig. collaterale ulnare:** from the Proc. styloideus ulnae to the Os triquetrum
- **Lig. radiocarpale dorsale:** runs diagonally from the dorsal side of the radius to the carpal bones located near the ulna, especially to the Os triquetrum
- **Lig. ulnocarpale palmare:** runs flatly from the Proc. styloideus ulnae to Os lunatum and Os triquetrum

Particularly palmar, but also dorsally the radial and ulnar ligament tensors together form the so-called **V-ligaments** in that they converge on the wrist joint.

Other joints of the wrist and middle hand

The Articulationes intercarpales in each row are functionally *amphiarthroses* because they are tautly tightened by ligaments on the palmar and dorsal side as well as by interosseous ligaments. In the same way, the Articulationes carpometacarpales II–IV as well as Articulationes intermetacarpales II–V are clamped to amphiarthroses. The Articulatio carpometacarpalis pollicis (*Carpometacarpal thumb joint*) occupies a special place with its good mobility.

As **ligaments between the carpal bones** (➤ Fig. 4.31) the ligament complexes can be divided into 3 levels (Ligg. intercarpalia dorsalia, palmaria and interossea). In principle, the ligaments are named according to the bone that they are connected to. Here only 3 major ligament structures are highlighted:
- The **Lig. carpi radiatum** radiates on the palmar side in a star shape from the Os capitatum in all directions.
- The so-called **Lig. carpi arcuatum** on the dorsal side connects the Os scaphoideum in an arch-like form over the Os lunatum with the Os triquetrum.
- The **Lig. pisohamatum** constitutes the continuation of the attachment tendon of the M. flexor carpi ulnaris to the hamate bone, into which the Os pisiform is incorporated.

Carpometacarpal joint of thumb (Articulatio carpometacarpalis pollicis)

As the German name suggests (*Daumensattelgelenk*), this joint is a classic example of a *saddle joint*. It articulates the concave articular surfaces of the Os trapezium and the Basis Ossis metacarpi I.

The wide joint capsule is reinforced by palmar and dorsal ligaments (**Ligg. carpometacarpalia palmaria and dorsalia**). Serving as the most important ligament for stabilising the joint, are fibrous connections that are referred to as the '**Lig. trapeziometacarpale palmare**', which define abduction of the thumb from palmar outwards (*radial abduction*).

> **Clinical remarks**
>
> Due to the loose ligament fastening of the carpometacarpal thumb joint **luxations** are very common (classical 'ski pole injury' by getting caught in a ski pole strap).

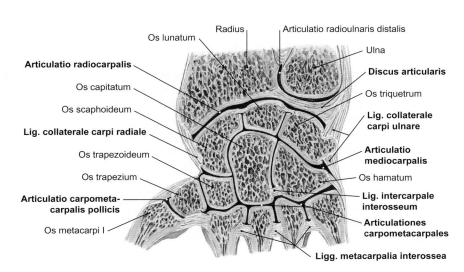

Os lunatum · Radius · Articulatio radioulnaris distalis · Ulna · Articulatio radiocarpalis · Discus articularis · Os capitatum · Os triquetrum · Os scaphoideum · Lig. collaterale carpi ulnare · Lig. collaterale carpi radiale · Articulatio mediocarpalis · Os trapezoideum · Os hamatum · Os trapezium · Lig. intercarpale interosseum · Articulatio carpometacarpalis pollicis · Articulationes carpometacarpales · Os metacarpi I · Ligg. metacarpalia interossea

Fig. 4.30 Joints of the wrist and middle hand, right.

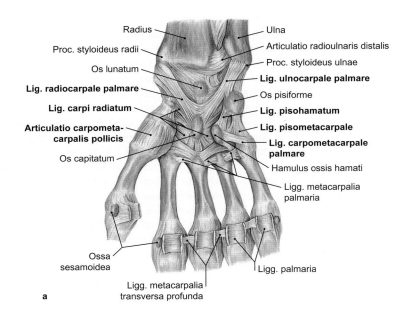

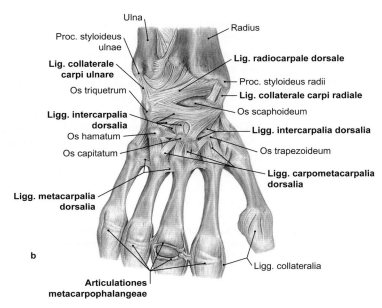

Fig. 4.31 Ligament systems of the hand, right. a Palmar view. **b** Dorsal view.

Carpometacarpal joints (Articulationes carpometacarpales) II–V and intermetacarpal joints (Articulationes intermetacarpales)

In these **joints** the distal row of the carpal bones articulates with the Ossa metacarpi and the bases of the metacarpal bones articulate amongst themselves. The tight **ligaments** allow Articulationes carpometacarpales II–IV and articulationes intermetacarpales to become *amphiarthroses*. Only the carpometacarpal joint of the small finger is slightly more flexible, which can be seen by the fact that the ball of the small finger on the intersection to the small finger can be deflected in a palmar direction roughly from the level of the palm. This reinforces the concavity of the palm, which is important for gripping a spherical object, e.g. a handball.

The carpometacarpal joints are stabilised by the **Ligg. carpometacarpalia palmaria and dorsalia** (➤ Fig. 4.31). The **Lig. pisometacarpale** is the continuation of the M. flexor carpi ulnaris tendon to the Ossa metacarpi IV and V. The **Ligg. metacarpalia palmaria, interossea and dorsalia** clamp the metacarpal bones to each other.

Finger joints (articulationes metacarpophalangeae and articulationes interphalangeae manus)

The **metacarpophalangeal joints** (Articulationes metacarpophalangeae) II–V are ball joints (➤ Fig. 4.32). Here they articulate the convex articular surfaces of the heads of the metacarpal bones with the articular surfaces of the base of the proximal finger bones that form the joint socket. As an anomaly, the metacarpophalangeal joint of the thumb forms a hinge joint, whereby only movements around one axis are possible.

Proximal and distal interphalangeal joints of the fingers (Articulationes interphalangeae manus) are hinge joints between the phalanges and accordingly have restricted flexion and extension movement capability.

The wide joint capsules of all finger joints are each stabilised by 2 **ligament systems** (➤ Fig. 4.33):

- **Ligg. collateralia** (both ulnar and radial)
- **Ligg. palmaria** (ventral)

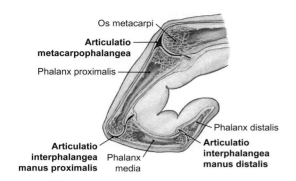

Fig. 4.32 Finger joints (Articulationes digiti), right. Lateral view.

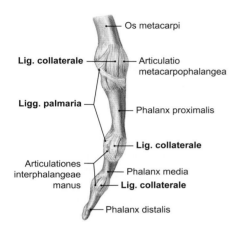

Fig. 4.33 Ligaments of the finger joints, right. Lateral view.

The Ligg. collateralia run diagonally from proximal/dorsal to distal/palmar. The Lig. palmare forms the base of the tendon sheaths of the long finger flexors.

The joint capsules of the metacarpal joints are also connected to each other by a diagonally running ligament, the **Lig. metacarpale transversum profundum** (➤ Fig. 4.31a).

4.5.8 Hand-joint mechanics

Proximal and distal wrist joints

Proximal and distal wrist joints do not move in isolation from each other, but functionally form a single unit. The range of movement is given in ➤ Fig. 4.34 and in ➤ Table 4.11.

In general **ulnar and radial abduction** as well as the greater part of **palmar flexion** occur in the *proximal wrist joint*, whilst the greater part of **dorsal extension** is carried out in the *distal wrist joint*. The movement of the individual carpal bones is, however, more complex. In the case of **palmar flexion** the proximal row of carpal bones rotates against the articular surface of the radius and the Discus articularis just like the distal row against the proximal one. Due to the stronger rotation in the proximal joint there is

Table 4.11 Range of movement from the proximal and distal carpal joint.

Movement	Range of movement
Dorsal extension/palmar flexion	60°–0°–60°
Ulnar abduction/radial abduction	30°–0°–30°

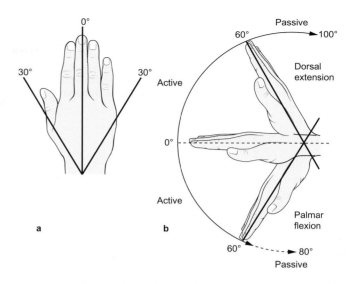

Fig. 4.34 Range of movement of the hand joints.

greater involvement of this joint in palmar flexion. It is the reverse in **dorsiflexion.** Here, the distal row of carpal bones rotates to a greater extent against the proximal row, so that the midcarpal joint carries out the greater part of dorsal extension.

Radial and ulnar abduction however, occurs around one axis, which runs from dorsal to palmar through the Os capitatum. In the neutral position the Os lunatum is in contact with both the radius and the Discus articularis. In ulnar abduction the proximal carpal bones slide radially, so that the Os lunatum is still only abutting the radius. Radial abduction, on the other hand, takes place mainly in the distal wrist joint; the Os lunatum remains in the proximal wrist largely in the central position. Due to the movement of the distal row of carpal bones against the proximal, the Os trapezium and the Os trapezoideum are moved onto the Os scaphoideum. In order to make room for the movement, the scaphoid bone tilts ventrally. In radial abduction from palmar outwards, this tilting is palpable beginning at the ball of the thumb; here one can feel the movement of the Os scaphoideum.

> **NOTE**
> **P**almar flexion as well as radial and ulnar abduction: mainly in the **p**roximal wrist joint.
> **D**orsal extension: mainly in the **d**istal wrist joint.

Carpometacarpal thumb joint

In the carpometacarpal thumb joint the following movements around 2 axes occur:

- **Abduction** (abduction of the thumb) and **adduction** (application of the thumb to the ring finger) around a slightly slanted dorsopalmar axis.
- **Flexion** (tilting thumb to palmar) and **extension** (thumb to dorsal) around one axis, which runs from the carpometacarpal thumb joint approximately to the top of the small finger.

A special feature in this joint is **opposition movement,** during which the tip of the thumb is drawn near to finger tips of the other fingers. In this case adduction and flexion movements are carried out in combination. In addition, there is a slight rotation around the longitudinal axis of the Os metacarpale I. In the process, the contact of the articular surfaces of the carpometacarpal thumb joint is partly neutralised.

The carpometacarpal thumb joint is designed by the form of its joint surfaces for movements around 2 axes. In an opposition movement, however, rotation also ensues, which increases stress to the articular surfaces. This non-physiological stress is seen as a reason why arthrosis **(rhizarthrosis)** often occurs in this joint.

Finger joints

In the **metacarpophalangeal joints** both flexion/extension movements as well as abduction (abduction of the fingers) and adduction (adduction of fingers II, IV and V to the middle finger) are possible due to their spherical shape (➤ Fig. 4.35, ➤ Table 4.12). The Lig. metacarpale transversum profundum limits larger abduction movements. With a stretched finger even a slight rotation is passively feasible at most. The collateral ligaments prevent a larger abduction of the fingers in a flexed position of the base joint.

In the **carpometacarpal thumb joint** only marginal abduction or adduction as well as rotation is possible. Here movement is limited to flexion and extension.

In the **interphalangeal joints** once again only flexion and extension are possible. Extension is inhibited by the Ligg. palmaria and the Ligg. collateria are also involved.

Table 4.12 Range of movement in the finger joints.

Movement	Base joints	Proximal joints	Distal joints
Dorsal extension/ palmar flexion	30°–0°–90°	0°–0°–100°	0°–0°–90
Ulnar abduction/ radial abduction	(20–40)°–0°–(20–40)°	–	–

NOTE

In each of the finger joints flexion to around 90° is possible. Significant extension, however, is only possible in the metacarpophalangeal joints. Hereby, extension movements in all base joints, especially those passively involved, vary very differently in their individual extents.

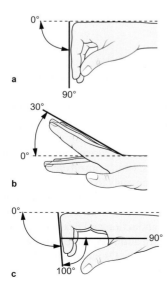

Fig. 4.35 Range of movement of the finger joints, right.

4.5.9 Muscles of the forearm and hand

A topographical distinction is made between forearm muscles and hand muscles. The **forearm muscles** are located with their muscle bellies on the forearm; however, many of them insert in the area of the carpus or the finger bones. Therefore, there are muscles that also move the fingers in addition to acting on the wrist joints. Since the superficial muscles originate from the Humerus, they are also involved in flexion of the elbow.

The displacement of the bellies of some stronger muscles for finger movement onto the forearm enables the delicate shape of the hand, thus creating the prerequisite for fine motor movements.

The **hand muscles**, on the other hand, have their origin at the hand bones and thus have no effect on movement of the hand compared to the forearm. Therefore, they only move the fingers.

Forearm muscles

On the forearm there are 19 muscles in total, making finely tuned movements of the hand and the individual fingers possible. These are divided into three groups:
- Ventral group
- Lateral (radial) group
- Dorsal group

The ventral and dorsal groups are each divided into a superficial and a deep layer. Due to its innervation the radial muscle group is often merged with the dorsal group on the forearm to the extensors of the wrist.

Ventral superficial group (sequence from radial to ulnar):
- M. pronator teres (proximal)
- M. flexor carpi radialis
- M. palmaris longus
- M. flexor digitorum superficialis
- M. flexor carpi ulnaris

Ventral deep group (from radial to ulnar):
- M. flexor pollicis longus
- M. flexor digitorum profundus
- M. pronator quadratus (distal)

Lateral (radial) group (from proximal to distal):
- M. brachioradialis
- M. extensor carpi radialis longus
- M. extensor carpi radialis brevis

Dorsal superficial group (from radial to ulnar):
- M. extensor digitorum
- M. extensor digiti minimi
- M. extensor carpi ulnaris

Dorsal deep group (from radial to ulnar):
- M. supinator (proximal)
- M. abductor pollicis longus
- M. extensor pollicis brevis
- M. extensor pollicis longus
- M. extensor indicis

In the case of the **flexor muscles** the division into superficial and deep muscles represents a simplification that occurs due to their common origins and their innervation. Here, the M. flexor digitorum superficialis lies under the remaining superficial muscles and forms a middle layer, whilst the M. pronator quadratus is located under the attachment tendons of the remaining deep flexors. Thus, there are a 4 layers in total.

Superficial flexors

All superficial flexors have at least one of their origins at the Epicondylus medialis humeri and lie ventral of the transverse axis of

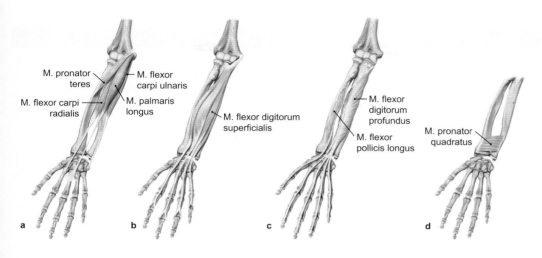

M. pronator teres
M. flexor carpi ulnaris
M. flexor carpi radialis
M. palmaris longus
M. flexor digitorum superficialis
M. flexor digitorum profundus
M. flexor pollicis longus
M. pronator quadratus

a b c d

Fig. 4.36 Ventral muscles of the forearm, right. Ventral view.

Table 4.13 Ventral superficial muscles of the forearm.

Innervation	Origin	Attachment	Function
M. pronator teres			
N. medianus	*Caput humerale:* Epicondylus medialis of the humerus *Caput ulnare:* Proc. coronoideus	Lateral in the middle of the radius	*Elbow joint:* pronation *(most important muscle)*, flexion
M. flexor carpi radialis			
N. medianus	Epicondylus medialis of the humerus, Fascia antebrachii	Palmar on Os metacarpi II	*Elbow joint:* flexion, pronation *Wrist:* palmar flexion, abduction radial
M. palmaris longus (inconstant muscle)			
N. medianus	Epicondylus medialis of the humerus	Aponeurosis palmaris	*Elbow joint:* flexion *Wrist:* palmar flexion, tension of palmar aponeurosis
M. flexor digitorum superficialis[1]			
N. medianus	• Caput humeroulnare: Epicondylus medialis of the humerus, Proc. coronoideus • Caput radiale: Facies anterior of the radius	With 4 long tendons at the middle phalanx of the 2nd –5th fingers	*Elbow joint:* flexion *Wrist:* palmar flexion *Finger joints (II–V):* flexion *(most important flexor of the middle joints)*
M. flexor carpi ulnaris			
N. ulnaris	Caput humerale: Epicondylus medialis of the humerus Caput ulnare: olecranon, proximal on the Margo posterior of the Ulna	Via the Os pisiforme and the Ligg. pisometacarpale and pisohamatum at the Basis of Os metacarpi V and of the Os hamatum	*Elbow joint:* flexion *Wrist:* palmar flexion, abduction to ulnar

[1] The tendons of these muscles are penetrated by the tendons of the M. flexor digitorum profundus shortly before their base.

the elbow joint (➤ Fig. 4.36, ➤ Table 4.13). Their main function is movement of the hand and fingers, but they also flex the elbow joint. All muscles apart from the M. flexor carpi ulnaris are innervated by the N. medianus.

The **M. flexor carpi ulnaris** serves as a guide for the N. ulnaris and is also innervated by it. Its end tendon does not run through the carpal tunnel, but on its ulnar side to the Os pisiform. There it continues into the Lig. pisohamatum to the Hamulus ossis hamati and into the Lig. pisometarcapale to the Basis ossis metacarpi V.

The **M. pronator teres** is the most important pronator (➤ Fig. 4.36). Its two heads are penetrated by the N. medianus, making it rare that initiation of this nerve occur.

The **M. flexor digitorum superficialis** runs to fingers II–V and is the most important flexor in the proximal interphalangeal joints. Its 4 end tendons each split into a radial and an ulnar string, each of which attaches laterally to the base of the Phalanx media of fingers II–V. Between each string there remains a gap, which is penetrated by an end tendon of the M. flexor digitorum profundus. The 4 muscle bellies are not on the same plane, but the two middle bellies of the middle and the ring finger cover the bellies of the index and the little finger.

The **M. palmaris longus** is inconsistent and in about 20% of the cases it is missing on one side (visible in a flexed hand position when only the tendon of the M. flexor carpi radialis protrudes at the distal forearm instead of 2 tendons). Apart from the M. flexor carpi ulnaris, the M. palmaris longus is the only one of the long flexors whose end tendon does not run through the carpal tunnel.

Deep flexors

The deep flexors originate at the radius, ulna and Membrana interossea antebrachii (➤ Fig. 4.36, ➤ Table 4.14). Therefore, they have no flexion function in the elbow joint. Like the superficial muscles, they are innervated by the N. medianus (albeit by its deep R. interosseus antebrachii anterior). An exception is the **M. flexor digitorum profundus,** which receives a double innervation whereby its 2 radial bellies (for index finger and middle finger) are innervated by the N. medianus, but the 2 ulnar bellies (for ring and small finger) by the N. ulnaris. The M. flexor digitorum profundus is similar to

Table 4.14 Ventral deep forearm muscles.

Innervation	Origin	Attachment	Function
M. flexor digitorum profundus			
N. ulnaris for the ulnar part, N. medianus for the radial part	Facies anterior of the Ulna, Membrana interossea	Distal phalanx of the 2nd–5th fingers	*Wrist:* palmar flexion *Finger joints (II–V):* flexion *(most important flexor of the distal finger joints)*
M. flexor pollicis longus			
N. medianus	Facies anterior of the radius	Distal phalanx of the thumb	*Wrist:* palmar flexion *Carpometacarpal thumb joint:* flexion, opposition *Thumb joints:* flexion
M. pronator quadratus			
N. medianus	Distal to the Facies anterior of the ulna	Facies anterior of the radius	*Radioulnar joints:* pronation

the M. flexor digitorum superficialis with 4 end tendons to fingers II–V; however, after it has traversed the forked end tendons of the M. flexor digitorum superficialis, it inserts to the base of the distal phalanges. It is the most important flexor in the distal interphalangeal joints (since it is the only one).

As the only one of the ventral forearm muscles, the **M. flexor pollicis longus** runs to the thumb and with its attachment to the distal phalanx of the thumb, it is also the only flexor in the carpometacarpal thumb joint. The **M. pronator quadratus** lies under all other muscles of the forearm. It is the only one to have an almost transverse fibre course and it supports the M. pronator teres during pronation.

Lateral/radial groups

The muscles of the lateral or radial group originate in the area of the Epicondylus lateralis and evolutionarily belong to the extensors (➤ Fig. 4.37, ➤ Table 4.15). Like all other extensors of the upper extremities, they are also innervated by the N. radialis. The term 'extensor' refers here again to their effect on the wrist joints; however, in the elbow joint all 3 muscles act as flexors.

The **M. brachioradialis** is the muscle which originates furthest to proximal and is the only one to lie against the Proc. styloideus radii thus having no effect on the wrist joints. Therefore, its main function is flexion in the elbow joint, where it is the most effective out of a middle flexed position. It is also involved in both supination

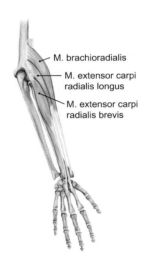

- M. brachioradialis
- M. extensor carpi radialis longus
- M. extensor carpi radialis brevis

Fig. 4.37 Lateral (radial) forearm muscles, right. Dorsal view.

Clinical remarks

In the case of **failure** or tendon rupture of the **M. flexor digitorum superficialis** flexion in the finger joints is restricted, but due to the **M. flexor digitorum profundus** still possible. If this is also affected, e.g. because of a deep laceration, then flexion in the proximal and also distal interphalangeal joints is impossible. If the cause is a **proximal (!) lesion of the N. medianus** then, due to the double innervation of the M. flexor digitorum profundus, it results in the image of an **ape hand.**

With the M. flexor digitorum superficialis there is sometimes also a permanent contraction (dystonia), which often affects just a single finger ('writer's cramp'). In these cases, the affected muscle belly must be treated by targeted injection of botulinum toxin, which inhibits synaptic transmission at the muscular end sheet.

In the case of **lesions of the M. pronator teres** pronation of the forearm is severely affected.

In case of **failure of the M. flexor pollicis longus** flexion in the distal interphalangeal joint of the thumb is no longer possible.

Table 4.15 Lateral (radial) forearm muscles.

Innervation	Origin	Attachment	Function
M. brachioradialis			
N. radialis	Margo lateralis of the humerus	Proximal of the Proc. styloideus of the radius	*Elbow joint:* flexion, pronation or supination (out from the opposite end positions)
M. extensor carpi radialis longus			
N. radialis	Crista supraepicondylaris lateralis to Epicondylus lateralis	Dorsal at Os metacarpi II	*Elbow joint:* flexion, slight pronation (out from the opposite end positions) *Wrist:* dorsal extension, abduction to radial
M. extensor carpi radialis brevis			
N. radialis	Epicondylus lateralis of the humerus	Dorsal at Os metacarpi III	*Elbow joint:* flexion, slight pronation (out from the opposite end positions) *Wrist:* dorsal extension, abduction to radial

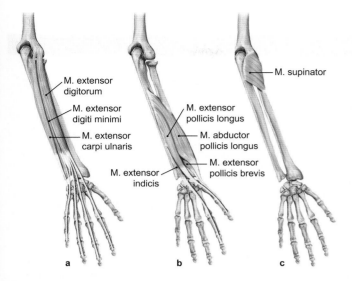

Fig. 4.38 Dorsal forearm muscles, right. Dorsal view.

(from a pronation position) and pronation (from a supination position).

The **Mm. extensor carpi radialis longus and brevis** run parallel, share the 2nd tendon compartment with their end tendons and insert side-by-side on the dorsal side of the Os metacarpale II and III. Since the M. extensor carpi radialis brevis, with its attachment to the Os metacarpale III, runs very closely to the abduction axis of the wrist joints, it has minimal involvement in radial abduction.

Superficial extensors

The largest superficial extensor, the **M. extensor digitorum,** inserts at the dorsal aponeuroses of fingers II–V and is supported in its extension effect at the little finger by the attached end tendon of the **M. extensor digiti minimi** (➤ Fig. 4.38a, ➤ Table 4.16). The **M. extensor carpi ulnaris**, with its attachment at the Os metacarpale V has no effect on the finger joints, but only serves ulnar abduction and extension of the wrist joints.

Deep extensors

All deep extensors are innervated by the R. profundus of the N. radialis. The **M. abductor pollicis longus** and the **M. extensor pollicis brevis** (➤ Fig. 4.38b, ➤ Table 4.17) are very easy to recognise due to their course. They stretch diagonally from radial and thereby overlap the muscles of the radial group in the distal third of the forearm.

The same applies for the **M. extensor pollicis longus** as for the M. flexor pollicis longus. It is the only muscle that is located at the distal phalanx of the thumb and therefore is the only extensor in the distal interphalangeal thumb joint.

The **M. supinator** runs from dorsal coming laterally around the radius and inserting at its ventral side (➤ Fig. 4.38c and ➤ Fig. 4.39). It is the *most important supinator in an extended elbow joint* (in flexion: M. biceps brachii). The muscle is penetrated by the R. profundus of the N. radialis (**supinator canal),** which switches to the dorsal side of the forearm after coming out of the elbow. The intersection point through the muscle is covered by a sickle-like reinforcement of muscle fascia (**FROHSE's arcade)** , at which the R. profundus can be damaged.

Clinical remarks

In the case of **failure of the Mm. extensor carpi radialis longus and brevis** a clinical image of **drop wrist** ensues, as both muscles serve especially to stabilise the wrist joints. If, however, the superficial and deep **extensors** of fingers and thumb fail, extension of the finger joints is severely impaired, but is still possible due to the effect of the Mm. lumbricales and Mm. interosseis at the proximal and distal interphalangeal joints of the fingers; however, at the thumb extension is no longer possible and abduction is also decreased. Since extension of the wrist joints is also necessary for prestretching of the finger flexors to counteract their active insufficiency, fist closure is also weakened when finger extensors fail. In the event of failure of the **M. supinator**, supination of the extended arm is no longer possible, but that of the flexed elbow is still possible because here the M. biceps brachii is the most important muscle.

Pronators and supinators of the forearm

The turning/rotational movement of the forearm is of great significance for the functioning of the upper extremity because it increases the range of movement (in conjunction with shoulder joint and movements of the shoulder girdle) so far that the palm can be rotated by 360° in total. In this respect, in the two radioulnar joints **pronation** (thumb to medial) and **supination** (thumb to lateral) of 90° from each respective normal position are possible.

Table 4.16 Superficial dorsal forearm muscles.

Innervation	Origin	Attachment	Function
M. extensor digitorum			
N. radialis (R. profundus)	Epicondylus lateralis of the humerus, Fascia antebrachii	Dorsal aponeuroses of the 2nd–5th fingers	*Elbow joint:* extension *Wrist:* dorsal extension *Finger joints (II–V):* extension *(most important extensor of the base and proximal joints)*
M. extensor digiti minimi			
N. radialis (R. profundus)	Lateral epicondyle of the humerus, antebrachial fascia	Dorsal aponeurosis of the 5th finger	*Elbow joint:* extension *Wrist:* dorsal extension *Finger joints (V):* extension *(most important extensor of the base and proximal joints)*
M. extensor carpi ulnaris			
N. radialis (R. profundus)	• Caput humerale: Epicondylus lateralis of the humerus • Caput ulnare: Olecranon, Facies posterior of the ulna, Fascia antebrachii	Dorsal at Os metacarpi V	*Elbow joint:* extension *Wrist:* dorsal extension, abduction to ulnar

Table 4.17 Dorsal deep forearm muscles.

Innervation	Origin	Attachment	Function
M. supinator			
N. radialis (R. profundus)	Epicondylus lateralis humeri, Crista musculi supinatoris of the ulna, Ligg. collaterale radiale and anulare radii	Facies anterior of the radius (proximal third)	Radioulnar joint: supination (*most important muscle of the flexed elbow*)
M. abductor pollicis longus			
N. radialis (R. profundus)	Facies posterior of Ulna and radius, Membrana interossea	Os metacarpi I	*Wrist:* dorsal extension *Carpometacarpal thumb joint:* abduction
M. extensor pollicis brevis			
N. radialis (R. profundus)	Facies posterior of ulna and radius, Membrana interossea	Base phalanx of the thumb	*Wrist:* dorsal extension *Carpometacarpal thumb joint:* abduction, reposition *Metacarpophalangeal thumb joint:* extension
M. extensor pollicis longus			
N. radialis (R. profundus)	Distal half of the Facies posterior of the ulna, Membrana interossea	Endphalanx distalis of the thumb	*Wrist:* dorsal extension *Carpometacarpal thumb joint:* extension, reposition *Thumb joint:* extension
M. extensor indicis			
N. radialis (R. profundus)	Distal quarter of the Facies posterior of the ulna, Membrana interossea	Dorsal aponeurosis of the index finger	*Wrist:* dorsal extension *Finger joints (II):* extension, adduction

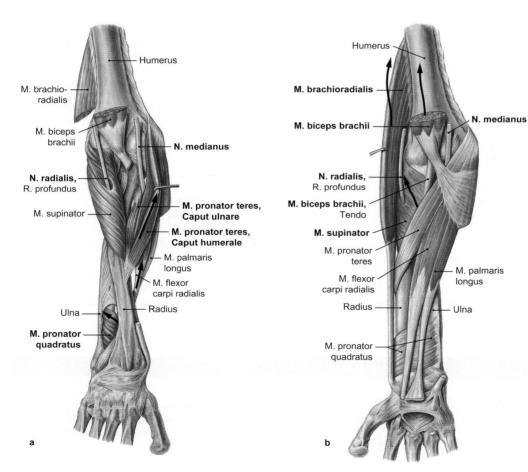

Fig. 4.39 Position of the forearm bones and involved muscles, right, ventral views. **a** Pronation position. **b** Supination position.

The **most important pronators** are(➤ Fig. 4.39a):
- M. pronator teres (strongest pronator!)
- M. pronator quadratus
- M. brachioradialis (only from supination position)

The **most important supinators** are (➤ Fig. 4.39b)
- M. biceps brachii (for flexed elbow)
- M. supinator (for extended elbow)
- M. brachioradialis (only from pronation position)

Although slightly weaker than the M. brachioradialis, the other two muscles of the radial group (Mm. extensor carpi radialis longus and brevis) can also act as pronators and supinators, if the forearm is in the respective opposite position and the muscles are thus brought into a position in which they intersect the diagonal axis of the forearm. In a similar way, the M. flexor carpi radialis and the M. palmaris longus support pronation (➤ Fig. 4.39a).

The muscles that are necessary for turning movements have 2 features in common:
- All muscles intersect the diagonal axis of the forearm (➤ Chap. 4.1, overview)
- All important pronators and supinators have their attachment at the radius

Hand muscles

Depending on their localisation the 11 hand muscles are divided into 3 groups:
- Muscles of the thenar eminence (Thenar)
- Muscles of the middle hand
- Muscles of the little finger eminence (Hypothenar)

All hand muscles (apart from the Mm. lumbricales) originate at the carpal or metacarpal bones. Innervation is either via the N. ulnaris or the N. medianus; the N. radialis does not supply any hand muscles. The muscles of the metacarpus are mainly located in the depth of the palm or between the finger rays (➤ Fig. 4.41 and ➤ Fig. 4.42), whilst the thenar and hypothenar muscles mostly run to palmar of the hand skeleton (➤ Fig. 4.40 and ➤ Fig. 4.41). They therefore raise the thenar and hypothenar eminences.

Thenar muscles:
- M. abductor pollicis brevis
- M. flexor pollicis brevis
- M. opponens pollicis
- M. adductor pollicis

Lumbrical muscles:
- Mm. lumbricales I–IV
- Mm. interossei palmares I–III
- Mm. interossei dorsales I–IV

Hypothenar muscles:
- M. abductor digiti minimi
- M. flexor digiti minimi brevis
- M. opponens digiti minimi
- M. palmaris brevis

At the **ball of the thumb** the M. abductor pollicis brevis, the M. flexor pollicis brevis and the M. adductor pollicis are ordered from radial to ulnar (➤ Fig. 4.41, ➤ Table 4.18). The M. opponens pollicis lies beneath the M. abductor pollicis brevis. The muscles are mostly innervated by the N. medianus. Exceptions are the M. adductor pollicis, as well as the Caput profundum of the M. flexor pollicis brevis, which are supplied by the R. profundus of the N. ulnaris.

At the **hypothenar eminence** the M. abductor digiti minimi, the M. flexor digiti minimi brevis and the M. opponens digiti minimi can be found in the order from radial to ulnar (➤ Table 4.19). All muscles of the hypothenar eminence are innervated by the N. ulnaris (R. profundus). The M. palmaris brevis, on the other hand, is a cutaneous muscle, which has no function for the joints of the little finger and is the only muscle to be innervated by the R. superficialis of the N. ulnaris.

The **muscles of the middle hand** (➤ Table 4.20) are mainly supplied by the N. ulnaris (exception: Mm. lumbricales I and II – N. medianus). The Mm. interossei palmares and dorsales together are the most important flexors in metacarpophalangeal joints II–V (➤ Fig. 4.42a, b). Due to their course on the sides facing the middle finger, the Mm. interossei palmares adduct fingers II, IV and V in the metacarpophalangeal joints ➤ Fig. 4.42c). In contrast, the interossei abduct in these joints.

The Mm. lumbricales similarly flex in the metacarpophalangeal joints (➤ Fig. 4.42d). Due to their distal radiation into the dorsal aponeurosis they are, however, the most effective extensors in the distal interphalangeal joints.

4.5.10 Auxiliary structures of the musculature in the area of the hand

In the area of the hand, because of the large strain and of the long course of the tendons, special auxiliary structures (**tendon sheaths**) are necessary. Likewise, there are supporting structures that prevent tendons shifting against or egressing out of the level of the palmar or dorsal side of the hand. The **Retinaculum musculo-**

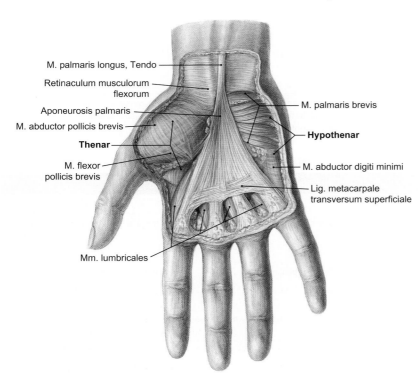

M. palmaris longus, Tendo
Retinaculum musculorum flexorum
Aponeurosis palmaris
M. abductor pollicis brevis
Thenar
M. flexor pollicis brevis
Mm. lumbricales
M. palmaris brevis
Hypothenar
M. abductor digiti minimi
Lig. metacarpale transversum superficiale

Fig. 4.40 Palmar muscles, Palma manus, right. Palmar view.

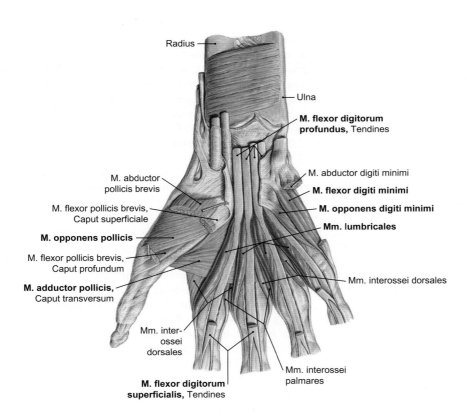

Radius

Ulna

**M. flexor digitorum
profundus,** Tendines

M. abductor
pollicis brevis

M. abductor digiti minimi

M. flexor digiti minimi

M. flexor pollicis brevis,
Caput superficiale

M. opponens digiti minimi

Mm. lumbricales

M. opponens pollicis

M. flexor pollicis brevis,
Caput profundum

M. adductor pollicis,
Caput transversum

Mm. interossei dorsales

Mm. inter-
ossei
dorsales

Mm. interossei
palmares

**M. flexor digitorum
superficialis,** Tendines

**Fig. 4.41 Middle layer of the
hand muscles, right.** Palmar
view.

Table 4.18 Muscles of the ball of the thumb (Thenar muscles).

Innervation	Origin	Attachment	Function
M. abductor pollicis brevis			
N. medianus	Retinaculum musculorum flexorum, Eminentia carpi radialis	Radial sesamoid bone of the thumb base joint, proximal phalanx of the thumb	*Carpometacarpal thumb joint:* abduction, opposition *Thumb base joint:* flexion
M. flexor pollicis brevis			
• Caput superficiale: N. medianus • Caput profundum: N. ulnaris (R. profundus)	• Caput superficiale: Retinaculum musculorum flexorum • Caput profundum: Ossa capitatum and trapezium	Radial sesamoid bone of the thumb base joint, proximal phalanx of the thumb	*Carpometacarpal thumb joint:* opposition, adduction *Thumb base joint:* flexion
M. opponens pollicis			
N. medianus	Retinaculum musculorum flexorum, Eminentia carpi radialis	Os metacarpi I	*Carpometacarpal thumb joint:* opposition
M. adductor pollicis			
N. ulnaris (R. profundus)	• Caput obliquum: Os hamatum, Ossa metacarpi II–IV • Caput transversum: Os metacarpi III	Ulnar sesamoid bone of the thumb base joint, proximal phalanx of the thumb	*Carpometacarpal thumb joint:* adduction, opposition *Thumb base joint:* flexion

Table 4.19 Muscles of the ball of the small finger (Hypothenar muscles).

Innervation	Origin	Attachment	Function
M. palmaris brevis			
N. ulnaris (R. superficialis)	Aponeurosis palmaris	Skin of the hypothenar eminence	Tenses the skin in the area of the hypothenar eminence
M. abductor digiti minimi			
N. ulnaris (R. profundus)	Os pisiforme, Retinaculum musculorum flexorum	Proximal phalanx	*Carpometacarpal joint (V):* opposition *Carpometacarpal joint (V):* abduction
M. flexor digiti minimi brevis			
N. ulnaris (R. profundus)	Retinaculum musculorum flexorum Hamulus ossi hamati	Proximal phalanx of the 5th finger	*Carpometacarpal joint (V):* opposition *Carpometacarpal joint (V):* flexion
M. opponens digiti minimi			
N. ulnaris (R. profundus)	Retinaculum musculorum flexorum Hamulus ossi hamati	Os metacarpi V	*Carpometacarpal joint (V):* opposition

Table 4.20 Muscles of the middle hand.

Innervation	Origin	Attachment	Function
Mm. lumbricales I–IV			
N. medianus (I, II); N. ulnaris (R. profundus) (III, IV)	Tendons II–IV of the M. flexor digitorum profundus (I + II from radial side; III + IV sides facing each other, two-headed)	Projecting radially into the dorsal aponeurosis (lateral tract) of fingers II–V	*Metacarpophalangeal joints (II–V):* flexion *Finger joints (II–V):* extension *(most important extensor of the metacarpophalangeal joints)*
Mm. interossei palmares I–III			
N. ulnaris (R. profundus)	Ulnar side of the Os metacarpi II, radial side of the Ossa metacarpi IV and V	Proximal phalanx and dorsal aponeurosis (lateral tract) of fingers II, IV and V	*Metacarpophalangeal joints (II, IV, V):* flexion *(most important flexor!),* adduction (to the middle finger) *Finger joints (II, IV, V):* extension
Mm. interossei dorsales I–IV (two-headed)			
N. ulnaris (R. profundus)	Sides facing each other of Ossa metacarpi I–V	Proximal phalanx and dorsal aponeurosis of fingers II–IV	*Metacarpophalangeal joints (II–IV):* flexion *(most important flexor!),* abduction (to the middle finger) *Finger joints (II–IV):* extension

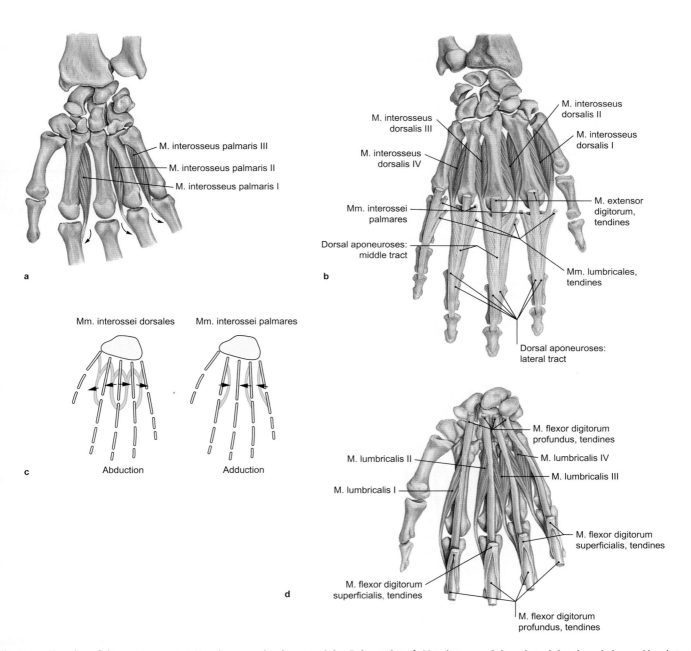

Fig. 4.42 Muscles of the metacarpus. a Mm. interossei palmares, right. Palmar view. **b** Mm. interossei dorsales, right, dorsal view. **c** Mm. interossei, diagram of their course and function. **d** Mm. lumbricales, right, palmar view.

rum extensorum on the dorsal side is once again divided into individual chambers, which are called tendon compartments. The **Retinaculum musculorum flexorum** forms the roof of the carpal tunnel (see also ➤ Chap. 4.10.5).

Tendon sheaths and ligamentous structures of the long flexors

The tendon of the M. palmaris longus is located at the **palmar aponeurosis**. This connective tissue sheet lies superficially directly under the cutaneous integument of the metacarpus, is fastened proximally to the Retinaculum musculorum flexorum, and tapers out into individual finger rays, which are fixed to the Lig. metacarpale transversum profundum (➤ Fig. 4.40). Diagonally running fibres proximal to the metacarpophalangeal joints are referred to as the Lig. metacarpale transversum superficiale.

Clinical remarks

Benign hardenings and node formations within the palmar aponeurosis can cause movement restrictions and flexion contractions of the finger joints, especially of the little and ring fingers. Largely unclear is the cause of **DUPUYTREN**'s **contraction**.

In order to reduce friction, the tendons of the
- Mm. flexor digitorum superficial and profundus,
- M. flexor pollicis longus and
- M. flexor carpi radialis

run in **tendon sheaths (Vaginae tendinum)** through the carpal tunnel (➤ Fig. 4.43). The tendon sheath of the M. flexor pollicis longus proceeds until the attachment point (radial tendinous sheath). The joint tendon sheath of M. flexor digitorum superficialis and profundus ends roughly at the level of the bases of the metacarpal bones and usually envelops just the tendons to the small fin-

ger up until their attachment (ulnar tendinous sheath). At the level of phalanges II–IV there are several tendon sheaths that only communicate with the ulnar tendinous sheath in exceptional circumstances.

Clinical remarks

Within the tendon sheaths bacterial infections can spread freely. Thus radiating from the little finger outwards all flexor tendons may be affected and, due to the geographical proximity between the ulnar and the radial tendon sheaths in the area of the wrist, inflammation can spread up to the distal interphalangeal joint of the thumb. This prospect of the **V-phlegmon** can lead to stiffening of the whole hand if treatment is insufficient.

The fibrous outer layer (Vagina fibrosa) of the tendon sheaths with ring and cross-shaped fibres (Pars anularis and Pars cruciformis), which are referred to *clinically* as **the annular and cruciate ligaments,** are fixed to the phalanges and joint capsules of the finger joints. This ensures the coupling of the end tendons onto the finger bone and avoids detachment during flexion.

Clinical remarks

Ruptures of the annular and cruciate ligaments of the tendon sheaths are especially common in climbing sports because these structures are put under tremendous pressure.

Tendon sheaths and ligament structures of the extensors

The **Retinaculum musculorum extensorum** secures the course of the extensor muscles of the hand. For this purpose, it is divided into 6 compartments that are numbered from radial from 1 to 6

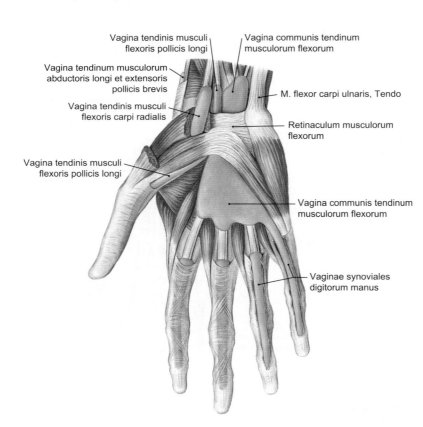

Vagina tendinis musculi flexoris pollicis longi

Vagina tendinum musculorum abductoris longi et extensoris pollicis brevis

Vagina tendinis musculi flexoris carpi radialis

Vagina tendinis musculi flexoris pollicis longi

Vagina communis tendinum musculorum flexorum

M. flexor carpi ulnaris, Tendo

Retinaculum musculorum flexorum

Vagina communis tendinum musculorum flexorum

Vaginae synoviales digitorum manus

Fig. 4.43 Tendon sheaths of the palmar side of the hand, right. Palmar view.

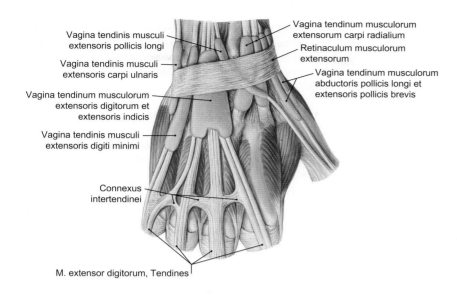

Vagina tendinis musculi extensoris pollicis longi

Vagina tendinis musculi extensoris carpi ulnaris

Vagina tendinum musculorum extensoris digitorum et extensoris indicis

Vagina tendinis musculi extensoris digiti minimi

Connexus intertendinei

M. extensor digitorum, Tendines

Vagina tendinum musculorum extensorum carpi radialium

Retinaculum musculorum extensorum

Vagina tendinum musculorum abductoris pollicis longi et extensoris pollicis brevis

Fig. 4.44 Dorsal tendon sheaths of the hand, right.

(➤ Fig. 4.44). (**Tip:** Dissection of the tendon compartments is useful because it makes it much easier to map the individual muscles!) The tendons of the following muscles pass through:

1. **Tendon compartment:** M. abductor pollicis longus, M. extensor pollicis brevis
2. **Tendon compartment:** Mm. extensores carpi radialis longus and brevis
3. **Tendon compartment:** M. extensor pollicis longus
4. **Tendon compartment:** M. extensor digitorum, M. extensor indicis
5. **Tendon compartment:** M. extensor digiti minimi
6. **Tendon compartment:** M. extensor carpi ulnaris

Similarly to the flexor muscles, the extensors run in short tendon sheaths through the compartments of the retinaculum.

The **dorsal aponeurosis** is a loose connective tissue ligament structure that runs on the dorsal side of each finger from the proximal to the distal phalanx. It is predominantly formed by the end tendons of the long finger extensors, the interossei and Mm. lumbricales (➤ Fig. 4.45) and consists of a medial and a lateral tract:

• The **medial tract** is primarily formed by the long finger extensors and inserts at the proximal and middle phalanges.
• The **lateral tract** consists primarily of the end tendons of the Mm. lumbricales and inserts at the distal phalanx.

Because of this configuration the Mm. lumbricales are the most effective extensors in the distal interphalangeal joints. Individual fi-

bres of the Mm. interossei radiate into the lateral tract, but they mainly stretch to the middle tract. Due to the diagonal fibre course of the Mm. interossei and Mm. lumbricales (from palmar of the rotational axis of the proximal joint to dorsal of the rotational axis of middle and distal joints) the muscles act as flexors on the proximal joints, but as extensors in the middle and end joints.

NOTE

The most important muscles for flexion and extension of the finger and thumb joints

• Flexion of the finger joints:
  – Base joints: Mm. interossei palmares and dorsales
  – Middle joints: M. flexor digitorum superficialis
  – End joints: M. flexor digitorum profundus
• Extension of the finger joints:
  – Base and middle joints: M. extensor digitorum, M. extensor indicis
  – End joints: Mm. lumbricales
• Thumb (each with a long and a short flexor and extensor)
  – Flexion of the base joint: M. flexor pollicis brevis
  – Flexion of the end joint: M. flexor pollicis longus
  – Extension of the base joint: M. extensor pollicis brevis
  – Extension of the end joint: M. extensor pollicis longus

Clinical remarks

Injuries to the dorsal aponeurosis are common due to its exposed position: In the case of a severance above the metacarpophalangeal joint the finger can no longer be stretched effectively in the metacarpophalangeal joint; however, extension in the proximal and distal interphalangeal joints (Mm. lumbricales and interossei, radiating from lateral), remains unaffected. In a severance of the medial tract above the proximal interphalangeal joint the lateral tract slips to palmar and flexion in the proximal interphalangeal joint and extension in the distal interphalangeal joint occur (**'boutonniere deformity'**). In a severance of the lateral tract in the area of the distal interphalangeal joint, the distal phalanx falls into a flexed position (because the Mm. lumbricales become ineffective). The other joints remain unaffected (**'mallet finger'**).

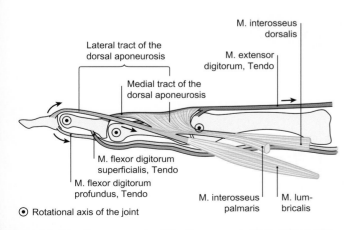

Lateral tract of the dorsal aponeurosis

Medial tract of the dorsal aponeurosis

M. flexor digitorum superficialis, Tendo

M. flexor digitorum profundus, Tendo

M. interosseus dorsalis

M. extensor digitorum, Tendo

M. interosseus palmaris

M. lumbricalis

⊙ Rotational axis of the joint

Fig. 4.45 Dorsal aponeurosis of the fingers and effect of finger flexors and extensors. [L126]

4.6 Nerves of the upper extremity

After working through this chapter you should be able to:
- explain the structure of the Plexus brachialis, show its structures on a specimen, and explain the symptoms associated with plexus lesions
- know the functions and failures of the shoulder nerves
- know the course, function and exact symptoms associated with failure of major nerves of the arm and show these on a specimen.

Spinal nerves **C4–T3** are involved in sensory innervation of shoulder and arm. The Rr. anteriores of spinal nerves **C5–T1** merge into the brachialis plexus (**Plexus brachialis**), out of which the actual nerves of the arm and shoulder region finally emerge.

4.6.1 Sensory innervation

The following nerves ensure sensory innervation of the skin of the arm (➤ Fig. 4.46a, b):
- N. axillaris
- N. radialis

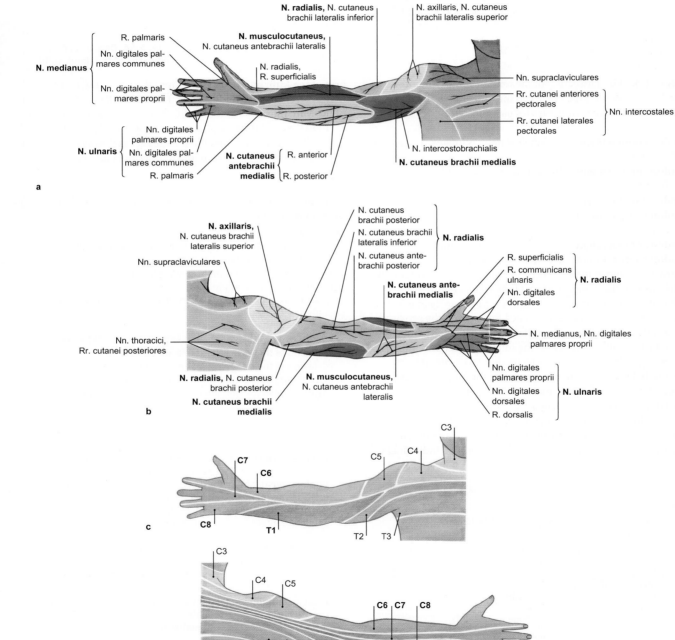

Fig. 4.46 Cutaneous nerves and segmental innervation of the upper extremity. a Cutaneous nerves, right, ventral view. **b** Cutaneous nerves, right, dorsal view. **c** Dermatomes, right, ventral view. **d** Dermatomes, right, dorsal view.

- N. musculocutaneus
- N. medianus
- N. ulnaris
- N. cutaneus brachii medialis
- N. cutaneus antebrachii medialis

In addition, individual fibres of the truncal nerves (**Nn. intercosto-brachiales** from T2 and T3) are involved in supplying the medial upper arm as they are attached to the N. cutaneus brachii medialis. An important point is that an area of skin is usually supplied in an overlapping fashion by several nerves. The part which is only innervated by a single nerve is usually rather small and is referred to as an **autonomic region**.

An area which is specifically supplied by the spinal nerve of a spinal cord segment is called a **dermatome** (➤ Fig. 4.46c, d). Whilst dermatomes on the torso are mostly arranged horizontally, on the arm they run along its longitudinal axis. As the comparison of ➤ Fig. 4.6 with ➤ Fig. 4.43c clearly shows, the torso dermatomes located at this point were 'lengthened' onto the arm during growth of the extremity buds.

Since the spinal nerves interlace within the Plexus brachialis and are positioned together with the nerves of the arm, the dermatomes do not correspond to the supply area of a nerve.

N O T E

The location of the dermatomes on the arm can be best remembered by imagining the arm abducting by 90° with the thumb directed upwards (➤ Fig. 4.46d). Here, the dermatomes are essentially arranged from cranial to caudal corresponding to the supplying spinal nerves segments:
From cranial to caudal:
- Shoulder height above the acromion: C4
- Skin above the M. deltoideus: C5
- Radial side of the arm and radial fingers (thumb!): C6
- Dorsal side of the arm and middle fingers: C7
- Dorsal side of the arm and ulnar fingers (little finger!): C8
- Medial side of the arm: distal: T1, proximal: T2
- Caudal sections of the axillary folds: T3
On the ventral side segments C7 and C8 only include the area from around the distal forearm.

Clinical remarks

Knowledge of the **dermatomes** is indispensable for diagnosing radiculopathy (damage of the spinal nerve root or the corresponding spinal section). In the case of intervertebral disc prolapses that can lead to compression of the spinal nerve root, sensory deficiencies or pain in the corresponding dermatomes usually enable the affected area to be well localised. Dermatomes C6–8 are of particular importance for diagnosis of herniated discs in the area of the cervical spine.
In addition to the mostly obvious loss of function of the supplied muscles, **injuries to the peripheral nerve** are recognised by sensory deficits particularly in the autonomic areas.

4.6.2 Structure of the Plexus brachialis

The Rr. anteriores of the spinal nerves of **C5–T1** form the Plexus brachialis (➤ Fig. 4.47). This serves as a 'distribution station' for the nerve supply of most parts of the arm, since in the arm spinal nerves are transferred to the nerves of the arm. It can be topographically subdivided into:
- **Pars supraclavicularis:** above the Clavicula
- **Pars infraclavicularis:** below the Clavicula
Individual nerves of the supraclavicular part also receive nerve fibres from segments C3 and C4.

Pars supraclavicularis

In the Pars supraclavicularis the Rr. anteriores of 5 spinal nerves amalgamate into **3 trunci (trunci)**:
- **Truncus superior:** receives fibres from **C5 and C6**
- **Truncus medius:** is only formed by **C7**
- **Truncus inferior:** forms from **C8 and T1**
The spinal nerves run together with the A. subclavia through the **'scalene hiatus'** between the M. scalenus anterior and M. scalenus medius to lateral, then unite into the trunci and enter caudally of the Clavicula and into the axillary cavity. Located ventral of this

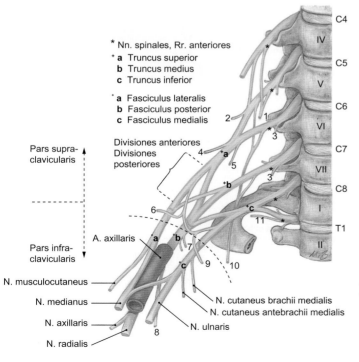

* Nn. spinales, Rr. anteriores
⁺ a Truncus superior
  b Truncus medius
  c Truncus inferior

˙ a Fasciculus lateralis
  b Fasciculus posterior
  c Fasciculus medialis

Divisiones anteriores
Divisiones posteriores

Pars supraclavicularis

Pars infraclavicularis

A. axillaris

N. musculocutaneus
N. medianus
N. axillaris
N. radialis
N. ulnaris
N. cutaneus brachii medialis
N. cutaneus antebrachii medialis

1 N. phrenicus (Plexus cervicalis)
2 N. dorsalis scapulae
3 Rr. musculares
4 N. suprascapularis
5 N. subclavius
6 N. pectoralis lateralis
7 N. subscapularis
8 N. thoracodorsalis
9 N. pectoralis medialis
10 N. thoracicus longus
11 N. intercostalis

Fig. 4.47 Brachial plexus, Plexus brachialis, right. Ventral view.

neurovascular bundle and in front of the M. scalenus anterior is the V. subclavia.

Lesions of the Plexus brachialis are characterised by injury (e.g. strain, bruising or tear) of one or more of the spinal nerve roots, which leads to severe functional deficiencies (➤ Fig. 4.48a). Cause are mostly accidents (typically motorcycle accidents or impacts on the shoulder with hyperextension of the nerve), birth complications or incorrect positioning on the operating table. There are two main types of plexus lesions:

• **Upper plexus paralysis** (type **ERB**, affect C5/C6 for the superior trunk. It causes failures in the proximal arm area (➤ Fig. 4.48b): abduction and lateral rotational weakness of the arm, failure of flexion in the elbow joint and of supination. Thus in the medial rotational position the arm (palms to posterior) the arm hangs flaccidly. In addition, sensory deficits, especially at the shoulder, can ensue.

• **Lower plexus paralysis** (type **KLUMPKE**, affects C8/T1 for the Truncus inferior). It causes failures in the area of the distal arm, especially of the long finger flexors and the hand muscles as well as sensory deficits mainly in the area of the ulnar area of the hand (➤ Fig. 4.46c). Because of the involvement of C8 and T1 and due to damage to preganglionic sym-

pathetic nerve fibres **HORNER's syndrome** can ensue (narrowing of the pupil, drooping upper eyelid, sinking of the eyeball) on the corresponding side.

Occasionally, a **lesion of segment C7** is referred to as a medial plexiform lesion, which is not very useful, because the lesion does not occur in isolation. Rather, segment C7 can be involved in an upper or lower lesion. Since the guide muscle for C7 is the M. triceps brachii, this usually fails. Depending on the extent of dermatome C7, sensation on the dorsal forearm and the middle fingers is affected. In the case of a **complete lesion** all parts of the Plexus brachialis are affected. Therapeutically, an attempt is made to reconnect the torn nerve roots with each other by suturing the fascicles of the nerves to their surrounding connective tissue.

A new procedure in hand surgery is **distal nerve transposition,** where in the case of upper plexiform lesions, e.g. a fascicle from the N. ulnaris is connected to the failed N. musculocutaneous.

In anaesthesia it is common to perform different operations using local anaesthesia whereby, e.g. the 3 fascicles of the Plexus brachialis are targeted via injections with local anaesthetics **(plexus blockade).**

From the **Pars supraclavicularis** of the Plexus brachialis the following 4 nerves as well as individual branches to cervical muscles originate at the level of the trunci (➤ Fig. 4.49):

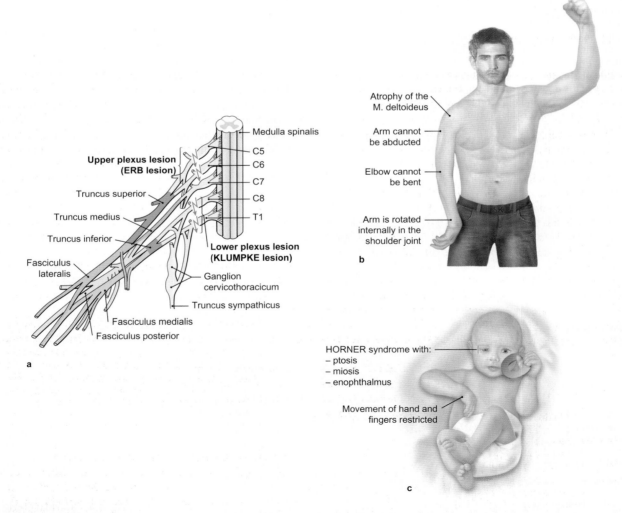

Fig. 4.48 Lesions of the Plexus brachialis. a Lesion forms, right. Front view. **b** Clinical remarks regarding upper plexus lesion (ERB's PALSY). **c** Clinical remarks regarding lower plexus lesion (KLUMPKE's PALSY). a [L126]; b and c [L238]

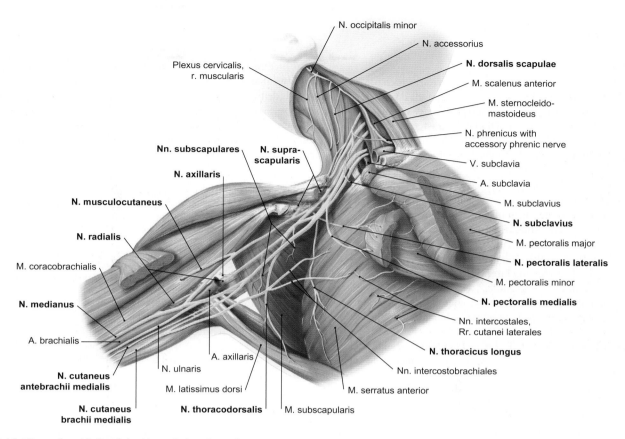

Fig. 4.49 Plexus brachialis, right. Ventral view. [L266]

- **N. dorsalis scapulae** (C3–C5): it penetrates and innervates the M. scalenus medius, then runs to the lower edge of the M. levator scapulae (guide muscle!) along the Margo medialis of the scapula. It innervates the M. levator scapulae and the Mm. rhomboidei.
- **N. thoracicus longus** (C5–C7): further caudal, the nerve penetrates the M. scalenus medius and runs behind the Clavicula and the Trunci to the anterior abdominal wall and runs on the M. serratus anterior, which it innervates.
- **N. suprascapularis** (C4–C6): after originating from the Truncus superior, the nerve runs together with the A. suprascapularis to the Incisura scapulae and under the Lig. transversum scapulae superius into the Fossa supraspinata and around the Spina scapulae under the Lig. transversum scapulae inferius into the Fossa infraspinata (> Fig. 4.72). There it innervates the M. supraspinatus and the M. infraspinatus.
- **N. subclavius** (C5–C6): short branch to the M. subclavius, which occasionally issues a branch to the N. phrenicus (so-called accessory phrenicus, > Fig. 4.49).
- **Muscle branches for the Mm. scaleni and the M. longus colli** (C5–C8).

Clinical remarks

Lesions of the shoulder nerves of the Pars supraclavicularis lead to the following failures:
- **N. dorsalis scapulae:** in the case of functional failure of the Mm. rhomboidei the scapula is shifted somewhat laterally and slightly elevated from the thorax. An isolated lesion is rare due to its protected location.
- **N. thoracicus longus:** if e.g. when carrying heavy loads (backpack palsy) the N. thoracicus longus under the Cla-

vicula becomes compressed or injured due to lacerations to the lateral thoracic wall, then the clinical image of **Scapula alata** ensues due to the failure of the M. serratus anterior (> Fig. 4.50): The scapula is shifted to medial and its medial border is raised from the ribcage. Patients are particularly affected by the fact that arm elevation is no longer possible.
- **N. suprascapularis:** a failure can occur due to compression in the Incisura scapulae or injuries in the lateral cervical region and due to the absence of the main functions of the M. supraspinatus and M. infraspinatus, lead to abduction and external rotation weaknesses.
- An isolated lesion of the **N. subclavius** is very rare and has no clear clinical symptoms.

The Trunci of the Plexus brachialis divide after rendering the supraclavicular branches into an anterior and a posterior part (**Divisiones anteriores and posteriores**). These then settle at the fasci-

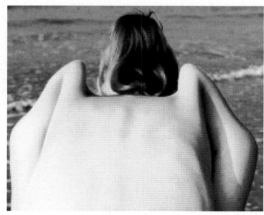

Fig. 4.50 Scapula alata. [O932]

cles of the Pars infraclavicularis of the Plexus brachialis (➤ Fig. 4.47).

Pars infraclavicularis

The Pars infraclavicularis includes the fascicles from which the main nerves of the Plexus brachialis then emerge. From the **3 fascicles** the Divisiones anteriores and posteriores of the 3 Trunci are formed:

- **Fasciculus posterior:** from the Divisiones posteriores of all 3 Trunci (C5–T1)
- **Fasciculus lateralis:** from the Divisiones anteriores of the trunci superior and medius (C5–C7)
- **Fasciculus medialis:** from the Divisio anterior of the Truncus inferior (C8–T1)

In their course the fascicles become attached to the A. axillaris so that, as reflected in their names, the Fasciculus posterior lies to posterior of the artery, the Fasciculus medialis medial and the Fasciculus lateralis lateral to the artery.

The fascicles have the following **lateral branches,** which each serve muscular innervation of the shoulder (➤ Fig. 4.49):

- **N. pectoralis lateralis** (C5–C7): originates from the lateral fascicle and passes through the Trigonum clavipectorale to the M. pectoralis major, which it mainly supplies.
- **N. pectoralis medialis** (C8–T1): runs from the medial fascicle via the M. pectoralis minor to the M. pectoralis major and supplies both muscles.
- **Nn. subscapulares** (C5–C7): usually 2 short branches from the posterior fascicle to the M. subscapularis, and more rarely also to the M. teres major.
- **N. thoracodorsalis** (C6–C8): it runs coming out of the posterior fascicle, with the A. thoracodorsalis to the M. latissimus dorsi, which it innervates together with the M. teres major.

Clinical remarks

Lesions of the shoulder nerves of the Pars infraclavicularis lead to the following failures:

- **Nn. subscapulares:** for example, with a proximal fracture of the humerus, muscle function failure of the eponymous muscles causes significant weakening of medial rotation in the shoulder joint.
- **N. thoracodorsalis:** adduction of the retroverted arm is disrupted. The arms can no longer be crossed behind the back. The rear axillary fold is sunken. Despite the size of the M. latissimus dorsi, the damage is minimal since it and the M. teres major are not particularly important for movement in the shoulder joint.
- **Nn. pectorales:** here, weakness in adduction and anteversion often ensues. The arms can no longer be crossed in front of the body.

Injuries to individual nerves are relatively rare due to their protected position.

The main nerves of the arm emerging distally from the fascicles are:

Fasciculus posterior:
- N. axillaris (C5–C6)
- N. radialis (C5–T1)

Fasciculus lateralis:
- N. musculocutaneus (C5–C7)
- N. medianus, radix lateralis (C6–C7)

Fasciculus medialis:
- N. medianus, Radix medialis (C8–T1)
- N. ulnaris (C8–T1)
- N. cutaneus brachii medialis (C8–T1)
- N. cutaneus antebrachii medialis (C8–T1)

4.6.3 N. axillaris

The N. axillaris (C5–C6) originates from the posterior fascicle and runs together with the A. circumflexa humeri posterior through the **lateral axillary space** (➤ Fig. 4.72). There it branches under the M. deltoideus, which it supplies together with the M. teres minor (➤ Fig. 4.51). A sensory branch, the N. cutaneus brachii lateralis superior, supplies the skin of the shoulder above the M. deltoideus. The skin nerve runs through the fascia at the posterior margin of the M. deltoideus.

NOTE

Autonomic region of the N. axillaris: skin above the M. deltoideus

---

Clinical remarks

A **lesion of the N. axillaris,** e.g. due to shoulder luxation or proximal fractures of the Humerus, is characterised by abduction weakness in the shoulder joint, a sunken shoulder region due to atrophy of the M. deltoideus (➤ Fig. 4.52) and a sensory deficiency above the M. deltoideus.

4.6.4 N. radialis

The N. radialis (C5–T1) continues the course of the Fasciculus posterior (➤ Fig. 4.53). It courses ventrally of the attachment tendon of the M. latissimus dorsi and runs with the A. profunda brachii through the **triceps groove** (between the Caput longum and Caput laterale of the M. triceps brachii). In the radial groove it then attaches to the humerus and in the radial tunnel between the M. brachialis and M. brachioradialis and runs laterally into the elbow. On its way at the upper arm from proximal to distal, it gives off the following branches:

- **N. cutaneus brachii posterior:** outlet in the area of the triceps groove to supply the skin of the posterior upper arm.
- **N. cutaneus brachii lateralis inferior:** outlet *before* attaching to the humerus in the Sulcus nervi radialis.

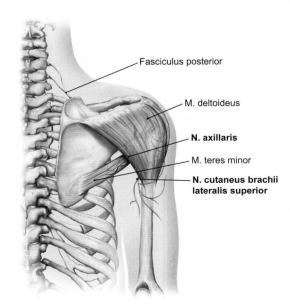

Fig. 4.51 N. axillaris, right. Dorsal view.

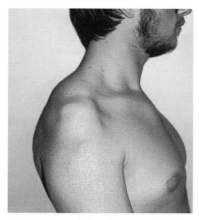

Fig. 4.52 Lesion of the N. axillaris, right. Lateral view.

- **Muscle branches to the M. triceps brachii:** outlet *before* the Sulcus nervi radialis.
- **N. cutaneus antebrachii posterior:** outlet *in the* Sulcus nervi radialis; runs between the attachment of the M. deltoideus and M. triceps brachii through the fascia and supplies the extensor side of the forearm.
- **Muscle branches for the radial group** of the forearm (M. brachioradialis, Mm. extensores carpi radialis longus and brevis).

The N. radialis enters laterally through the **radial tunnel** (between the M. brachioradialis and M. brachialis) into the elbow and divides into its 2 terminal branches:
- R. superficialis
- R. profundus

R. superficialis

The purely sensory branch follows the course of the N. radialis further. Together with the A. radialis, it runs along the M. brachioradialis (guide muscle!). Then it runs through the Tabatière ('Fovea radialis', between the tendons of the Mm. extensor pollicis longus and brevis) onto the dorsal side of the wrist, the radial side of which it supplies. Here, it dispatches the R. communicans ulnaris to the N. ulnaris. The R. superficialis divides into 5 Nn. **digitales**, out of which 2 each provide sensory supply to the radial and ulnar dorsal side of the thumb and of the forefinger and one supplies the radial dorsal side of the middle finger (**radial 2½ fingers on the dorsal side**); however, this supply area only covers the skin over the proximal and intermediate phalanges; the dorsal side of the distal phalanges is innervated by the terminal branches of the N. medianus from ventral outwards.

NOTE

Autonomic region of the N. radialis: skin on the dorsal side between thumb and index finger (first interdigital space).

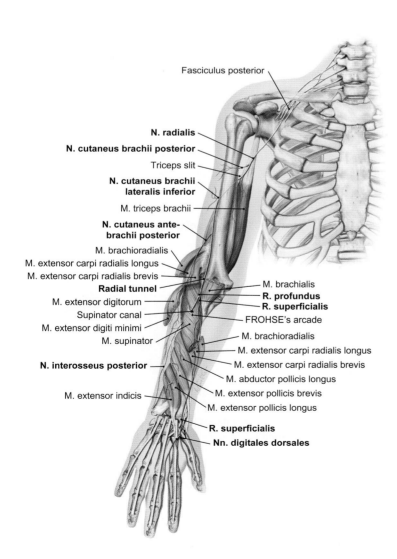

Fasciculus posterior

N. radialis
N. cutaneus brachii posterior
Triceps slit
N. cutaneus brachii lateralis inferior
M. triceps brachii
N. cutaneus antebrachii posterior
M. brachioradialis
M. extensor carpi radialis longus
M. extensor carpi radialis brevis
Radial tunnel
M. extensor digitorum
Supinator canal
M. extensor digiti minimi
M. supinator
N. interosseus posterior
M. extensor indicis

M. brachialis
R. profundus
R. superficialis
FROHSE's arcade
M. brachioradialis
M. extensor carpi radialis longus
M. extensor carpi radialis brevis
M. abductor pollicis longus
M. extensor pollicis brevis
M. extensor pollicis longus
R. superficialis
Nn. digitales dorsales

Fig. 4.53 Course and innervation area of the N. radialis, right. Anterior view.

R. profundus

The R. profundus penetrates the M. supinator somewhat distal of the elbow (**supinator canal**). At its entrance, the canal is covered by a crescent-shaped reinforcement of muscle fascia (**FROHSE's arcade**). Then the R. profundus loops around the radius onto the dorsal side of the forearm and runs between the deep and superficial layers of the extensor muscles distally. On its way it supplies all the extensor muscles of the forearm and tapers out into the sensory **N. interosseus antebrachii posterior**, which is involved in the innervation of the wrist joint.

Clinical remarks

The N. radialis emits branches over the entire length of the arm. In the case of injuries to the nerve, symptoms thus depend on the location of the injury (➤ Fig. 4.54).

There are 3 lesion locations, which have their own clinical characteristics:

- **Proximal lesion** (1 in ➤ Fig. 4.54): the damage in the area of the axilla can be caused by crutches, upon which the weight of the body in the axillary cavity is supported. A more common cause is incorrect positioning during an operation. It leads to paralysis of all of the muscles supplied by the N. radialis. The following movements are not or only weakly possible:
  - Extension in the elbow joint (failure of the M. triceps brachii)
  - Supination of the extended arm (failure of the M. supinator and of the M. brachioradialis)
  - Extension in the wrist and Base/Middle joints (failure of all dorsal forearm muscles and of the radial group). It causes an image of **drop wrist** (➤ Fig. 4.55): The hand cannot be raised against gravity.
  - A strong closed fist is not possible because, due to the active insufficiency of the finger flexors, dorsal extension in the wrist joints is necessary.
  - Sensory deficiencies are also possible on the back of the upper arm and forearm, in the first interdigital space and at the dorsal 2½ fingers.
- **Medial lesion** (2a and 2b in ➤ Fig. 4.54): a cause of damage between axilla and forearm can be a pressure sore due to lying on one's side ('park bench palsy'), but also fractures of the upper arm or a compression while passing through the supinator.
  - If the nerve in the Sulcus nervi radialis is damaged (most commonly, 2a in ➤ Fig. 4.54), there is no loss of extension in the elbow joint or sensory deficits on the dorsal side of the upper arm because the corresponding branches lead off beforehand. The rest of the clinical image corresponds to that of a proximal lesion.
  - In the case of damage in the area of FROHSE's arcade (2b in ➤ Fig. 4.54) only the R. profundus is affected. Sensory loss of the hand does not appear (R. superficialis intact, the supply of the wrist joint through the R. profundus is of little relevance), and drop hand is also not detectable because the branches to the Mm. extensor carpi radialis muscles lead off before the M. supinator and these muscles suffice to prevent a drop of the hand against gravity. A loss of extension in the fingers is noticeably present; however, the strength in fist closure is also lessened.
- **Distal lesion** (3 in ➤ Fig. 4.54): with a lesion of the forearm or wrist, e.g. due to a laceration or a distal radial fracture, only the R. superficialis is affected. There are no motor deficits and, therefore, no drop hand. The sensory deficit extends to the skin in the first interdigital space and over the dorsal 2½ fingers.

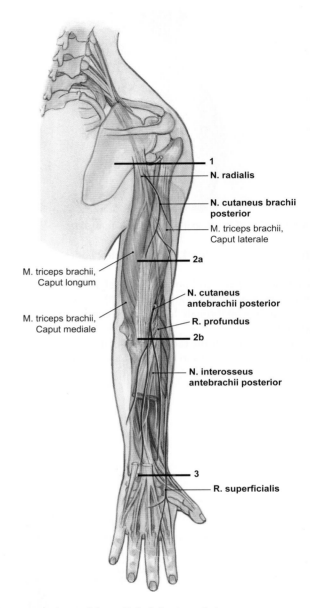

Fig. 4.54 Lesions of the radial, right. Dorsal view.

Labels:
1
N. radialis
N. cutaneus brachii posterior
M. triceps brachii, Caput laterale
2a
M. triceps brachii, Caput longum
N. cutaneus antebrachii posterior
R. profundus
2b
M. triceps brachii, Caput mediale
N. interosseus antebrachii posterior
3
R. superficialis

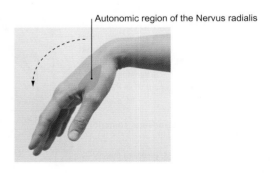

Autonomic region of the Nervus radialis

Fig. 4.55 Clinical aspects of proximal lesion of the N. radialis ('wrist drop').

4.6.5 N. musculocutaneus

The N. musculocutaneus (C5–C7) branches off from the lateral fascicle. It usually penetrates the M. coracobrachialis and runs distally between the M. brachialis and the M. biceps brachii (➤ Fig. 4.56).

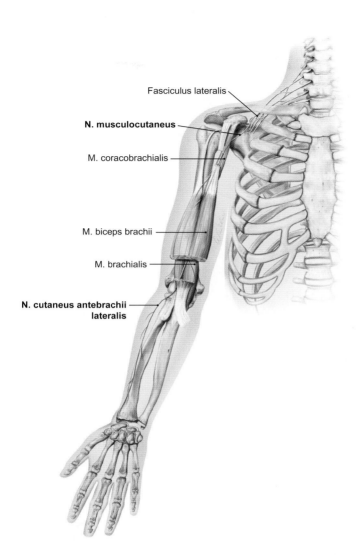

Fasciculus lateralis

N. musculocutaneus

M. coracobrachialis

M. biceps brachii

M. brachialis

N. cutaneus antebrachii lateralis

Fig. 4.56 Course and innervation area of the N. musculocutaneous, right. Ventral view.

There it penetrates the fascia laterally somewhat above the elbow with its sensory terminal branch, the **N. cutaneus antebrachii lateralis**, and supplies the skin at the lateral forearm up to the wrist joints. The N. musculocutaneus issues (in this order) motor branches to supply the **M. coracobrachialis, M. biceps brachii** and **M. brachialis.** Therefore, it supplies all the ventral upper arm muscles.

Clinical remarks

The N. musculocutaneus is endangered in shoulder luxation. As a result of the nerve injury, supination of the flexed elbow and flexion in the elbow joint are extremely restricted. Weak flexion is still possible because the superficial flexors of the forearm (innervated by the N. medianus) and the radial muscle group (innervated by the N. radialis) also carry out this function. There can be slight sensory deficit on the forearm because the innervation areas of the 3 cutaneous nerves overlap here.

4.6.6 N. medianus

The N. medianus (C6–T1) is formed by an amalgamation of the Radix lateralis of the lateral fascicle and the Radix medialis of the

medial fascicle on the ventral side of the A. axillaris (➤ Fig. 4.57). This formation is referred to as the median fork. The amalgamated nerve branch courses distally in the Sulcus bicipitalis medialis on the Septum intermusculare brachii mediale and then runs medially of the A. brachialis on the M. brachialis into the elbow. There it runs between the two **heads of the M. pronator teres** and further between the Mm. flexores digitorum superficialis and profundus up to the wrist joints, where it runs via the **carpal tunnel** (Canalis carpi, bottom: Ossa carpi, roof: Mm. flexores digitorum superficialis and profundus) and further under the palmar aponeurosis to the fingers (➤ Fig. 4.73).

Clinical remarks

The very common compression of the N. medianus in its course through the Canalis carpi (➤ Fig. 4.73) is called **carpal tunnel syndrome.** After failure of conventional treatment (protection, rest), treatment consists of a division of the Retinaculum musculorum flexorum.

NOTE

Autonomic region of the N. medianus: distal phalanges of index and middle fingers.

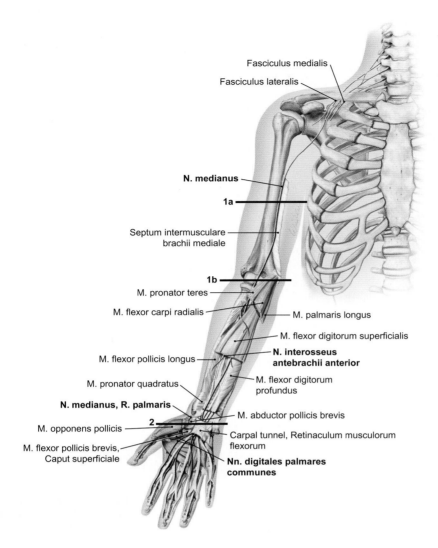

Fasciculus medialis
Fasciculus lateralis

N. medianus

1a

Septum intermusculare
brachii mediale

1b

M. pronator teres
M. flexor carpi radialis
M. palmaris longus
M. flexor digitorum superficialis
M. flexor pollicis longus
N. interosseus
antebrachii anterior
M. pronator quadratus
M. flexor digitorum
profundus
N. medianus, R. palmaris
M. abductor pollicis brevis
M. opponens pollicis
2
M. flexor pollicis brevis,
Caput superficiale
Carpal tunnel, Retinaculum musculorum
flexorum
Nn. digitales palmares
communes

Fig. 4.57 Course and innervation areas of the N. medianus, right. Ventral view.

The N. medianus first gives off branches at the forearm, thus it has no effect at the upper arm. These branches are:
- **Rr. musculares** run to nearly all ventral forearm muscles (except the M. flexor carpi ulnaris and ulnar muscle bellies of the M. flexor digitorum profundus).
- **N. interosseus antebrachii anterior:** it courses with the A. interossea anterior on the Membrana interossea to the M. pronator quadratus. It provides motor innervation to all deep flexor muscles of the forearm (apart from the two ulnar muscle bellies of the M. flexor digitorum profundus) and from palmar it provides sensory innervation to the wrist joints.
- **R. palmaris:** this cutaneous branch supplies the eminence of the thumb and the radial side of the palm.
- **Nn. digitales palmares communes:** they emerge after the N. medianus has passed through the carpal tunnel and divide again into the sensory **Nn. digitales palmares proprii**. In each case 2 of these terminal branches supply the palmar surface of the thumb, index and middle fingers, and a 7th branch stretches to the radial side of the ring finger. These branches additionally innervate the distal sections of the dorsal palms. Therefore, the branches of the N. medianus provide sensory innervation to the **palmar parts of the 3½ radial fingers** and their end sections on the dorsal side. Its motor innervation areas are:
  - most thenar muscles (apart from the M. adductor pollicis and Caput profundum of the M. flexor pollicis brevis)
  - the Mm. lumbricales I and II

- **Distal lesion:** this damage in the area of the wrist joints (2 in ➤ Fig. 4.57) is usually the result of **carpal tunnel syndrome,** e.g. due to swelling of the tendon sheaths when overburdened, rheumatic diseases or during pregnancy or due to lacerations (cutting the 'arteries'). The symptoms are similar to those of a proximal lesion; however, no ape hand occurs, because the muscular branches for the innervation of the long flexors exit before the carpal tunnel!

4.6.7 N. ulnaris

Der N. ulnaris (C8–T1) is the thickest branch of the medial fascicle. It runs in the Sulcus bicipitalis medialis to the forearm (➤ Fig. 4.59). In contrast to the N. medianus, it penetrates the Septum intermusculare mediale in the middle of the upper arm and runs dorsally onto the extensor side, where it attaches to the Epicondylus medialis of the humerus in the **Sulcus nervi ulnaris (cubital tunnel).** On the forearm it runs back on the flexion side in order to then run together with the A. ulnaris along the M. flexor carpi ulnaris (guide muscle!) to the wrist joints and further through the **GUYON's canal** (base: Retinaculum musculorum flexorum, roof: separation from the flexor, sometimes referred to as the 'lig. carpi palmare') to the palm.

> **NOTE**
>
> In jolting of the elbow, the N. ulnaris can become compressed in the Sulcus nervi ulnaris. This results in pain and pins and needles in the sensory innervation area of the nerve **(funny bone).**
> **GUYON's canal** is bordered on both sides by parts of the Retinaculum flexorum and therefore lies superficially of the carpal tunnel on the ulnar side of the wrist (➤ Fig. 4.73). The GUYON's canal is traversed by the A., V. and N. ulnaris. The nerve, in particular, can be damaged here by compression.

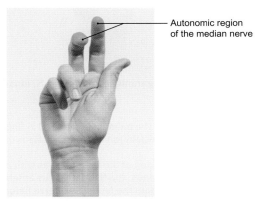

Autonomic region of the median nerve

Fig. 4.58 Clinical remarks regarding proximal lesion of the N. medianus ('ape hand').

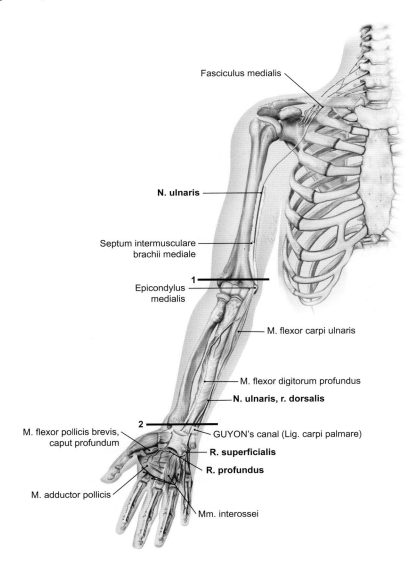

Fasciculus medialis

N. ulnaris

Septum intermusculare brachii mediale

1

Epicondylus medialis

M. flexor carpi ulnaris

M. flexor digitorum profundus

N. ulnaris, r. dorsalis

2

M. flexor pollicis brevis, caput profundum

GUYON's canal (Lig. carpi palmare)

R. superficialis

R. profundus

M. adductor pollicis

Mm. interossei

Fig. 4.59 Course and innervation areas of the N. ulnaris, right. Ventral view.

Like the N. medianus, the N. ulnaris does not give off any branches on the upper arm. On the forearm 4 branches diverge:
- **R. articularis cubiti:** to the elbow joint.
- **Rr. musculares** for the M. flexor carpi ulnaris and the two ulnar bellies of the M. flexor digitorum profundus.
- **R. dorsalis:** it originates half way along the forearm, runs to the dorsal side and divides into the **Nn. digitales dorsales,** which supply the back of hand from the ulnar side as well as the **dorsal side of the 2½ ulnar finger**.
- **R. palmaris:** this small branch supplies the skin above the wrist and the hypothenar eminence.

In GUYON's canal (➤ Fig. 4.73) the N. ulnaris divides into its two terminal branches:
- **R. profundus**
- **R. superficialis**

R. profundus

This runs under the M. flexor digiti minimi brevis of the palmar arch to the **M. adductor pollicis** and to the **M. flexor pollicis brevis**. On its way, it supplies the short muscles of the hand that are not innervated by the N. medianus:
- All hypothenar muscles
- All Mm. interossei palmares and dorsales
- Mm. lumbricales III and IV
- M. adductor pollicis
- Caput profundum of the M. flexor pollicis brevis

R. superficialis

The predominantly sensory branch (supplies only the M. palmaris brevis) runs over the M. flexor digiti minimi brevis distally and branches further into 2 Nn. **digitales palmares communes,** which each divide into the **Nn. digitales palmares proprii**.
In this way the ulnar 1½ fingers are supplied from the palmar side as well as their distal phalanges dorsally.

> **NOTE**
> Autonomic region of the N. ulnaris: distal phalanx of the little finger

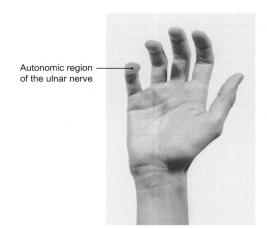
Autonomic region of the ulnar nerve

Fig. 4.60 Clinical remarks regarding lesions of the N. ulnaris ('claw hand').

- Sensory deficiences on the palmar side in the 1½ fingers on the ulnar side and especially on the distal phalanx of the little finger.

In the case of proximal lesion of the N. ulnaris, as with a proximal lesion of the N. medianus, the N. interosseus antebrachii anterior can be diverted onto the respective nerve before entering into the M. pronator quadratus in order to remedy the loss of function (distal nerve transposition).

4.6.8 N. cutanei brachii and antebrachii medialis

Both nerves are purely sensory and originate from the medial fascicle (C8–T1). They run in the Sulcus bicipitalis medialis. Fibres of the thoracic wall out of T2 and T3 are attached to the very thin and short **N. cutaneus brachii medialis** via the Nn. intercostobrachiales and supply the skin of the axillary cavity and the medial upper arm. The **N. cutaneus antebrachii medialis** penetrates with the V. basilica into the upper arm fascia and divides into an R. anterior and an R. posterior. It supplies the skin of the ulnar forearm up to the wrist.

4.7 Arteries of the upper extremity

> ┌─ **Skills** ──────────────
> After working through this chapter, you should be able to:
> - identify all arteries of the upper extremity on a specimen
> - explain the vessel anastomoses of the shoulder and the upper arm

The **A. subclavia** is the main vessel that supplies the arm (➤ Fig. 4.61). The A. axillaris continues the course of the A. subclavia from rib I and merges at the lower edge of the M. pectoralis major into the artery of the upper arm, the A. brachialis. This runs within the Sulcus bicipitalis medialis and is divided within the elbow into the A. radialis and the A. ulnaris. These two arteries then run on both the radial and the ulnar side of the ventral forearm to the hand and join together in the palmar hand surface via the deep and superficial palmar arterial arch (➤ Fig. 4.61).

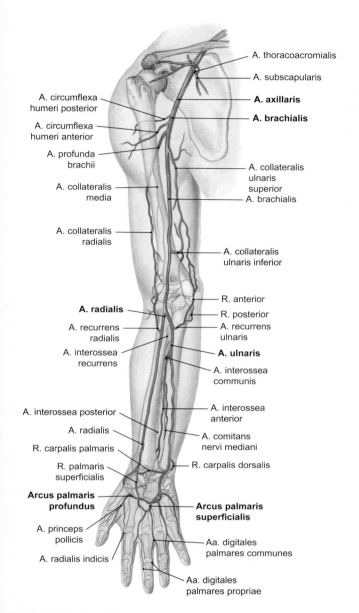

A. circumflexa humeri posterior

A. circumflexa humeri anterior

A. profunda brachii

A. collateralis media

A. collateralis radialis

A. radialis

A. recurrens radialis

A. interossea recurrens

A. interossea posterior

A. radialis

R. carpalis palmaris

R. palmaris superficialis

Arcus palmaris profundus

A. princeps pollicis

A. radialis indicis

A. thoracoacromialis

A. subscapularis

A. axillaris

A. brachialis

A. collateralis ulnaris superior

A. brachialis

A. collateralis ulnaris inferior

R. anterior

R. posterior

A. recurrens ulnaris

A. ulnaris

A. interossea communis

A. interossea anterior

A. comitans nervi mediani

R. carpalis dorsalis

Arcus palmaris superficialis

Aa. digitales palmares communes

Aa. digitales palmares propriae

Fig. 4.61 Arteries of the arm

4.7.1 A. subclavia

The A. subclavia originates on the right-hand side from the Truncus brachiocephalicus (1st branch of the aortic arch); on the left side, it is a direct outflow (3rd branch) of the aorta (➤ Fig. 4.62). On its way through the scalene hiatus between the Mm. scaleni anterior and medius it traverses the pleural cupula and then merges at rib I into the A. axillaris. In addition to supplying the arm, with its branches the A. subclavia supplies the neck region and the organs located there, parts of the ventral thoracic wall and parts of the brain. This vessel is attached caudally in the scalene hiatus to the Plexus brachialis, but runs dorsally of the V. subclavia. The A. subclavia usually has 4 branches:

- **A. vertebralis:** it exits medially of the M. scalenus anterior in a cranial direction (Pars prevertebralis), moves into the Foramen transversarium of the VI cervical vertebra, usually passes through the other Foramina intertransversaria upwards (Pars transversaria), and then lies on the posterior arch of atlas (Pars atlantica). It then penetrates the Membrana atlantooccipitalis

and the Dura mater and passes through the Foramen magnum into the cranial cavity (Pars intracranialis), where, after merging with the reciprocal artery to the A. basilaris, it is involved in supplying the brain stem, cerebellum and posterior parts (Lobus occipitales and temporalis) of the cerebrum.

- **A. thoracica interna:** it emerges caudally and runs about 1 cm laterally of the edge of the sternum between the Fascia endothoracica and caudally to the ribs. At the level of the VI rib it splits into its two terminal branches (A. musculophrenica and A. epigastrica superior). Its branches are:
  - **Rr. tracheales and bronchiales,** Rr. thymici and Rr. mediastinales: fine branches to the respective organs and the Mediastinum
  - **A. pericardiacophrenica:** runs with the N. phrenicus between the pericardium and Pleura mediastinalis to the diaphragm, which it supplies along with the pericardium
  - **Rr. sternales** to the sternum
  - **Rr. perforantes** to the chest muscles, they form the **Rr. mammarii mediales** to the chest
  - **Rr. intercostales anteriores** (1–6), which anastomose with the Aa. intercostales posteriores and supply ICS 1–6
  - **A. musculophrenica:** runs along the costal arch to the diaphragm and gives off the Rr. intercostales anteriores 7–10.
  - **A. epigastrica superior:** it continues the course, passes through the Trigonum sternocostale of the diaphragm and anatomises with the A. epigastrica inferior
  - **Tip:** take care when lifting the A. thoracica interna from the ribs because on its way to the diaphragm it easily ruptures!
- **Truncus thyrocervicalis:** this usually strong vessel trunk branches off cranially, runs medially in front of the M. scalenus anterior and divides into 4 branches:
  - **A. thyroidea inferior:** this is the strongest branch of the Truncus thyrocervicalis, which runs coiled medially with the Rr. glandulares to the caudal sections of the thyroid gland. On its way, it gives off the Rr. pharyngeales to the Hypopharynx, Rr. oesophageales to the Pars cervicalis of the Oesophagus and Rr. tracheales to the trachea. A stronger branch, the **A. laryngea inferior,** supplies the larynx from a caudal direction.
  - **A. cervicalis ascendens:** it runs as a thin vessel on the M. scalenus anterior cranially to supply the muscles of the neck. Gives off the Rr. spinales to the spinal cord.
  - **A. transversa colli (A. transversa cervicis):** it runs laterally and divides into two branches:
    – R. profundus: traverses the fascia of the Plexus brachialis and becomes attached (now called the **A. dorsalis scapulae**) to the Margo medialis of the scapula, where it runs caudally to supply the superficial back muscles. Anastomises on the dorsal side of the scapula with the A. suprascapularis and the A. circumflexa scapulae.
    – R. superficialis: traverses the Plexus brachialis and runs to the lower side of the M. trapezius.
  - **A. suprascapularis:** this usually rather strong vessel runs over the Plexus brachialis and attaches to the N. suprascapularis. It runs over the Lig. transversum scapulae superius and under the Lig. transversum scapulae into the Fossa supraspinata to supply the muscles located there (➤ Fig. 4.64). An R. acromialis runs to the acromion. The A. suprascapularis usually anastomoses with the A. circumflexa scapulae and often via fine branches with the A. dorsalis scapulae (shoulder blade anastomoses).
- **Truncus costocervicalis:** this short branch runs caudally and divides behind the M. scalenus anterior into 2 terminal branches:

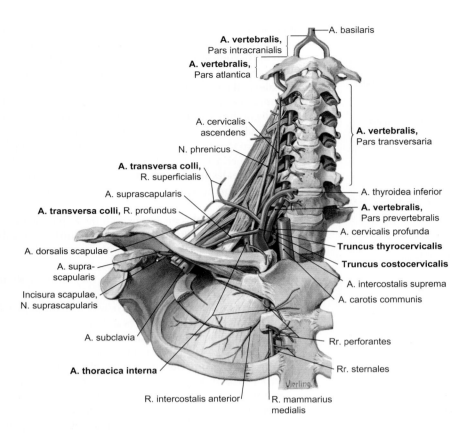

Fig. 4.62 Branches of the A. subclavia. [S010-2-16]

- **A. intercostalis suprema:** to the 1st and 2nd ICS
- **A. cervicalis profunda:** runs dorsally into the depths to the prevertebral neck muscles
- **Tip:** the Truncus costocervicalis can be best demonstrated in dissection from caudal via the pleural cupola.

NOTE

The **A. subclavia,** with its outlets, in particular the Truncus thyrocervicalis is **very variable.** Therefore, the A. transversa cervicis can be missing and instead the R. superficialis emerges directly (then called the A. cervicalis superficialis). The R. profundus is then, as the A. dorsalis scapulae, also a direct branch of the Truncus or originates from the A. subclavia. The A. thyroidea inferior is also often a direct branch of the A. subclavia.

4.7.2 A. axillaris

The A. axillaris starts at the lateral margin of the thorax at the level of the I rib and traverses the axillary cavity between the M. pectoralis major and the end tendon of the M. latissimus dorsi (➤ Fig. 4.63). On the lower edge of the M. pectoralis major it merges into the A. brachialis. The outlets of the A. axillaris supply the area of the shoulder, its muscles and parts of the anterior abdominal wall. The following 6 branches can be distinguished:

- **A. thoracica superior:** this inconsistently thin vessel stretches to the Mm. pectorales major and minor and also supplies them as parts of the M. serratus anterior.

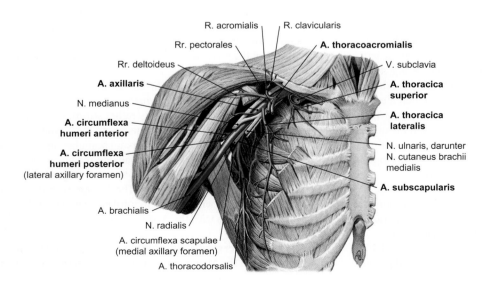

Fig. 4.63 Branches of the A. axillaris. [S010-2-16]

- **A. thoracoacromialis:** the short, strong vessel runs in a ventral-cranial direction and divides within the Trigonum clavipectorale into the following branches:
  - R. clavicularis to the Clavicula
  - R. acromialis laterally to the acromion
  - R. deltoideus to the M. deltoideus
  - Rr. pectorales to the Mm. pectorales
- **A. thoracica lateralis:** it runs on the M. serratus anterior and lateral to the M. pectoralis minor and caudally and gives off the **Rr. mammarii laterales** to supply the mammary glands.
- **A subscapularis:** the short, strong vessel runs along the Margo lateralis of the scapula and is divided into 2 terminal branches:
  - The **A. circumflexa scapulae** passes through the **medial axillary space** onto the back of the shoulder blade into the Fossa infraspinata and anastomoses there with branches of the A. suprascapularis and often via thin branches with the A. dorsalis scapulae (➤ Fig. 4.64).
  - The **A. thoracodorsalis** continues the course of the A. subscapularis, accompanies the N. thoracodorsalis and runs anteriorly on the M. serratus anterior to the M. latissimus dorsi. Both muscles are supplied by this artery.
- **A. circumflexa humeri anterior:** it runs as a thin vessel forwards around the proximal humeral shaft to the humeral head, which it supplies.
- **A circumflexa humeri posterior:** this artery is once again stronger, passes through the **lateral axillary space** (➤ Fig. 4.72) behind the humeral shaft and divides underneath the M. deltoideus, which it also supplies. It anastomoses with the A. circumflexa humeri anterior.

The branches of the A. axillaris are also relatively variable. The variations here generally affect the A. thoracoacromialis and the A. subscapularis, from which e.g. the Aa. circumflexae humeri anterior and posterior can branch off.

On the dorsal side of the scapula, 2 branches of the A. subclavia anastomose with 1 branch of the A. axillaris (➤ Fig. 4.64). The **A. suprascapularis** (branch of Truncus thyrocervicalis) runs above the Lig. scapulare transversum superius into the Fossa suprascapularis and receives inflows from the **A. dorsalis scapulae** that runs along the Margo medialis of the scapula. (branch of the A. transversa cervicis from the Truncus thyrocervicalis; * in ➤ Fig. 4.64). Both vessels then anastomose with the **A. circumflexa scapulae** (branch of the A. subscapularis) (** in ➤ Fig. 4.64), which runs through the medial axillary space stretching onto the dorsal side of

the Scapula. The R. acromialis of the A. thoracoacromialis can also be involved in the formation of these bypass circulation (*** in ➤ Fig. 4.64).

4.7.3 A. brachialis

The A. brachialis follows the course of the A. axillaris (➤ Fig. 4.65). It runs on the inner side of the arm distally (Sulcus bicipitalis medialis) in the neurovascular pathway of the upper arm between the flexors and extensors. Here it is accompanied by the N. medianus and two Vv. brachiales. The A. brachialis then rotates onto the M. brachialis ventrally and runs radially of the N. medianus under the aponeurosis of the M. biceps brachii into the depth of the elbow, where it branches into the A. radialis and the A. ulnaris. The A. brachialis supplies the humeral shaft and the distal epiphysis, the muscles of the upper arm, and the elbow joint. It gives off 3 large branches:

- **A. profunda brachii:** it usually exits a few centimetres after the A. circumflexa humeri posterior and rotates dorsally. Between the lateral and the medial head of the M. triceps brachii it attaches to the N. radialis and accompanies it within the Sulcus nervi radialis of the humerus. Its branches are:
  - **A. collateralis media:** it penetrates the M. triceps brachii and divides dorsally within a vascular network on the elbow joint (Rete articulare cubiti).
  - **A collateralis radialis:** it continues the course of the A. profunda brachii on the lateral side of the upper arm and participates in the Rete articulare cubiti.
- **A. collateralis ulnaris superior:** this consists of one or more arteries along the N. ulnaris to the Rete articulare cubiti.
- **A. collateralis ulnaris inferior:** it originates far distally on the upper arm and stretches to the Rete articulare cubiti.

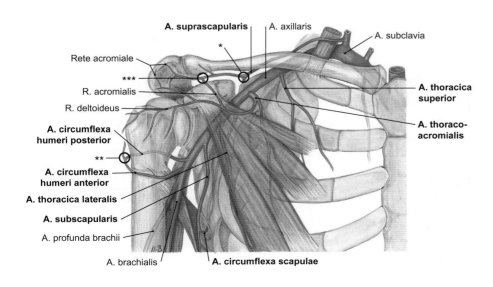

Fig. 4.64 Anastomoses between A. subclavia and A. axillaris, right. Ventral view; * anastomosis between A. suprascapularis and A. dorsalis scapulae, ** further anastomosis with the A. circumflexa scapulae, *** R. acromialis of the A. thoracoacromialis.

Labels: A. suprascapularis · A. axillaris · A. subclavia · Rete acromiale · R. acromialis · R. deltoideus · A. circumflexa humeri posterior · A. circumflexa humeri anterior · A. thoracica lateralis · A. subscapularis · A. profunda brachii · A. brachialis · A. circumflexa scapulae · A. thoracica superior · A. thoraco-acromialis

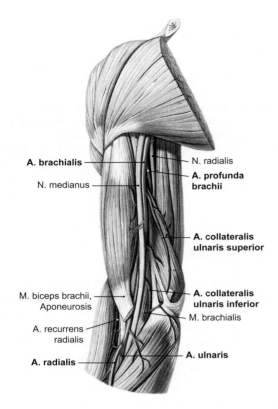

Fig. 4.65 Branches of the A. brachialis. [S010-2-16]

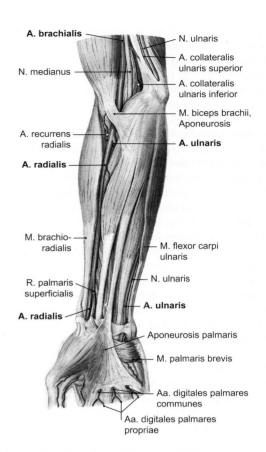

Fig. 4.66 Branches of the A. radialis. [S010-2-16]

4.7.4 A. radialis

In the elbow the A. brachialis forks into the A. ulnaris and the A. radialis (➤ Fig. 4.66, ➤ Fig. 4.67, ➤ Fig. 4.68). The A. radialis lies in the elbow radially to the M. pronator teres and then runs together with the R. superficialis of the N. radialis distally along the M. brachioradialis. The pulse of the artery can be felt at the distal end of the radius by using the bone as a bearing. Here, the A. radialis rotates dorsally and moves into the 'tabatière' on the radial side of the carpus, to then pass through the M. interosseus dorsalis I into the palm to form the deep palmar arch (Arcus palmaris profundus).

NOTE

The **tabatière** (French: snuff box, also referred to as the 'Fovea radialis') is a depression in the area of the metacarpal bones that is especially visible in an abducted thumb and is formed by the end tendons of the M. extensor pollicis brevis on one side, and on the other by the M. extensor pollicis longus. The Os scaphoideum forms the floor. In addition to the A. and V. radialis the R. superficialis of the N. radialis also traverse this area proximally.

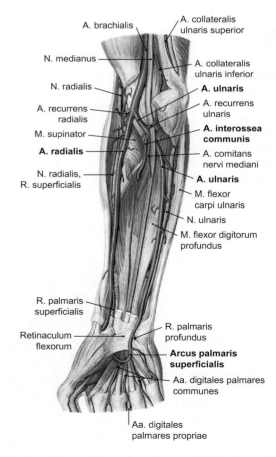

Fig. 4.67 A. radialis and A ulnaris with superficial palmar arch. [S010-2-16]

The A. radialis shares the blood supply of the entire forearm and the hand with the A. ulnaris. It usually gives of 7 branches:

- **A. recurrens radialis:** it is the only branch at the proximal forearm, runs on the radial side beneath the M. brachioradialis to the Rete articulare cubiti and supplies the surrounding muscles.
- **R. carpalis palmaris:** it runs into the carpal channel and supplies it.
- **R. palmaris superficialis:** together with the A. ulnaris it forms the superficial palmar arterial arch under the palmar aponeurosis (Arcus palmaris superficialis).
- **R. carpalis dorsalis:** this branch essentially feeds the Rete carpale dorsale in the area of the Retinaculum musculorum extensorum. Originating from the Rete carpale dorsale are the **Aa. metacarpales dorsales**, which each divide into 2 **Aa. digitales dorsales** to supply the posterior side of the fingers.
- **A. princeps pollicis:** it originates as the A. radialis passes through the M. interosseus dorsalis I and supplies the palmar surface of the thumb.
- **A. radialis indicis:** it runs along the radial side of the index finger.
- **Arcus palmaris profundus** ➤ Fig. 4.68): below the M. adductor pollicis it overlies the bases of the 2nd 4th metacarpal bones and connects to the R. palmaris profundus of the A. ulnaris. The Arcus palmaris profundus gives off 3 **Aa. metacarpales palmares** to supply the Mm. interossei, which connect distally with the digital arteries.

--- Clinical remarks ---

Due to their superficial position and the many bony abutments, the distal sections of the **A. radialis are very vulnerable to injury; h**owever, an **arterial puncture** here (e.g. for blood gas analysis) is also easily possible. Due to its good accessibility, the A. radialis is increasingly also the access route of choice for angiographic examination of the coronary arteries ('coronary catheter').

4.7.5 A. ulnaris

After exiting from the A. brachialis, the A. ulnaris runs under the N. medianus and the M. pronator teres to the ulnar side of the forearm (➤ Fig. 4.67). Here it attaches to the N. ulnaris and runs along the M. flexor carpi ulnaris to the hand. There it runs between the Os pisiforme and Hamulus ossis hamati into the GUYON's canal and then turns off into the palm to form the superficial palmar arch (Arcus palmaris superficialis). It has 5 branches:

- **A. recurrens ulnaris:** it runs proximally under the M. pronator teres to the N. ulnaris and the Rete articulare cubiti.
- **A. interossea communis:** as the most powerful branch of the A. ulnaris, it medially runs a short section distally on the M. flexor digitorum profundus until it divides into the following branches:
  - **A. interossea anterior:** it runs on the Membrana interossea antebrachi and penetrates far distally to discharge into the Rete carpale dorsale.
  - **A. comitans nervi mediani:** this usually thin vessel accompanies the N. medianus (can also be strongly formed as an embryonic relic and connect to the palmar arches).
  - **A. interossea posterior:** it runs through a proximal gap in the Membrana interossea antebrachii and runs on the dorsal side of the membrane together with the R. profundus nervi radialis to the Rete carpale dorsale. Under the M. anconeus, the **A. interossea recurrens** reaches the Rete articulare cubiti.
- **R. carpalis dorsalis:** this branch runs to the dorsal side of the wrist and discharges into the Rete carpale dorsale; however, it is much weaker than the corresponding radial vessel.
- **R. palmaris profundus:** it branches off in the GUYON's canal and penetrates the hypothenar muscles to run to the Arcus palmaris profundus.
- **Arcus palmaris superficialis:** it lies under the palmar aponeurosis on the tendons of the long finger flexor, is fed mainly from the A. ulnaris and anastomoses with the R. palmaris superficialis of the A. radialis. Originating from the superficial palmar arch are the **Aa. digitales palmares communes**, which branch into 2 **Aa. digitales palmares propriae** along the finger edges.

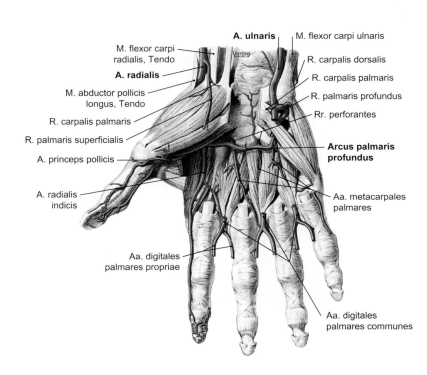

M. flexor carpi radialis, Tendo
A. radialis
M. abductor pollicis longus, Tendo
R. carpalis palmaris
R. palmaris superficialis
A. princeps pollicis
A. radialis indicis
Aa. digitales palmares propriae
A. ulnaris
M. flexor carpi ulnaris
R. carpalis dorsalis
R. carpalis palmaris
R. palmaris profundus
Rr. perforantes
Arcus palmaris profundus
Aa. metacarpales palmares
Aa. digitales palmares communes

Fig. 4.68 A. ulnaris and A. radialis with deep palmar arch.
[S010-2-16]

In a clinical examination the following **pulses** can be palpated on the arm: the pulse of the A. radialis on the radial side of the wrist (ulnar of the tendon of the M. brachioradialis), the pulse of the A. ulnaris on the ulnar side of the wrist (radial of the tendon of the M. flexor carpi ulnaris). In addition, the pulse of the A. axillaris can be palpated in the distal axillary cavity and the A. brachiali can be palpated in the Sulcus bicipitalis medialis , which, however, is less commonly used.

NOTE

The A. ulnaris forms the Arcus palmaris superficialis, the A. radialis forms the Arcus palmaris profundus.

4.8 Veins of the upper extremity

Skills

After working through this chapter, you should be able to:
- understand the basic principles of the venous outflow of the upper extremity
- know the large epifascial veins and show them on a specimen

On the arm a system of deeply located veins, which accompany the arteries, is differentiated from a superficial system that runs in the subcutaneous adipose tissue. (➤ Fig. 4.69).

4.8.1 Superficial veins

The superficial veins designated as cutaneous veins always lie over the fascia of the upper arm and forearm, Fascia brachii and Fascia antebrachii. A distinction is made between 2 large cutaneous vein branches (➤ Fig. 4.69a):

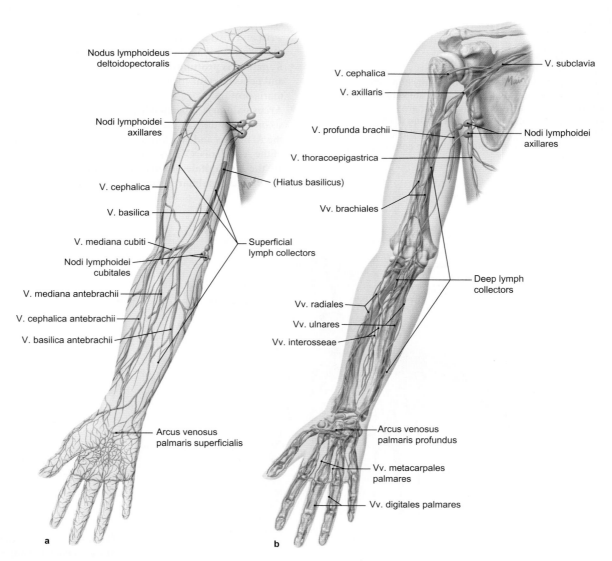

Fig. 4.69 Veins and lymphatic pathways of the arm, right. Ventral view. **a** Superficial system. **b** Deep system.

- **V. basilica:** it courses proximally as a strong vessel in the Sulcus bicipitalis medialis, penetrates the Fascia brachii at variable heights on the upper arm, and discharges into the Vv. brachiales.
- **V. cephalica:** this generally relatively thin vein runs laterally on the upper arm proximally, traverses the upper arm fascia and runs in the gap between the M. deltoideus and M. pectoralis major. It discharges within the Trigonum clavipectorale (Fossa infraclavicularis, MOHRENHEIM groove) into the V. axillaris.

The superficial venous outflow of the hand is focused on the dorsal side of the Rete venosum dorsale manus. In the palmar direction there is usually an Arcus venosus palmaris superficialis. The V. cephalica antebrachii collects blood on the radial side of the hand, runs radially on the extension side of the forearm proximally, and carries the blood of the V. cephalica. The V. basilica antebrachii runs on the ulnar edge of the arm and merges into the V. basilica. The **V. mediana cubiti** connects the V. cephalica with the V. basilica in the elbow. In addition to the superficial vessel networks, there are often even larger vein branches (e.g. the **V. mediana antebrachii** in the middle of the flexion side of the forearm). The superficial veins are connected via their connecting vessels (Vv. perforantes) to the deep veins.

N O T E

The superficial veins of the arm are very variable. Therefore, e.g. the V. cephalica or the V. mediana cubiti can be missing or additional cutaneous veins may be present. Due to the exposed location in the subcutaneous adipose tissue, the vessels are very suitable for **blood collection** or for **intravenous administration of drugs.** For this purpose, the large calibre V. mediana cubiti in the elbow is particularly used; however, by palpation in the elbow for a pulse it is essential that a superficially routed A. brachialis must be excluded (variation in approximately 8% of people).

4.8.2 Deep veins

In the case of the deep veins, typically 2 veins accompany 1 artery (➤ Fig. 4.69b). These veins are often connected to each other in the form of a rope ladder via cross-bridges. Since there are only artery-accompanying veins in the deep system, they are named after the respective artery. The V. axillaris and the V. subclavia are usually only present once on each side of the body. Both veins are located in front of their arterial counterparts. Whilst the A. subclavia passes through the scalene hiatus, the V. subclavia runs ventrally to the M. scalenus anterior.

Clinical remarks

Since the V. subclavia is superficial and lies in front of the A. subclavia, it is preferentially used to apply a **central venous catheter (CVC).** As a guiding structure for the route of the puncture cannula, the lower edge of the clavicula is used. The risk of incorrect puncture of the A. subclavia is very low, but following the puncture a breach of the rib cage must be excluded by a chest x-ray examination.

The deep veins of the arm are equipped with many **venous valves**. These allow a blood flow directed towards the heart in any position of the arm.

4.9 Lymphatic vessels of the upper extremity

Skills

After working through this chapter, you should be able to:
- know the principles of lymphatic drainage of the upper extremity
- explain the lymph node stations in the axillary cavity and their clinical relevance

4.9.1 Epifascial and subfascial lymph vessels

Similar to the veins, the lymph vessels run either epifascially or subfascially (➤ Fig. 4.69).

The **superficial collectors** form 3 bundles in the forearm (radial, ulnar and medial bundle), which in the elbow predominately converge to the medial collector bundle of the upper arm around the V. basilica. This finally discharges into the axillary lymph nodes. The dorsolateral bundle around the V. cephalica enables a second drainage path on the upper arm, the lymph vessels of which ultimately flow into the supraclavicular nodes and partially into the axillary lymph nodes. Individual lymph nodes can be installed into this bundle as an initial filter station, e.g. the Lnn. cubitales in the elbow.

The **subfascial collectors** accompany the large venous branches and also flow into the axillary lymph nodes. Here again, individual regional lymph nodes, such as e g. the Lnn. brachiales can be integrated into the deep collectors.

4.9.2 Lymph nodes of the axilla

The lymph nodes of the axilla drain almost the entire lymphatic system of the upper extremity, as well as the upper quadrants of the ventral and dorsal abdominal walls. Of high clinical relevance is that fact that up to 50 lymph nodes can receive lymph from large parts of the mammary glands (➤ Fig. 4.70). The lymph nodes are divided into three levels and into different groups relative to their position to the M. pectoralis minor.
- **Level I:** *lateral* to the M. pectoralis minor
  - Lnn. paramammarii (at the lateral border of the mammary gland)
  - Lnn. axillares pectorales (along the A. thoracica lateralis)
  - Lnn. axillares subscapulares (around the A. subscapularis)
  - Lnn. axillares laterales (lateral to the A. axillaris)
- **Level II:** *ventral and/or dorsal* to the M. pectoralis minor
  - Lnn. interpectorales (between the two Mm. pectorales)
  - Lnn. axillares centrales (under the M. pectoralis minor on the A. axillaris)
- **Level III:** *medial* to the M. pectoralis minor
  - Lnn. axillares apicales (in the area of the Trigonum clavipectorale = Fossa infraclavicularis = MOHRENHEIM groove)

The lymph initially flows mostly into the lymph nodes of levels I and II, to then be conducted further to those of level III. Afterwards, the lymph flows into the Truncus subclavius. Thus, **abnormal cells,** e.g. in tumours of the mammary gland, can be found in the temporal course often initially in levels I and II and only later in level III. From level III, they enter via the subclavian trunk into the Ductus thoracicus or directly into the left venous angle or on the right side via the Ductus lymphaticus dexter into the right venous angle.

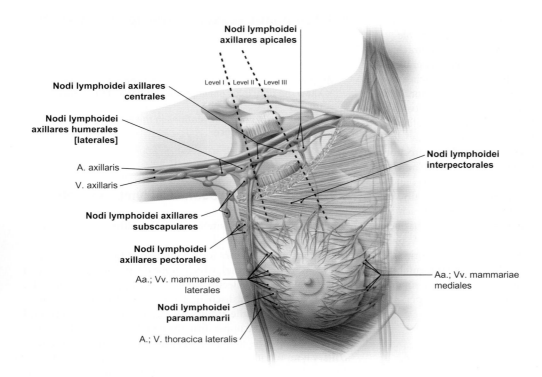

Nodi lymphoidei
axillares apicales

Nodi lymphoidei axillares
centrales

Nodi lymphoidei
axillares humerales
[laterales]

A. axillaris

V. axillaris

Nodi lymphoidei axillares
subscapulares

Nodi lymphoidei
axillares pectorales

Aa.; Vv. mammariae
laterales

Nodi lymphoidei
paramammarii

A.; V. thoracica lateralis

Level I Level II Level III

Nodi lymphoidei
interpectorales

Aa.; Vv. mammariae
mediales

Fig. 4.70 Lymph nodes of the axilla.

Clinical remarks

Precise knowledge of the various lymph node stations is decisive, e.g. in the case of tumours of the mammary gland **(breast cancer)**. Due to the frequency (most frequent malignant tumour in women, every 10th woman suffers from breast cancer, but men can also be affected) breast cancer must thus be addressed and ruled out in the case of any enlargement of the axillary lymph nodes. The number and location of affected lymph nodes is thereby important for tumour staging and thus also determines treatment. In the past, all 3 levels, including the pectoral muscles were resected, which was extremely disfiguring. For a long time it was standard to remove level I with the breast in order to analyse the lymph nodes. Today, treatment is more sophisticated. Often treatment can preserve the breast and lymph node metastasis can be excluded by means of scintigraphic representation of a sentinel lymph node. In the case of complete removal of the lymph nodes (axillary lymphadenectomy) oedema in the arm can form due to the lack of removal of tissue fluid via the lymph.

4.10 Topographically important aspects of the arm

Skills

After working through this chapter, you should be able to:
- know the vascular, lymphatic and nervous systems that traverse the MOHRENHEIM groove
- name the boundaries of the axillary spaces, and define the penetrating structures and locate them on a specimen
- define the course of the vascular, lymphatic and nervous systems in the elbow
- explain the composition and penetrating structures of the carpal tunnel and GUYON's canal.

4.10.1 Trigonum clavipectorale

The Trigonum clavipectorale (Fossa infraclavicularis, MOHRENHEIM groove) is a triangular depression of the ventral abdominal wall (➤ Fig. 4.71). It is bordered laterally by the M. deltoideus, medially by the M. pectoralis major and cranially by the Clavicula. The MOHRENHEIM groove is used by various vascular, lymphatic and nervous systems as a passageway through the Fascia clavipectoralis:
- Nn. pectorales medialis and lateralis: to the M. pectoralis major and M. pectoralis minor
- A. thoracoacromialis: divides here into its terminal branches
- V. cephalica: enters here into the depths into the V. axillaris
- Lnn. axillares apicales

4.10.2 Axillary cavity

The axillary cavity (Fossa axillaris) is a cavity somewhat pyramidal in shape when the arm is hanging down loosely and filled with fat and connective tissue. This is traversed by all vascular, lymphatic and nervous systems that supply the arm (exception: V. cephalica with surrounding lymphatic pathways). The skin of the axillary cavity forms the bottom of the pyramid, the tip extends to the shoulder joint. The anterior axillary fold is formed by the M. pectoralis major and the posterior axillary fold by the M. latissimus dorsi.

Within the Fossa axillaris the 3 fascicles of the Plexus brachialis run dorsally, medially and laterally to the A. axillaris. The V. axillaris is located ventrally of this neurovascular bundle. In addition to a large number of axillary lymph nodes, there are also the corresponding efferent and afferent lymphatic vessels.

The vascular, lymphatic and nervous systems exit the axilla via the axillary space dorsally.

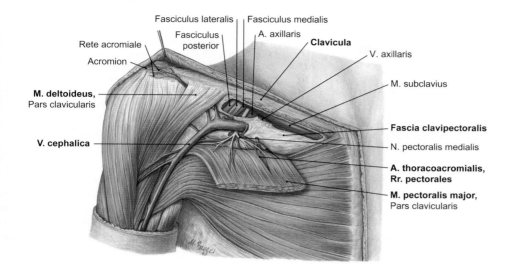

Fig. 4.71 Trigonum clavipec-torale, right. Ventral view.

4.10.3 Axillary spaces and triceps groove

There are 2 axillary spaces (➤ Fig. 4.72):
- **Medial axillary space** (triangular)
- **Lateral axillary space** (quadrangular)

Caudal of the lateral axillary space is the **triceps groove,** through which the N. radialis runs in order to become attached to the humerus in the Sulcus nervi radialis (➤ Table 4.21).

4.10.4 Elbow

The elbow (Fossa cubitalis) lies ventrally between the upper and the lower arm and is bordered on the radial side by the M. brachioradialis and by the M. pronator teres on the ulnar side. The base is formed by the attachment tendons of the M. biceps brachii and the M. brachialis.

Many vascular, lymphatic and nervous systems branch in the elbow on their way to the forearm. Found in the depth of the elbow from radial to ulnar are:

Table 4.21 Delineating and permeating structures of axillary spaces and triceps groove.

Medial axillary space	Lateral axillary space	Triceps groove
Delineation		
• M. teres minor • M. teres major • Caput longum of the M. triceps brachii	• M. teres minor • M. teres major • Caput longum of the M. triceps brachii • Humerus	• Caput longum of the M. triceps brachii • Caput laterale of the M. triceps brachii
Penetrating vascular, lymphatic and nervous systems		
• A. circumflexa scapulae • V. circumflexa scapulae	• A. circumflexa humeri posterior • V. circumflexa humeri posterior • N. axillaris	• A. profunda brachii • N. radialis

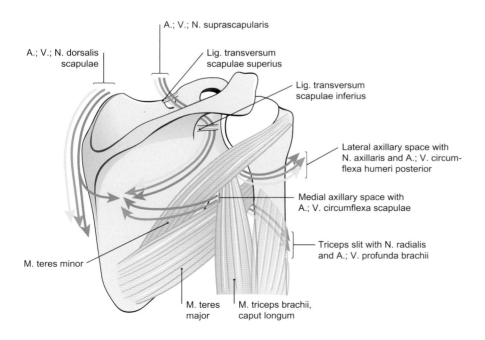

Fig. 4.72 Diagram of axillary cavities and the triceps groove, right. Dorsal view. [L126]

- **N. radialis** with the A. collateralis radialis. Division into R. profundus and R. superficialis
- **A. brachialis**. Division into A. radialis and A. ulnaris. The latter gives off the A. interossea communis.
- **N. medianus,** penetrates between the heads of the M. pronator teres and traverses the A. ulnaris.

The deep compartment is terminated towards the surface anatomy by the M. bicipital aponeurosis. Running very variably over the aponeurosis in its place are the V. cephalica antebrachii and the V. basilica antebrachii as well as the V. mediana cubiti as their connection.

Clinical remarks

Improperly taken venous blood (puncture too deep) can injure both the arterial vessels and the N. medianus (runs over the A. ulnaris) below the M. bicipital aponeurosis. In this case the N. ulnaris is not in danger because it is protected in the Sulcus nervi ulnaris on the dorsal side of the Epicondylus medialis.

4.10.5 Carpal tunnel and GUYON's canal

On the wrists, a distinction is made between 2 spaces, which are used as passage points by the vascular, lymphatic and nervous systems to the palm of the hand (➤ Fig. 4.73):
- Carpal tunnel (Canalis carpi), deep
- GUYON's canal, superficial

Clinical remarks

In both spaces, the nerves can be damaged, e.g. because of compression or lacerations (distal lesion of the N. medianus or the N. ulnaris). Because various muscle tendons in their tendon sheaths run through the carpal tunnel, **carpal tunnel syndrome** can also be caused by a tenosynovitis after overload of the muscles, rheumatic diseases or oedema in pregnancy. If there is no improvement after conservative treatment, treatment is by partitioning of the enveloping ligaments.

The base of the **carpal tunnel** is formed by the carpal bones. The proximal bones (Os scaphoideum and Os trapezium) also form the radial wall of the carpal tunnel. The ulnar wall is formed by the Os pisiforme and a protrusion of the hamate bone (Hamulus ossis hamati). In this way a groove is formed, referred to as the Sulcus carpi. As a roof, the Retinaculum musculorum flexorum closes the groove to the carpal tunnel, through which the **tendons of the long finger flexors** and also the **N. medianus** pass.

The **GUYON's canal** is located ventrally on the ulnar side of the wrist and is thus superficial of the carpal tunnel. Its base is the Retinaculum musculorum flexorum, which, due to a partition ('Lig. carpi palmare') also forms the roof. Running through the GUYON's canal is the **N. ulnaris** together with the **A./V. ulnaris.**

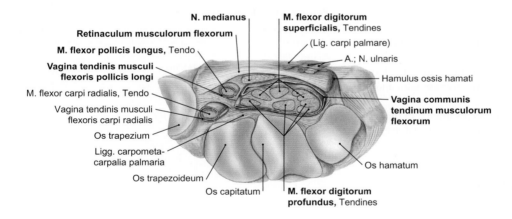

Fig. 4.73 Carpal tunnel and penetrating structures as well as GUYON's CANAL, right. Distal view.

5 Lower extremity

Volker Spindler, Jens Waschke

Rupture of an Achilles tendon

Medical history

A 56-year-old man is brought by friends into the Accident and Emergency department of the clinic. He says that every Wednesday night, he plays volleyball with his team. On taking a powerful jump from a squatting position, he suddenly felt an impact on the back of his right leg. At the same time, a loud clicking noise was heard. Since then he has had severe pain and is only able to limp. He is an avid runner, and enjoys sport on a regular basis. He says that for a few days, after long runs he occasionally has pain in the back of his leg.

Examination findings

The patient is completely conscious and the vital parameters are within the normal range. There is a noticeable swelling of the distal third of the right leg. During the examination an indentation about 1 cm long and the width of a palm could be felt above the calcaneus. The patient is unable to stand on tiptoe on the right leg. On examination, the ankle joint is normal.
The ultrasound examination shows a rupture of the Achilles tendon. The gap between the two torn ends of the tendon is 8 mm wide. An x-ray image in lateral beam projection reveals no evidence of avulsion of a bone fragment at the attachment of the tendon onto the calcaneal tuberosity, or of any fractures.

Diagnosis

Right side Achilles tendon rupture.

Treatment

After comprehensively informing the patient, a conservative approach is decided on. The patient receives a therapeutic shoe adapted with 3 cm heel lift, so that the foot is fixed in 20° plantar flexion position. It is immediately possible to place all his weight on the leg. The patient is discharged with the instruction to wear the shoe day and night for 12 weeks. The foot must also be maintained in a plantar flexed position if the shoe is removed, for example, for showering.

Subsequent progression

After 3 weeks, physiotherapy is started. The heel wedges are gradually reduced to 2 cm and 1 cm high. After 12 weeks, the patient is pain-free without the therapeutic shoe.

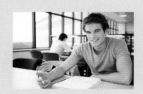

You have just started your internship and the first patient to be presented is waiting to see the senior consultant. Fortunately, you are allowed to choose a patient for this, and since you are also a passionate volleyball player, the decision about which patient is easy.
You make you some notes about history, admission status, previous investigations and, so that nothing can go wrong, notes about treatment.

The head doctor visit – Take 1
Hx: 56-year-old patient, Achilles tendon rupture on right
Trigger: jump from squatting position in volleyball games, resulting in impact lower leg rear right, noticed snapping noise.
Anamnestic after prolonged exercise (jogging)
Pain in the back of lower leg area for a couple of days
Admission status: swelling distal third right lower leg,
depression of approx. 1 cm, 1 hand width above heel bone,
Not possible to stand on the tips of the right toes, ankle unobtrusive
Further differential diagnosis: Sono: **Rupture of the Achilles tendon**, gap of 8 mm
x-ray: no evidence of a vulsion bone fragment or fractures
Treatment: local decongestive measures, in the course of conservative procedure with fixation of the foot in 20° plantar-flexion position

5.1 Overview

The upper and lower extremities are basically similar; however, they have different characteristics in their construction in order to adapt to their different functions. The arm is a gripping tool designed to ensure maximum freedom of movement for interacting with the environment (e.g. by enabling turning movements of the forearm, or by the high mobility of the thumb). Conversely, the lower limbs with evolutionary transition to walking upright, have adopted the role of **running and support organs.** The stability needed to carry the body is ensured by the fixed coupling of the hips to the spine and by more bulky bones. Solid ligaments stabilise the joints and limit movements in such a way that it is possible to stand without becoming tired, as well as preserving mobility to enable running. In contrast to the upper limbs, the muscles of the leg and especially those of the foot are more designed for stability (e.g. by bracing the plantar arch), rather than for fine motor skills. Despite this stable construction, degenerative joint diseases such as osteoarthritis and traumatic injuries (for example, fractures of the neck of the femur) are extremely common and are therefore relevant for all doctors.

The lower extremities (Membrum inferius) are subdivided into the pelvic girdle (Cingulum pelvicum) and the leg (➤ Fig. 5.1). The leg is subdivided into the thigh (Femur), lower leg (Crus) and foot (Pes). The longitudinal axes of the upper and lower thigh bones laterally form the exterior knee angle of 174°.

The weight of the body is not exactly borne by the longitudinal axis of the long leg bones, instead the pressure is placed on the connecting line between the hip and the centre of the ankle joint (MIKULICZ's line) (➤ Fig. 5.2). Ideally, this axis, which is designated as an axis line of the leg, runs largely through the centre of the knee joint. Deviations from this line of the knee joint in the frontal plane are called **knock knees (Genu valgum)** or **bow legs (Genu varum):**

- In **knock knees,** the knee joint is medial of the axis line, so the exterior angle of the knee is reduced. The distance between the right and left knee is reduced. In Genu valgum, the lateral compartment of the knee joint carries a heavier load than the medial one.
- In **bow legs,** this situation is reversed so that the knee joint is positioned lateral to the axis line, the exterior angle of the knee is greater and the distance between the two knee joints increases. In Genu varum, the medial compartment is affected as a result of greater pressure.

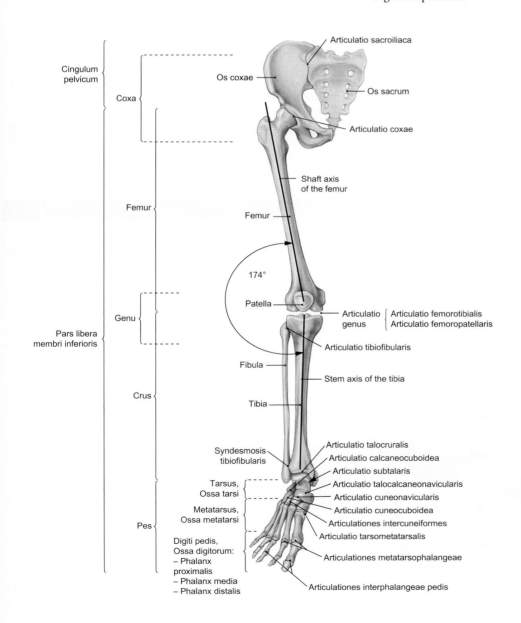

Fig. 5.1 Bones and joints of the lower extremity, Membrum inferius, right side. Ventral view.

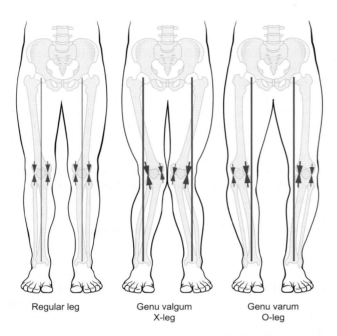

Fig. 5.2 The axis line of the leg (MIKULICZ's line). Ventral view. Normal knee joint (left), Genu valgum (centre) and Genu varum (right).

If the axis line runs through the centre of the knee joint, the right and left sides of the knee joint are evenly loaded (indicated by arrows in ➤ Fig. 5.2).

Clinical remarks

Deviations of the knee joint from the axis line are very common and not abnormal during growth. Thus in infants, in physiological terms a Genu varum can be observed, which often becomes a Genu valgum after a few years have elapsed. As a rule, these deformities are 'grown out of' within the first decade of life. Severe deformities in adults can, however, lead to arthritis of the knee joint due to the ongoing incorrect loading of the knee joint surfaces and the menisci (gonarthrosis). In the case of severe deformities, to ensure correction during growth a part of the growth plate such as the growth plate of the femur is clamped (temporary epiphysiodesis, prevents the growth of the lateral or medial bone end). Better centring of the axis line in adults may be achieved by removing a wedge of bone (osteotomy).

5.2 Pelvis

Skills

After working through this chapter, you should be able to:
- indicate the composition and the main structures of the pelvis, and explain the differences between the male and female pelvis,
- demonstrate the connections of the pelvic bone with each other and to the vertebral column and, in doing so, explain the course and the function of the ligaments involved,
- explain the function of the pelvic ring for the stability of the upright gait.

5.2.1 Structure and form

The pelvis (syn.: pelvic girdle, Cingulum pelvicum) forms the connection between the legs and the torso. It is composed of the right and left hip bone (**Os coxae**) and the sacrum (**Os sacrum**) (➤ Fig. 5.3). The two hip bones are attached ventrally via a synarthrosis, the pubic symphysis (**Symphysis pubica**). The right and left hip bone are united dorsally with the sacrum via an amphiarthrosis, the sacroiliac joint (**Articulatio sacroiliaca**). This means that there is a stable ring of bone, but still with a degree of flexibility.

Cranially, the greater pelvis can be distinguished (Pelvi major) from the lesser pelvis (Pelvis minor) caudally. The transition from the greater to lesser pelvis is the Linea terminalis. This runs from the Symphysis pubica via the Pecten ossis pubis and the Linea arcuata to the Promontorium of the Sacrum. The lesser pelvis forms a bony 'canal' with an upper opening, the Apertura pelvis superior, and a lower opening, the Apertura pelvis inferior.

Table 5.1 Internal female pelvis dimensions (➤ Fig. 5.4a).

Name	Course	Size
Diameter vera	Rear of the pubic symphysis to Promontorium	11 cm
Diameter anatomica	Upper margin of the pubic symphysis to Promontorium	11.5 cm
Diameter diagonalis	Lower margin of the pubic symphysis to Promontorium	12.5 cm
Diameter transversa	Largest transversal diameter between the two terminal lines	13.5 cm

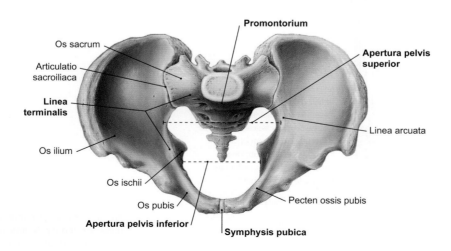

Fig. 5.3 Pelvis. Ventral cranial view.

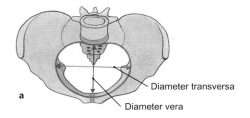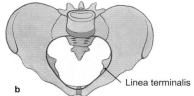

a — Diameter transversa
Diameter vera

b — Linea terminalis

Fig. 5.4 Pelvis.
a Female pelvis.
b Male pelvis.

The pelvis of males and females differs in shape. In women, the largest diameter of the plane of the arch of the pelvis is located horizontally (➤ Fig. 5.4a), whereas in men it is in a sagittal position (➤ Fig. 5.4b). Therefore, in men the aperture is slightly heart-shaped, and in women it is horizontally oval. In men, the lower pubic branches meet the symphysis at a relatively sharp angle (Angulus subpubicus). In women, however, this angle is flat and is therefore referred to as the Arcus pubicus. In women the iliac wings are also larger and more protruding.

The **internal dimensions** of the pelvis provide information about the width of the lesser pelvis (➤ Fig. 5.4a). In women, this is important for assessing whether a normal birth is possible. To do so, the dimensions provided in ➤ Table 5.1 can be used.

Clinical remarks

In **normal vaginal birth** the child passes through the lesser pelvis which represents the narrowest point of the birth canal. A disparity between the size of the child (the diameter of its head is relevant here) and the size of the pelvis can make normal birth impossible. What is decisive here is primarily the **Diameter vera** (clinically known as Conjugata vera), since this represents the shortest distance between the walls of the lesser pelvis. During pregnancy the sacroiliac joint and Symphysis pubica are relaxed by hormones (e.g. relaxin). This leads to an enlargement of the Diameter vera by about 1 cm. In cases where there is a suspected disparity between the pelvis and the child's head, the pelvic dimensions can be determined before birth by magnetic resonance imaging (MRI). If a failure of birth progression makes a **caesarean section** (Sectio

caesarea) necessary, the pelvis can be directly measured during the operation. This means that for a subsequent pregnancy, a decision can be taken in time as to whether a vaginal birth is possible or if a planned caesarean section would be sensible.

5.2.2 Bones of the pelvis

The pelvis is made up of the sacrum (**Os sacrum,** ➤ Chap. 3.3.2) and 2 hip bones (**Ossae coxae**). The hip bone (Os coxae) is made up of 3 bone portions (➤ Fig. 5.5, ➤ Fig. 5.6):
* Iliac bone (**Os ilium**): forms the upper part of the hip bone
* Ischium (**Os ischii**): is positioned caudally and dorsal
* Pubic bone (**Os pubis**): is located ventrally and caudal

The initially existing cartilage plates between the individual bones ossify between the ages of *13 and 18 years*.

Os ilium

The Os ilium forms the wing of the ilium (**Ala ossis ilii**). Medially this has a concave shape (➤ Fig. 5.5). The front section of the medial side is indented by the **Fossa iliaca**, which forms the origin of the M. iliacus. On the dorsal side of the Fossa iliaca is the **Facies sacropelvica**, which with the **Facies auricularis** is located on the articular surface of the sacrum. The **Tuberositas iliaca** is an important attachment point for the ligaments of the sacroiliac joint (Articulatio sacroiliaca). At the cranial end of the iliac bone is the **Crista iliaca**. The respective abdominal muscles are attached at its Labium internum, the Linea intermedia and the Labium externum. To the

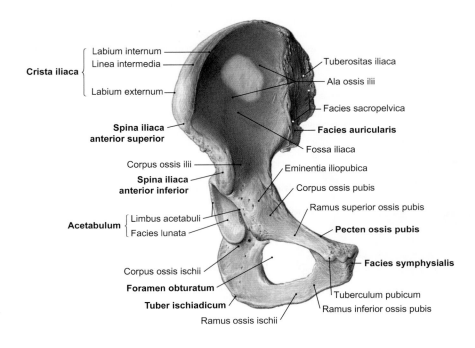

Crista iliaca {
Labium internum
Linea intermedia
Labium externum
}

Tuberositas iliaca
Ala ossis ilii
Facies sacropelvica
Facies auricularis
Fossa iliaca

Spina iliaca anterior superior

Corpus ossis ilii
Spina iliaca anterior inferior

Eminentia iliopubica
Corpus ossis pubis
Ramus superior ossis pubis
Pecten ossis pubis

Acetabulum {
Limbus acetabuli
Facies lunata
}

Facies symphysialis

Corpus ossis ischii
Foramen obturatum
Tuber ischiadicum
Ramus ossis ischii

Tuberculum pubicum
Ramus inferior ossis pubis

Fig. 5.5 Hip bone, Os coxae, right. Ventral view.

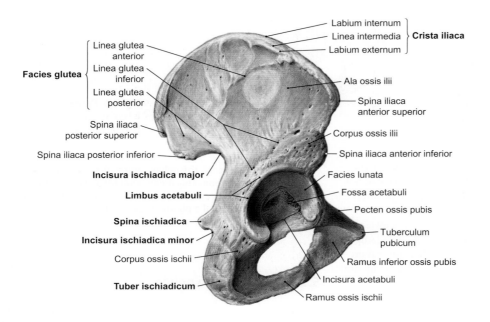

Labium internum
Linea intermedia **Crista iliaca**
Labium externum

Facies glutea
Linea glutea anterior
Linea glutea inferior
Linea glutea posterior

Ala ossis ilii

Spina iliaca anterior superior

Spina iliaca posterior superior

Corpus ossis ilii

Spina iliaca posterior inferior

Spina iliaca anterior inferior

Incisura ischiadica major

Facies lunata

Limbus acetabuli

Fossa acetabuli

Pecten ossis pubis

Spina ischiadica

Incisura ischiadica minor

Tuberculum pubicum

Corpus ossis ischii

Ramus inferior ossis pubis

Tuber ischiadicum

Incisura acetabuli

Ramus ossis ischii

Fig. 5.6 Hip bone, Os coxae, right. Lateral view.

front and rear, the Crista iliaca tapers into the **Spina iliaca anterior superior** and **Spina iliaca posterior superior.** Correspondingly, caudal of each of these two structures there is another projection, the **Spina iliaca anterior inferior** and **Spina iliaca posterior inferior.** Under the Spina iliaca posterior inferior the Incisura ischiadica major is grooved in. On the lateral side (**Facies glutea**) of the wings of ilium the Linea glutea anterior, Linea glutea inferior and Linea glutea posterior are important origins for the dorsolateral hip muscles (➤ Fig. 5.6).

Os ischii
The Os ischii bears the **Tuber ischiadicum.** The ischium (**Corpus ossis ischii**) runs cranially into the **Spina ischiadica** and caudally connects the **Ramus ossis ischii** with the Os pubis. Under the Spina ischiadica is the Incisura ischiadica minor (➤ Fig. 5.6).

Os pubis
The Os pubis is divided into **Corpus, Ramus inferior** and **Ramus superior** and, together with the Facies symphysialis forms the connection to the opposite side. Close to this joint surface, the Tuberculum pubicum serves as the attachment for the **Lig. inguinale,** which is anatomically represented as bands of connective tissue

originating from the Spina iliaca anterior superior (➤ Fig. 5.7). The inguinal ligament is therefore not a ligament in the real sense of the word; in fact it is produced by the uniting of the M. obliquus externus abdominis with the fascia of the M. iliopsoas. It is an important limitation for 2 places where vessels and nerves pass through:
- The floor of the inguinal canal (Canalis inguinalis): the passage from the abdominal cavity to the external genitalia (➤ Chap. 3.1.4)
- The roof of the Lacuna musculorum and Lacuna vasorum (➤ Chap. 5.10.1)

On the **Ramus superior,** there is a pronounced bony ridge, the **Pecten ossis pubis,** which continues from the Linea arcuata in the direction of sacroiliac joint.

The **Acetabulum** is the socket of the hip joint and receives the head of the femur. It is formed from parts of all 3 bones of the hip. The depression (**Fossa acetabuli**) is almost completely covered by a crescent-shaped area, the Facies lunata. This is only interrupted caudally on the **Incisura acetabuli.** In the **Limbus acetabuli** the acetabulum is externally elevated in a ring shape.

Caudally of the Fossa acetabuli, the ramus and body of the Os ischii, as well as the Ramus superior and Ramus inferior of the Os pubis,

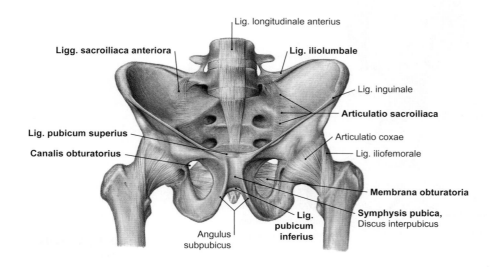

Lig. longitudinale anterius

Ligg. sacroiliaca anteriora

Lig. iliolumbale

Lig. inguinale

Articulatio sacroiliaca

Articulatio coxae

Lig. pubicum superius

Lig. iliofemorale

Canalis obturatorius

Membrana obturatoria

Symphysis pubica, Discus interpubicus

Angulus subpubicus

Lig. pubicum inferius

Fig. 5.7 Joints and ligaments of the pelvis. Ventral view.

form a bony ring around the largest opening in the pelvic bone, the **Foramen obturatum.** This is filled by a plate of connective tissue (Membrana obturatoria), which serves as the origin of the muscles bearing the same name (Mm. obturatorii internus and externus). An opening (Canalis obturatorius) serves as an exit point for vessels and nerves (A./V. obturatoria, N. obturatorius) from the small pelvis to the leg (➤ Chap. 5.10.2).

Clinical remarks

The Crista iliaca can also be easily palpated even in obese people, because it is located just below the surface of the skin. Since even in the elderly population blood-forming red bone marrow is still present, in the case of disorders of blood formation or suspected diseases of the blood cells in the bone marrow (e.g. in the case of leukaemia) a punch biopsy is taken from the iliac crest **(bone marrow puncture).** The bone marrow is histologically processed and then assessed by a pathologist.

5.2.3 Pelvic joints and ligament attachments

Three joints from the bones of the pelvis form a stable ring (➤ Fig. 5.7):
- **Articulatio sacroiliaca** dorsal to the right and left
- **Symphysis pubica** ventral

The Articulationes sacroiliacae are a diarthrosis; conversely the Symphysis pubica is a synarthrosis.

In the **Articulatio sacroiliaca** the Facies auricularis of the hip is attached to the Facies auricularis of the sacrum. The arch-shaped joint surfaces are held very tight by ligaments and as an amphiarthrosis the joint has only very limited mobility.

The **Symphysis pubica** is formed by the two Facies symphysiales of both hips (to be more precise: the pubic bone). Both bones are connected by the Discus interpubicus, which is made up of fibrous cartilage.

The following **ligaments** secure the **Articulatio sacroiliaca:**
- **Lig. sacroiliacum anterius,** spans the joint space ventrally
- **Lig. sacroiliacum interosseum**
- **Lig. sacroiliacum posterius,** runs like the Lig. sacroiliacum interosseum dorsal of the joint space between Tuberositas iliaca and the Sacrum

While the anterior ligaments bridge the joint space ventrally, the interosseous and posterior ligaments form a powerful ligamentous apparatus at the dorsal side of the joint (➤ Fig. 5.8).

In addition, the **Lig. iliolumbale** joins the Procc. costales of the two lower lumbar vertebrae with the Crista iliaca and is attached to parts of the Lig. sacroiliacum anterius.

Caudal of the sacroiliac joint there are 2 more strong ligaments:
- **Lig. sacrotuberale:** the sacrotuberal ligament goes from the dorsal side of the Sacrum descending to the Tuber ischiadicum and Ramus inferior of the pubic bone.
- **Lig. sacrospinale:** this ligament runs horizontally from the dorsal side of the sacrum to the Spina ischiadica, and divides the opening between the hip bones (Incisurae ischiadicae major and minor), the sacrum and Lig. sacrotuberale into a cranial Foramen ischiadicum majus and a caudal Foramen ischiadicum minus (➤ Fig. 5.9).

The **Symphysis pubica** is held in place by 2 ligaments:
- The **Lig. pubicum superius** connects the two pubic bones on the upper side of the joint.
- The **Lig. pubicum inferius** is located on the lower side (➤ Fig. 5.7).

5.2.4 Mechanics of the pelvic joints

The pelvis forms a ring with its three bones. It is connected by the joints and ligaments so that, on one hand, *stability* is ensured, allowing transfer of the body's weight onto the legs, while on the other hand also ensuring a certain springy *mobility*. This is especially important for dynamic movements such as running or jumping, to cushion the power surges that arise.

The **sacroiliac joint** must transfer the full load of the upper half of the body to the hip bones. This occurs due to the strong ligaments of an amphiarthrosis making only minor movements possible. These slight movements (maximum 10°) are used to mitigate the effect of strong peak loads on the joint. As can be seen from the V-shaped position of the sections of the powerful ligamentous apparatus of the Lig. sacroiliacum posterius (➤ Fig. 5.8), the sacrum is suspended between the right and left Facies sacropelvica. Therefore, the sacrum does not press the body's weight down onto the hip bones; instead it is 'suspended' by means of the ligaments. This allows a distribution of force over the entire Tuberositas sacroiliaca, which is subjected to tension. Simultaneously the hip bone is pressed onto the sacrum by this tension, which, together with the ligaments, prevents the sacrum from sliding caudally.

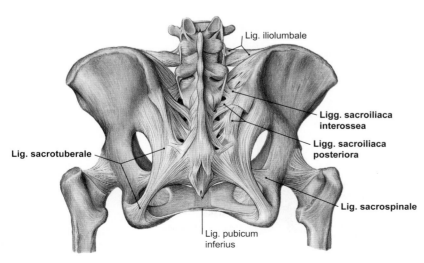

Lig. iliolumbale

Ligg. sacroiliaca interossea

Ligg. sacroiliaca posteriora

Lig. sacrotuberale

Lig. sacrospinale

Lig. pubicum inferius

Fig. 5.8 Joints and ligaments of the pelvis. Dorsal view.

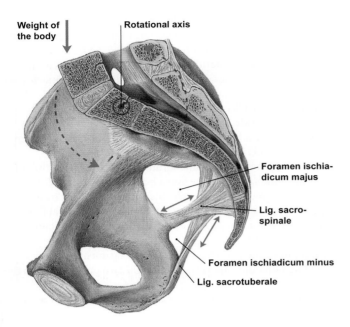

Fig. 5.9 Joints and ligaments of the pelvis in an infant; mid-sagittal section. Medial view.

Placing a load on the Os sacrum and sacroiliac joint leads to tensile forces being exerted at the **Symphysis pubica.** A separation of the fibre cartilage is prevented by the Ligg. pubica which run transversally. The Lig. iliolumbale performs the same function for the sacroiliac joint.

When standing, the body's **centre of gravity** is located ventral of the sacroiliac joint. This could lead to the rotation of the sacrum in the transverse axis so that the sacrum is transferred dorsally upwards and the body would tip ventrally (➤ Fig. 5.9, dotted arrows). This rotation is prevented by the Lig. sacrospinale and the Lig. sacrotuberale. The Ligg. sacroiliaca cannot do this alone due to their smaller lever arm.

NOTE
The **Ligg. sacroiliaca** prevent the sacrum from sliding caudally, while the **Lig. sacrospinale and sacrotuberale** prevent rotation in the transverse axis.

5.3 Thigh

Skills

After working through this chapter, you should be able to:
* explain the structure of the femur and its blood supply, in particular of a neck and head of the femur
* explain the structure and function of the hip joint as well as the course and the function of the hip joint ligaments and show them on the skeleton
* know all the hip muscles with their origins, attachment and function and demonstrate their course on a skeleton or dissected specimen

5.3.1 Thigh bone

The thigh bone (**Femur**) is the largest bone in the human body (➤ Fig. 5.10). It is divided into a head (**Caput**), a neck (**Collum**) and a shaft (**Corpus**).

A small depression at the **head,** the Fovea capitis femoris serves to attach the Lig. capitis femoris. The head tapers towards the neck of the femur, which merges into the shaft in the area of the two tro-

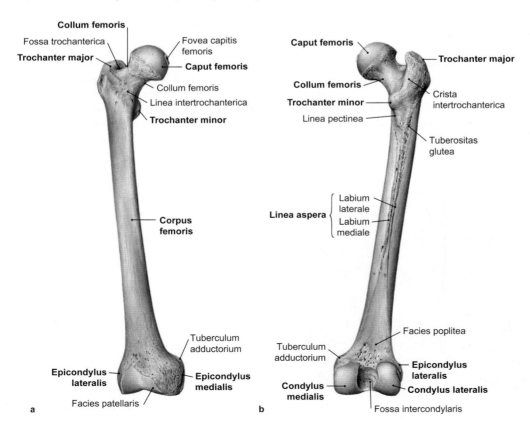

Fig. 5.10 Thigh bone, femur, right. a Ventral view, **b** dorsal view.

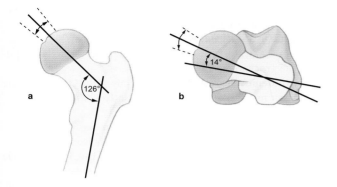

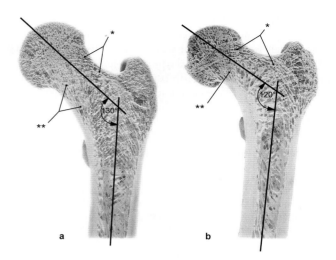

Fig. 5.11 Proximal end of the femur, right. a Representation of the CCD angle, dorsal view. **b** Representation of the angle of antetorsion, proximal view.

Fig. 5.12 Section through the proximal end of the femur, right side. Illustration of the structure of the spongiosa and the CCD angle. **a** Coxa valga. **b** Coxa vara. * 'tension bundle', ** 'pressure bundle'

chanters. The greater trochanter (**Trochanter major**) faces dorso-laterally, the lesser trochanter (**Trochanter minor**) faces dorsomedially. The trochanters act as an attachment point for muscles that make the hip joint move. Between the Trochanter major and Trochanter minor, the **Linea intertrochanterica** passes on the ventral side. On the dorsal side, the **Crista intertrochanterica** is more elevated. Below the lesser trochanter, the **Linea pectinea** is positioned as the attachment of the M. pectineus. Lateral from this is the **Tuberositas glutea,** the attachment for the M. gluteus maximus.
The **femoral shaft** is largely circular in diameter; only on the dorsal side is there a bony ridge called the **Linea aspera** with a Labium mediale and a Labium laterale. Distally the shaft widens to the Epicondylus medialis and lateralis and ends in the two cylindrically-shaped joint surfaces of the knee joint (**Condyli medialis and lateralis**). Between the two condyles there is a recess for the cruciate ligaments of the knee joint, the **Fossa intercondylaris.** The front surface of the femoral condyles is called the **Facies patellaris;** on the rear surface is the **Facies poplitea** (➤ Fig. 5.10).
At the femur 2 **angular dimensions** can be distinguished:

- **Centrum-Collum-Diaphyseal angle** (CCD angle) between the neck of the femur and femoral shaft (➤ Fig. 5.11a).
- **Antetorsion angle:** between the connecting line of the two condyles (equivalent to approximately the transverse axis of the knee) and the longitudinal axis of the neck of the femur (➤ Fig. 5.11b).

The **CCD angle** depends on age and is approximately 126° in adults. It is 150° in newborn babies, decreasing throughout life to 120° in old age. If the angle is *more than 130°,* it is referred to as a **Coxa valga** (➤ Fig. 5.12a), with an angle *less than 120°* as a **Coxa vara** (➤ Fig. 5.12b).
As can be seen in ➤ Fig. 5.2, the axis line of the leg does not run along the longitudinal axis of the shaft of the femur. Through the neck of the femur, the proximal parts of the shaft are displaced lateral of the axis line, so that only the distal end of the femur remains in the axis line. This lateralisation is important, providing the small gluteal muscles (running from the pelvic ring to the trochanter major) with a larger lever arm. This is required, for example, to prevent the pelvis from dropping down to the contralateral side when standing on one leg; however, the 'position' of the Trochanter major has the disadvantage that the femoral shaft and, most importantly the neck of the femur, does not bear its load axially, but at an angle. In the neck of the femur, this means that there are areas primarily subjected to compressive loading (** in ➤ Fig. 5.12), and areas which are primarily subjected to tension (* in ➤ Fig. 5.12). In order to compensate for this loading, the spongious trabaeculae are longitudinally aligned to the arising forces (the trajectories).

Therefore, there is a trajectorial orientation of the trabeculae, which are either under tension or subject to pressure.
In the case of a **Coxa vara,** the neck of the femur to the shaft has a greater bend, resulting in a higher tensile loading of the spongious trabeculae in the upper sections of the neck of the femur(* in ➤ Fig. 5.12b). Correspondingly, in the case of a **Coxa valga,** the trabeculae in the lower part of the neck of the femur are increasingly subject to pressure (** in ➤ Fig. 5.12a).
The **antetorsion angle** means the twisting of the shaft in relation to the knee joint axis. The neck of the femur, compared to this axis, is rotated by approximately 14° to the front, i.e. in an antetorsion position. This angle also varies according to age. In infants it is even more pronounced at 30°. The torsion causes the kneecap to point somewhat medially. With increased antetorsion the toes point further inwards while running, and where there is low antetorsion, they point outwards.

Clinical remarks

CCD and antetorsion angles are highly pathophysiologically significant. Variations of this angle lead to altered power transfer in the hip joint. Due to incorrect loading on the cartilage, this leads to increased wear and often contributes to the development of **coxarthrosis (osteoarthritis of the hip).**
The oblique loading of the neck of the femur predisposes it to fractures ('femoral neck fractures'). These are very common, especially in older people, in combination with osteoporosis. Typically, these fractures are triggered by falls. In order to avoid long immobilisation of the patient, femoral neck fractures are often treated by the use of an **artificial hip joint** (total endoprosthesis = TEP). A TEP consists of joint cup and joint head with an artificial femoral head. The femoral head and neck are fixed in place in the femoral shaft by the two trochanters.

5.3.2 Hip joint

The hip joint (**Articulatio coxae**) is a *ball joint* with 3 degrees of freedom. The cup is formed by the Os coxae, with the head of the femur as its counterpart.
The Facies lunata is lined with joint cartilage. A connective tissue lip, the Labrum acetabuli, expands the articular surface and extends

over the Incisura acetabularis with the Lig. transversum acetabuli. This joint lip extends over the equator of the femoral head, so that approximately two-thirds of the surface area of the ball are covered by the joint cup. This is a special type of ball joint called a *cotyloid joint* (Articulatio cotylica, enarthrosis). As with the covering of the socket, the majority of the joint head is lined with cartilage.

Clinical remarks

The joint socket only reaches its final depth after birth. It is important that the femoral head is already located in the centre of the flat cup in infancy. Therefore, in infants the position of the femoral head is examined using ultrasound. If there is a deformity, at this stage a simple correction can be carried out, just using splints for example. If **hip dysplasias** like these (no covering of the femoral head by the Os coxae) remain uncorrected, this can often result in osteoarthritis of the hip joint. The femoral head can even exit the socket (hip dislocation) and lead to the development of a new but functionally inefficient articular surface above the acetabulum.

The **joint capsule** originates from the Limbus acetabuli and spans the femoral head and the largest part of the femoral neck. It is inserted at the front of the Linea intertrochanterica and behind it is attached a little further proximally. Three ligaments reinforce the joint capsule from outside and stabilise the hip joint (➤ Fig. 5.13):

- **Lig. iliofemorale:** originates distally from the Spina iliaca anterior inferior and runs to the Linea intertrochanterica and the Trochanter major (strongest ligament in the human body!)
- **Lig. pubofemorale:** runs from the Ramus superior of the Os pubis to the Trochanter minor
- **Lig. ischiofemorale:** runs from the corpus of the Os ischii to the Trochanter major (Pars superior) and the Trochanter minor (Pars inferior)

The **Lig. capitis femoris** on the other hand, has no holding function. It passes within the joint cavity from the Incisura acetabuli to the Fovea capitis femoris. The **R. acetabularis of the A. obturatoria** runs within this ligament to the femoral head and plays a role in blood supply. In small children it is responsible for the majority of the blood supply, but in adults only about 20–30 %. The main blood supply is shared between the A. circumflexa femoris medialis and the A. circumflexa femoris lateralis (➤ Fig. 5.14), which emerge from the A. profunda femoris:

- The **A. circumflexa femoris medialis** runs on the dorsal side of the neck, giving rise to several branches running between the joint capsule and the periosteum to the femoral head. It supplies the back of the femoral neck and the majority of the femoral head.
- The **A. circumflexa femoris lateralis** runs on the ventral side of the femoral neck, which it mainly supplies, and also provides small branches to the femoral head.

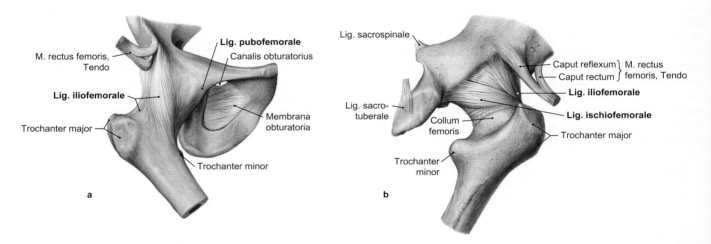

Fig. 5.13 Hip joint, Articulatio coxae, with ligaments, right. a Ventral view. **b** Dorsal view.

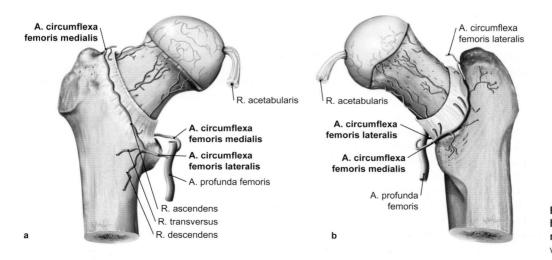

Fig. 5.14 Blood supply to the hip joint, Articulatio coxae, right. a Ventral view. **b** Dorsal view.

The **hip socket** is supplied by arteries coming from the lesser pelvis. Branches of the A. obturatoria and the A. glutea superior are involved. Both vessels arise from the A. iliaca interna.

— **Clinical remarks** ——————————————

The fact that the femoral head is mainly supplied by blood vessels from the femoral neck is clinically highly relevant. In the case of fractures, particularly of the femoral neck or dislocations of the joint, these vessels are frequently damaged. This can therefore result in the destruction of bone tissue and **femoral head necrosis** due to insufficient blood supply to the femoral head. This complication is also a reason why with femoral head fractures, a total endoprosthesis is usually implanted.

5.3.3 Mechanics of the hip joint

The hip joint can be moved in 3 axes (➤ Fig. 5.15, ➤ Table 5.2):
- **Flexion** and **extension** in the transverse axis, bending and stretching of the thigh
- **Abduction** and **adduction** in the sagittal axis, stretching or pulling of the leg
- **Internal rotation** and **external rotation** around the longitudinal axis, internal rotation (kneecap pointing more medially) and external rotation (kneecap pointing laterally) of the thigh.

In particular, extension can only be precisely defined with a fixed contralateral hip joint. When trying to move the leg as far as possible dorsally when standing, the contralateral hip joint is always bent. Therefore, the extension is defined best in the prone position.

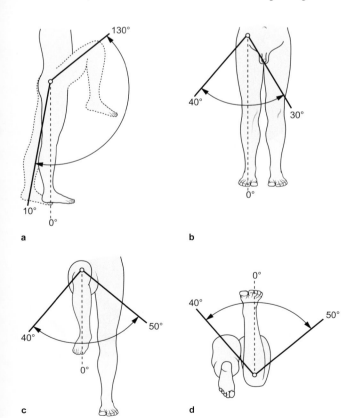

Fig. 5.15 Range of movement in the hip joint. a Extension/flexion. **b** Abduction/adduction. **c, d** External rotation/internal rotation.

Table 5.2 Range of movement in the hip joint.

Movement	Range of movement
Extension/flexion	10°–0°–130°
Abduction/adduction	40°–0°–30°
External rotation/internal rotation	50°–0°–40°

Table 5.3 Functions of the hip joint ligaments.

Movement	Inhibition by
Extension	• Lig. iliofemorale • Lig. pubofemorale • Lig. ischiofemorale
Abduction	Lig. pubofemorale
Adduction	Lig. ischiofemorale
Lateral rotation	Lig. pubofemorale
Medial rotation	Lig. ischiofemorale

Internal and external rotation must be assessed with the knee joint in a flexed position. By doing this, the possibility of additional rotation in the other leg joints is eliminated.

The hip joint can only be very slightly extended (important for stability when standing), but can be flexed very well (important for walking). This is achieved with the **ligaments of the hip joint,** which are all tensed in **extension,** but relaxed during flexion, (➤ Table 5.3). This function can be explained by the spiral track of the ligaments around the femoral head (➤ Fig. 5.13). In addition, the ligaments prevent excessive adduction and abduction, as well as extreme internal and external rotation.

Securing the extension is also important when standing for longer periods. This pushes the hip slightly forwards, tightening the ligaments due to the slight extension that takes place in the hip. When standing for a long time, these ligaments provide support, and this saves a great deal of energy.

5.3.4 Muscles of the hip joint

There are 4 groups of muscles which affect the movement of the hip joint:
- **Ventral muscles**
  - M. iliacus (part of the M. iliopsoas)
  - M. psoas major (part of the M. iliopsoas)
  - M. psoas minor (part of the M. iliopsoas, variable)
- **Dorsolateral muscles**
  - M. gluteus maximus
  - M. gluteus medius
  - M. gluteus minimus
  - M. tensor fasciae latae
- **Pelvitrochanteric (medial) muscles**
  - M. piriformis
  - M. obturatorius internus
  - M. gemellus superior
  - M. gemellus inferior
  - M. quadratus femoris
  - M. obturatorius externus
- **Adductor group**
  - M. pectineus
  - M. gracilis
  - M. adductor brevis
  - M. adductor longus
  - M. adductor magnus

Table 5.4 Ventral muscles of the hip joint.

Innervation	Origins	Attachment	Function
M. iliopsoas (consists of M. iliacus and M. psoas major)			

Plexus lumbalis (Rr. musculares)	• M. iliacus: Fossa iliaca
	• M. psoas major:
	  – *Superficial layer:* Facies lateralis of the body of the XIIth thoracic to the IVth Intervertebral discs
	  – *Deep layer:* Proc. costalis of Ist–IVth lumbar vertebrae
		Trochanter minor	*Lumbar spine:*
			• Lateral flexion
			Hip joint:
			• Flexion *(most important muscle)*
			• Lateral rotation from medial rotation position

M. psoas minor (interictal muscle)			
Plexus lumbalis (Rr. musculares)	Body of the XIIth thoracic and Ist lumbar vertebrae	Fascia of the M. iliopsoas, Arcus iliopectineus, iliopectineal arch	*Lumbar spine:* • Lateral flexion

The adductor group also belongs to the thigh muscles, because they are located medially of the femur. Other muscles of the thigh also move the hip joint; however, since in contrast to the adductor group, their main function is the movement of the knee they will be dealt with there.

Ventral muscles

All the ventral muscles together form the **M. iliopsoas** (➤ Fig. 5.16, ➤ Table 5.4). Their joint terminal tendon is inserted at the trochanter minor of the Femur. The muscles run ventral to the hip joint, so their main function is the flexion of the joint. The M. iliopsoas is the most important muscle for doing this. The muscle also plays a role in external rotation, especially when flexing the thigh.

--- Clinical remarks ---

Failure of the M. iliopsoas leads to discomfort when walking, as flexion in the hip joint is compromised. Furthermore, in the case of bilateral paralysis of the muscle, straightening of the upper body with the hip joint from the reclined position is no longer possible.

Dorsolateral muscles

The dorsolateral muscles form the superficial muscle group of the gluteal region. The bulky **M. gluteus maximus** (➤ Fig. 5.17, ➤ Table 5.5) is responsible for the expression of the relief of the gluteal region. All of its fibres run dorsal to the transverse axis of the hip

joint, making it the *most important extensor* and essential for extension from the flexed position. The cranial parts cross the hip joint above the sagittal axis, while the caudal part crosses underneath it. Therefore, the top half of the muscle carries out abduction movements, whereas the bottom half takes part in adduction. Due to its location on the dorsal side of the longitudinal axis, the M. gluteus maximus is the *most important external rotator.* In addition to its attachment to the femur, the M. gluteus maximus is also attached to the Tractus iliotibialis. This is a reinforcement of the thigh fascia (Fascia lata) on the lateral side, which inserts below the Condylus lateralis of the tibia. The Tractus iliotibialis is tasked with reducing the flexural stresses that act on the femoral neck, like a tension spring.

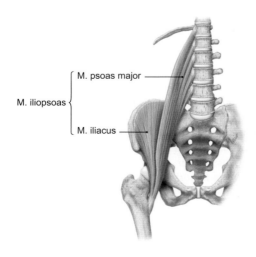

Fig. 5.16 Ventral muscles of the hip joint. Ventral view.

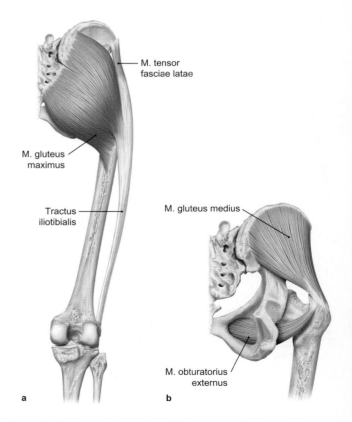

Fig. 5.17 Dorsolateral muscles of the hip joint. Dorsal view. **a** Superficial layer. **b** Deep layer.

In the case of **paralysis of the M. gluteus maximus** extension in the hip joint is extremely limited. This is particularly evident when climbing stairs, because here the leg needs to be stretched out from the flexed position. In the event of the muscle malfunctioning, this is no longer possible because it is vital to lift the entire body weight.

The **M. gluteus medius** and the **M. gluteus minimus** form a functional unit and are also referred to as the 'small gluteals' (➤ Fig. 5.17, ➤ Fig. 5.18, ➤ Table 5.5). They originate to the front of and cranial to the Facies glutea of the hip and pull forward laterally to the Trochanter major below. This makes them the most important abductors. As a majority of the fibres are located ventral to the longitudinal axis, these muscles are also the most important medial rotators.

The muscles are essential for walking upright. When walking, one leg remains stable on the ground (standing leg), while the other leg

swings forward (free leg). When doing so, the M. gluteus medius and M. gluteus minimus prevent the hip from descending down to the free leg, in order for the pelvic ring to remain horizontally aligned.

A **lesion of the N. gluteus superior** can arise when an intramuscular injection is administered incorrectly into the gluteal region leading to failure of the M. gluteus medius and M. gluteus minimus. Weakening of the muscles is the long-term effect of hip dysplasia with luxation (see above). The muscles are usually actively insufficient as they cannot be shortened enough due to the femoral head being positioned too high. This prevents powerful abduction. In these cases, the patients are not able to stand on the leg of the injured side (biomechanically impossible) and when walking, they suffer primarily from a disturbed movement pattern. The hip descends towards the side of the contralateral (!) free leg side since, due to muscle failure, the pelvic ring can no longer be kept in the horizontal plane (TRENDELENBURG's sign). In order to compensate for this descent when walking, the trunk flexes to the side of the lesion laterally, in order to shift the body's centre of gravity and prevent the hip from descending. This characteristic gait is called the 'DUCHENNE limp'.

The **M. tensor fasciae latae** has a short muscle belly ending in the Tractus iliotibialis (➤ Fig. 5.17, ➤ Table 5.5). Thus, the M. tensor fasciae latae not only acts on the hip joint (flexion, abduction, internal rotation), but also stabilises the knee in the extended position and supports tensing.

Pelvitrochanteric (medial) muscles
The pelvitrochanteric muscles lie caudal to the M. gluteus medius and M. gluteus minimus (➤ Fig. 5.18, ➤ Table 5.6). They are all lateral rotators of the hip joint, because they run behind the longitudinal axis. Their course is sometimes very complicated. The **M. obturatorius internus** arises on the medial side of the hip bone at

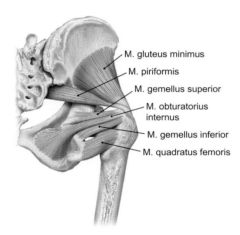

Fig. 5.18 Pelvitrochanteric muscles. Dorsal view.

- M. gluteus minimus
- M. piriformis
- M. gemellus superior
- M. obturatorius internus
- M. gemellus inferior
- M. quadratus femoris

Table 5.5 Dorsolateral muscles of the hip joint.

Innervation	Origins	Attachment	Function
M. gluteus maximus			
N. gluteus inferior	• Facies glutea of the Os ilium dorsal to the Linea glutea posterior • Facies posterior of the Os sacrum • Fascia thoracolumbalis • Lig. sacrotuberale	• Cranial part: Tractus iliotibialis • Caudal part: Tuberositas glutea	*Hip joint:* • Extension *(most important muscle)*, external rotation *(most important muscle)* • Cranial part: abduction • Caudal part: adduction *Knee joint:* • Stabilisation in the extended position • Tensing of the femur
M. gluteus medius and minimus			
N. gluteus superior	Facies glutea of the Os ilium: • M. gluteus medius: between the Lineae gluteae anterior and posterior • M. gluteus minimus: between the Lineae gluteae anterior and inferior	Tip of the Trochanter major	*Hip joint:* • Abduction *(most important muscle)* • Ventral portion: flexion, internal rotation *(most important muscle)* • Dorsal part: extension, external rotation
M. tensor fasciae latae			
N. gluteus superior	Spina iliaca anterior superior	Via Tractus iliotibialis, tibia below the Condylus lateralis	*Hip joint:* • Flexion • Abduction • Medial rotation *Knee joint:* • Stabilisation in the extended position • Tensing of the femur

the Membrana obturatoria. It enters through the Foramen ischiadicum minus, redirected at the Corpus ossis ischii in the area of the Incisura ischiadica minor and inserts at the Trochanter major. The **Mm. gemelli** adhere to it.

An important orientation mark is the **M. piriformis.** It is always recognisable due to its conical shape, after dissecting the M. gluteus maximus. Above and below the muscle there are 2 openings, the Foramen suprapiriforme and Foramen infrapiriforme, which are used by various vessels and nerves as an exit point from the lesser pelvis (➤ Chap. 5.10.3). The cranially lying M. piriformis is abducted in the hip joint while the caudally located **M. quadratus femoris** and the **M. obturatorius externus** are involved in adduction. The M. obturator externus is assigned in developmental terms to the adductor group (see below) and therefore is the only muscle innervated by the Plexus lumbalis.

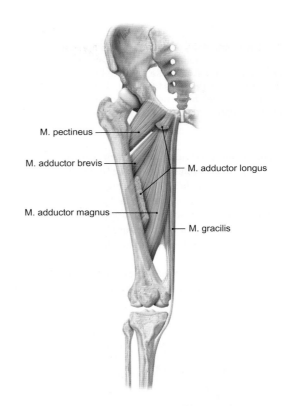

N O T E

All pelvitrochanteric muscles are for external rotation. Hence **failure of these muscles** results in weakened movement; however, the most important external rotator is the M. gluteus maximus.

Adductor group

The **adductor muscles with their origin** occupy the entire lower portions of the hip bones around the Foramen obturatum (➤ Fig. 5.19, ➤ Table 5.7). In addition to their main function, the adduction of the hip joint, all the muscles contribute to flexion and external rotation, because they run ventrally and medially over the hip joint to the rear of the femur. Only the dorsal portions of the M. adductor magnus are behind the transverse axis, so that they stretch into the hip joint. The **M. gracilis** is the only twin-articulated muscle of this group so that it also operates the knee joint (flexion, internal rotation). The adductor group has an important function for balance when standing on one leg. The forces which are exerted by the abductors are balanced out, and are therefore also essential when walking.

The **various muscles** of the adductor group are not easy to differentiate. Furthest lateral and cranial is the small M. pectineus. Medial and caudal from it is the M. adductor longus, followed by the M. gracilis. Behind the M. adductor longus are the M. adductor brevis (cranial) and the M. adductor magnus (caudal). Between the

Fig. 5.19 Adductor muscles of the hip joint. Ventral view.

two attachments of the M. adductor magnus (Labium mediale of the Linea aspera and medial femoral epicondyle) there is an opening. This **Hiatus adductorius** is used by the A. and V. femoralis as the passage to the hollow of the knee.

┌─ **Clinical remarks** ──────────────────

The adductor muscles can be irritated and injured by sudden, extreme abduction movements (e. g. lunging tackle in football), which is often referred to as **'groin strain'**. Permanent

Table 5.6 Pelvitrochanteric muscles of the hip joint.

Innervation	Origins	Attachment	Function
M. piriformis			
Plexus sacralis (Rr. musculares)	Facies pelvica of the Os sacrum	Tip of the Trochanter major	*Hip joint:* • Lateral rotation • Abduction
M. obturatorius internus			
Plexus sacralis (Rr. musculares)	Bony margin of the Foramen obturatum, medial fascia of the Membrana obturatoria	Tip of the Trochanter major	*Hip joint:* • External rotation
Mm. gemelli superior and inferior			
Plexus sacralis (Rr. musculares)	• M. gemellus superior: Spina ischiadica • M. gemellus inferior: Tuber ischiadicum	Tendon of the M. obturatorius internus	*Hip joint:* • External rotation
M. quadratus femoris			
Plexus sacralis (Rr. musculares)	Tuber ischiadicum	Crista intertrochanterica	*Hip joint:* • External rotation • Adduction
M. obturatorius externus			
N. obturatorius	Bony margin of the Foramen obturatum, Facies lateralis of the Membrana obturatoria	Fossa trochanterica	*Hip joint:* • External rotation • Adduction

Table 5.7 Adductor of the hip joint.

Innervation	Origins	Attachment	Function
M. pectineus			
N. femoralis and N. obturatorius	Pecten ossis pubis	Trochanter minor and Linea pectinea of the femur	*Hip joint:* • Adduction • Flexion • External rotation
M. gracilis			
N. obturatorius	Corpus ossis pubis, Ramus inferior ossis pubis	Condylus medialis of the tibia ('Pes anserinus superficialis')	*Hip joint:* • Adduction • Flexion • External rotation *Knee joint:* • Flexion • Inner rotation
M. adductor brevis			
N. obturatorius	Ramus inferior ossis pubis	Proximal third of the Labium mediale of the Linea aspera	*Hip joint:* • Adduction • Flexion • External rotation
M. adductor longus			
N. obturatorius	Os pubis up to the symphysis	Middle third of the Labium mediale of the Linea aspera	*Hip joint:* • Adduction • Flexion • External rotation
M. adductor magnus[1]			
• Main part: N. obturatorius • Dorsal part: tibial portion of the N. ischiadicus	• Main part: Ramus inferior ossis pubis, Ramus ossis ischii • Dorsal part: Tuber ischiadicum	• Proximal two thirds of the Labium mediale of the Linea aspera, • Epicondylus medialis of the femur, • Septum intermusculare vastoadductorium	*Hip joint:* • Adduction • External rotation • Main part: flexion • Dorsal part: extension

[1] *An incomplete proximal splitting of the M. adductor magnus is known as the M. adductor minimus*

contraction (spastic paralysis) of the adductor muscles can be observed, e.g. after neonatal brain damage (e. g. LITTLE's disease). This results in standing and walking no longer being possible.

5.3.5 Fascia lata and Tractus iliotibialis

The **Fascia lata** surrounds the muscles of the gluteal region and the thigh. This very stable connective tissue sheath is attached proximally at the pubic bone, at the inguinal ligament, iliac crest and on the sacrum. It extends distally over the knee joint and passes over the muscle fascia of the lower leg, the Fascia cruris. On the outside it is reinforced by the radiation of the end tendons of the M. gluteus maximus and M. tensor fasciae latae. This cord, called the **Tractus iliotibialis,** inserts lateral to the tibia and works on the principle of tension (see above).

Two strong septa of connective tissues as part of the Fascia lata divide the flexor side from the extensor side on the upper thigh: the Septum intermusculare femoris mediale is located medially, the Septum intermusculare femoris laterale forms the septum on the outside. The end tendon of the M. adductor magnus radiates into the Septum intermusculare vastoadductorium which is involved in the limitation to the adductor canal (➤ Chap. 5.10.2).

5.4 Lower leg

Skills

After working through this chapter, you should be able to:
• show the bony structures of the leg as well as the structure and function of the knee joint in a dissected specimen
• describe the course of internal and external ligaments of the knee joint and their positioning to the joint capsule, as well as the symptoms and principles of clinical tests in cases of damage to these ligaments
• explain the functions of the ligaments in relation to the position of the knee joint
• understand the design, function and blood supply of the menisci as well as their relationship with the collateral ligaments
• show all of the muscles of the knee joint with their origin, attachment and function on a skeleton or dissected specimen

5.4.1 Bones of the leg

As on the forearm, the skeleton of the lower leg (Crus) is formed by 2 bones (➤ Fig. 5.20):
• Shin bone **(Tibia)**
• Fibula

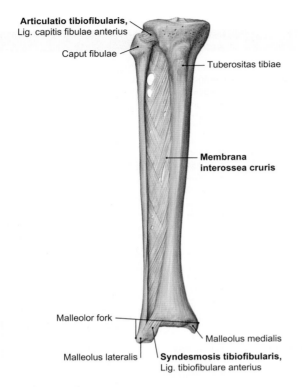

Articulatio tibiofibularis,
Lig. capitis fibulae anterius

Caput fibulae

Tuberositas tibiae

Membrana
interossea cruris

Malleolor fork

Malleolus medialis

Malleolus lateralis

Syndesmosis tibiofibularis,
Lig. tibiofibulare anterius

Fig. 5.20 Bones of the lower leg and joint connections. Ventral view.

Proximally, both bones are connected by the Articulatio tibiofibularis, and distally connected by the Syndesmosis tibiofibularis. Both bones come together to form the ankle joint (Articulatio talocruralis).

Tibia

The tibia is in cross-section a triangular bone, which is flat and runs proximally. On the shaft (**Corpus**) 3 surfaces can be distinguished, (**Facies lateralis, medialis and posterior**) and 3 edges (**Margines anterior, lateralis and interosseus**). The Facies medialis and the Margo anterior lie just beneath the skin and are easily palpated. The Tuberositas tibiae acts as the attachment of the M. quadriceps femoris via the Lig. patellae. There is a crest located on the Facies posterior with the **Linea musculi solei** as the origin for the M. soleus. The **'tibial plateau'** is formed by both tibial condyles (**Condylus medialis and lateralis**). On the upper side there is an elevation, the **Eminentia intercondylaris** with the Tuberculum intercondylare mediale and laterale. In the front middle of the plateau lies the **Area intercondylaris anterior,** behind the **Area intercondylaris posterior.** Both condyles together bear the Facies articularis superior at the top as a joint surface for the knee joint. At the distal end of the tibia, the articular surface for the ankle (Facies articularis inferior) is found. Medially, the inner ankle (**Malleolus medialis**) can be well palpated; its Facies articularis malleoli medialis also plays a role in the structure of the ankle joint.

Fibula

The fibula like the tibia, has 3 sides and 3 edges (**Facies lateralis, medialis** and **posterior; Margines anterior, posterior** and **interosseus**). Proximal of the corpus there is a neck section (**Collum fibulae**) and the fibular head (**Caput fibulae**). This articulates with the Condylus lateralis of the tibia. The distal end of the fibula is formed by the outer ankle (**Malleolus lateralis**), which bears the Facies articularis malleoli lateralis of the upper ankle joint.

Clinical remarks

The superficial position of the tibia is used in emergency medicine to administer fluids via an **intraosseous access.** If large calibre venous access is not possible, in an emergency the tibia distal to the Tuberosita tibiae, can be drilled into and a cannula can be inserted. The fibula is used as a **bone substitute material** in oral and maxillofacial surgery. Since the fibula is not a part of the knee joint and the axial line of the leg generally only passes through the tibia, the proximal and middle sections are expendable. For example, these can be used to substitute parts of the lower jaw, which have to be removed due to a carcinoma of the oral cavity.

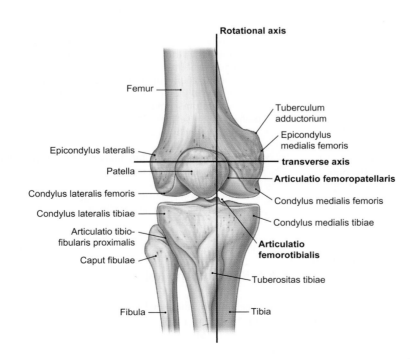

Rotational axis

Femur

Epicondylus lateralis

Patella

Condylus lateralis femoris

Condylus lateralis tibiae

Articulatio tibio-
fibularis proximalis

Caput fibulae

Fibula

Tuberculum
adductorium

Epicondylus
medialis femoris

transverse axis

Articulatio femoropatellaris

Condylus medialis femoris

Condylus medialis tibiae

**Articulatio
femorotibialis**

Tuberositas tibiae

Tibia

Fig. 5.21 Knee joint, Articulatio genus, right. Ventral view. [E460]

5.4.2 Attachments between the Tibia and Fibula

Proximally, the tibia and fibula are linked via a true joint, the **Articulatio tibiofibularis** (➤ Fig. 5.20). Due to its 2 ligaments **(Ligg. capitis fibulae anterius and posterius)** this joint is an *amphiarthrosis* and does not have a wide range of movement.

The tibia and fibula are coupled with each other via the flat **Membrana interossea cruris.** This spans the two Margines interosseae of both bones. The distal end of the membrane closes the gap at the contact surface between the tibia and fibula, called the **distal tibiofibular joint.** Therefore, this is a syndesmosis **(Syndesmosis tibiofibularis).** This is also reinforced by 2 ligaments, the **(Ligg. tibiofibularia anterius and posterius)** by the connection of the ankle to the 'fork' of the malleolus.

5.4.3 Knee joint

In the knee (Articulatio genus) joint one of the femoral condyles is articulated with the tibial condyles and the other with the rear surface of the Patella. Thus the knee joint can be divided into 2 parts, referred to as the **Articulatio femorotibialis** and **Articulatio femoropatellaris** (➤ Fig. 5.21). The joint capsule encloses both parts of the joint.

The cylindrical **femoral condyles** are not round when viewed from the side, they are horizontally ovoid (➤ Fig. 5.22). The curvature of the articular surface is towards dorsal. This means that in the extended position, the contact area towards the tibia is greater than in a flexed position.

The joint surfaces of the two **tibial condyles** are shaped differently. The Condylus medialis is slightly recessed (concave), whereas the Condylus lateralis is flat or even slightly convex in shape.

This poor fit (congruence) between the curved joint surfaces of the femur and its counterpart of the 'tibial plateau' is balanced out by the menisci composed of fibrous cartilage (➤ Fig. 5.22).

Knee cap (Patella)

The patella is shaped somewhat like a tear drop, with its tip pointing distally (Apex patellae) and a proximally located curved Basis patellae (➤ Fig. 5.21). The posterior side has a **Facies articularis** in order to connect with both condyles of the femur. With its **Facies anterior** it is embedded in the terminal tendon of the M. quadriceps femoris. Distally from the patella, the tendon is referred to as the Lig. patellae, which is attached to the Tuberositas tibiae. Thus the patella is a *sesamoid bone* and serves as a hypomochlion for the tendon of the M. quadriceps femoris. Thus, it gains greater distance from the transverse axis of the knee joint, so the torque of the muscle is significantly increased by the extended virtual lever arm. When standing, the patella is positioned on the Facies patellae of the femoral condyles and thus largely above the joint gap between the femur and the tibia.

Joint capsule

The joint capsule surrounds the cartilage-coated parts of the joint surfaces of the femur and tibia, creating a space of a few millimetres around it. The knee cap with the Lig. patellae is embedded in the front wall of the capsule. The capsule extends ventrally upwards under the tendon of the M. quadriceps femoris **(Recessus suprapatellaris).** Strictly speaking, this is a bursa (Bursa suprapatellaris), but is usually found directly connected with the joint capsule. The **Membrana fibrosa and Membrana synovialis** are points not closely linked at all points; instead they are separated by large sections (➤ Fig. 5.23). At the front beneath the patella, the space between the two layers is filled by a fat body (Corpus adiposum infrapatellare, HOFFA's fat pad). Outwardly this has folds (Plicae alares) and is connected via the strap-shaped Plica infrapatellaris to the anterior cruciate ligament. Also dorsally the two sheets of the joint capsule differ from each other. The **Membrana synovialis** passes deep into the joint up to the anterior cruciate ligament. Thus, the **cruciate ligaments** are positioned *extrasynovially* between the two sheets of the joint capsule.

Clinical remarks

Knee joint effusion, i.e. increased fluid in the joint capsule, is relatively common. It can exist, for example, due to acute injury (fractures, meniscal lesions), inflammation (e.g. rheumatoid arthritis) or degenerative processes (arthrosis). In order to confirm joint effusion by clinical examination, firstly the Recessus suprapatellaris is stretched out from proximal to distal. Where large amounts of fluid have collected, this leads to the phenomenon of the 'floating patella' (➤ Fig. 5.24). When applying pressure on the kneecap, momentary resistance is felt as the patella 'swims' on the articular effusion. Smaller effusions can be detected reliably by ultrasound.

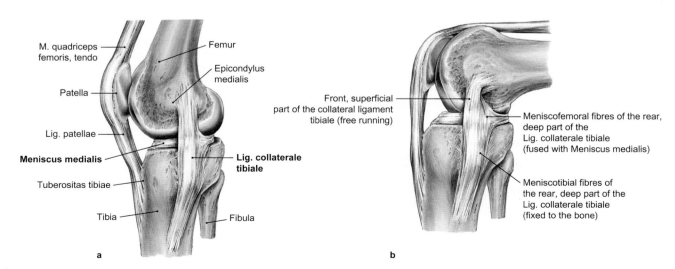

Fig. 5.22 Knee joint, Articulatio genus, right. Medial view. **a** Extended position, **b** flexed position.

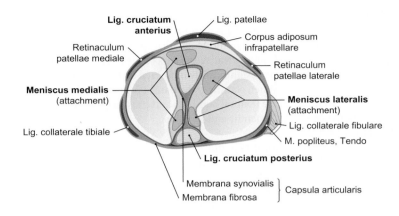

Fig. 5.23 Schematic representation of the joint capsule of the knee joint. Proximal view. [L126]

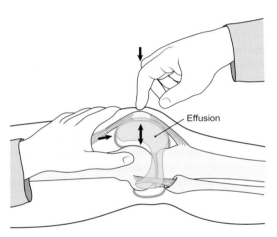

Fig. 5.24 Clinical examination of an articular effusion of the knee Lateral view. [L126]

Menisci

The menisci, primarily made up of fibrous cartilage, are designed to reduce irregularities between the joint surfaces of the knee. From a proximal view the **Meniscus medialis** is somewhat oval and shaped like a big 'C', whereas the smaller **Meniscus lateralis** is more rounded (➤ Fig. 5.25). Viewed in *cross-section*, the menisci are wedge-shaped, with the thicker edged zone on the outside running into the flat internal zone. The thickness of the lateral meniscus is largely the same; however the medial meniscus in its rear sections (posterior horn) is much thicker than at the front (anterior horn). The ends of the medial meniscus are attached to the Tubercula intercondylaria of the Eminentia intercondylaris and to the Areae intercondylaria. The corresponding fibres are also referred to as 'Ligg. meniscotibialia anterius and posterius'. The **medial meniscus** is also fused together with the **medial collateral ligament** of the knee joint. The **lateral meniscus** with its horns is also attached to the Areae intercondylaria and via the Ligg. meniscofemoralia

anterius and posterius by the cruciate ligaments. It is *not* fused with the lateral collateral ligament of the knee. On the ventral side, both menisci are joined by the Lig. transversum genus.

The 'tibial plateau' is enlarged into a joint surface by menisci joined together by ligaments, and has 2 cup-like indentations.

The menisci are supplied by branches of the **A. poplitea** (➤ Fig. 5.26a). The Aa. inferiores lateralis and medialis genus and the A. media genus are of particular significance here. The vessels and its branches form a perimeniscal vascular network which enters from the outside into the meniscus. The vessels particularly supply the thicker edge zone of the menisci, whereas the internal sections are fed by diffusion via the synovial fluid (arrows in ➤ Fig. 5.26b).

Clinical remarks

Due to its strong attachment and its inhomogeneous shape, the internal meniscus is more susceptible to injury. Typically, **injuries** arise due to a sudden rotation in the flexed position (e.g. the twisting of skis in a squatting position on the slopes), in which the stronger fixed inner meniscus cannot deal with the sliding movement needed for the rotation. This creates new fissures or pre-existing degenerative changes increase to become fissures (➤ Fig. 5.27). Less commonly, even whole fragments may shear off and for example, can prevent the extension of the joint by becoming trapped between the joint bodies. Knee arthroscopy is required to remove the fragments. When the inner meniscal lesion is combined with other injuries, these are often lesions of the internal ligaments and the anterior cruciate ligament and referred to as the 'unhappy triad'. Transverse and longitudinal tears can also appear due to **degenerative changes.** Small tears may become bigger over time. If there is a tear in the well-perfused marginal zone, it is often still possible for spontaneous healing to take place. In the more poorly-supplied internal areas, this is more unlikely. Meniscal lesions may lead to osteoarthritis of the knee joint (gonarthrosis); however, in the case of degenerative changes, whether an operation to (partially) remove the menisci improves clinical outcomes is still currently under discussion.

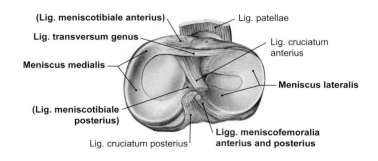

Fig. 5.25 Menisci. Proximal view.

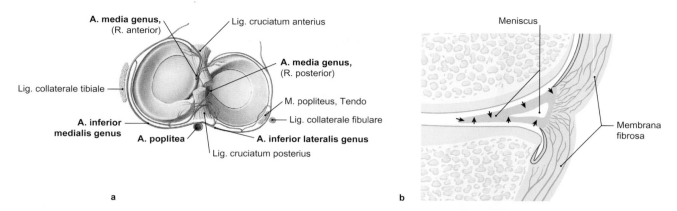

Fig. 5.26 Blood supply to the menisci. a Proximal view. **b** Cross-section. [L126]

Ligaments of the knee joint
Differentiation is made between 3 groups of ligaments:
- Cruciate ligaments (inner ligaments)
- Collateral ligaments (outer ligaments)
- Additional ligaments to strengthen the capsule

Cruciate ligaments
The cruciate ligaments (Ligg. cruciata) are positioned within the joint gap between the femur and tibia (➤ Fig. 5.28); however, they are not freely exposed within the joint cavity but are surrounded by the Membrana synovialis of the joint capsule. Thus they are positioned between the two sheets of the joint capsule. Therefore, its position is referred to as intracapsular but extrasynovial (➤ Fig. 5.23).

The **anterior cruciate ligament (Lig. cruciatum anterius)** runs from the inner surface of the lateral femoral condyle to the Area intercondylaris anterior to the tibia and, therefore, runs from the rear lateral above to ventromedial below (like a hand in a coat pocket).
The **posterior cruciate ligament (Lig. cruciatum posterius)** runs from the inner surface of the medial femoral condyle to the Area intercondylaris posterior of the tibia therefore, from frontal medial above to rear lateral below.

> **N O T E**
> Course of the cruciate ligaments:
> - Lig. cruciatum anterius: 'Like a hand in the coat pocket' (posterior lateral top to ventromedial below)
> - Lig. cruciatum posterius: in the opposite direction (ventromedial top to posterior lateral below)

Collateral ligaments
The collateral ligaments (Ligg. collateralia) are located on the outside of the knee (➤ Fig. 5.29).
The **Lig. collaterale tibiale** (inner ligament, medial ligament) is relatively wide and runs from the Epicondylus medialis of the femur to the medial surface of the tibial plateau (also ➤ Fig. 5.22). It is joined both to the joint capsule and to the interior meniscus.
The narrow **Lig. collaterale fibulare** (outer ligament, lateral ligament) connects the lateral epicondyle of the femur with the head of the fibula. In contrast to the medial collateral ligament, it is joined neither to the meniscus nor to the joint capsule. The gap between capsule and the ligament is filled by the M. popliteus and the Lig. popliteum arcuatum (➤ Fig. 5.23). An additional ligament from the lateral epicondylus of the femur to the Condylus lateralis of the tibia is called the anterolateral ligament (ALL).

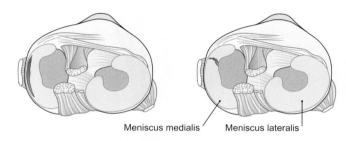

Fig. 5.27 Lesions of the inner meniscus. Proximal view. [L126]

Additional ligaments to strengthen the capsule
Multiple ligaments reinforce the Membrana fibrosa of the joint capsule:
- The **Lig. patellae** extends the tendon of the M. quadriceps femoris tibae from the patella to the Tuberositas tibae.
- The **Retinacula patellae** (mediale and laterale) are split-offs from the tendon of the M. quadriceps femoris on each side of the patella (➤ Fig. 5.29) and have superficial longitudinal and deep transverse parts.
- The **Lig. popliteum obliquum** is a split-off from the terminal tendon of the M. semimembranosus and runs on the dorsal side of the capsule from medial above to lateral below.
- The **Lig. popliteum arcuatum** also runs in an arched shape on the rear wall of the capsule to the Caput fibulae.

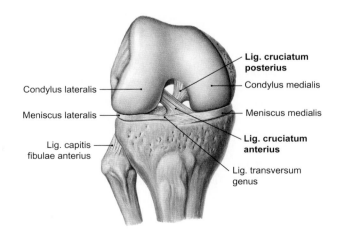

Fig. 5.28 Cruciate ligaments, Ligg. cruciata, right. Ventral view in knee flexion.

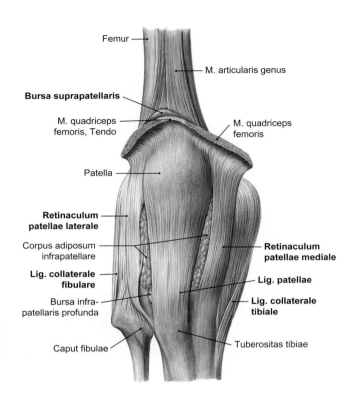

Fig. 5.29 Lateral ligaments, Ligg. collateralia, right. Ventral view.

Bursae of the knee joint

In the knee region there are many synovial bursae (Bursae synoviales) (➤ Fig. 5.30). These bursae serve as bearings and as a rule underpin the tendons of the muscles. Some are associated with the joint capsule, such as the **Bursa suprapatellaris** under the tendon of the M. quadriceps femoris or the **Bursa subpoplitea** beneath the M. popliteus. Additionally, other bursae act as shock absorbers when bearing a load, e.g. when kneeling (Bursa subfascialis prepatellaris in front of the patella or the Bursa infrapatellaris profunda under the Lig. patellae) or as slide bearings for origin and attachment tendons (Bursa m. semimembranosi, Bursae subtendineae musculi gastrocnemii medialis and lateralis).

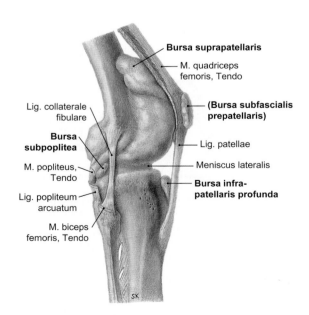

Fig. 5.30 Bursae of the knee joint, right side. Lateral view.

> ## Clinical remarks
>
> Heavy loads placed on the knee, e.g. jobs requiring frequent kneeling (tilers, road construction etc.) can lead to inflammation of the synovial bursae **(bursitis)**. Chronic bursitis is recognised as an occupational disease. Also chronic joint inflammation such as that found in rheumatic diseases can cause enlargement or the fusion of bursae, which appear as swollen masses in the popliteal fossa as **(BAKER's cysts)**.

5.4.4 Mechanics of the knee joint

The knee joint is a bicondylar joint. Movements in the joint is possible in 2 different axes (➤ Fig. 5.31a, ➤ Table 5.8):
- **Transversal axis:** flexion/extension
- **Longitudinal axis:** internal/external rotation

This means that functionally it is a *hinge-pivot joint*. Unlike the hip joint, flexion here does not mean bending ventrally but dorsally. When rotated externally the toes point laterally and when they are rotated inwards, medially.

The **bending** movement is a combination of rolling and turning. At the beginning of bending (for example, for the first 25°) the femorial condyles roll on the tibia (like a car tyre on tarmac). Thus the femur moves backwards in relation to the tibia. In the case of strong flexion, the femoral condyle then turns on the spot (like a 'spinning' tyre). The result of this combination of sliding and rotational motion is that during the deflection movement the transverse axis does not stay in its position and moves backwards (➤ Fig. 5.31c). As the radius of curvature of the femoral condyles is smaller dorsally than ventrally, ultimately an arc-shaped displacement of the axis occurs. Further dorsal displacement of the femoral is prevented by the cruciate ligaments (➤ Table 5.9). Particularly in a flexed position, the lateral portions of the cruciate ligaments are stretched. The collateral ligaments are relaxed (➤ Fig. 5.32b). During flexion both menisci glide dorsally together with the femur condyles on the plateau. Here, the lateral meniscus travels the largest distance.

The movements of the femur in relation to the tibia are not the same in both compartments. In the lateral condyle, rolling predominates and the medial condyle primarily performs a twisting motion. This is also a result of the more strongly fixed medial meniscus (fused at the medial collateral ligament) reducing the sliding movement dorsally.

The shape of the joint surfaces should make an **extension** possible without any problem. The two outer ligaments ➤ Table 5.9 are the primary reason for the very small range of extension (5°). Because these pass behind the transverse axis with their major attachments, they are stretched to the maximum in the extended position due to the larger ventral radius of curvature of the femoral condyles, so preventing overextension, and additionally, they prevent abduction and adduction movement and rotation (see below) (➤ Fig. 5.31, ➤ Fig. 5.32a). At the same time, the medial components of the cruciate ligaments are stretched. An extension of over 5° is referred to as 'Genu recurvatum' and can be caused, for example, by weak ligaments.

Table 5.8 Range of movement in the knee joint.

Movement	Range of movement
Extension/flexion	5°–0°–140°
External rotation/internal rotation	30°–0°–10°

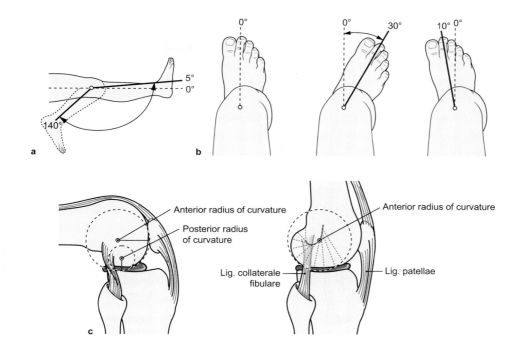

Fig. 5.31 **Range of movement in the knee joint. a** Extension/flexion. **b** External rotation/internal rotation. **c** Displacement of the transverse axis.

The rotational axis of the knee joint runs somewhat eccentrically through the Tuberculum intercondylare mediale (➤ Fig. 5.21). No rotation can be carried out in the extended position as the collateral ligaments effectively prevent this from occurring; however, in a flexed position the collateral ligaments are slack due to the smaller dorsal radius of curvature of the femoral condyles, making rotation possible.

In **internal rotation** the cruciate ligaments wrap tightly around each other and in **external rotation** away from each other. Therefore, the scope of external rotation is wider than medial rotation. The collateral ligaments are only tensed in the case of major external rotation, and prevent any further rotation (➤ Table 5.9).

Where there is complete stretching in the knee joint, so-called **final rotation** can occur. Here parts of the anterior cruciate ligament tighten, and the tibia rotates outwards by approximately 5–10°.

whereas increased mobility dorsally (posterior drawer) indicates an (old) rupture of the posterior cruciate ligament. **Examination of the collateral ligaments** must be carried out in the extended position, because the collateral ligaments must be held under tension. Adduction (enlargement of the exterior knee angle, lateral tilt) is indicative of a lesion of the Lig. collaterale fibulare. Conversely, strengthened abduction (reduction of the knee exterior angle with a medial tilt) indicates a lesion of the Lig. collaterale tibiale (➤ Fig. 5.33b).

Table 5.9 Functions of the ligaments of the knee joint.

Movement	Inhibition by
Extension	• Collateral ligaments • Cruciate ligaments (medial parts)
Flexion	• Cruciate ligaments (lateral parts)
Medial rotation	• Cruciate ligaments • Collateral ligaments (in the extended knee)
External rotation	• Collateral ligaments (in the extended and flexed knee)

Clinical remarks

A simple method for the **functional testing of the cruciate ligament** is the drawer test (LACHMAN test). With the knee in a slightly flexed position (to relax the collateral ligaments) and the foot in a fixed position, the examiner moves the proximal calf forward or backward in relation to the femur (➤ Fig. 5.33a). An abnormal ability to relocate forwards (anterior drawer) indicates an (old) injury to the anterior cruciate ligament

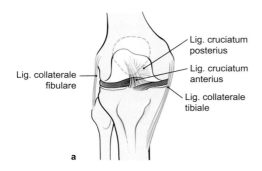

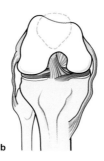

Fig. 5.32 **Stabilisation of the knee joint by cruciate and collateral ligaments, right.** Ventral view. Tensed parts of ligaments are shown in red. **a** Extended position. **b** Flexed position. [L126]

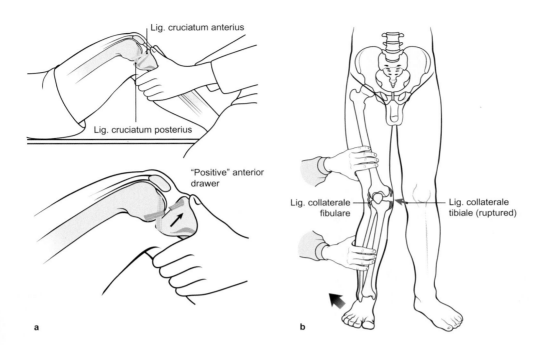

Fig. 5.33 Clinical tests to investigate the functioning of the ligaments at the knee joint.
a Examination of the anterior cruciate ligament (drawer signs). **b** Examination of the internal ligament. [L126]

5.4.5 Muscles of the knee joint

The muscles for movement in the knee joint are positioned at the thigh mainly ventrally or dorsally. Only the M. popliteus and parts of the M. triceps surae are located on the lower leg. In the latter muscle, its main function is seen in the movement of the foot, hence the M. triceps surae will be discussed there.

Ventral muscles
The ventral group is made up of only 2 muscles (➤ Fig. 5.34, ➤ Table 5.10):
- M. quadriceps femoris
- M. sartorius

The most important movement performed by the **M. quadriceps femoris** is the extension of the knee. It is the only muscle capable of performing this function. Its 4 sections make up the majority of the thigh's muscle mass. It is inserted predominantly via its terminal

tendons attached to the patella and the Lig. patellae to the Tuberositas tibiae. In addition, attachments are located over the Retinacula patellae lateral to the Tuberositas tibiae. Only one part of the M. quadriceps femoris, the **M. rectus femoris,** is a double-hinged muscle, and in addition, performs flexion in the hip joint.

> **NOTE**
> Since the **M. quadriceps femoris** is mainly supplied by spinal cord segment **L3** , it is a **reference muscle** for damage to this segment. In addition, if the patellar reflex is reduced, an impact onto the Lig. patellae will trigger an extension movement in the knee.

The **M. sartorius** is a long lean muscle, which goes from lateral above at an oblique angle to medially down to the Condylus medialis of the tibia (➤ Fig. 5.34, ➤ Table 5.10). Together with a muscle coming from dorsal, the M. semitendinosus, and the M. gracilis (from the adductor group), its end tendon forms a tendon com-

Table 5.10 Ventral muscles of the knee joint.

Innervation	Origins	Attachment	Function
Quadriceps femoris			
N. femoralis	*M. rectus femoris:* • Spina iliaca anterior inferior • Cranial edge of the acetabulum *M. vastus medialis:* • Labium mediale of the Linea aspera *M. vastus lateralis:* • Trochanter major • Labium laterale of the Linea aspera *M. vastus intermedius:* • Facies anterior of the femur	• Patella • Tuberositas tibiae over Lig. patellae • Areas to the side of the Tuberositas tibiae over Retinacula patellae	F: *Hip joint* (only M. rectus femoris): flexion *Knee joint:* extension *(sole extensor!)*
M. sartorius			
N. femoralis	Spina iliaca anterior superior	Condylus medialis of the tibia ('Pes anserinus superficialis')	*Hip joint:* • Flexion • External rotation • Abduction *Knee joint:* • Flexion • Medial rotation

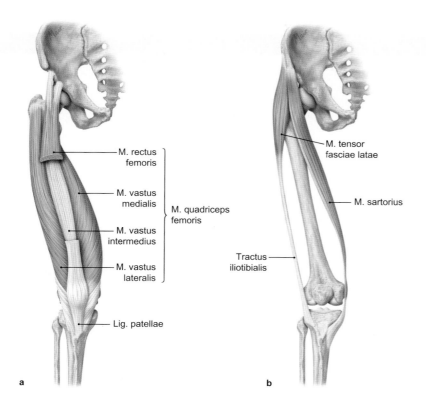

a

b

Fig. 5.34 Ventral muscles of the knee joint, right. Ventral view.
a M. quadriceps femoris.
b M. sartorius.

partment, also known as the *Pes anserinus superficialis*. Through its oblique course it crosses over all the movement axes of the hip and knee joints. It flexes and abducts in the hip joint and rotates externally. In the knee joint it plays a role in flexion and medial rotation.

Clinical remarks

In the case of **a malfunction of the M. quadriceps femoris** it is no longer possible to flex the knee. This is particularly evident in climbing stairs, as this cannot be performed. Even a slight drop of the knee cannot be stopped and the patient buckles backwards in an uncontrolled way. Impaired function of the M. sartorius is functionally insignificant, as for all of the movements it performs there are stronger muscles available.

Dorsal muscles

On the dorsal side there are 4 muscles (➤ Fig. 5.35, ➤ Table 5.11):
- M. biceps femoris
- M. semitendinosus
- M. semimembranosus
- M. popliteus

The M. biceps femoris (Caput longum), M. semitendinosus and M. semimembranosus are double-hinged muscles which run from the Tuber ischiadicum to the lower leg. Therefore, they are also referred to collectively by the term **ischiocrural muscles.** All 3 muscles bend in the hip joint and flex in the knee joint. The M. biceps femoris runs lateral to the Caput fibulae, and is the most effective external rotator. The M. semitendinosus and M. semimembranosus run medially to the Condylus medialis of the tibia. Both muscles are also medial rotators, with the M. semimembranosus being the strongest. The broad attachment of this muscle is also known as *Pes anserinus profundus*. The **M. popliteus** is also considered as one of the deep muscles of the leg (➤ Fig. 5.50b) due to its innervation by the tibial nerve; however, it only affects the knee and here is a medial rotator. It can also stretch the joint capsule, as its tendon is embedded in the Membrana fibrosa.

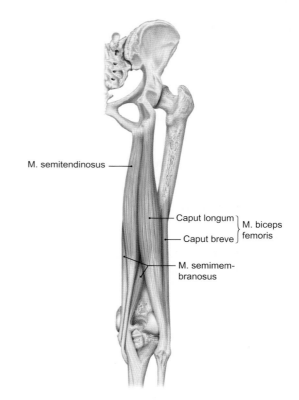

Fig. 5.35 Dorsal muscles of the knee joint, right side. Dorsal view.

Clinical remarks

When there is a **functional failure of the ischiocrural muscles,** bending and external rotation of the knee are impaired. Walking, standing and climbing stairs are however possible as long as the M. gluteus maximus is not affected (most important ex-

Table 5.11 Dorsal muscles of the knee joint.

Innervation	Origins	Attachment	Function
M. biceps femoris			
• Caput longum (twin-articulated): tibial part of the N. ischiadicus • Caput breve (single-articulated): fibular part of the N. ischiadicus	• Caput longum: Tuber ischiadicum • Caput breve: Labium laterale of the Linea aspera	Caput fibulae	*Hip joint:* • Extension • External rotation (most important muscle), adduction *Knee joint:* • Flexion • External rotation
M. semitendinosus			
Tibial portion of the N. ischiadicus	Tuber ischiadicum	Condylus medialis of the tibia ('Pes anserinus superficialis')	*Hip joint:* • Extension • Medial rotation *Knee joint:* • Flexion • Medial rotation
M. semimembranosus			
Tibial portion of the N. ischiadicus	Tuber ischiadicum	Condylus medialis of the tibia ('Pes anserinus profundus')	*Hip joint:* • Extension • Medial rotation *Knee joint:* • Flexion *(most important muscle)* • Medial rotation *(most important muscle)*
M. popliteus			
Tibial portion of the N. ischiadicus	Condylus lateralis of the femur, posterior horn of the outer meniscus	Facies posterior of the tibia above the Linea musculi solei	*Knee joint:* • Medial rotation • Prevents the meniscus from getting trapped

tensor in the hip); however, use of the M. quadriceps femoris preponderantly on the ventral side results in overstretching in the knee joint, Genu recurvatum.

In summary, the following muscles are involved in the respective movements of the knee joint (most important muscle in bold type):
- Extension:
  - **M. quadriceps femoris**
- Flexion:
  - **M. semimembranosus**
  - M. semitendinosus
  - M. biceps femoris
  - M. gracilis
  - M. sartorius
- External rotation:
  - **M. biceps femoris**
  - M. tensor fasciae latae
- Internal rotation
  - **M. semimembranosus**
  - M. semitendinosus
  - M. popliteus
  - M. sartorius
  - M. gracilis

NOTE

The **M. quadriceps femoris** is the only extensor of the knee joint. All **ischiocrural muscles** bend in the knee joint and flex in the hip joint. All muscles that have their attachment medially in the lower leg rotate inwards in the knee joint. All muscles which attach laterally rotate outwards.

5.5 Foot

Skills

After working through this chapter, you should be able to:
- indicate the bones of the foot skeleton with its main structures
- explain the construction, range of movement and mechanics of the ankle joint and the other joints of the foot
- explain the course and the function of ligaments for securing the ankle and the basic characteristics of the ligaments of the other joints of the foot
- know the structure and the importance of the arch of the foot, including the necessary ligaments and muscles
- know the muscles of the leg with origin, attachment and function, and also show them on the skeleton or dissected specimen, and name the short foot muscles and their innervation

On the foot a differentiation is made between the tarsus (**Tarsus**), the mid-foot (**Metatarsus**) and the toes (**Digiti pedis**).

The big toe is called the Hallux (Digitus primus [I]). The other toes are numbered accordingly. The second toe is the Digitus secundus (II), the third is Digitus tertius (III), the fourth is Digitus quartus (IV) and the little toe is referred to as the Digitus minimus (V). The sole of the foot (Planta pedis) has a concave shape in relation to the floor. A distinction is made between a longitudinal arch and a transverse arch. The characteristics of the arches involve the shape of the bones, the tensor ligament systems, as well as tension by muscles.

5.5.1 Bones of the foot

The skeleton of the foot is divided into the tarsal bones (**Ossa tarsi**), the metatarsal bones (**Ossa metatarsi**) and the toe bones (**Ossa digitorum, Phalanges**) (➤ Fig. 5.36). Just as in the wrist, a proximal and a distal row can be distinguished in the tarsal bones:

- Proximal row (2 bones):
  - Ankle bone (**Talus**)
  - Heel bone (**Calcaneus**)
- Distal row (5 bones):
  - **Os naviculare**
  - 3 sphenoid bones:
    - **Os cuneiforme mediale**
    - **Os cuneiforme intermedium**
    - **Os cuneiforme laterale**
  - Cuboid bone (**Os cuboideum**)

The **talus** is part of both the upper ankle joint and a joint body for the lower ankle. Above it bears the talar dome (**Trochlea tali**) as the articular surface for the upper ankle. The head (**Caput**), neck (**Collum**) and body (**Corpus**) can be distinguished. Below is the Sulcus tali, the dividing line between the front and rear chamber of the lower ankle joint. At the front on the head is the Facies articularis navicularis, below are the Facies articularis anterior and Facies articularis media, and dorsal the Facies articularis posterior, all providing joint surfaces for the lower ankle joint.

The rear section of the elongated **calcaneus** is called the **Tuber calcanei**. It has 2 raised areas, the Proc. lateralis tuberis calcanei and the Proc. medialis tuberis calcanei. The Sulcus calcanei, together with the Sulcus tali located directly above forms a tunnel, the Sinus tarsi. Medially a protrusion stands out, the **Sustentaculum tali.** The calcaneus has a total of 4 joint surfaces: at the front is the Facies articularis cuboidea, top ventral the Facies articularis talaris anterior and facies articularis talaris media and top dorsal, the Facies articularis talaris posterior.

The **Os naviculare** lies medially and articulates distally with the 3 sphenoid bones and laterally with the cuboid bone which, in turn, articulates with the calcaneus bone. The narrow end of the sphenoid bones faces plantar, creating an important requirement for the formation of the transverse arch of the foot.

With the 5 **metatarsal bones** (Ossa metatarsi) the toes are numbered from medial to lateral, from I–V. As with the hand, a distinction is made between the Basis, Corpus and Caput. A special feature is that underneath Os metatarsi I, there are typically 2 sesamoid bones located under the metatarsal bones. The Tuberositas ossis metatarsi I serves as an attachment for the M. tibialis anterior; the Tuberositas ossis metatarsi V forms the attachment for the M. fibularis brevis.

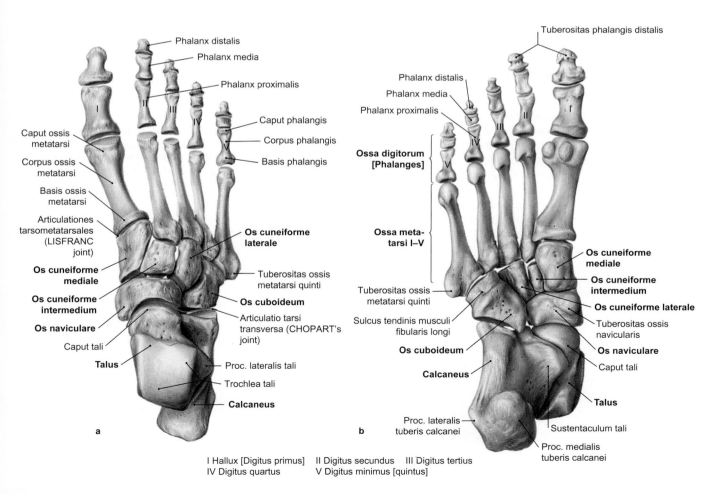

Fig. 5.36 Skeleton of the foot, right. a Dorsal view. **b** Plantar view.

I Hallux [Digitus primus]   II Digitus secundus   III Digitus tertius
IV Digitus quartus   V Digitus minimus [quintus]

A disease often occurring in pubescent girls is **KÖHLER's** disease II, in which an aseptic necrosis of generally the 2nd or 3rd metatarsal head occurs. Necrosis of the Os naviculare is called KÖHLER's disease I.

The **Hallux** consists of the proximal phalanx and distal phalanx (Phalanx proximalis and Phalanx distalis), whereas toes II–V, as with the fingers of the hand, are made up of 3 bones (Phalanx proximalis, Phalanx media and Phalanx distalis). Here, too for, each phalanx basis, corpus and caput can be distinguished.

5.5.2 Joints of the foot

The two large joints of the foot are
- Upper ankle (**Articulatio talocruralis**)
- Lower ankle (consisting of the **Articulatio subtalaris** and the **Articulatio talocalcaneonavicularis**)

Clinically, these two joints are abbreviated to UAJ and LAJ. The other joints of the tarsus and of the midfoot are referred to by the interrelated bones (Articulatio talonavicularis, Articulatio calcaneocuboidea, Articulatio cuneonavicularis, Articulationes intercuneiformes, Articulatio cuneocuboidea, Articulationes tarsometatarsales and Articulationes intermetatarsales).

The **Articulatio tarsi transversa** (between the proximal and distal rows of tarsal bones) is also known as **CHOPART's joint line.** The **Articulationes tarsometatarsales** between the tarsus and midfoot form **LISFRANC's joint line** (➤ Fig. 5.36a). The lines have a certain relevance in amputations.

The toe joints are referred to as:
- **Articulationes metatarsophalangeae**
- **Articulationes interphalangeae pedis**

Upper ankle joint

The upper ankle joint (**Articulatio talocruralis**) is the connection between the lower leg and the foot. Here the Malleolus medialis of the tibia and the Malleolus lateralis of the fibula and the distal end of the tibia articulate with the talus. The talus is slightly wider ventrally than dorsally, which is important for the stability of the ankle joint.

A differentiation is made between the **medial and lateral ligaments,** which stabilise the upper ankle joint. Located *medial* is the wide **Lig. collaterale mediale;** It is often referred to as the deltoid ligament (**Lig. deltoideum**) (➤ Fig. 5.37). It has 4 parts:
- Pars tibionavicularis
- Pars tibiocalcanea
- Pars tibiotalaris anterior
- Pars tibiotalaris posterior

On the *lateral side,* there are 3 weaker individual ligaments (➤ Fig. 5.38):
- **Lig. talofibulare anterius**
- **Lig. talofibulare posterius**
- **Lig. calcaneofibulare**

They are collectively known as the Lig. collaterale laterale, but in contrast to the deltoid ligament, do not represent a single unit. Strictly speaking, a secure attachment is only made by the ligament parts between the tibia and the fibula and the tibia and the talus except for the upper ankle. The other ligaments also stretch over the lower ankle, thus providing additional stability.

The interlocking of the tibia and fibula via the Membrana interossea cruris and the Ligg. tibiofibularia is also crucial for the stability of the upper ankle joint.

Fractures in the region of the joint surfaces of the UAJ are among the 5 most common fractures. They often affect the distal end of the fibula. The commonly used **classification according to WEBER** (➤ Fig. 5.39) categorises the breaks according to the position of the fracture of the fibula in relation to the distal tibiofibular joint (Syndesmosis tibiofibularis):
- **WEBER A:** fracture in the outer ankle distal of the syndesmosis; syndesmosis intact
- **WEBER B:** fracture at the level of the syndesmosis with injury to the tibiofibular ligaments; even the syndesmosis itself can be injured
- **WEBER C:** fracture proximal to the syndesmosis, tear in the Membrana interossea, generally including the dislocation of the syndesmosis.

Additional fractures, e.g. of the talus and the distal tibia, can also occur.

The severity of injury increases from A to C. WEBER A fractures can often be treated conservatively with just a splint. It is essential to have a stable upper ankle (joint space in the x-ray image is of the same width, ability to stand on tip-toe).

WEBER C fractures on the other hand, are highly unstable and must always be treated by an operation.

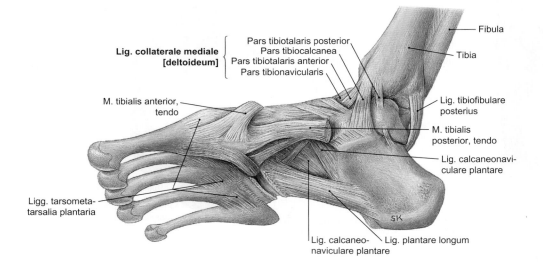

Fig. 5.37 labels: Lig. collaterale mediale [deltoideum] — Pars tibiotalaris posterior, Pars tibiocalcanea, Pars tibiotalaris anterior, Pars tibionavicularis; Fibula; Tibia; M. tibialis anterior, tendo; Lig. tibiofibulare posterius; M. tibialis posterior, tendo; Lig. calcaneonaviculare plantare; Ligg. tarsometatarsalia plantaria; Lig. calcaneonaviculare plantare; Lig. plantare longum

Fig. 5.37 Upper ankle with ligaments, right. Medial view.

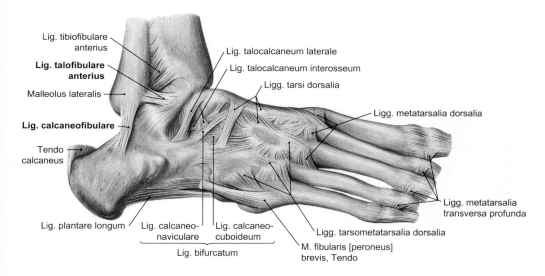

Fig. 5.38 Upper ankle with ligaments, right. Lateral view.

Lower ankle joint

The lower ankle joint is articulated by the talus, calcaneus and the Os naviculare. The joint is complicated and consists of 2 individual joints, which are separated by the Sinus tarsi (➤ Fig. 5.40):
- Articulatio subtalaris (dorsal)
- Articulatio talocalcaneonavicularis (ventral)

In the **Articulatio subtalaris** the Facies articularis calcanea posterior of the talus meets the Facies articularis talaris posterior of the calcaneus. This joint is separated from the anterior joint by the Lig. talocalcaneum interosseum, which fills the Sinus tarsi.

The **Articulatio talocalcaneonavicularis** has 3 articulating bony joint surfaces:
- Facies articularis navicularis of the talus with the Os naviculare
- Facies articulares calcanea anterior and media of the talus with the Facies articularis talaris anterior and media of the calcaneus

When observing the skeleton of the foot from plantar (➤ Fig. 5.36b), it becomes clear that there is a gaping bony gap between the calcaneus and the Os naviculare. The two bones are connected by the **socket ligament (Lig. calcaneonaviculare plantare)**. This completes the socket of the lower ankle joint (➤ Fig. 5.40). As this ligament forms part of the articular surface, its upper surface is covered with cartilage like the other bony joint surfaces.

The lower ankle is partially stabilised by the ligaments of the upper ankle joint and by the ligaments that connect the talus and calcaneus together (➤ Fig. 5.37, ➤ Fig. 5.38).

Other joints of the foot

The remaining joints of the tarsus are mainly *amphiarthroses* and are tightly braced. The corresponding ligaments generally run between two adjacent bones and so are named after these bones. Put

simply, a distinction is made between the ligaments on the dorsal side (**Ligg. tarsi dorsalia**), and on the plantar side (**Ligg. tarsi plantaria**) and the ligaments between the bones (**Ligg. tarsi interossea**). The **Lig. bifurcatum** is bifurcated (➤ Fig. 5.38) and bridges the CHOPART's joint line (Lig. calcaneonaviculare and Lig. calcaneocubideum).

Dorsal, plantar and interosseous ligaments can also be distinguished at the amphiarthroses between the tarsus and midfoot as well as between the metatarsal bones.

The toes are stabilised by plantar ligaments and collateral ligaments running along the sides.

5.5.3 Mechanics of the ankle joints

The **upper ankle joint** is a *hinge joint* (➤ Fig. 5.41). Only movements around *one axis* are possible, which runs through the tips of the two ankle bones. The corresponding movements are referred to as dorsal extension and plantar flexion. Instead of 'dorsal extension' in some books the term dorsiflexion can also be found. The upper ankle does not have equal stability in all positions. This results mainly from the differing width of the trochlea as the lower articular surface. This is wider ventrally compared to dorsally by up to 5 mm. In the *dorsiflexion position* the malleolar fork is located over the wider anterior end of the talus. The joint surfaces of the Malleolus lateralis and Malleolus medialis sit firmly on the talus on both sides. To do this, the Ligg. tibiofibularia must also yield somewhat and the 'dovetailing' of the forks are slightly spread. In the *plantarflexion position* the malleolar fork is located over the narrower dorsal end of the Trochlea tali. The joint surfaces are no longer held

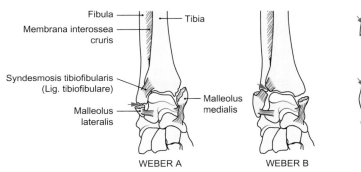
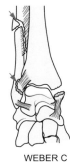

Fig. 5.39 WEBER classification of fibular fractures with involvement of the ankle joint. From left to right WEBER A, WEBER B and WEBER C fracture.

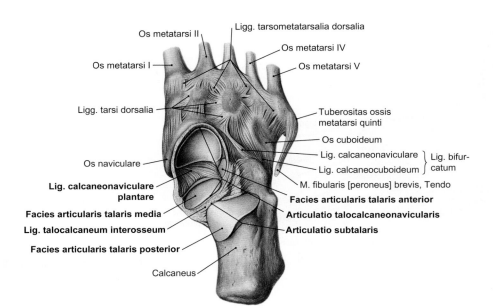

Os metatarsi II
Ligg. tarsometatarsalia dorsalia
Os metatarsi IV
Os metatarsi I
Os metatarsi V
Ligg. tarsi dorsalia
Tuberositas ossis metatarsi quinti
Os cuboideum
Os naviculare
Lig. calcaneonaviculare
Lig. calcaneocuboideum
} Lig. bifur-catum
Lig. calcaneonaviculare plantare
M. fibularis [peroneus] brevis, Tendo
Facies articularis talaris media
Facies articularis talaris anterior
Articulatio talocalcaneonavicularis
Lig. talocalcaneum interosseum
Articulatio subtalaris
Facies articularis talaris posterior
Calcaneus

Fig. 5.40 Lower ankle joint, distal surface, right. Proximal view.

taut on the talus, allowing a little more play. Stability is reduced by the poor closure of the joint in this position.

Clinical remarks

Injuries of the upper ankle joint are very common. Usually this is the classical **'sprained ankle'**, whereby the joint is 'twisted' laterally. Due to its poor stability, this 'twisting' frequently takes place in the plantar flexion position, such as when walking down hills or wearing high-heeled shoes. Here external ligaments are frequently damaged (especially the **Lig. talofibulare anterius**). Depending on the severity of injury, conservative treatment is sufficient, otherwise the ligament injury must be surgically treated.

Movement in the **lower ankle joint** always takes place in both compartments at the same time, functionally fitting together to make a unit (➤ Fig. 5.41, ➤ Table 5.12). The joint has one degree of freedom. The *axis* runs forwards and medially from the front to the rear through the Os naviculare and Talus posterior laterally

through the Tuber calcanei (➤ Fig. 5.41c). Functionally, the joint is therefore best described as an *atypical pivot joint.* Movement around this oblique axis is referred to as **inversion** and **eversion.** When looking at the axis from the rear, inversion means turning clockwise, with the rear foot being medially rotated. Conversely, eversion, means anticlockwise rotation with lateral rotation of the foot.

Inversion and eversion are not to be confused with **pronation** and **supination** (➤ Fig. 5.41). Pronation means the lifting of the lateral margin of the foot, while supination is the lifting of the medial margin of the foot. Whereas inversion/eversion only occurs around the axis of the lower ankle joint, for pronation/supination, additional movements are required in the other, mostly tightly compressed joints of the tarsus and midfoot. The Articulatio tarsi transversa ('CHOPART's joint') is not an amphiarthrosis but has greater mobility.

These additional joints as a whole allow the foot to twist in the sagittal axis (e.g. through the second toe ray). This means that the front and rear sections of the foot can easily be turned against each other. In addition, there is an elastic bone plate which exists as a

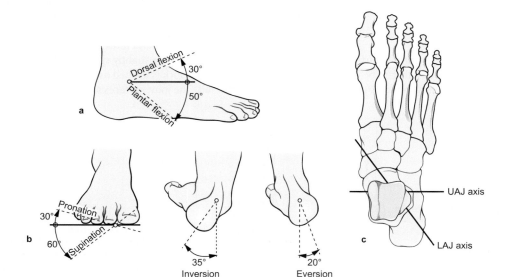

Fig. 5.41 Axes and ranges of movement of the upper and lower ankle joints.
a Dorsal flexion/plantar flexion. **b** Pronation/supination and eversion/inversion. **c** Axes of the upper and lower ankle.

Table 5.12 Range of movement in the ankle joints.

Joint	Movement	Range of movement
Upper ankle	Dorsal extension/plantar flexion	30°–0°–50°
Lower ankle	Eversion/inversion	20°–0°–35°
Lower ankle and other joints of the tarsus and metatarsus	Pronation/supination	30°–0°–60°

result of the tightly securing ligaments of this joint, especially in the area of the metatarsus, which is also able to compensate for uneven floors.

The metatarsophalangeal **joints** are *ball joints;* however, due to the tightly securing ligaments, movement is only possible in 2 axes (➤ Fig. 5.42, ➤ Table 5.13), no rotation takes place:
- Dorsal flexion/plantar flexion
- Abduction/adduction

Abduction, means spreading of the toes, whereas with adduction, the movement of the toes is to the midline of the foot. Especially in the base joint of the hallux, dorsiflexion is possible and at least passively very far (often over 90°). This is important for the rolling movement when walking.

The **middle and distal interphalangeal joints of the toes** are hinge joints. The movement is limited to relatively limited dorsiflexion and plantarflexion (➤ Fig. 5.42, ➤ Table 5.13).

Clinical remarks

Hallux valgus is a common deformity of the big toe (➤ Fig. 5.43). It leads to a valgus position in the first metatarsophalangeal joint, i.e., the angle between the longitudinal axis of metatarsal I and the Phalanx proximalis of the big toe increases. This goes hand in hand with an enlargement of the angle between the longitudinal axis of Os metatarsi I and II. Thus, the head of the metatarsal protrudes painfully medially and the tip of the big toe overlays or underlays the second toe. Often this deformity is triggered by a predisposition and the continuous wearing of footwear which is too tight with a widened forefoot (generally because of splayed foot). The modified muscle structure assists the pathology even more by the tension of the long muscle tendon of the big toe reinforcing the valgus position. As a result of lateralisation of the medial sesamoid bone, the M. abductor pollicis may even become an adductor in the base joint. Larger deformities and resulting pain must be treated by an operation.

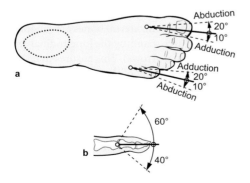

Fig. 5.42 Range of movement of the toe joints. a Abduction/adduction. **b** Dorsal flexion/plantar flexion.

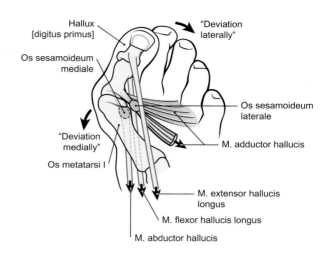

Fig. 5.43 Distal foot with Hallux valgus, right. Dorsal view. [L126]

Table 5.13 Scope of movement of the toe joints.

Movement	Range of movement
Dorsal flexion/plantar flexion	60°–0°–40°
Abduction/adduction	10°–0°–20°

5.5.4 The arch of the foot

When standing, the weight of the body is transferred via the ankle to the remaining part of the foot skeleton. Put simply, a **medial and lateral strand** can be distinguished, and these spread the load (➤ Fig. 5.44). The talus acts as a distributor, because the entire weight is placed on it via the upper ankle joint and the Trochlea tali. The medial metatarsal bones radiate out and run over the Os naviculare, Ossa cuneiforma and Ossi metatarsi I–III to the first three toes. The 4th and 5th metatarsal bones form the lateral strand through the calcaneus, the Os cuboideum and the Ossa metatarsi bones IV and V to the two outer toes.

The midfoot and tarsus are curved in a concave sense in a plantar direction. Whereas the heads of the Ossa metatarsi are positioned largely flatly, the Corpus and Basis rise up towards the tarsal bones. The apex of the **longitudinal arch** is the talus. The calcaneus, the anterior attachments of which are also raised, descends dorsally to form the posterior end of the arch. Viewed in **cross-section** an arch is most strongly formed in the area of the cuneiform bones and the cuboid bone (apex of the **transverse arch:** Os cuneiforme intermedium). These arches mean that in the normal position, only 3 bone points are in contact with the ground (➤ Fig. 5.44b):
- Tuber calcanei
- Head of the Os metatarsi I
- Head of the Os metatarsi V

The arches of the foot are formed in the course of growth with increasing requirements for standing and walking. In infants, the arch is only very slightly pronounced. Only during the first years of life does the foot skeleton elevate and completely form the transverse and longitudinal arches.

The arches of the foot are maintained in place both passively by ligaments and actively by muscles (➤ Fig. 5.45, ➤ Fig. 5.46). The **longitudinal arch** is stabilised by 3 ligament systems arranged in layers:
- **Upper layer: socket ligament** (Lig. calcaneonaviculare plantare); from the Sustentaculum tali to the Os naviculare

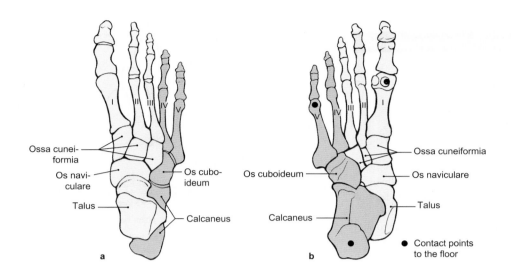

Fig. 5.44 **Bone of the arch, right. a** Dorsal view. **b** Plantar view.

a

b

● Contact points to the floor

Ossa cunei-formia

Os navi-culare

Talus

Os cubo-ideum

Calcaneus

Ossa cuneiformia

Os cuboideum

Os naviculare

Talus

Calcaneus

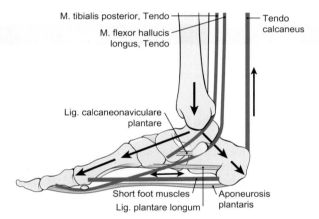

M. tibialis posterior, Tendo

M. flexor hallucis longus, Tendo

Tendo calcaneus

Lig. calcaneonaviculare plantare

Short foot muscles

Lig. plantare longum

Aponeurosis plantaris

Fig. 5.45 **Longitudinal arch of the foot, right side.** Medial view. [L126]

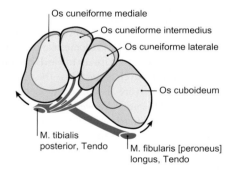

Os cuneiforme mediale

Os cuneiforme intermedius

Os cuneiforme laterale

Os cuboideum

M. tibialis posterior, Tendo

M. fibularis [peroneus] longus, Tendo

Fig. 5.46 **Transverse arch of the foot, right.** [L126]

- **Middle layer: Lig. plantare longum;** from underneath the calcaneus to the Os cuboideum and the bases of Ossi metatarsi II–V
- **Lower layer: plantar aponeurosis** (Aponeurosis plantaris); stretches between the Tuber calcanei and the heads of the Ossi metatarsi

The short foot muscles on the plantar side are important for the active tension on the longitudinal arch (➤ Fig. 5.45). Also the tendons of all deep lying calf muscles (M. flexor hallucis longus, M. flexor digitorum longus and M. tibialis posterior) work against flattening of the longitudinal arch (➤ Table 5.14). The opposing muscle here is the M. triceps surae which, by tensing via the Achilles

Table 5.14 Stabilisation of the arch of the foot.

Passive stabilisation	Active stabilisation
Longitudinal arch	
• Lig. calcaneonaviculare • Lig. plantare longum • Plantar aponeurosis	• M. flexor hallucis longus • M. flexor digitorum longus • M. tibialis posterior • Short foot muscles
Transverse arch	
Short plantar ligaments between the bones of the tarsus and metatarsus	• M. fibularis longus • M. tibialis posterior • M. adductor hallucis

tendons at the Tuber calcanei, counteracts the calcaneus from being in an excessively steep position (and thereby strengthening the longitudinal arch). Thus, it is possible by actively tensing the muscles to fine tune the arch and make adjustments to loadings.

The **transverse arch** is passively held in place by the short ligaments between the bones of the tarsus and the midfoot on the plantar side. Also contributing to its active support are the M. fibularis longus and the M. tibialis posterior (➤ Fig. 5.46) as well as the individual short foot muscles of the M. adductor hallucis (➤ Table 5.14). The M. fibularis longus is deflected at the lateral side of the cuboid bone towards the sole of the foot. It crosses underneath the foot at an angle and sets the radius of curvature at the medial ray of the foot ray so that its tension reinforces the transverse arch.

By the formation of the arch, the **load transferred** to the talus is shared and transferred to the support points. This is particularly clear in the example of the longitudinal arch, where the forces in the Tuber calcanei and the metatarsal bones are dissipated (➤ Fig. 5.45). Thus, the structures spanning the longitudinal arch are held under tension (horizontal arrows). This ensures that the arch of the foot performs a certain amount of the shock absorber function, and thus can absorb force peaks.

Clinical remarks

Flattened sections of the arch due to a failure of passive and active tension mechanisms are common diseases, which, due to incorrect weight bearing leading to a reduction in shock absorber function, can lead to severe pain and degenerative changes. A **flattening of the longitudinal arch** leads to falling of the calcaneus and the talus, referred to as **flat feet or fallen arches** (Pes planus). Often in this case, the talus buckles medially, **splay foot** (Pes valgus).

A **flattening the transverse arch** is due to the descent of the Ossi metatarsalia II–IV. This leads to a broadening of the forefoot (**splay foot,** Pes transversoplanus). In addition to the often painful additional stress of the middle metatarsal bone, it often results in Hallux valgus (see above). A strong curvature of the foot is referred to as **Pes cavus** (Pes excavatus).

A congenital club foot is the most common **foot malformation** (Pes equinovarus). Here the unstressed foot remains in the plantarflexion position and is supinated. This is the normal intrauterine position but up to the time of birth the foot generally reverts to the position found in normally developed feet.

5.5.5 Muscles of the lower leg and foot

Muscles of the talocalcaneonavicular joint
The muscles that move the foot in the joints are located in the lower ankle. Here, **three groups** can be distinguished:
- Ventral group (dorsal extensors)
- Lateral group (fibularis or peroneus group, pronators)
- Dorsal group (plantar flexors)

In the plantar flexors a superficial group is differentiated from a deep group:
- **Ventral group** (from medial to lateral)
  - M. tibialis anterior
  - M. extensor hallucis longus
  - M. extensor digitorum longus
- **Lateral group** (from proximal to distal)
  - M. fibularis longus
  - M. fibularis brevis
- **Dorsal superficial group**
  - M. triceps surae
  - M. plantaris
- **Dorsal deep group** (from medial to lateral)
  - M. flexor digitorum longus
  - M. tibialis posterior
  - M. flexor hallucis longus

Each group runs in a separate osteofibrous canal, referred to in its entirety as the Compartimenta cruris. These muscle compartments are made up of the lower leg fascia (Fascia cruris), its divisions, as

well as the bones of the leg. In particular, the extensor compartment (Compartimentum anterius) is very taut and does not allow much extra expansion.

All the long muscles pass over the upper and lower ankle joint, with most of them being inserted into the front sections of the tarsus. Thus all the muscles contribute to both flexion/extension (upper ankle joint) as well as in pronation and supination movements (lower ankle and other joints of the foot). So the function of each muscle is dependent on the course of its end tendon (➤ Fig. 5.47).

NOTE
All muscles with end tendons coursing ventral of the flexion/extension axis of the upper ankle joint are **dorsal extensors** (left figure in ➤ Fig. 5.47, red). Muscles whose tendons course dorsally to this axis are **plantar flexors** (left figure in ➤ Fig. 5.47, blue). Muscles that course medial to the axis of the lower ankle joint, are **supinators** (lifting the medial margin of the foot, right figure in ➤ Fig. 5.47, blue). All muscles whose end tendons course laterally to the axis act as **pronators** (lifting the lateral margin of the foot) (right figure in ➤ Fig. 5.47, red).

Ventral group
The most important of all the **extensors** is the **M. tibialis anterior** (➤ Fig. 5.48, ➤ Table 5.15). It originates from the lateral side of the tibia and therefore has to overlap the tibia in its distal course. Due to its attachment medial to the skeleton of the foot, it is also a supinator. Conversely, the terminal tendons of the other muscles course further laterally, so they are pronators (➤ Fig. 5.47, ➤ Table 5.15).

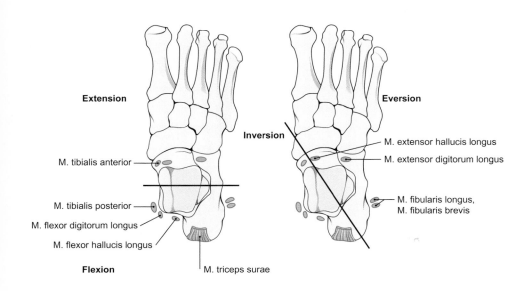

Fig. 5.47 Effect of the muscles of the lower leg on the ankle joints. Dorsal view. Course of the end tendons for the axis of the ankle joint (left) and of the lower ankle joint (right). [L126]

Table 5.15 Ventral group of the lower leg muscles.

Innervation	Origins	Attachment	Function
M. tibialis anterior			
N. fibularis profundus (N. ischiadicus)	Facies lateralis of the tibia, Fascia cruris, Membrana interossea	Os metatarsi I, Os cuneiforme mediale	• Upper ankle joint: dorsal extension *(most important muscle)* • Lower ankle: supination (weak)
M. extensor hallucis longus			
N. fibularis profundus (N. ischiadicus)	Facies medialis of the fibula, Membrana interossea, Fascia cruris	Distal phalanx of the Hallux	• Upper ankle: dorsal extension • Lower ankle: pronation (weak) • Joints of the big toe: extension
M. extensor digitorum longus			
N. fibularis profundus (N. ischiadicus)	Condylus lateralis of the tibia, Margo anterior of the fibula, Membrana interossea cruris, Fascia cruris	Dorsal aponeurosis of the 2nd–5th toes	• Upper ankle: dorsal extension • Lower ankle: pronation • Toe joints: extension

The M. extensor hallucis longus and M. extensor digitorum longus are primarily responsible for dorsal flexion in the toe joints. An occasionally occurring separation of the M. extensor digitorum longus muscle with an attachment to the Os metatarsi V is referred to as the M. fibularis tertius.

NOTE

The **M. tibialis anterior** is a **reference muscle** for segment **L4** and the **M. extensor hallucis longus** for spinal cord segment **L5**. In the case of injury to L5 (e.g. as a result of a hernia), this leads to a weakening of extension of the Hallux.

Clinical remarks

When there is damage to the muscles of the ventral group, dorsiflexion is no longer possible and the foot hangs down slackly **(equine foot position)**. Patients have to compensate by raising the thigh higher when walking, in order to avoid dragging the slack foot on the floor **(drop foot gait)**.

Lateral group

The **M. fibularis longus** derives proximally on the fibula and is located dorsal to the **M. fibularis brevis** (> Fig. 5.49, > Table 5.16). Both muscles run dorsally from the outer ankle to the foot. The M. fibularis longus in the area of the Os cuboideum transfers from the lateral margin of the foot to the sole of the foot, crosses (as viewed from plantar) under all the muscles running there and is inserted at the medial margin of the foot skeleton. It is the *strongest pronator*

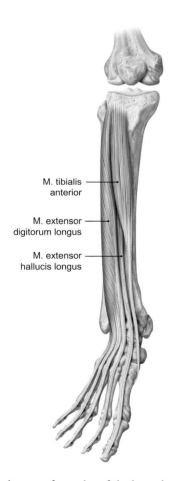

M. tibialis anterior

M. extensor digitorum longus

M. extensor hallucis longus

Fig. 5.48 Ventral group of muscles of the lower leg, right side. Ventral view.

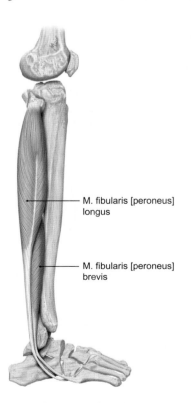

M. fibularis [peroneus] longus

M. fibularis [peroneus] brevis

Fig. 5.49 Lateral group of muscles of the leg, right side. Lateral view.

Table 5.16 Lateral group of the lower leg muscles.

Innervation	Origins	Attachment	Function
M. fibularis (peroneus) longus			
N. fibularis superficialis (N. ischiadicus)	Caput fibulae, proximal two thirds of the fibula, Fascia cruris	Tuberositas ossis metatarsi I, Os cuneiforme mediale	• Upper ankle: plantar flexion • Lower ankle: pronation *(most important muscle)*
M. fibularis (peroneus) brevis			
N. fibularis superficialis (N. ischiadicus)	Distal half of the fibula	Tuberositas ossis metatarsi V	• Upper ankle: plantar flexion • Lower ankle: pronation

and due to its course crossing over the sole area, it is involved in tension of the transverse arch. In addition to pronation, both muscles contribute to plantar flexion.

Clinical remarks

A malfunction in the fibularis group leads to the **supination position** of the foot due to the predominance of the antagonistic muscles.

Dorsal group

The calf muscles are positioned dorsally. The dorsal superficial compartment is largely enclosed by the muscle bellies of the **M. triceps surae,** made up of the two heads of the M. gastrocnemius and the M. soleus (➤ Fig. 5.50a, ➤ Table 5.17). All the end tendons converge to the **Achilles tendon (Tendo calcaneus).** This is the

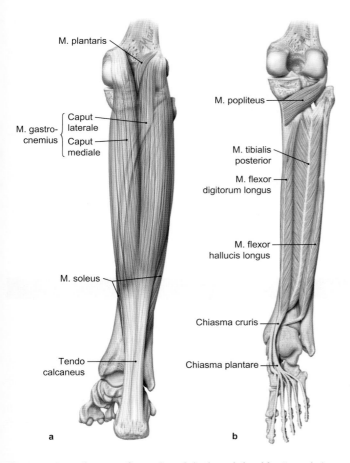

M. plantaris

M. gastrocnemius
{ Caput laterale
  Caput mediale

M. soleus

Tendo calcaneus

a

M. popliteus

M. tibialis posterior

M. flexor digitorum longus

M. flexor hallucis longus

Chiasma cruris

Chiasma plantare

b

Fig. 5.50 Dorsal group of muscles of the leg, right side. Dorsal view. **a** Superficial plantar flexors. **b** Deep plantar flexors.

strongest and thickest tendon of the human body. It is twisted in a spiral and inserts flatly onto the bottom edge of the Tuber calcanei. A bursa (**Bursa tendinis calcanei**) supports the tendon in its course along the rear edge of the calcaneus.

The M. triceps surae is the *strongest plantar flexor* and also the *strongest supinator* (the Achilles tendon inserts medial to the axis of the lower ankle joint!).

NOTE

The **M. triceps surae** is the **reference muscle** for the **S1** segment. When this segment is injured, the Achilles tendon reflex fails soon afterwards. Normally, hitting the Achilles tendon with a reflex hammer results in the contraction of the Triceps surae and hence, plantar flexion.

Its largest part, the **M. gastrocnemius,** originates at the thigh bone and can therefore also flex in the knee joint. The lateral portion of the **M. soleus** originates at the fibula, and its medial part at the tibia. Both origins are connected by a tendinous arch (Arcus tendineus m. solei), under which dorsal vessels and nerves of the leg (A./V. posterior tibialis and N. tibialis) course.

The **M. plantaris,** which is sometimes absent, only has a very short muscle belly and a long end tendon, which also radiates into the Achilles tendon. It also originates from the femur, which is why it is able to bend the knee joint weakly (➤ Table 5.17). Due to its exceptional wealth of muscle spindles (receptors for the measuring the length of a muscle) it is accorded a role in the orientation of the body in space (proprioception).

Clinical remarks

A failure of the M. triceps surae alone occurs with the **rupture of the Achilles tendon.** A chronically damaged Achilles tendon, after suffering many small injuries, can often tear under acute stress (e.g. jumping up high when playing badminton), which can clearly be heard as a bang.

In the event of malfunction of the M. triceps surae walking is difficult. In particular, **standing on tip-toe** is no longer possible, as this cannot be compensated for by the deep flexors. In addition, the arch of the foot is reinforced by the predominance of the muscles located on the sole of the foot (**Pes cavus**).

After removal of the superficial group, the relatively slender **deep flexor group** (in comparison to the M. triceps surae) is visible between the tibia and fibula (➤ Fig. 5.50b, ➤ Table 5.18). The M. flexor digitorum longus originates furthest medially, in the middle is the M. tibialis posterior and lateral the M. flexor hallucis longus. The M. flexor hallucis longus and the M. flexor digitorum longus flex all the phalangeal joints. The M. tibialis posterior is a strong supinator and braces the longitudinal and transverse arch of the foot.

Table 5.17 Dorsal superficial group of lower leg muscles.

Innervation	Origins	Attachment	Function
M. triceps surae[1]			
N. tibialis (n. ischiadicus)	• M. gastrocnemius, Caput mediale: Condylus medialis of the femur • M. gastrocnemius, Caput laterale: Condylus lateralis of the femur • M. soleus: proximal third of the fibula, Facies posterior of the tibia (Linea musculi solei), Arcus tendineus musculi solei	Tuber calcanei	• Knee joint flexion (only M. gastrocnemius) • Upper ankle joint: plantar flexion (*most important muscle*) • Lower ankle joint: supination (*most important muscle*)
M. plantaris			
N. tibialis (N. ischiadicus)	Condylus lateralis of the femur	Tuber calcanei	• Knee joint: flexion • Upper ankle joint: plantar flexion • Lower ankle joint: supination

[1] The broad tendon of the M. triceps surae is known as the ACHILLES tendon (Tendo calcaneus).

Clinical remarks

A **malfunction of the M. tibialis posterior** (e.g. as a result of a ruptured tendon) results in the foot being in a pronation position, because the supinator's counterbalance to the pronators is reduced.

A **malfunction of all flexors** (deep and superficial) leads to a rise in the tip of the foot due to the predomination of the dorsal extensors **(Pes supinatus).** Walking and standing are more difficult, rolling up of the foot is no longer possible. Patients can only move forwards on the calcaneus. When standing, it is even impossible to crouch slightly, since the failure of the flexors means that it is not possible to halt the descending movement.

All deep flexors run along the medial side of the leg and behind the inner ankle to the sole of the foot. On the way they cross over each other (➤ Fig. 5.50b): at the distal lower leg (as seen from the dorsal side) the M. flexor digitorum longus crosses over the M. posterior tibialis **(Chiasma crurale).** At the sole of the foot it then crosses over the M. hallucis longus **(Chiasma plantare).** Before attaching to the final phalanges, the M. flexor digitorum perforates the divided attachment tendons of the M. flexor digitorum brevis.

NOTE

Chiasma crurale: M. flexor **dig**itorum longus crosses over M. **tib**ialis posterior

Chiasma plantare: M. flexor **dig**itorum longus crosses over the M. flexor **hall**ucis longus.

To summarise, the following muscles are involved in the respective movements of the ankle (most important muscle highlighted in bold):

Dorsal extension:
- **M. tibialis anterior**
- M. extensor digitorum longus
- M. fibularis tertius
- M. extensor hallucis longus

Plantar flexion:
- **M. triceps surae**
- M. flexor hallucis longus
- M. tibialis posterior
- M. flexor digitorum longus
- M. fibularis longus
- M. fibularis brevis

Supination:
- **M. triceps surae**
- M. tibialis posterior
- M. tibialis anterior
- M. flexor digitorum longus
- M. flexor hallucis longus

Pronation:
- **M. fibularis longus**
- M. fibularis brevis
- M. extensor digitorum longus
- M. fibularis tertius
- M. extensor hallucis longus

Table 5.18 Dorsal deep group of the lower leg muscles.

Innervation	Origins	Attachment	Function
M. tibialis posterior			
N. tibialis (N. ischiadicus)	Membrana interossea, tibia and fibula	Tuberositas ossis navicularis, plantar aspect of the Ossa cuneiformia I–III, Ossa metatarsi II–IV	• Upper ankle joint: plantar flexion • Lower ankle joint: supination
M. flexor digitorum longus			
N. tibialis (N. ischiadicus)	Facies posterior to the tibia	Distal phalanx of the 2nd–5th toes	• Upper ankle joint: plantar flexion • Lower ankle joint: supination • Toe joints: flexion
M. flexor hallucis longus			
N. tibialis (N. ischiadicus)	Distal facies posterior to the fibula, Membrana interossea	Distal phalanx of the big toe	• Upper ankle joint: plantar flexion • Lower ankle joint: supination • Joints of the big toe: flexion

Short muscles of the foot

The short foot muscles originate at the foot skeleton and have no function in the ankle joints. Their main function is seen less in the movement of the toes than in the bracing of the plantar arch. This is clearly different in the hand where the short muscles of the hand are essential for the fine motor skills of the fingers.

The short foot muscles can be differentiated into **4 groups:**
- Muscles of the dorsum of the foot (➤ Table 5.19)
- Muscles of the big toes (➤ Table 5.20)
- Muscles of the centre of the sole of the foot (➤ Table 5.21)
- Muscles of the little toes (➤ Table 5.22)

The individual muscles of each group can be taken from the muscle tables. The functions of the toes generally correspond to the name of their respective muscle.

The **muscles of the dorsum of the foot** assist dorsiflexion in the toe joints (➤ Fig. 5.51), but do not run to the little toe. All **plantar muscles** assist with plantar flexion of the toe joints and prevent tipping forward in the toe joints when the upper body is bent forwards (➤ Fig. 5.52). In addition, they can adduct or abduct. The muscles of the foot, in their course, function and innervation, correspond to those of the hand; however, the Mm. interossei plantares run to toes 3–5 (and not 2, 4 and 5, as in the hand), and the Mm. interossei dorsales insert on both sides of the 2nd toe (instead of on the 3rd finger).

Conversely there are two muscles that do not have an equivalent in the hand:
- **M. flexor digitorum brevis:** it runs from the Tuber calcanei to the middle phalanges 2–5, thus corresponding to the M. flexor digitorum superficialis in the forearm.
- **M. quadratus plantae:** it runs from the calcaneus in the rear half of the sole of the foot to the tendon of the M. flexor digitorum longus, and supports it.

5.5.6 Support facilities of the musculature in the region of the lower leg and foot

As in the hand, the long muscles of the foot are also guided by strengthening bands (**Retinacula**) of muscle fascia, in this case the Fascia cruris. The retinacula prevent the muscle tendons from detaching from their base. In addition, the long foot muscles with their final tendons run in **tendon sheaths.** These are formed particularly in the area of the retinacula.

The **Retinaculum musculorum extensorum** spans the muscles of the extensor compartments ventrally at the level of the ankle joint, each of which is surrounded by its own tendon sheath (➤ Fig. 5.51).

Table 5.19 Muscles of the instep (dorsum) of the foot.

Innervation	Origins	Attachment	Function
M. extensor digitorum brevis			
N. fibularis profundus (N. ischiadicus)	Facies dorsalis of the calcaneus	Dorsal aponeurosis of the 2nd–4th toes	Toes II–IV: extension
M. extensor hallucis brevis			
N. fibularis profundus (N. ischiadicus)	Facies dorsalis of the calcaneus	Phalanx proximalis of the big toe	First metatarsophalangeal joint: extension

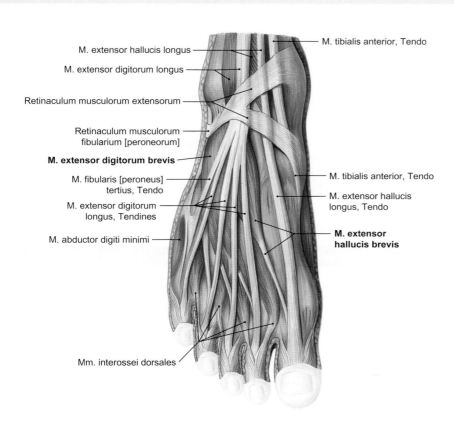

M. extensor hallucis longus
M. extensor digitorum longus
Retinaculum musculorum extensorum
Retinaculum musculorum fibularium [peroneorum]
M. extensor digitorum brevis
M. fibularis [peroneus] tertius, Tendo
M. extensor digitorum longus, Tendines
M. abductor digiti minimi
Mm. interossei dorsales

M. tibialis anterior, Tendo
M. tibialis anterior, Tendo
M. extensor hallucis longus, Tendo
M. extensor hallucis brevis

Fig. 5.51 Muscles of the dorsum of the foot. Dorsal view.

Table 5.20 Medial muscles of the sole of the foot.

Innervation	Origins	Attachment	Function
M. abductor hallucis			
N. plantaris medialis (N. tibialis)	Proc. medialis of the Tuber calcanei, Aponeurosis plantaris, Retinaculum musculorum flexorum	Medial sesamoid bone of the first metatarsophalangeal joint, proximal phalanx of the big toe	First metatarsophalangeal joint: abduction, flexion, tensing of the medial longitudinal curvature of the foot
M. flexor hallucis brevis			
• Caput mediale: N. plantaris medialis (N. tibialis) • Caput laterale: N. plantaris lateralis (N. tibialis)	Plantar aspect of the Ossa cuneiformia, plantar ligaments	• Caput mediale: medial sesamoid bone of the first metatarsophalangeal joint, proximal phalanx of the big toe • Caput laterale: lateral sesamoid bone of the first metatarsophalangeal joint, Phalanx proximalis of the big toe	First metatarsophalangeal joint: flexion, tensing of the medial longitudinal curvature of the foot
M. adductor hallucis			
N. plantaris lateralis (N. tibialis)	• Caput obliquum: Os cuboideum, Os cuneiforme laterale, plantar ligaments • Caput transversum: capsules of the base joints of the 3rd–5th toes, Lig. metatarsale transversum profundum	Lateral sesamoid bone of the capsule of the first metatarsophalangeal joint, base phalanx of the big toe	Base big toe joint: adduction for 2nd toe, flexion, tension of the longitudinal foot and transverse arch

Table 5.21 Muscles of the centre of the sole of the foot.

Innervation	Origins	Attachment	Function
M. flexor digitorum brevis[1]			
N. plantaris medialis (N. tibialis)	Plantar surface of the Tuber calcanei, Aponeurosis plantaris	Middle phalanx of the 2nd–5th toes	Base and middle joints of the toes: flexion, extension of the longitudinal curvature of the foot
M. quadratus plantae			
N. plantaris lateralis (N. tibialis)	Plantar surface of the calcaneus, Lig. plantare longum	Lateral margin of the tendon of the M. flexor digitorum longus	Supports the M. flexor digitorum longus
Mm. lumbricales pedis I–IV			
Nn. plantares mediales (I) and lateralis (II–IV) (N. tibialis)	M. lumbricalis pedis: tendons of the M. flexor digitorum longus • I: single-headed • II–IV: double headed	Medial side of the proximal phalanx of the 2nd–5th toes	Base joints of the toes: flexion, adduction
Mm. interossei plantares pedis I–III			
N. plantaris lateralis (N. tibialis)	Plantar surface of the Ossa metatarsi III–V, Lig. plantare longum	Medial side of the proximal phalanx of the 3rd–5th toes	Base joints of the toes: flexion, adduction to the 2nd toes
Mm. interossei dorsales pedis I–IV (twin-headed muscles)			
N. plantaris lateralis (N. tibialis)	Facing sides of the Ossa metatarsi I–V, Lig. plantare longum	Proximal phalanx of the 2nd–4th toes (2nd on both sides, 3rd and 4th toes laterally)	Base joints of the toes: flexion, abduction of the 2nd toe medially, the 3rd and 4th toes laterally

[1] The tendons of this muscle are perforated by the tendons of the M. flexor digitorum longis shortly before their attachment

Table 5.22 Lateral plantar muscles.

Innervation	Origins	Attachment	Function
M. abductor digiti minimi			
N. plantaris lateralis (N. tibialis)	Proc. lateralis of the Tuber calcanei, Aponeurosis plantaris	Tuberositas ossis metatarsi V, proximal phalanx of the 5th toe	Proximal joint of the 5th toe: abduction, flexion, tensing of the longitudinal curvature of the foot
M. flexor digiti minimi brevis			
N. plantaris lateralis (N. tibialis)	Base of the Os metatarsi V, Lig. plantare longum	Proximal phalanx of the 5th toe	Proximal joint of the 5th toe: flexion, tensing of the longitudinal curvature of the foot
M. opponens digiti minimi (inconstant muscle)			
N. plantaris lateralis (N. tibialis)	Base of the Os metatarsi V, Lig. plantare longum	Os metatarsi V	Proximal joint of the 5th toe: opposition, flexion, tensing of the longitudinal curvature of the foot

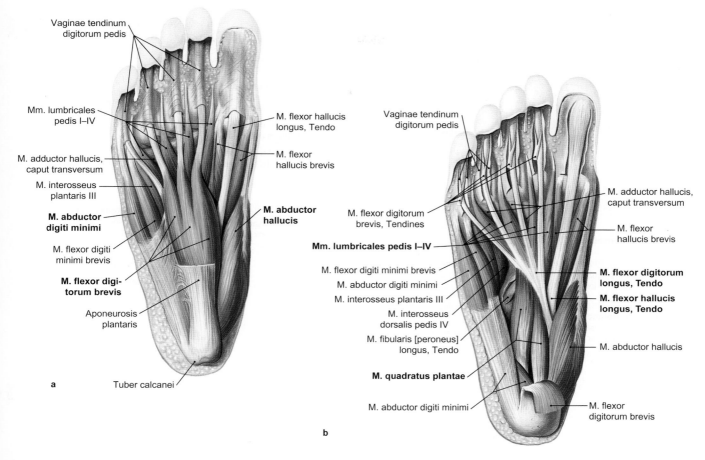

Fig. 5.52 Plantar muscles, right. Plantar view. **a** After removal of the plantar aponeurosis. **b** After removal of the M. flexor digitorum brevis.

Laterally, the **Retinaculum musculorum fibularium** spans the distance between the outer ankle and the calcaneus, and fixes the two fibularis muscles together, mostly in a common tendinous sheath. On the medial side the **malleolar canal** forms a tunnel (tarsal tunnel), which originates as a result of the bridging of the gap between the inner ankle and calcaneus by the **Retinaculum musculorum flexorum.** The 3 deep plantar flexors pass through this, also in their own tendon sheaths, along with the vessels and nerves of the sole of the foot (A./V. tibialis posterior, N. tibialis).

5.6 Nerves of the lower extremity

― Skills ―

After working through this chapter, you should be able to:
- explain the structure of the Plexus lumbosacralis and explain the symptoms associated with plexus lesions
- know the course, function and the exact symptoms associated with loss of major nerves in the lower extremity and show these on a dissection specimen

The innervation of the lower limbs involves the **spinal nerves T12–S4.** The Rr. anteriores of the spinal nerves **T12–L4** form the **Plexus lumbalis,** which is amalgamated with the **Plexus sacralis (L4–S5, Co1)** into the **Plexus lumbosacralis.**

The actual nerves of the leg, the pelvic floor and the caudal sections of the abdominal wall arise from this plexus.
The following nerves ensure the **sensory innervation** of the skin of the lower limbs and the perineal region (➤ Fig. 5.53a and b):
- Plexus lumbalis:
  - N. iliohypogastricus
  - N. ilioinguinalis
  - N. genitofemoralis
  - N. cutaneus femoris lateralis
  - N. femoralis
  - N. obturatorius
- Plexus sacralis:
  - N. cutaneus femoris posterior
  - N. ischiadicus
  - N. pudendus

In addition, the lateral branches of the Rr. posteriores of segments L1–L3 as the **Nn. clunium superiores,** and segments S1–S3 as the **Nn. clunium medii,** sensorily innervate the buttock area. As in the arm, the skin areas on the leg are usually innervated by the overlapping skin branches of a variety of nerves.
Also the **dermatomes of the leg** (➤ Fig. 5.53c and d) run in a similar way to the arm along the longitudinal axis. The dermatomes of the lumbar spinal nerves on the ventral side of the leg run from lateral descending obliquely to medial. The dorsal side of the leg, together with the lateral margin of the foot, is innervated by the sacral spinal nerves. The dermatomes run almost longitudinally here.

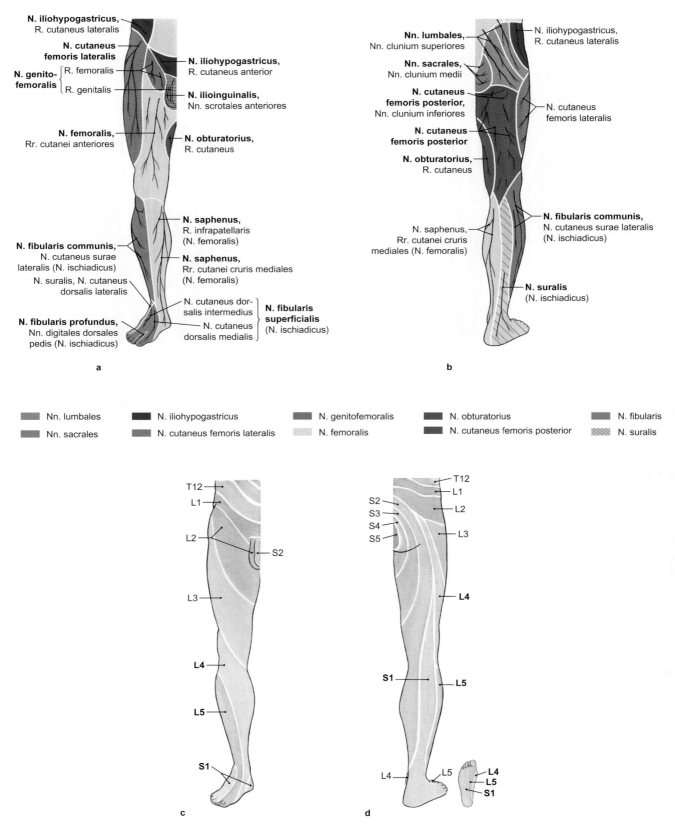

Fig. 5.53 Cutaneous nerves and segmental innervation of the lower extremity. a Cutaneous nerves, right, ventral view. **b** Cutaneous nerves, right, dorsal view. **c** Dermatomes, right, ventral view. **d** Dermatomes, right, dorsal view.

- Ventral side of the leg: L1–L5 (descending obliquely from the inguinal ligament to the foot)
- Medial margin of the foot: L4
- Big toe and the second toe: L5
- Little toe and the lateral margin of the foot: S1
- Dorsal side of the leg: S1–S5 (from the lateral margin of the foot ascending longitudinally to the buttocks)

Clinical remarks

Slipped discs occur principally in the discs between the 4th and 5th lumbar vertebrae and between the 5th lumbar vertebra and the sacrum. After a rupture of the Anulus fibrosus, the Nucleus pulposus protrudes forwards into the vertebral canal and compresses one or more nerve roots. In addition to pain in the area of the lesion, this results in discomfort in the respective dermatome and malfunctioning of the reference muscle of the corresponding nerve root. When there is compression of L5, it is typical for there to be pain symptoms radiating into the leg as far as the foot. This is accompanied by a loss of sensitivity of the skin and a weakness when extending the big toe **(reference muscle L5: M. extensor hallucis longus).**

5.6.1 Plexus lumbosacralis

The **Plexus lumbalis (T12 – L4)** and the **Plexus sacralis (L4–S5, Co1)** are amalgamated to form the **Plexus lumbosacralis.** The spinal nerves of L4 and L5 form the Truncus lumbosacralis, constituting the connection between the two nerve plexus. The branches of the Plexus lumbalis run ventral to the hip joint and course to the anterior side of the leg. Conversely, the branches of the Plexus sacralis are dorsal to the hip joint and run to the back of the leg.

Clinical remarks

The Plexus lumbosacralis can be damaged by tumours (e.g. of the uterus), by bruising (haematomas in the fascia of the M. iliopsoas) or by fractures of the pelvis. A **plexus lesion** should be considered if the clinical picture is not limited to the malfunction of a single nerve:
- Where there is a lesion of the **Plexus lumbalis** (T12–L4), there is pain and disruption to the sensory system on the front side of the thigh (➤ Fig. 5.54a). Bending and adduction are affected in hip and knee extensions. Standing and walking are difficult.

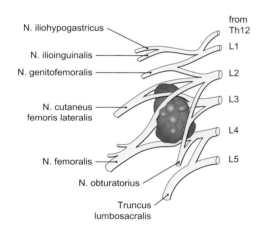

N. iliohypogastricus
N. ilioinguinalis
N. genitofemoralis
N. cutaneus femoris lateralis
N. femoralis
N. obturatorius
Truncus lumbosacralis

from Th12
L1
L2
L3
L4
L5

a

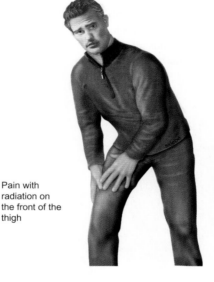

Pain with radiation on the front of the thigh

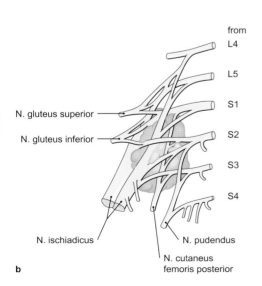

N. gluteus superior
N. gluteus inferior
N. ischiadicus
N. pudendus
N. cutaneus femoris posterior

from L4
L5
S1
S2
S3
S4

b

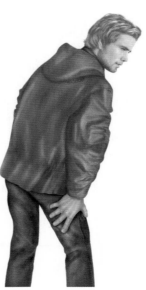

Pain with radiation on the back of the thigh

Fig. 5.54 Structure of the Plexus lumbosacralis and symptoms associated with lesions.
a Tumour in the Plexus lumbalis.
b Lesion in the Plexus sacralis.
left [L126]; right [L238]

- Lesions of the **Plexus sacralis** (L4–S5, Co1) are recognisable due to pain and sensory deficits in the dorsal thigh (➤ Fig. 5.54b) as well as in the lower leg. It damages extension and abduction (TRENDELENBURG's signs positive, see below) in the hip, as well as flexion of the knee, and all the muscles of the lower leg and the foot. Autonomic disturbances can arise because the branches of the Plexus sacralis parasympatheticaly supply the pelvic viscera and the external genitalia. This may result in loss of erection in the penis or impaired filling of the erectile tissue of the clitoris. A malfunction in the innervation of the pelvic floor can be expressed as urinary and faecal incontinence.

An isolated lesion of both plexus attachments is however rare. In most cases, both the Plexus lumbalis and Plexus sacralis are affected.

Plexus lumbalis

The Rr. anteriores of the spinal nerves of **T12–L4** form the Plexus lumbalis (➤ Fig. 5.55). They exit through the Foramina intervertebralia between the origins of the M. psoas major and form the following nerves:

The **Rr. musculares** (T12–L4) are short, purely motor branches to the M. iliopsoas and M. quadratus lumborum and Mm. intertransversarii.

The **N. iliohypogastricus** (L1, ➤ Fig. 5.53a, b, ➤ Fig. 5.55) runs behind the kidneys, penetrates the M. transversus abdominis, and courses forwards between here and the M. obliquus internus abdominis along the inguinal ligament. Its Rr. musculares innervate the M. obliquus internus abdominis and M. transversus abdominis. The R. cutaneous lateralis supplies the skin above the iliac crest, and the R. cutaneus anterior supplies an area of skin medially above the inguinal ligament.

The **N. ilioinguinalis** (L1, ➤ Fig. 5.53a, ➤ Fig. 5.55) runs further caudal than the N. iliohypogastricus and innervates the same abdominal muscles. Its terminal branch is attached to the spermatic cord (runs outside) and runs with it through the inguinal canal. It supplies the skin of the external genitalia via the Rr. scrotales and Rr. labiales anteriores.

The **N. genitofemoralis** (L1–L2, ➤ Fig. 5.53a, ➤ Fig. 5.55) penetrates the M. psoas major and runs downwards on the anterior side (important identification sign). It crosses underneath the ureter and is divided into:

- **R. genitalis:** it courses medially through the inguinal canal and runs in the spermatic cord to the scrotum. In men, it innervates the M. cremaster, and together with the N. ilioinguinalis, sensorily innervates the anterior parts of the external genitalia.

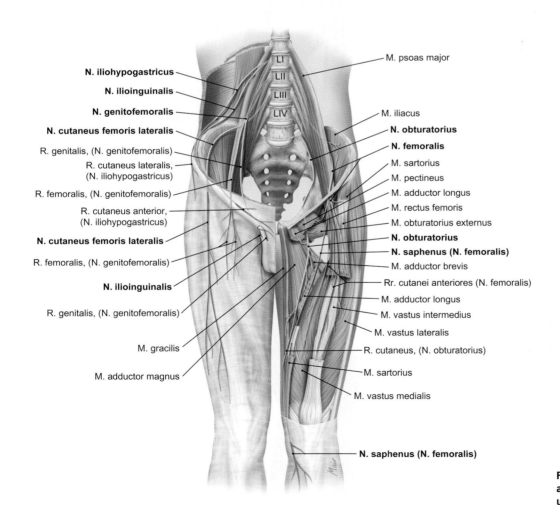

N. iliohypogastricus
N. ilioinguinalis
N. genitofemoralis
N. cutaneus femoris lateralis
R. genitalis, (N. genitofemoralis)
R. cutaneus lateralis, (N. iliohypogastricus)
R. femoralis, (N. genitofemoralis)
R. cutaneus anterior, (N. iliohypogastricus)
N. cutaneus femoris lateralis
R. femoralis, (N. genitofemoralis)
N. ilioinguinalis
R. genitalis, (N. genitofemoralis)
M. gracilis
M. adductor magnus

LI
LII
LIII
LIV

M. psoas major
M. iliacus
N. obturatorius
N. femoralis
M. sartorius
M. pectineus
M. adductor longus
M. rectus femoris
M. obturatorius externus
N. obturatorius
N. saphenus (N. femoralis)
M. adductor brevis
Rr. cutanei anteriores (N. femoralis)
M. adductor longus
M. vastus intermedius
M. vastus lateralis
R. cutaneus, (N. obturatorius)
M. sartorius
M. vastus medialis
N. saphenus (N. femoralis)

Fig. 5.55 Course and target areas of the nerves of the Plexus lumbalis.

- **R. femoralis:** it runs in the Lacuna vasorum below the inguinal ligament lateral to the vessels and sensorily supplies the skin below the inguinal ligament.

The **N. cutaneus femoris lateralis** (L2–L3, ➤ Fig. 5.53a, b, ➤ Fig. 5.55) is the only purely sensory nerve of the Plexus lumbalis and courses laterally through the Lacuna muscularum, exits medial to the Spina iliaca anterior superior and supplies the skin of the lateral thigh.

Clinical remarks

Lesions of the N. genitofemoralis lead to malfunction of the cremaster muscle reflex when brushing the medial thigh. The wearing of overtight trousers and overtightened belts may lead to **Meralgia paraesthetica** ('Skinny jeans syndrome'). Here, compression of the N. cutaneus femoralis lateralis under the inguinal ligament causes pain and discomfort at the lateral thigh (➤ Fig. 5.56).

The **N. femoralis** (L2–L4, ➤ Fig. 5.53a, b, ➤ Fig. 5.55) innervates the ventral muscle group of the thigh and supplies sensory innervation to the front of the entire leg. It lies medial in the Lacuna musculorum to the Trigonum femorale, where it splits into its terminal branches approximately 5 cm below the inguinal ligament:

- **Rr. musculares:** innervate the M. iliopsoas, M. sartorius, M. pectineus and M. quadriceps femoris
- **Rr. cutanei anteriores:** sensorily innervate the anterior aspect of the thigh
- **N. saphenus:** this terminal branch of the N. femoralis accompanies the A. femoralis into the adductor canal and breaches the Septum intermusculare vastoadductorium, to course epifascially with the V. saphena magna towards the foot. With a R. infrapatellaris, it supplies the skin below the knee cap, and with the Rr. cutanei cruris mediales supplies the medial side of the lower leg.

Clinical remarks

As the **N. femoralis** divides immediately beneath the inguinal ligament, complete malfunctions (e.g. due to incision wounds on the thigh) are rare. It can still be damaged before it branches, e.g. during hernia operations. Sensory deficits can be seen on the front of the thigh and on the medial side of the leg. Deficits also arise during flexion in the hip joint (most important muscle: M. iliopsoas) as well as during extension of the knee joint (single muscle: M. quadriceps femoris).

The **N. obturatorius** (L2–L4, ➤ Fig. 5.53a, b, ➤ Fig. 5.55) innervates the medial adductor group at the thigh and supplies sensory innervation to a small area of skin medially above the knee. It courses medially to the M. psoas major and downwards slightly below the ovary, then passes through the obturator canal (Canalis obturatorius) to the inside of the thigh. It innervates the M. obturatorius externus and is divided into:

- **R. anterior:** runs in front of the M. adductor brevis and provides motor innervation to the M. pectineus, M. gracilis and Mm. adductor brevis and longus and sensory innervation to the medial skin of the thigh (**R. cutaneus**) down to the knee
- **R. posterior:** is located behind the M. adductor brevis and innervates the M. adductor magnus as well as the knee joint capsule

Clinical remarks

Tumours or inflammatory processes of the ovaries can lead to deficits of the **N. obturatorius** due to their physical proximity and pain in the inner thigh and the knee (ROMBERG's knee phenomenon). An injury to the nerve is also possible in pelvic fractures or femoral hernia. Where there is a complete failure, adduction is no longer possible in the hip joint; the legs cannot be crossed on top of each other.

Plexus sacralis

The Rr. anteriores of the spinal nerves of **L4–S5 , Co1** form the sacral plexus (➤ Fig. 5.57). They pass through the Foramina intervertebralia (L4–L5) via the Truncus lumbosacralis or via the Foramina sacralia anterioria of the Sacrum to the lesser pelvis where they form the plexus. The branches of the plexus largely exit the lesser pelvis through the Foramen ischiadicum majus to the Regio glutealis. The following branches are formed:

Muscle branches to the pelvitrochanteric muscles (M. piriformis, M. obturatorius internus and Mm. gemelli superior and inferior,

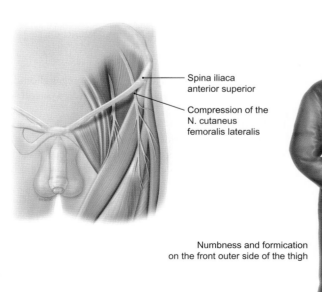

Spina iliaca anterior superior

Compression of the N. cutaneus femoralis lateralis

Numbness and formication on the front outer side of the thigh

Fig. 5.56 Meralgia paraesthetica. [L238]

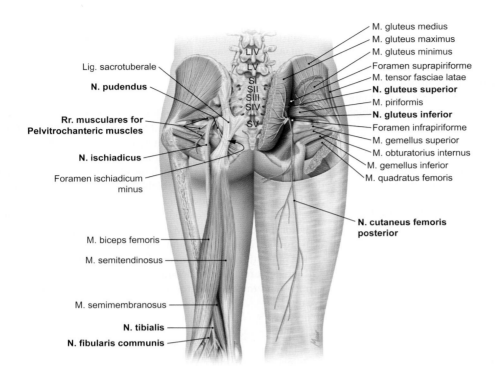

M. gluteus medius
M. gluteus maximus
M. gluteus minimus
Foramen suprapiriforme
M. tensor fasciae latae
N. gluteus superior
M. piriformis
N. gluteus inferior
Foramen infrapiriforme
M. gemellus superior
M. obturatorius internus
M. gemellus inferior
M. quadratus femoris

N. cutaneus femoris posterior

Lig. sacrotuberale
N. pudendus
Rr. musculares for Pelvitrochanteric muscles
N. ischiadicus
Foramen ischiadicum minus
M. biceps femoris
M. semitendinosus
M. semimembranosus
N. tibialis
N. fibularis communis

Fig. 5.57 Course and target area of the nerves of the Plexus sacralis.

M. quadratus femoris) reach the muscles through the Foramen infrapiriforme.

The **N. gluteus superior** (L4–S1, ➤ Fig. 5.57) runs through the Foramen suprapiriforme between the Mm. gluteus medius and gluteus minimus and innervates them. In addition, it supplies the M. tensor fasciae latae.

The **N. gluteus inferior** (L5–S2, ➤ Fig. 5.57) passes through the Foramen infrapiriforme and innervates the M. gluteus maximus.

Clinical remarks

Both Nn. glutei can be damaged by an incorrectly performed intramuscular injection:
- A **failure of the N. gluteus superior** leads to TRENDELEBURG's sign. When standing on the leg on the injured side, the pelvis drops to the opposing, healthy side, as it can no longer be held in the horizontal plane due to failure of the Mm. gluteus maximus et minimus. When walking this leads to the DUCHENNE limp where the trunk of the patient leans to the affected side, in order to compensate for the drop.
- A **failure of the N. gluteus inferior** results in severe impairment of extension and lateral rotation of the hip joint. Climbing stairs and getting up from a squatting position are impossible since the M. gluteus maximus is the most important extensor of the hip joint.

The **N. cutaneus femoris posterior** (S1–S3, ➤ Fig. 5.53b, ➤ Fig. 5.57) exits through the Foramen infrapiriformis and provides the Nn. clunium inferiores for sensory innervation of the lower buttock region and the Rr. perineales for the perineal region. It courses subfascially up to the middle of the posterior thigh, passes through the fascia here and supplies the skin of the back of the thigh.

The **N. ischiadicus** (L4–S3) is the strongest nerve in the human body (➤ Chap. 5.6.2).

The **N. pudendus** (S2–S4, ➤ Fig. 5.57) exits through the Foramen infrapiriforme and then runs through the Foramen ischiadicum

minus under the Lig. sacrotuberale in the Fossa ischioanalis. Here it runs on the M. obturator internus, ventrally covered by its fascia (= ALCOCK's canal). It has three branches:
- Nn. rectales inferiores: supply the M. sphincter ani externus and the perianal skin
- Nn. perineales:
  - Nn. scrotales/labiales posteriores to the skin of the external genitalia
  - Rr. musculares to supply the perineal musculature (Mm. transversus perinei profundus and superficialis, M. bulbospongiosus, M. ischiocavernosus)
- N. dorsalis penis/clitoridis for the sensory supply of the penis or clitoris.

Clinical remarks

The **failure of the N. pudendus** is characterised by urinary and faecal incontinence (failure of the voluntary sphincter muscles) as well as by disorders in sexual function.

The **Nn. splanchnici pelvici** (S2–S4) are preganglionic parasympathetic nerve fibres supplying the pelvic viscera (sacral section of the parasympathetic nervous system).

The **Rr. musculares** (S3–S4) innervate the pelvic floor muscles (M. levator ani and M. ischiococcygeus).

Small **sensory branches** (S2–S5, Co1) innervate the skin over the Tuber ischiadicum (N. cutaneus perforans) and the skin between the anus and coccyx (N. coccygeus).

5.6.2 N. ischiadicus

The thickest nerve of the human body supplies all of the dorsal muscles of the upper and lower leg and foot muscles; it sensorily innervates the calf and the entire foot. It passes through the Foramen infrapiriforme and, initially covered by the M. gluteus maximus, passes over the pelvitrochanteric muscles and then continues distally under the M. biceps femoris. **It divides** mostly at the transition to the distal femur into:

- The **N. fibularis communis** (L4–S2)
- The **N. tibialis** (L4–S3)

Even before the bifurcation two separate parts are present and these are connected only by a sheath of connective tissue. Therefore, the corresponding **innervation areas** above the division point can also be distinguished:

- **Fibularis portion:** innervates the Caput breve of the M. biceps femoris
- **Tibialis portion:** supplies the remaining ischiocrural muscles (M. semitendinosus, M. semimembranosus, Caput longum of the M. biceps femoris) and the dorsal part of the M. adductor magnus

The division of the N. ischiadicus can also occur far proximally (before leaving the Foramen infrapiriforme) (**high division** in approximately 10% of cases). Here, the N. fibularis communis mostly penetrates the M. piriformis, whereas the N. tibialis takes the standard route.

Clinical remarks

The **N. ischiadicus,** like the N. gluteus superior, can be damaged by wrongly administered injections. A **lesion** leads to a malfunction in the ischiocrural muscles (loss of extension in the hip joint, loss of flexion and rotation in the knee joint) and in addition, to symptoms of failure in the terminal branches of the N. tibialis and the N. fibularis communis (see below).

The **high division** of the N. ischiadicus can cause irritation when passing through the M. pirifomis and cause symptoms similar to those of a slipped disc.

An intense pain in the supply area of the N. ischiadicus occurs during **LASÈGUE's test.** The examiner raises the extended leg of the supine patient, creating tension on the N. ischiadicus. The resulting pain sensation can indicate a slipped disc with compression of L5 or S1, as well as an infection of the meninges (meningitis).

N. fibularis communis

After the division, the N. fibularis communis runs along the M. biceps femoris at the edge of the hollow of the knee and the head of the Fibula (➤ Fig. 5.58). It delivers the **N. cutaneus surae lateralis** for the sensory innervation of the lateral calf and has a connection to the N. cutaneus surae medialis (N. tibialis) via the **R. communicans fibularis.** It then runs underneath the M. fibularis longus and divides again into:

- **N. fibularis superficialis:** it runs distally in the fibularis compartment and with its Rr. musculares, it supplies the Mm. fibulares longus and brevis. It penetrates the fascia at the distal lower leg and, as the N. cutaneus dorsalis medialis and intermedius supplies the *skin of the dorsum of the foot.*
- **N. fibularis profundus:** enters the extensor compartment and with its Rr. musculares, it supplies the ventral muscles of the ankle joint. Its sensory terminal branch penetrates the fascia far distal on the dorsum of the foot, supplying only the *skin between the big toe and the second toe.*

Clinical remarks

The most common issues are **lesions of the N. fibularis communis** in the region of the fibular head. This can be easily palpated directly under the skin, so the highly exposed nerve can be very easily damaged here. Typically, this occurs in fractures of the fibula or due to chronic pressure injury arising from constant crossing of the legs ('crossed legs palsy').

A failure of the N. fibularis communis leads to the equine foot position due to loss of the extensors with compensatory drop foot (stronger hip flexion when walking, in order to avoid dragging the foot on the floor). A malfunction in the fibularis group leads to the supination position. Sensory innervation of the skin of the dorsum of the foot and the lateral calf is compromised.

An isolated **lesion of the N. fibularis profundus** occurs with compartment syndrome of the extensor compartment (see above) with equinus foot position and drop foot. A malfunction of the sensors in the first toe is often the first indication of the onset of a compartment syndrome, but it can also arise due to compression beneath the Retinaculum musculorum extensorum **('anterior tarsal tunnel syndrome'),** with no misalignment of the foot. This means that the sensitivity in this area must be regularly checked following surgery on the lower leg or after placing the lower leg in a plaster cast! The sensitivity of the rest of the foot remains normal.

An isolated **lesion of the N. fibularis superficialis** is very rare, since the nerve is protected between the two fibularis muscles. What is conspicuous here is the supination position of the foot, as well as the non-operational sensors of the dorsum of the foot (apart from the first toe!).

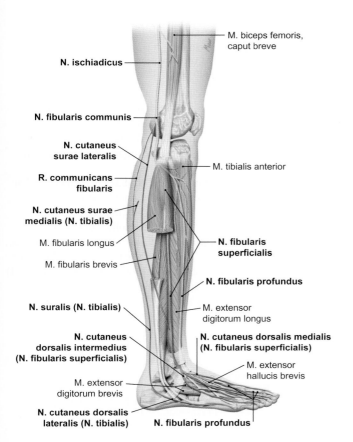

Labels:
- M. biceps femoris, caput breve
- N. ischiadicus
- N. fibularis communis
- N. cutaneus surae lateralis
- M. tibialis anterior
- R. communicans fibularis
- N. cutaneus surae medialis (N. tibialis)
- M. fibularis longus
- M. fibularis brevis
- N. fibularis superficialis
- N. fibularis profundus
- N. suralis (N. tibialis)
- M. extensor digitorum longus
- N. cutaneus dorsalis intermedius (N. fibularis superficialis)
- N. cutaneus dorsalis medialis (N. fibularis superficialis)
- M. extensor digitorum brevis
- M. extensor hallucis brevis
- N. cutaneus dorsalis lateralis (N. tibialis)
- N. fibularis profundus

Fig. 5.58 Course of the N. fibularis communis, right. Lateral view.

N. tibialis

The N. tibialis continues the course of the N. ischiadicus through the hollow of the knee (➤ Fig. 5.59). It runs superficially from the A. and V. poplitea, passes *between* the heads of the M. gastrocnemius and *under* the tendinous arch of the M. soleus distally, and runs in the lower leg between the superficial and deep calf muscles

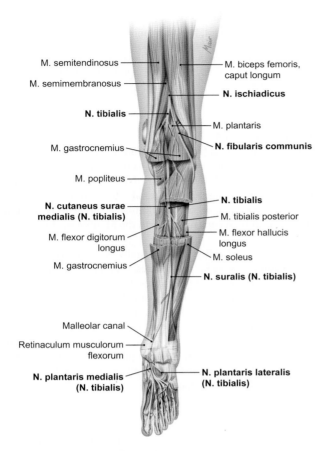

M. semitendinosus

M. semimembranosus

N. tibialis

M. gastrocnemius

M. popliteus

N. cutaneus surae
medialis (N. tibialis)

M. flexor digitorum
longus

M. gastrocnemius

Malleolar canal

Retinaculum musculorum
flexorum

N. plantaris medialis
(N. tibialis)

M. biceps femoris,
caput longum

N. ischiadicus

M. plantaris

N. fibularis communis

N. tibialis

M. tibialis posterior

M. flexor hallucis
longus

M. soleus

N. suralis (N. tibialis)

N. plantaris lateralis
(N. tibialis)

Fig. 5.59 Course of the N. tibialis, right. Dorsal view.

along with the A./V. tibialis posterior. Distal of the medial malleolus it divides into two branches for the sole of the foot.
In its course, the N. tibialis divides into a total of 5 branches:
- **Rr. musculares** for the innervation of all calf muscles
- **N. interosseus cruris:** runs distally on the Membrana interossea and together with the Rr. calcanei mediales supplies the skin over the inner ankle and heel
- **N. cutaneus surae medialis:** skin branch, runs together with the V. saphena parva and, together with the R. communicans fibularis (from the N. fibularis communis), forms the **N. suralis.** This supplies the skin of the dorsal lower leg, with the Rr. calcanei laterales supplies the skin above the outer ankle and with the R. cutaneous dorsalis lateralis supplies the *skin of the lateral margin of the foot.*

While still in the **malleolar canal,** the N. tibialis splits into its 2 terminal branches:
- **N. plantaris medialis:** is positioned in the centre of the sole along the M. quadratus plantae and is divided into 3 Nn. digitales plantares communes each with 2 Nn. digitales plantares propriae. It supplies sensory innervation to the plantar side of the **medial 3½ toes** and the skin over the corresponding distal phalanges. Hence the nerve corresponds to the N. medianus on the hand. It supplies the motor function to the following muscles:
  - Most of the muscles of the big toe (except for M. adductor hallucis and the lateral head of the M. flexor hallucis brevis)
  - the M. lumbricalis I
  - the M. flexor digitorum brevis
- **N. plantaris lateralis:** runs to the lateral side of the sole of the foot and divides again into R. superficialis and R. profundis. The superficial branch forms the Nn. digitales plantares communes and Nn. digitales plantares propriae for supplying the plantar

side of the **lateral 1½ toes** and their distal phalanges dorsally. It corresponds to the N. ulnaris on the hand. It innervates the motor functions of:
- all the muscles of the little toe
- at the big toe, the M. adductor hallucis and the Caput laterale of the M. flexor hallucis brevis
- the Mm. lumbricales II–IV
- M. quadratus plantae

The N. plantaris medialis and lateralis innervate together the entire short foot muscles on the plantar side.

Clinical remarks

A **high lesion of the N. tibialis** (e.g. in the hollow of the knee) leads to failure of all of the flexors of the leg. If the foot is extended dorsally (Pes supinus) and in the pronation position, standing on tip-toe is impossible.
A claw foot is formed due to a malfunction of the plantar muscles. There is no sensitivity at the medial calf, the heel, the sole of the foot and the lateral margin of the foot. The nerve is also often injured at the distal lower leg when passing through the malleolar canal under the Retinaculum flexorum (**'posterior tarsal tunnel syndrome'**) or in the event of the ankle joint being damaged. Here, the symptoms are limited to the malfunction of sensors on the sole of the foot and paralysis of the short foot muscles.

5.7 Arteries of the lower extremity

Skills

After working through this chapter, you should be able to:
- know all the arteries of the lower extremity and identify them on dissection specimens
- know the right places to take the pulse
- explain vascular anastomoses in the hip region

The lower extremities are supplied with blood by the **A. iliaca communis.** The buttock region and the intestines mainly receive blood from the parietal branches of the A. iliaca interna. As it is also responsible for supplying the pelvic organs, it is discussed in (➤ Chap. 8.8.2).
The artery responsible for the leg is the **A. iliaca externa** (➤ Chap. 5.7.1). After it passes underneath the inguinal ligament, it continues into the **A. femoralis** (➤ Fig. 5.60, ➤ Chap. 5.7.2). This changes to the dorsal side of the leg to the hollow of the knee, where it becomes the **A. poplitea** (➤ Chap. 5.7.3). As it continues, it is divided into an artery for supplying the front side of the lower leg and the dorsum of the foot (**A. tibialis anterior,** ➤ Chap. 5.7.4) and an artery supplying the back and the sole of the foot (**A. tibialis posterior,** ➤ Chap. 5.7.5).

Clinical remarks

The **pulse** can be palpated in the following places on the leg:
- A. femoralis: in the groin
- A. poplitea: in the hollow of the knee
- A. dorsalis pedis: at the dorsum of the foot lateral to the tendons of the M. extensor hallucis longus
- A. tibialis posterior: behind the inner ankle

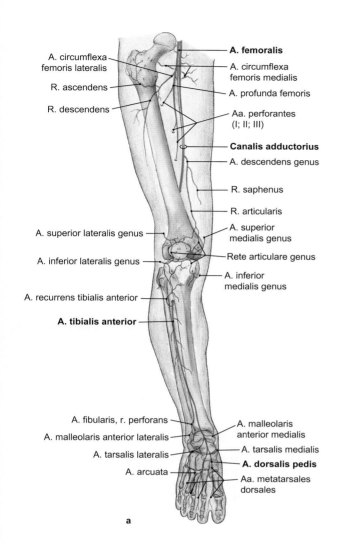

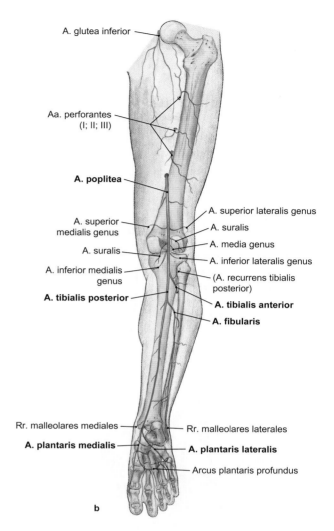

Fig. 5.60 Overview of the arteries of the leg, right. a Ventral view. **b** Dorsal view.

Palpation of the pedal pulse provides important evidence about which section of the leg arteries has succumbed to a blockage of an artery, for example due to arteriosclerosis or a blood clot.

5.7.1 A. iliaca externa

The vessel is formed from the A. iliaca communis after branching into the A. iliaca interna (➤ Fig. 5.61). The A. iliaca externa runs medial to the M. psoas major to the inguinal ligament, which it crosses underneath the Lacuna vasorum. Prior to this, it delivers 2 branches:

- **A. epigastrica inferior:** it runs cranially along the rear of the M. rectus abdominis in a fold which is visible from the abdominal cavity (**Plica umbilicalis lateralis**). It anastomoses with the A. epigastrica superior (A. thoracica interna).
  - R. pubicus: a medial branch which enters into an anastomosis with the A. obturatorius along with the R. obturatorius
  - A. cremasterica: a thin artery in men for the testicular sheath, passes through the inguinal canal
  - A. ligamenti teretis uteri: corresponding artery in women, passes through the inguinal canal along with the Lig. teres uteri

- **A. circumflexa ilium profunda:** it runs on the inside at the inguinal ligament and laterally at the iliac crest and anastomoses with the A. iliolumbalis (from the A. iliaca interna).

Clinical remarks

If the anastomosis between the A. epigastrica inferior and A. obturatoria is highly developed, it can be damaged during inguinal or femoral hernia operations. Since in earlier times, this was often fatal due to heavy bleeding, this variant was referred to as '**Corona mortis**'. In 20% of cases, the A. obturatoria does not originate from the A. iliaca interna, but from the A. epigastrica inferior.

5.7.2 A. femoralis

The **A. femoralis** begins after leaving the Lacuna vasorum beneath the inguinal ligament (➤ Fig. 5.61). Here it runs between the N. femoralis (lateral) and V. femoralis (medial). The vessel runs through the adductor canal and switches to the dorsal side of the leg. The A. femoralis divides into 5 branches (➤ Fig. 5.62):

- The **A. epigastrica superficialis** runs epifascially as a thin vessel cranially over the inguinal ligament.

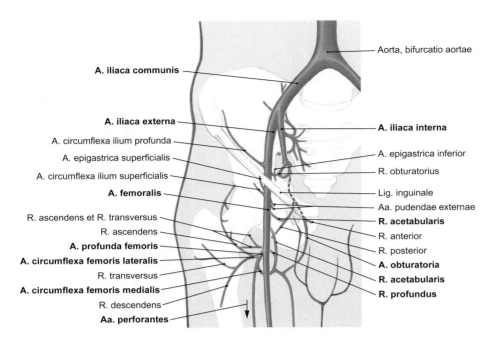

Fig. 5.61 **Arteries of the pelvis, right.** Ventral view.

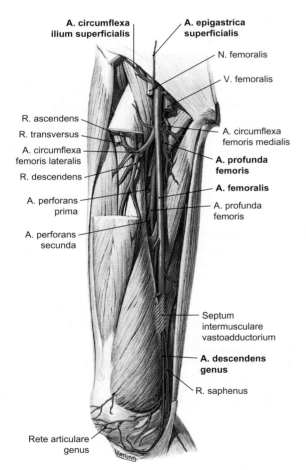

Fig. 5.62 **A. femoralis.** Ventral view after removal of M. sartorius and parts of the M. rectus femoris. [S010-2-16]

- The **A. circumflexa ilium superficialis** also runs epifascially under the inguinal ligament laterally to the Spina iliaca anterior superior.
- The **Aa. pudendae externae** run medially and supply the external genitalia (Rr. labiales/scrotales anteriores).
- The **A. profunda femoris** is the strongest branch (see below).

- The **A. descendens genus** branches off into the adductor canal and forms Rr. articulares to the knee joint and a R. saphenus, which accompanies the N. saphenus approximately to the knee.

Clinical remarks

The A. femoralis is easily accessed due to its superficial position under the inguinal (palpable pulse!). It is therefore used, like the A. radialis in the arm, to draw blood for an arterial **blood gas analysis.** It is also a standard access route for **cardiac catheterisation.**

A profunda femoris

The **A. profunda femoris** is the most important vessel for supplying the thigh, including the femoral head. It enters approximately 5 cm below the inguinal ligament into the depths and continues distally, running parallel to the A. femoralis. On its way it divides into 3 branches (➤ Fig. 5.62):

- **A. circumflexa femoris medialis:** it runs medial and posterior, and continues to divide into:
  - R. ascendens for the anterior parts of the adductors
  - R. profundus to the posterior portions of the adductors, the ischiocrural muscles and the femoral head
  - R. acetabularis to the hip joint; connects to the R. acetabularis of the A. obturatoria and runs in the Lig. capitis femoris to the femoral head
- **A. circumflexa femoris lateralis:** it runs laterally under the M. rectus femoris and has the following branches:
  - R. ascendens proximally to the gluteal muscles and the femoral neck; anastomoses with the A. circumflexa femoris medialis and the Aa. glutae superior and inferior
  - R. transversus laterally to the M. vastus lateralis
  - R. descendens to the M. quadriceps femoris
- **Aa. perforantes** (typically 3): at right angles to the course of the A. profunda femoris, they penetrate the adductor muscles and the ischiocrural muscles, supplying these and the femoral shaft.

In approximately 20% the Aa. circumflexae femoris medialis and lateralis each originate directly from the A. femoralis. They form an arterial ring around the neck of the femur (also ➤ Fig. 5.14) and supply these and large parts of the femoral head. This creates an anastomosis network made up of branches of the A. iliaca interna (Aa. glutea superior and inferior, A. obturatoria) and branches of the A. profunda femoris (A. circumflexa femoris medialis) (➤ Fig. 5.63).

─ Clinical remarks ───────────────────

These vascular anastomosis networks vary enormously in their characteristics, and they can ensure the supply of the leg in the case of acute occlusions or constriction of the A. femoris proximal to branching of the A. profunda femoris.

N O T E

The **A. profunda femoris** supplies the thigh, both front and back!

5.7.3 A. poplitea

With the exit from the adductor canal in the Hiatus adductorius, the A. femoralis extends to the A. **poplitea** (➤ Fig. 5.64a). This transverses the hollow of the knee (Fossa poplitea) until it divides at the level of the tibial condyles into the **Aa. tibiales anterior and posterior**. It gives up another 6 branches and forms a vessel network with these anterior to the knee joint (Rete articulare genus):

- **A. superior medialis and lateralis genus** around the medial/lateral femoral condyle
- **A. media genus** to the knee joint
- **A. inferior medialis and A. lateralis genus** around the proximal tibia/the head of the fibula
- **Aa. surales** to the calf muscles

─ Clinical remarks ───────────────────

Despite their many tributaries, the anastomoses of the Rete articulare genus are not usually sufficient to be able to ensure the supply of the leg if the A. poplitea is compromised.

5.7.4 A. tibialis anterior

The vessel penetrates the Membrana interossea cruris and runs along this in the extensor compartment distally (➤ Fig. 5.64b). It is then accompanied by the N. fibularis profundus. It forms the A. dorsalis pedis at the level of the ankle joint. At the lower leg the A. tibialis anterior divides into 4 branches:

- **Aa. recurrentes tibialis anterior and posterior:** run before and after the passage through the Membrana interossea back to the knee joint
- **Aa. malleolares anteriores medialis and lateralis** to the vascular network on the inner and outer ankle

A. dorsalis pedis

It continues the direction of the A. tibialis anterior to the medial side of the dorsum of the foot, and divides into a total of 4 branches (➤ Fig. 5.64b):

- **Aa. tarsales medialis and lateralis** to the medial and lateral margin of the foot.
- **A. arcuata:** it arches over the bases of the metatarsal bones and divides into the Aa. metatarsales dorsales, which are involved in supplying the toes via the Aa. digitales dorsales.
- **A. plantaris profunda:** it penetrates the first interphalangeal space and anastomoses with the Arcus plantaris profundus of the sole of the foot.

─ Clinical remarks ───────────────────

A non-palpable pulse of the **A. dorsalis pedis** with simultaneous palpable pulse of the A. poplitea and the A. tibialis posterior indicates an occlusion of the A. tibialis anterior. This can be caused by arteriosclerosis, as well as by compartment syndrome of the extensor compartment (see above).

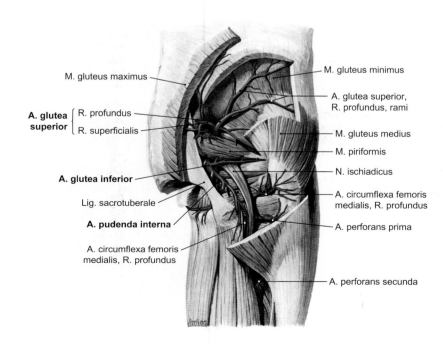

M. gluteus maximus

A. glutea superior { R. profundus / R. superficialis }

A. glutea inferior

Lig. sacrotuberale

A. pudenda interna

A. circumflexa femoris medialis, R. profundus

M. gluteus minimus

A. glutea superior, R. profundus, rami

M. gluteus medius

M. piriformis

N. ischiadicus

A. circumflexa femoris medialis, R. profundus

A. perforans prima

A. perforans secunda

Fig. 5.63 Parietal branches of the A. iliaca interna right, anastomosis region with branches of the A. femoralis. Lateral view after removal of parts of the Mm. gluteus maximus and medius. [S010-2-16]

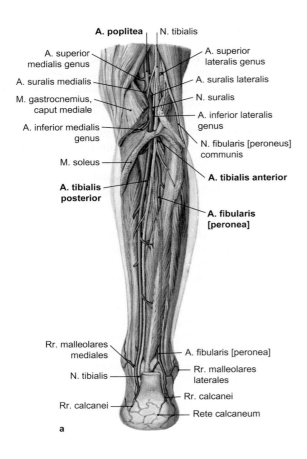

A. poplitea — N. tibialis

A. superior medialis genus

A. suralis medialis

M. gastrocnemius, caput mediale

A. inferior medialis genus

M. soleus

A. tibialis posterior

A. tibialis posterior

Rr. malleolares mediales

N. tibialis

Rr. calcanei

A. superior lateralis genus

A. suralis lateralis

N. suralis

A. inferior lateralis genus

N. fibularis [peroneus] communis

A. tibialis anterior

A. fibularis [peronea]

A. fibularis [peronea]

Rr. malleolares laterales

Rr. calcanei

Rete calcaneum

a

A. superior lateralis genus

A. inferior lateralis genus

M. extensor digitorum longus

A. fibularis [peronea], R. perforans

A. malleolaris anterior lateralis

A. tarsalis lateralis

A. arcuata

Aa. digitales dorsales

Rete articulare genus

A. recurrens tibialis anterior

M. tibialis anterior

A. tibialis anterior

M. extensor hallucis longus

A. dorsalis pedis

Aa. tarsales mediales

A. plantaris profunda

Aa. metatarsales dorsales

b

Fig. 5.64 Arteries of the leg, right. a Dorsal view. **b** Ventral view. [S010-2-16]

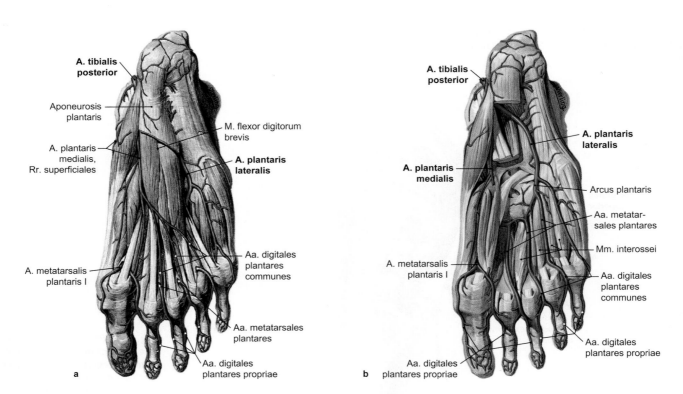

A. tibialis posterior

Aponeurosis plantaris

A. plantaris medialis, Rr. superficiales

A. metatarsalis plantaris I

M. flexor digitorum brevis

A. plantaris lateralis

Aa. digitales plantares communes

Aa. metatarsales plantares

Aa. digitales plantares propriae

a

A. tibialis posterior

A. plantaris medialis

A. metatarsalis plantaris I

Aa. digitales plantares propriae

A. plantaris lateralis

Arcus plantaris

Aa. metatarsales plantares

Mm. interossei

Aa. digitales plantares communes

Aa. digitales plantares propriae

b

Fig. 5.65 Arteries of the sole of the foot, right. Plantar view. **a** Superficial vessels following removal of the plantar aponeurosis. **b** Deep vessels following removal of the long and short flexors. [S010-2-16]

5.7.5 A. tibialis posterior

The A. **tibialis posterior** continues the course of the A. poplitea (➤ Fig. 5.64a). It accompanies the N. tibialis between the deep and superficial calf muscles distally behind the inner ankle, which it supplies with **Rr. malleolares mediales,** and divides into the **Rr. calcanei** to the medial side of the heel. It runs through the neurovascular passageway of the **malleolar canal** towards the sole of foot The main branch is the:

- **A. fibularis:** it runs along behind the Fibula parallel to the A. tibialis posterior distally and divides into the Rr. malleolares laterales to the external ankle and Rr. calcanei to the lateral side of the heel.

On the sole of the foot, the A. tibialis posterior is divided into its two terminal branches:

- **A. plantaris medialis** (➤ Fig. 5.65a): it runs medial to the M. flexor digitorum brevis and connects to the Arcus plantaris profundus.
- **A. plantaris lateralis:** it runs underneath the M. flexor digitorum brevis and forms the Arcus plantaris profundus (➤ Fig. 5.65b). This deep arch (a superficial arch is not usually formed) is located below the bases of the Ossi metatarsi and divides into the Aa. metatarsales plantares. With the Aa. digitales plantares communes and the Aa. digitales plantares propriae, they supply the underside of the toes.

5.8 Veins of the lower extremity

─ Skills ─────────────────────────────────

After working through this chapter, you should be able to:
- understand the basic principle of the venous outflow of the lower extremity
- know the large epifascial veins and show them on a dissection specimen

The venous blood of the lower extremity drains via the V. iliaca communis into the inferior vena cava. **Blood from the hip region**

is carried by branches of the V. iliaca interna (➤ Chap. 8.8.3) and by branches of the V. iliaca externa into the V. iliaca communis. The branches of the V. iliaca externa (V. epigastrica inferior and V. circumflexa ilium profunda) correspond to the arteries in terms of their name and course.

The **blood from the whole leg** is collected via the **V. femoralis.** Here, a distinction is made between a superficial system (epifascial) and a deep system (that accompanies the artery). Both systems are connected by perforans veins (Vv. perforantes) (➤ Fig. 5.66). These veins have valves, which only allow blood to flow from the superficial to the deep system. Ultimately therefore, the majority of the blood from the leg (85%) travels through the deep system. Among the numerous **perforating veins,** 3 groups are clinically significant:

- DODD veins: on the medial side of the thigh
- BOYD veins: on the inner side of the proximal lower leg
- COCKETT veins: on the medial side of the distal lower leg

The **veins of the deep system** accompany the arteries. Therefore, as with the arm, the arteries and veins have the same name (➤ Fig. 5.67). On the lower leg and foot, typically 2 veins accompany the corresponding artery. The V. poplitea as well as the veins of the thigh, generally only occur as single veins.

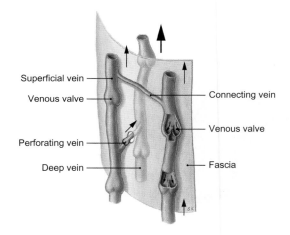

Fig. 5.66 Classification principle of the venous outflow in the leg, superficial and deep leg veins with valves.

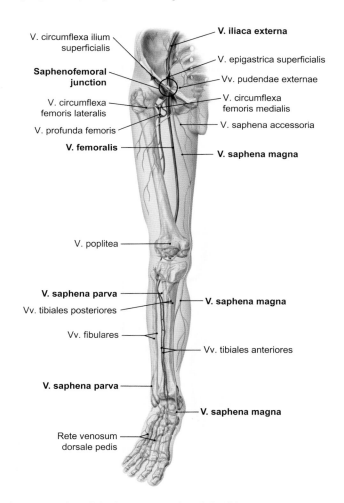

Fig. 5.67 Veins of the lower extremity, right side. Ventral view.

In **deep vein thrombosis,** a blood clot blocks a vein of the deep system (➤ Fig. 5.68). The V. poplitea, V. femoralis at the confluence of the V. saphena magna or the iliac veins are frequently involved. Possible causes are coagulation disorders (intensified coagulation of the blood), immobilisation (long plane journeys, being bed ridden, operation) and oral contraceptives ('the pill', particularly in combination with smoking). In 30% of cases it leads to a life-threatening **pulmonary embolism.** When this occurs, parts of the thrombus in the veins of the legs will break off and are then transported via the right ventricle of the heart into the pulmonary circulation, blocking a branch of the A. pulmonalis. A blockage of major arteries causes right cardiac stress (acute Cor pulmonale), which can lead to heart failure and death. Due to under-perfusion of the lungs, acute respiratory distress almost always occurs.

The **superficial system** consists of 2 large vein stems and a wide variety of side branches (➤ Fig. 5.67)
- **V. saphena magna**
- **V. saphena parva**

Both veins start at the foot and are fed primarily by vessels of the dorsum of the foot (Rete venosum dorsale pedis and Arcus venosus dorsalis pedis). Further on their course, the blood vessels pass through subcutaneous fat until they penetrate through the fascia and culminate in the deep vein system.

The **V. saphena magna** is formed at the medial margin of the foot, runs in front of the inner ankle to the lower leg and continues proximally on the medial side of the leg. It enters an opening in the Fascia lata (Hiatus saphenus) just below the inguinal ligament in the depth and culminates in the V. femoralis. This arch-shaped confluence is clinically referred to as 'cross'. At the Hiatus saphenus the V. saphena magna or the veins of the front hip region include what are known as **'venous star':**
- V. epigastrica superficialis
- V. cirumflexa ilium superficialis
- V. saphena accessoria
- Vv. pudendae externae

The **V. saphena parva** originates at the lateral margin of the foot and passes behind the outer ankle to the rear of the lower leg. Here it runs epifascially further proximally and penetrates the Fascia cruris in order to flow into the V. poplitea in the hollow of the knee.

If the **venous valves** cease to function the blood returning to the torso in an upright posture is reduced. The resulting knotty, enlarged veins of the superficial system are known as **varicose veins** (varicosis). In cases of failure of the valves of the perforating veins or relocation of the deep veins after a deep vein thrombosis, this may cause flow reversal in these vessels (the blood then flows from the deep vessels to the superficial system), and this can contribute to varicosis of the superficial veins.

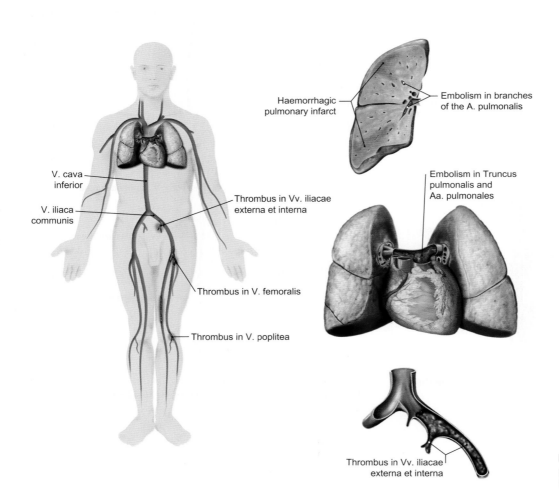

Haemorrhagic pulmonary infarct

Embolism in branches of the A. pulmonalis

V. cava inferior

V. iliaca communis

Thrombus in Vv. iliacae externa et interna

Embolism in Truncus pulmonalis and Aa. pulmonales

Thrombus in V. femoralis

Thrombus in V. poplitea

Thrombus in Vv. iliacae externa et interna

Fig. 5.68 Deep vein thrombosis possibly resulting in an embolism. [L266]

5.9 Lymph vessels of the lower extremity

5.9.1 Lymph vessels

The large lymph vessels (collectors) of the lower extremity mainly run along the large veins. Therefore, here also the superficial (epifascial) system can be differentiated from the deep (subfascial) system. Accordingly, superficial and deep lymph node groups can be found on the leg.

The majority of lymph from the leg is transported by the **superficial system.** It consists of 2 large collector bundles (➤ Fig. 5.69):
- The **ventromedial bundle** runs along the V. saphena magna to the superficial lymph nodes in the area of the linguinal ligament (**Nodi lymphodei inguinales superficiales**). These transfer the lymph further into the deep inguinal lymph nodes (**Nodi lymphoidei inguinales profundi**). The ventromedial collector bundle drains the majority of the lymph of the leg, apart from the dorsal lower leg and the lateral side of the foot.

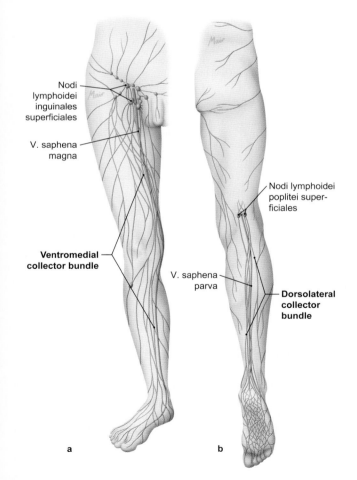

Fig. 5.69 Superficial lymph vessels of the leg, right. a Ventral view. **b** Dorsal view.

- The **dorsolateral bundle** runs along with the V. saphena parva proximally and culminates in the superficial lymph nodes in the area of the hollow of the knee (**Nodi lymphoidei poplitei superficiales**) and also via the **Nodi lymphoidei poplitei profundi** to the deep system and the deep inguinal lymph nodes. The dorsolateral bundle drains the dorsal lower leg and the outer margin of the foot.

The **deep system** drains the lymph of the deep leg regions directly into the deep popliteal and inguinal lymph nodes. The collectors share their course with the major vessels. Because there are so few lymph vessels, less lymph is carried via the deep lymph system than the superficial system.

> **N O T E**
> The epifascial system (via the superficial inguinal lymph nodes) and the subfascial system run together in the Nodi lymphoidei inguinales profundi. This means that almost the entire lymph of the free lower extremity is routed through the deep inguinal lymph nodes!

5.9.2 Inguinal lymph nodes

The lymph nodes are divided into the epifascial Nodi lymphoidei inguinales superficiales and the subfascial Nodi lymphoidei inguinales profundi.

There are up to 25 **superficial lymph nodes** on the Fascia lata, positioned lateral and medial on the inguinal ligament (superolateral and superomedial group) as well as in the area of the Hiatus saphenus (inferior group) (➤ Fig. 5.70). In addition to the lymph of the leg, in the superficial lymph nodes, there is also the lymph from the lower parts of the abdomen and back, from the external genitalia, the perineum as well as the lower segments of the vagina and the anal canal (➤ Fig. 5.70). In addition, in women the lymph vessels are connected via the Lig. teres uteri from the cranial sections of the uterus (Fundus uteri and the 'tube angle'), to the superficial inguinal lymph nodes. Efferent lymph vessels transfer the lymph, especially to the deep inguinal lymph nodes.

┌─ Clinical remarks ─────────────────────

Enlargement of the superficial lymph nodes can be caused by many different things. These include injury to or inflammation of the leg, as well as deep-seated rectal and anal carcinomas or even tumours of the external genitalia or the uterus (endometrial cancer). A thorough palpation of the inguinal region for enlarged lymph nodes must be part of all clinical examinations.

The 1–3 **deep inguinal lymph nodes** are below the Fascia lata in the area of the Hiatus saphenus and transport the lymph to the pelvic lymph nodes in the area of the V. iliaca externa (Nodi lymphodei iliaci externi).

5.9.3 Pelvic lymph nodes

Along the major vessels in the pelvis, there are 3 lymph node stations (➤ Table 5.23) into which the lymph from the pelvic region, as well as the lymph from the leg, is transported (➤ Chap. 8.8.4):
- **Nodi lymphoidei iliaci externi** along the V. iliaca externa, receive the lymph from the deep inguinal lymph nodes as well as from the viscera of the lesser pelvis.
- **Nodi lymphoidei iliaci interni** along the V. iliaca interna also drain the pelvic viscera.

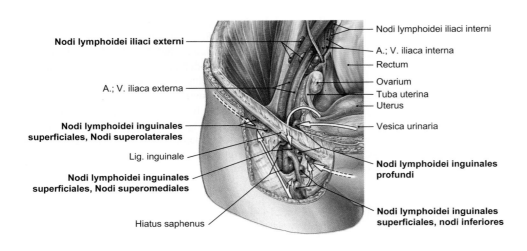

Nodi lymphoidei iliaci externi

A.; V. iliaca externa

Nodi lymphoidei inguinales superficiales, Nodi superolaterales

Lig. inguinale

Nodi lymphoidei inguinales superficiales, Nodi superomediales

Hiatus saphenus

Nodi lymphoidei iliaci interni

A.; V. iliaca interna

Rectum

Ovarium

Tuba uterina

Uterus

Vesica urinaria

Nodi lymphoidei inguinales profundi

Nodi lymphoidei inguinales superficiales, nodi inferiores

Fig. 5.70 Superficial inguinal lymph nodes and drainage areas, right.

Table 5.23 drainage areas and drainage passages of the lymph nodes of the lower extremity, from distal to proximal.

Nodi lymphoidei	Drainage area	Main drainage to
Nodi lymphoidei poplitei superficiales	Superficial sections of the • Dorsal lower leg • Lateral margin of the foot	Nodi lymphoidei poplitei profundi
Nodi lymphoidei poplitei profundi	Deep sections of • Lower leg • Foot	Nodi lymphoidei inguinales profundi
Nodi lymphoidei inguinales superficiales	• Superficial portions of the leg, with the exception of the dorsal calf and the outer side of the foot • Lower abdominal wall • Lower back • Perineal region, gluteal region • Lower anal canal • External genitalia • Female: lower sections of the vagina and the Fundus uteri	Nodi lymphoidei inguinales profundi
Nodi lymphoidei inguinales profundi	• Deep regions of the leg • Superficial parts of the leg via Nodi lymphoidei inguinales superficialis and Nodi lymphoidei poplitei	Nodi lymphoidei iliaci externi
Nodi lymphoidei iliaci externi	• Pelvic viscera • Nodi lymphoidei inguinales profundi	Nodi lymphoidei iliaci communes
Nodi lymphoidei iliaci interni	• Pelvic viscera • Pelvic wall including the gluteal muscles • Deep perineal region	Nodi lymphoidei iliaci communes
Nodi lymphoidei iliaci communes	• Nodi lymphoidei iliaci externi • Nodi lymphoidei iliaci interni	Nodi lymphoidei lumbales

• **Nodi lymphoidei iliaci communes** around the V. iliaca communis receive the lymph of the Nodi lymphoidei illiaci interni and externi and transfer it to the lumbar lymph nodes (Nodi lymphoidei lumbales). From there, the lymph is transported via the Trunci lumbales into the Ductus thoracicus, as the body's main lymphatic duct (➤ Chap. 8.8.4).

5.10 Topographically important aspects of the leg

• explain the structure of the gluteal region, and identify the vessels and nerves penetrating the Foramina suprapiriforme and infrapiriforme
• explain the structure of the hollow of the knee and the arrangement of the vessels and nerves that run through it

5.10.1 Lacuna musculorum and Lacuna vasorum

The **inguinal ligament (Lig. inguinale)** runs from the Spina iliaca anterior superior to the Tuberculum pubicum directly next to the symphysis (➤ Fig. 5.71). The rough connective tissue structure is formed from the aponeurosis of the M. obliquus externus abdominis and the M. iliopsoas by the radiation of different fascia of the abdominal wall (Fascia transversalis) and the leg and pelvic region (Fascia lata, Fascia pelvis parietalis).

In the gap between the inguinal ligament and hip bone, the vessels and nerves exit from the pelvis on their way to the front side of the

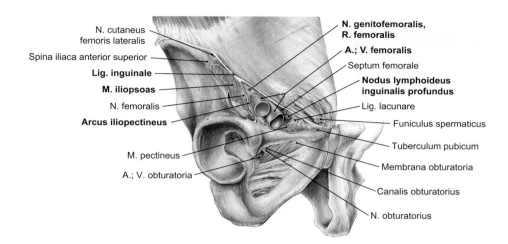

N. cutaneus femoris lateralis
Spina iliaca anterior superior
Lig. inguinale
M. iliopsoas
N. femoralis
Arcus iliopectineus
M. pectineus
A.; V. obturatoria

N. genitofemoralis, R. femoralis
A.; V. femoralis
Septum femorale
Nodus lymphoideus inguinalis profundus
Lig. lacunare
Funiculus spermaticus
Tuberculum pubicum
Membrana obturatoria
Canalis obturatorius
N. obturatorius

Fig. 5.71 Lacuna vasorum and Lacuna musculorum, right. Ventral view.

Table 5.24 Content of Lacuna vasorum and Lacuna musculorum.

Lacuna vasorum (from medial to lateral)	Lacuna musculorum (from medial to lateral)
• Deep inguinal lymph nodes and lymph vessels • V. femoralis • A. femoralis • R. femoralis of the N. genitofemoralis	• N. femoralis • M. iliopsoas • N. cutaneus femoris lateralis

thigh. The Arcus iliopectineus (a reinforcement of the fascia of the M. iliopsoas) separates the *lateral* **Lacuna musculorum** beneath the inguinal ligament from the *medially* located **Lacuna vasorum** (➤ Fig. 5.71, ➤ Table 5.24).

NOTE

The abbreviation **mVAN** can help the sequence of vessels and nerves to be remembered
• **m**edial
• **V**ein → V. femoralis in Lacuna vasorum
• **A**rtery → A. femoralis in Lacuna vasorum
• **N**erves → R. femoralis of the N. genitofemoralis in Lacuna vasorum, N. femoralis in Lacuna musculorum, N. cutaneus femoris lateralis in Lacuna musculorum

Between the V. femoralis and the medial limit of the Lacuna vasorum (Lig. lacunare, split off from the inguinal ligament) there is a gap which is sealed by a layer of connective tissue (Septum femorale). This is breached by the lymph vessels of the leg, and even some of the deep inguinal lymph nodes are located there.

Clinical remarks

The Lacuna vasorum is the breach point for **femoral hernias.** Thus, the Septum femorale is breached and an opening is formed, which in a similar way to the inguinal canal, is referred to as a femoral ring ('Anulus femoralis'). Unlike inguinal hernias, femoral hernias do not breach above the inguinal ligament but below. Femoral hernias are the most common hernias in women. They are difficult to diagnose, because only very large hernias can be palpated beneath the inguinal ligament.

5.10.2 Femoral triangle and adductor canal

Femoral triangle

The femoral triangle (**Trigonum femoris**) is a triangular area on the front of the thigh, in which the penetrating vessels and nerves passing under the inguinal ligament (in the Lacuna vasorum and Lacuna musculorum, see above) can continue or be divided (➤ Fig. 5.72a). It is delimited *at the top* by the inguinal ligament, *laterally* by the M. sartorius and *medially* by the M. gracilis (➤ Table 5.25). The *floor* is formed medially by the M. pectineus and laterally by the M. iliopsoas.

When the M. pectineus is removed, underneath it (and thus dorsal of the femoral triangle), the N. obturatorius and the A./V. obturatoria become visible, having exited the pelvis through the **Canalis obturatorius,** a gap in the Membrana obturatoria.

The N. femoralis is separated in the femoral triangle into its terminal branches and here the A. femoralis delivers the A. profunda femoris to supply the thigh. Just below the inguinal ligament, the epifascial veins form the 'venous star', from which the V. saphena magna passes into the Hiatus saphenus into the depths and flows into the V. femoralis.

Adductor canal

The A. and V. femoralis run distally at the thigh together with the N. saphenus (sensory terminal branch of the N. femoralis) through the **adductor canal** (Canalis adductorius) to the hollow of the knee. The canal is delimited *ventrally* by the Septum intermusculare vastoadductorium and the M. sartorius, *dorsally* by the M. adductor longus, *laterally* by the M. vastus medialis, and *medially* by the M. adductor magnus (➤ Table 5.26). The Septum intermuscululare vastoadductorium is an aponeurosis attachment of the

Table 5.25 Limitation and contents of the femoral triangle.

Limitation	Contents
• Cranial: inguinal ligament • Caudal: M. sartorius • Medial: M. gracilis • Dorsal: M. iliopsoas and M. pectineus	• Lacuna vasorum and musculorum • Branching of the N. femoralis • Branching of the A./V. femoralis with venous star • Inguinal lymph nodes

Table 5.26 Limitation and content of the adductor canal.

Limitations	Contents
• Ventral: Septum intermusculare vastoadductorium (covered by the M. sartorius) • Dorsal: M. adductor longus • Lateral: M. vastus medialis • Medial: M. adductor magnus	• A./V. femoralis • N. saphenus • A. descendens genus

M. adductor magnus, runs to the M. vastus medialis and so completes the adductor canal to a tunnel. The N. saphenus breaks through the Septum and continues to run epifascially to the lower leg. In contrast, the Vasa femoralia run medially past the thigh bone dorsally and under the **Hiatus adductorius** into the hollow of the knee. The Hiatus adductorius is a tendinous arch of the M. adductor magnus between its attachments to the Labium mediale of the Linea aspera and the Epicondylus medialis.

5.10.3 Gluteal region

The gluteal region (Regio glutealis) is located behind the hip joint between the iliac crest and the Sulcus glutealis; when standing, there is a visible, palpable groove in the skin, running horizontally. This is caused by taut connective tissue and therefore does not correspond to the lower margin of the M. gluteus maximus. After removal of this muscle, the M. gluteus medius and the pelvitrochan-teric muscles, the Lig. sacrotuberale and the vessels and nerves are exposed (➤ Fig. 5.72b). The M. gluteus minimus is located dorsal to the M. gluteus medius and is only visible if this is detached. The M. piriformis, positioned caudally to the M. gluteus medius is always easily recognisable; caudal from it is the triplet consisting of the M. obturatorius internus and the two Mm. gemelli ('M. triceps coxae'). Further below is the square-shaped M. quadratus femoris which needs to be removed in order to demonstrate the M. obturatorius externus.

The M. piriformis divides the **Foramen ischiadicum majus** above the Lig. sacrospinale into 2 gaps: **Foramen suprapiriforme** and the **Foramen infrapiriforme.** Both gaps are used as passages for the vessels and nerves of the gluteal region, the perineal region of the external genitalia and of the leg (➤ Table 5.27).

> **Clinical remarks**
>
> The Regio glutealis is still commonly used for **intramuscular injections,** although for most injections, the M. deltoideus is better suited. The injection should not be carried out in the M. gluteus maximus to protect the vessels and nerves, but should be performed ventrally in the M. gluteus medius. Using the VON HOCHSTETTER technique, the index finger of the left hand is placed on the Spina iliaca anterior superior, and the middle finger is braced. The injection is carried out between the index and middle fingers.

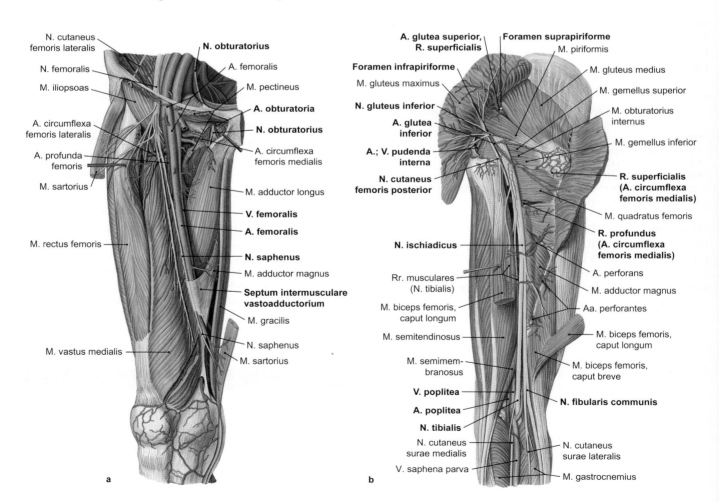

Fig. 5.72 Topography of the hip, femur and knee joint, right. a Ventral view. **b** Dorsal view.

Table 5.27 Foramen isciadicum majus and minus and penetrating pathways.

Foramen		Location	Pathways
Foramen ischiadicum majus	Foramen supra-piriforme	Between M. gluteus medius/minimus and M. piriformis	• N. gluteus superior • A./V. glutea superior
	Foramen infra-piriforme	Between M. piriformis and M. gemellus superior	• N. ischiadicus • N. gluteus inferior • N. pudendus • N. cutaneus femoris posterior • Muscle branches to pel-vitrochanteric muscles • A./V. glutea inferior • A./V. pudenda interna
Foramen ischiadicum minus		Between Lig. sacrospinale and Lig. sacrotuberale	• N. pudendus • A./V. pudenda interna

5.10.4 Hollow of the knee

The hollow of the knee (Fossa poplitea) is a diamond-shaped area behind the knee joint (➤ Fig. 5.72b). At the *top* it is *laterally* delimited by the M. biceps femoris and *medially* by the M. semimembranosus and the M. semitendinosus. The *lower margin* is formed by the

Table 5.28 Limitation and content of the hollow of the knee.

Limitations	Content (from superficial to deep)
• Cranial lateral: M. biceps femoris • Cranial medial: M. semitendinosus and M. semimembranosus • Caudal: M. gastrocnemius	• N. fibularis communis (lateral) • N. tibialis (central) • V. poplitea • A. poplitea

two heads of the M. gastrocnemius (➤ Table 5.28). The major vessels and nerves from the thigh pass through the hollow of the knee on their way to the lower leg (➤ Table 5.28):

- Most superficially positioned are the N. tibialis (middle) and the N. fibularis communis (lateral).
- Below this is the V. poplitea.
- The most deep-seated is the A. poplitea. Here, it also gives rise to branches to supply the knee joint. Due to its deep position, the pulse of the A. poplitea is often difficult to palpate.

NOTE

The vessels and nerves in the knee rank from superficial to deep as follows:
- **N.** tibialis and N. fibularis communis
- **V.** poplitea
- **A.** poplitea
Mnemonic: '**NiVeA**'

INTERNAL ORGANS

6 Chest viscera

Daniela Kugelmann, Jens Waschke

Myocardial infarction (acute coronary syndrome)

Case study

The emergency physician is called to attend 73-year-old Klaus M., who is retired. Mr. M. reports that in the morning after breakfast he felt an acute onset of chest pain that radiated to the neck and left arm. In addition there was shortness of breath, sweating and tightness of the chest. The pain was so strong, not improving with complete rest, that he called the emergency doctor. Medical history indicates known arterial hypertension, otherwise no previous cardiac disease is known. Mr. M. indicates he is a heavy smoker and therefore frequently has problems with his lungs. The emergency doctor immediately brings the patient to hospital.

Examination results

Cold sweating, dyspnoeic patient (respiratory rate 15/min) with mainly retrosternal chest pain radiating to the left in the throat area and arm. The heart rate is elevated at 120/min, blood pressure is low at 100/60 mmHg. On auscultation a systolic murmur with point of maximum impulse above the aortic valve was determined. The lungs are inconspicuous.

Diagnostics

Troponin T, myoglobin, creatine kinase (CK and CK-MB) and C-reactive peptide (CRP) are elevated.
The ECG indicates pronounced signs of ischemia over the anterior wall (ST elevation in I, aVL and V_1-V_6).

Preliminary diagnosis

Diagnostically everything suggests an acute coronary syndrome. Acute coronary syndrome includes myocardial infarction (heart attack) with or without ST elevation in the ECG and unstable angina. Because the cell necrosis markers myoglobin and creatine kinase and the heart muscle-specific enzyme troponin are increased, unstable angina pectoris is ruled out. The ST elevation in the ECG indicates an ST elevation myocardial infarction. The clinical examination is most compatible with a closure of the R. interventricularis anterior of the A. coronaria sinistra (RIVA). Differential diagnosis must exclude angina pectoris, aortic dissection, pulmonary embolism and heart defects.

Treatment

The cardiac catheterisation with percutaneous transluminal coronary angioplasty (PTCA) provides an angiographic confirmation of vascular stenosis. The R. interventricularis anterior is expanded with a balloon catheter during the same examination and a stent is implanted.

Further course

The coronary artery can be dilated with the stent. Later the ischemia markers decline and there are no complications. After 2 weeks the patient can be referred to follow-up treatment with antithrombotic therapy. Overall, this is a very favourable course after myocardial infarction.

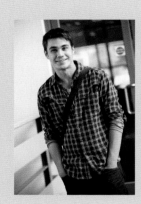

During your internship in A&E, you come across the following case. For the report you have to write about the internship, you make the following notes:

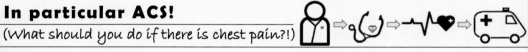

In particular ACS!
(What should you do if there is chest pain?!)

_Hx.:_ 73 year-old patient, acute chest pain since the morning, radiating in left arm and throat area. Shortness of breath, sweating, thoracic tightness; no complete recovery when resting Smoker (problems with lung!), arterial hypertension (AHT)

_CE:_ cold sweats, dyspnoea, HR 120/min, RR 100/60 mmHg systolic with

p.m. over aortic valve, lungs free

_DD.:_ Tropic positive, myoglobin, CK, CK-MB and CRP ↑

ECG: ST elevation in I, aVL and V1 – V6 (esp. STEMI!!)

_TX:_ heart catheter with PTCA and Stent (RIVA)

Proc.: platelet aggregation inhibition!

6.1 Heart

Skills

After working through this chapter, you should be able to:
- Explain the development of the heart with any possible malformations in main features
- Explain the change from foetal to post-natal circulation
- Explain on a specimen and using an x-ray the location, orientation and projection of the heart with edge-forming structures
- Describe on a specimen the inner and outer structures of the heart chambers
- Explain the wall layers of the heart and pericardial sac
- Describe the location, structure and function of the heart skeleton
- Explain on a specimen the structure, function and projection of the various heart valves
- Deduce heart sounds and murmurs and indicate their auscultation type
- Show on a specimen the conduction system with accurate localisation of sinu-atrial and AV nodes and understand the anatomical basis of the ECG
- Explain the autonomic innervation of the heart
- Indicate on a specimen the coronary arteries with all important branches and describe their importance in the development, diagnosis and treatment of coronary artery disease
- Specify the main features of the veins and lymph vessels of the heart

6.1.1 Overview

The heart (Cor) is a Cone-shaped, four-chambered, muscular hollow organ. The size is roughly equivalent to the fist of the respective person and the weight is on average 250–300 g (0.45 % of body weight, i.e. in men 280–340 g and in women: 230–280 g). The heart is divided into a left and a right half by the cardiac septum. The two halves of the heart are each divided into a right and left atrium (Atrium dextrum and sinistrum) as well as a right and left ventricle (Ventriculus dexter and sinister). The atria have blind ending ap-

pendages, known as auricles (Auricula dextra and sinistera). The heart is absolutely essential for life as the superordinate organ of the cardiovascular system. Its significance in medicine can, amongst other things, be recognised in that in addition to general practitioners and primary care physicians, multiple disciplines, such as cardiologists and cardiac surgeons have specialised in heart diseases.

Clinical remarks

Above a **heart weight of 500 g** blood flow to the heart muscles by its own supply vessels (coronary vessels) is not enough. This increases the risk of blood flow deprivation (ischemia) and therefore death of cardiac tissue (heart attack). This weight is known as the **critical heart weight.** Some pathological conditions may cause the heart to weigh up to 1100 g, a condition referred to as **Cor bovinum** (ox heart).

6.1.2 Function

The heart drives the blood circulation, which can be divided into a small circulation (pulmonary circulation) and a large circulation (systemic circulation). The circulation serves to transport blood and distribute it throughout the body. Therefore, its functions are identical to those of the blood.

The **most important functions** of the cardiovascular system are:
- Oxygen and nutrient supply of the organism (transport of respiratory gases and nutrients) respectively metabolism end products
- Thermal regulation (heat transfer in blood)
- Defence function (transport of immune cells and antibodies)
- Hormonal control (transport of hormones)
- Haemostasis (transport of blood platelets and coagulation factors).

Both circulations form a closed system, with the heart at the centre functioning as a muscular suction and pressure pump as the driving force. The heart is responsible for continuous blood circulation and beats at an average of 70 times per minute. This allows blood

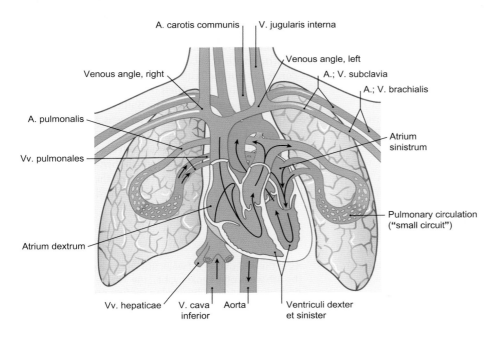

A. carotis communis | V. jugularis interna | Venous angle, left | A.; V. subclavia | A.; V. brachialis | Venous angle, right | A. pulmonalis | Vv. pulmonales | Atrium sinistrum | Atrium dextrum | Pulmonary circulation ("small circuit") | Vv. hepaticae | V. cava inferior | Aorta | Ventriculi dexter et sinister

Fig. 6.1 Blood flow through the heart and lungs as part of the cardiovascular system; blue = blood low in oxygen, red = oxygenated blood. [L126]

low in oxygen from the systemic circulation to first reach the right atrium and then the right ventricle via the V. cava inferior and V. cava superior. From there, the blood is pumped into the pulmonary circulation via the Truncus pulmonalis and enriched with oxygen. Saturated with oxygen, it flows through the Vv. pulmonales back into the left atrium and, from there, via the left ventricle and aorta back into the systemic circulation (➤ Fig. 6.1).

6.1.3 Development of the heart and blood vessels

The cardiovascular system is the first functioning organ system of the embryo (from the 3rd week of development!).

Development of the blood vessels
The cardiovascular system develops out of the **mesoderm.** The first blood vessels are formed in the *3rd week* initially in the yolk sac and the body stalk and 2 days later also in the embryo (splanchnic and somatic layer). Hemangioblasts initially develop out of the mesoderm as precursor cells of blood vessel endothelium and red blood cells **(vasculogenesis)** and form blood islands. New vessels sprout from the first simple blood vessel **(angiogenesis).** At first arteries and veins have no structural differences, but are only distinguished based on the direction of blood flow in relation to the heart:
- Arteries: carry the blood from the heart
- Veins: carry the blood to the heart

Initially 3 paired vein stems are formed that combine to form the Sinus venosus of the heart (➤ Fig. 6.2):
- **V. umbilicalis:** brings oxygenated blood from the placenta back to the embryo (also ➤ Chap. 8.6.6)
- **Yolk sac veins** (Vv. vitellinae): transport blood low in oxygen from the yolk sac
- **Cardinal veins** (Vv. cardinales communes superiores and inferiores, Vv. subcardinales and supracardinales): collect the deoxygenated blood from the upper and lower body, which then form the Vena cavae (Vv. cavae superior and inferior) with their tributaries as well as the V. azygos and V. hemiazygos

The pharyngeal arch arteries originate from the **Saccus aorticus,** which transport the blood into the initially paired aorta, which then combine to form the Aorta dorsalis (➤ Fig. 6.2). **3 types of arteries** issue from the aorta:
- **Aa. umbilicales** (Aa. umbilicales): transport deoxygenated blood to the placenta
- **Yolk sac arteries** (Aa. vitellinae): after the yolk sac is included they form the vessels for the 3 intestinal segments in the intestinal tube (Truncus coeliacus for the foregut, A. mesenterica superior for the midgut, A. mesenterica inferior for the hindgut)
- **Intersegmental arteries** (Aa. intersegmentales): these form the Aa. vertebrales, the intercostal and lumbar arteries as well as the arteries for the extremities systems

The **pharyngeal arch arteries** supply the pharyngeal arches, which form in the 4th–5th week. Of the 6 pairs of pharyngeal arch arteries the first two and the 5th degenerate. Derivatives of the 3rd, 4th and 6th pharyngeal arch arteries are:
- A. carotis communis (3rd pharyngeal arch artery)
- A. subclavia (right) and aortic arch (left) (4th pharyngeal arch artery)
- Pulmonary arteries (on both sides) and Ductus arteriosus (left) (6th pharyngeal arch artery)

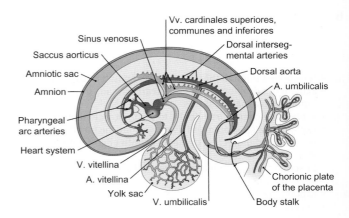

Fig. 6.2 Early embryonic blood circulation In the 4th week (day 26). [E347-09]

Development of the heart
Formation of the cardiac tube and heart loop
In the *3rd week (18th day)* a vascular plexus arises from the horseshoe-shaped cardiogenic plate in the mesoderm of the upper pole of the embryonic disc, the branches of which combine to form the unpaired **endocardial** tube. Gaps around the endocardial tube dorsal to the cardiac system lead to the formation of the pericardial cavity (➤ Chap. 6.5.5).
The inner layer (intra-embryonic coeloma) of the pericardium solidifies into the **myocardium,** which surrounds the endocardium and forms a cardiac tube, which contracts rhythmically from the end of the 3rd week. The tube is divided into (➤ Fig. 6.3; ➤ Fig. 6.4):
- A primitive atrium with Sinus venosus as an inflow segment
- A ventricle with Truncus arteriosus as an outflow segment

The connection of the Truncus arteriosus to the Saccus aorticus is controlled by cells at the outlets of the pharyngeal arch arteries (secondary cardiogenic field). The Bulbus cordis bulges out of between the ventricle and Truncus arteriosus, the distal portion of which is called the Conus cordis.
The **epicardium** arises from a small cell area on the outside of the Sinus venosus (proepicardium), which then surrounds the whole cardiac tube. Through the cranial folding the heart shifts caudally and ventrally to the foregut into the pericardial cavity together with the Septum transversum (➤ Fig. 6.3).

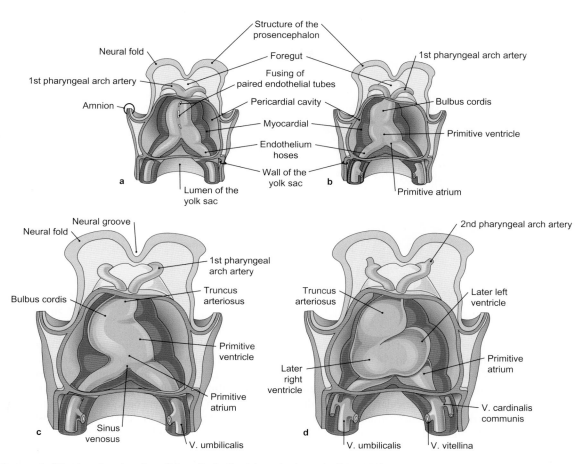

Fig. 6.3 Development of the heart and pericardial cavity in the 4th and 5th week. [E347-09]

In the *4th–5th week* what will later be the right ventricle grows faster than the other sections, creating an S-shaped **heart loop** (➤ Fig. 6.3c, d; ➤ Fig. 6.4). In doing so, the atrium and Sinus venosus shift cranially and dorsally, so that the inflow and outflow channels now face upwards. The Sinus venosus extends towards the right and left sinus horns and has sinus valves that are designed to prevent the backflow of blood. The mouth of the sinus venosus increasingly shifts towards the right. Hereby, the **right sinus horn** becomes larger and is incorporated into the right atrium, where it forms the **Sinus venarum cavarum.** This smooth-walled part of the right atrium is divided from the rest of the atrium by the Crista terminalis (cranial part of the right sinus valve), which emerges from the primitive atrium together with the Auricula dextra and has muscle blocks (Mm. pectinate). The **left sinus horn** becomes the **Sinus coronarius,** which, just like the mouth of the V. cava inferior, has a separate valve (caudal part of the right sinus valve). Similar to that on the right side, the primitive pulmonary vein is incorporated into the left atrium up to the point where it branches, so that now 4 Vv. pulmonales separately enter the smooth-walled atrium. Only the left auricle originates from the primitive atrium.

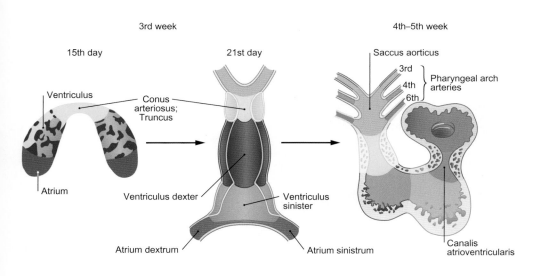

Fig. 6.4 Stages of heart development in the 3rd–5th week.

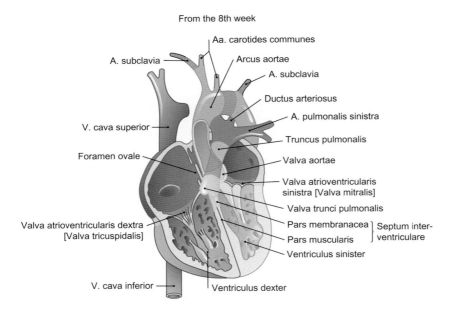

From the 8th week

Aa. carotides communes

A. subclavia

Arcus aortae

A. subclavia

Ductus arteriosus

A. pulmonalis sinistra

V. cava superior

Truncus pulmonalis

Foramen ovale

Valva aortae

Valva atrioventricularis sinistra [Valva mitralis]

Valva trunci pulmonalis

Valva atrioventricularis dextra [Valva tricuspidalis]

Pars membranacea ⎫ Septum inter-
Pars muscularis ⎭ ventriculare

Ventriculus sinister

V. cava inferior

Ventriculus dexter

Fig. 6.5 Septation of ventricle in the 5th–7th week.

During the contraction of the heart the cells of the Sinus venosus have a pacemaker function and after integration of the right atrium form the **sinus nodes** and **AV nodes.**

The connection between atrium and ventricle is narrowed to form the atrioventricular canal (Canalis atrioventricularis), which is diverted into the centre line and divided by endocardial cushions into a right and a left atrioventricular opening (➤ Fig. 6.4). The endocardial cushions arise from the cardiac jelly that is formed between the endocardium and the myocardium and later develops into the **cuspid valves.**

During its development the heart increasingly loses its connection to the dorsal wall of the pericardial cavity (Mesocardium dorsale), until it is reduced to the folding of the epicardium into the pericardium. The **Sinus transversus pericardii** forms between them.

Septation of the heart

In the *5th–7th week* the **interventricular septum** (Septum interventriculare) develops. In a caudal position close to the tip of the heart, first the muscular part of the septum forms (Pars muscularis), which incompletely separates the two ventricles. They continue to communicate with each other until the end of the 7th week via a **Foramen interventriculare,** until the Pars membranacea of the septum completely separates the two ventricles (➤ Fig. 6.5).

In the *5th week* the Conus cordis and Truncus arteriosus are also separated by bulges that are formed by proliferation of neural crest cells (➤ Fig. 6.6). These bulges join together, forming the **Septum aorticopulmonale,** which spirally divides the outflow tract and, together with the adjacent Saccus aorticus, forms the **Truncus pulmonalis** and the **aorta.** In the Truncus arteriosus 3 endocardial cushions form the semilunar valves of the pulmonary and aortic valve.

Septation of the atrium also occurs in the *5th–7th week* and begins with the formation of the **Septum primum,** that grows in dorsally from above and initially leaves the Ostium/Foramen primum free (➤ Fig. 6.7a). Within the upper part of the Septum primum, the Ostium/Foramen secundum is created through programmed cell death (apoptosis) (➤ Fig. 6.7b). The **Septum secundum** then develops to the right of the Septum primum, and merges with the left sinus valve (➤ Fig. 6.7c, e). Both septa fuse and together enclose the **Foramen ovale** (➤ Fig. 6.7d, f).

The Septum primum forms the Valvula foraminis ovalis that enables directional flow of the blood from the right atrium into the left atrium. After birth the Valvula foraminis ovalis closes the Foramen ovale due to the increased blood pressure in the left atrium. From the septum secundum the Limbus fossae ovalis remains.

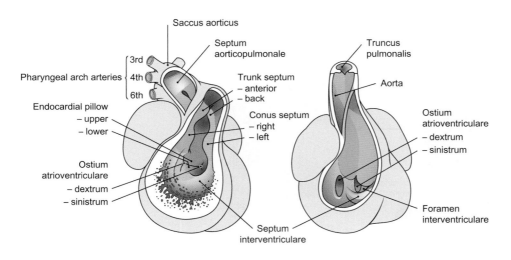

Saccus aorticus

Septum aorticopulmonale

Truncus pulmonalis

Pharyngeal arch arteries ⎧ 3rd
⎨ 4th
⎩ 6th

Trunk septum
– anterior
– back

Aorta

Endocardial pillow
– upper
– lower

Conus septum
– right
– left

Ostium atrioventriculare
– dextrum
– sinistrum

Ostium atrioventriculare
– dextrum
– sinistrum

Foramen interventriculare

Septum interventriculare

Fig. 6.6 Septation of the outflow tract. [L126]

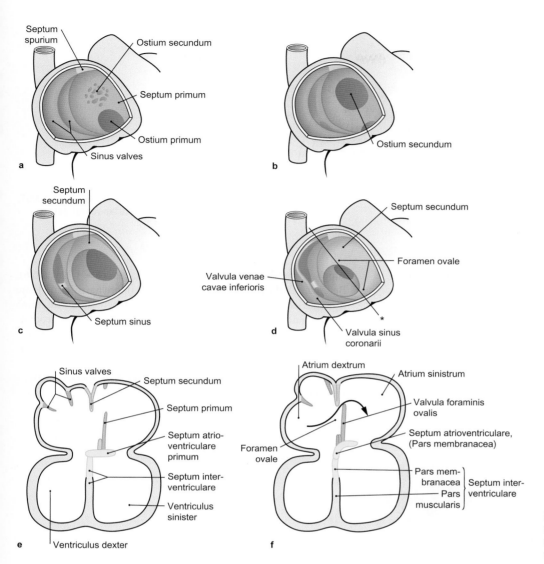

Fig. 6.7 Septation of the atria.
a, b in the 5th week. **c, e** In the 6th week. **d, f** In the 7th and 8th week; * cutting plane in e and f.

Clinical remarks

Congenital heart defects occur in 0.75% of all newborn babies and are thus the most common developmental disorders. Not all heart defects require treatment because they are often not functionally relevant and some close spontaneously. Pathophysiologically, the most common heart defects can be divided into three groups:

- **Defects with left to right shunt** are among the most common congenital heart defects: ventricular septal defects 25% (most frequent congenital heart defect [➤ Fig. 6.8b]), atrial septal defects 12%, open (persistent) Ductus arteriosus 12% (➤ Chap. 6.1.4). Due to the increased pressure in the systemic circulation the blood flows from left to right into the pulmonary circulation. If no operative remedial action is taken, pulmonary hypertension will lead to right heart insufficiency.
- **Defects with right to left shunt:** Tetralogy of FALLOT 9% (➤ Fig. 6.8a), transposition of the great vessels 5%. These defects are characterised by a bluish tinge of the skin (cyanosis) because deoxygenated blood is transported from pulmonary circulation to the systemic circulation.
- **Defects with obstruction:** Pulmonary valve stenosis 6%, aortic valve stenosis 6%, aortic coarctation 6% (➤ Chap. 6.1.4, ➤ Fig. 6.11). This leads to hypertrophy of the respective ventricle.

The **tetralogy** of **FALLOT** is the most common cyanotic heart defect and makes up 65 % of all congenital cyanotic heart defects (➤ Fig. 6.8). It is a combination of:
- Pulmonary artery stenosis
- 'Overriding' aorta
- Right ventricular hypertrophy
- Ventricular septal defect

Due to the asymmetrical septation of the Conus arteriosus, the pulmonary valve is too narrow and in contrast the aorta is too wide and displaced over the septum ('overriding'). The narrow pulmonary valve causes right ventricular hypertrophy, which is responsible for the right to left shunting through the ventricular septal defect and thus the cyanosis.

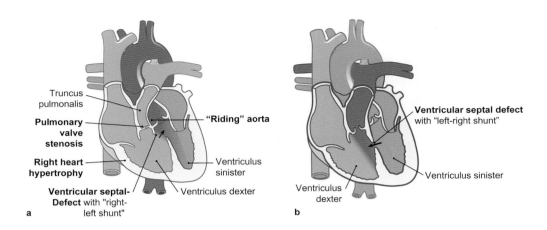

a
Truncus pulmonalis
Pulmonary valve stenosis
Right heart hypertrophy
Ventricular septal-Defect with "right-left shunt"
"Riding" aorta
Ventriculus sinister
Ventriculus dexter

b
Ventricular septal defect with "left-right shunt"
Ventriculus sinister
Ventriculus dexter

Fig. 6.8 a Tetralogy of FALLOT, b ventricular septal defect. [L126]

6.1.4 Prenatal and postnatal blood circulation

Prenatal circulation

The development of the heart and blood vessels is described in ➤ Chap 6.1.3.

The prenatal circulation has various unusual features, which are based on the fact that various organs are not yet fully developed and do not have their final functions. The lungs are not yet fully unfolded because it is still filled with amniotic fluid and the oxygen supply of the child is undertaken by the placenta (➤ Chap. 8.6.6). Before birth the pulmonary vessels are therefore narrow and there is no gas exchange in the lungs. The capillary bed of the still immature liver also has a high flow resistance. These organs are separated from the prenatal circulation by bypass pathways, so all of the blood does not have to pass through the organs. This is why there is a **physiological right to left shunt** in the atrium and the large vessels of the heart, and a bypass of the liver, that opens directly into the V. cava inferior (➤ Fig. 6.9).

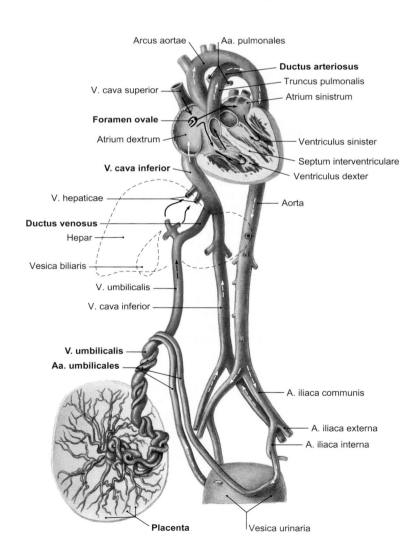

Arcus aortae
Aa. pulmonales
Ductus arteriosus
V. cava superior
Truncus pulmonalis
Atrium sinistrum
Foramen ovale
Atrium dextrum
Ventriculus sinister
Septum interventriculare
Ventriculus dexter
V. cava inferior
V. hepaticae
Aorta
Ductus venosus
Hepar
Vesica biliaris
V. umbilicalis
V. cava inferior
V. umbilicalis
Aa. umbilicales
A. iliaca communis
A. iliaca externa
A. iliaca interna
Placenta
Vesica urinaria

Fig. 6.9 Prenatal circulation.

The 3 most important structures of the **prenatal bypass circulation** are:

- The Foramen ovale: shunt at the atrial level
- The Ductus arteriosus BOTALLI: shunt between the great heart vessels
- The ductus venosus (clinically ARANTII): vessel bypassing the liver

The oxygenated blood flows from the placenta into the V. umbilicalis of the umbilical cord through the navel (Umbilicus) to the liver. A part of the blood is sent directly to the capillaries of the liver, but the vast majority bypasses it due to the high flow resistance of the liver and is transferred via the **Ductus venosus** (clinically ARANTII) directly to the inferior vena cava (V. cava inferior) and further into the right atrium (liver bypass). In the V. cava inferior oxygen-rich blood from the placenta is already mixed with the blood from the lower body. The valve at the bottom of the confluence of the V. cava inferior (Valvula venae cavae inferioris) guides the blood into the right atrium directly to the Foramen ovale. The **Foramen ovale** is a direct bypass connection in the septum between the right and left atrium, so that the blood can be transported directly via the aorta into the systemic circulation, bypassing the lungs. A part of the blood, especially the blood from the upper half of the body, which flows into the right atrium via the superior vena cava (V. cava superior), enters the right ventricle. The majority of this blood flows through the **Ductus arteriosus,** a direct connection between the Truncus pulmonalis and the aorta, into the systemic circulation. 65% of the blood flows through the Aa. umbilicales back to the placenta. The remaining 35% remains in the organs of the lower half of the body.

Postnatal circulation

After birth the placental circulation is interrupted by clamping the umbilical cord. The partial pressure of CO_2 in the blood of the newborn increases. The respiratory centre is stimulated and the lungs assume their function. The bypass connections must now be interrupted (➤ Fig. 6.10):

- As a result of the pressure increase in the left atrium the **Foramen ovale** is functionally closed. Later the Valvula foraminis ovalis grows together with the Septum secundum. The Fossa ovalis remains as a relic.
- The **Ductus arteriosus** is actively closed by smooth muscle contraction, which is triggered by the high level of oxygen. Four days after birth it has usually closed completely. In adults the Ligamentum arteriosum can be found as a relic.
- The **Ductus venosus** obliterates after birth into the Ligamentum venosum.
- The **V. umbilicalis** obliterates to the Lig. teres hepatis between the liver and abdominal wall.
- The two **Aa. umbilicales** also contract to prevent blood loss. The distal part of the A. umbilicalis becomes the medial umbilical ligament on both sides, which both form the basis of the Plica umbilicalis medialis on the inner relief of the abdominal wall.

> N O T E
> After the change from prenatal circulation
> • the Foramen ovale becomes the Fossa ovalis
> • the Ductus arteriosus becomes the Lig. arteriosum
> • the Ductus venosus becomes the Lig. venosum
> • the Vv. umbilicalis becomes the Lig. teres hepatis
> • the A. umbilicalis (distal portion) becomes the Lig. umbilicale mediale

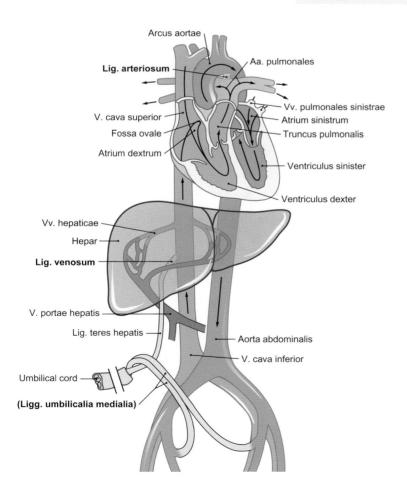

Fig. 6.10 Postnatal circulation.

Patent Ductus arteriosus: if the Ductus arteriosus does not close, it creates a patent ductus arteriosus. It is more common in females. If it is not blocked, blood from the aorta can get into the Truncus pulmonalis. This creates a left to right shunt. Since prostaglandin E_2 has a diluting effect on the ductus, an inhibitor of prostaglandin synthesis may cause a closure and possibly help avoid an operation. However, since these active substances are used to some extent as anti-inflammatory agents and analgesics, they can also cause a premature closure of the foetal Ductus arteriosus in a pregnant woman.

Opening in the Foramen ovale: Approximately 20% of the adult population have a residual opening in the area of the Foramen ovale. This is usually functionally irrelevant and therefore not to be confused with an atrial septal defect. The opening, however, can lead to thrombi in the form of emboli from the leg veins entering the systemic circulation and there causing organ infarction and stroke in the brain (paradoxical embolism).

Aortic coarctation: When the occlusion of the Ductus arteriosus encroaches upon the surrounding sections of the aortic arch, a coarctation of the aorta ensues (➤ Fig. 6.11). This results in hypertrophy of the left heart with high blood pressure (hypertension) in the upper part of the body. In contrast, pressure in the lower half of the body is too low. What stands out diagnostically is a systolic cardiac murmur between the shoulder blades as well as radiographically visible rib defects (erosions) due to bypass circulations of the intercostal arteries to the A. thoracica interna. The stenosis must be corrected via an operation or by dilation, because otherwise heart failure and strokes can ensue even at a young age.

6.1.5 Location and projection

The heart lies in the pericardium between the pleural cavity in the inferior middle mediastinum (➤ Chap. 6.5.2) in the pericardial cavity (Cavitas pericardiaca) (➤ Fig. 6.12). It is rotated round its longitudinal axis, so that the right heart faces the ventral thoracic wall and the left heart more towards the left side and to the back. Two thirds of the heart project left of the median plane, the last third to the right of it. In the membrane-free triangle (Trigonum pericardiacum) a part of the cardiac sac lies directly on the ventral thoracic wall.

Cardiac dullness describes a weakened sound over the heart on percussion (tapping) of the chest. A distinction is made between **absolute cardiac dullness,** which corresponds to the percussion sound directly above the membrane-free triangle and relative cardiac dullness. With **relative cardiac dullness,** the percussion sound is less reduced due to the lungs (Recessus costomediastinalis) lying over the heart. Relative cardiac dullness can be used to determine the size of the heart.

The direct location of the heart in the thorax can be used for intracardiac injections in the 4th–5th intercostal space (ICS) and operative access to the heart. The location of the heart directly on the chest is advantageous for cardiac massage (➤ Fig. 6.13). Here the heart can be compressed by the chest.

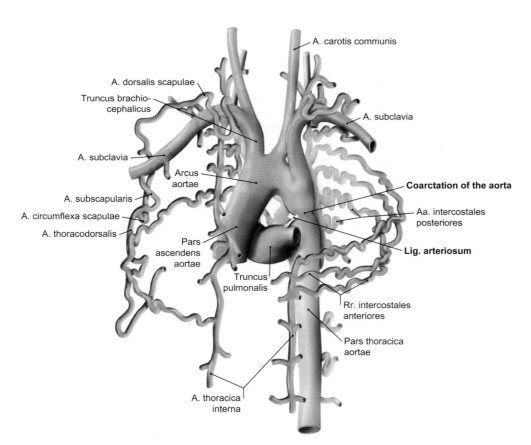

A. carotis communis
A. dorsalis scapulae
Truncus brachio-cephalicus
A. subclavia
A. subclavia
Arcus aortae
Coarctation of the aorta
A. subscapularis
Aa. intercostales posteriores
A. circumflexa scapulae
A. thoracodorsalis
Pars ascendens aortae
Lig. arteriosum
Truncus pulmonalis
Rr. intercostales anteriores
Pars thoracica aortae
A. thoracica interna

Fig. 6.11 Coarctation of the aorta. Stenosis causes the formation of bypass circulations between the branches of the A. subclavia and the Aorta descendens. The convoluted course of dilated intercostal vessels is characteristic (rib erosion in the x-ray image). [L266]

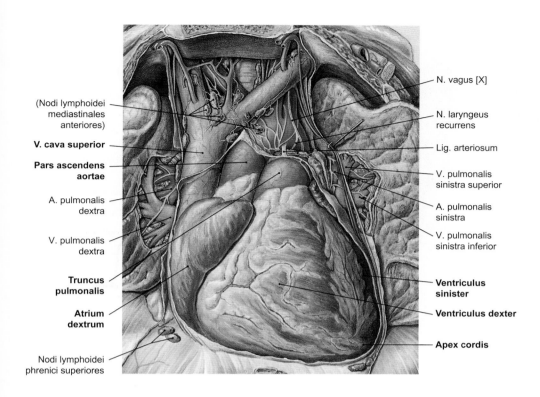

(Nodi lymphoidei mediastinales anteriores)

V. cava superior

Pars ascendens aortae

A. pulmonalis dextra

V. pulmonalis dextra

Truncus pulmonalis

Atrium dextrum

Nodi lymphoidei phrenici superiores

N. vagus [X]

N. laryngeus recurrens

Lig. arteriosum

V. pulmonalis sinistra superior

A. pulmonalis sinistra

V. pulmonalis sinistra inferior

Ventriculus sinister

Ventriculus dexter

Apex cordis

Fig. 6.12 Situs cordis; location of the heart in the thorax. Ventral view, after the opening of the pericardium.

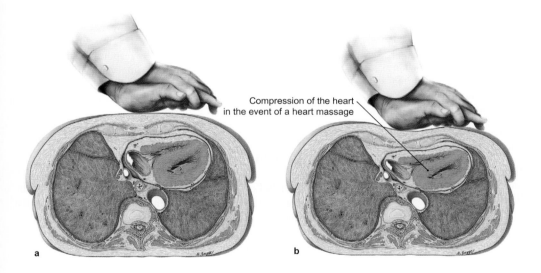

Compression of the heart in the event of a heart massage

a b

Fig. 6.13 Cardiac massage. By applying pressure to the chest, the ventricles are also compressed so that blood is ejected into the great vessels and blood circulation can be maintained. For cardiac massage, both hands are initially placed loosely on the chest **(a)**, then the heart is alternately compressed by pressure on the chest **(b)** and then released again **(a)** in order to maintain blood circulation. [L266]

The **right border of the heart** is located approximately 2 cm beside the right sternal border, starting from the 3rd–6th costal cartilage. The **left coronary border** projects onto a connecting line between the lower border of the 3rd rib (2–3 cm parasternal, left) to the 5th ICS in the medioclavicular line (MCL). The apex beat can be tested in the 5th midclavicular ICS. From the centre of the base of the heart to the apex a 12 cm long **longitudinal axis (anatomical cardiac axis)** can be described. It passes along the thorax diagonally from dorsal right top to ventral left bottom and normally creates an angle of approximately 45° to all 3 main planes of the space. The anatomical cardiac axis may differ depending on the type of constitution. Knowledge of the **marginal structures** is of major clinical importance in the interpretation of x-ray images (➤ Fig. 6.14). In the sagittal (posterior–anterior) projection, the following structures are marginal:

- Right border of the heart (from top to bottom):
  - V. cava superior
  - Right atrium (Atrium dextrum)
- Left border of the heart (from top to bottom):
  - Aortic arch (Arcus aortae)
  - Truncus pulmonalis
  - Left auricle (Auricula sinistra)
  - Left ventricle (Ventriculus sinister)

N O T E

In an x-ray image with sagittal projection (posterior–anterior) the right ventricle does not form a margin. In a lateral x-ray image the right atrium does not form a margin.

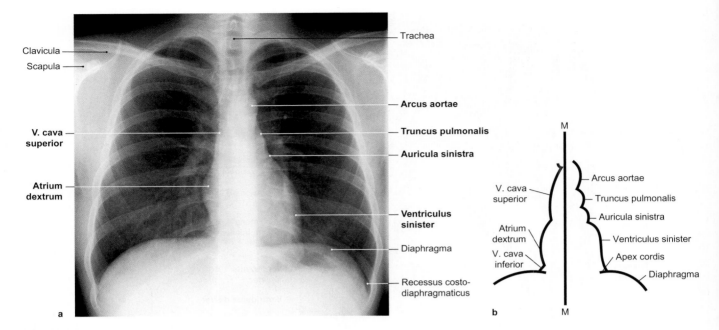

Fig. 6.14 Cardiac contours in the chest x-ray.

Based on the relative positions various **surfaces of the heart** can be distinguished:
- **Facies sternocostalis:** ventral location and mostly formed by the right ventricle
- **Facies diaphragmatica:** (under)side lying on the diaphragm, consisting of parts of the right and left ventricle; the Facies diaphragmatica corresponds to the clinical 'posterior wall'
- **Facies pulmonales dextra and sinistra:** adjacent to the pleural cavities on each side; on the right it is formed by the right atrium, on the left by the left atrium and ventricle

The heart has the **form** of a reversed cone:
- **Basis cordis** (base of the heart): cranial, corresponds to the valve level. This is where the great vessels (aorta, Truncus pulmonalis) originate. The Truncus pulmonalis issuing from the right ventricle is enlarged directly at the outlet to the Conus arteriosus. The aorta issues from the left ventricle and has a spiral course, so that its origin behind the Truncus pulmonalis is not visible from the outside. The base of the heart is elastically fixed by the great vessels and pulmonary veins and Membrana bronchopericardiaca.

- **Apex cordis** (apex of the heart): is mainly formed by the left ventricle and is directed to the bottom left

At the ventral Facies sternocostalis, the location of the interventricular septum (Septum interventriculare) at the **Sulcus interventricularis anterior** can be observed through which the R. interventricularis anterior of the A. coronaria sinistra runs. On the bottom side (Facies diaphragmatica) this limit corresponds to the **Sulcus interventricularis posterior** with the R. interventricularis posterior. The distinction between atria and ventricles is formed by the **Sulcus coronarius,** through which, among others, the A. coronaria dextra and the Sinus coronarius run.

6.1.6 Atria and ventricles

The heart is a hollow muscle with 4 separate spaces that can be divided into a right heart with right atrium and right ventricle and a left heart with left atrium and left ventricle:

Right atrium (Atrium dextrum)
The V. cava inferior and the V. cava superior as well as the Sinus coronarius enter into the right atrium (➤ Fig. 6.15) and drain venous blood from the systemic circulatory system as well as from the heart's own supply (Vasa privata). Small cardiac veins from the Vasa privata discharge directly into the right atrium (Foramina venarum minimarum). The right atrium is separated laterally from the left atrium by the **Septum interatriale,** where the sealed Foramen ovale is located in the form of the **Fossa ovalis,** the edge of which is raised to form the limbus fossae ovalis. In the right atrium is the **atrial sinus (Sinus venarum cavarum),** which developmentally originated from the sinus horn and has a smooth surface anatomy. It is located between the V. cava inferior and V. cava superior. In contrast, in the rest of the atrium, especially in the **auricle (Auricula dextra),** the inner surface is lined with Mm. pectinati. From the outside this transition can be recognised at the **Sulcus terminalis cordis** and on the inside this corresponds to the **Crista terminalis.** Subepicardially at the sulcus terminalis lies the pacemaker of the conduction system, the sinus node. At the confluence of the V. cava

inferior the rudimentary formed **Valvula venae cavae inferioris** protrudes. A second 'valve' is located on the opening of the Sinus coronarius, the **Valvula sinus coronarii.** The extension of the Valvula venae cavae inferioris leads to **TODARO's TENDON.** Together with the Ostidum of the Sinus coronarius and the edge of the septal cusp of the tricuspid valve they form the boundaries of **KOCH's triangle,** in which the atrioventricular node (AV node, Nodus atrioventricularis) of the cardiac conduction system is found (➤ Chap. 6.1.9). The Ostium atrioventriculare dextrum, where the tricuspid **right atrioventricular valve (Valvula tricuspidalis)** lies, separates the right atrium from the right ventricle.

Right ventricle (Ventriculus dexter)
The musculature of the right ventricle consists of two layers and raised by trabeculae (Trabeculae carneae). The wall thickness is 3–5 mm (➤ Fig. 6.15). There are **3 papillary muscles** in the ventricle (M. papillaris anterior, M. papillaris posterior, M. papillaris septalis) at which the tendinous cords (**Chordae tendineae**) of the tricuspid valve are fixed. They are part of the active cuspid attachment apparatus and prevent retrogression of the cuspids during systole. The ventricle can be divided into inflow and outflow streams, which are divided by a myocardial crest, the **Crista supraventricularis.** The inflow stream also includes the **Trabecula septomarginalis** (moderator band described by Leonardo da Vinci) extending from the intermuscular septum (Septum intermusculare) to the anterior papilllary muscle. In this regularly occurring trabecula there are fibres of the conducting system. The outflow stream crosses the Conus arteriosus to the Truncus pulmonalis.

Left atrium (Atrium sinistrum)
In the left atrium the 4 pulmonary veins issue; 2 right and 2 left Vv. pulmonales. They transport oxygenated blood from the lungs to the heart. The opening of the Vv. pulmonales has a smooth wall, otherwise Mm. pectinati can be found, especially in the **left auricle** **(Auricula sinistra).** In the **Septum interatriale** the valve of the Valvula foraminis ovalis can be recognised, the edge of the original Septum primum, which is fused with the Septum secundum.

Left ventricle (Ventriculus sinister)
The Ostium atrioventriculare sinistrum contains the **left atrioventricular valve (mitral valve/Valva mitralis)** with 2 cusps and represents the connection from the atrium to the left ventricle. The mitral valve is connected to **2 papillary muscles** (M. papillaris anterior, M. papillaris posterior) via tendinous cords (**Chordae tendineae**). Because of the higher pressure the wall of the left ventricle is three times as strong as the right ventricle and is thus 8–12 mm thick (➤ Fig. 6.16). The musculature of the left ventricle has three layers (➤ Fig. 6.16) and is elevated by trabeculae (Trabeculae carneae). The **Septum interventriculare** functionally belongs to the left ventricle. The predominantly smooth outflow part leads the blood into the Vestibulum aortae.

> **NOTE**
> The muscles of the left ventricle are three times as strong as the right ventricle (➤ Fig. 6.16).

Clinical remarks

The wall thickness of the right ventricle should not be more than 5 mm, and of the left ventricle not more than 15 mm. If there is an enlargement of the myocardium, this is called **cardiac hypertrophy.** A right ventricular hypertrophy can, for example, be caused by stenosis of the pulmonary valve or chronic obstructive pulmonary disease (pulmonary hypertension). A left ventricular hypertrophy may be caused by underlying arterial hypertension or aortic valve stenosis. In this case the left heart has to generate higher pressure during the ejection phase and becomes hypertrophic.

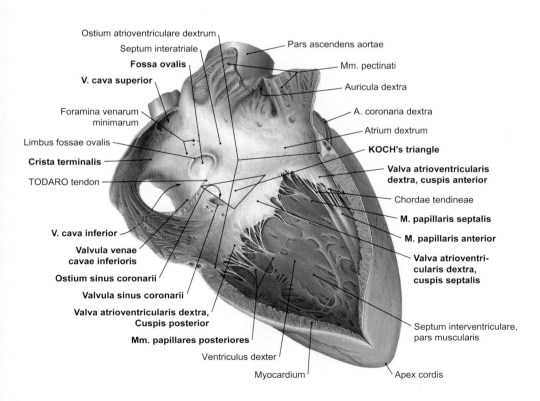

Fig. 6.15 Right atrium and right ventricle.

Labels:
Ostium atrioventriculare dextrum
Septum interatriale
Fossa ovalis
V. cava superior
Foramina venarum minimarum
Limbus fossae ovalis
Crista terminalis
TODARO tendon
V. cava inferior
Valvula venae cavae inferioris
Ostium sinus coronarii
Valvula sinus coronarii
Valva atrioventricularis dextra, Cuspis posterior
Mm. papillares posteriores
Ventriculus dexter
Myocardium

Pars ascendens aortae
Mm. pectinati
Auricula dextra
A. coronaria dextra
Atrium dextrum
KOCH's triangle
Valva atrioventricularis dextra, cuspis anterior
Chordae tendineae
M. papillaris septalis
M. papillaris anterior
Valva atrioventricularis dextra, cuspis septalis
Septum interventriculare, pars muscularis
Apex cordis

6.1.7 Heart wall and pericardium

Heart wall

The heart wall consists of three layers (➤ Fig. 6.16):

- **Endocardium:**
  - Inner surface, which is made up of endothelial cells and connective tissue
  - Cuspid and semilunar valves are duplicates of the endocardium
- **Myocardium:**
  - Cardiac muscle consists of individual cardiomyocytes; the fibre bundles run in diagonal, circular and longitudinal lines, which enables concentric contraction and longitudinal shortening of the longitudinal axis
  - In the atria and the right ventricle there is a dual layered structure; in the left ventricle the myocardium is made up of three layers.
  - In the area of the apex of the heart the muscles form a vortex (Vortex cordis).
- **Epicardium (Lamina visceralis pericardii):**
  - The epicardium consists of a single layer of epithelium as well as connective and adipose tissue. The adipose tissue contains the blood vessels and nerves of the heart.
  - The epicardium corresponds to the Lamina visceralis of the Pericardium serosum (see below) and is therefore a part of the heart sac.

Pericardium (heart sac)

For the development of the pericardial cavity ➤ Chap. 6.5.5
The pericardium, with a volume of 700–1100 ml including the heart serves to aid low-friction contraction of the heart and gives it stability. In the **pericardial cavity** (Cavitas pericardiva) there are 10–20 ml of serous fluid. The heart sac consists of:
- **Pericardium fibrosum** (outside), close-fitting connective tissue
- **Pericardium serosum** (inside), a serous membrane (Tunica serosa)
  - The section of the pericardium directly inside the Pericardium fibrosum, is referred to as the parietal sheet (Lamina parietalis). This folds over the large blood vessels (Aorta, Truncus pulmonalis, V. cava superior) on the front side to form the visceral sheet (Lamina visceralis).
  - The visceral sheet corresponds to the Epicardium of the heart wall (see above). At the weak points of the heart muscle, especially the atria, the Lamina parietalis is very strong.

The enveloping folds of the epicardium and pericardium create a vertical fold on the back of the atrium between the V. cava inferior and the V. cava superior and a transverse fold between the 4 pulmonary veins. This T-shaped arrangement creates 2 dorsal extensions to the pericardial cavity:
- **Sinus transversus pericardii:** above the horizontal fold between the V. cava superior and Aorta or Truncus pulmonalis, respectively
- **Sinus obliquus pericardii:** below the horizontal and to the left of the vertical fold, and therefore between the 4 openings of the pulmonary veins

> **NOTE**
> The epicardium forms the visceral sheet (Pericardium serosum) of the pericardial cavity, and its parietal sheet lies adjacent to the Pericardium fibrosum of the heart sac (pericardium).

The pericardium is fixed at 3 points:
- Centrum tendineum of the diaphragm, where it broadly adheres

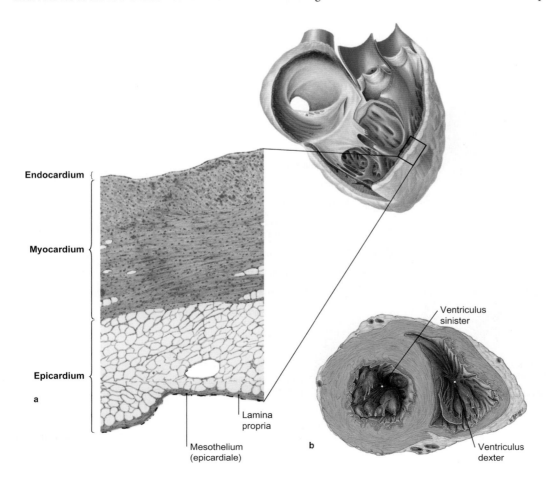

Fig. 6.16 Muscles of the cardiac wall. [S010-2-16]

Endocardium

Myocardium

Epicardium

a

Lamina propria

Mesothelium (epicardiale)

b

Ventriculus sinister

Ventriculus dexter

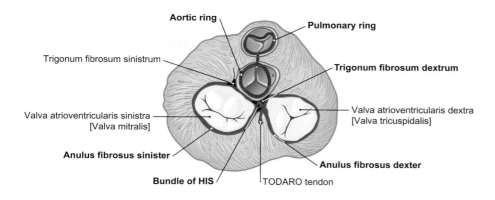

Fig. 6.17 Cardiac skeleton.

• Posterior side of the sternum via the Ligg. sternopericardiaca
• Bifurcatio tracheae via the Membrana bronchopericardiaca

Clinical remarks

In cases of heart failure or inflammation of the pericardium (pericarditis) fluid can accumulate in the pericardium **(pericardial effusion)** and affect cardiac activity.

In the case of rupture of the heart wall, e.g. after a heart attack or due to injury (knife stab), the pericardium fills with blood **(cardiac tamponade).** The cardiac activity is inhibited by the blood. Progression is usually fatal.

6.1.8 Cardiac skeleton and heart valves

Cardiac skeleton

The atria and ventricles are separated by close-fitting, collagen-based connective tissue, known as the cardiac skeleton (➤ Fig. 6.17). This forms the **fibrous rings** around the 4 heart valves. Because they are all on the same plane, which corresponds to the Sulcus coronarius on the outside, this level is also referred to as the valve level (➤ Fig. 6.18):

• The tricuspid valve lies in the Anulus fibrosus dexter.
• The mitral valve lies in the Anulus fibrosus sinister.
• Aortic and pulmonary valves are surrounded by the aortic and pulmonary ring, respectively. The aortic ring is connected via the Tendo infundibuli with the fibrous ring of the Truncus pulmonalis.

At 2 triangular points the cardiac skeleton is slightly wider (Trigonum fibrosum dextrum and sinistrum).

In addition to stabilisation of the valves, the cardiac skeleton probably enables the **electrical insulation** of the atrial and ventricular musculature. Conduction from the atria to the ventricles therefore only takes place via a portion of the cardiac conduction system, the HIS bundle, which passes through the cardiac skeleton at the Trigonum fibrosum dextrum. This ensures the insulated contraction of atria and ventricles, to ensure regular filling of the ventricles.

N O T E

The function of the cardiac skeleton is to isolate the atrial and ventricular muscles and to stabilise the heart valves.

Heart valves

The heart valves are essential for the directional blood flow. In the heart, a distinction is made between 2 types of valves (➤ Fig. 6.18):

• **Atrioventricular valves** (Valvae atrioventriculares) between atria and ventricles:
  – **Tricuspid valve** (Valva tricuspidalis, Valva atrioventricularis dextra) between right atrium and right ventricle
  – Bicuspid **mitral valve** (Valva mitralis, Valva atrioventricularis sinistra) between the left atrium and left ventricle
• **Semilunar valves** (Valvae semilunares) between ventricles and large vessels
  – **Pulmonary valve** (Valva trunci pulmonalis) at the junction of the right ventricle to the Truncus pulmonalis
  – **Aortic valve** (Valva aortae) at the transition from the left ventricle into the aorta

The **atrioventricular valves** (➤ Table 6.1) are closed during systole, when the myocardium of the ventricle contracts and prevent return flow of blood to the atrium **(passive valve-supporting system).** The bases of the cusps (Cuspes) are adhered to the fibrous ring of the cardiac skeleton. The cusps are connected to the papillary muscles via tendinous cords (Chordae tendineae). By contraction of the muscles during systole, inversion of the cusps into the atrium is prevented **(active valve-supporting system).** During diastole (filling phase) the atrioventricular valves open.

The **semilunar valves** (➤ Table 6.1) are located at the transition from the ventricles to the major vessels (Truncus pulmonalis, aorta). The pulmonary and aortic valves each consist of 3 semilunar valves (Valvae semilunares). On their free edges (Lunulae) a small, central thickened areas (Noduli) seals the valve completely when closed. The valves open in response to the pumping action of the ventricles and close again when the blood flows black when the pressure in the circulation rises above the pressure in the ventricle.

Table 6.1 Heart valves.

Type	Valve	Components
Cuspid valves	Valva atrioventricularis dextra, Valva tricuspidalis	• Cuspis anterior, Cuspis posterior, Cuspis septalis • M. papillaris anterior, M. papillaris posterior, M. papillaris septalis with Chordae tendineae
	Valva atrioventricularis sinistra, Valva mitralis	• Cuspis anterior, Cuspis posterior • M. papillaris anterior, M. papillaris posterior with Chordae tendineae
Semilunar valves	Valva trunci pulmonalis	• Valvula semilunaris dextra • Valvula semilunaris sinistra • Valvula semilunaris anterior
	Valva aortae	• Valvula semilunaris dextra • Valvula semilunaris sinistra • Valvula semilunaris posterior

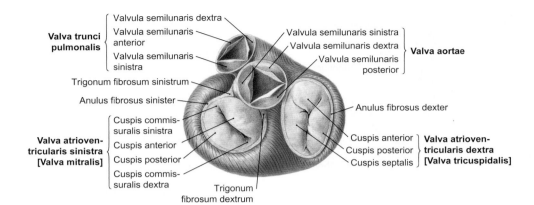

Fig. 6.18 Heart valves.

After a **heart attack** that also includes the papillary muscles, the Chordae tendinae may become detached. The leaflets recoil into the atrium during systole **(active valve insufficiency)** and blood flows back into the atrium.

NOTE
During systole the semilunar valves open; during diastole the atrioventricular valves open.

On **auscultation of the heart,** heart sounds (physiological) and heart murmurs (pathological) need to be distinguished:
- The **first heart sound** is created at the beginning of the systole by ventricular contraction and the cuspidal valves snapping shut.
- The **second heart sound** is generated at the beginning of the diastole by the closure of the semilunar valves.
- **Heart murmurs** are only created when the valves are damaged.

Table 6.2 Anatomical projection and auscultation of the heart valves.

Heart valve	Anatomical projection	Auscultation site
Pulmonary valve	3. ICS left sternal border	2nd ICS left parasternal
Aortic valve	3. ICS left sternal border	2nd ICS right parasternal
Tricuspid valve	5th rib cartilage on the dorsal side of the sternum	5th ICS right parasternal
Mitral valve	4th–5th costal cartilage left	5th ICS midclavicula

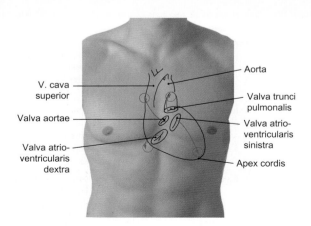

Fig. 6.19 Projection of the heart contours and the heart valves with auscultation sites onto the ventral thoracic wall

The heart sounds and heart murmurs are carried along by the bloodstream. This means that the auscultation sites of the heart valves do not correspond to their anatomical location (➤ Table 6.2, ➤ Fig. 6.19).

Clinical remarks

Congenital or acquired disorders (such as bacterial colonisation of the heart valves with endocarditis or rheumatic diseases) can damage the valves. Possible consequences are **valve stenosis or valve insufficiency** (➤ Fig. 6.20). Failures are usually acquired and can also be caused by heart attacks, if the papillary muscles, which anchor the cuspidal valves are damaged.
These damages are heard as **heart murmurs** on auscultation. These are most noticeable at the auscultation sites of the respective valves (➤ Fig. 6.19). If over more than one **atrioventricular valve**
- a noise occurs during **systole** (between the 1st and 2nd heart sounds), this suggests insufficiency, because the valve should be closed during this phase
- a noise occurs during **diastole,** this suggests stenosis, as the valve should be open in the filling phase.
With the **semilunar valves** it is exactly the opposite.

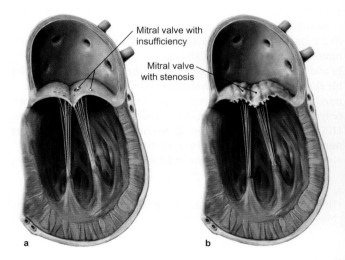

Fig. 6.20 Valve insufficiency and stenosis using the example of the mitral valve, e g. due to inflammatory changes underlying bacterial or rheumatic endocarditis. **a** Mitral insufficiency. **b** Mitral stenosis. [L266]

6.1.9 Conduction system and innervation of the heart

Electrical stimulation and conduction system of the heart

The heart has an autonomous electrical stimulation and conduction system that is independent of the nervous system (➤ Fig. 6.21). It is formed by specialised heart muscle cells. The stimulus follows the following pathway:

- **Sinus node** as a pacemaker (Nodus sinuatrialis, KEITH–FLACK node)
- **AV node** (Nodus atrioventricularis, ASCHOFF-TAWARA node)
- **Atrioventricular bundle** (Fasciculus atrioventricularis, bundle of HIS)
- **Bundle branches** (Crus dextrum and sinistrum, bundles of TAWARA)

The electrical stimulation is created in the pacemaker, the **sinus node** (3 × 10 mm) by spontaneous depolarisation. It lies subepicardially in the right atrium at the mouth of the V. cava superior at the height of the Crista terminalis. Starting from the sinus node, the stimulus is transferred via the **atrial myocardium to the AV node.** Here, excitation transfer to the ventricle is delayed by 60–120 ms. This delay ensures separate contraction of atria and ventricles. If the sinus node fails, there is a possibility of the AV node taking over the pacemaker function as a secondary pacemaker with a lower frequency. The AV node (3 × 5 × 1 mm) is located in the triangle of KOCH in the right atrium (➤ Fig. 6.15), which is bordered by the following:

- Tendon of TODARO
- Edge of the septal leaflet of the tricuspid valve
- Ostium of the Sinus coronarius

Starting from the AV node, the stimulus can be transferred to the ventricular myocardium at one point only: the **atrioventricular bundle** passes through the Trigonum fibrosum dextrum of the cardiac skeleton. (HIS bundle; 4 × 20 mm) to the ventricular muscles. In the Pars membranacea of the Septum interventriculare the bundle of HIS divides into the **bundle branches (TAWARA).** The right bundle branch (Crus dextrum) stimulates the right ventricle and has individual fibres that lead to the Trabecula septomarginalis on to the right M. papillaris anterior. The left bundle branch (Crus

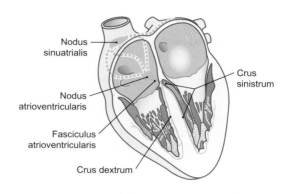

Fig. 6.21 Electrical stimulation and conduction system of the heart.

Labels: Nodus sinuatrialis; Nodus atrioventricularis; Fasciculus atrioventricularis; Crus dextrum; Crus sinistrum

sinistrum) passes through the Pars membranacea of the Septum interventriculare into the left ventricle, where it divides into **3 fascicles:**

- The front fascicle leads to the M. papillaris anterior and the apical ventricular septum.
- The middle fascicle leads towards the apex of the heart.
- The rear fascicle leads to the M. papillaris posterior and the ventricular myocardium.

The specialised heart muscle cells of the individual fascicles pass under the endocardium (Rr. subendocardiales) and occasionally between the trabeculae of the heart wall through the ventricular lumen.

The spread of the stimulus through the heart can be revealed by the **ECG (electrocardiogram)** (➤ Fig. 6.22):

- **P-wave:** spread of stimulation in the atria.
- **PQ interval:** spread of the stimulus from the AV node to the ventricle; during this interval there is no change in the excitation level (isoelectric), because the atrium is already completely depolarised and the ventricles have not yet been depolarised.
- **QRS complex:** spread of stimulation in the ventricles at the same time, invisible repolarisation of the atria.
- **ST segment:** full depolarisation of the ventricles.
- **T wave:** repolarisation in the ventricles (spreads from the apex to the base of the heart).

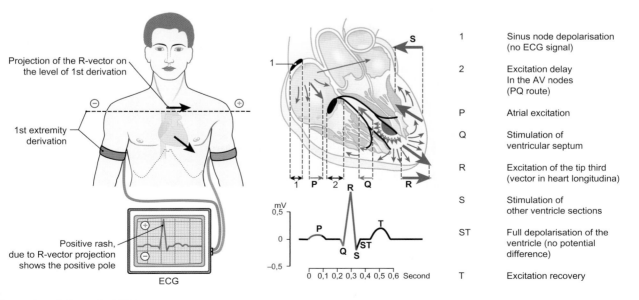

1	Sinus node depolarisation (no ECG signal)
2	Excitation delay In the AV nodes (PQ route)
P	Atrial excitation
Q	Stimulation of ventricular septum
R	Excitation of the tip third (vector in heart longitudina)
S	Stimulation of other ventricle sections
ST	Full depolarisation of the ventricle (no potential difference)
T	Excitation recovery

Left diagram labels: Projection of the R-vector on the level of 1st derivation; 1st extremity derivation; Positive rash, due to R-vector projection shows the positive pole; ECG

Fig. 6.22 Formation of the typical ECG.

The ECG allows **arrhythmia** of various etiologies to be verified, where the heart beats too quickly (tachycardia >100/min.), too slowly (bradycardia <60/min.) or simply irregularly (arrhythmia). A possible cause of cardiac arrhythmia are atrial fibres that bypass the AV node and connect directly to the HIS bundle or the ventricular muscles. If the resulting arrhythmias (WOLFF-PARKINSON-WHITE syndrome, WPW syndrome) become unpleasantly symptomatic and cannot be treated with medicinal products, cardiac catheterisation is required in which the accessory conduction bundles are interrupted. In addition, in the case of coronary heart diseases (e.g. **heart attack**) circulation disorders and other diseases such as inflammation of the myocardium affect stimulus propagation. The ECG is of particular importance for the identification of myocardial infarction.

Innervation

Cardiac output can adapt to the current individual performance of the body. The autonomic nerves of the heart (**Plexus cardiacus,** ➤ Fig. 6.23, ➤ Table 6.3) can impact frequency (chronotropic), force development (inotrope), conduction (dromotropic), excitability (bathmotropic), the laxity (lusitropy) as well as cardiomyocyte cohesion (adhesiotropy). The cardiac plexus contains parasympathetic (N. vagus) and sympathetic fibres (postganglionic nerve fibres of the cervical and upper chest ganglia of the sympathetic trunk). Near the base of the heart are up to 550 usually only microscopically visible ganglia (Ganglia cardiaca) with the cell bodies of postganglionic parasympathetic neurons.

Table 6.3 Innervation of the heart.

Autonomic innervation (Plexus cardiacus)	Afferent innervation
• N. vagus (parasympathetic) – Rr. cardiaci cervicales superiores and inferiores – Rr. cardiaci thoracici • Sympathetic (from the ganglia cervicalia superius, media and cervicothoracicum; T1–T4) – Nn. cardiaci cervicales superior, medius and inferior – Nn. cardiaci thoracici	• N. phrenicus – R. pericardiacus

The **parasympathetic nervous system** leads to a reduction of cardiac output and has a negative chronotropic, dromotropic and bathmotropic effect on the heart and a negative inotropic effect on the atria. The **sympathetic nervous system** leads to an increase in cardiac output and therefore has a positive chronotropic, dromotropic, inotropic, lusitropic and adhesiotropic effect. The **phrenic nerve** only sensitively innervates the pericardium and therefore is not counted as part of the cardiac plexus.

An increased sympathetic tonus, as in stress situations, is accompanied by increased heart rate **(tachycardia)** and elevated arterial blood pressure **(hypertension).** Damage of the parasympathetic nerve fibres can also lead to tachycardia. The escalation of cardiac output increases the oxygen requirements of the cardiomyocytes and with narrowing of the coronary vessels (coronary heart disease) can lead to angina pectoris and myocardial infarction.

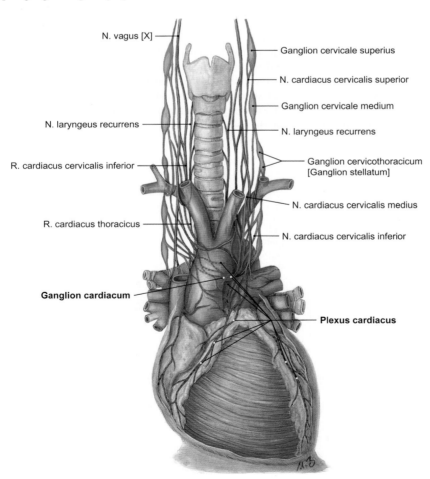

N. vagus [X]

Ganglion cervicale superius

N. cardiacus cervicalis superior

Ganglion cervicale medium

N. laryngeus recurrens

N. laryngeus recurrens

R. cardiacus cervicalis inferior

Ganglion cervicothoracicum [Ganglion stellatum]

N. cardiacus cervicalis medius

R. cardiacus thoracicus

N. cardiacus cervicalis inferior

Ganglion cardiacum

Plexus cardiacus

Fig. 6.23 Autonomic innervation.

6.1.10 Coronary blood vessel

The coronary blood vessels (➤ Fig. 6.24) are the Vasa privata of the heart and ensure the heart's own supply. There are 2 coronary arteries:

- A. coronaria sinistra
- A. coronaria dextra

The coronary arteries are functional terminal arteries. Both coronary arteries originate from the ascending aorta above the aortic valve.

The **A. coronaria dextra** (➤ Table 6.4) originates from the right Sinus aortae, runs through the Sulcus coronarius along the right atrium to the lower edge of the heart (Margo dexter) and extends across the underside (Facies diaphragmatica), where it usually ends in the **R. interventricularis posterior** as a terminal branch.

The **A. coronaria sinistra** (➤ Table 6.4) issues from the left aortic valve sinus. After only 1 cm it divides into the **R. interventricularis anterior** and the **R. circumflexus**. The R. interventricularis anterior runs forwards through the Sulcus interventricularis anterior above the Septum interventriculare on the Facies sternocostalis and issues another major branch, the R. lateralis, along its trajectory. The **R. circumflexus** runs through the Sulcus coronarius around the left margin of the heart to the back and normally issues the R. posterior ventriculi sinistri.

NOTE

Normally the **A coronaria sinistra** supplies the left atrium, the left ventricle, the anterior two thirds of the ventricular septum and portions of the right front ventricular wall. The **A. coronaria dextra** supplies parts of the underside of the left ventricle, the right atrium and right ventricle as well as most of the conduction system.

Table 6.4 Branches of the coronary arteries.

Branches of the A. coronaria dextra	Branches of the A. coronaria sinistra

• R. coni arteriosi: runs to the Conus arteriosus
• R. nodi sinuatrialis (two thirds of all cases): approx. 1 mm thick artery, that stretches to the **sinus node** (in some cases also 2 arteries)
• Rr. atriales and Rr. atrioventricularis: small branches for the atrium and ventricle
• R. marginalis dexter: stretches along the Margo dexter of the right ventricle
• R. polsterolateralis dexter: inconsistant
• R. nodi atrioventricularis: to the **AV node** (usually)
• R. interventricularis posterior (usually) with Rr. interventriculares septales (supplies the **HIS bundle**)
	• R. interventricularis anterior:
	  – R. coni arteriosi to the Conus arteriosus
	  – R. lateralis for the front and side wall of the left ventricle
	  – Rr. interventriculares septales for the anterior two thirds of the Septum interventriculare (in some cases also involved in supply of the AV node)
	• R. circumflexus
	  – R. nodi sinuatrialis (one third of all cases): to the sinoatrial node
	  – R. marginalis sinister
	  – R. posterior ventriculi sinistri to the Facies diaphragmatica of the left ventricle

Clinical remarks

In clinical practice the description of the coronary arteries is different from the Nomina Anatomica. The following names are common:

- A. coronaria sinistra corresponds to the LCA (**l**eft **c**oronary **a**rtery)
  - **R. i**nter**v**entricularis **a**nterior corresponds to the RIVA or LAD (**l**eft **a**nterior **d**escending coronary artery)
  - **R. c**ircumfle**x**us corresponds to the RCX
- A. coronaria dextra corresponds to the RCA (**r**ight **c**oronary **a**rtery)
  - R. interventricularis posterior corresponds to the RPD (**r**ight **p**osterior **d**escending coronary artery)

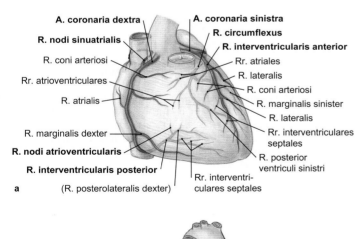

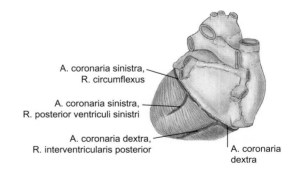

Fig. 6.24 Coronary arteries, Aa. coronariae. a Cranial view. **b** Normal supply type. **c** Left supply type. **d** Right supply type.

The previously described normal case only occurs in about two thirds to three quarters of the population. Therefore, in addition to the normal supply types additional **supply types** are distinguished (➤ Fig. 6.24):

- **Normal supply type:** (approx. 55–75 %) the R. interventricularis posterior from the A. coronaria dextra supplies the right ventricle whereas the back of the left ventricle is supplied by the R. posterior ventriculi sinistri of the A. coronaria sinistra.
- **Left supply type:** (approx. 11–20 %) the R. interventricularis posterior (and also the R. nodi atrioventricularis) derive from the A. coronaria sinistra. Both issue from the R. circumflexus. In this case, the entire septum is supplied by the A. coronaria sinistra.
- **Right supply type:** (approx. 14–25 %) the A. coronaria dextra issues the R. interventricularis posterior (and also the R. nodi atrioventricularis) and, via an additional branch called the R. posterior ventriculi sinistri, supplies parts of the back of the left ventricle as well as most of the Septum interventriculare.

Especially in clinical practice, the term '**dominance**' is used in addition to supply types. The dominant artery is the vessel that issues the R. interventricularis posterior, i.e., for the normal supply type and the right supply type this is the A. coronaria dextra.

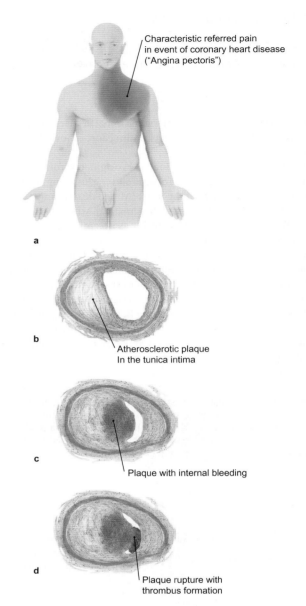

Fig. 6.25 Coronary heart disease (CHD). a Tightness in the chest with characteristic radiating pain. **b–d,** The cause is usually atherosclerosis of the coronary arteries, which starts with plaque formation due to lipid deposits (**b**) that are enlarged by bleeding (**c**) and in the case of rupture can completely close the lumen due to formation of a blood clot (thrombus, **d**). [L266]

Labels on figure:
- Characteristic referred pain in event of coronary heart disease ("Angina pectoris")
- a
- b
- Atherosclerotic plaque In the tunica intima
- c
- Plaque with internal bleeding
- d
- Plaque rupture with thrombus formation

Clinical remarks

Coronary heart disease (CHD) is one of the most common causes of death in the Western world. Coronary artery disease (CAD) is caused by stenosis of the coronary arteries resulting from arteriosclerosis (➤ Fig. 6.25). Due to the lack of blood circulation this may lead to pain in the chest (**Angina pectoris**) that radiates into the arm (mostly on the left) or into the neck. In the case of a complete occlusion muscle tissue dies (**heart attack**). As the coronary arteries are functional terminal arteries, an occlusion of individual branches leads to certain infarction patterns (➤ Fig. 6.26). These can often already be determined in the various leads in an ECG. The most certain confirmation method is achieved by cardiac catheter examination using x-ray contrast media. In **posterior wall myocardial infarction** the perfusion of the AV node is typically also impaired because the perfusing artery usually originates at the outlet of the R. interventricularis posterior. This can result additionally in bradycardiac arrhythmias. Mostly (in the case of balanced and right supply type) the R. interventricularis posterior is the terminal branch of the A. coronaria dextra. Since the muscle wall of the right ventricle has a lower oxygen demand than that of the left ventricle due to pressure conditions, a proximal occlusion of the A. coronaria dextra often results in an isolated posterior myocardial infarction. In this case, the bradycardia can be very pronounced due to insufficient perfusion of the SA node.

If the narrowing of the coronary artery cannot be resolved by balloon dilatation or implantation of a stent, a bypass circulation must be created. The A. thoracica interna or epifascial leg veins are often used for this purpose (➤ Fig. 6.27). Since the supply areas of the coronary arteries can vary in size depending on supply type, the extent of the damage and the clinical picture can also vary enormously between patients.

NOTE

Infarction patterns and their most affected arteries are (➤ Fig. 6.26):
- Anterior wall myocardial infarction: R. interventricularis anterior
- Lateral myocardial infarction: R. lateralis or proximal branches of the R. circumflexus
- Front wall myocardial infarction: A. coronaria sinistra
- Posterior wall myocardial infarction (Facies diaphragmatica): A. coronaria dextra (conduction defects) or distal branches of the R. circumflexus

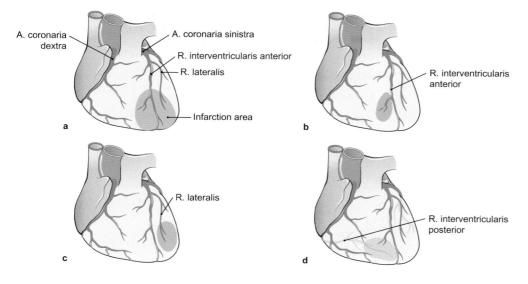

Fig. 6.26 Areas of infarction. a Anterior wall myocardial infarction in the case of occlusion of the R. interventricularis anterior. **b** Apical infarction in the case of distal occlusion of the R. interventricularis anterior. **c** Small lateral myocardial infarction in the case of closure of the R. lateralis (from the R. interventricularis anterior). **d** Posterior wall myocardial infarction in the case of occlusion of the R. interventricularis posterior.

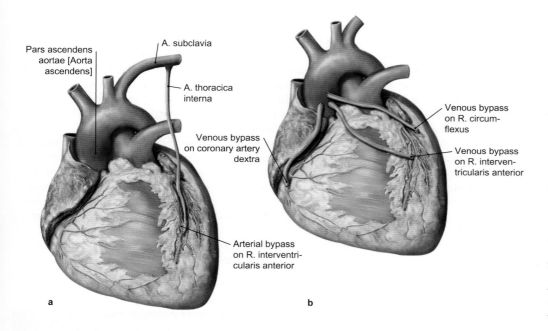

Fig. 6.27 Bypasses. a For arterial bypasses the A. thoracica interna is attached distal to the stenosis. **b** In venous bypasses epifascial leg veins (V. saphena magna or parva) are attached from the ascending aorta to the respective narrowed branches of the coronary arteries. Several bypasses can be attached to this site. [L266]

6.1.11 Veins and lymphatic vessels of the heart

Veins of the heart

The venous drainage (➤ Fig. 6.28) of the heart occurs via 3 venous systems (➤ Table 6.5):

- Coronary sinus system
- Transmural system
- Endomural system

Two thirds of the venous blood are taken up by the **Sinus coronarius** and drained through the Ostium sinus coronariis into the right atrium. 3 main veins lead to the Sinus coronarius:

- The **V. cardiaca magna** corresponds to the supply area of the A. coronaria sinistra.
- The **V. cardiaca media** runs around the R. interventricularis posterior.
- The **V. cardiaca parva** is a small vessel which drains the rest of the supply area of the A. coronaria dextra but it is only present in 50% of cases.

Table 6.5 Cardiac veins (vv. cordis).

Venous system	Veins

Sinus coronarius system	• V. cardiaca magna: corresponds to the supply area of the A. coronaria sinistra
	   – V. interventricularis anterior
	   – V. marginalis sinistra
	   – Vv. ventriculi sinistri posteriores
	 • V. cardiaca media: in the Sulcus interventricularis posterior
	 • V. cardiaca parva: in the right coronary groove, present in 50% of cases
	 • V. obliqua atrii sinistri (vein of MARSHALL)

Transmural system	• Vv. ventriculi dextri anteriores • Vv. atriales
Endomural system	• Vv. cardiacae minimae (Vasa THEBESII)

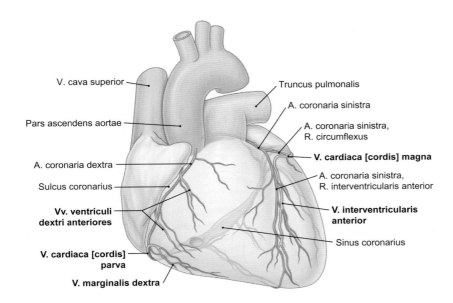

V. cava superior

Pars ascendens aortae

A. coronaria dextra

Sulcus coronarius

Vv. ventriculi dextri anteriores

V. cardiaca [cordis] parva

V. marginalis dextra

Truncus pulmonalis

A. coronaria sinistra

A. coronaria sinistra, R. circumflexus

V. cardiaca [cordis] magna

A. coronaria sinistra, R. interventricularis anterior

V. interventricularis anterior

Sinus coronarius

Fig. 6.28 Cardiac veins, Vv. cordis Ventral view. [E402]

The final third of the venous blood reaches the atria and ventricles directly via the **transmural** and **endomural systems.**

Lymph vessels

The lymph of the heart flows endocardially, myocardially and epicardially over larger collectors along the coronary arteries in small, usually only microscopically visible lymph nodes that are located ventral to the aorta and Truncus pulmonalis. From there it is transferred via the Nodi lymphoidei tracheobronchiales and other mediastinal lymph nodes.

For the pericardium the **Nodi lymphoidei prepericardiaci** and **Nodi lymphoidei pericardiaci laterales** drain in Nodi lymphoidei parasternales and other mediastinal lymph nodes.

6.2 Trachea and lungs

┌─ Skills ─

After working through this chapter, you should be able to:
- explain the structuring of the lower airway with development from the foregut
- explain the sections from the trachea to the tracheal bifurcation with wall construction on a specimen
- indicate on a specimen the projection of the lungs and their division into lobes and segments
- explain the systematics of the bronchial tree and structures of the lung hilum on a specimen
- describe Vasa publica and privata of the lungs including origin, course and function
- describe the lymph vessel systems and the autonomic innervation of the lungs

6.2.1 Overview and function

The trachea and the two lungs (Pulmones) as well as the larynx belong to the lower respiratory tract (➤ Fig. 6.29, ➤ Table 6.6). The **trachea** connects the larynx with the main bronchi (Bronchus principalis dexter and sinister). It is one of the air conducting parts of the respiratory system and serves to transport the inhaled air, humidify and warm it. The trachea is like the upper respiratory tract, the bronchi and most of the bronchioles of the lungs part of the **anatomical dead space** (150–170 ml). This means that these portions of the respiratory system are *not* involved in gas exchange. **Gas exchange** itself (uptake of oxygen from the inhaled air, elimination of carbon dioxide) during breathing takes place in the lungs. Therefore the **lungs** are one of the absolutely vital organs. The anatomy of the respiratory tract is therefore also of medical importance because respiratory diseases in Germany are among the most common diseases. Acute upper respiratory tract infections with bacteria or viruses are the most common cause of treatment in paediatric medical practices (paediatrics). If this no longer involves the presence of a minor infection, which can be treated by general practitioners, a pulmonologist must be consulted. Disorders requiring surgery are treated by a thoracic surgeon.

Table 6.6 Respiratory system.

Upper respiratory tract	Lower respiratory tract
- Nasal cavity (cavitas nasi) - Throat (pharynx)	- Larynx - Trachea - Lungs (Pulmones): the right lung (Pulmo dexter) has 3 lobes, the left lung (Pulmo sinister) has 2 lobes

┌─ Clinical remarks ─

The volume of the **anatomical dead space** has an important practical relevance for resuscitation. During ventilation the volume of oxygenated air needs to exceed 170 ml to effectively reach the alveoli and avoid just moving the air column within the conducting part. Therefore, it is preferable to ventilate slowly with more volume than quickly with too little volume.

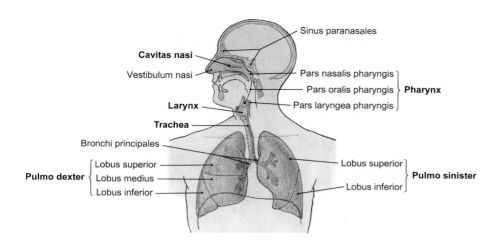

Fig. 6.29 Upper and lower respiratory tract. Ventral view.

6.2.2 Development of trachea and lungs

The epithelial tissues of the larynx, trachea and lungs develop from the *4th week* from the **entoderm** of the foregut. Connective tissue, smooth muscles, and blood vessels are derived from the surrounding **mesoderm**. First, a **laryngotracheal groove** forms on the inside of the foregut, that bulges outwards to form the **lung bud** (➤ Fig. 6.30). By extension, a **laryngotracheal tube** is formed, from the lowest sections of which form **bronchial buds,** the predecessors of the main bronchi. The bronchial buds fold medially into the **coelomic ducts** (Ductus pericardiacoperitoneales), which later expand to form the pleural cavities (➤ Fig. 6.53). The medial septum of the coelomic ducts forms the visceral pleura (Pleura visceralis), the lateral septum the parietal pleura (Pleura parietalis).

During the *4th–5th week* mesenchymal folds form on both sides, which join to form the **tracheoesophageal septum** and thus separate the lower respiratory tract system from the oesophagus (➤ Fig. 6.31).

In due course the bronchial buds start to branch and create the bronchial tree of the lungs. In **lung development** a distinction is made between **4 phases,** which partially overlap (➤ Fig. 6.32):

- **Pseudoglandular phase** (6th-16th week): formation of the air-conducting bronchial tree

- **Canalicular phase** (16th–26th week): early development of gas exchanging bronchial tree with formation of first primitive alveoli
- **Saccular phase** (26th week until birth): proliferation of capillary network with formation of the blood–air barrier. Increase in surfactant production
- **Alveolar phase** (32nd week–8th year): formation of the alveoli

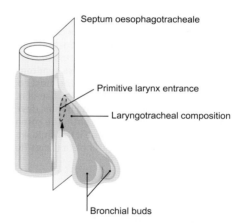

Fig. 6.31 Development of the Septum tracheoesophageale. [E581]

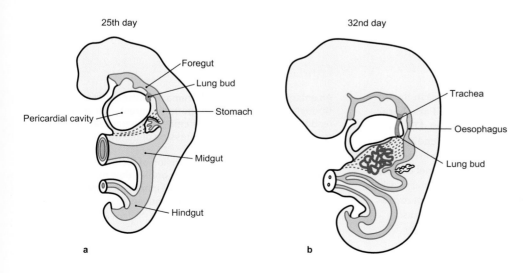

Fig. 6.30 Development of the lower respiratory tract. a 4th week of development (25th day). **b** 5th week of development (32nd day).

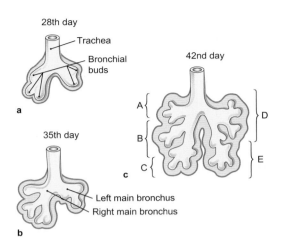
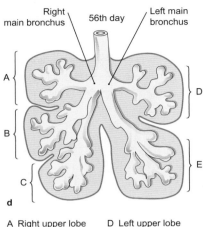

A Right upper lobe   D Left upper lobe
B Right middle lobe E Left middle lobe
C Right lower lobe

Fig. 6.32 Stages of lung development. [E581]

Clinical remarks

A disorder in the separation of the oesophagus and trachea can lead to the formation of a shunt **(tracheaoesophageal fistulas),** often with a blind ending oesophagus **(oesophageal atresia).**

From the 20th week onwards **surfactant** is produced in the alveoli, which reduces the surface tension of the alveoli. From the 35th week onwards, surfactant production is usually sufficient to enable spontaneous breathing. Insufficient surfactant production results in **respiratory distress syndrome** (Respiratory Distress Syndrome, RDS), which is the most common cause of death in newborn infants. In the case of birth before the 30th week up to 60% of premature babies develop RDS. Since the lungs are filled with air at birth, the coroner can use the **lung floatation test** to determine if the child was born dead (lungs submerge) or died after birth (lungs float).

6.2.3 Topography and structure of the trachea and main bronchi

The **trachea** is 10–13 cm long; however, due to its flexibility can extend up to 5 cm during deep inspiration. It joins to the cricoid cartilage of the larynx and projects onto the 7th cervical vertebrae, and higher when lying down. It ends at the **Bifurcatio tracheae** at the level of the 4th-5th thoracic vertebra in the two **main bronchi (Bronchi principales).** A distinction is made between 2 parts:

- Cervical section (Pars cervicalis)
- Thoracic section (Pars thoracica)

The **Pars cervicalis** lies ventral and lateral on both sides to the thyroid. In the chest cavity, the thymus lies ventral to the **Pars thoracica.** The trachea here runs in the superior mediastinum. Directly ventral to the bifurcation is the aortic arch with its ascending vessels. The left V. brachiocephalica crosses the trachea and receives the V. thyroidea inferior lying in front of it. In the channel between the trachea and the oesophagus the recurrent laryngeal nerve arises on both sides in the direction of the larynx. Throughout its trajectory the dorsal trachea is accompanied by the oesophagus.

The lumen of the trachea is kept open by the 16–20 horse-shoe-shaped **cartilage rings (tracheal cartilage)** (➤ Fig. 6.33). The cartilage rings consist of hyaline cartilage, but are elastically deformable. They are connected by the **Ligg. anularia** made of collagen fibres and elastic fibres, which gives them flexibility and enables changes in length. On the rear wall of the trachea, the ends of the cartilage rings are connected to elastic fibres (**Paries membranaceus**) via a connective tissue plate, in which smooth muscles (**M. trachealis**) are embedded. This membranous portion of the trachea allows an enlargement of the tracheal diameter. The M. trachealis is always minimally contracted at rest and ensures that the Paries membranaceus is taught, making the diameter of the trachea approx. 16–18 mm. For inspiration, the muscle tone is reduced and the lumen increases slightly. At the **fork of the trachea** dividing it into the two main bronchi, at the level of the 4th thoracic vertebra, corresponding to the sternal attachment of the 3rd rib, is a ridge projecting into the lumen from the last tracheal cartilage (**Carina tracheae**). Here, the air is divided into the left (Bronchus principalis sinister) and right main bronchi (Bronchus principalis dexter). At this point, turbulence may occur that are heard as breathing sounds during auscultation.

The **angle between the main bronchi** is 55°–65°. The distribution of the trachea is asymmetrical: the right main bronchus is stronger, 1–2.5 cm long and almost vertical, whereas the left main bronchus is almost twice as long and the diameter is narrower and angled (➤ Fig. 6.33). The further division of the bronchial tree (Arbor bronchialis) is dichotomous (➤ Chap. 6.2.6).

Clinical remarks

An enlarged thyroid gland (**struma** or **goitre**), that extends through the upper thoracic aperture (retrosternal goitre), can lead to pressure-induced softening of the tracheal cartilage (tracheomalacia) to full compression of the trachea, resulting in shortness of breath.

Because of the asymmetrical division of the trachea, during inspiration **(aspiration)** of foreign bodies they more frequently enter the **right lung.** In the event of imminent suffocation this knowledge can bring a crucial time advantage!

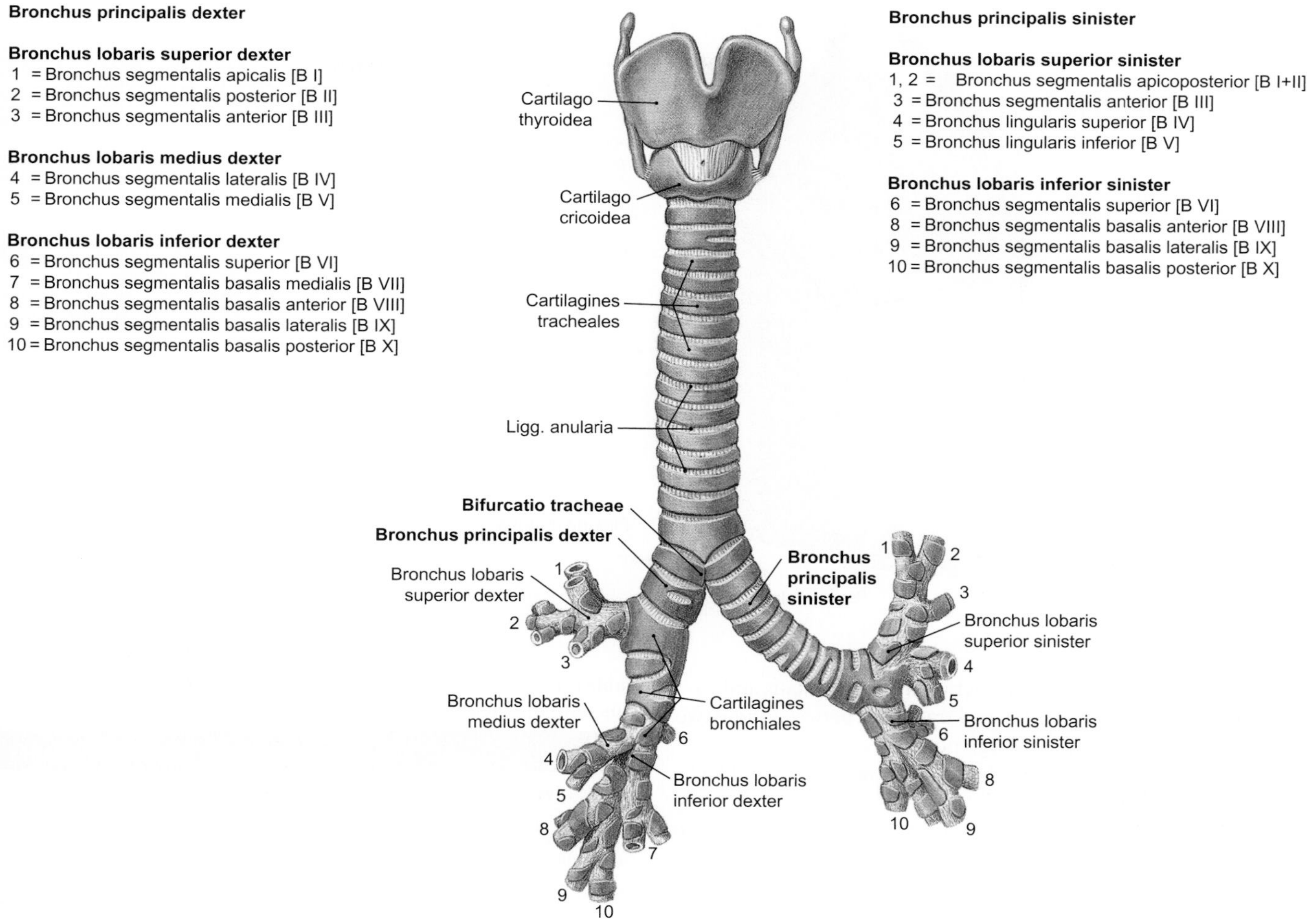

Bronchus principalis dexter

Bronchus lobaris superior dexter
1 = Bronchus segmentalis apicalis [B I]
2 = Bronchus segmentalis posterior [B II]
3 = Bronchus segmentalis anterior [B III]

Bronchus lobaris medius dexter
4 = Bronchus segmentalis lateralis [B IV]
5 = Bronchus segmentalis medialis [B V]

Bronchus lobaris inferior dexter
6 = Bronchus segmentalis superior [B VI]
7 = Bronchus segmentalis basalis medialis [B VII]
8 = Bronchus segmentalis basalis anterior [B VIII]
9 = Bronchus segmentalis basalis lateralis [B IX]
10 = Bronchus segmentalis basalis posterior [B X]

Bronchus principalis sinister

Bronchus lobaris superior sinister
1, 2 = Bronchus segmentalis apicoposterior [B I+II]
3 = Bronchus segmentalis anterior [B III]
4 = Bronchus lingularis superior [B IV]
5 = Bronchus lingularis inferior [B V]

Bronchus lobaris inferior sinister
6 = Bronchus segmentalis superior [B VI]
8 = Bronchus segmentalis basalis anterior [B VIII]
9 = Bronchus segmentalis basalis lateralis [B IX]
10 = Bronchus segmentalis basalis posterior [B X]

Cartilago thyroidea

Cartilago cricoidea

Cartilagines tracheales

Ligg. anularia

Bifurcatio tracheae
Bronchus principalis dexter

Bronchus lobaris superior dexter

Bronchus principalis sinister

Bronchus lobaris superior sinister

Bronchus lobaris medius dexter

Cartilagines bronchiales

Bronchus lobaris inferior sinister

Bronchus lobaris inferior dexter

Fig. 6.33 Lower respiratory tract. Ventral view.

6.2.4 Vessels and nerves of the trachea and main bronchi

Vessels and nerves of the trachea and main bronchi are:
- **Arterial blood supply**
  - **Pars cervicalis** of the trachea: Rr. tracheales of the A. thyroidea inferior.
  - **Pars thoracica of the trachea and Bronchi principales:** Rr. tracheales and Rr. bronchiales of the A. thoracica interna and the Aorta thoracica, 3rd–4th A. intercostalis.
- **Venous drainage**
  - **Pars cervicalis** of the trachea: the venous blood of the trachea collects in the Plexus thyroideus impar and flows from there into the V. thyroidea inferior.
  - **Pars thoracica of the trachea and Bronchi principales:** drainage occurs in the veins of the oesophagus or via the Vv. bronchiales into the V. azygos/hemiazygos.
- **Lymphatic drainage**
  - **Pars cervicalis** of the trachea: the Nodi lymphoidei paratracheales drain via the Nodi lymphoidei cervicales profundi into the Truncus jugularis.
  - **Pars thoracica of the trachea and Bronchi principales:** the Nodi lymphoidei tracheobronchiales and paratracheales drain into the Truncus bronchomediastinalis.

- **Innervation**
  - Parasympathetic innervation: Rr. tracheales from the N. laryngeus recurrens (N. vagus).
  - Sympathetic innervation: sympathetic trunk.

6.2.5 Projection of the lungs

The right and left lungs (Pulmo dexter and sinister) lie in the thorax and are separated by the mediastinum in the two pleural cavities (Cavitates pleurales, ➤ Chap 6.5.3). The lungs have the shape of a rounded off cone (➤ Fig. 6.34). The upper convex portion of the lungs (**Apex pulmonis**) reach above the upper thoracic aperture by approx. 5 cm, while the concave base of the lungs broadly covers the diaphragmatic dome (**Facies diaphragmatica**). The **Facies costalis** lying laterally on the ribs is the largest area of the lungs. In the medially lying **Facies mediastinalis,** that separates the lungs towards the mediastinum, is the lung hilum (**Hilum pulmonis**) (➤ Fig. 6.35).

Between the 3 areas of the lungs, lie the **lung margins** (➤ Fig. 6.34), which, however, just like the depressions created by the various surrounding structures, are only visible in lungs fixed in situ and therefore regarded as artefacts:

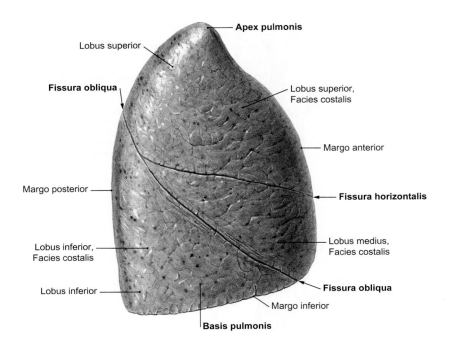

Fig. 6.34 Right lung, lateral view.

- **Margo anterior:** lying ventrally between Facies costalis and Facies mediastinalis. The blunt dorsal transition between these two areas is often referred to as 'Margo posterior'.
- **Margo inferior:** lying caudally between Facies costalis and Facies diaphragmatica

The main bronchi and the vessels and nerves of the lungs (Aa. pulmonales, Vv. pulmonales, Rr. bronchiales, Vv. bronchiales, lymph vessels and nodes, autonomic nerve fibres) run in and out of the **Hilum pulmonis** and form the 'root of the lungs'. In the fixed lung, the topographic relationships to adjacent organs can be understood based on the impressions generated. On the right lung there are impressions of the V. azygos, the oesophagus and the heart (Impressio cardiaca); the cardiac impression is bigger on the

Table 6.7 Projection of the lung boundaries in resting expiratory position; the pleural boundaries each lie one rib lower.

Body line	Right lung boundaries	Left lung boundaries
Sternal line	6th rib	4th rib
Midclavicular line (MCL)	6th rib parallel	6th rib
Midaxillary line	8th rib	8th rib
Scapula line	10th rib	10th rib
Paravertebral line	11th rib	11th rib

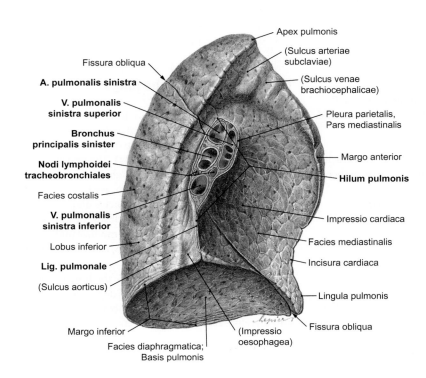

Fig. 6.35 Left lung, medial view.

left due to the shape of the heart. On the left lung there are impressions of the aortic arch and Aorta thoracica.

NOTE

Directly on the hilum of the lung a distinction is made between the following location of in-going and out-going structures:
- On the **right lung** the right main bronchus (or upper lobe bronchus) lies cranial to the A. pulmonalis.
- In the hilum of the **left lung,** the left main bronchus enters caudal to the A. pulmonalis.

The Vv. pulmonales are always facing forward, below the previously mentioned structures (➤ Fig. 6.35).

During the clinical examination, the **projection of the lung boundaries** is assessed (➤ Table 6.7) to obtain a first impression of the lung volume and volume changes during breathing. It has to be noted that the projection of the lung boundaries depends on diaphragmatic excursion. This means the lungs are lower during inspiration and higher during expiration.

Clinical remarks

The movement of the lung boundaries during breathing is determined in clinical investigations by **percussion (tapping).** Usually there should be a two finger-width distance between deep inspiration and expiration.

6.2.6 Structure of the lungs

The lungs weigh approximately 800 g (without blood 550 g). The total volume of the lungs is 2–3 L and during inspiration 5–8 L. Through the left shift of the mediastinum, the left lung has about a 10-20% lower volume.

The tissue of the lungs is formed by the dichotomously branching **bronchial tree** and its accompanying blood vessels. The **main bronchi** each divide into the **lobar bronchi (Bronchi lobares),** of which the right lung has 3 and the left lung 2 (➤ Fig. 6.34, ➤ Fig. 6.35). Accordingly, the **right lung** has 3 lung lobes (**Lobi**), an upper lobe (**Lobus superior**), a middle lobe (**Lobus medius**) and a lower lobe (**Lobus inferior**).

In contrast, due to the mediastinum dilating predominantly to the left, the **left lung** only has 2 lobes, an upper lung lobe (**Lobus superior**) and a lower lobe (**Lobus inferior**). The lingula of the left lung (Lingula pulmonis sinistri), that runs below the Incisura cardiaca, corresponds to the middle lobe of the right lung.

The lobes of the lungs are separated from each other by **fissures,** which allow the lobes to expand against each other. Both lungs are transversed by the sloping **Fissura obliqua.** It starts dorsal above at the level of the 4th rib and follows this to the midaxillary line. Then it rises steeply to the 6th rib, which it reaches in the midclavicular line. On the right lung the Fissura obliqua separates the upper from the middle lobe dorsally and the lower lobe from the middle lobe ventrally. On the left lung it runs between the upper and lower lobe.

On the right lung is additionally there is the **Fissura horizontalis,** which extends the trajectory along the 4th rib and separates the upper lobe from the middle lobe.

The lobe bronchi are split into the **segmental bronchi** (Bronchi segmentales), that correspond to one **lung segment** each (➤ Fig. 6.36, ➤ Table 6.8). The right lung has 10 segments. In the left lung

Table 6.8 Segments of the lungs.

Pulmo dexter	Pulmo sinister
Lobus superior (3 segments)	**Lobus superior (5 segments)**
• Segmentum apicale [S I]	• Segmentum apicoposterius [S I + II]
• Segmentum posterius [S II]	• Segmentum anterius [S III]
• Segmentum anterius [S III]	• Segmentum lingulare superius [S IV]
Lobus medius (2 segments)	• Segmentum lingulare inferius [S V]
• Segmentum laterale [S IV]	**Lobus inferior (4 segments)**
• Segmentum mediale [S V]	• Segmentum superius [S VI]
Lobus inferior (5 segments)	• Segmentum basale anterius [S VIII]
• Segmentum superius [S VI]	• Segmentum basale laterale [S IX]
• Segmentum basale mediale (cardiacum) [S VII]	• Segmentum basale posterius [S X]
• Segmentum basale anterius [S VIII]	
• Segmentum basale laterale [S IX]	
• Segmentum basale posterius [S X]	

the 7th segment (mediobasal segment) is not formed at all or only in rudimentary fashion due to the predominant expansion of the heart, so that there are only 9 segments. The segments form a functional unit and are only separated from each other by connective tissue. Macroscopically this distinction is not visible.

Clinical remarks

The classification of the lungs into individual segments is clinically important as this means that during, for example, **bronchoscopy,** tissue samples can be assigned to individual segments.
Since a lung segment is supplied by a corresponding segmental bronchus with associated segmental artery and segmental vein, the segment forms a functional unit. Surgically, this creates the option of **segment resection.** This means that in the case of lung metastases, for example, multiple segments from all lobes can be excised, without endangering the function of the lungs. In the case of lung tumours (lung carcinoma), at least the whole affected lobe of a lung is resected.

Table 6.9 Distribution of the bronchi.

Bronchial tree	Lung unit	Function	Comment
Bronchi principales (main bronchi)	Lung	Conductive	
Bronchi lobares	Lung lobes	Conductive	
Bronchi segmentales	Lung segments	Conductive	
Bronchi		Conductive	
Bronchioli	Lung lobules	Conductive	No cartilage and no glands in the wall
Bronchioli terminales	Acinus	Conductive	Only microscopically visible
Bronchioli respiratorii	Alveoli	Respiratory (gas exchanging)	Only microscopically visible
Ductus alveolares, Sacculi alveolares	Alveoli	Respiratory (gas exchanging)	Only microscopically visible

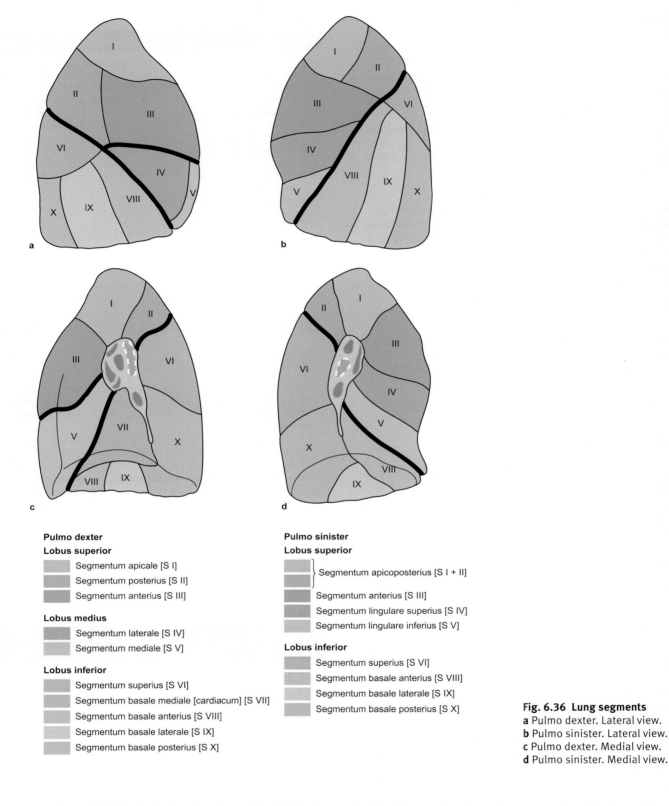

Pulmo dexter
Lobus superior

	Segmentum apicale [S I]
	Segmentum posterius [S II]
	Segmentum anterius [S III]

Lobus medius

| | Segmentum laterale [S IV] |
| | Segmentum mediale [S V] |

Lobus inferior

	Segmentum superius [S VI]
	Segmentum basale mediale [cardiacum] [S VII]
	Segmentum basale anterius [S VIII]
	Segmentum basale laterale [S IX]
	Segmentum basale posterius [S X]

Pulmo sinister
Lobus superior

	}Segmentum apicoposterius [S I + II]
	Segmentum anterius [S III]
	Segmentum lingulare superius [S IV]
	Segmentum lingulare inferius [S V]

Lobus inferior

	Segmentum superius [S VI]
	Segmentum basale anterius [S VIII]
	Segmentum basale laterale [S IX]
	Segmentum basale posterius [S X]

Fig. 6.36 Lung segments
a Pulmo dexter. Lateral view.
b Pulmo sinister. Lateral view.
c Pulmo dexter. Medial view.
d Pulmo sinister. Medial view.

The segmental bronchi divide 6–12 times into **bronchi,** which in turn divide into the already cartilage-free **bronchioles,** the primary division of which form the **pulmonary lobules (Lobuli pulmonis)** (➤ Table 6.9). The lobules are separated incompletely from connective tissue. Macroscopically, these polygonal fields are made visible by retention of carbon dust particles from the air in the subpleural connective tissue along the lymph vessels. In the lung lobules the bronchioles divide another 3–4 times to form the **Bronchioli ter-**

minales. This ends the air-conducting portion of the bronchial tree. From the Bronchioli terminales, the **Bronchioli respiratorii** issue, which branch into Ductus and Sacculi alveolares, where gas exchange takes place.

The air conduction section comprises a volume of 150–170 ml. This volume (**anatomical dead space**) does not take part in the gas exchange and must therefore first be filled before the alveoli can be ventilated.

6.2.7 Vessels and nerves of the lungs

Vessels

The lungs serve the total organism. Therefore, in vessel supply, a distinction is made between the **Vasa publica,** that correspond to the smaller circulation (pulmonary circulation) the purpose of which is oxygenation of the blood and therefore the oxygen supply of the whole body, and the **Vasa privata,** which are responsible for the lung's own supply. Both vessel networks are connected by shunts.

Vasa publica

The **Aa. pulmonales** transfer blood low in oxygen (deoxygenated blood) from the heart to the lungs. They run along the bronchi in the pulmonary tissue and follow the division of the bronchi down to the small blood vessels of the terminal vascular bed (microcirculation) (➤ Fig. 6.37).
The **Vv. pulmonales** do not follow the bronchi, but lie intersegmentally in the connective tissue, i.e. between the individual lung segments. They transfer the oxygen-rich (oxygenated) blood from the lungs back to the heart (➤ Fig. 6.37).

Vasa privata

The Vasa privata course with the bronchi.
- **Arterial blood supply: Rr. bronchiales** originate on the left directly from the aorta but on the right mostly from the 3rd intercostal artery
- **Venous outflow: Vv. bronchiales** carry the blood into the V. azygos, V. hemiazygos. The further peripherally located Vv. bronchiales drain directly into the Vv. pulmonales.

The bronchial vessels also supply the Pleura visceralis around the Hilum pulmonale.

Anastomoses between Vasa publica and Vasa privata

Direct shunts exist between the A. pulmonalis and the Rr. bronchiales. Normally, these arteries are closed (contractile arteries), but may open in the case of reduced blood pressure in the pulmonary artery.

Lymphatic drainage

Lymphatic drainage is ensured by **2 lymphatic drainage systems:** the subpleural and septal as well as the periarterial or peribronchial lymphatic systems. Both lymph vessel systems run together at the hilum (➤ Fig. 6.38).
In the **peribronchial lymphatic system** 3 lymph node stations are arranged in series in the lung tissue:
- Nodi lymphoidei intrapulmonales (at the branching of lobar and segmental bronchi)
- Nodi lymphoidei bronchopulmonales (located in the hilum)
- Nodi lymphoidei tracheobronchiales superiores and inferiores (lymph node clusters at the tracheal bifurcation)

The **subpleural lymph vessel system** is only joined with the peribronchial system at the hilum and therefore has the Nodi lymphoidei trachebronchiales as the first lymph node station. The further outflow of the lymph from the lungs is carried out by the Nodi lymphoidei paratracheales or directly into the Trunci bronchome-

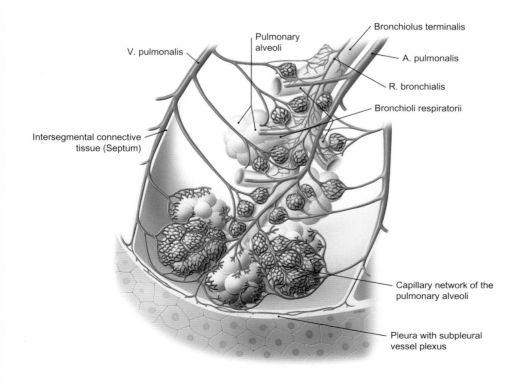

V. pulmonalis

Pulmonary alveoli

Bronchiolus terminalis

A. pulmonalis

R. bronchialis

Bronchioli respiratorii

Intersegmental connective tissue (Septum)

Capillary network of the pulmonary alveoli

Pleura with subpleural vessel plexus

Fig. 6.37 Blood supply to the lungs.

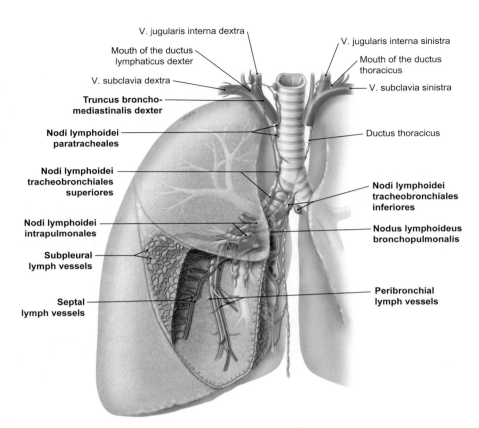

V. jugularis interna dextra

Mouth of the ductus lymphaticus dexter

V. subclavia dextra

Truncus broncho-mediastinalis dexter

Nodi lymphoidei paratracheales

Nodi lymphoidei tracheobronchiales superiores

Nodi lymphoidei intrapulmonales

Subpleural lymph vessels

Septal lymph vessels

V. jugularis interna sinistra

Mouth of the ductus thoracicus

V. subclavia sinistra

Ductus thoracicus

Nodi lymphoidei tracheobronchiales inferiores

Nodus lymphoideus bronchopulmonalis

Peribronchial lymph vessels

Fig. 6.38 Lymphatic drainage from the lungs.

diastinales or below the main bronchi also directly into the Ductus thoracicus. The connection to the paratracheal lymph nodes and the Trunci bronchiomediastinales is crossed, so that lymph from one lung is transferred into the Truncus bronchomediostinalis of the opposite side.

> ### Clinical remarks
>
> Clinicians usually collectively call all lymph nodes of the lungs **hilar lymph nodes.** This is deceptive as the Nodi lymphoidei (intra)pulmonales are spread relatively widely into the lung parenchyma. This linguistic inexactitude can lead to mass lesions in the parenchyma being prematurely considered as independent disease processes and not as enlargements of the lymph nodes, so that unnecessary diagnostic steps for their clarification are initiated.
> The crossed over lymphatic drainage from the Nodi lymphoidei paratracheales has the consequence that lymph node metastases from **lung carcinoma** in the diagnostics are not limited to the respective pleural cavity, but have already spread to both sides of the mediastinum. This means that healing by surgical removal of a lung is usually no longer possible.

Innervation

The **autonomic innervation** of the lungs, whether afferent or efferent, takes place via the **Plexus pulmonalis,** that lies ventral and dorsal to the main bronchi.

The **sympathetic nervous system** runs fibres (Rr. pulmonales) from the Ganglion cervicale inferius and from the 1st–4th thoracic ganglion to the Plexus pulmonalis. Activation of the sympathetic nervous system leads to expansion of the bronchi (bronchodilation).

The **parasympathetic nervous system** feeds the pulmonary plexus via branches of the N. laryngeus recurrens and the N. vagus (Rr. bronchiales). The parasympathetic nervous system leads to narrowing of the bronchi (bronchoconstriction).

Afferent, sensory fibres run through the N. vagus. The perikarya originate from the sensitive ganglia of the nerve (Ganglion superius [jugulare] and Ganglion inferius [nodosum]) and are used for the transmission of pain and stretch stimuli.

6.3 Oesophagus

> ### Skills
>
> After working through this chapter, you should be able to:
> • indicate on a specimen the sections of the oesophagus with their positional relationships
> • localise narrowing of the oesophagus
> • describe the closure mechanisms of the proximal and distal oesophagus and their clinical significance
> • explain the vessels and nerves of the different sections of the oesophagus including the relationship of the veins to the portal venous system

6.3.1 Overview, function and development

The oesophagus is a 25–30 cm long, elastically deformable muscle tube. It is used to transport food from the throat (pharynx) into the stomach (Gaster) (➤ Fig. 6.39).

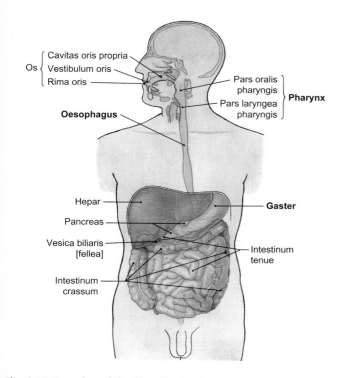

Os
- Cavitas oris propria
- Vestibulum oris
- Rima oris

Pars oralis pharyngis
Pars laryngea pharyngis

Pharynx

Oesophagus

Hepar
Pancreas
Vesica biliaris [fellea]
Intestinum crassum

Gaster

Intestinum tenue

Fig. 6.39 Overview of the digestive tract.

Diseases of the oesophagus fall into the field of gastroenterology. If surgery is required, a visceral surgeon is consulted.

The epithelium and glands of the oesophagus are formed as of the *4th week* from the **entoderm** of the foregut, connective tissue and muscle from the surrounding **mesoderm** (➤ Fig. 6.30). Since only the distal part of the foregut has its own artery in the Truncus coeliacus, the oesophagus is supplied by various blood vessels in its various sections.

As of the *4th–5th week,* the oesophagus is separated by a **tracheoesophageal septum** from the lower respiratory tract, which also originates from the from the foregut (➤ Fig. 6.31). Only the distal part of the oesophagus (Pars abdominalis) is surrounded by the expanding peritoneal cavity and has a coating of visceral peritoneum just like the stomach and adjacent segments of the intestine. The proximal parts in the area of the neck (Pars cervicalis) and in the mediastinum of the thoracic cavity (Pars thoracica) have no contact with the sections of the abdominal cavity and therefore only have a connective tissue coating (Tunica adventitia) (➤ Fig. 6.52).

Clinical remarks

A disorder in the separation of the oesophagus and trachea can lead to the formation of a shunt **(tracheoesophageal fistulas),** often with a blind ending oesophagus **(oesophageal atresia).** Breast milk is spat out after intake and can lead to breathing difficulties due to aspiration in the lungs.

6.3.2 Structure and projection

The oesophagus begins at the bottom of the cricoid cartilage (Cartilago cricoidea) 15 cm from the front row of teeth, at the level of the **6th cervical vertebra.** It runs behind the trachea, between the sheets of the middle and deep cervical fascia from the superior mediastinum into the rear mediastinum and passes through the diaphragm at the Hiatus oesophageus. It ends at the entrance to the stomach (Cardia) at the level of the **10th thoracic vertebra.**

Clinical remarks

The projection of the oesophagus makes is easy to understand why inflammation caused by gastric juice **(gastroesophageal reflux disease)** causes pain and retrosternal burning in a similar location as during a heart attack. From the two organs the afferent nerve fibres go into the same spinal cord segments as neurons of the anterior thoracic wall, so that the brain cannot properly differentiate whether the pain stems from the body surface or from one of the internal organs. Such organ-related areas of skin are referred to as a HEAD's zones. The distance from the front row of teeth to the stomach entrance is approximately 40 cm. This is extremely important for the placement of a gastric tube or for carrying out a **gastroscopy (oesophagogastroduodenoscopy)** because it is possible to estimate the location of pathological abnormalities based on the length of the tube.

6.3.3 Classification

The oesophagus is macroscopically divided into 3 parts:
- Pars cervicalis
- Pars thoracica
- Pars abdominalis

The **Pars cervicalis** is 5–8 cm long, joins to the pharynx and reaches to the upper thoracic aperture. Here, the oesophagus lies behind the trachea and directly in front of the cervical spine.

The **Pars thoracica** is the longest section of the oesophagus measuring 16 cm. On its trajectory to the diaphragm it increases its distance to the spine and runs to the right of the aorta, whereby the aortic arch crosses over the oesophagus and constricts it. In the chest part the oesophagus lies next to the left atrium of the heart, separated only by the pericardium. In the thoracic part the lumen of the oesophagus is usually open because of prevailing negative pressure.

The **Pars abdominalis** is 1–4 cm long and extends from the passage through the oesophageal hiatus up to the stomach entrance (Cardia). The abdominal part is covered by visceral peritoneum (Tunica serosa) and therefore lies in an intraperitoneal position. At rest the Pars abdominalis is closed and opens only during swallowing. The transition of mucosa from the oesophagus to the stomach is macroscopically visible, e.g. during gastroscopy, as a jagged line (Z-line) (➤ Fig. 6.41). This lies in an area 0.75 cm proximal to 1.3 cm distal of the externally assumed border between the oesophagus and stomach. In 70% of cases, it is present only in the area of the oesophagus and in 20% it extends to the Cardia.

NOTE
The oesophagus is separated from the left atrium only by the pericardium.

6.3.4 Constrictions of the oesophagus

The oesophagus is constricted by neighbouring structures in 3 places (➤ Fig. 6.40):

- Cricoid cartilage constriction
- Aorta constriction
- Diaphragm constriction

The first, uppermost constriction at the level of the cricoid cartilage **(cricoid cartilage constriction)** is projected on the 6th cervical

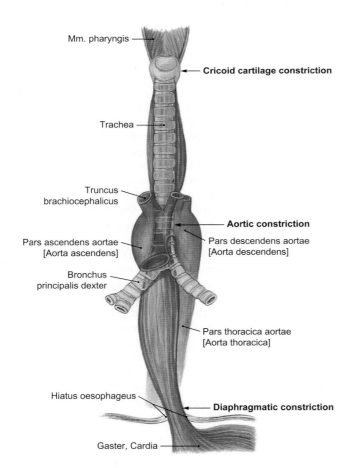

Mm. pharyngis

Cricoid cartilage constriction

Trachea

Truncus brachiocephalicus

Aortic constriction

Pars ascendens aortae [Aorta ascendens]

Pars descendens aortae [Aorta descendens]

Bronchus principalis dexter

Pars thoracica aortae [Aorta thoracica]

Hiatus oesophageus

Diaphragmatic constriction

Gaster, Cardia

Fig. 6.40 Narrowing of the oesophagus. Ventral view.

vertebrae. It is located at the entrance of the oesophagus in the area of the upper oesophageal sphincter. It is the narrowest point with a diameter of 1.5 cm. At rest the upper constriction is closed. The closure is ensured by a true sphincter (➤ Chap. 6.3.5).

The **aortic constriction** is located approximately 10 cm caudal to the uppermost constriction at the height of the 4th thoracic vertebra. Here, the oesophagus is constricted by the left main bronchus and the aortic arch, which are located dorsal and left, respectively. The Pleura parietalis and the main bronchus are connected here to the oesophagus via smooth muscle fibres, but do not contribute to its constriction.

The **diaphragmatic constriction** lies at the passage through the Hiatus oesophageus of the diaphragm at the level of the 10th thoracic vertebra. Here, the oesophagus is fixed by elastic fibres (Lig. phrenoesophageale) and the musculature of the diaphragm (➤ Fig. 6.41). There is no true sphincter here only an angiomuscular extension closure which functionally results in closure (➤ Chap. 6.3.5).

6.3.5 Closing mechanisms

Upper oesophageal sphincter

At the **cricoid cartilage constriction** circular muscle fibres of the lower pharyngeal constrictor muscle (M. constrictor pharyngis inferior) and circular muscle fibres of the oesophagus, together with the submuscular venous plexus form a *true sphincter* (upper oesophageal sphincter). The venous plexus ensures the airtight sealing of the oesophagus, which is opened with an audible sound during burping, for example.

Lower sphincter

Caudally, at the transition of the oesophagus to the stomach, there is *no true sphincter*. Closure is achieved functionally via several mechanisms:

- **Angiomusuclar extension closure** (➤ Fig. 6.42):
  - Under physiological conditions, the oesophagus is under strong **longitudinal elastic tension.** This means that at rest it is closed in the area of the neck and abdomen and only slightly opened in the chest area. The spirally arranged muscles fibres of the muscular layer (Tunica muscularis) are subject to contraction and longitudinal tension (due to gastric torsion during development) and provide a 'screw cap closure' in a physiological position. Food is transported by the peristaltic waves: the longitudinal tension is reduced locally by an arriving peristaltic wave, which means that the longitudinal musculature contracts and the lumen is widened so that the food can pass through.
  - The oesophageal **venous plexus** under the mucosa acts as a cavernous body and, amongst other things, ensures the closure is airtight.
- **Mucosal fold in the angle** of **HIS** (➤ Fig. 6.41, ➤ Fig. 6.42): at the gastro-oesophageal junction a steep angle (65°) is formed between the gastric orifice (Cardia) and gastric fundus in the Incisura cardialis (angle of HIS). Apparently a mucosal fold created by the notch prevents reflux of the stomach contents.

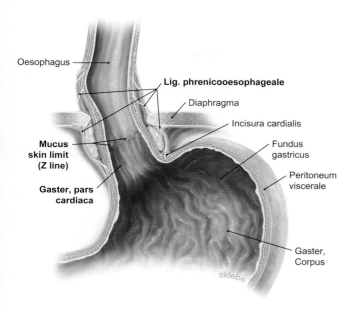

Fig. 6.41 Anchoring of the oesophagus in the Hiatus oesophageus. [L238]

- **Lig. phrenicoesophageale** (➤ Fig. 6.41): anchoring of the oesophagus in the diaphragm (Lig. phrenicoesophageale) and the tone of the diaphragm musculature also ensure a fixation of the oesophagus in the slit in the diaphragm and a narrowing of the lumen.
- **Different pressure gradients** in the abdomen and thorax: in the abdomen there is a higher pressure than in the chest cavity. This pressure gradient is especially high during inspiration resulting in a stronger closure.

Clinical remarks

If the closing mechanisms at the lower oesophagus fail, the result is reflux of gastric acid into the oesophagus, which causes an inflammation of the mucosa **(oesophageal reflux disease).** The consequences can be a BARRETT's oesophagus and malignant degeneration (oesophageal cancer). A possible cause is the lack of stabilisation in the diaphragmatic slit with loosening of the oesophagus. This means that the Pars abdominalis and even parts of the stomach may gain access to the chest area via the oesophageal hiatus **(hiatal hernia).** This supports the development of reflux where gastric acid can attack the mucosa of the oesophagus. Surgically this can be corrected by restoring the angle of HIS. For this purpose, the fundus of the stomach is placed around the oesophagus and sewed into the front wall of the stomach (fundoplication). The formation of pouches (diverticula) of the entire oesophageal wall can occur at different points:
- **ZENKER's diverticulum** is the most common (70%). These diverticula penetrate through KILLIAN's dehiscence of the hypopharynx and are erroneously attributed to the oesophageal diverticula. The cause is a defective weakening of the lower pharyngeal constrictor muscle and therefore the upper oesophageal sphincter.
- **Traction diverticula** (22%) are phylogenetically caused by a defective separation of oesophagus and trachea.
- **Epiphrenic diverticula** (8%) are believed to be evoked by a disturbed function of the lower angiomuscular oesophageal sphincter.

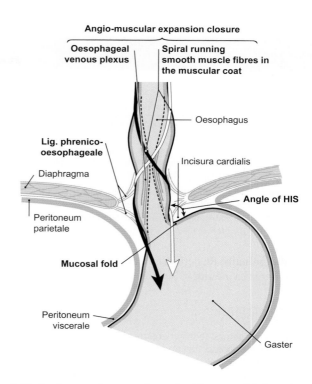

Fig. 6.42 Angiomuscular oesophageal sphincter and HIS angle at the terminal oesophagus. [L126]

6.3.6 Vessels and nerves of the oesophagus

Arteries

The oesophagus does not have its own arteries, but is supplied from the surrounding vessels (➤ Fig. 6.43, ➤ Table 6.10):
- **Pars cervicalis:** Rr. oesophageales of the A. thyroidea inferior
- **Pars thoracica:** Rr. oesophageales of the Aorta thoracica and from right intercostal arteries

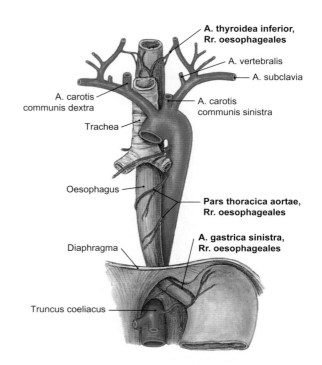

Fig. 6.43 Arterial blood supply of the oesophagus.

Table 6.10 Vessels and nerves of the oesophagus.

Oesophagus section	Vessels and nerves
Pars cervicalis	• A. thyroidea inferior • V. thyroidea inferior • Nodi lymphoidei cervicales profundi
Pars thoracica	• Rr. oesophageales of the aorta thoracica and right inter-costal arteries • V. azygos/hemiazygos • Nodi lymphoidei paratracheales, Nodi lymphoidei tracheo-bronchiales, Nodi lymphoidei mediastinales posteriores
Pars abdomina-lis	• A. gastrica sinistra, A. phrenica inferior • V. gastrica dextra and sinistra in V. portae • Nodi lymphoidei gastrici and Nodi lymphoidei phrenici inferiores

• **Pars abdominalis:** Rr. oesophageales of the A. gastrica sinistra and A. phrenica inferior

---
Clinical remarks

Because, in contrast to other organs of the gastrointestinal tract, the oesophagus has no dedicated arteries but is supplied by blood vessels from the surrounding organs, it is not easy to operate on, which is why **oesophageal surgery** is considered as challenging.

Veins

The venous blood flows through a very strong venous plexus under the mucosa and the Tunica adventitia. These venous plexuses are also part of the angiomuscular extension closure in the lower oesophagus (➤ Fig. 6.44). Drainage takes place via the **Vv. oesophageales** (➤ Table 6.10):
• **Pars cervicalis:** to the V. thyroidea inferior
• **Pars thoracica:** into the V. azygos/V. hemiazygos
• **Pars abdominalis:** via the Vv. gastrica dextra and sinistra, which are connected to the portal vein system (V. portae hepatis) and can therefore act as **portocaval anastomoses** (➤ Chap. 7.3.11).

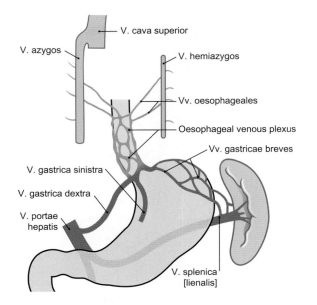

Fig. 6.44 Veins of the oesophagus with portocaval anastomoses.
[L126]

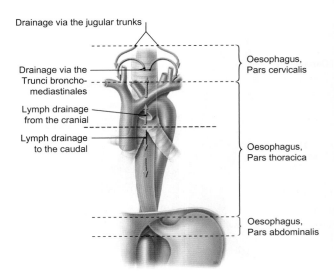

Fig. 6.45 Lymphatic drainage of the oesophagus.

Similar to the lymphatic drainage, the tracheal bifurcation appears to be a landmark for venous drainage: above, the blood is drained in a cranial direction and below the bifurcation caudally (➤ Fig. 6.45).

Clinical remarks

When the pressure in the portal vein system increases **(portal hypertension)**, e.g. because the flow resistance in the liver is increased by scarred reorganisation (liver cirrhosis), blood is fed in via short circulatory connections of the superior and inferior venae cavae **(portocaval anastomoses)**. The most clinically important portocaval anastomoses are the connections via the gastric veins to the oesophagus since these can cause expansion of the submucous veins **(oesophageal varices)**. Rupture of these varices is associated with a mortality of approximately 50 % and is, therefore, the most frequent cause of death in patients with liver cirrhosis. In the case of rupture inwards, the stomach is usually filled with black blood; in rarer ruptures the blood flows outside into the abdominal cavity. Therefore, oesophageal varices are prophylactically ligated (rubber band ligation) or injected with vascular cauterising substances.

Lymph

The lymph is drained into the local lymph nodes of the oesophagus **(Nodi lymphoidei juxtaoesophageales),** which transfers the lymph accordingly (➤ Table 6.10):
• Pars cervicalis: via **Nodi lymphoidei cervicales profundi** to the Truncus jugularis
• Pars thoracica: **Nodi lymphoidei paratracheales, Nodi lymphoidei tracheobronchiales and Nodi lymphoidei mediastinales posteriores** into the Truncus bronchomediastinalis
• Pars abdominalis: via **Nodi lymphoidei gastrici** and **Nodi lymphoidei phrenici inferiores** into the Trunci intestinales and lumbales

Drainage occurs above the tracheal bifurcation mainly in a cranial direction, below the bifurcation in a caudal direction (➤ Fig. 6.45).

Innervation

The oesophagus has an independently functioning **enteral nervous system,** which is modulated by the parasympathetic and sympathetic nervous systems: the parasympathetic nervous system promotes peristalsis and gland secretion, the sympathetic nervous system inhibits both processes.

- The **parasympathetic innervation** occurs cranially via the N. laryngeus recurrens and in the thoracic and abdominal sections via the N. vagus. Below the Bifurcatio tracheae both N. vagus trunks lie alongside the oesophagus and form the Plexus oesophageus in the adventitia, which in the distal part issues the Trunci vagales anterior and posterior. Both trunks pass through the oesophageal hiatus of the diaphragm together with the oesophagus. Due to the extension of the stomach, the left N. vagus lies on the front and the right N. vagus on the back of the stomach.
- The **sympathetic innervation** results from post-ganglionic sympathetic fibres from the cranial cervical and upper thoracic sympathetic ganglia (2nd–5th).

Sensitive afferent information, such as stretch and pain stimuli in particular are also centrally transferred via the N. vagus.

6.4 Thymus

6.4.1 Overview, function and development

The thymus is located in the Trigonum thymicum in the superior mediastinum (➤ Fig. 6.46). It is located behind the sternum and extends from the upper sternal border up to the pericardium (height of 4th rib cartilage). On the side it is covered by the mediastinal part of the Pleura parietalis. The large vessels and nerves run behind the thymus: aortic arch and Vv. brachiocephalicae with their unification into the V. cava superior.

The thymus, together with bone marrow, is one of the **primary lymphatic organs,** because the thymus is the location of maturation of T-lymphocytes. From the bone marrow the lymphocytes wander via the blood vessels to the thymus. This is where maturation (imprinting) and proliferation as well as selection of the T-lymphocytes takes place. Then, the T-lymphocytes reach the secondary lymphatic organs (spleen, lymph nodes, tonsils and mucosa-associated lymphatic tissue) via the blood, where the actual specific immune response takes place.

The **entoderm of the 3rd pharyngeal pouch** forms a ventral bud on both sides, which from the *6th week* both move medially and together form the two lobes of the thymus.

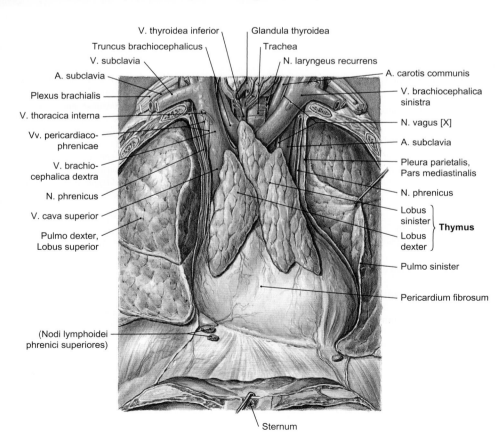

Fig. 6.46 Overview of the thymus.

The DiGEORGE syndrome describes a thymus aplasia. The thymus is formed but does not develop. The reason for this is a malformation of the 3rd pharyngeal pouch. This leads to a loss of cellular immunity. The patients are affected by recurrent infections and require a sterile environment.

N O T E

Thymus and bone marrow are part of the **primary lymphatic organs.** Their purpose is the production and maturation (**DiGEORGE syndrome** imprinting) of immune cells. Here, the mature cells gain the ability to distinguish between own body cells and foreign bodies. The actual immune reaction takes place in the secondary lymphatic organs.

6.4.2 Structure

The thymus consists of **2 asymmetric lobes (lobi),** each of which is surrounded by a dedicated connective tissue capsule. Septa made up of connective tissue divide the lobes into microscopically visible **lobules (Lobuli thymici),** which in turn can be divided into a **cortex** and **medulla.** After puberty the thymus experiences involution. The cortex is significantly reduced and replaced by fat tissue (**retrosternal fat body**). In older people only microscopically detectable remnants of the thymus tissue are left, which however can be used in an immune response if necessary. Here thymus tissue with a high percentage of fatty tissue and higher blood vessel density is characteristic. Macroscopically, these remnants can only be identified by the small arterial branches of the A. thoracica interna and venous connections to the Vv. brachiocephalicae.
At the neck accessory thymus lobules may occur.

6.4.3 Vessels and nerves of the thymus

* **Arterial blood supply:** Rr. thymici of the A. thoracica interna
* **Venous drainage:** Vv. thymicae to the V. brachiocephalica
* **Lymph vessels:** only efferent lymph vessels to the mediastinal lymph nodes
* **Innervation:** predominantly sympathetic via the neck ganglia of the sympathetic trunk; parasympathetic: N. vagus

6.5 Thoracic cavity

Skills

After working through this chapter you should be able to:
* describe the structure of the thoracic cavity and the contents of the mediastinum on a specimen
* show the sections of the pleural cavity with its recesses and explain the vessels and nerves of the pleura
* explain the processes during respiration and demonstrate the function of the respiratory muscles
* understand the principles of development of the abdominal cavities and the diaphragm

6.5.1 Overview

The chest cavity (Cavitas thoracis) is surrounded by the rib cage (Cavea thoracis). It is divided into 2 **pleural cavities** (Cavitates pleurales), that each contain one lung. Between them lies the **mediastinum,** which represents a connective tissue space between the sternum and thoracic spine (➤ Fig. 6.48).

6.5.2 Mediastinum

The mediastinum (Lat.: what stands in the middle) is a connective tissue space between the sternum and spine, that is filled with an individually very different amount of fat. The mediastinum is divided into different sections relative to the location of the heart (➤ Fig. 6.47):
Mediastinum superius, above the heart
Mediastinum inferius, where the heart is. The lower mediastinum is divided into:
* **Mediastinum anterius** (in front of the heart)
* **Mediastinum medium** (with the pericardium)
* **Mediastinum posterius** (between heart and spine)
The **upper mediastinum** contains the thymus, the trachea up to its bifurcation, the oesophagus, as well as the major arterial and venous blood vessels of the heart (aortic arch, Truncus pulmonalis, V. cava superior with tributaries), the mediastinal lymph nodes and lymphatic trunks as well as various nerves that run from the neck through the chest cavity (N. phrenicus, N. vagus, Truncus sympathicus with branches) (➤ Table 6.11).

Table 6.11 Content of the mediastinum.

Content of the superior mediastinum	Content of the inferior mediastinum
• Thymus • Trachea • Oesophagus • Aortic arch and Truncus pulmonalis • Vv. brachiocephalicae and V. cava superior • Lymphatic pathways: lymphatic trunks (Ductus thoracicus, Trunci bronchiomediastinales) and mediastinal lymph nodes • Autonomic nervous system (Truncus sympathicus, N. vagus [X] with N. laryngeus recurrens) • N. phrenicus	• **Mediastinum anterius:** retrosternal lymphatic drainage of the mammary glands • **Mediastinum medium:** pericardium with vessels around the heart, N. phrenicus with Vasa pericardiacophrenica • **Mediastinum posterius:** Aorta descendens, oesophagus with Plexus oesophageus of the N. vagus, Ductus thoracicus, Truncus sympathicus with Nn. splanchnici, V. azygos and V. hemiazygos as well as intercostal vessels and nerves

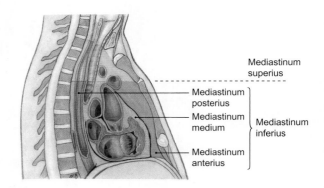

Fig. 6.47 **Structure of the mediastinum.**

Mediastinum superius
Mediastinum posterius
Mediastinum medium
Mediastinum anterius
Mediastinum inferius

The **front lower mediastinum** contains only the retrosternal lymph outflows of the mammary gland (the A./V. thoracica interna are, however, included in the abdominal wall). The **middle lower mediastinum** is filled completely by the pericardium, on which the N. phrenicus and A./V. pericardiacophrenica run. In the pericardium are the heart and the Aorta ascendens. The **rear lower mediastinum** in contrast has a complex structure and is crossed by the oesophagus, the Aorta descendens, the azygos venous system, the N. vagus and the sympathetic trunk with branches, the Ductus thoracicus as well as the intercostal vessels and nerves (➤ Table 6.11).

6.5.3 Pleural cavities

The **pleural cavities (Cavitas pleuralis)** are lined by the parietal pleura **(Pleura parietalis)** that is divided according to its 3 areas:
- Pars costalis (inside on the ribs)
- Pars mediastinalis (on the mediastinum)
- Pars diaphragmatica (on the diaphragm)

The enveloping folds push medially between the Pleura costalis and Pleura mediastinalis on both sides so far between the mediastinum and sternum that they touch. Only in 2 small areas do they stay apart, so that the mediastinum directly comes into contact with the sternum (➤ Fig. 6.48):
- **Trigonum thymicum** (cranial), contains the thymus
- **Trigonum pericardiacum** (caudal), in which the pericardium lies adjacent to the sternum with varied levels of expansion and corresponds to the field of 'absolute cardiac dullness'

At the **top** the pleural cavities extend over the thoracic aperture with the pleural dome **(Cupula pleurae)** by up to 5 cm (!).

At the **hilum** of the lungs, the Pleura parietalis continues into the visceral pleura **(Pleura visceralis),** which covers the external surface of the lungs. The enveloping fold may extend caudally to varying degrees as the pulmonary ligament.

Both pleural membranes form a capillary cleft space that contains a total of 5 ml of serous fluid, which mediates the adhesion of the lungs to the wall of the torso, so that during breathing the lungs can mirror the volume change of the rib cage.

Clinical remarks

When inserting a **central venous catheter** (CVC) into the **V. subclavia,** the distension of the pleural dome must be considered. In doing so the catheter is inserted in bottom edge of the front convexity of the clavicle in the direction of the sternoclavicular joint. If the cannula is positioned too steeply, the Cavitas pleuralis may be injured which can result in collapse of the lungs **(pneumothorax)** by an inflow of air into the Cavitas pleuralis.

The pleural cavities have 4 paired reserve spaces **(Recessus pleurales)** into which the lungs expand during deep inspiration:
- **Recessus costodiaphragmaticus:** lateral, in the mid-axillary line up to 5 cm deep; it stretches in a caudal direction to the right behind the right lobe of the liver and to the left behind the stomach and spleen and can also extend on both sides behind the upper renal pole (➤ Fig. 6.48)
- **Recessus costomediastinalis:** bilateral, ventral between mediastinum and chest wall; corresponds to the area of 'relative cardiac dullness', because here the air-filled lung is located between pericardium and chest wall and thus does not reduce the percussion sound as much as in the area of 'absolute cardiac dullness' (➤ Fig. 6.48)
- **Recessus phrenicomediastinalis:** caudal, between diaphragm and mediastinum
- **Recessus vertebromediastinalis:** dorsal, adjacent to the vertebral column

While the **Pleura visceralis** is also supplied by the vessels and nerves of the lungs and is not sensitive to pain, the 3 sections of the

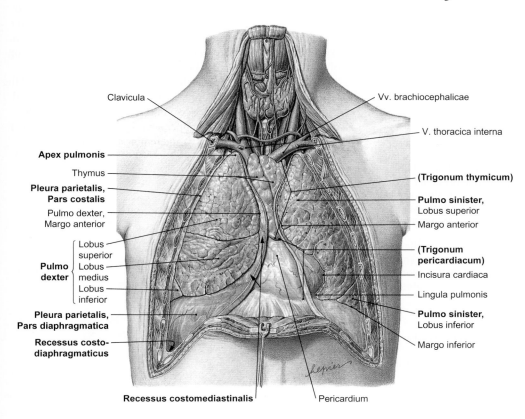

Clavicula

Vv. brachiocephalicae

V. thoracica interna

Apex pulmonis

Thymus

Pleura parietalis, Pars costalis

Pulmo dexter, Margo anterior

(Trigonum thymicum)

Pulmo sinister, Lobus superior

Margo anterior

Lobus superior

Pulmo dexter Lobus medius

Lobus inferior

(Trigonum pericardiacum)

Incisura cardiaca

Lingula pulmonis

Pleura parietalis, Pars diaphragmatica

Recessus costodiaphragmaticus

Pulmo sinister, Lobus inferior

Margo inferior

Recessus costomediastinalis

Pericardium

Fig. 6.48 Pleural cavities and mediastinum of an adolescent. Ventral view after removal of the chest wall and fat tissue of the mediastinum.

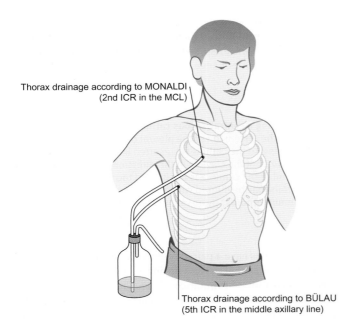

Thorax drainage according to MONALDI
(2nd ICR in the MCL)

Thorax drainage according to BÜLAU
(5th ICR in the middle axillary line)

Fig. 6.49 Chest drainage according to MONALDI in the 2nd ICS in the midclavicular line (MCL) or according to BÜLAU in the 5th ICS in the middle axillary line. The trapped air or liquid is removed from the pleural cavity using the drainage system. [L126]

Pleura parietalis are supplied by the surrounding vessels and nerves. It therefore also has somatic innervation and is sensitive to pain:

- **Pars costalis:**
  - Aa./Vv. intercostales posteriores (back)/Rr. intercostales anteriores (front)
  - Nodi lymphoidei intercostales (back) and parasternales (front)
  - Nn. intercostales
- **Pars mediastinalis and diaphragmatica:**
  - A./V. pericardiacophrenica, A./V. musculophrenica, A./V. phrenica superior
  - Nodi lymphoidei mediastinales and Nodi lymphoidei phrenici superiores
  - N. phrenicus

Clinical remarks

Increased fluid in the pleural cavity **(pleural effusion)** may occur during pneumonia (pleuritis), by tailback due to heart failure or tumours of the lungs or the pleura. In addition, there is chylous pleural effusion, in which lymph bursts out of the Ductus thoracicus into the pleural cavity. Pleural effusions cause a dull knocking sound. They are punctured in the Recessus costodiaphragmaticus to clarify the cause and to improve respiration.

For **thorax drainage** the pleural cavity is punctured, either to allow the lungs to expand by removing the air that has entered, as in the case of a pneumothorax or to remove blood in the case of haemothorax (➤ Fig. 6.49). The access routes chosen in emergency medicine are:

• for MONALDI drainage the 2nd ICS in the midclavicular line or
• for the BÜLAU drainage the 5th ICS in the middle axillary line.

For the BÜLAU drainage puncture of the liver on the right side must be avoided, as it can extend underneath the diaphragmatic dome to the 4th ICS.

Since only the parietal pleura is pain-sensitive, lung diseases are only painful once the **Pleura parietalis** is affected. In the case of irritation of the Pleura costalis, the pain is felt in the respective ICS of the abdominal wall; in the case of involvement of the diaphragmatic pleura, however, pain is felt via the N. phrenicus in the area of the shoulder (referred pain). **Lung cancer** only becomes noticeable through pain when the disease is advanced and has invaded the costal pleura; before the symptoms are unspecific.

6.5.4 Breathing

The human body meets its energy needs predominantly through oxidative breakdown of nutrients. All cells therefore require sufficient oxygen and emit carbon dioxide as a waste product. These gases are conveyed by the blood in the pulmonary circulation to the lungs, where they are exhaled to the outside air. The lungs thereby passively follow the volume changes of the pleural cavities in the chest cavity.

During **inspiration** the volume of the pleural cavity can be increased by 2 mechanisms (➤ Fig. 6.50):

- In **diaphragmatic breathing** ('abdominal breathing') the pleural cavity is enlarged in a caudal direction by contraction of the diaphragm (the most important respiratory muscle), on which the diaphragmatic part of the pleura rests.
- In **rib cage breathing** ('chest breathing') the pleural cavity is enlarged in a ventral, dorsal and lateral direction by lifting of the ribs via the Mm. intercostales externi and Mm. scaleni ventrally, dorsal and laterally.

Inhalation requires the use of the muscles of the thorax and therefore active. Accessory respiratory muscles support inspiration during forced breathing (➤ Table 6.12).

Expiration on the other hand, is mostly passive, as the diaphragm relaxes and the cartilaginous parts of the ribs that were deformed during inspiration, the ligaments of the rib cage and the elastic tissue of the lung tissue return to their original position. In addition, exhalation is supported by various muscles, that all lead to sinking of the ribs (➤ Fig. 6.50, ➤ Table 6.12).

The **antagonistic function** of the Mm. intercostales externi and the lateral portions of the Mm. intercostales interni, can be explained by the torque the muscles create on the ribs. Since the Mm. intercostales externi run from an upper lateral position to a lower medial position, the virtual lever of caudal muscles to the axis of rota-

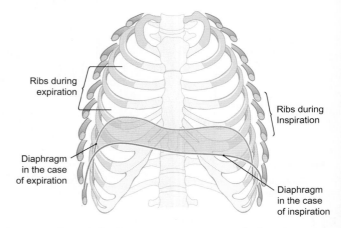

Ribs during expiration

Ribs during Inspiration

Diaphragm in the case of expiration

Diaphragm in the case of inspiration

Fig. 6.50 Ribs and diaphragm during inspiration (red) and expiration (blue). [L126]

Table 6.12 Muscles for breathing and accessory breathing muscles.

Inspiration	Expiration
Effective during **inspiration:** • The diaphragm (most important respiratory muscle!) • Mm. intercostales externi • Parasternal portions of the Mm. intercostales interni ('Mm. intercartilaginei') • Mm. scaleni **Inspiratory accessory respiratory muscles:** • M. sternocleidomastoideus (when head is fixed by neck musculature) • Mm. serrati posteriores superior and inferior (by fixing the ribs) • M. pectoralis major (with supported arm) • M. pectoralis minor (with supported arm) • M. serratus anterior (with supported arm)	Rffective during **expiration:** • Mm. intercostales interni and intimi • Mm. subcostales • M. transversus thoracis **Expiratory accessory respiratory muscles:** • M. transversus abdominis • Mm. obliqui externus and internus abdominis • Mm. latissimus dorsi ('cough muscle') • M. iliocostalis (lateral tract of autochthonous back muscles)

tion is enlarged by the neck of the ribs, as well as the torsional movement, so that the muscles lift the caudal ribs in particular. The Mm. intercostales interni (and intimi), on the other hand, have an opposite trend and therefore more strongly depress the cranial ribs.

Clinical remarks

Since the diaphragm is the most important respiratory muscle, bilateral **diaphragmatic insufficiency,** e.g. due to traumatic or surgical wounding of the Nn. phrenici is not compatible

with life. Since the Nn. phrenici issue from the Plexus cervicalis are predominantly supplied by the C4 spinal cord segment, injuries of these segments in **paraplegia** can lead to suffocation. Lesions caudal to C4 that still can lead to a complete paralysis of the extremities, do not endanger breathing.

6.5.5 Development of the visceral cavities

The **chest cavity (Cavitas thoracis),** together with the **abdominal cavity (Cavitas abdominalis,** ➤ Chap. 7.7.1) and the **pelvic cavity (Cavitas pelvis,** ➤ Chap. 8.7.1) form the 3 large visceral cavities of the trunk. In these visceral cavities 3 abdominal cavities develop, lined with a **serous membrane (Tunica serosa):**
• In the thoracic cavity the **pericardial cavity (Cavitas pericardiaca)** and **pleural cavity (Cavitates pleurales),** develop
• In the abdominal and pelvic cavities, the **peritoneal cavity (Cavitas peritonealis)** develops.

The serous skin derives from the mesoderm whereas the **parietal sheet** (parietal sheet of the Pericardium serosum, Pleura parietalis, Peritoneum parietale) is derived from the abdominal wall (so-called somatopleural mesenchyme) and covers it. The **visceral sheet** (epicardium, Pleura visceralis, Peritoneum viscerale), on the other hand, is derived from the mesoderm of the gut wall (so-called splanchopleural mesenchyme) and covers the surface of the organs.

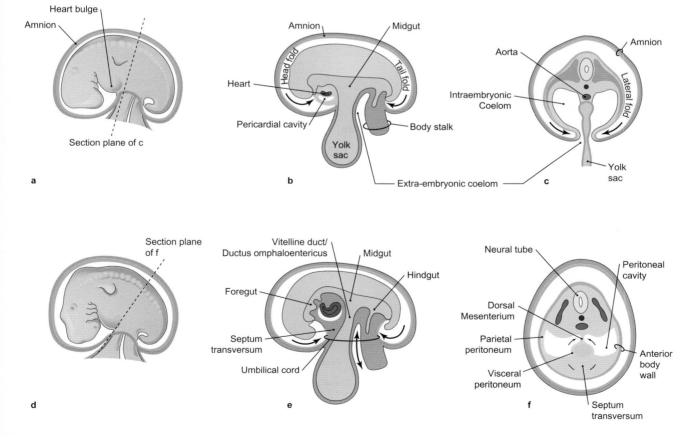

Fig. 6.51 Embryonic cleavage in the 4th week of development. a Side view of an embryo in the 4th week (26th day). **b** Sagittal section of the embryo at the same time. **c** Transverse section through the section plane specified in **a. d** Side view of the embryo at the end of the 4th week (28th day). **e** Sagittal section of the embryo at the same time. **f** Transverse section through the section plane specified in **d.** [E347-09]

The **abdominal cavity (Coelom)** is formed by the merging of the gaps in the mesoderm. The coelom consists of an extra-embryonic portion **(extra-embryonic coelom, chorionic cavity),** that develops between the intermediate trophoblast and yolk sac, and an **intra-embryonic coelom** in the mesoderm between the endoderm and ectoderm of the germ disc. While these two sections first communicate with each other, the extra-embryonic coelom later degenerates, while the intra-embryonic coelom is divided into pericardial, pleural and peritoneal cavities.

Initially at the end of the *3rd developmental week* the horseshoe-shaped **pleuropericardial cavity,** is formed, the cranial portion of which later becomes the pericardial cavity in the region of the heart, whereby the two caudal legs are the attachments for the pleural cavities (➤ Fig. 6.51). Caudal the **division of the coelom,** starts to form which communicates laterally with the extra-embryonic coelom, creating the attachment for the peritoneal cavity. The pleuropericardial cavity is now connected to the division in the coelom, so that through these **coelom ducts (Ductus pericardia-** **coperitoneales)** a continuous intra-embryonic abdominal cavity is first formed (➤ Fig. 6.52), which is separated later into sections. In the *4th developmental week* embryonic folding begins in both a craniocaudal as well as lateral direction (➤ Fig. 6.51c, e), so that the navel is formed and the widely spaced connection between the intra-embryonic intestinal system and the extra-embryonic yolk sac to the **vitelline duct** (Ductus omphaloentericus/Ductus vitellinus) is narrowed (➤ Fig. 6.51e). As a result, the intestinal attachment is divided into 3 sections that are cranial, caudal and at the level of the Ductus omphaloentericus, representing the foregut, hindgut and midgut. The lateral folding results in an enlargement of the peritoneal cavity on both sides of the intestinal tube, so that it is connected to the dorsal wall of the trunk only by a small line of connective tissue **(dorsal mesentery)** (➤ Fig. 6.51f ➤ Fig. 6.52d). The mesenterium is therefore covered by peritoneum on both sides (peritoneal duplication), which as the **Peritoneum viscerale** covers the surface of the intestinal system and in the form of the **Peritoneum parietale** lines the peritoneal cavity (➤ Fig. 6.52e).

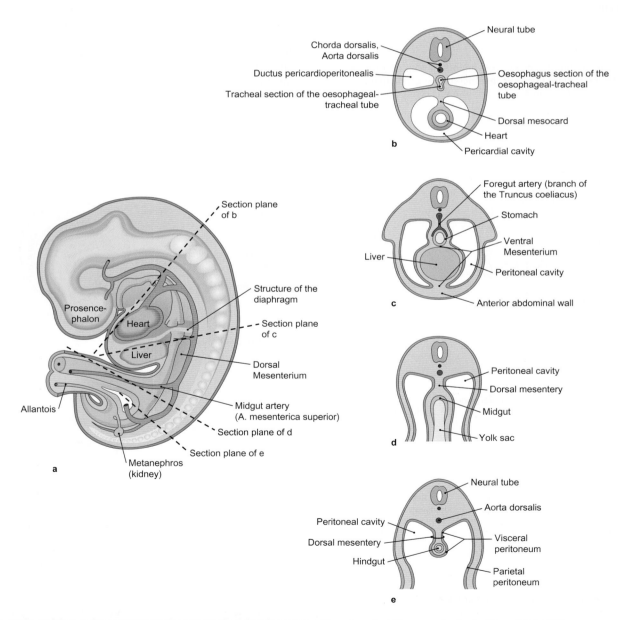

Fig. 6.52 Body cavities and mesentery in the 5th week of development. a Overview. **b–e** Planes as indicated in **a.** [E347-09]

A **ventral mesentery** only forms in the area above the navel, i.e. at the foregut, because the developing liver here has a connection to the ventral trunk wall by being embedded in the Septum transversum (➤ Fig. 6.52c). The **Septum transversum** is a mesenchymal plate between pericardial cavity and Ductus omphaloentericus and therefore the initial separation between pericardial and peritoneal cavities (➤ Fig. 6.51e, f). The peritoneal cavity communicates with the extra-embryonic coelom in the umbilicus even up to the *10th week,* until this degenerates during regression of the gut.

The cranial parts of the coelomic ducts extend to the pleural cavity and extend ventrally on both sides of the pericardial cavity, from which they are separated in the *7th week* by the **pleuropericardial membranes** (➤ Fig. 6.53b). The pericardial cavity is incorporated in the mesenchyme in the vicinity of the foregut, which later becomes the **mediastinum** (➤ Fig. 6.53c, d). The folds in the serosa at the caudal aspect of the pleura separate these at the *end of the 2nd month* as **pleuroperitoneal membranes** from the pericadial cavity, by combining ventrally with the Septum transversum and dorsally with the mesentery of the oesophagus. This happens earlier on the right than on the left, perhaps because the liver has already been formed here.

N O T E

The coelom arises from gaps in the mesoderm and is later divided into the pericardial, pleural and peritoneal cavities. These are lined by serous skins, also originating from the mesoderm.

By division into the pleural and peritoneal cavities the **diaphragm** is also formed, the Centrum tendineum of which is derived from the Septum transversum (➤ Fig. 6.51e). Since this occurs first at the height of the cervical somites and is only displaced to the height of the thoracic somites (descensus) due to the fast growth of the back of the embryo, it becomes obvious why the muscle precursor cells entering the Septum transversum are innervated by the cranial spinal cord segments, the nerve fibres of which later form the N. phrenicus (plexus cervicalis, C3–5). The largest parts of the diaphragm that surround the central tendon (**Partes sternalis, costalis and lumbalis**) are largely derived from the adjacent parts of the body wall. Only the **diaphragmatic leg of the Pars lumbalis** are a relic of the dorsal mesentery of the oesophagus. The **pleuroperitoneal membranes** degenerate to a large extent and only form a small area of the diaphragm near the Trigonum lumbocostale (BOCHDALEK's triangle).

N O T E

The diaphragm is made up of 4 parts:
• Centrum tendineum: from the Septum transversum
• Partes sternalis, costalis and lumbalis (largest part): from the adjacent abdominal wall
• Diaphragmatic leg: from the dorsal mesentery of the oesophagus
• Small section at the Trigonum lumbocostale: from the pleuroperitoneal membranes
The muscle cells and their innervation (N. phrenicus) originate from the cervical somites.

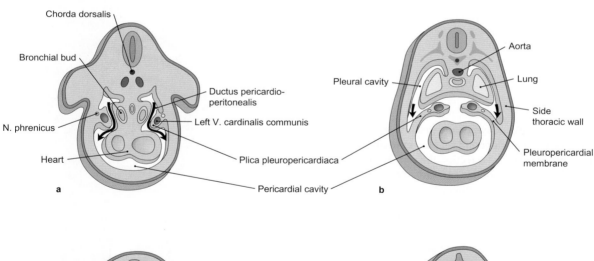

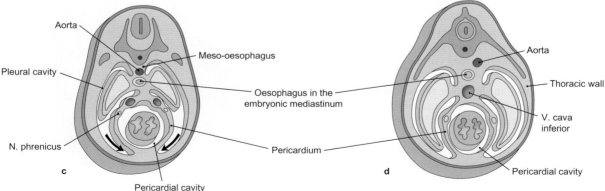

Fig. 6.53 Division of the body cavity between 5th and 8th developmental week. a At the end of the 5th week, the arrows show the connections between pleural and pericardial cavities. **b** 6th week: formation of pleuropericardial membrane. **c** 7th week: expansion of the pleural cavity ventrally. **d** 8th week. [E347-09]

The complicated development of the diaphragm explains why congenital malformations can occur. The most common is the **posterolateral diaphragmatic hernia,** in which closure of the pleuroperitoneal membrane is usually missing. This defect is also known as congenital BOCHDALEK's hernia, although there is no hernial sac. Due to the relocation of the stomach, spleen and small intestine sections in the thoracic cavity, a frequent result is underdevelopment of the lungs (pulmonary hypoplasia) leading to shortness of breath, blue discolouration of the skin (cyanosis) and increase in heart rate (tachycardia) after birth.

6.6 Vessels and nerves of the thoracic cavity

Skills

After working through this chapter, you should be able to:
* understand the basic structure of the vessels and nerves of the thoracic cavity, so that you can see the origin of the vessels and nerves in the individual organs
* show the sections of the aorta in the chest with its branches in a specimen
* name the V. cava superior with tributaries, the azygos vein system and cavocaval anastomoses and understand their clinical relevance
* explain lymph node groups and systematics of lymphatic trunks in the thoracic cavity and describe the course of the Ductus thoracicus in detail on a specimen
* show the trajectory and supply area of the N. phrenicus
* explain the organisation of the autonomic nervous system in the thoracic cavity as well as demonstrate the construction of the sympathetic trunk and trajectory and branches of the Nn. vagi on a specimen

6.6.1 Overview

The major arterial, venous and lymphatic vascular trunks of the body are positioned in the **upper** and **rear lower mediastinum of the thoracic cavity.** In a cranial direction the vessels and nerves protrude through the upper thoracic aperture into the connective tissue area of the neck. In a caudal direction they protrude through the diaphragm and continue into the **retroperitoneal space** of the abdominal cavity (➤ Chap. 8.7).

The **aorta** is divided into Aorta ascendens, aortic arch (Arcus aortae) and the thoracic section of the Aorta descendens (Pars thoracica aortae), which each issue various branches.

The **superior vena cava (V. cava superior)** transports the blood of the upper half of the body to the heart. It receives the veins of the **azygos vein system,** the inflows of which correspond to the supply area of the aorta.

The main lymphatic trunk of the body, the **thoracic duct (Ductus thoracicus),** ascends in front of the spine, crosses the left pleural dome and exits in the left venous angle. In addition, the mediastinum contains a variety of lymph nodes.

As parts of the somatic **nervous system** the intercostal nerves, which innervate the abdominal wall (➤ Chap. 3.2.3), and the N. phrenicus are in the mediastinum. The autonomic nervous system consists of the thoracic section of the sympathetic trunk (Truncus sympathicus) and the N. vagus.

6.6.2 Arteries of the thoracic cavity

In the superior mediastinum the ascending aorta (Aorta ascendens) flows into the aortic arch (Arcus aortae) and then continues as the descending leg (Aorta descendens) of the thoracic aorta (Aorta thoracica) (➤ Fig. 6.54).

The coronary arteries (A. coronaria dextra and sinistra) issue from the **Aorta ascendens** still in the pericardium.

The **aortic arch** traverses the Bifurcatio tracheae and arrives at the left side of the trachea, oesophagus and spine. It issues the following branches (➤ Fig. 6.55, ➤ Fig. 6.56):
* **Truncus brachiocephalicus,** which branches into the A. subclavia dextra and the A. carotis communis
* **A. carotis communis sinistra**
* **A. subclavia sinistra**
* **(A. thyroidea ima):** an unpaired lowest thyroid artery is present in up to 10% of all cases, but typically branches off from the

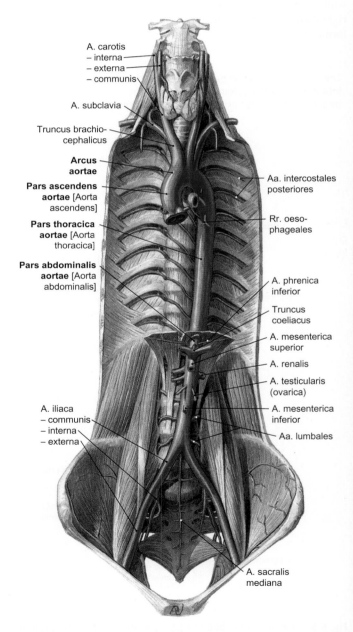

Fig. 6.54 Sections of the aorta with outlets of the great arteries from the aortic arch. [S010-2-16]

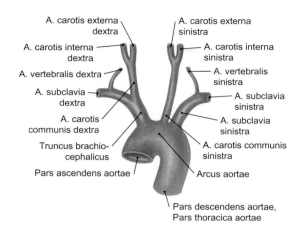

Fig. 6.55 Aortic arch with branches.

Truncus brachiocephalicus or an A. carotis communis and therefore not directly from the aorta.

Table 6.13 Branches of the Pars thoracica aortae.

Parietal branches to the thoracic wall	Visceral branches to the thoracic viscera
• Aa. intercostales posteriores: 9 pairs (the first two are branches of the Truncus costocervicales from the A. subclavia) • A. subcostalis: the last pair under the 12th rib • A. phrenica superior: to the upper side of the diaphragm	• Rr. bronchiales: Vasa privata of the lungs (on the right side mostly from the A. intercostalis posterior dextra III) • Rr. oesophageales: 3–6 branches to the oesophagus • Rr. mediastinales: small branches to the mediastinum and pericardium

---

Clinical remarks

In rare cases (< 1%), the A. subclavia dextra can issue from the aortic arch as the last independent branch and then extend behind the oesophagus to the right arm. As the oesophagus is constricted in this case between the A. subclavia dextra (also known as A. lusoria) and the aortic arch, swallowing disorders may occur (**Dysphagia lusoria**).

6.6.3 Veins of the thoracic cavity

The **superior vena cava (V. cava superior)** is 5–6 cm long and forms to the right of the spine behind the 1st sternocostal joint through unification of the V. brachiocephalica dextra and sinistra (➤ Fig. 6.57). On entering the pericardium on the right side the azygos vein flows into it at the height of the 4th–5th thoracic vertebra. The V. cava superior and Vv. brachiocephalicae have no valves. The **Vv. brachiocephalicae** originate in the V. jugularis interna and the V. subclavia in the **venous angle,** which is placed directly behind the sternoclavicular joint and have very different trajectories on either side (➤ Fig. 6.57). *On the right* the vein is short and merges almost vertically into the superior vena cava. Clinicians also refer to this as 'V. anonyma' and use it for the introduction of a central venous catheter (CVC). *On the left,* on the other hand, the vein traverses the branches of the aortic arch and trachea practically horizontally and includes 2 unpaired vessels:
• V. thyroidea inferior
• V. hemiazygos accessoria
Bilaterally the following are conjoined:
• V. vertebralis
• V. thoracica interna
• V. intercostalis suprema

The **Aorta descendens** lies left ventral of the spine in the posterior mediastinum (**Aorta thoracica**) and issues various parietal branches to the abdominal wall and the diaphragm as well as visceral branches for the lungs, oesophagus and mediastinum (➤ Table 6.13, ➤ Fig. 6.54).

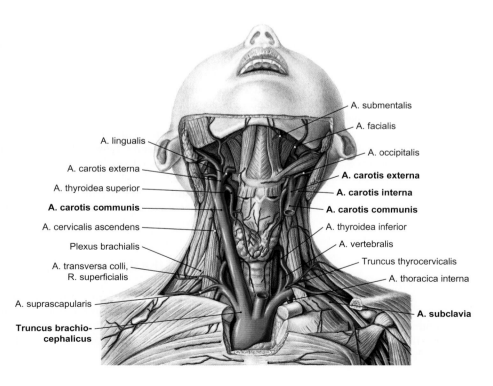

Fig. 6.56 Aorta with branches.
[S010-2-16]

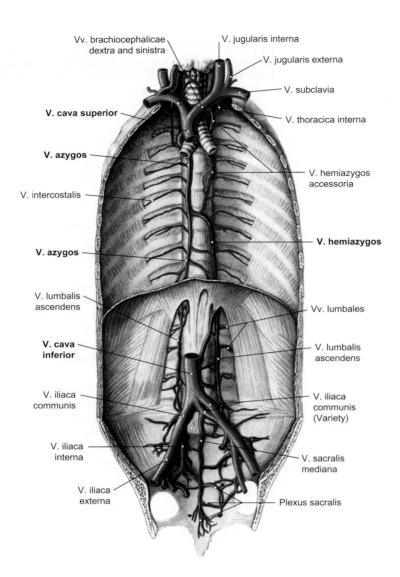

Vv. brachiocephalicae dextra and sinistra

V. jugularis interna

V. jugularis externa

V. subclavia

V. cava superior

V. thoracica interna

V. azygos

V. hemiazygos accessoria

V. intercostalis

V. hemiazygos

V. azygos

V. lumbalis ascendens

Vv. lumbales

V. cava inferior

V. lumbalis ascendens

V. iliaca communis

V. iliaca communis (Variety)

V. iliaca interna

V. sacralis mediana

V. iliaca externa

Plexus sacralis

Fig. 6.57 Vv. cavae superior and inferior with tributaries and azygos system. [S010-2-16]

The **azygos venous system** is located on both sides of the spine and its tributaries are equivalent to the branches of the thoracic aorta. The **V. azygos** ascends on the *right side* of the spine, crosses the main bronchi and pulmonary vessels and exits at the level of the IVth/Vth thoracic vertebra dorsally into the V. cava superior. *On the left* it corresponds to the **hemi-azygos vein,** which, for its part, exits between the Xth and VIIth thoracic vertebrae into the V. azygos. From the upper intercostal veins, the blood is received by a **V. hemiazygos accessoria,** which in addition to the V. hemiazygos has a cranial connection to the V. brachiocephalica sinistra. Since the V. azygos is the strongest vessel and in the lower half of the posterior mediastinum often runs ventral to or even to the left of the spine, the venous system is usually not symmetrical. The azygos veins have the following inflows:

- **Visceral inflows:** Vv. mediastinales: of the organs of the mediastinum (Vv. oesophageales, Vv. bronchiales, Vv. pericardiacae)
- **Parietal inflows:**
  - Vv. intercostales posteriores and V. subcostalis: from the posterior abdominal wall
  - Vv. phrenicae superiores: from the diaphragm

Below the diaphragm a V. lumbalis ascendens continues the course of the azygos veins left and right and connects into the V. cava inferior. The azygos system therefore forms part of the bypass circuit

that indirectly connects the upper and lower vena cava (**Cavocaval anastomoses**) and makes it possible to divert the blood if one or both of the vessels are occluded or compressed. The 4 most important **cavocaval anastomoses** are:

- **V. epigastrica superior** with **V. epigastrica inferior** (at the ventral wall posterior to the M. rectus abdominis)
- **V. epigastrica superficialis** with **V. thoracoepigastrica** (at the ventral trunk wall in the subcutaneous fat)
- **Vv. lumbales** with **V. azygos/hemiazygos** (on the inside of the posterior abdominal wall in the retroperitoneum and the rear mediastinum)
- **Plexus venosus vertebralis** with **azygos vein** and **V. iliaca interna** (outside of the vertebrae and in the vertebral canal with an expansion from the pelvis to the skull)

6.6.4 Lymph vessels of the thoracic cavity

The different groups of lymph nodes in the mediastinum are categorised into **parietal** lymph nodes (drainage of the thoracic walls) and **visceral** lymph nodes (drainage of the chest viscera) (➤ Fig. 6.58). From these lymph node groups the lymph flows into the major lymphatic trunks.

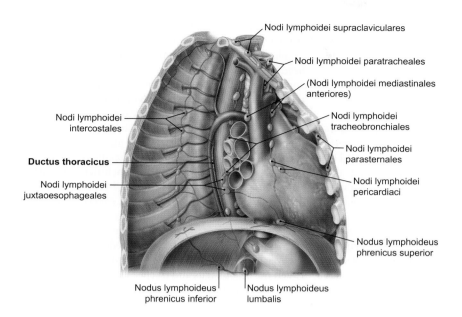

Nodi lymphoidei supraclaviculares

Nodi lymphoidei paratracheales

(Nodi lymphoidei mediastinales anteriores)

Nodi lymphoidei tracheobronchiales

Nodi lymphoidei parasternales

Nodi lymphoidei pericardiaci

Nodi lymphoidei intercostales

Ductus thoracicus

Nodi lymphoidei juxtaoesophageales

Nodus lymphoideus phrenicus superior

Nodus lymphoideus phrenicus inferior

Nodus lymphoideus lumbalis

Fig. 6.58 Lymph vessels and lymph nodes of the mediastinum. View from the right ventrolateral side after removal of the lateral chest wall. (according to [S010-2-16])

Parietal lymph nodes are:
- **Nodi lymphoidei parasternales:** They lie adjacent to the sternum on both sides and receive lymph from the anterior thoracic wall, the mammary glands, and the diaphragm. From them, the lymph passes into the Truncus subclavius.
- **Nodi lymphoidei intercostales:** They lie between the ribs and filter lymph from the posterior chest wall. The efferent lymph vessels drain directly into the Ductus thoracicus.

Visceral lymph nodes with connection to the Trunci bronchomediastinales are:
- **Nodi lymphoidei mediastinales anteriores:** They are located on both sides of the great vessels, receive inflows from lungs and pleura, diaphragm (Nodi lymphoidei phrenici superiores), the heart and the pericardium (Nodi lymphoidei pericardiaci) and thymus.
- **Nodi lymphoidei mediastinales posteriores:** They lie on the bronchi and trachea (Nodi lymphoidei tracheobronchiales and paratracheales) and oesophagus (Nodi lymphoidei juxta-oeso-phageales).

The Trunci bronchomediastinales also receive inflow from lymph vessels of the other half of the body. The lymph vessels of the individual organs and their regional lymph nodes are dealt with in the individual organs of the thoracic cavity.

The **Ductus thoracicus** (thoracic duct) is the **main lymphatic trunk** of the body. It has a total length of 38–45 cm and is 5 mm thick up to its usually enlarged outlet. It is formed underneath the diaphragm through the merging of the two lumbar trunks with the intestinal trunks and therefore carries the lymph of all of the lower body from there (➤ Chap. 8.8.4). At the level of the XIIth thoracic vertebra, the Ductus thoracicus protrudes **dorsal and to the right of the aorta** through the Hiatus aorticus of the diaphragm and ascends in the posterior mediastinum between aorta (left), V. azygos (right) and oesophagus (front) on the spine to the VIIth cervical vertebra. It crosses the pleural dome behind the left A. subclavia and issues dorsally into the **left venous angle** (between V. subclavia and V. jugularis interna). As it does so, it crosses over the first outflows of the V. subclavia, as well as the sympathetic trunk and the N. phrenicus, but remains dorsal to the N. vagus and V. jugularis interna. Shortly before draining, it receives the Truncus bronchomediastinalis sinister, which courses independently in the medias-

tinum, and also the Truncus subclavius sinister (from the arm) and the Truncus jugularis sinister (from the neck).

On the right side, a short (1 cm) **Ductus lymphaticus dexter** connects the respective lymphatic trunks and enters the **right venous angle.** The lymphatic trunks can also enter the venous angle separately on both sides. At the mouth of the lymphatic trunks are flaps that reduce reflux of blood; however, after death the blood that has been introduced may result in them being confused with veins.

Clinical remarks

Injuries of the Ductus thoracicus can be caused by malignant tumours in the mediastinum, such as malignant lymphomas (cancer of the lymph nodes) or during surgery of the oesophagus. This may result in an extension of the mediastinum or the formation of fatty pleural effusion **(chylothorax)** as well as a nutrient deficiency, because most lipids from food are transported via the lymph. Conservative therapy therefore aims to reduce the lymph flow through a low fat diet, and enable spontaneous closure. If this therapy is unsuccessful, the Ductus thoracicus can be disabled by surgery or, recently, embolysed by radiological intervention after puncture.

The systematics of the major lymphatic trunks also explain why malignant tumours of abdominal organs (e.g. gastric cancer) or pelvic viscera (e.g. ovarian cancer) can lead to lymph node metastasis in the area of the left venous angle. These lymph node swellings in the *left* supraclavicular fossa are named after their initial descriptors **VIRCHOW**'s **node** and means the doctor always has to check for tumours in the abdominal and pelvic cavities.

6.6.5 Nerves of the thoracic cavity

The thoracic cavity is innervated by parts of the somatic and autonomic nervous systems.

N. phrenicus

The N. phrenicus (C3–5) is a nerve of the Plexus cervicalis, which due to the developmental connection of the diaphragm in the cervical area was transferred with the diaphragm into the thoracic cavity. It innervates the **diaphragm** in terms of motor function and throughout its trajectory the **pericardium, Pleura** (costalis and diaphragmatica) in terms of sensitive function and with its terminal branches (Rr. phrenicoabdominales) the **peritoneum** on the underside of the diaphragm as well as on the liver and gallbladder. The N. phrenicus first descends on the neck on the M. scalenus anterior and then runs behind the venous angle over the pleural dome into the upper mediastinum. It extends right onto the V. brachiocephalica dextra and to the left over the aortic arch to the pericardium in the lower middle mediastinum, where, accompanied by the A./V. pericardiacophrenica, it extends to the diaphragm. Its terminal branches extend through the foramen V. cava on the right, and left on their own through an opening at the apex of the heart.

Autonomic nervous system

The autonomic nervous system of the thoracic cavity is formed from the **sympathetic trunk** (of the sympathetic nervous system [Truncus sympathicus]) and from the **N. vagus** (of the parasympathetic nervous system) (for the organisation of the autonomic nerve plexuses of the abdominal organs ➤ Chap. 7.8.5).

The **sympathetic trunk** in the posterior mediastinum is made up of **12 thoracic ganglia,** which are located in the respective ICS on both sides of the spinal cord (paravertebral) and are connected to each other by Rr. interganglionares (➤ Fig. 7.52). It continues on directly behind the pleural dome through the upper aperture of the thorax into the connective tissue area of the neck and through the diaphragm into the retroperitoneal space. The first ganglion is usually fused with the lower cervical ganglion forming the **Ganglion cervicothoracicum (stellatum),** through which the nerve fibres of the C8–T3 segments reach the head via the cervical sympathetic trunk and the arm via the Plexus brachialis. The preganglionic neurons of the sympathetic nervous system are located in the **lateral horns (C8 – L3)** of the spinal cord and exit the spinal canal with the spinal nerves and reach the **ganglia of the Truncus sympathicus** via their Rr. communicantes albi. This is the location of the perikarya of the postganglionic neurons, with which they are connected via synapses. Their axons return to the spinal nerves and their branches via the Rr. communicantes grisei and therefore reach the abdominal walls in the thoracic region or run from the 2nd-5th thoracic ganglion to the heart and lungs (Rr. cardiaci thoracici/Rr. pulmonales thoracici), to innervate them sympathetically. On the abdominal wall and arm (via the Ganglion stellatum) the sympathetic nervous system causes narrowing of the blood vessels (vasoconstriction/vasomotor), activates the sweat glands (sudomotor activation) and induces 'goose bumps' (pilomotor reflex) by making hair stand on end.

In the sympathetic trunk neurons can also rise or descend several segments. The nerve fibres of T2–7, for example rise to the stellate ganglion and extend sudomotor neurons to the sweat glands of the head, neck and arm.

Some preganglionic neurons are not switched in the sympathetic trunk, but instead run with the **Nn. splanchnici** through the diaphragm to the ganglia in the nerve plexuses on the Aorta abdominalis (prevertebral) where the switch happens. These neurons are used for the innervation of the abdominal organs. The **N. splanchnicus major** is formed from the preganglionic neurons of the spinal cord segments T5–9, the **N. splanchnicus minor** from T10–11. Sometimes a **N. splanchnicus imus** (T12) is present.

The **N. vagus** runs right across the A. subclavia and left between A. subclavia and the A. carotis communis behind the V. brachiocephalica in the upper mediastinum. On the left, it crosses the aortic arch. It issues an N. laryngeus recurrens, which winds right around the A. subclavia and left around the aortic arch and then rises between the oesophagus and trachea.

The preganglionic parasympathetic neurons approach the heart and lungs (Rr. cardiaci thoracici and Rr. bronchiales) as well as the oesophagus behind the root of the lungs via the **vagus nerves** and form the **Plexus oesophageus.** 2 trunks form from this **(Trunci vagales anterior and posterior),** which traverse the diaphragm with the oesophagus to the autonomic nerve plexuses of the abdominal aorta. Here, however, there is no interconnection, as the postganglionic neurons are usually found in the vicinity of the respective organs.

Clinical remarks

The trajectory of the sympathetic neurons can be clinically relevant:

- Sympathetic nerve fibres for the head run from the spinal cord segments C8–T3 via the stellate ganglion, which is located directly behind the pleural dome, to the neck. Lung cancer from the upper sections of the lungs (so-called PANCOAST tumours) can damage these nerve fibres and lead to **HORNER's syndrome,** which with symptoms of the eyes, such as pupil constriction (myosis), drooping eyelids (ptosis) and backward placement of the eyeball (enophthalmus), damage to the cervical sympathetic nervous system must always be considered.

- In the case of a tendency to increased **sweating** in the face and hands, there is the possibility of severing the sympathetic trunk below the 1st ICS **(endoscopic thoracic sympathectomy).**

7 Abdominal viscera

Jens Waschke

Acute appendicitis

Case study

A 24-year-old female student presents at the outpatient department of the surgical clinic. She reports that she has had severe stomach pain for 2 days, first of all spread through the upper abdomen and since yesterday stronger pain in the right lower abdomen. Since yesterday she has vomited twice due to nausea and was not able to leave her bed because of the abdominal pain; there have, however, been no instances of diarrhoea. It was noted that the pain subsided if the right leg was bent slightly when lying down. She measured her temperature as being 38°C.
Menstruation is regular and most recently ended 1 week ago. There is no history of pre-existing conditions and no previous surgery in the abdominal cavity has taken place.

Examination results

The patient has severe pain. Heart-rate (70/min), respiratory rate (20/min) and blood pressure (120/80 mmHg) are regular, rectal temperature 38°C, axillary temperature 37°C; weight approx. 56 kg and 165 cm in height; bowel sounds in all 4 quadrants sparse. The pain in the right lower abdomen is greatest when pressure is applied, but also occurs when the pressure is reduced again in the left lower abdomen (cross release pain). Raising the right leg against resistance also increases the pain. The rectal examination is normal.

Diagnosis

Except for leukocytosis (> 11,000 white blood cells/μl), all laboratory results are normal. A medical sonography of the abdomen is not clear due to excessive flatulence.
A pregnancy test is negative.

What is the preliminary diagnosis?

The clinical evidence most likely suggests an acute inflammation of the appendix (appendicitis). Typical for this, in addition to the spread of pain, is pain on application of pressure, especially above McBURNEY's point and a little less pain over LANZ's point as well as the crossed BLUMBERG's release sign. Pain dependent on the movement and position of the right leg indicates a positive psoas sign, by which irritation of the muscular fascia is painful when straining and tensioning the M. iliopsoas. Differential diagnoses include an acute gastrointestinal infection and for women, inflammation of the ovaries or pregnancy where there has been an incorrect implantation of the embryo (ectopic pregnancy). Also an inflammation of MECKEL's diverticulum and a kidney stone in the ureter might be possible.

Treatment

Removal of the appendix by means of a laparoscopy (laparoscopic appendectomy). Here, the appendix is very red and swollen in a retrocaecal position, which is sent to the pathology department to confirm the diagnosis.

Subsequent progression

The patient shows rapid improvement in the evening after the procedure and she is discharged the following day.

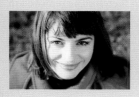

You're doing a rotational placement in the emergency admission. It is Friday afternoon and there is a lot going on. Your senior consultant sends you to the examination room because he himself has other patients he is looking at. You have already carried out a medical history and physical examination and consider what you should report to the senior consultant later.

The most stressful day in the outpatient clinic ever... ▽ Mc Burney, Lanz,
⫶ Blumberg

Hx.: *24-year-old patient, student, for 2 days*
severe abdominal pain, first diffuse, now right bowel,
also nausea and 2x vomiting, diarrhoea, Temp. 38 °C
less pain when lying down and with right leg bent
Menstr. regular, last 1 week ago, pre-existing conditions and procedures.
CE: *strong pressure pain in the right bowel, cross release-*
pain, pain when lifting the right leg against resistance.
Bowel sounds across all four quadrants sparse, rectal examination normal
Proc.: *blood taken, pregnancy test negative.*
  → abdominal scan
in particular acute appendicitis!!

7.1 Stomach

7.1.1 Overview

The stomach (Gaster) together with the intestines (often referred to as the gastrointestinal tract), the anterior sections of the oral cavity, pharynx, and oesophagus as well as the digestive glands (salivary glands, pancreas, liver and bile ducts) forms the digestive system (➤ Fig. 7.1, ➤ Table 7.1). In the digestive tract, a distinction is made between the head and torso bowels which differ in terms of histological wall construction.

As a hollow organ, the stomach serves to temporarily store food and to initiate digestion. It is located **intraperitoneally** in the left epigastrium between the left lobe of the liver and spleen and takes up differing amounts of space depending on the extent to which it is filled ('between liver and spleen there should still be room for a

Table 7.1 Structure of the digestive system.

Section	Components
Digestive tract	
Head bowel	• Oral cavity (Cavitas oris) (➤ Chap. 9.7.1) • Throat (Pharynx) (➤ Chap. 10.7)
Torso bowel	• Gullet (Oesophagus) (➤ Chap. 6.3) • Stomach (Gaster) • Small intestine (Intestinum tenue) (➤ Chap. 7.2) • Large intestine (Intestinum crassum) (➤ Chap. 7.2)
Digestive glands	
Salivary glands	• Oral salivary glands (Glandulae salivariae majores) (➤ Chap. 9.7.9) • Pancreas (➤ Chap. 7.5)
Liver (Hepar)	• ➤ Chap. 7.3
Bile ducts	• Gall bladder (Vesica biliaris) (➤ Chap. 7.4) • Bile ducts (Ductus hepaticus communis, Ductus cysticus, Ductus choledochus) (➤ Chap. 7.4)

beer'). Like the rest of the digestive system, the stomach is of great importance for various medical fields, such as gastroenterologists and visceral surgeons, as well as general medical practitioners and family physicians. While the construction and location are important for radiologists and internists, particularly for the diagnosis of various diseases, a visceral surgeon needs additional detailed knowledge about the vessels and nerves and precise topographical conditions.

7.1.2 Functions of the stomach

The stomach has various functions that are largely fulfilled by the cells of the gastric glands. Like most hollow organs, the stomach is not, however, absolutely essential and can therefore be removed in whole or in part.

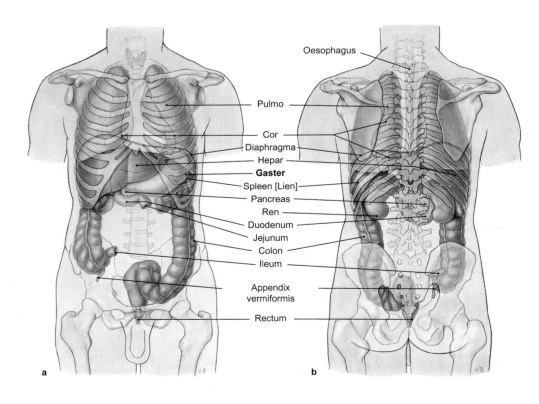

Fig. 7.1 Projection of the stomach and the rest of the internal organs onto the body surface.
a Ventral view. **b** Dorsal view.

Oesophagus
Pulmo
Cor
Diaphragma
Hepar
Gaster
Spleen [Lien]
Pancreas
Ren
Duodenum
Jejunum
Colon
Ileum
Appendix vermiformis
Rectum

a

b

The functions of the stomach include:

- Intermediate storage and breaking down of food
- Denaturation and digestion of proteins
- Killing of micro-organisms
- Formation of the 'intrinsic factor' for the absorption of vitamin B_{12}
- Secretion of messenger substances (e. g. histamine) and hormones (e. g. gastrin) to regulate the formation of gastric acid.

Once the food has passed through the oesophagus, it is stored in the stomach and broken down through its peristaltic movements. Through the **hydrochloric acid** formed in the glands in the stomach body, proteins are also denatured and the chyme is acidified so that the enzyme precursors produced by the glands are activated to form pepsin. Pepsin initiates the digestion of protein by splitting the proteins. Gastric acid also serves to kill most of the micro-organisms ingested with the food. The glands of the stomach body therefore also form the **'intrinsic factor'**, a protein that binds in the stomach with vitamin B_{12} and which is necessary for its reabsorption at a later stage in the small intestine (terminal Ileum).

7.1.3 Development of stomach, Bursa omentalis, Omentum minus and Omentum majus

The stomach develops from the lower section of the **foregut**. At the time at which embryonic cleavage takes place in the *4th week*, a part of the yolk sac is included in the body and, together with the endoderm, forms the intestinal system. The link to the yolk sac around the navel is thus narrowed to form the vitelline duct (Ductus omphaloentericus /Ductus vitellinus). As a result, the intestinal system is divided into 3 sections (foregut, midgut and hindgut), each served by their own unpaired artery, departing from the abdominal section of the aorta.

Since the stomach emerges from the foregut, it is supplied with blood from the branches of the Truncus coeliacus (> Fig. 7.2). During development only the epithelium of the stomach is derived from the **entoterm** of the foregut, while connective tissue and smooth muscles are formed from the surrounding **mesoderm**. In contrast to the lower sections of the intestine, the stomach and duodenum, as derivatives of the foregut, are not only connected over a wide surface with the posterior wall of the peritoneal cavity through the **dorsal mesentery (Mesogastrium dorsale)**, but also through the **ventral mesentery (Mesogastrium ventrale)** with the anterior abdominal wall. The ventral connection is as a result of the Septum transversum being sited here as an appendage to the diaphragm, in which the liver and gall bladder systems are embedded (> Fig. 7.3a). Through the liver, the Mesogastrium ventrale is divided into the Mesohepaticum ventrale (between the ventral wall and liver) and the Mesohepaticum dorsale (between the liver and stomach). Through this suspension via mesenteries on the front and back of the peritoneal cavity, the stomach is completely intraperitoneal and is covered on all sides with Peritoneum viscerale.

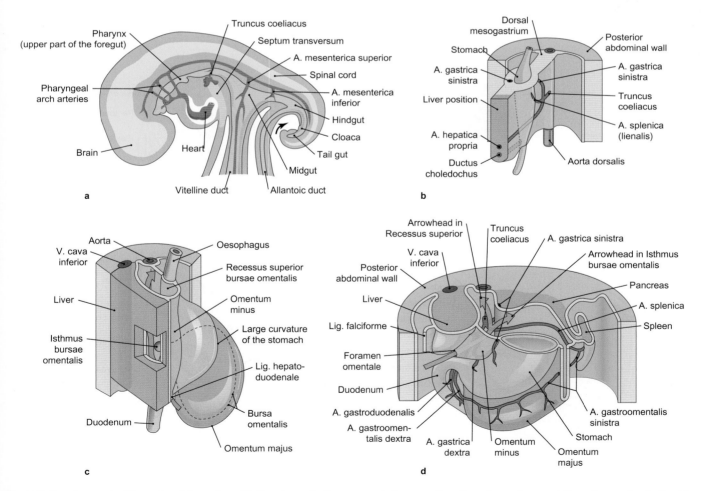

Fig. 7.2 Development of the epigastric region with the stomach, Bursa omentalis, as well as Omentum minus and Omentum majus in the 4th and 5th weeks of development. **a** Sagittal section through an embryo at the end of the 4th week (28th day). **b–d** Representation of rotation of the stomach on the 26th day (**b**), 32nd day (**c**) and 52nd day (**d**). [E347-09]

The further development of the stomach and the entire upper abdominal region in the 5th week is determined by **stomach rotation**. First of all, the rear of the stomach system grows faster than the front and appears increasingly more saggy. This creates the large and the small stomach curvatures. Then the stomach revolves **clockwise** around a longitudinal axis at **90°** (view from cranial); since the left stomach wall grows faster than the right, the large stomach curvature is now directed to the left and the small curvature to the right (➤ Fig. 7.3). This also twists the Trunci vagales, which accompany the oesophagus through the diaphragm as terminal branches of the N. vagus. Therefore the right N. vagus predominantly innervates the back surface of the stomach via the Truncus vagalis posterior, and the left N. vagus innervates the front surface of the stomach as the Truncus vagalis anterior. In addition, the stomach rotates around the sagittal axis, so that the stomach entrance (Cardia) is shifted to the left and the stomach exit (Pylorus) is shifted to the right. Parallel to the stomach rotation the **Bursa omentalis** also develops in the *4th and 5th week* in the dorsal mesogastrium as a recess (Recessus) of the peritoneal cavity (➤ Chap. 7.7.3). First, an invagination of the right surface anatomy of the Mesogastrium dorsale forms and extends cranially as a narrow tube into the site of the lungs. Therefore, this enlargement is initially called the pneumatoenteric recess. During the stomach rotation, the gap spreads along the posterior side of the stomach and thus forms the Bursa omentalis as a serosa-lined adjoining space of the peritoneal cavity between the stomach and the developing pancreas (➤ Fig. 7.3c, d). Through the stomach rotation and the formation of the Bursa omentalis, the Mesogastrium ventrale and the Mesogastrium dorsale are extruded as thin layers and thus form the Omentum majus and minus.

From the Mesogastrium ventrale dorsal to the liver (Mesohepaticum dorsale), the **lesser omentum (Omentum minus)** develops with its two parts:
- Lig. hepatogastricum (between the liver and stomach)
- Lig. hepatoduodenale (between the liver and duodenum)

As a result of the stomach rotation, the lesser omentum extends as a frontal peritoneal duplicature. The Lig. hepatoduodenale is the free lower edge of the former ventral mesentery, which was only formed in the area of the foregut. Under this ligament the **Foramen omentale** remains the only access to the Bursa omentalis. Through the Bursa omentalis, the dorsal mesogastrium sags and forms the **greater omentum (Omentum majus)** (➤ Fig. 7.3d) with its large apron-shaped section. Since the spleen is also formed in the dorsal mesogastrium, this part of the Omentum majus is also described as the **Lig. gastrosplenicum** (➤ Fig. 7.3c), while the parts running further to the dorsal torso wall are the **Lig. gastrophrenicum**. Because the greater omentum thus originates from the stomach curvature, it is also supplied by the vessels and nerves of the greater curvature of the stomach (➤ Chap. 7.7.2).

N O T E

The development of the stomach with stomach rotation is decisive for the entire formation of the epigastric region:
- The Omentum minus develops from the Mesogastrium ventrale.
- The Omentum major arises from the Mesogastrium dorsale.
- The liver and gall bladder systems are found in the Mesogastrium ventrale.
- The Bursa omentalis, pancreas and spleen arise in the Mesogastrium dorsale.

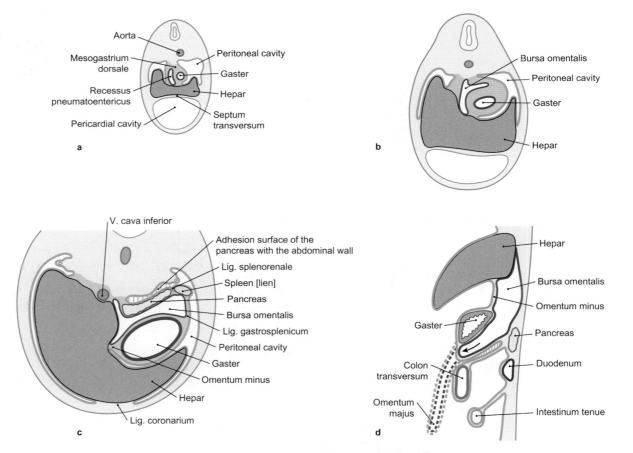

Fig. 7.3 Development of the epigastric region; Peritoneum (green); peritoneum of the pneumatoenteric recess and the Bursa omentalis (dark red) (according to [S010-1-16]). **a** End of the 4th week, transverse section. **b** Beginning of the 5th week, transverse section. **c** Beginning of the 7th week, transverse section. **d** Paramedian section.

7.1.4 Projection of the stomach

The projection of the stomach is relevant in the event of clinical examinations undertaken to assign discomfort or examination findings to the stomach. While the **body** of the stomach (Corpus) is highly variable depending on the size and the extent to which it is filled and extends caudally to the level of the II–III. lumbar vertebrae, the stomach entrance (Cardia) and stomach exit (Pylorus) are relatively constant as a result of the fixing of the oesophagus and duodenum. The **stomach entrance** (Cardia) is projected caudally in the lower constriction of the oesophagus during its passage through the diaphragm at approximately the height of the XI. thoracic vertebra and therefore lies directly below the Proc. xiphoideus of the breastbone. The easiest way is to understand the position of the pylorus in the patient. The **pylorus** is relatively constant 1–2 cm to the right of the midpoint of a line between the pubic symphysis (Symphysis pubica) and the jugular fossa (Fossa jugularis) and thus projects approximately over the I. lumbar vertebra.

N O T E

Projection of the sections of the stomach on the skeleton and the anterior abdominal wall:
- Cardia: XI. thoracic vertebra, below the Proc. xiphoideus
- Body of the stomach: II.–III. lumbar vertebrae
- Pylorus: I. lumbar vertebra, to the right of the midpoint of the line between the pubic symphysis and the jugular fossa

7.1.5 Structure and sections of the stomach

The stomach has a volume capacity of 1,000–1,500 ml (one to one-and-a-half Bavarian glasses of beer!) and is divided into **3 sections** (➤ Fig. 7.4):
- Stomach entrance: Pars cardiaca (Cardia)
- Main part: Corpus gastricum with Fundus gastricus
- Stomach exit: Pars pylorica

The stomach is almost positioned head-on due to the stomach rotation that takes place during development. Therefore, its large areas form a **front (Paries anterior)** and a **rear wall (Paries posterior)**. The two edges between these areas are curved and are called **curvatures**. The lesser curvature (Curvatura minor) is to the right, the greater curvature (Curvatura major) is to the left.

The **Cardia** starts at the lower end of the oesophagus. The limit can be seen on the greater curvature as a notch (Incisura cardialis). This creates an angle between the stomach and oesophagus (HIS angle), which is normally less than 80°. Through this angle, a fold of mucous skin is formed inside that prevents the reflux of stomach acid into the oesophagus and thus functionally contributes to the closure mechanisms of the oesophagus (➤ Chap. 6.3.5). On the inside, the mucosal transition is located between the oesophagus and stomach in an area 0.75 cm proximal and 1.5 cm distal of the borders defined by the Incisura cardialis and forms a jagged line (**Z-line**). Thereby the mucosal transition is predominantly (approx. 70%) exclusively in the Pars abdominalis of the oesophagus, whereas it is rare (10%) to be completely below the HIS angle. The Cardia itself forms a thin mucous membrane strip that is only 1–3 cm wide and can only be separated histologically from the main part of the stomach.

Clinical remarks

If the HIS angle is lost, e.g. as a result of erroneous fixing in the diaphragm (axial hiatal hernia), it can result in reflux of gastric juice with inflammation of the oesophagus **(gastro-esophageal reflux disease)**. If drug therapy for reducing acid production with proton pump blockers fails, an operation leads to improved closure whereby the fundus of the stomach is looped around the oesophagus (NISSEN fundoplication). A **tumour in the transition from the oesophagus to the stomach** must be categorised either as oesophageal or gastric cancer and then either the oesophagus or the stomach is removed. Therefore, various classifications have been developed for tumours in this transition area, whereby currently the first gastric mucosal fold is considered to be the border. This subdivision is necessary because stomach acid reflux may lead to an expansion of gastric mucosa in the oesophagus, in which adenocarcinoma frequently form that are treated clinically as oesophageal cancer. In this case, the visible mucosal limit (Z-line) is shifted in an oral direction.

The **main part** of the stomach contains the typical gastric glands that are, e.g. responsible for the formation of gastric acid. It begins with a Fundus gastricus, the upper pole of which is known as the Fornix gastricus.

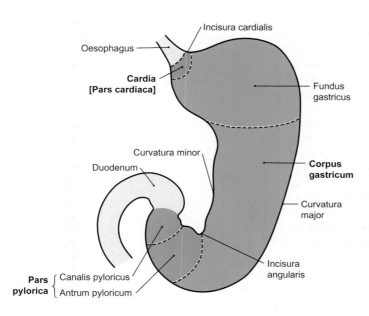

Fig. 7.4 Structure of the stomach. Schematic drawing. (according to [S010-1-16])

The transition to the **Pars pylorica** is visible at the lesser curvature as an angular notch (Incisura angularis) and, in turn, differs histologically from the main part. The following section is known as the Antrum pyloricum and continues into the Canalis pyloricus, which is surrounded by the sphincter of the stomach (M. sphincter pyloricus).

7.1.6 Surface enlargement of the stomach lining

The gastric mucosa has a characteristic relief that serves to enlarge the surface anatomy; however, macroscopically, only the gastric folds (Plicae gastricae) are seen, which are longitudinally oriented (gastric folds) (➤ Fig. 7.5). With a magnifying glass, plot-like fields (Areae gastricae) are visible on these folds. Depressions emanate from the surface anatomy, at the bottom of which the gastric glands open.

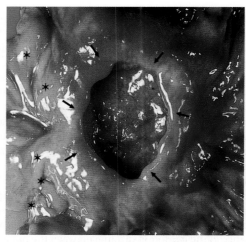

Fig. 7.6 Stomach ulcer (Ulcus ventriculi); Asterisks mark the pyloric ring, arrows mark the borders of the ulcer. [R236]

┌─ Clinical remarks ──────────────────────────────

Gastric ulcers are substance defects that affect the entire stomach lining (➤ Fig. 7.6). Therefore, it is understandable why this can lead to perforations into the abdominal cavity. More than 80% of all **gastric and duodenal ulcers** are caused by the bacterium *Helicobacter pylori*. In addition, there can be increased gastric acid production or reduced formation of surface mucus, e.g. after taking pain medication containing the active substance acetylsalicylic acid, which promotes the formation of gastric ulcers. Accordingly, treatment involves removing bacteria with antibiotics, together with inhibiting the secretion of gastric acid. In addition to a perforation in adjacent organs or the abdominal cavity with the risk of life-threatening peritonitis, erosion of a gastric artery is also possible, which can lead to heavy bleeding. In the case of these complications, surgical treatment is indicated.

therefore mostly covered by the left costal arch but a small area is directly adjacent to the ventral **abdominal wall**.

Contact surfaces of the stomach with adjacent organs are:
- ventral: liver, diaphragm, abdominal wall
- dorsal: spleen, kidneys, adrenal glands, pancreas, Mesocolon transversum

The contact surfaces are highly variable, because the stomach is well supported in comparison to adjacent organs. Even an altered stomach filling can change the contact surfaces.

┌─ Clinical remarks ──────────────────────────────

The stomach field is clinically used in terms of nutrition to insert a **PEG tube** (percutaneous endoscopic gastrostomy). In the case of a gastroscopy, the light passing through the abdominal wall is used for orientation on the body surface in order to introduce the probe through the skin.

The gastric contact surfaces are of clinical relevance, as stomach ulcers or gastric tumours may lead to a **perforation into adjacent organs**, which can lead to organ damage and associated symptoms or can complicate the removal of tumours.

7.1.7 Topography

The stomach is positioned **intraperitoneally** in the left epigastrium between the left lobe of the liver and the spleen. The stomach is

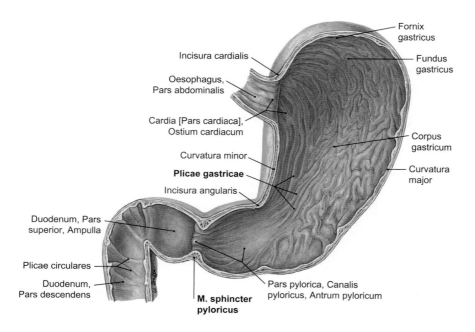

Fornix gastricus
Incisura cardialis
Fundus gastricus
Oesophagus, Pars abdominalis
Cardia [Pars cardiaca], Ostium cardiacum
Corpus gastricum
Curvatura minor
Curvatura major
Plicae gastricae
Incisura angularis
Duodenum, Pars superior, Ampulla
Plicae circulares
Duodenum, Pars descendens
M. sphincter pyloricus
Pars pylorica, Canalis pyloricus, Antrum pyloricum

Fig. 7.5 Stomach and duodenum. Ventral view.

The stomach is connected by various peritoneal duplicatures with the adjacent organs, which are referred to as ligaments (Ligamenta) and which partially surround the various vessels and nerves of the stomach. The course of these ligaments can be understood from looking at the development (➤ Chap. 7.1.3):
- **Lesser curvature** (part of the Omentum minus):
  - Lig. hepatogastricum
- **Greater curvature** (part of the Omentum majus):
  - Lig. gastrocolicum
  - Lig. gastrosplenicum
  - Lig. gastrophrenicum

At the lesser curvature, the **Lig. hepatogastricum** links the stomach with the Facies visceralis of the liver. The ligament extends caudally into the **Lig. hepatoduodenale**, with which it forms the **lesser omentum (Omentum minus)**. Under the Lig. hepatoduodenale is the entrance to the **Bursa omentalis** (Foramen omentale), a peritoneum-lined recess of the abdominal cavity (➤ Chap. 7.7.3). The largest part of the Bursa omentalis is located dorsal to the Omentum minus and extends behind the stomach.

The ligaments on the greater curvature form the **Omentum majus** with a free, apron-shaped section (➤ Chap. 7.7.2). The **Lig. gastrocolicum** is thereby only a narrow bridge to the Colon transversum and continues left into the **Lig. gastrosplenicum**, which is positioned on the spleen. The cranial continuation of the Omentum majus into the diaphragm is known as the **Lig. gastrophrenicum**. In anatomical terminology, many other peritoneal duplicatures are named and assigned to the two omenta. Since this is not useful in a medical sense, we will forgo it here.

7.1.8 Arteries of the stomach

All three main branches of the Truncus coeliacus (A. gastrica sinistra, A. hepatica communis, A. splenica) collectively give rise to **six gastric arteries** (➤ Table 7.2, ➤ Fig. 7.7).

The gastric arteries form **vascular arcades** at both curvatures in the Omentum majus and Omentum minus, in which the arteries of both sides are joined by anastomoses. The branches to the anterior and posterior of the stomach (Rr. gastrici) emerge from the arcades. At the lesser curvature, the **A. gastrica sinistra** is significantly stronger in structure than the **A. gastrica dextra** and usually forms an anterior and posterior main stem. Conversely, it is positioned in the greater curvature where the **A. gastroomentalis dextra** is the dominant vessel and therefore on its course in the Lig. gastrocolicum also supplies the largest part of the Omentum majus (Rr. omentales),

Table 7.2 Arteries of the stomach.

Anatomical structure	Arterial blood supply
Lesser curvature	• A. gastrica sinistra (directly from the Truncus coeliacus) • A. gastrica dextra (from the A. hepatica propria)
Greater curvature	• A. gastroomentalis sinistra (from the A. splenica) • A. gastroomentalis dextra (from the A. gastroduodenalis of the A. hepatica communis) These vessels also supply the Omentum majus!
Fundus	Aa. gastricae breves (in the area of the hilum of the spleen from the A. splenica)
Posterior side	A. gastrica posterior (present in 30–60% of cases, originates behind the stomach from the A. splenica)

while the **A. gastroomentalis sinistra** is somewhat thinner. The A. gastrica sinistra, after its origin from the Truncus coeliacus, first produces the Plica gastropancreatica that delimits the atrium from the main space of the Bursa omentalis. After the distribution of branches for the Pars abdominalis of the oesophagus (Rr. oesophageales) and occasionally (20%) for the left hepatic lobe, it then reaches the stomach in the Lig. hepatogastricum. The fundus receives 5–7 of its own **Aa. gastricae breves**, which, in addition to the **A. gastrica posterior**, exit into an inconstant vessel in the middle of the posterior wall from the A. splenica. The A. gastroomentalis sinistra and the Aa. gastricae breves run in the Lig. gastrosplenicum.

Clinical remarks

Since the gastric arteries run directly to and, in some cases, also in the stomach wall, **gastric ulcers** (Ulcera ventriculi) can sometimes cause fatal **gastric haemorrhages**.

In the case of a surgical removal of the oesophagus due to oesophageal cancer, the stomach is most often selected as a replacement **(gastric pull-up)**. In this case a stomach tube is formed for which the A. gastroomentalis dextra alone is sufficient for supply.

7.1.9 Veins of the stomach

The veins correspond to the arteries and support them along the curvature of the stomach; however, they differ in their connection to the portal vein: only the Vv. gastricae dextra and sinistra drain di-

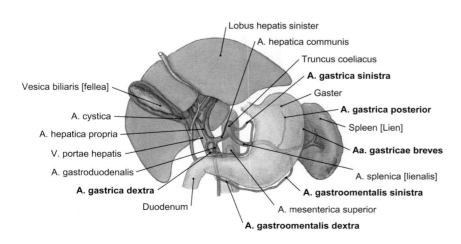

Fig. 7.7 Arteries of the stomach. Ventral view.

Table 7.3 Veins of the stomach.

Receiving vessel	Inflows
Confluence directly into the portal vein	• V. gastrica sinistra • V. gastrica dextra and over this V. prepylorica (inconstant), which cross the pylorus ventrally
Confluence into V. splenica	• V. gastroomentalis sinistra (from the V. splenica) • Vv. gastricae breves • V. gastrica posterior (inconstant, usually present if artery is formed)
Confluence into V. mesenterica superior	• V. gastroomentalis dextra

rectly into the portal vein, while all other veins lead the blood into the main stems of the portal vein (➤ Table 7.3).

— Clinical remarks —

In the case of high-pressure in the portal vein (portal hypertension), e.g. in the case of cirrhosis of the liver, **portocaval anastomoses** can form from the connections of the V. gastrica sinistra to the oesophageal veins, which in turn are connected via the Azygos vein to the superior vena cava. These connections are highly dangerous because the widened oesophageal veins (oesophageal varices) burst and can lead to life-threatening bleeding.

7.1.10 Lymph vessels of the stomach

The stomach has 3 lymphatic drainage areas and 3 lymphatic drainage stations arranged in series (➤ Fig. 7.8):
Lymphatic drainage areas are:
• Cardia area and lesser curvature: **Nodi lymphoidei gastrici** directly to the lesser curvature
• Upper left quadrant: **Nodi lymphoidei splenici** at the hilum of the spleen
• Bottom two thirds of the greater curvature and pylorus: **Nodi lymphoidei gastroomentales** and **Nodi lymphoidei pylorici**

The lymph flows from these regional lymph nodes along the curvature through 2 more stations, before they are guided through the Trunci intestinales to the Ductus thoracicus.
Thus, in the 3 major lymphatic areas are 3 **lymphatic drainage stations** in series:
• First station (➤ Fig. 7.8, green): regional lymph nodes of the 3 drainage areas
• Second station (➤ Fig. 7.8, yellow): lymph nodes along the branches of the Truncus coeliacus
• Third station (➤ Fig. 7.8, blue): lymph nodes at the exit of the Truncus coeliacus (Nodi lymphoidei coeliaci]; from there, the lymph flows via the Truncus intestinalis into the Ductus thoracicus

— Clinical remarks —

The lymphatic drainage stations (➤ Fig. 7.8) of the stomach are of clinical relevance in the **surgical treatment of gastric cancer** (D-level of surgeons). The lymph nodes of the first and second stations are usually removed together with the stomach, which is known as a D2 gastrectomy. If, however, during surgery it is detected that the lymph nodes of the third station with the surrounding retroperitoneal lymph nodes along the Aorta and the V. cava inferior (D3 level) are affected, no cure is possible. Hence in this case, the patient should be spared the removal of the stomach. The decision on which the patient's life depends must be made by the surgeon at the operating table. This example very clearly illustrates how important knowledge of the lymphatic drainage pathways is in some organs.

N O T E
The stomach has 6 arteries of its own and 3 lymphatic drainage areas with 3 lymphatic drainage stations.
In accordance with its development from the Mesogastrium dorsale the Omentum majus is supplied by the vessels and nerves on the greater curvature of the stomach and therefore belongs to the stomach, not the colon.

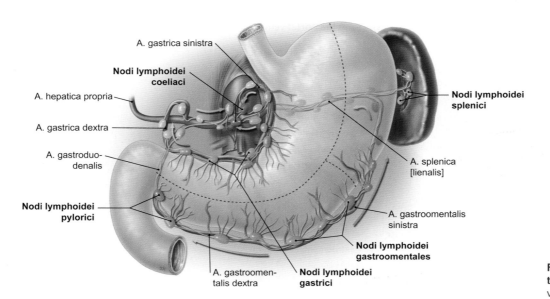

A. gastrica sinistra
Nodi lymphoidei coeliaci
A. hepatica propria
A. gastrica dextra
A. gastroduodenalis
Nodi lymphoidei pylorici
A. gastroomentalis dextra
Nodi lymphoidei gastrici
Nodi lymphoidei splenici
A. splenica [lienalis]
A. gastroomentalis sinistra
Nodi lymphoidei gastroomentales

Fig. 7.8 Lymph drainage stations of the stomach. Ventral view. (according to [S010-1-16])

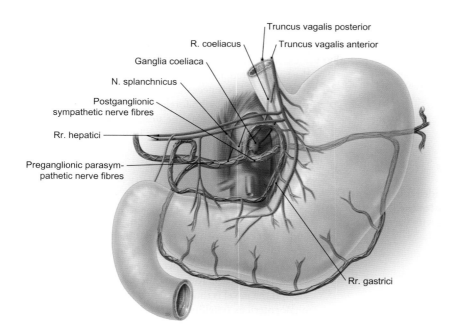

Truncus vagalis posterior

Truncus vagalis anterior

R. coeliacus

Ganglia coeliaca

N. splanchnicus

Postganglionic
sympathetic nerve fibres

Rr. hepatici

Preganglionic parasym-
pathetic nerve fibres

Rr. gastrici

Fig. 7.9 Autonomic innervation of the stomach (Gaster); sympathetic innervation (green), parasympathetic innervation (purple) (according to [S010-1-16]).

7.1.11 Innervation of the stomach

The stomach is innervated both sympathetically and parasympathetically (➤ Fig. 7.9):

- The **parasympathetic nervous system** promotes gastric acid production as well as peristalsis and gastric emptying.
- The **sympathetic nervous system** acts antagonistically to the parasympathetic nervous system by reducing gastric acid secretion, peristalsis and blood circulation and preventing gastric emptying by activating the M. sphincter pyloricus.

The autonomic nerve fibres form nerve plexuses (Plexus gastrici) on the anterior and posterior of the stomach.

Sympathetic nerve fibres from the Nn. splanchnici to the Ganglia coeliaca run along the arteries after switching over. Preganglionic sympathetic fibres act as Nn. splanchnici major and minor on both sides through the lumbar branches of the diaphragm and reach the Ganglia coeliaca at the exit of the Truncus coeliacus, where they are switched to postganglionic neurons. They reach the various sections of the stomach along with the preganglionic parasympathetic nerve fibres as periarterial plexus along the gastric arteries. The sympathetic nervous system also has afferent pain fibres. The zone of the transmitted pain in the abdominal wall (HEAD zone) corresponds with the dermatomes T5–8 in the left epigastric region, in which the stomach lies in the stomach field of the ventral wall.

Parasympathetic fibres reach the small curvature, as well as the posterior and anterior of the stomach as the Trunci vagales but reach the greater curvature indirectly through the Plexus coeliacus as periarterial plexus. Preganglionic parasympathetic fibres reach the stomach as Trunci vagales descending anterior and posterior along the oesophagus and run along the lesser curvature. From there, the Rr. gastrici radiate over the posterior and anterior wall of the stomach and supply the majority of the corpus and fundus. Due to the stomach rotation at the time of development, the Truncus vagalis anterior is predominantly derived from the left **N. vagus [X]** and the Truncus vagalis posterior from the right. The Pars pylorica is innervated by its own branches (Rr. pylorici), that initially proceed with the Rr. hepatici from the Truncus vagalis anterior to the liver and then move into the pyloric region in the Omentum minus. Individual nerve fibres go to the greater stomach curvature from the Truncus vagalis posterior and take a detour via the Plexus coeliacus, where they are not switched but join the gastric arteries from the Truncus coeliacus.

The postganglionic parasymphatic neurons are located mostly in the stomach wall and are not therefore depicted in the dissection. For general organisation of the autonomic nervous system in the abdomen see ➤ Chap. 7.8.5.

Clinical remarks

Previously, severance of the N. vagus **(vagotomy)** was the only effective way to reduce acid secretion in the event of stomach ulcers. A former therapy in patients with peptic ulcers was to sever the entire N. vagus [X] inferior to the diaphragm **(total vagotomy)** or its branches to the stomach **(selective vagotomy)** to reduce the production of gastric acid. The course of the nerve fibres explains why this often leads to disruption of gastric emptying (Rr. pylorici) and the formation of gallstones (Rr. hepatici); however, since the option of blocking acid with medication and the removal of the triggering *Helicobacter pylori* bacteria with antibiotics, this procedure has become significantly less important.

7.2 Intestines

Skills

After working through this chapter you should be able:
- to show the sections of the small and large intestines on the dissection and explain their structural features
- to explain the origin of the individual intestinal segments, including the boundaries of their innervation and vascular supply and the positional changes they undergo during development
- to understand the positional relationships of the individual sections of the intestines with respect to the other abdominal organs in a dissected specimen and in the case of the appendix in particular, the projection on the surface of the body in terms of clinical importance

- to illustrate the blood supply to the individual intestinal sections in detail on the dissection specimen and recognise clinically important anastomoses of arteries
- to explain the venous and lymph node drainage areas, as well as the innervation areas of individual sections of the intestine on the dissection specimen.

7.2.1 Overview

The intestines join to the stomach and are divided into **the small intestine (Intestinum tenue)** and **the large intestine (Intestinum crassum)**, which each show different sections with varying positional relationships (➤ Fig. 7.10).

7.2.2 Functions of the intestine

While the small intestine in essence serves the digestion and absorption of nutrients, particularly in the large intestine a thickening of the food bolus and controlled excretion through faecal matter takes place. Therefore, it is understandable why at least a part of the small intestine (approx. 1 m) is essential for life, while the large intestine is not essential. In clinical terms, the English names are used for the two parts of the intestine, while the Latin terms are predominantly used for the individual sections.
Functions of the intestine are:
- Transport and breaking down of food
- Digestion of food and absorption of nutrients
- Immune defence
- Distribution of messenger substances and hormones for regulation of digestion
- Thickening of the food bolus
- Intermediate storage and controlled excretion of faecal matter
After gastric emptying, the chyme is further transported through the **peristaltic movement** of the intestine and broken down. In the first section of the small intestine, the **enzymes** of the pancreas and the bile acids from the gall bladder are added to the duodenum and cause the digestion of nutrients that are then absorbed by the cells of the mucosa. After this **resorption**, the nutrients travel in the blood and reach the portal vein and lymph vessels of the liver, the central metabolic organ of the body. In the large intestine **fluid is extracted** from the chyme and is used to thicken the faecal matter. In the last sections of the large intestine (rectum and anal canal), the faecal matter is then stored and released in a controlled manner.

In addition to the resorption, the cells of the intestinal mucosa have additional functions. Especially in the small intestine many **messenger substances** and **hormones** are formed, which enable the coordinated interaction of the stomach, liver, gall bladder and pancreas, which is necessary for digestion. Through food, the body is constantly faced with foreign substances and pathogens, which are rendered harmless in the stomach, but still require that the cells of the immune system mount an **immune defence** in the intestinal mucosa if necessary.

7.2.3 Development

The intestinal system develops in the *4th week* from the **entoderm** and a part of the **yolk sac**, which is included in the body at the time of embryonic cleavage. Thereby the entoderm forms the epithelium of the intestine, while connective tissue and smooth muscles are formed from the surrounding **mesoderm**. The link to the yolk sac around the navel is thus restricted to the vitelline duct (Ductus omphaloentericus /vitelline duct) (➤ Chap. 6.5.5). As a result, the intestinal system is divided into three sections, each of which are supplied by their own artery and later form different sections of the small and large intestines:
- **Foregut** (cranial to the vitelline duct, supplied by the **Truncus coeliacus**): forms the proximal half of the duodenum
- **Midgut** (at the level of the vitelline duct, supplied by the **A. mesenterica superior**): forms the remaining sections of the small intestine, as well as the proximal large intestine including the Colon transversum
- **Hindgut** (caudal to the vitelline duct, supplied by the **A. mesenterica inferior**): forms the large intestine from the Colon descendens to the proximal half of the anal canal. The distal half of the anal canal is everted from the ectoderm of the anal depression (Proctodeum).

The result of this is that the 3 parts and thus also the innervation and supply areas of the 3 arteries and other vascular, lymphatic and nervous systems do not correspond to the final intestinal sections. There are therefore 3 clinically important areas in terms of the small and large intestines, which the innervation and supply areas of the vessels and nerves switch:
- Transition between **proximal and distal duodenum** (border between the foregut and midgut, not visible in the intestine): **BÜHLER**'s **anastomosis** connects the innervation and supply areas of the Truncus coeliacus and A. mesenterica superior

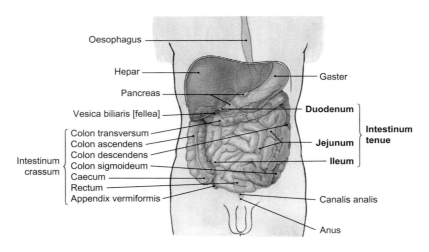

Fig. 7.10 Projection of the intestinal sections onto the body surface. Ventral view.

- **Left colic flexure** (border between midgut and hindgut): **RIOLAN**'s **anastomosis** connects the innervation areas of the Aa. mesentericae superior and inferior
- **Linea pectinata** (clinically: Linea dentata) at the transition between proximal and distal anal canal (border between behind hindgut and anal depression). Here, the A. mesenterica inferior communicates with the flow area of the A. iliaca interna from the pelvis.

The proximal duodenum arises from the last section of the **foregut** and therefore has a ventral mesentery in addition to a dorsal mesentery, which later develops to the **Lig. hepatoduodenale** as part of the Omentum minus. The distal intestinal sections are only anchored to the dorsal wall of the peritoneal cavity by a dorsal mesentery. All intestinal sections are therefore initially intraperitoneal and are, apart from the attachment of the Mesenterium, covered by a serous membrane (Tunica serosa), on the surface of which the **Peritoneum viscerale** forms. The Mesenterium is a peritoneal duplicature, from which the serosa of the intestinal surface passes through to the **Peritoneum parietale** of the abdominal cavity wall. During the switching processes of intestinal sections, individual sections later become closely adjacent to the dorsal torso wall and

receive a secondary retroperitoneal location. With the duodenum, this already happens in the 5th week in the context of the stomach rotation. A special feature here is that in the *5th and 6th week* the lumen of the duodenum is closed by excess epithelial proliferation and is only re-channelled at the end of the embryonic period.

The development of the **midgut** is determined by the intestinal rotation (➤ Fig. 7.11). First, the midgut undergoes rapid growth and in the *5th week* forms a ventrally oriented umbilical loop, the sagittal axis of which forms the A. mesenterica superior and from its peak the Ductus omphaloentericus branches off (➤ Fig. 7.11a). The midgut rotates around this axis by a total of 270° counterclockwise. In the late foetal period the caecum, which was formed in the *6th week* as the caecum bud at the distal leg of the umbilical loop, descends and extends to the right lower abdomen. Due to the lack of space in the 6th week the umbilical loop is relocated in the body stalk (development-related umbilical hernia) by the navel and only returns in the *10th week* into the abdominal cavity (reposition; ➤ Fig. 7.12). Since the Mesenterium is reformed at an early stage in the area of the later Colon ascendens and Colon descendens, these sections achieve a secondary retroperitoneal position.

The **hindgut** forms the left-sided colon and ends in the cloaca, in which the genitourinary canal flows. The cloaca reaches the cloacal depression (Proctodeum), which represents an invagination of the ectoderm and which is initially closed by the cloacal membrane. In the *7th week* the cloaca and the cloacal membrane are divided by a

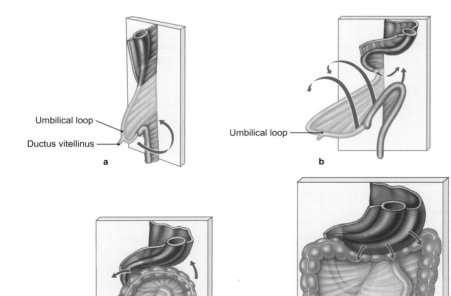

Umbilical loop

Ductus vitellinus

a

Umbilical loop

b

c

d

Fig. 7.11 Intestinal rotation. Schematic representation, View from the left side. Intestinal segments and their mesenteries are highlighted in different colours: stomach and mesogastrium (purple), duodenum and mesoduodenum (blue), jejunum and ileum with associated mesenteries (orange), colon and mesocolon (ochre) (according to [S010-1-16]). Rotation and displacement of the midgut between the 6th (**a**) and 11th (**c**) developmental weeks, as well as in the late foetal period (**d**).

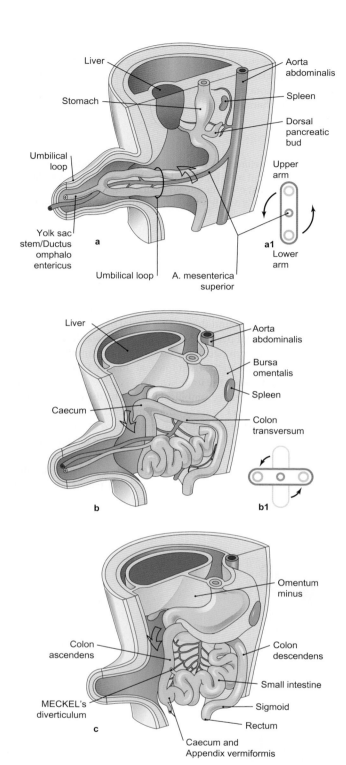

Fig. 7.12 Rotation of the midgut; View from the left side. **a** Sagittal section (start of the 6th week): the umbilical loop has not yet rotated and has already entered the body stalk. **a1** Schematic cross-section through the umbilical loop before intestinal rotation takes place. **b** 11th week: intestinal rotation has been completed and the intestine has already shifted back into the body. **b1** Schematic cross-section through the umbilical loop upon completion of the intestinal rotation. **c** Late foetal period: the caecum is relegated to its final position [E347-09].

Septum urorectale into the ventral Sinus urogenitalis (precursor of urinary bladder and urethra) and the dorsally located rectum and upper anal canal. The rear part of the cloacal membrane becomes the anal membrane which ruptures in the *8th week*, so that now the

cloacal depression communicates with the hindgut and forms the distal anal canal.

Clinical remarks

In the event of disturbances of the intestinal rotation, a **malrotation** can occur (hyporotation and hyperrotation). This can cause an intestinal obstruction (ileus), but also leads to an abnormal positioning of the various intestinal segments, which can, e.g. complicate the diagnosis of appendicitis. In the event of **Situs inversus** all of the organs are reversed (mirror image). If the repositioning of the intestine is incomplete, newborns can be born with an **umbilical hernia (omphalocele)**. In addition to the intestinal sections, the hernial sac can also contain other abdominal organs, such as the liver and spleen, which have been secondarily displaced. The hernial sac is not covered by skin, but only by the amniotic membrane of the umbilical cord. In contrast, a **navel hernia** occurs in the first month after birth if the navel does not close completely. It contains the Omentum majus and intestinal sections that are covered by skin on the outside. Navel hernias usually resolve spontaneously.

Remnants of the Ductus omphaloentericus can remain as a MECKEL's diverticulum. This is a common occurrence (3% of the population) and is usually located in the part of the small intestine that is located approximately 100 cm cranial of the ileocecal valve. Because they often contain dispersed gastric mucosal or pancreatic tissue, the inflammation and bleeding often presents an incorrect clinical picture of appendicitis.

If the Septum urorectale deviates dorsally, an **anal stenosis** can occur. An **imperforate anus** is when the anal membrane does not break down.

7.2.4 Structure and projection of the small intestine

The small intestine is usually 4–6 m long and is divided into **3 sections** (➤ Fig. 7.10):
- Duodenum (25–30 cm) with Pars superior (5 cm), descendens (10 cm), horizontalis (10 cm), ascendens (2.5 cm)
- Jejunum (approx. 2 m)
- Ileum (approx. 3 m)

The sections of the small intestine have different topographical relationships in the abdominal cavity and are therefore covered to various degrees with peritoneum (➤ Chap. 7.7.1).

Intraperitoneal (i.e. in the peritoneal cavity of the abdominal cavity) are found the Pars superior of the duodenum, jejunum and ileum. **Secondarily retroperitoneal** (in the dorsal wall of the peritoneal cavity, the retroperitoneum) are the Pars descendens, Pars horizontalis and the Pars ascendens of the duodenum.

The **duodenum** is the shortest section at 25–30 cm (➤ Fig. 7.13). It is relatively fixed in its position because only the first part (Pars superior) is located intraperitoneally and is connected here by a peritoneum duplicature (Lig. hepatoduodenale) with the liver, while the following parts (Partes descendens, horizontalis and ascendens) are in a secondary retroperitoneal position and therefore surrounded by connective tissue. The duodenum therefore creates a C-shaped loop that encompasses the head of the pancreas. The **Pars superior** is often extended (ampulla or bulbus) and is therefore projected like the pylorus of the stomach onto the I. lumbar vertebra. It passes into the Flexura duodeni superior in the **Pars descendens**. Connected to the Flexura duodeni inferior runs the **Pars horizontalis** at the level of the III. lumbar vertebra, before the **Pars ascendens** runs up to the II. lumbar vertebra again. Here, together with the Flexura duodenojejunalis is the transition into the following small intestine bundle of the jejunum (approximately two fifths of the total length and the ileum (approximately three fifths of the total length). These two sections are located intraperitoneally and have no sharp boundary in relation to each other. The ileum ends at the ileocecal valve 'Valva ileocaecalis' (BAUHIN's valve) at which it joins the caecum as the first section of the large intestine.

The most important section is the Pars descendens. Here, the **bile duct (Ductus choledochus)** opens out together with the excretory duct of the pancreas, **Ductus pancreaticus** (Ductus WIRSUNGIANUS), to a mucosal elevation (Papilla duodeni major, Papilla VATERI), which is located 8–10 cm from the pylorus. Shortly before the papilla, the mucous membrane often runs into a longitudinal mucosal fold (Plica longitudinalis duodeni). In most cases, 2 cm proximal of the Papilla VATERI is a smaller **Papilla duodeni minor**, on which the **Ductus pancreaticus accessorius** (Ductus SANTORINI) emits secretions.

Clinical remarks

An obstruction of the bile ducts may occur as a result of a **gallstone**, which is stuck to the Papilla VATERI, or **jaundice (icterus)** that can occur as a result of **tumours** of the pancreas and bile ducts in which the bile fluid can flow back into the liver and the bile pigment (bilirubin) enters the blood vessel system. For diagnostic evaluation and removal of gallstones, endoscopic retrograde cholangiopancreatography (ERCP) is carried out, as part of which the papilla is examined and the excretory ducts are represented using x-ray contrast agent. Here, the Plica longitudinalis duodeni can be used as a landmark for the identification of the papilla.

The adjacent intraperitoneal parts of the small intestine bundle of the **Jejunum** and **Ileum** are fixed over a peritoneal duplication, the **mesentery**), in the form of 14–16 intestinal loops at the dorsal abdominal wall. Within the mesentery can be found the vessels and nerves. Due to the length of the small intestine, the origin of the mesentery, the mesenteric root (**Radix mesenterii**), is much shorter than the attachment to the intestines. The latter is not sharply defined and an approx. 30 cm long section of the small intestine is known as the terminal Ileum (Pars terminalis). This is where sections of the intestine's immune system frequently occur (PEYER's plaques) and only specific absorption functions are found here, such as the uptake of vitamin B_{12} and bile acids.

Clinical remarks

The terminal ileum is often affected by **CROHN**'s **disease**, a chronic inflammatory disease of the intestine with autoimmune components, which may cause anaemia due to a vitamin B_{12} deficiency.

7.2.5 Structure and projection of the large intestine

The large intestine is about 1.5 m long and is divided into **4 sections** (➤ Fig. 7.14):
- Caecum (appendix) 7 cm with Appendix vermiformis, 8–9 cm
- Colon with Colon ascendens (15 cm), Colon transversum (50 cm), Colon descendens (15 cm) and Colon sigmoideum (35–45 cm)
- Rectum, 12 cm
- Canalis analis (anal canal), 3–4 cm

The sections of the large intestine alternate strictly in relation to their position in the abdominal cavity.
- **Intraperitoneal** (in the peritoneal cavity of the abdominal cavity) are:
  – Caecum with appendix (mostly)
  – Colon transversum
  – Colon sigmoideum
- **Secondary retroperitoneal** (in the dorsal wall of the peritoneal cavity, the retroperitoneum) are:
  – Colon ascendens
  – Colon descendens
  – Rectum (proximal)
- **Subperitoneal** (in the connective tissue below the peritoneal cavity) are:
  – Rectum (distal)
  – Anal canal

The **appendix (Caecum)** is usually approximately 7 cm long and is joined at the **ileocecal valve** 'Valva ileocaecalis' (BAUHIN's valve) to the ileum (➤ Fig. 7.15, ➤ Fig. 7.16): the opening (Ostium ileale) is limited by 2 lips, which after coming together, continue as

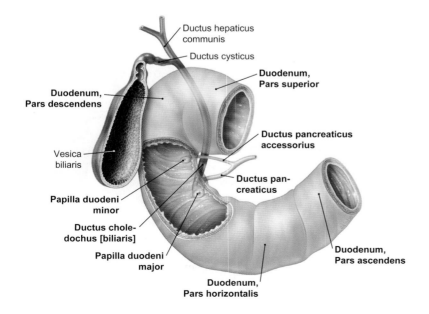

Ductus hepaticus communis

Ductus cysticus

Duodedum, Pars superior

Duodenum, Pars descendens

Ductus pancreaticus accessorius

Vesica biliaris

Ductus pancreaticus

Papilla duodeni minor

Ductus choledochus [biliaris]

Papilla duodeni major

Duodenum, Pars ascendens

Duodenum, Pars horizontalis

Fig. 7.13 Sections of the duodenum; extrahepatic bile ducts and excretory ducts of the pancreas. Ventral view.

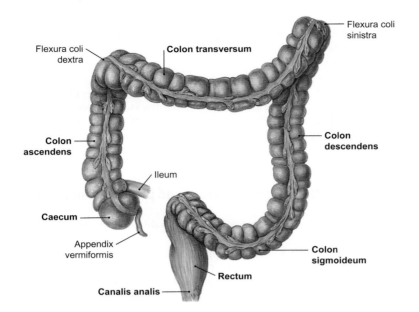

Fig. 7.14 Structure of the large intestine (Intestinum crassum). Ventral view.

the Frenulum ostii ilealis. The valve has a sympathetically activated circular musculature and can prevent the reflux of chyme to a certain degree; a real sphincter is not yet formed. The caecum projects onto the lumbar vein or the Os sacrum.

At the blind end of the caecum (hence the German name *Blinddarm),* approximately 2–3 cm below the junction with the Ileum, hangs the mostly 8–9 cm long **vermiform appendix (Appendix vermiformis)**, which is frequently erroneously called the 'Blinddarm' (even by doctors). Since the 3 taenia of the Caecum come together at the exit of the appendix, it is usually easy to locate during an operation. The appendix (in an intraperitoneal position of the caecum) usually has its own mesentery (Mesoappendix) in which the vessels and nerves run.

Clinical remarks

Appendicitis is a common disease in the 2nd and 3rd decades of life. It is an endogenous infection, mostly caused by the covering of the lumen by faeces or (rarely) other foreign bodies or the passage through the wall by bacteria from the intestinal flora. A perforation with life-threatening peritonitis can be a consequence.

Of particular importance, therefore, are the **location and projection of the appendix** (➤ Fig. 7.16):

- The appendix is mostly (65%) tilted backwards to the caecum (retrocaecal).
- With the second most frequent variant (30%) the appendix stretches down and reaches the small pelvis and therefore in women, lies in the immediate vicinity of the ovarian and fallopian tube (pendulous).

These positional variants have an impact on the projection of the appendix onto the abdominal wall. The base of the Appendix vermiformis projects onto McBURNEY's point (located in the right third of a line connecting the Spina iliaca anterior superior and the navel). The tip of the hanging Appendix vermiformis projects onto LANZ's point (located in the right third of a line connecting both sides of the Spinae iliacae anteriores superiores).

Clinical remarks

Diagnosis of appendicitis (in German often referred to incorrectly as 'inflammation of the *Blinddarm')* is a clinical diagnosis that the surgeon must make mainly dependent on the findings because other signs, such as an increased number of white blood cells or ultrasound findings, are often unclear. The diagnosis is often difficult as pain in the right lower abdomen can be a result of enteritis, or in women can be caused by inflammation of the ovaries and fallopian tubes. On the other hand, a correct diagnosis is important because in a case of missed appendicitis, perforation with potentially fatal peritonitis may occur but it is also best to avoid unnecessary surgery with possible complications or subsequent adhesions. Therefore, **pressure pain** at McBURNEY's point or LANZ's point is a very important clue in diagnosis.

NOTE

McBURNEY's point and LANZ's point are important projection points of the appendix on the abdominal wall. Your examination is important for the diagnosis of appendicitis and should be part of every complete physical examination of the abdominal region.

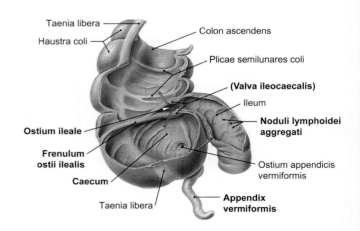

Fig. 7.15 Caecum with vermiform appendix (Appendix vermiformis) and terminal Ileum. Ventral view after removal of the anterior parts of the wall.

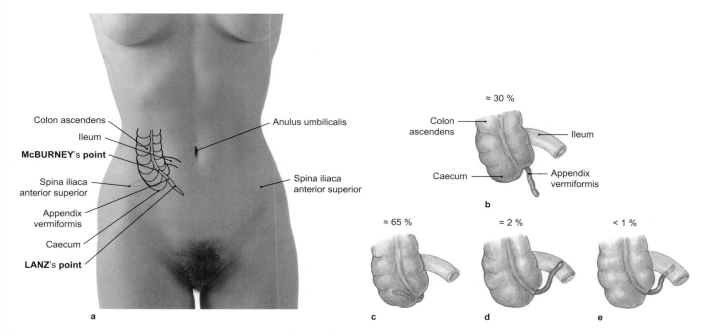

Fig. 7.16 Projection of the appendix (caecum) and Appendix vermiformis onto the ventral torso wall. Positional variants of the Appendix veri-formis. Ventral view. **a** and **b** Appendix descending into the small pelvis (pendulous). **c** Retroceceal appendix (most frequent case). **d** Pre-ileal appendix. **e** Retro-ileal appendix.

The caecum continues without borders into the **Colon ascendens**, which rises in a secondary retroperitoneal position and passes be-low the liver in the right colic flexure (Flexura coli dextra) and merges into the **Colon transversum** that runs intraperitoneally. It is anchored by its transverse mesocolon and then after connect-ing to the left colic flexure (Flexura coli sinistra) descends as the **Colon descendens** which again is in a secondarily retroperitoneal position. The right colic flexure is usually projected over the I–II. lumbar vertebrae but the left colic flexure is higher (XI.–XII). thoracic vertebrae).

The border to the **Colon sigmoideum** is, however, easy to discern because this section resembles an S-shaped course (hence the name) and has its own Mesocolon sigmoideum. The transition to the rectum at the level of the II–III. sacral vertebrae can be rec-ognised since it varies at various points from the construction fea-tures of the colon (see below).

The various sections of the large intestine surround the small intes-tine like a picture frame surrounds a picture; however, the length of the sections and the position of the colon flexure, and thus also the shape of the large intestine, are very variable. The left flexure usual-ly extends further cranially and, due to the change in the course of direction of the intestine by almost 180°, can be difficult to over-come when performing enteroscopy. In addition, the Colon ascen-dens and Colon descendens can also lie intraperitoneally and then have their own Mesocolon ascendens and Mesocolon descendens. **The Rectum and anal canal** lie in the pelvis and due to various pe-culiarities in topography, their structure and vessels and nerves will be covered along with the pelvic organs in (➤ Chap. 8.4).

7.2.6 Structural features of the small and large intestines

The intestinal mucosa has an inner relief that differs depending on the individual sections. The inner relief of the **small intestine** has circular folds (Plicae circulares, KERCKRING's folds; ➤ Fig. 7.17);

however, the folds of the large intestine do not include the entire lumen of the intestine, but are more crescent-shaped (Plicae semi-lunares).

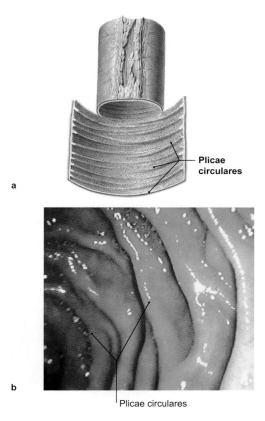

Fig. 7.17 Small intestine mucosa. a Section from the jejunum. **b** Plicae circulares in an endoscopic image of the small intestine.

The majority of the **large intestine** (caecum and colon) can therefore be clearly distinguished from the small intestine by 4 structural features (➤ Fig. 7.18):

- **Larger diameter** (it is 'large' whereas the small intestine is 'small')
- **Taenia:** the longitudinal muscle layer is reduced to three bands. Of these the Taenia libera is visible, while the Mesocolon transversum is attached to the Taenia mesocolica and the Omentum majus is attached to the Taenia omentalis.
- **Sacculations of the colon and Plicae semilunares:** the sacculations (Haustra coli) are protrusions that are caused by contractions of the Plicae semilunares.
- **Appendices epiploicae:** adhesions from the adipose tissue contained in the Tela subserosa

The vermiform appendix, rectum and anal canal differ from the other sections of the large intestine:

- No taenia, but rather a closed longitudinal muscular layer
- No Haustra coli
- Folds: not present in the appendix but in the rectum as 3 irregular horizontal folds (Plicae transversae recti), in the anal canal as longitudinal folds (Columnae anales)
- No Appendices epiploicae

7.2.7 Topography of small and large intestines

Topography of the small intestine

The **Pars superior** of the of the duodenum is located behind the neck of the gall bladder and is in direct contact with the Facies visceralis of the liver, with which it is also connected via the **Lig. hepatoduodenale**. The Lig. hepatoduodenale contains the vessels and nerves of the liver as well as the extrahepatic bile ducts and borders the entrance to the Bursa omentalis (Foramen omentale/epiploicum). The Ductus choledochus runs dorsal to the Pars superior duodeni.

Behind the **Pars descendens** of the duodenum, albeit separated by their different fascial systems, are the right kidney and adrenal gland. The pancreatic head adjoins its medial surface, which is oriented to the left. The Colon ascendens ascends lateral to the Pars descendens.

The **Pars horizontalis** of the duodenum crosses the spine below the pancreatic head, the aorta and the V. cava inferior with the right Vasa testicularia/ovarica and the right ureter. The Pars horizontalis is thereby covered ventrally by the jejunum and ileum, the Colon transversum and the mesenteric root (with A. and V. mesenterica superior).

The **Pars ascendens** rises to the Flexura duodenojejunalis and is fixed via a peritoneal duplicature (Lig. suspensorium duodeni,

TREITZ ligament) at the exit of the A. mesenterica superior. The TREITZ ligament can also contain striated and smooth muscles (M. suspensorius duodeni, TREITZ muscle). Bulges of the peritoneal cavity often occur here (Recessus duodenales superior and inferior). Behind the Pars ascendens are the left kidney with its ureter, as well as the left Vasa testicularia/ovarica.

The **jejunum** and the **ileum** have a positional relationship to both kidneys and different sections of the large intestine and lie on the pelvis of the urinary bladder and in women, the intraperitoneal sections of the internal genitalia (womb, ovaries and fallopian tube). The **Radix mesenterii** is approx. 12–16 cm long and extends from the Flexura duodenojejunalis up to the iliac fossa (Fossa iliaca). It crosses over the duodenum and the right ureter.

Topography of the large intestine

The **caecum** is in the right Fossa iliaca (➤ Fig. 7.19a). In the transition area between the caecum and the terminal ileum, there are often bulges in the peritoneal cavity (Recessus ileocaecales superior and inferior). The **Appendix vermiformis** usually lies in the Recessus retrocaecalis. The caecum and appendix lie on the right M. iliopsoas and thus have a positional relationship to various nerves of the Plexus lumbalis (N. cutaneus femoris lateralis, N. femoralis and N. genitofemoralis) as well as the A. testicularis/ovarica. In this area, the pendulous type of Appendix vermiformis may come in close proximity to the ovaries and fallopian tubes.

The **Colon ascendens** then rises, covered by the small intestine convolute and in front of the Nn. cutanei femoris lateralis, iliohypogastricus and ilioinguinalis up to the lower surface of the right lobe of the liver, thereby also touching the fundus of the gall blad-

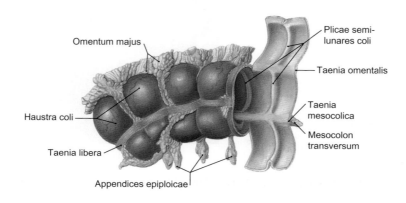

Omentum majus

Plicae semi-lunares coli

Taenia omentalis

Taenia mesocolica

Mesocolon transversum

Haustra coli

Taenia libera

Appendices epiploicae

Fig. 7.18 Structural features of the large intestine (Intestinum crassum) exemplified by the transverse colon. Ventral caudal view.

der at the right colic flexure (also called the hepatic flexure). Behind the right colic flexure (Flexura colica dextra) is the right kidney and medial thereof the Pars descendens of the duodenum (➤ Fig. 7.19a).

The **Colon transversum** is connected via the Mesocolon transversum with the posterior abdominal wall and via the Lig. gastrocolicum with the stomach. The Mesocolon transversum lies on the posterior wall of the stomach and thereby limits the main space of the Bursa omentalis both to the rear and below (➤ Fig. 7.3d). From

the Taenia omentalis of the Colon transversum hangs the apron-shaped section of the Omentum majus and covers the small and large intestines. Behind the Colon transversum to the right lies the Pars descendens of the duodenum and the pancreatic head, in the middle the small intestine convolute from the jejunum and ileum, and the Flexura duodenojejunalis to the right.

The **left colic flexure** (Flexura colica sinistra; ➤ Fig. 7.19b) is usually further cranial and dorsal than the right colic flexure and is generally at more of an acute angle. It is connected via the Lig. phren-

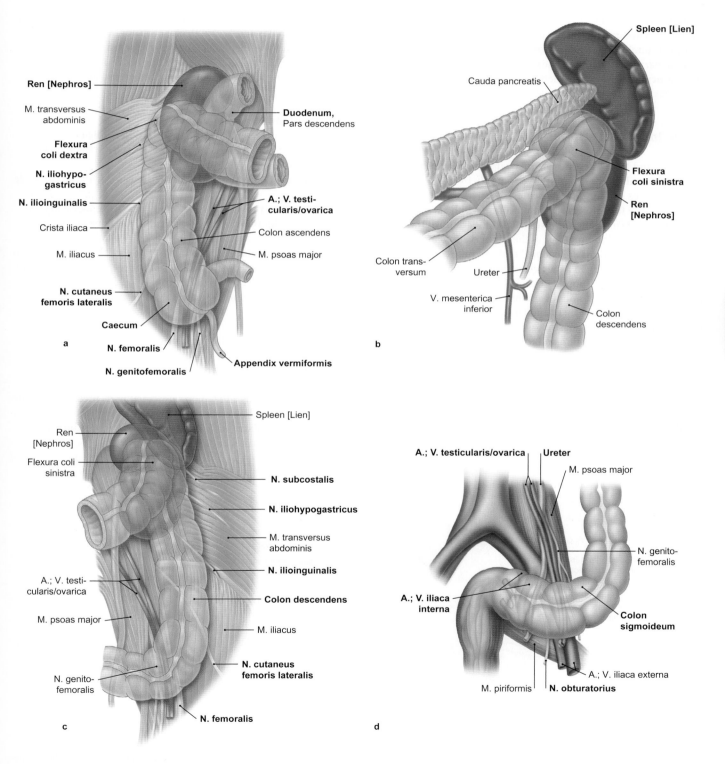

Fig. 7.19 Positions of the various sections of the colon. a Caecum, Colon ascendens and right colic flexure **b** Colon transversum and left colic flexure **c** Colon descendens **d** Colon sigmoideum [G210].

icocolicum with the abdominal wall and in the thus formed splenic niche, is in direct contact with the Facies visceralis of the spleen (in English therefore 'splenic flexure'). Behind the left colic flexure are the pancreatic tail and, separated by their sheaths, the left kidney. The **Colon descendens** then rises ventral to the kidney into the left Fossa iliaca and thereby crosses the nerves of the Plexus lumbalis (➤ Fig. 7.19c).

In the left lower abdomen the **Colon sigmoideum** bulges outwards with its Mesocolon sigmoideum variably deep into the peritoneal cavity of the pelvis and makes contact with the small intestine and urinary bladder (➤ Fig. 7.19a); in women, contact is also made with the intraperitoneal internal genital organs (uterus, ovarian and fallopian tube). In doing so, it forms a Recessus intersigmoideus that can vary greatly in size. The Colon sigmoideum crosses the left Vasa testicularia/ovarica, the left N. obturatorius, the ureter, as well as the Vasa iliaca externa and interna.

7.2.8 Intestinal arteries

The small and large intestines are made up of the **3 major unpaired visceral arteries** that emerge ventrally from the abdominal aorta (Truncus coeliacus, A. mesenterica superior, A. mesenterica inferior). Since the arteries can communicate with each other through well-formed anastomoses (BÜHLER's and RIOLAN's anastomoses) at the boundaries of their innervation and supply areas, **bypass circulations** are enabled that can fully compensate for the closure of an artery in a particular instance. The innervation and supply areas correspond to the evolutionary divisions of the intestine in the foregut, midgut and hindgut and not the macroscopic divisions into the small and large intestines. It is therefore easy to understand why anastomoses are found between the vessels in the area of the duodenum and the left colic flexure.

Arteries of the duodenum

The blood supply of the duodenum takes a **double vascular arch**, ventrally and dorsally that is fed cranially and caudally, respectively (BÜHLER's anastomosis; ➤ Fig. 7.20):

- **Aa. pancreaticoduodenales superiores anterior and posterior**, which represent the terminal branches of the A. gastroduodena-

lis from the catchment area of the Truncus coeliacus from cranial. The A. gastroduodenalis runs directly behind the Pars superior duodeni (various small branches of the A. gastroduodenalis above and below the Pars superior duodeni are known as A. supraduodenalis and Aa. retroduodenales).
- **A. pancreaticoduodenalis inferior** (with R. anterior and R. posterior) from the A. mesenterica superior from caudal.

Arteries of the jejunum and ileum

The small intestine convolute of jejunum and ileum is supplied by the **A. mesenterica superior** which runs with its branches (usually 4–5 **Aa. jejunales** and 12 **Aa. ileales**) within the mesentery of the small intestine (➤ Fig. 7.21). The vessels form a series of 3 (jejunum) to 5 arcades (ileum) in descending order of size along the intestine, from which the vascular branches extend up to the intestine wall.

Arteries of the large intestine

- Caecum and Appendix vermiformis: **A. ileocolica** as the end section of the A. mesenterica superior results in the following branches:
  - **R. ilealis** to the terminal ileum (connected with the last A. ilealis)
  - **R. colicus** (proximally connected with the A. colica dextra)
  - **A. caecalis anterior** and **A. caecalis posterior** ventral and dorsal to the caecum
  - **A. appendicularis**, which almost always (99%) runs dorsal to the ileum before it enters the mesoappendix, via which it supplies the Appendix vermiformis
- Colon ascendens and Colon transversum:
  - **A. colica dextra** with an ascending and descending branch (for Colon ascendens)
  - **A. colica media** with a right and left branch (for Colon transversum)

Both arteries originate (often with a common stem) from the A. mesenterica superior and anastomose with each other
- Colon descendens and Colon sigmoideum: **A. mesenterica inferior** with the following branches:
  - **A. colica sinistra** with an ascending and descending branch for the Colon descendens

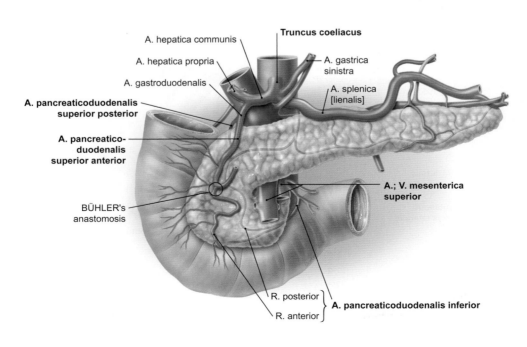

Fig. 7.20 Arteries of the duodenum. Ventral view. (according to [S010-1-16])

A. hepatica communis
A. hepatica propria
A. gastroduodenalis
A. pancreaticoduodenalis superior posterior
A. pancreaticoduodenalis superior anterior
BÜHLER's anastomosis
R. posterior
R. anterior
A. pancreaticoduodenalis inferior
Truncus coeliacus
A. gastrica sinistra
A. splenica [lienalis]
A.; V. mesenterica superior

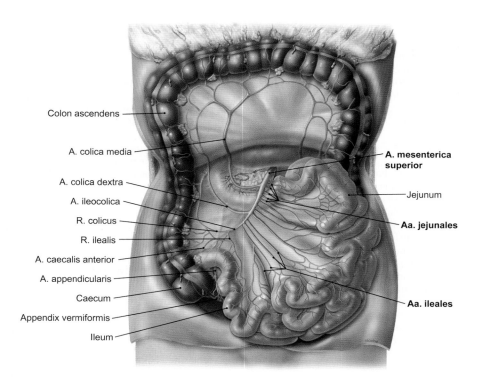

Fig. 7.21 Arteries of the jejunum and ileum. Ventral view. Colon transversum folded upwards. (according to [S010-1-16])

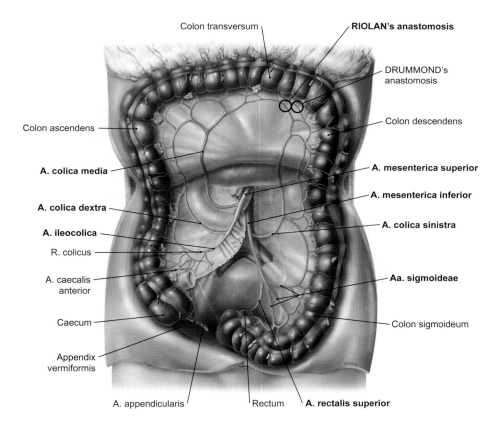

Fig. 7.22 Arteries of the large intestine. Ventral view. Colon transversum folded upwards. (according to [S010-1-16])

– **Aa. sigmoideae** (2–5) for the Colon sigmoideum
– **A. rectalis superior**, supplies the rectum and the upper anal canal

Between the left third of the Colon transversum and the left colic flexure the innervation and supply areas of the Aa. mesentericae superior and inferior do not end abruptly, but the A. colica media almost always has a connection to the A. colica sinistra (**RIOLAN's anastomosis;** ➤ Fig. 7.22). Occasionally, the mostly available

(93%) connection in one of the arcades close to the intestines is referred to as DRUMMOND's anastomosis. This designation is, however, seldom used in clinical practice in English and the term 'DRUMMOND's artery' is not specifically used for vascular connections on the left colic flexure, but refers to the vessels as the marginal artery (A. marginalis coli) which directly flows from the different sections of the large intestine (therefore also, e.g. the Colon ascendens).

Clinical remarks

The **short circuit connections** between the A. colica media and A. colica sinistra, which in clinical terms are usually collectively known as RIOLAN's anastomosis, take on a role in the event of circulatory disorders, e.g. with arteriosclerosis or displaced blood clots (emboli). Similar connections exist in the area of the duodenum and the rectum. Even complete occlusion of one of the 3 unpaired abdominal arteries (Truncus coeliacus, A. mesenterica superior, and A. mesenterica inferior) can largely be compensated for without intestinal infarction occurring. Circulatory disorders of the intestine are usually characterised by abdominal pain which occurs after eating (postprandial pain). The collateral circulations through the rectum not only serve to supply the large intestine but at the closure of the distal aorta or the A. iliaca communis can also maintain a certain amount of blood supply to the legs via the A. mesenterica inferior (and its A. rectalis media) and via the A. iliaca interna.

In the case of **colon cancer** a **hemicolectomy** is usually carried out. In the case of a tumour in the Colon descendens, within the context of a left-sided hemicolectomy, the Colon descendens, together with the entire A. mesenterica inferior is removed. In contrast, in a right-sided hemicolectomy for treatment of a tumour in the Colon ascendens, the intestine with the entire A. mesenterica superior will not be removed, since these also supply the largest part of the small intestine. Accordingly, in addition to the Colon ascendens, only the A. colica dextra, and in the event of an extended right-sided hemicolectomy, the Colon transversum with the A. colica media will also be resected.

7.2.9 Veins of the intestine

The veins correspond to the arteries and drain into the main tributaries of the portal vein (V. portae hepatis) (➤ Fig. 7.31). The **V. mesenterica superior** joins behind the pancreatic neck with the V. splenica to the V. portae hepatis. It has the following branches:
- V. gastroomentalis dextra
- Vv. pancreaticoduodenales (the V. pancreaticoduodenalis superior posterior drains directly into the portal vein)
- Vv. pancreaticae
- Vv. jejunales and ileales
- V. ileocolica
- V. colica dextra
- V. colica media

The **V. mesenterica inferior** mostly drains (70% of cases) into the V. splenica, in some cases (30%) into the V. mesenterica superior or the origin of the portal vein. Branches of the V. mesenterica inferior are:
- V. colica sinistra
- Vv. sigmoideae
- V. rectalis superior: drains the majority of the blood from the rectum and the upper anal canal – the vein is connected to the V. rectalis media and to the V. rectalis inferior, which lead blood into the V. cava inferior

Clinical remarks

In the case of high pressure in the portal vein (portal hypertension), e.g. in cirrhosis of the liver, connections to the drainage area of the V. cava superior and V. cava inferior (**portocaval anastomosis**) can open up or be formed (➤ Fig. 7.32). This also includes connections of the V. rectalis superior to the V. rectalis media and V. rectalis inferior, which take blood to the V. cava inferior. These do not lead, as was previously assumed, to the formation of haemorrhoids; however, when using suppositories, it must be borne in mind that active ingredients can be administered via the inferior veins of the rectum and into the systemic circulation in order to avoid the portal vein and thus the liver, which partially breaks down and eliminates the active substances.

7.2.10 Lymph vessels of the intestine

The intestine has **2 large drainage areas,** in which 100–200 lymph nodes in multiple lymphatic drainage stations are connected in series (➤ Table 7.4, ➤ Fig. 7.23).

The lymph from the entire intraperitoneal small intestine convolute, as well as from the 'right-sided colon' (Caecum, Colon ascendens and transversum) ultimately lead to the **Nodi lymphoidei mesenterici superiores** along the A. mesenterica superior, before they are carried via the Trunci intestinales to the Ductus thoracicus.

In contrast, the 'left-sided colon' (Colon descendens and Colon sigmoideum, proximal rectum) drain to the **Nodi lymphoidei mesenterici inferiores**, of which the lymph arrives via the two Trunci lumbales in the Ductus thoracicus.

In contrast, the lymph from the duodenum is routed via the **Nodi lymphoidei pancreaticoduodenales** and the **Nodi lymphoidei hepatici** along the respective arteries either to the Nodi lymphoidei coeliaci or even the Nodi lymphoidei mesenterici superiores.

Clinical remarks

The **lymphatic drainage** plays a role in the diagnosis of **colon carcinomas** since the therapeutic approach depends on the stage of the disease (staging). In the case of a tumour in the Colon ascendens or in the Colon transversum, lymph nodes in the drainage area of the Nodi lymphoidei mesenterici superiores should be looked for; however, for tumours in the Colon descendens, the lymph nodes in the drainage area of the inferior mesenteric lymph nodes are relevant, which, based on the retroperitoneal course of the A. mesenterica inferior along which they lie, frequently prove to connect to other retroperitoneal lymph nodes (Nodi lymphoidei lumbales).

7.2.11 Innervation of the intestine

The intestine is, like most viscera, innervated both by the sympathetic nervous system as well as the parasympathetic nervous system. The **parasympathetic nervous system** promotes the peristaltic movement and the secretion of the glands of the intestinal mucosa. The **sympathetic nervous system**, on the other hand, inhibits this function, as well as the circulation of the mucosa and thus nutrient absorption, but activates the muscles of the ileocecal valve. The intestine is innervated by the **Plexus coeliacus** as well as the **Plexus mesenterici superior and inferior** (Plexus aorticus abdominalis with sympathetic ganglions). The plexus contains sympathetic

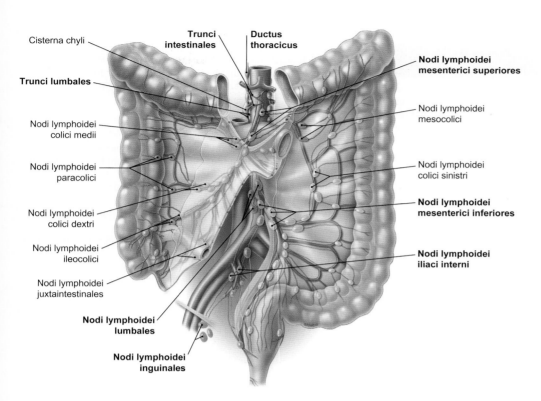

Fig. 7.23 Lymph vessels and regional lymph nodes of the small intestine and the large intestine. The individual groups of lymph nodes are coloured differently according to their catchment areas. (according to [S010-1-16])

Table 7.4 Lymphatic drainage stations of the intestine.

Drainage station	Location
Lymphatic drainage stations of the duodenum	
Nodi lymphoidei pancreaticoduodenales	At the pancreas head
Nodi lymphoidei hepatici	Along the A. hepatica
'Nodi lymphoidei gastroduodenales'	Along the A. gastroduodenalis
Nodi lymphoidei coeliaci	Retroperitoneal
Nodi lymphoidei mesenterici superiores	Along the A. mesenterica superior to the outlet (predominantly intraperitoneal)
Lymphatic drainage stations from the Jejunum and Ileum	
Nodi lymphoidei juxtaintestinales	Directly at the attachment of the mesentery on the intestines
Nodi lymphoidei superiores centrales	Along the A. mesenterica superior
Nodi lymphoidei mesenterici superiores	Along the A. mesenterica superior to the outlet (predominantly intraperitoneal)
Lymphatic drainage stations from the caecum, appendix, Colon ascendens and Colon transversum	
Nodi lymphoidei paracolici	At the vascular arcade directly on the intestines
Nodi lymphoidei precaecales	At the vascular arcade directly on the intestines
Nodi lymphoidei retrocaecales	At the vascular arcade directly on the intestines
Nodi lymphoidei appendiculares	At the vascular arcade directly on the intestines
Nodi lymphoidei ileocolici	Along the A. ileocolica
Nodi lymphoidei colici dextri	Along the A. colica dextra
Nodi lymphoidei colici medii	Along the A. colica media
Nodi lymphoidei mesocolici	On the Mesocolon transversum
Nodi lymphoidei superiores centrales	Along the A. mesenterica superior
Nodi lymphoidei mesenterici superiores	Along the A. mesenterica superior to the outlet (predominantly intraperitoneal)
Lymphatic drainage stations from Colon descendens and Colon sigmoideum and proximal rectum	
Nodi lymphoidei paracolici	At the vascular arcade directly on the intestines
Nodi lymphoidei rectales superiores	At the vascular arcade directly on the intestines
Nodi lymphoidei mesenterici inferiores	At the trunk and exit of the A. mesenterica inferior (retroperitoneal)

Table 7.5 Innervation of the intestine.

Section of the intestine	Innervation
Duodenum	Sympathetic (T5–12) and parasympathetic (N. vagus) via the Plexus coeliacus and Plexus mesentericus superior (Partes superior and descendens up to the Papilla duodeni major directly from the Truncus vagalis anterior via the Rr. hepatici)
Jejunum to Colon transversum	Sympathetic (T5–12) and parasympathetic (N. vagus) via the Plexus mesentericus superior
Colon descendens to upper anal canal	Sympathetic (L1–2) via the Plexus mesentericus inferior, parasympathetic (S2–4) via the Plexus hypogastricus inferior

and parasympathetic fibres, whereby the sympathetic fibres are switched to postganglionic fibres in the ganglia of the same name (Ganglia coeliaca, Ganglia mesenterica superius and inferius), while the parasympathetic nerve fibres are preganglionic and only encounter postganglionic neurons (➤ Fig. 7.52) in the nerve plexuses within the intestinal wall (**enteral nervous system**).

While the sympathetic neurons descend from the Plexus coeliacus to the Plexus mesentericus superior from cranial to caudal and for the Plexus mesentericus inferior also receive additional nerve fibres from the Nn. splanchnici lumbales, the innervation and supply area of the N. vagus (cranial parasympathetic nervous system) ends on the left colic flexure and, therefore, with the Plexus mesentericus superior (traditionally known as the CANNON's point).

The left-sided colon sections receive nerve fibres from the sacral parasympathetic nervous system (S2–4) where they leave as **Nn. splanchnici pelvici** and then in the **Plexus hypogastricus inferior** in the vicinity of the rectum are switched to postganglionic neurons. Only a small part of the postganglionic nerve fibres ascend to the Plexus mesentericus inferior, as the majority arrive as direct branches to the Colon descendens and Colon sigmoideum and the proximal rectum (➤ Fig. 7.52). The perivascular nerve plexus then reach the respective intestinal sections (➤ Table 7.5).

Sympathetic and parasympathic nervous systems also have **afferent nerve fibres**. The zone of the transmitted pain in the abdominal wall (HEAD zone) for the small intestine corresponds to dermatome T10 and for the large intestine, dermatomes T11–L1; however, pain localisation is usually very vague in the periumbilical and epigastric region, and with the Colon ascendens and Colon descendens more to the right or left.

For the general organisation of the autonomic nervous system in the abdomen see ➤ Chap. 7.8.5.

Clinical remarks

The Plexus coeliacus is the strongest plexus on the Aorta abdominalis and is also colloquially known as the 'solar plexus'. A blow to the abdomen can mean that visceral reflexes lead to a **drop in blood pressure and shortness of breath**.

For the diagnosis of **appendicitis**, the typical changes to the projection of pain are important. Initially, the pain will diffuse periumbilically or in the central epigastrium because the mapping of vegetative afferents to specific sections of the abdominal wall is very vague. If subsequently the parietal peritoneum on the fascia of the M. iliopsoas is irritated, the pain shifts into the right lower abdomen.

The positional relationship to the M. iliopsoas also explains **'psoas signs'**, which depending on movement, mostly due to tension of the muscle during hip flexion, can lead to an increase

in pain. Accordingly, diseases in the Colon descendens and Colon sigmoideum, e.g. inflammation of bulges in the intestinal wall **(diverticulitis)**, which are very common in older people, can lead to pain radiating into the left lower abdomen and via the Plexus lumbalis, to the front of the left thigh.

NOTE

In terms of developmental history, there is a necessary switch to the **left colic flexure** of the innervation and supply areas of all vessels and nerves:
- Blood vessels: A. and V. mesenterica superior ↔ A. and V. mesenterica inferior
- Lymph nodes: Nodi lymphoidei mesenterici superiores ↔ Nodi lymphoidei mesenterici inferiores
- Sympathetic innervation: Plexus mesentericus superior ↔ Plexus mesentericus inferior
- Parasympathetic innervation: N. vagus ↔ N. splanchnici pelvici (CANNON's point)

7.3 Liver

Skills

After working through this chapter you should be able to:
- identify the vital importance of the liver with its different functions
- show the location of the liver and its peritoneal duplication in the epigastrium and to describe the development
- show the differences between the anatomical and functional structure of the liver, including the liver segments on a specimen and explain the clinical significance
- know the arterial, lymphatic and autonomic supply to the liver
- explain the sensory innervation of the liver capsule
- set out in detail the portal vein system with portocaval anastomoses and their clinical significance

7.3.1 Overview

The **liver (Hepar)** is the main metabolic organ, the largest digestive organ and the largest gland (1200–1800 g) in the body.

It is located **intraperitoneally** in the right epigastrium (➤ Fig. 7.24), is divided into two large lobes and is brown in colour. Due to its size, structure and, last but not least, the way it is fixed into the surroundings, it determines the entire site of the upper abdomen. Due to the adhesion with the diaphragm, it follows the respiratory movements.

7.3.2 Functions of the liver

The liver has a wide range of functions and is absolutely essential. Functions:
- Central metabolic organ and nutrient storage (glycogen, fats, amino acids, vitamins, metals)
- Detoxification and excretion function
- Production of bile (exocrine gland)
- Production of plasma proteins (coagulation, oncotic pressure, hormones)
- Formation of hormones (endocrine gland)
- Immune defence
- Breakdown of red blood cells (in the event of haemolysis), as well as formation of blood (foetal period)

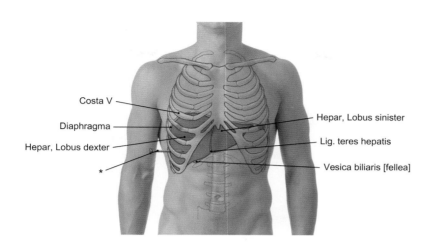

Costa V

Diaphragma

Hepar, Lobus dexter

*

Hepar, Lobus sinister

Lig. teres hepatis

Vesica biliaris [fellea]

Fig. 7.24 Projection of the liver on the ventral torso wall in central respiratory position;* Position of the needle during liver puncture.

The liver takes up the nutrients absorbed in the intestines, which are predominantly transported via the portal vein (glucose, amino acids, fatty acids, vitamins) or in the same way as lipids are transported as lipoproteins by way of the systemic blood circulation. The importance of the liver as the central metabolic organ is also evident from the fact that some metabolic processes (e.g. the urea cycle) take place exclusively in the liver.

Glucose is converted into glycogen as needed, which is how various vitamins (vitamin A, vitamin B_{12}, folic acid) and iron and copper are **stored**.

A wide variety of plasma proteins, such as albumin, blood coagulation factors, hormones and their precursors, and complement proteins of the non-specific immune system, are **synthesised** from the amino acids. The liver converts lipoproteins from the intestine so that they can be used by the tissues of the body and is also the central formation point for cholesterol that is formed depending on the food intake.

Cholesterol is also converted to bile acids , which as the main components of **bile** undertake diverse tasks. After discharge into the bile duct, bile is stored in the gallbladder and in the case of food intake, it is emptied into the intestine. As a result, it is possible for the body to distribute cholesterol and, at the same time to support fat digestion.

In addition to the kidneys, the liver is the second major **excretory organ**. Some substances generated within the body (e. g. bilirubin) or exogenous substances (e. g. medications) are detoxified and discharged via the bile into the intestine or are discharged into the blood for excretion via the kidneys.

In addition to plasma proteins, there are also specific cell types in the liver (e. g. KUPFFER cells) that are involved in regulation of the **immune system**. The liver can, under special circumstances, also be involved in the formation and breakdown of blood cells. In this way it can provide support if there is an increase in red blood cells (erythrocytes) that are to be broken down or in the case of deficiency can assist the bone marrow in **blood formation**. Normally, the liver is like the spleen responsible for the formation of the blood but only during the foetal period.

7.3.3 Development of the liver and gall bladder

The epithelial tissues of the liver (hepatocytes) and gall bladder are derived from the **entoderm** of the foregut at the level of the future duodenum. In the *4th week* the entoderm forms a ventrally-oriented

bud (hepatic diverticulum), which divides into a superior liver primordium and an inferior **primordium for the bile system** (gall bladder and Ductus cysticus; ➤ Fig. 7.25). The stalk of the liver diverticulum becomes the **Ductus choledochus**. The epithelium of the liver system continues to grow into the Septum transversum, which provides the connective tissue of the liver and the islets for blood formation. The blood vessels formed are connected to the umbilical vein (V. umbilicalis), which carries the oxygenated blood from the placenta.

The liver is then gradually displaced into the Mesogastrium ventrale, which initially corresponds to the Septum transversum and is thus divided into a Mesohepaticum ventrale and a Mesohepaticum dorsale. As a result of stomach rotation, the **Mesohepaticum dorsale** is drawn out to the **Omentum minus**, which binds the liver with the stomach and duodenum. Since the abdominal cavity also increases, the liver separates largely from the ventral wall, so that the **Mesohepaticum ventrale** is also extended into a thin peritoneal duplicature. The liver is thereby largely covered by Peritoneum viscerale and only remains fused cranially with its Area nuda at the diaphragm, which partly emerges from the Septum transversum. The **Lig. falciforme hepatis** forms from the Mesohepaticum ventrale as a connection to the anterior torso wall, in which the V. umbilicalis is embedded under the lower free edge, which later obliterates to the Lig. teres hepatis.

7.3.4 Projection of the liver

The liver lies in an **intraperitoneal** position and takes up the majority of the right upper abdomen (➤ Fig. 7.24). On the left side the liver and the left hepatic lobe reaches as far as the left epigastrium (approximately up to the left midclavicular line, MCL) where it lies anterior to the stomach.

When the diaphragm is in a normal position, which the liver directly lies underneath, the upper edge of the right hepatic lobe projects onto the 4th intercostal space (ICS) and the left lies somewhat deeper on the Vth rib. Because of the domed shape of the diaphragm, the anterior and posterior sides of the liver are covered in part by the pleural cavity. With a normal anatomy the lower edge of the liver is covered by the costal arch up to the right MCL.

Overall, it has to be noted that the position of the liver is dependent on breathing as a result of its adhesion to the diaphragm (it lowers on inhalation and rises on exhalation).

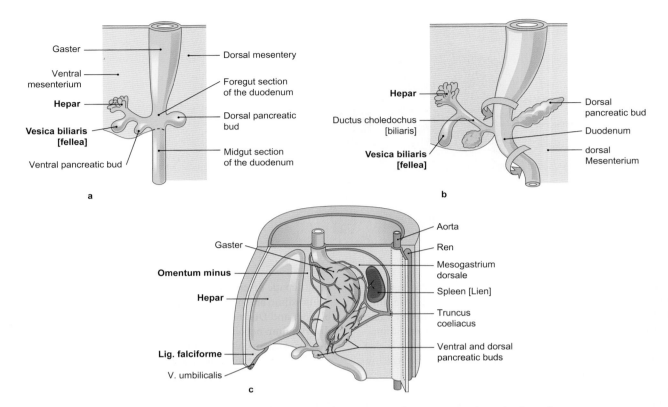

Fig. 7.25 Developmental stages of the liver (Hepar) and gall bladder (Vesica biliaris) in the 4th–5th weeks. [E581]

The examination of the liver with **determination of the liver size** is part of every complete physical examination, as its consistency and size can provide the first evidence of abnormal changes, e.g. fatty liver (in the case of obesity, diabetes mellitus, alcohol abuse), inflammation (hepatitis) in the case of infection with hepatitis virus or alcohol abuse or liver cirrhosis as a pathological end stage of most chronic liver diseases. Determination of the position of the lower liver margin alone is not sufficient for estimation of the size of the liver, since the size of the lungs and the position of the diaphragm influence the position of the liver margins. If the lungs are enlarged, e.g. in the case of pulmonary emphysema in smokers, the liver may be palpable without it being enlarged. Therefore, on examination not only the bottom edge of the liver should be checked by touching (palpation) when breathing in, but also the upper edge of the liver by tapping (percussion) of the chest. When estimating the size of the liver, as a rule of thumb the liver in the right MCL should not have a craniocaudal diameter of more than 12 cm.

The projection of the liver is also important for diagnostic procedures, such as **liver puncture**, in which it must be ensured that other organs such as the lungs and kidneys are not accidentally damaged.

N O T E

The liver is located intraperitoneally in the right upper abdomen and in a central respiratory position with **normal anatomy**, is not **palpable** under the right costal arch. Its position is still largely influenced by the size of the lungs and the position of the diaphragm, so an enlargement of the liver does not always need to be present if the liver is palpable.

7.3.5 Structure

The liver is divided into a large right and a small left hepatic lobe (**Lobus hepatis dexter** and **Lobus hepatis sinister**), that are separated anteriorly by the **Lig. falciforme hepatis**. On the bottom edge of the Lig. falciforme, which runs to the front of the abdominal wall, lies the **Lig. teres hepatis** (relic of the V. umbilicalis). A differentiation is made between the upper side lying underneath the diaphragm (Facies diaphragmatica) and the lower side facing down towards the viscera (Facies visceralis), which anteriorly is delimited by the inferior margin (Margo inferior) (➤ Fig. 7.26). The **Facies diaphragmatica** is partially fused to the diaphragm and is not covered with Peritoneum viscerale (Area nuda).

On the **Facies visceralis**, the incision (Fissura ligamenti teretis) caused by the Lig. teres hepatis continues up to the hepatic porta (Porta hepatis).

In the **Porta hepatis** the right and left main tributaries of the vessels and nerves of the liver mostly enter or leave in the following order:
- Ductus hepaticus communis (right ventral arrangement)
- A. hepatica propria (left ventral)
- V. portae hepatis (dorsal)

The Lig. venosum (remnant of the Ductus venosus of foetal circulation) continues the course of the Lig. teres hepatis in a cranial direction.

On the right side of the Porta hepatis the V. cava inferior is located above in a groove and the **gall bladder (Vesica biliaris)** is located below in the gall bladder fossa (Fossa vesicae biliaris). This close relationship of the V. cava inferior and its afferent hepatic veins is important for the stability of the liver. The Lig. teres hepatis, Lig. venosum, V. cava inferior and gall bladder create an H-shaped structure, whose horizontal beams represents the Porta hepatis. Ventral and dorsal of the Porta hepatis, 2 approximately square areas

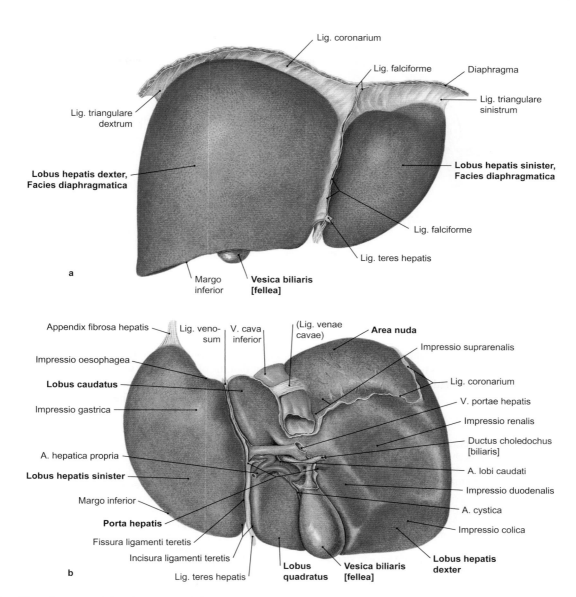

Fig. 7.26 Liver (Hepar). a Ventral view. **b** Dorsocaudal view.

are defined on the underside of the right hepatic lobe, which are designated ventrally as the **Lobus quadratus** and dorsally as the **Lobus caudatus**. These designations are misleading, since they are more a continuation rather than an independent lobe.

The liver is not covered by peritoneum in 4 larger areas:

- Area nuda
- Porta hepatis
- Gall bladder bed
- Groove of the V. cava inferior

7.3.6 Parts and segments of the liver

The liver is divided into **8 functional segments**. Thereby, the 3 vertically running hepatic veins (Vv. hepaticae; ➤ Fig. 7.27), which together with their surrounding connective tissue are referred to as fissures, divide the liver into four adjacent divisions. The **Divisio lateralis sinistra** corresponds to the left anatomical lobe of the liver and reaches as far as the Lig. falcifome hepatis, behind which the left hepatic vein runs into the Fissura umbilicalis. The **Divisio medialis sinistra** extends between the Lig. falciforme and the gall bladder, at which height the middle hepatic vein lies in the Fissura

portalis principalis. Then to the right side follow the **Divisio medialis dextra and the Divisio lateralis dextra**, which are separated by the right hepatic vein in the Fissura portalis dextra but there is no visible landmark for this on the outer surface.

These 4 vertical divisions are divided by the branches of the **liver triad** (V. portae hepatis, A. hepatica propria, Ductus hepaticus communis) into **8 liver segments**. Segment I corresponds to the Lobus caudatus, segments II and III the anatomical left hepatic lobe, segment IV the Divisio medialis sinistra and segments V–VIII the rest of the anatomical right hepatic lobe, where the latter are numbered in a clockwise direction. The Lobus quadratus is a part of segment IVb. Subsequently, a ninth segment, which lies between segment VIII and I could be described, but is so far hardly taken into account in surgery.

In functional terms it is important that **segments I–IV** are supplied by the left branches of the liver triad and, therefore, in contrast to the macroscopically visible hepatic lobes, collectively belong to the left part of the liver (Pars hepatis sinistra), while **segments V–VIII** are dependent on the right branches of the liver triad and represent the functional right side of the liver (Pars hepatis dextra). Only segment I is regularly supplied from the branches of both sides.

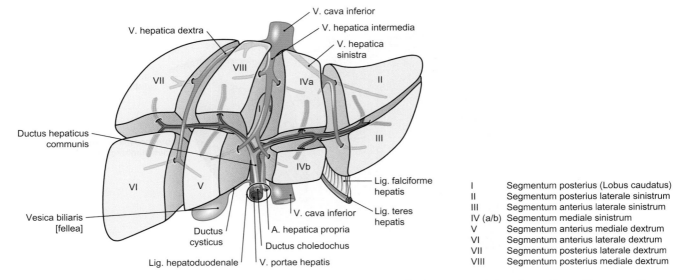

Fig. 7.27 Liver segments and their relationship with the intrahepatic vessels and bile ducts. Ventral view. (according to [S010-1-16])

I	Segmentum posterius (Lobus caudatus)
II	Segmentum posterius laterale sinistrum
III	Segmentum anterius laterale sinistrum
IV (a/b)	Segmentum mediale sinistrum
V	Segmentum anterius mediale dextrum
VI	Segmentum anterius laterale dextrum
VII	Segmentum posterius laterale dextrum
VIII	Segmentum posterius mediale dextrum

Thus, the border between the functional right and the functional left part of the liver in the sagittal plane is between the V. cava inferior and the gall bladder (**'Cava gall bladder plane'**) and not at the level of the Lig. falcifome hepatis.

> **NOTE**
>
> The liver is divided into **8 segments,** of which segments **I–IV** in line with their blood supply, belong to the functional **left** part of the liver and segments V–VIII to the functional **right** part. Thus, the functional left part of the liver is greater than the anatomical left hepatic lobe.

> **Clinical remarks**
>
> The liver segments have a great clinical significance in **visceral surgery**, as they make it possible to carry out resections of individual parts of the liver with little loss of blood, as long as the segment borders are observed. This means that in pathological processes, e.g. liver metastases, several individual segments in different parts of the liver can be resected without compromising the liver function as a whole. In practical terms, the surgeon proceeds in the removal of the segments by ligating individual branches of the afferent vessels in order to be able to clearly identify the dependent liver segments by their discoloration due to the reduced blood flow.

7.3.7 Fine structure of the liver

Tip: The following brief explanation of the histology serves to understand the blood flow through the liver and the understanding of how a portal hypertension occurs when it stops working: the hepatic parenchyma is divided into hepatic lobules (➤ Fig. 7.28). At the corners are the **periportal fields,** in which the terminal branches of the liver triad are found. In the centre of the liver lobules the **V. centralis**, which collects the blood from the blood vessels of the liver triad again after it has flowed past the liver cells (hepatocytes) and carries it via the Vv. sublobulares to the Vv. hepaticae. This allows the hepatocytes to extract nutrients and substances to be eliminated from the blood and to secrete synthesised substances,

such as plasma proteins into the blood. It should be taken into account that the blood flows to the centre of the lobules and therefore flows in the reverse direction to bile, which is routed between the hepatocytes to the periphery where it flows into the intrahepatic bile ducts in the periportal field.

> **Clinical remarks**
>
> The blood flow in the hepatic lobules is extremely important for maintenance of the liver function. If the structure of the lobules in the event of **liver cirrhosis** are destroyed by nodular, connective tissue reorganisation (pseudo-lobules), the blood flow is impaired. The high parenchymal resistance in the liver results in an increased blood pressure in the portal vein (**portal hypertension**). As a result, bypass circuits can form (**portocaval anastomoses**, ➤ Chap. 7.3.11) (➤ Fig. 7.29).

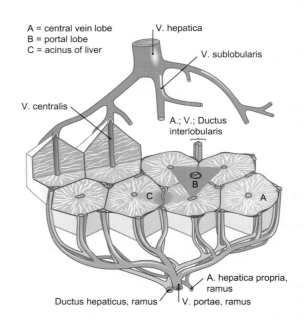

A = central vein lobe
B = portal lobe
C = acinus of liver

Fig. 7.28 Lobular subdivision of the liver parenchyma. [L126]

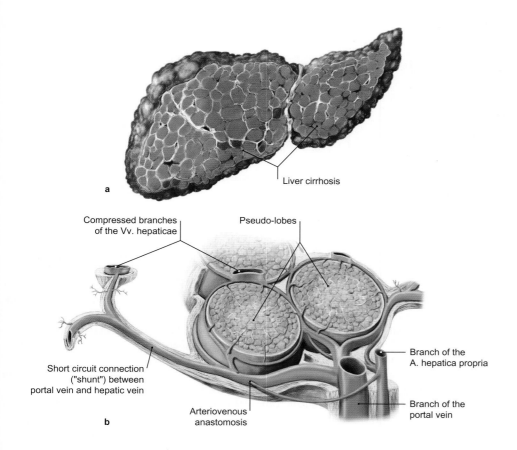

Liver cirrhosis

Compressed branches
of the Vv. hepaticae

Pseudo-lobes

Branch of the
A. hepatica propria

Short circuit connection
("shunt") between
portal vein and hepatic vein

Arteriovenous
anastomosis

Branch of the
portal vein

a

b

Fig. 7.29 Liver cirrhosis. [L266]
a Section through the liver.
b Formation of pseudo-lobules.
[L266]

7.3.8 Topography

In vivo the liver is malleable and adjusts to the shape of the surrounding organs. In a fixed state the adjacent organs leave marks (impressions), which are regarded as fixation artefacts and are not significant; however, they provide information about the positions of the liver. The liver has direct **positional links** to the following adjacent organs (➤ Fig. 7.26):

- Right hepatic lobe: kidneys, adrenal glands, duodenum, colon
- Left hepatic lobe: oesophagus, stomach

The liver is connected through a series of peritoneal duplicatures, which are referred to as ligaments (Ligamenta), above with the diaphragm near the Area nuda, anteriorly with the abdominal wall and caudally with the neighbouring organs. These ligaments originate from the ventral 'Meso' of the intestine (Mesogastrium ventrale). On the Facies diaphragmatica the **Lig. falciforme hepatis** continues cranially to the **Lig. coronarium**. This surrounds the Area nuda and runs on the right and left each into a **Lig. triangulare** as a connection to the diaphragm. The Lig. triangulare sinistrum runs over into the peak-shaped Appendix fibrosa hepatis. Below the **Lig. teres hepatis** (a relic of the V. umbilicalis from the foetal circulation) joins the Lig. falciforme. Both ligaments run to the ventral wall and contain fine arteries, veins (Vv. paraumbilicales) and lymph vessels, via which the liver connects to the vessels and nerves of the anterior torso wall.

outflow. Vice versa, cleavage of the Lig. triangulare dextrum or Lig. triangulare sinistrum enables mobilisation of the respective hepatic lobes when access to the V. cava inferior, the oesophagus or diaphragm is necessary. Due to the arterial connections between segment IV and the supply area of the A. thoracica interna in the Lig. teres hepatis, this ligament must generally be ligated or coagulated in all operations in the right upper abdomen that require mobilisation of the liver, in order to avoid bleeding.

The origin of the lesser omentum (**Omentum minus**), is on the Facies visceralis, which after its attachment, is divided into a Lig. hepatogastricum and a Lig. hepatoduodenale. In the Lig. hepatogastricum the parasympathetic Rr. hepatici run from the Trunci vagales to the liver and in this way the Rr. pylorici to the stomach. In the **Lig. hepatoduodenale** the components of the liver triad run in the following arrangement to the liver:

- right: Ductus choledochus
- left: A. hepatica propria
- dorsal: V. portae hepatis
- in addition: lymph vessels, lymph nodes and autonomic nerves (Plexus hepaticus)

Under the Lig. hepatoduodenale is the entrance to the Bursa omentalis (Foramen omentale/epiploicum), which represents a recess (Recessus) of the peritoneal cavity behind the Omentum minus or the stomach.

7.3.9 Arteries of the liver

The liver is supplied with blood by the **A. hepatica propria** (➤ Fig. 7.30). This is the continuation of the A. hepatica communis, a main branch of the Truncus coeliacus. After branching of the A. gastrica

---

Clinical remarks

The **liver connections** are of great importance in surgery. The Lig. triangulare sinistrum stabilises the left hepatic lobe if the (functional) right half of the liver must be removed and there by prevents a rotation of the lobe and disruption of the venous

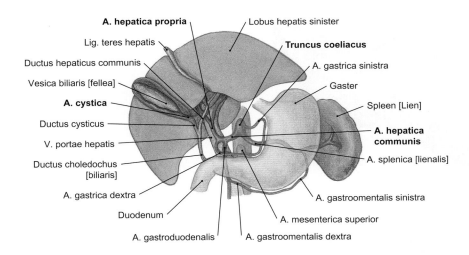

Fig. 7.30 Arteries of the liver (Hepar) and the gall bladder (Vesica biliaris).

Labels: A. hepatica propria · Lobus hepatis sinister · Lig. teres hepatis · Truncus coeliacus · Ductus hepaticus communis · A. gastrica sinistra · Vesica biliaris [fellea] · Gaster · A. cystica · Spleen [Lien] · Ductus cysticus · A. hepatica communis · V. portae hepatis · A. splenica [lienalis] · Ductus choledochus [biliaris] · A. gastrica dextra · A. gastroomentalis sinistra · Duodenum · A. mesenterica superior · A. gastroduodenalis · A. gastroomentalis dextra

dextra, the A. hepatica propria runs in the Lig. hepatoduodenale together with the V. portae hepatis and the Ductus choledochus to the hepatic portal. There it is normally divided into a **R. dexter** and a **R. sinister** for the two **functional liver parts.**

In 10–20% of cases, the A. mesenterica superior contributes to the blood supply of the right hepatic lobe, and the A. gastrica sinistra contributes to the supply of the left hepatic lobe (**accessory hepatic arteries**). Rarely, the entire A. hepatica communis or propria originates from the A. mesenterica superior (3%).

> ### Clinical remarks
>
> The variations of the arterial liver supply are of clinical importance:
> - Accessory hepatic arteries can be injured during surgical procedures in the right upper abdomen and can cause **bleeding** (e.g. the right accessory artery, in surgery of the pancreatic head or left accessory artery during cleavage of the Omentum minus, in which it runs).
> - Accessory hepatic arteries can be decisive for survival in patients with **bile duct carcinoma**, as they are further away from the main stems of the Ductus hepaticus communis and are therefore not infiltrated by the tumour.
> - For **liver transplantations** the supply pattern must be known.

7.3.10 Veins of the liver

The liver has an afferent and an efferent venous system.
- The **portal vein** (V. portae hepatis) leads the nutrient-rich blood from the unpaired abdominal organs (stomach, intestines, pancreas, spleen) *to the liver* (➤ Fig. 7.31).
- The 3 **hepatic veins** (Vv. hepaticae) transport the blood *from the liver* to the V. cava inferior.

The **portal vein** is approximately 7 cm long and has 3 main tributaries (V. mesenterica superior, V. splenica, V. mesenterica inferior):
- The **V. mesenterica superior** joins with the **V. splenica** behind the pancreatic neck to become the V. portae hepatis.
- The **V. mesenterica inferior** mostly drains (70% of all cases) into the V. splenica, in some cases (30%) into the V. mesenterica superior or the confluence of the main stems.

After the joining of its main stems, the portal vein initially runs secondarily retroperitoneally behind the pancreas and duodenum and after the entry into the Lig. hepatoduodenale intraperitoneal.

In the area of the hepatic porta the portal vein divides into its right and left main stem.

Branches of the V. splenica (collect blood from the spleen and from parts of the stomach and pancreas):
- Vv. gastricae breves
- V. gastroomentalis sinistra
- V. gastrica posterior (inconstant)
- Vv. pancreaticae (from the tail and body of the pancreas)

Branches of the V. mesenterica superior (collect blood from parts of the stomach and pancreas, from the entire small intestine, the Colon ascendens, and Colon transversum):
- V. gastroomentalis dextra with Vv. pancreaticoduodenales
- Vv. pancreaticae (from the head and body of the pancreas)
- Vv. jejunales and ileales
- V. ileocolica
- V. colica dextra
- V. colica media

Branches of the V. mesenterica inferior (collect blood from the Colon descendens and the upper rectum):
- V. colica sinistra
- Vv. sigmoideae
- V. rectalis superior: the vein is connected to the V. rectalis media and the V. rectalis inferior, which belong to the catchment area of the V. cava inferior.

In addition, there are also **veins** which drain **directly into the portal vein** after the main venous branches have merged:
- V. cystica (from the gall bladder)
- Vv. paraumbilicales (via veins in the Lig. teres hepatis from the abdominal wall around the umbilicus)
- Vv. gastricae dextra and sinistra (from the small stomach curvature)
- V. pancreaticoduodenalis superior posterior (dorsal from the pancreatic head)

7.3.11 Portocaval anastomoses

Connections of the V. portae hepatis to the drainage area of the Vv. cavae superior and inferior are referred to as portocaval anastomoses. These vascular connections are clinically important (and extremely relevant for examinations).

There are 4 possible bypass circulations through portocaval anastomoses:
- **V. gastrica dextra** and **V. gastrica sinistra** connected through oesophageal veins and azygos veins to the V. cava superior. In

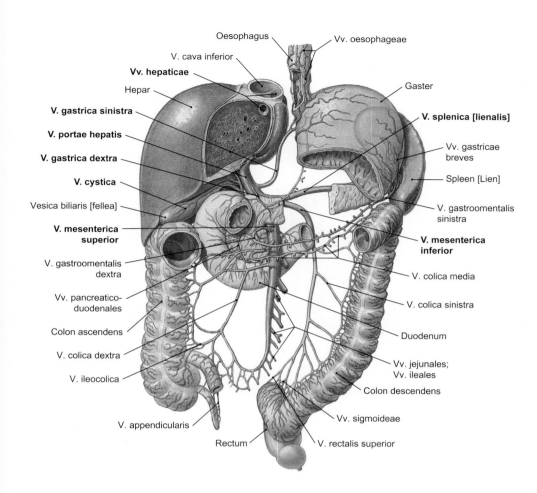

Oesophagus
Vv. oesophageae
V. cava inferior
Vv. hepaticae
Hepar
Gaster
V. gastrica sinistra
V. splenica [lienalis]
V. portae hepatis
Vv. gastricae breves
V. gastrica dextra
V. cystica
Spleen [Lien]
Vesica biliaris [fellea]
V. gastroomentalis sinistra
V. mesenterica superior
V. mesenterica inferior
V. gastroomentalis dextra
V. colica media
Vv. pancreatico-duodenales
V. colica sinistra
Colon ascendens
Duodenum
V. colica dextra
Vv. jejunales; Vv. ileales
V. ileocolica
Colon descendens
Vv. sigmoideae
V. appendicularis
Rectum
V. rectalis superior

Fig. 7.31 Veins of the liver (Hepar) and the gall bladder (Vesica biliaris). Ventral view.

this case, expansion of the submucosal veins of the oesophagus **(oesophageal varices)** can occur.

- **Vv. paraumbilicales** are connected via the veins of the anterior torso wall (deep: V. epigastrica superior and V. epigastrica inferior; superficial: V. thoracoepigastrica and V. epigastrica superficialis) to the superior and inferior vena cava. The dilation of the superficial veins may lead to **Caput medusae**.
- **V. rectalis superior** via veins of the lower rectum and the V. iliaca interna to the V. cava inferior. Rarely, varicosities form around the anus and so this must not be confused with haemorrhoids.
- **Retroperitoneal anastomoses** via the V. mesenterica inferior to the V. testicularis/ovarica with connection to the V. cava inferior.

Clinical remarks

In the case of high pressure in the portal vein circulation (portal hypertension), e.g. in cirrhosis of the liver, the connections to the drainage area of the V. cava superior and V. cava inferior **(portocaval anastomosis)** can become opened up or dilated (➤ Fig. 7.32). Clinically important are the connections to the **oesophageal veins** because rupture of oesophageal varices may result in life-threatening haemorrhaging, the most common cause of death in patients with liver cirrhosis. The connections to superficial veins of the ventral abdominal wall are only of diagnostic value. Although a **Caput medusae** is rare, the appearance is so characteristic that liver cirrhosis cannot be overlooked. In contrast, the retroperitoneal connections and anastomoses between the veins of the rectum are not clinically significant.

In terms of treatment, a ligature and sclerotherapy of oesophageal varices in the event of high portal hypertension is possi-

ble. Alternatively, a balloon catheter can be introduced from the V. cava inferior through the liver tissue to establish a connection between the Vv. hepaticae and the blocked branches of the portal vein (transjugular intrahepatic portosystemic shunt, TIPS).

7.3.12 Lymph vessels of the liver

The liver has 2 lymphatic vascular systems (➤ Fig. 7.33):
- the superficial subperitoneal system on the surface of the liver
- the deep intraparenchymatous system that follows the components of the hepatic triad to the hepatic porta.

With respect to the regional lymph nodes, there are 2 **major lymph drainage routes:**
- **Caudally to the hepatic porta** (most important drainage route) via the Nodi lymphoidei hepatici on the hepatic porta and from there through lymphatic vessels in the Lig. hepatoduodenale to the Nodi lymphoidei coeliaci at the outlet of the Truncus coeliacus and from there to the Trunci intestinales.
- **Cranially through the diaphragm** (through the Foramen v. cavae and the Hiatus oesophageus) via the Nodi lymphoidei phrenici inferiores and superiores in the Nodi lymphoidei mediastinales, which connect to the Trunci bronchiomediastinales. In this way, liver carcinomas can also result in thoracic lymph node metastases. Individual lymphatic vessels within the Lig. coronarium and the Ligg. triangularia can also draw directly into the Ductus thoracicus.

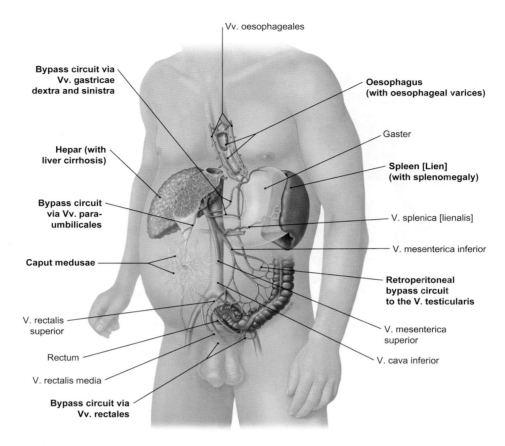

Fig. 7.32 Clinical aspects of formation of portocaval anastomoses. The oesophageal varices and the Caput medusae are significant. The enlargement of the spleen (splenomegaly) is a result of a build up of blood due to the portal hypertension. [L238]

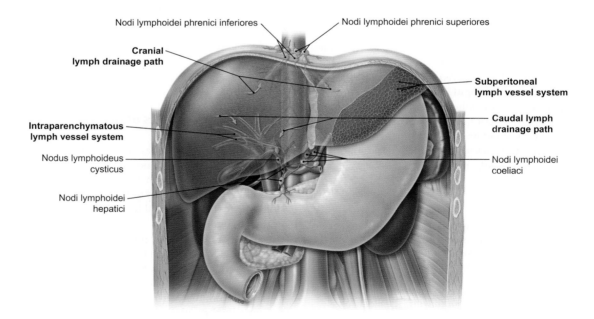

Fig. 7.33 Lymph vessels and lymph nodes of the liver and bile duct system. The green arrows depict the direction of lymph drainage from the parenchyma via the cranial or caudal route.

── Clinical remarks ──────────────

Liver tumours can also lead to the formation of lymph node metastases in the chest cavity.

7.3.13 Innervation of the liver

The **liver** is innervated by the **Plexus hepaticus** a separate autonomic nerve plexus around the A. hepatica propria, which represents a continuation of the Plexus coeliacus:

- **Sympathetic:** postganglionic nerves, whose nerve bodies sit in the Ganglia coeliaca (under exertion these nerves initiate a breakdown of glycogen in order to increase the level of blood sugar and the secretion of the bile is throttled)
- **Parasympathetic:** preganglionic nerves, which additionally branch out as Rr. hepatici in the Omentum minus from the Trunci vagales and are switched in the Plexus hepaticus (these nerve fibres convey the production of bile on food intake)
- **Sensory:** the peritoneum on the surface of the liver capsule is innervated by the right N. phrenicus (R. phrenicoabdominalis) and the lower intercostal nerves.

For general organisation of the autonomic nervous system in the abdomen, see ➤ Chap. 7.8.5.

> ### Clinical remarks
>
> Due to the sensory innervation of the liver capsule by the N. phrenicus (Plexus cervicalis), in the event of a **liver puncture** or **rupture of the liver capsule** this can lead to pain sensations on the right side of the abdominal wall, as well as in the right shoulder (projection pain).

7.4 Gall bladder and bile ducts

> ### Skills
>
> After working through this chapter, you should be able to:
> - explain the location and the projection of the gall bladder on a dissection specimen
> - illustrate the structure of the gall bladder and bile ducts with their exact course
> - describe the opening and the closure mechanisms of the Ductus choledochus
> - locate the vessels and nerves of the gall bladder and bile ducts
> - illustrate the topography of CALOT's triangle on a dissection specimen and explain its clinical relevance

7.4.1 Overview and function

The **gall bladder (Vesica biliaris)** is located **intraperitoneally** in the right upper abdomen directly under the liver, where it merges into the gall bladder bed (Fossa vesicae biliaris). It is connected with the liver and duodenum via the bile ducts.

The gall bladder is used for the **storage** and the **concentration** of the **bile** produced by the liver. It is remarkable that the gall bladder is filled by backflow when the sphincter at the opening into the duodenum is closed. Therefore, the gall bladder, in contrast to the liver, is not essential to life.

For the development of the gall bladder, see ➤ Chap. 7.3.3.

7.4.2 Projection and topography of the gall bladder

The fundus of the gall bladder overlies the lower edge of the liver and projects onto the IX. rib (➤ Fig. 7.24). Here it lies immediately on the abdominal wall. The gall bladder is only palpable if it is significantly enlarged as a result of a build-up of bile. The fundus of the gall bladder is in contact with the right flexure of the colon; the body and neck area lie ventrally to the duodenum.

> ### Clinical remarks
>
> Due to their close relationships with the duodenum and colon, during an inflammation of the gall bladder **(cholecystitis)** caused by gall-stones **(Cholecystolithiasis),** these gall-stones can enter the intestine through perforations in the wall and are then excreted or lead to a blockage **(gall-stone ileus).**

7.4.3 Construction of gall bladder and extrahepatic bile ducts

The gall bladder is 7–10 cm long and is divided into the **body of gall bladder** (Corpus vesicae biliaris) with a **fundus** (Fundus vesicae biliaris) and a **neck portion** (Collum vesicae biliaris). It usually holds approximately 40–70 ml of bile. At the neck, it joins the 3–4 cm long excretion duct **(Ductus cysticus)** which, by means of a fold (Plica spiralis HEISTER) is closed before it merges with the main bile duct of the liver (Ductus hepaticus communis) into the Ductus choledochus (➤ Fig. 7.34). The Ductus hepaticus communis is formed in the Porta hepatis from its right and left main stem (Ductus hepatici dexter and sinister). At the neck there is a peritoneal duplicature to the liver, in which the A. cystica runs.

The **Ductus choledochus** is on average 6 cm long and 0.4–0.9 cm in diameter. The length is very variable and depends on the height of the Ductus cysticus which joins the Ductus hepaticus communis. In rare cases, the Ductus cysticus can be duplicated or even missing. The Ductus choledochus initially runs ventrally and right of the portal vein in the Lig. hepatoduodenale then behind the Pars superior of the duodenum to finally reach the Pars descendens of the duodenum via the head of the pancreas. The confluence is located in the **Papilla duodeni major** (Papilla VATERI; ➤ Fig. 7.35), which lies 8–10 cm away from the pylorus of the stomach on the dorsomedial wall in the middle third of the Pars descendens of the

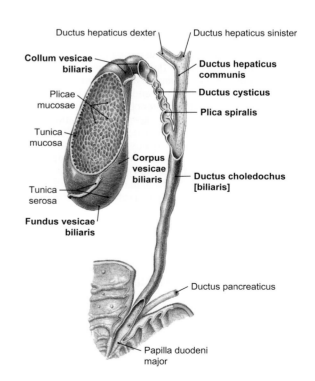

Fig. 7.34 Gall bladder (Vesica biliaris) and extrahepatic bile ducts. Ventral view.

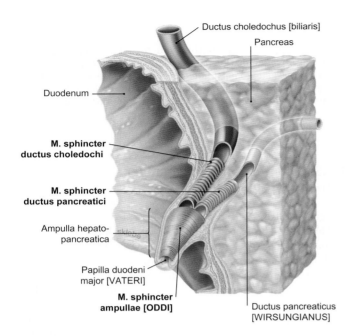

Fig. 7.35 Confluence of the Ductus choledochus and Ductus pancreaticus into the duodenum. Ventral view. [L238]

duodenum. Before the confluence, the Ductus choledochus mostly (in 60% of cases) combines with the Ductus pancreaticus to the **Ampulla hepatopancreatica**. The smooth muscles of the wall form a M. sphincter ductus choledochi, whose lower section, the **M. sphincter ampullae (ODDI)** also includes the ampulla and their confluence. Together with the M. sphincter ductus pancreatici this forms a sphincter complex 3 cm in length.

> **Clinical remarks**
>
> As the Ductus choledochus runs through the pancreatic head and a bottleneck is formed at the Papilla duodeni major by the M. sphincter ampullae ODDI, in cases of pancreatic cancer (mostly painless), this can lead to bile backflow **(cholestasis)** into the blood, just as a gall-stone trapped in the papilla (usually painful with biliary colic). Due to the deposition of the bile pigment bilirubin in the connective tissue, there is usually a yellowing of the sclera of the eye and later the skin **(jaundice, icterus)**. In these cases, the efferent bile ducts are examined with ultrasound or x-ray contrast agent for clarification (endoscopic retrograde cholangiopancreatography, ERCP). An enlargement of the Ductus choledochus of over 1 cm in diameter is indicative for cholestasis. Due to the amalgamation of the Ductus choledochus with the Ductus pancreaticus, it can simultaneously lead to a backflow of pancreatic secretions with **inflammation of the pancreas (pancreatitis)**, which is caused by partial self-digestion of the organ.

7.4.4 Pathways of the gall bladder and bile ducts

Arterial supply of the gall bladder
The **A. cystica** usually originates (63–75%) from the R. dexter of the A. hepatica propria and is divided into a superficial branch for the gall bladder itself and a deep branch to the gall bladder bed, the branches of which anastomose with each other. In addition, fine branches of the liver tissue (from the branches of the R. dexter of the A. hepatica propria to liver segment V) to the body of the gall

bladder. The A. cystica can also originate from other branches or the stem of the A. hepatica propria or the A. gastroduodenalis (4%). In 80% of cases there is only one A. cystica but in up to 20% an **accessory A. cystica** occurs. This good supply explains why necrosis of the gall bladder is rare.

Arterial blood supply to the bile ducts
Whereas the **Ductus hepaticus communis** is only supplied by branches of the A. cystica and from the R. dexter of the A. hepatica propria, the **Ductus choledochus** additionally has ascending arteries to complement these two descending arteries, which originate from the A. gastroduodenalis. The distal third, as well as the **Papilla duodeni major** are fed from a vascular plexus from the A. pancreaticoduodenalis superior posterior (➤ Fig. 7.36).

> **Clinical remarks**
>
> Due to the variations in the origin of the A. cystica, in the event of a gall bladder removal **(cholecystectomy)** a high degree of preparatory care is necessary. The existence of a second A. cystica should always be ruled out in order to avoid bleeding. The good perfusion of the Papilla duodeni major explains why in the event of surgical removal of a trapped gallstone **(papillotomy)** heavy bleeding from the A. pancreaticoduodenalis superior posterior may occur.

Venous drainage
The **V. cystica** runs along the peritoneal side of the gall bladder and enters directly into the portal vein. On the side facing the liver, there are many small branches, which also drain the proximal sections of the bile ducts. The blood from the distal sections flows via the **veins at the pancreatic head** to the portal vein.

Lymph vessels
On the gall bladder there is usually an individual **Nodus lymphoideus cysticus** at the neck portion from which the lymph flows via the lymph nodes of the hepatic porta to the **Nodi lymphoidei coeliaci**. The lymph vessels from the portions of the gall bladder adjoining the liver, on the other hand, enter the liver tissue and connect here with the lymph drainage channels of the liver. The lymph from the **Ductus choledochus** also passes from the proximal section to the Nodus lymphoideus cysticus, distal to the lymph nodes on the pancreatic head.

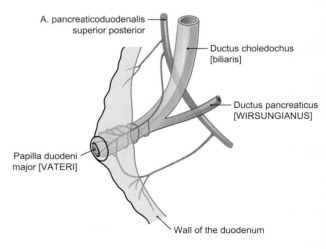

Fig. 7.36 Arteries of the Ductus choledochus. [L126]

Innervation

The innervation corresponds to the supply of the liver:
- **Sympathetic and parasympathetic** via the Plexus hepaticus. The parasympathetic-mediated contraction supports the hormone-induced contraction of the gall bladder wall musculature, inhibits the M. sphincter ampullae and thus promotes emptying of bile. The sympathetic nervous system has antagonistic functions.
- **Sensory:** the peritoneum on the surface away from the liver is innervated by the right N. phrenicus (R. phrenicoabdominalis). For general organisation of the autonomic nervous system in the abdomen ➤ Chap. 7.8.5.

> ### Clinical remarks
>
> As with the liver, pain can radiate into the right shoulder on inflammation of the gall bladder (**cholecystitis**) due to the sensory innervation of the liver capsule through the N. phrenicus (Plexus cervicalis).

7.4.5 CALOT's triangle

The Ductus cysticus, Ductus hepaticus communis, and inferior surface of the liver together form the cystohepatic triangle, also referred to as CALOT's triangle. (➤ Fig. 7.37). Its limits are:
- Ductus cysticus
- Ductus hepaticus communis
- Inferior surface of the liver

In 75% of cases, the A. cystica originates in the CALOT's triangle from the R. dextra of the A. hepatica propria and runs posteriorly through this triangle to reach the Ductus cysticus and the neck of the gall bladder. In the remaining cases there are different origins and course patterns of the A. cystica.

> ### Clinical remarks
>
> CALOT's triangle is an important orientation point for every **removal of the gall bladder**. Prior to removal of the gall bladder

all relevant structures are identified before the A. cystica and the Ductus cysticus are ligated. This makes it possible to reduce the risk of erroneously inhibiting the Ductus choledochus, which would cause a bile backflow (cholestasis).

7.5 Pancreas

> ### Skills
>
> After working through this chapter, you should be able to:
> - know the vital importance and explain the function of the exocrine and endocrine pancreas
> - show the classification of the pancreas on the dissection specimen and explain the development, including malformations
> - describe the topography of the individual sections of the pancreas and explain the relationship with the adjacent organs
> - describe the system of ducts with confluence into the duodenum
> - explain the different supply of the sections of the pancreas by arteries, veins, lymph vessels and autonomic nerves and, as far as possible, to demonstrate on the dissection specimen

7.5.1 Overview

The **pancreas** is a combined exocrine and endocrine gland of the digestive system and in living people, is salmon pink in colour. Due to rearrangement processes during development, the pancreas is **secondarily retroperitoneal** in the central upper abdomen. This position, the confluence behaviour of the excretory ducts of the exocrine gland section, and the supply patterns for the respective vessels and nerves are of major clinical relevance (➤ Fig. 7.38).

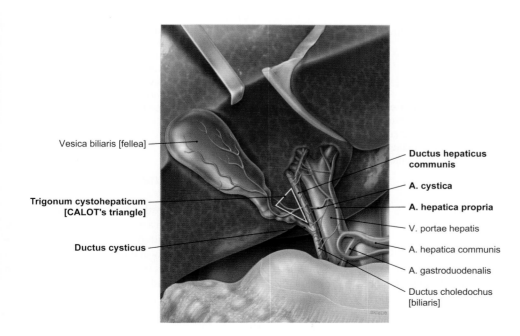

Vesica biliaris [fellea]

Trigonum cystohepaticum [CALOT's triangle]

Ductus cysticus

Ductus hepaticus communis

A. cystica

A. hepatica propria

V. portae hepatis

A. hepatica communis

A. gastroduodenalis

Ductus choledochus [biliaris]

Fig. 7.37 CALOT's triangle (cystohepatic triangle). Caudal view. (according to [S010-1-16])

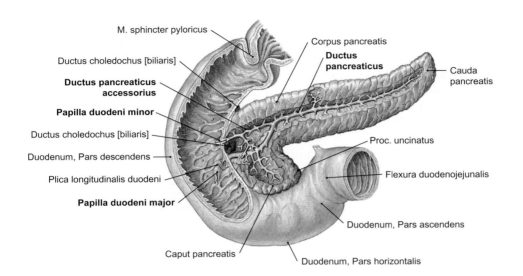

M. sphincter pyloricus

Ductus choledochus [biliaris]

Ductus pancreaticus accessorius

Papilla duodeni minor

Ductus choledochus [biliaris]

Duodenum, Pars descendens

Plica longitudinalis duodeni

Papilla duodeni major

Caput pancreatis

Corpus pancreatis

Ductus pancreaticus

Cauda pancreatis

Proc. uncinatus

Flexura duodenojejunalis

Duodenum, Pars ascendens

Duodenum, Pars horizontalis

Fig. 7.38 Structure and excretory duct system of the pancreas. Ventral view; Ductus pancreaticus after opening of the pancreas and duodenum.

7.5.2 Functions of the pancreas

The pancreas is a gland that has both **exocrine** (90% of organ weight) as well as **endocrine** (10%) sections. The endocrine cell groups are distributed as islets in the organ (Islets of LANGERHANS) and are especially common in the tail section.

The production of the hormone insulin that is essential for the regulation of blood sugar levels and metabolism, makes the pancreas an essential and vital organ. Functions of the pancreas are:

- Formation of **digestive enzymes**, which are predominantly emitted as inactive precursors (exocrine pancreatic section)
- Secretion of **hormones** for regulation of blood sugar levels, metabolism and digestion (endocrine pancreatic section)

As soon as the chyme passes from the stomach into the duodenum, it will hormonally stimulate the release of the **exocrine** pancreatic secretions, which are released via the two excretory ducts of the pancreas into the duodenum. The alkaline pancreatic juice contains mainly enzyme precursors, which are first activated in the intestinal lumen. This is a protection mechanism to prevent the destruction of pancreatic tissue.

The **endocrine** pancreas forms different hormones and releases them into the blood through veins. The release of the blood sugar regulating hormones insulin and glucagon are controlled directly by the blood sugar level.

Clinical remarks

The function of the pancreas makes it easy to understand why tissue destruction (necrosis) of the pancreas, e.g. if inflammation occurs (**pancreatitis**), can lead to digestive disorders culminating in diarrhoea, and in the case of extensive damage (loss of 80–90% of the tissue) can also lead to diabetes mellitus as a result of reduced insulin production.

7.5.3 Development

At the end of the *4th week* at the level of the duodenum, a ventral and a dorsal pancreatic bud emerge from the **entoderm of the foregut** (➤ Fig. 7.39). Together with the stomach rotation, the ventral pancreatic bud folds to the left behind the duodenum and fuses there in the *6th–7th week* with the dorsal pancreatic bud. The **dorsal bud** thereby forms the upper part of the head and the entire body and tail of the pancreas; the **ventral bud**, however, only forms the lower part of the head and the Proc. uncinatus.

The **excretory duct** of the pancreas (Ductus pancreaticus) arises from the union of the distal duct portion of the dorsal pancreatic bud with the ventral pancreatic duct and confluences at the Papilla duodeni major. The proximal section of the dorsal pancreatic duct predominantly (65%) opens into the accessory pancreatic duct (Ductus pancreaticus accessorius), which leads into the Papilla duodeni minor in the duodenum.

Clinical remarks

The development of the pancreas is clinically very important because it leads to disease-relevant malformations:

- **Pancreas anulare:** when the pancreatic tissue grows in a circular form around the duodenum, occlusion of the intestine **(ileus)** with vomiting may occur, particularly in newborns (➤ Fig. 7.40a). In this case, the duodenum has to be severed and sewn back next to the pancreas system.
- **Pancreas divisum:** as a general rule (65%) there are 2 excretory ducts that connect but enter the duodenum separately. The accessory duct can (35%) also be very thin and only lead into the Ductus pancreaticus (➤ Fig. 7.40b and c). If the two systems do not completely merge and the excretory ducts do not connect (10% of cases), the accessory duct can be too narrow for secretions to be delivered or for the dorsal system duct of the main excretory duct to be formed (➤ Fig. 7.40d, e); in both of these instances, a build-up of secretions can cause recurrent inflammation **(pancreatitis)**.

7.5.4 Projection and structure of the pancreas

The pancreas is a 14–20 cm long (mostly 16 cm), parenchymatous organ with a lobular structure and an average weight of approx. 70 g (40–120 g). Due to its well-fixed position in the retroperitoneum, the pancreas projects relatively constantly in the central upper abdomen on the I.–II. lumbar vertebrae and is surrounded by the duodenum. The pancreas is divided into the **head** (Caput pancreatis), **neck** (Collum pancreatis), **body** (Corpus pancreatis) and **tail** (Cauda pancreatis) (➤ Fig. 7.38). The head runs downwards into a process that surrounds the A. and V. mesenterica superior. Due to its

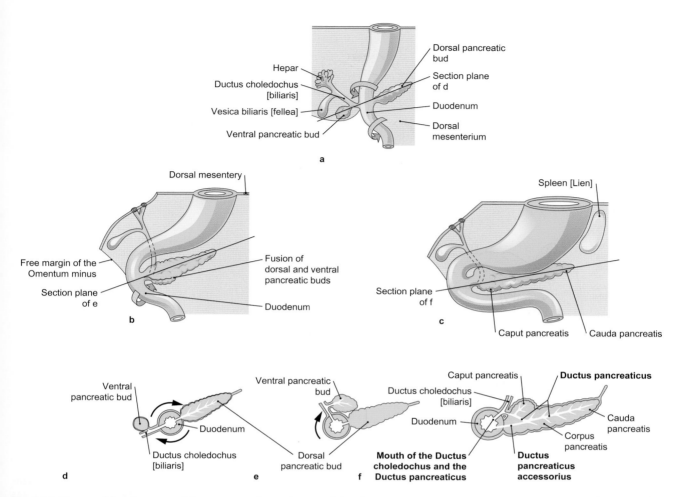

Fig. 7.39 Stages of development of the pancreas, in weeks 5–8 of development. a–c Fusion of both pancreatic buds; view from the left side. **d–f** Formation of the excretory ducts from both buds and representation of the confluence into the duodenum; schematic cross-sections through the pancreatic system and duodenum. [E581]

shape, it is referred to as a hook process (Proc. uncinatus). It is separated from the pancreas body by a notch (Incisura pancreatis). To the left, the head merges into the neck, which represents a narrow transition area (2 cm) to the body. The body is approximately triangular. The upper and lower edges (Margines superior and inferior) limit the anterior and posterior sides, whereby the anterior side is additionally divided into an upper and a lower section (Facies anterosuperior, anteroinferior and posterior) by an anterior border (Margo anterior), which is not always clearly visible.

7.5.5 Excretory duct system of the pancreas

In general (65%), the pancreas has **2 excretory ducts** (➤ Fig. 7.38):
- **Ductus pancreaticus** (Ductus WIRSUNGIANUS): the main excretory duct transfers pancreatic secretions from the body and tail and together with the bile duct (Ductus choledochus), conjoins with the Papilla duodeni major (Papilla VATERI) in the Pars descendens of the duodenum. Before the confluence the Ductus choledochus mostly (in 60% of cases) combines with the Ductus pancreaticus to the Ampulla hepatopancreatica and also the sphincter muscle (M. sphincter ductus pancreatici), which continues as the M. sphincter ampullae (ODDI) to the ampulla.
- **Ductus pancreaticus accessorius** (Ductus SANTORINI): the accessory duct conducts the secretions from the pancreas head and confluences 2 cm further orally on the Papilla duodeni minor.

Clinical remarks

The behaviour of the confluence of the excretory ducts has an impact on the progression of diseases of the pancreas. In addition to alcohol abuse, gall-stones in the Papilla duodeni major are the most common cause of inflammation of the pancreas **(pancreatitis)**, which is caused by a tailback of secretions with self-digestion. A Ductus pancreaticus accessorius with a separate confluence, which is formed in 65% of cases, can then prove to be useful when it communicates with the main duct, permitting an outflow of the digestive secretions.

NOTE

The presence of a main and an accessory duct, as well as the joining of the main excretory duct with the Ductus choledochus, is the norm and not the exception. The behaviour of the joining and confluence is of functional and clinical relevance.

7.5.6 Topography

The pancreas is **secondarily retroperitoneal** in the central upper abdomen. The **pancreatic head** is covered at the top by the Pars superior of the duodenum and adjoins the medial side of the Pars descendens of the duodenum (➤ Fig. 7.38). Here, the head is penetrated by the Ductus choledochus before joining with the Ductus

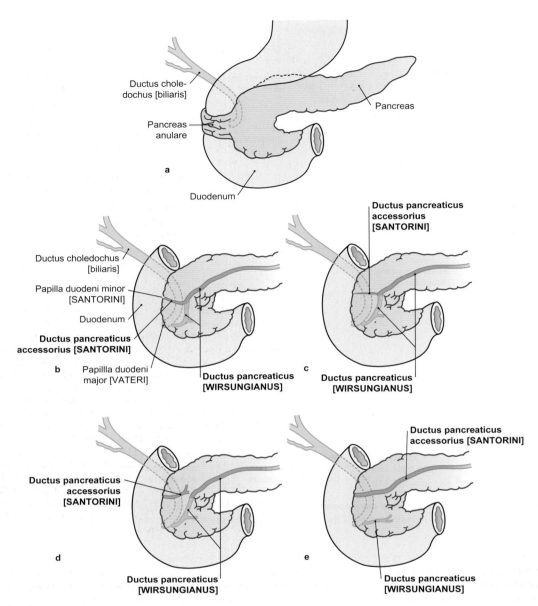

a

Ductus chole-
dochus [biliaris]

Pancreas
anulare

Pancreas

Duodenum

b

Ductus choledochus
[biliaris]

Papilla duodeni minor
[SANTORINI]

Duodenum

**Ductus pancreaticus
accessorius [SANTORINI]**

Papillla duodeni
major [VATERI]

**Ductus pancreaticus
[WIRSUNGIANUS]**

c

**Ductus pancreaticus
accessorius
[SANTORINI]**

**Ductus pancreaticus
[WIRSUNGIANUS]**

d

**Ductus pancreaticus
accessorius
[SANTORINI]**

Ductus pancreaticus
[WIRSUNGIANUS]

e

**Ductus pancreaticus
accessorius [SANTORINI]**

Ductus pancreaticus
[WIRSUNGIANUS]

Fig. 7.40 Malformations of pancreatic development. a Pancreas annulare: annular formation, which can lead to disorders of passage as a result of repositioning of the duodenum. **b–e** Normal (**b, c**) and incomplete (**d, e**) association of excretory ducts (Pancreas divisum). [L126]

pancreaticus. In front of the head is the Colon transversum. The **Proc. uncinatus** is appended downwards and encompasses the A. and V. mesenterica superior, which are accompanied by the lymphatic Trunci intestinales and pass behind the vessels (➤ Fig. 7.41). The head continues to the left in the **pancreatic neck**, which lies in front of the Vasa mesenterica superior. The portal vein is formed behind the neck by fusion of its main tributaries (V. mesenterica superior and V. splenica, which previously usually integrate the V. mesenterica inferior).

The **pancreatic body** then transverses the aorta and the vertebral column behind it and bends into the Bursa omentalis, which forms the posterior wall of the pancreas. This bulging is also called the Tuber omentale. The front side of the pancreas is covered by peritoneum and thus has a broad contact surface with the rear of the stomach, which forms the front wall of the Bursa omentalis (➤ Fig. 7.3). The posterior side of the pancreas is located on the right side directly on the V. cava inferior and has connections to the right V. renalis and the right A. and V. testicularis/ovarica, as well as to the adrenal glands on the left and the left lymphatic Trunci lumbales. The V. splenica is often embedded in the glandular parenchyma. At the top right edge of the body of the pancreas, the A. hepatica communis runs to the right, and the A. splenica to

the left. On the lower edge the Pars horizontalis of the duodenum is positioned on the left side.

The body runs left to the **pancreatic tail** and makes contact here with the hilum of the spleen behind the left colic flexure (➤ Fig. 7.42). On the dorsal side are the left renal blood vessels and the anterior side of the left kidney, separated by their different sheath systems.

Clinical remarks

As the Ductus choledochus runs through the head of the pancreas to the duodenum, this can result in a bile tailback with jaundice (icterus) in the event of a pancreatic carcinoma in the head of the gland. Tumours in other sections do not usually cause symptoms for a long time, so the prognosis on diagnosis is therefore often poor.

The close positional relationship of the pancreatic head to the A. and V. mesenterica superior and to the portal vein also harbours the danger that in the event of an **endoscopic examination of the Papilla duodeni major** for removal of a gall-stone or by contrast agent imaging of the biliary and pancreatic ducts (endoscopic retrograde cholangiopancreatography, ERCP) these vessels can be damaged, a situation that can normally only be resolved by emergency surgery.

7.5.7 Vessels and nerves of the pancreas

Arterial and venous supply

The pancreas is supplied via **2 separate arterial systems**, one for the head and the other for the body and tail (➤ Fig. 7.41):

- **Head and neck:** the double vascular ring consists of the **Aa. pancreaticoduodenales superiores anterior and posterior** (from the A. gastroduodenalis and thus the supply area of the Truncus coeliacus) and the **A. pancreaticoduodenalis inferior** with R. anterior and R. posterior (from the A. mesenterica superior, BÜHLER's anastomosis)
- **Body and tail: Rr. pancreatici** from the A. splenica, which form the A. pancreatica dorsalis behind the pancreas and the A. pancreatica inferior on the lower edge of the pancreas.

This intensive perfusion makes it clear why infarcts of this vital gland are rare.

The **veins** correspond to the arteries and form a vessel arcade ventrally and dorsally. These drain via the V. mesenterica superior and the V. splenica into the hepatic portal vein. The V. pancreaticoduodenalis superior posterior connects directly to the portal vein and does not open into one of the preceding main stems.

Lymph vessels

The different sections of the pancreas have **3 groups of regional lymph nodes** (➤ Fig. 7.42). From there, the lymph flows into the Nodi lymphoidei coeliaci and Nodi lymphoidei mesenterici superiores, before feeding into the Ductus thoracicus via the Trunci intestinales. The retroperitoneal location with its close proximity to various groups of lumbar lymph nodes (Nodi lymphoidei lumbales) and the left Trunci lumbares necessitates that there are extensive connections to other lymph nodes.

- Head and neck: **Nodi lymphoidei pancreaticoduodenales** along the same arteries (Aa. pancreaticoduodenales superiores anterior and posterior), connect from there via the Nodi lymphoidei hepatici to the Nodi lymphoidei coeliaci or directly to the Nodi lymphoidei mesenterici superiores.
- Body: **Nodi lymphoidei pancreatici superiores and inferiores** at the lower and upper edge of the organ and thus along the A. and V. splenica, and from there to the Nodi lymphoidei coeliaci and the Nodi lymphoidei mesenterici superiores.
- Tail: drainage to the **Nodi lymphoidei splenici** and from there to the Nodi lymphoidei coeliaci.

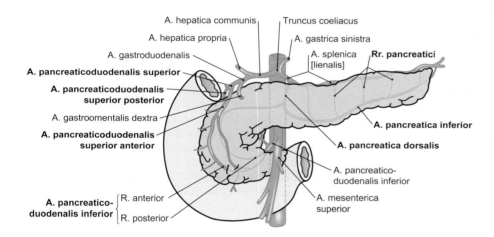

Fig. 7.41 Arteries of the pancreas. (according to [S010-1-16])

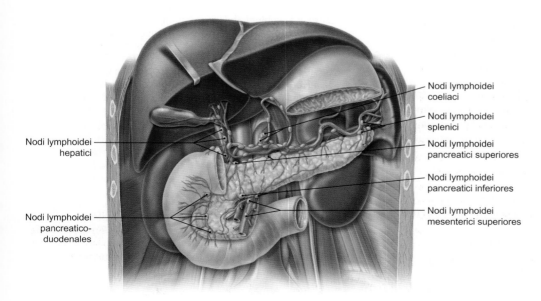

Fig. 7.42 Lymphatic drainage paths of the pancreas. Ventral view.

337

The diverse lymphatic drainage pathways explain why in cases of **pancreatic carcinoma** extensive **lymph node metastases** usually exist at the time of diagnosis. Because they usually cannot be completely removed, surgical treatment is rarely possible.

Innervation

The pancreas is innervated by the sympathetic and parasympathetic nervous systems. The parasympathetic nervous system promotes the formation of digestive enzymes, which results in secretions and insulin formation, while the sympathetic nervous system inhibits these functions.

Sympathic nervous system: the postganglionic nerve fibres, once switched, pass through the Plexus coeliacus as perivascular plexus, together with the various arteries, to the pancreas.

Parasympathetic nervous system: preganglionic nerve fibres sometimes reach the pancreas via perivascular plexus from the **Plexus coeliacus**, and sometimes directly from the **Truncus vagalis posterior** (and anterior) for the head.

The sympathetic and parasympathetic nervous systems also include afferent nerve fibres. The zone of the transmitted pain in the torso wall is not precisely localised. Pain will often be felt radiating like a belt around the central and left upper abdomen and if the retroperitoneal structures are involved, this is often dorsal to the left of the lower thoracic vertebral column.

For general organisation of the autonomic nervous system in the abdomen, see ➤ Chap. 7.8.5.

7.6 Spleen

After working through this chapter, you should be able to:
- understand the various functions of the spleen
- demonstrate the location and projection of the spleen on a dissection specimen and to know its classification in segments
- demonstrate the vessels and nerves of the spleen and explain their supply function for the surrounding organs

7.6.1 Overview

The spleen (or Lien) is located intraperitoneally in the left upper abdomen (➤ Fig. 7.43) and belongs to the secondary **lymphatic organs** together with all lymph nodes, the pharyngeal tonsils and the mucosa-associated lymphoid tissue, e.g. in the intestines.

7.6.2 Functions of the spleen

Out of the different functions of the spleen, the most important is the defence function:
- Immune defence against pathogens in the blood
- Degradation of defective and aging erythrocytes
- Storage of blood cells (thrombocytes)
- Blood formation (foetal period)

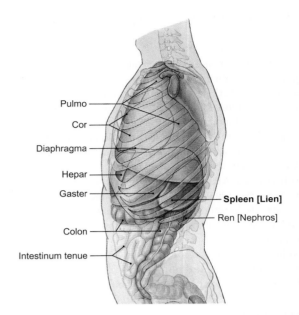

Fig. 7.43 Projection of the spleen on the body surface. View from the left side.

The **defence function** is undertaken by the 'white pulp', which is visible on the cut surface as white nodules. The initiation of a specific immune defence system against pathogens that have already reached the bloodstream, makes the spleen a very important organ. The spleen is not absolutely essential, but removing it predisposes to life-threatening infections. In addition, the spleen also has various functions with respect to **renewal of blood cells**, which are undertaken by the 'red pulp', the blood-filled parenchyma. Here, just as in bone marrow and the liver, old and in particular defective red blood cells (erythrocytes) are broken down. Although the spleen is very well supplied with blood, in humans it is not used to store larger quantities of blood but stores up to 30% of all platelets (thrombocytes) in the body. Together with the liver, it is responsible for **blood formation** during the foetal period and this can also support life in the event of bone marrow insufficiency.

The functions explain why injuries to the spleen (**splenic rupture**), e.g. in blunt abdominal trauma, can lead to life-threatening bleeding. In contrast to previously, attempts are made to preserve the spleen or at least parts of it since the risk of life-threatening infections (sepsis) significantly increases after its removal. Manipulation of the spleen, e.g. while being removed, can release large quantities of thrombocytes into the circulation, so that the risk of blood clots (**thrombi**) needs to be prevented as these can lead to a stroke or heart attack.

7.6.3 Development

Connective tissue and capsule of the spleen are formed in the *5th week* from the **Mesogastrium dorsale** from where it receives its coating from the Peritoneum viscerale (➤ Fig. 7.3). The connection to the stomach becomes the Lig. gastrosplenicum. The lymphocytes settle in the spleen in the 4th month.

7.6.4 Projection, construction and topography of the spleen

The spleen is reddish-grey to blueish-purple in colour in living people, is approximately 11 cm long, 7 cm wide and 4 cm thick, and weighs 150 g (80–300 g). It is located in the left upper abdomen and is well protected **intraperitoneally** by the costal arch in a separate compartment, which is known as the **splenic niche** (➤ Fig. 7.43). Here, the spleen sits on the Lig. phrenicocolicum, which connects the left colic flexure with the diaphragm. The position of the spleen is strongly dependent on breathing as a result of its position under the diaphragm and it projects in a respiratory central position onto the IXth–XIth ribs, from where it follows the Xth rib with its longitudinal axis. Therefore, the spleen is only palpable if enlarged.

The spleen has a convex Facies diaphragmatica (➤ Fig. 7.44), which has contact to the diaphragm, and a concave Facies visceralis with **contact to various organs:**
- to the posterior gastric wall (Facies gastrica, posterior, above), separated by the Recessus splenicus of the Bursa omentalis
- to the left colic flexure (Facies colica, anterior, above)
- to the lateral margin of the kidneys (Facies renalis, below)
- to the pancreatic tail (Facies pancreatica, at the hilum)

The edge facing upwards (Margo superior), which separates these two areas is usually irregular while the bottom edge (Margo inferior) appears smooth. From their position in the upper abdomen, one pole is directed forwards (Extremitas anterior) and the other directed backwards (Extremitas posterior). The Facies visceralis is divided into two halves by the **Hilum splenicum**, the point at which the peritoneal duplicatures insert and the vessels and nerves enter and exit. The **Lig. gastrosplenicum**, as part of the Omentum majus, connects the spleen forwards with the stomach, while the **Lig. phrenicosplenicum** and the **Lig. splenorenale** connect backwards with the diaphragm and kidney, from which they are separated by their sheaths (➤ Fig. 7.3).

A special feature is the existence in 5–30% of cases of an **accessory spleen** that is separated from the main organ, which is mostly located close to the hilum in one of the peritoneal duplicatures.

> **Clinical remarks**
>
> On removal of the spleen (**splenectomy**) investigations should be carried out to determine the existence of an accessory spleen. An accessory spleen can undertake the functions of the main organ on its removal, which may prevent the loss of the defence function; however, if the reason for the splenectomy is defective red blood cells, because they have been abnormally broken down in the spleen and have therefore caused anaemia, any possible accessory spleen must also be removed.

7.6.5 Vessels and nerves of the spleen

Arterial and venous supply

The **A. splenica** is the only supplying vessel and originates as a branch of the Truncus coeliacus. It follows a winding path at the upper edge of the pancreas along to the hilum of the spleen, where it branches into 2–3 main branches and then several terminal branches (➤ Fig. 7.42). On the way, the A. splenica supplies the pancreas (Rr. pancreatici) and the stomach (A. gastrica posterior, Aa. gastricae breves, A. gastroomentalis sinistra).

The terminal branches of the A. splenica are functional terminal arteries and subdivide the spleen into 3–6 variable, wedge-shaped arranged segments. (➤ Fig. 7.45).

The **V. splenica** has tributaries that correspond to the arteries, which run in the Lig. splenorenale and then on the posterior side of the pancreas to its neck area, where it joins with the V. mesenter-

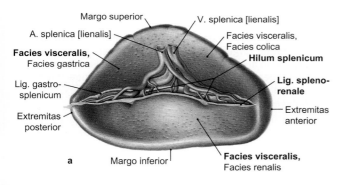
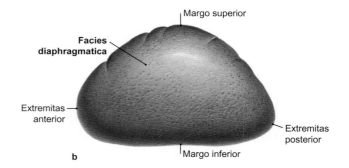

Fig. 7.44 Spleen. a Medial ventral view. **b** Cranial lateral view.

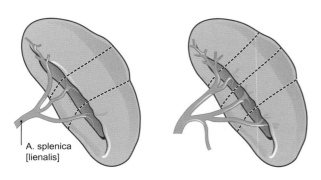
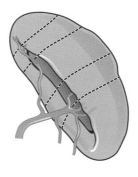

Fig. 7.45 Segments of the spleen. Schematic representation of 3, 4 or 5 segments. [L126]

ica superior to the portal vein. In the majority of cases (70%) it previously receives the V. mesenterica inferior.

Lymph vessels

The regional lymph nodes are the **Nodi lymphoidei splenici** on the hilum of the spleen, which also receive lymph from the fundus of the stomach and the pancreatic tail. From there, the lymph flows via the **Nodi lymphoidei coeliaci** and the Trunci intestinales into the Ductus thoracicus.

Innervation

The spleen is largely innervated by the **sympathetic nervous system** but also by the **parasympathetic** nervous system (**Plexus splenicus**). After switching in the Plexus coeliacus, the postganglionic sympathetic nerve fibres continue as a perivascular network together with the preganglionic parasympathetic fibres of the A. splenica. The sympathetic nervous system throttles the perfusion, otherwise little is known about autonomic regulation.

The sympathic and parasympathic nervous systems also have **afferent nerve fibres**. The zone of the transmitted pain on the torso wall is diffuse and projects onto the central or left upper abdomen, on dermatomes T8–9.

For general organisation of the autonomic nervous system in the abdomen, see ➤ Chap. 7.8.5.

7.7 Peritoneal cavity

Skills

After working through this chapter, you should be able to:
- explain the structure of the abdominal cavity and elucidate the peritoneal relationships of the individual abdominal organs on a dissection specimen
- describe the construction of the Omentum majus and Omentum minus with functions and vessels and nerves
- illustrate the recesses of the peritoneal cavity and to explain their clinical relevance
- know the location and structure of the Bursa omentalis in detail and to illustrate it on a dissection specimen

7.7.1 Overview

The **abdominal cavity** (Cavitas abdominalis) is divided by the Colon transversum into the upper and lower abdomen. In accordance with its positional relationships, the abdominal cavity is divided into a **peritoneal cavity** (Cavitas peritonealis), which is lined with peritoneum and an **extraperitoneal space** (Spatium extraperitoneale) between the Peritoneum parietale and the torso wall. Dorsally, the extraperitoneal space is expanded to the **retroperitoneum** (Spatium retroperitoneale), which continues caudally into the pelvic cavity in the **subperitoneal space** (Spatium extraperitoneale pelvis) (➤ Chap. 8.7.1). This results in different positional relationships for the organs.

Intraperitoneal organs are covered on their entire surface by Peritoneum viscerale, which represents the Tunica serosa of the respective organs. The organs have small suspensory ligaments (mesentery and ligaments) that contain the supplying vessels and nerves as peritoneal duplicatures; at their root, the Peritoneum viscerale of the organs changes into the Peritoneum parietale of the abdominal cavity wall.

The individual peritoneal duplicatures are described with respect to the respective organs. For the development of the peritoneal cavity, see ➤ Chap. 6.5.5.

Intraperitoneal are:
- Pars abdominalis of the oesophagus
- Stomach
- Pars superior of the duodenum
- Jejunum
- Ileum
- Caecum
- Appendix vermiformis
- Colon transversum
- Colon sigmoideum
- Liver
- Gall bladder
- Spleen

as well as the pelvic organs:
- Body of the uterus
- Adnexe (Ovarium and Tuba uterina)

Retroperitoneal organs are mostly only covered on their anterior side by the Peritoneum parietale. These organs can also be created as a primary retroperitoneal organs outside of the abdominal cavity, such as:
- Kidneys
- Adrenal glands

The primary retroperitoneal organs and subperitoneal located organs are described in ➤ Chap. 8. In contrast, the **secondary retroperitoneal organs** are only shifted to the dorsal torso wall during development. These include:
- Other parts of the duodenum
- Colon ascendens
- Colon descendens
- Proximal Rectum (up to Flexura sacralis)
- Pancreas

The secondary retroperitoneal organs can be bluntly separated from the primary retroperitoneal organs in the preparation.

Clinical remarks

This differences in location are important in terms of **access routes during surgery** because an organ situated retroperitoneally is also accessible from the dorsal side without opening the peritoneal cavity. This allows the risk of infection of the abdominal cavity (peritonitis) or postoperative adhesions to be reduced.

NOTE

Intraperitoneal:
- are located in the peritoneal cavity (Cavitas peritonealis) of the abdominal cavity or of the pelvis
- covered from all sides with Peritoneum viscerale
- secured with peritoneal duplicatures (mesentery and ligaments)

Extraperitoneal:
- are located outside the peritoneal cavity in the retroperitoneal space of the abdominal cavity (Spatium retroperitoneale) or the subperitoneal space of the pelvis (Spatium extraperitoneale pelvis)
- are not or only partially covered by Peritoneum parietale

The abdominal cavity is subdivided by the Colon transversum with its Mesocolon transversum into the upper and the lower abdomen. The **upper abdomen** ('glandular abdomen') is occupied to the right by the liver and the gallbladder and to the left by the stomach which

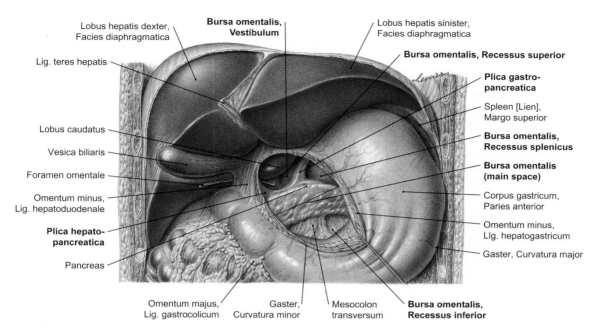

Lobus hepatis dexter, Facies diaphragmatica
Bursa omentalis, Vestibulum
Lobus hepatis sinister, Facies diaphragmatica
Bursa omentalis, Recessus superior
Lig. teres hepatis
Plica gastro-pancreatica
Spleen [Lien], Margo superior
Lobus caudatus
Vesica biliaris
Bursa omentalis, Recessus splenicus
Foramen omentale
Bursa omentalis (main space)
Omentum minus, Lig. hepatoduodenale
Corpus gastricum, Paries anterior
Plica hepato-pancreatica
Omentum minus, Llg. hepatogastricum
Pancreas
Gaster, Curvatura major
Omentum majus, Lig. gastrocolicum
Gaster, Curvatura minor
Mesocolon transversum
Bursa omentalis, Recessus inferior

Fig. 7.46 Location of the viscera in the upper abdomen. Ventral view.

continues in the Pars superior of the duodenum. Behind the stomach is the spleen and the pancreas in the retroperitoneum. Between the liver and stomach/duodenum extends the Omentum minus as a frontal peritoneal duplication (➤ Fig. 7.46).

The **lower abdomen** ('intestinal abdomen') contains the other sections of the small and large intestines and is overlaid to the front by the large Omentum majus that originates on the stomach. In addition to the various sections of duodenum and large intestine, also located in the retroperitoneum are the kidneys and adrenal glands.

7.7.2 Omentum majus and Omentum minus

Omentum majus

The Omentum majus is an apron-shaped peritoneal duplicature with an area of approximately 1 m², which overlays the organs of the lower abdomen. Depending on the type of constitution, different amounts of fat are stored in the network, so that its colour varies from translucent to yellowish. The Omentum majus consists of four parts:

- Lig. gastrocolicum
- Lig. gastrosplenicum
- Lig. gastrophrenicum
- Apron-shaped section

The most important peritoneal duplicature is the Lig. gastrocolicum, which connects the large curvature of the stomach with the Taenia omentalis of the Colon transversum. This ligament is the origin of the Omentum majus, which develops dorsally in the Mesogastrium and contains the supplying vessels and nerves. To the left it continues in the Lig. gastrosplenicum and up into the Lig. gastrophrenicum. The apron-shaped part is highly variable in its extent and can take up very different positions.

Functions of the Omentum majus:
- Secretion and absorption of peritoneal fluids
- Immune defence: arteriovenous anastomoses ('milk stains') for the outflow of leukocytes
- Mechanical protection
- Thermal insulation

Vessels and nerves of the Omentum majus:
The Omentum majus is supplied by the vessels and nerves along the greater stomach curvature:

- **Aa. and Vv. gastroomentales dextra** (predominantly with 5–8 Rr. omentales) **and sinistra** (usually only one branch)
- **Nodi lymphoidei gastroomentales dextri and sinistri**, from here via lymph nodes along the branches of the Truncus coeliacus to the Nodi lymphoidei coeliaci
- **Sympathetic** and **parasympathetic nervous systems** from the **Plexus coeliacus** via the periarterial plexus

Clinical remarks

The apron-shaped section can cover inflammation or perforation of the stomach and intestines and thus prevent **inflammation of the abdominal cavity (peritonitis)**.

Due to the large surface and thus very effective turnover of peritoneal fluid, in the event of kidney failure or poisoning by the repeated introduction of electrolyte solutions **peritoneal dialysis** can be used to removed toxins from the blood.

As a result of its developmental history, the Omentum majus belongs to the stomach and is supplied by the vessels and nerves at the greater curvature of the stomach. It must therefore, e.g. in the case of a colonisation of tumour cells **(peritoneal carcinomatosis)** be separated at the stomach and not at the colon.

Omentum minus

The Omentum minus is a frontal peritoneal duplicature, which connects the liver with the stomach and duodenum and forms the anterior wall of the Bursa omentalis (see below). Parts of the Omentum minus are:

- Lig. hepatogastricum to the small curvature of the stomach
- Lig. hepatoduodenale to the Pars superior of the duodenum

The **Lig. hepatogastricum** contains the vessels and nerves, making it the largest part of the omentum minus. Under the Lig. hepatoduodenale is the opening of the Bursa omentalis (Foramen omentale/ epiploicum).

In the **Lig. hepatoduodenale** the liver triad runs in the following order to the liver:

- Ductus choledochus (right)
- A. hepatica propria (left)
- V. portae hepatis (posterior)
- Lymph vessels, lymph nodes and autonomic nerves (Plexus hepaticus)

The Omentum minus is supplied by the **vessels and nerves** along the lesser stomach curvature:

- **Aa. and Vv. gastricae dextra and sinistra**
- **Nodi lymphoidei gastrici dextri and sinistri**, from here via lymph nodes along the branches of the Truncus coeliacus to the Nodi lymphoidei coeliaci
- **Sympathetic** and **parasympathetic** nerve fibers from the **Plexus coeliacus** via the periarterial plexus. The Truncus vagalis anterior gives up the Rr. hepatici to the Plexus hepaticus, from which the Rr. pylorici reach the pylorus of the stomach.

In anatomical terminology, many other peritoneal duplicatures are optionally named and assigned to the two omenta. Since this is not useful in a medical sense, we will forgo it here.

7.7.3 Recessus of the peritoneal cavity

The peritoneal duplicatures, which raise up the relief of the rear wall of the peritoneal cavity as folds (Plicae) and ligaments (Ligamenta), form the various **recesses (Recessus)** that represent the bulges of the peritoneal cavity. Due to their clinical relevance, the main recesses are described briefly (➤ Fig. 7.47).

Recessus of the epigastrum (supramesocolic compartment)

The largest and in terms of its extent, the most complex of these recesses, is the **Bursa omentalis**. The Bursa omentalis is a sliding space between the stomach and the pancreas, which only communicates with the abdominal cavity via the Foramen omentale (Foramen epiploicum) under the Lig. hepatoduodenale. Due to its extent, the Bursa omentalis is also referred to as the lesser sac of the peritoneal cavity.

The Bursa omentalis is divided into 4 sections (➤ Fig. 7.46):

- **Foramen omentale** (Foramen epiploicum): the entrance to the Bursa omentalis has a diameter of approximately 3 cm and is surrounded at the front by the Lig. hepatoduodenale, above by the Lobus caudatus of the liver, below by the Pars superior of the duodenum and behind by the V. cava inferior.
- **Vestibulum:** the front of the Vestibulum is delimited by the Omentum minus and with a **Recessus superior** reaches behind the liver.
- **Isthmus:** the narrowing between the first and main space is delimited by two peritoneal folds, on the right side through the Plica hepatopancreatica, which is raised by the A. hepatica communis, and on the left through the Plica gastropancreatica, in which the A. gastrica sinistra runs.
- **Main space:** it lies between the stomach (in front) and the pancreas or the parietal peritoneum of the abdominal wall (behind).

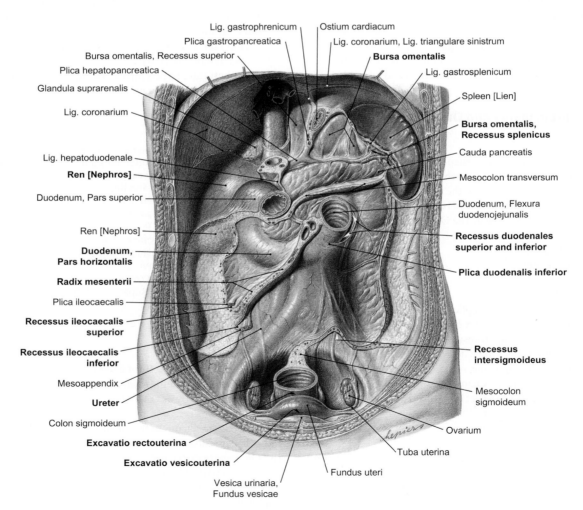

Fig. 7.47 Dorsal wall of the peritoneal cavity with recess spaces (Recessus). Ventral view.

Lig. gastrophrenicum
Plica gastropancreatica
Bursa omentalis, Recessus superior
Plica hepatopancreatica
Glandula suprarenalis
Lig. coronarium
Lig. hepatoduodenale
Ren [Nephros]
Duodenum, Pars superior
Ren [Nephros]
Duodenum, Pars horizontalis
Radix mesenterii
Plica ileocaecalis
Recessus ileocaecalis superior
Recessus ileocaecalis inferior
Mesoappendix
Ureter
Colon sigmoideum
Excavatio rectouterina
Excavatio vesicouterina
Vesica urinaria, Fundus vesicae

Ostium cardiacum
Lig. coronarium, Lig. triangulare sinistrum
Bursa omentalis
Lig. gastrosplenicum
Spleen [Lien]
Bursa omentalis, Recessus splenicus
Cauda pancreatis
Mesocolon transversum
Duodenum, Flexura duodenojejunalis
Recessus duodenales superior and inferior
Plica duodenalis inferior
Recessus intersigmoideus
Mesocolon sigmoideum
Ovarium
Tuba uterina
Fundus uteri

The **Recessus splenicus** stretches to the left until the hilum of the spleen and the **Recessus inferior** under the Lig. gastrocolicum up to the attachment of the mesocolon at the Colon transversum.

Under the diaphragm above the Facies diaphragmatica of the liver is the **Recessus subphrenicus**, which is divided by the Lig. falciforme hepatis into a right and left section, and by the Lig. triangulare dextrum/sinistrum into an upper and lower section. At the bottom right section, the **Recessus subhepaticus** follows, behind which in the upper section is the right kidney. This part is also known as the **Recessus hepatorenalis**.

Recessus of the lower abdomen (inframesocolic compartment)

This compartment is divided by the mesenteric root of the small intestine into a right and left infracolic space below the Mesocolon transversum (➤ Fig. 7.47). Lateral of the Colon ascendens and descendens are the paracolic trenches (**Sulci paracolici**) and below the Mesocolon sigmoideum of the **Recessus intersigmoideus**. The right paracolic trench is directly connected to the Recessus subhepaticus and the right Recessus subphrenicus, while on the left, the Lig. phrenicocolicum represents a barrier.

At the Flexura duodenojejunalis the Plicae duodenales superior and inferior form 2 recessed areas (**Recessus duodenales superior and inferior**) (➤ Fig. 7.47). There are further recesses at the confluence of the ileum, into the Caecum (**Recessus ileocaecales superior and inferior**) and the **Recessus retrocaecalis**, in which the Appendix vermiformis is usually raised behind the Caecum. In the pelvic section of the peritoneal cavity, there are various recesses in front of the rectum, dependention sex. In women, the space is limited anteriorly by the uterus. This **Excavatio rectouterina** (DOUGLAS pouch) is the lowest point of the female peritoneal cavity (➤ Fig. 7.47). The **Excavatio vesicouterina** located in front between the bladder and uterus does not go quite as far caudally. In men there is only one recess, which reaches at the front as far as the bladder and is accordingly known as the **Excavatio rectovesicalis**.

Clinical remarks

The **Bursa omentalis** is, like the rest of the peritoneal cavity recesses, of clinical significance as pathological processes can occur here:
- Spreading of tumours (peritoneal carcinomatosis)
- Inflammation of the peritoneum (peritonitis)
- Entrapment of the small intestinal loops (internal hernias)

Therefore, during operations of the abdomen, the surgeon inspects the Bursa omentalis in order to avoid overlooking any symptoms.

During operations on the upper abdomen, e.g. procedures on the pancreas, the surgeon has recourse to 3 **access paths** in the Bursa omentalis:
- through the Omentum minus
- through the Lig. gastrocolicum
- through the Mesocolon transversum

In the **Recessus duodenalis inferior** (and superior) most frequently (over 50%) of all recesses, entrapment of small intestinal sections occurs (TREITZ hernias). The incarceration can cause a blockage (ileus) and bowel infarction.

In an upright position inflammatory exudate or pus can accumulate in the deepest recesses of the peritoneal cavity, the **Excavatio rectovesicalis** in men and the **Excavatio vesicouterina** (DOUGLAS pouch) in women if there is inflammation in the lower abdomen, which can be detected in sonography as free liquid. In bedridden patients, inflammatory secretions

accumulate as a result of cranially oriented circulation of peritoneal fluid, especially in the right **Recessus subphrenicus** and the **Recessus subhepaticus.** On the left side, the circulation should be limited by the Lig. phrenicocolicum. With operations in the left upper abdomen, e.g. on the spleen, accumulation of fluid in the left recessus subphrenicus is very common. Inflammatory exsudates must be removed using sonographic or CT-guided drainage, as otherwise treatment resistant inflammation centres (**peritoneal collections of pus** or **abscesses**) may form.

7.8 Vessels and nerves of the peritoneal cavity

Skills

After working through this chapter, you should be able to:
- understand the system of vessels and nerves of the peritoneal cavity so that you can understand the origin of the supply in the individual organs
- recognise the visceral branches of the abdominal aorta with their supply areas and identify them on a dissection specimen
- explain the organisation of the autonomic nervous system in the peritoneal cavity and understand the origin of the nerve fibres in the individual organs

---

7.8.1 Overview

The vessels and nerves of the **abdominal cavity** serve to supply the viscera and also the dorsal abdominal wall. The major arterial, venous and lymphatic vessels run in the **retroperitoneum** and continue caudally to the pelvic cavity into the **subperitoneal space** as well as cranially to the **dorsal mediastinum of the thoracic cavity**. The plexus of the autonomic nervous system that innervate the organs of the abdomen and pelvic floor lie ventrally on the aorta and are caudally connected with the ligaments in the connective tissue of the pelvis. The branches of the vascular stems and autonomic nerve plexus run dorsally via the peritoneal duplicatures (**mesenteries**) into the **peritoneal cavity** and supply the respective organs.

In this chapter only the vessels and nerves of the peritoneal cavity are described in the overview. The individual vascular branches and their paths are explained alongside the vascular and nervous of the respective organs.

The large vascular stems are dealt with alongside the vessels and nerves of the retroperitoneal space and pelvic cavity (➤ Chap. 8.8) and presented in their cranial continuation in the chapter on the thoracic cavity (➤ Chap. 6.6).

7.8.2 Arteries of the peritoneal cavity

The abdominal viscera are supplied by the **3 unpaired arterial branches** that originate ventrally from the abdominal section of the aorta (Pars abdominalis aortae):
- Truncus coeliacus
- A. mesenterica superior
- A. mesenterica inferior

The 3 arteries, together with the branches of the A. iliaca interna, enter vascular connections (**anastomoses**) one below the other. 3 anastomoses are important:

- Connections between **Truncus coeliacus** and **A. mesenterica superior** via the Aa. pancreaticoduodenales (BÜHLER's anastomosis)
- Connections between the **Aa. mesentericae superior and inferior:** RIOLAN's anastomosis between the A. colica media and sinistra
- The plexus of the rectal arteries: this connects the A. rectalis superior from the **A. mesenterica inferior** with the Aa. rectales media and inferior from the supply area of the **A. iliaca interna**, which is part of the arteries of the pelvic cavity.

> **Clinical remarks**
>
> The **anastomoses** can prevent an **intestinal or pancreatic infarction** in the case of an occlusion of a vessel. In addition, the blood vessels around the rectum can also maintain a certain amount of blood supply to the legs if the blood supply is impaired by a narrowing of the distal abdominal aorta or the proximal iliac arteries.

Truncus coeliacus

The Truncus coeliacus originates as the first unpaired branch of the aorta (➤ Fig. 7.48).While still in the retroperitoneal space behind the Bursa omentalis the short stem (mostly 2–3 cm long) divides into the **3 major branches** that supply the organs of the upper abdomen (stomach, duodenum, liver, gall bladder, pancreas and spleen):

- **A. gastrica sinistra:** runs to the upper left and gives up the Plica gastropancreatica in the rear wall of the Bursa omentalis. The vessel is usually stronger than the A. gastrica dextra which it anastomoses with on the small stomach curvature

- **A. hepatica communis:** turns right and forms the Plica hepatopancreatica of the Bursa omentalis, before dividing into its main branches:
  - **A. hepatica propria:** gives off the A. gastrica dextra then supplies the liver and gall bladder (A. cystica)
  - **A. gastroduodenalis:** descends behind the pylorus or duodenum, divides into the A. gastroomentalis dextra for the greater stomach curvature and into the A. pancreaticoduodenalis superior anterior and posterior, which anastomose with the A. pancreaticoduodenalis inferior from the A. mesenterica superior and supplies the pancreatic head and duodenum. Various small branches of the A. gastroduodenalis on and behind the Pars superior duodeni are described as A. supraduodenalis and Aa. retroduodenales
- **A. splenica:** runs to the bottom left and on the upper margin of the pancreas, and on its way to the spleen gives off the following branches:
  - **Rr. pancreatici** to the pancreas
  - **A. gastrica posterior** to the stomach (in 30–60%)
  - **A. gastroomentalis sinistra:** runs from the left to the greater stomach curvature and anastomoses with the A. gastroomentalis dextra
  - **Aa. gastricae breves:** short branches to the fundus of the stomach
  - **Rr. splenici:** terminal branches to the spleen

A. mesenterica superior

The A. mesenterica superior originates unpaired from the aorta directly below the Truncus coeliacus (1–2 cm), initially runs retroperitoneally behind the pancreas and then into the Mesenterium (➤ Fig. 7.49). It supplies parts of the pancreas and duodenum, the entire small intestine, and the large intestine up to the left colic flexure.

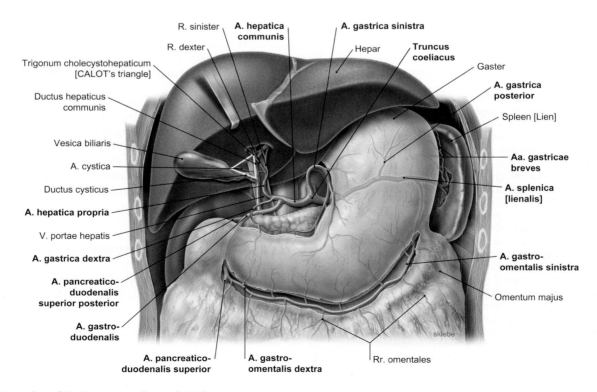

Fig. 7.48 Branches of the Truncus coeliacus. [L238]

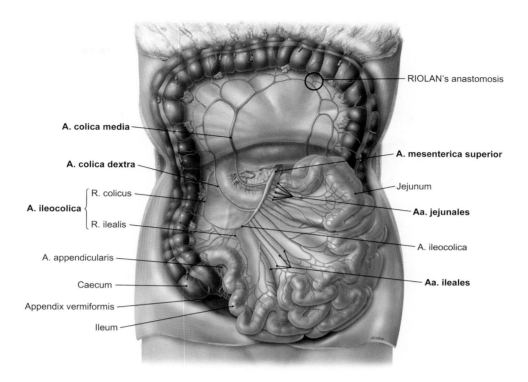

Fig. 7.49 A. mesenterica superior. Ventral view. Colon transversum folded upwards. (according to [S010-1-16])

Branches of the A. mesenterica superior:
- **A. pancreaticoduodenalis inferior:** usually goes off to the upper right; R. anterior and R. posterior anastomose with the Aa. pancreaticoduodenales superiores anterior and posterior from the supply area of the Truncus coeliacus (A. gastroduodenalis)
- **Aa. jejunales** (4–5) and **Aa. ileales** (12): originate to the left from the main vessel
- **A. colica media:** originates from the right side, anastomises with the A. colica dextra and the A. colica sinistra (RIOLAN's anastomosis) from the A. mesenterica inferior
- **A. colica dextra:** runs to the Colon ascendens
- **A. ileocolica:** supplies the distal ileum, caecum and Appendix vermiformis. Branches:
  - **R. ilealis** to the terminal ileum (connected with the last A. ilealis)
  - **R. colicus** (anastomoses with the A. colica dextra)
  - **A. caecalis anterior** and **A. caecalis posterior** on both sides of the Caecum
  - **A. appendicularis**, supplies the Appendix vermiformis

A. mesenterica inferior
The A. mesenterica inferior originates unpaired from the Aorta to the left, 6–7 cm below the A. mesenterica inferior branches off 6–7 cm below the A. mesenterica superior and 3–5 cm above the aortic bifurcation and then descends, whereby it runs retroperitoneally on the left colonic flexure except for a short end portion. It supplies the Colon descendens and Colon sigmoideum, the rectum and the upper anal canal. After 3–4 cm, the artery divides into an ascending and a descending main branch.

Branches of the A. mesenterica inferior
- **A. colica sinistra:** rises on the Colon descendens, anastomises with the A. colica media from the A. mesenterica superior (RIOLAN's anastomosis) ➤ Fig. 7.50
- **Aa. sigmoideae:** several (2–5) branches to the Colon sigmoideum

- **A. rectalis superior:** extends from above to the rectum, which predominantly supplies it and also feeds the cavernous body in the upper section of the anal canal, which is a part of the continence organ

7.8.3 Veins of the peritoneal cavity

In contrast to the arterial branches, which originate from the abdominal section of the aorta, the veins of the individual abdominal organs are not connected to the lower vena cava inferior (V. cava inferior) in the retroperitoneum, but join together with the **hepatic portal vein (V. portae hepatis)**, which carries the nutrient-rich blood from the intestine and the liver (➤ Fig. 7.31). The V. mesenterica superior is joined with the V. splenica behind the neck of the pancreas, which mostly (70%) has previously received the V. mesenterica inferior.

7.8.4 Lymph vessels of the peritoneal cavity

The 3 stations of the **collecting lymph nodes**, which receive all the lymph of the intraperitoneal and secondary retroperitoneal abdominal organs, are in the retroperitoneal space at the outlets of the 3 large unpaired abdominal arteries (➤ Fig. 7.48). They thereby drain the following organs:
- **Nodi lymphoidei coeliaci:** stomach, duodenum and pancreas, liver, gall bladder, spleen
- **Nodi lymphoidei mesenterici superiores:** duodenum and pancreas, 'right-sided large intestine' (caecum, appendix, Colon ascendens and Colon transversum)
- **Nodi lymphoidei mesenterici inferiores:** 'left-sided large intestine' (Colon descendens and Colon sigmoideum, proximal rectum)

The lymph flows from the collecting lymph nodes via the **Trunci intestinales**, which run in the Radix mesenterii together with the

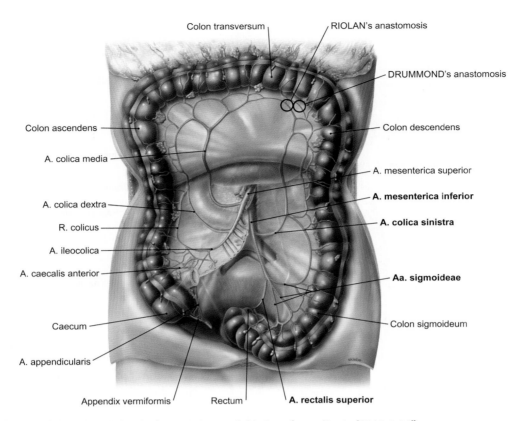

Fig. 7.50 **A. mesenterica inferior.** Ventral view. Colon transversum folded up. (according to [S010-1-16])

A. and V. mesenterica superior, as well as the exit of the Truncus coeliacus and join the retroperitoneum dorsal right of the aorta with the Trunci lumbales to the **Cisterna chyli** from which the **Ductus thoracicus** emerges cranially a main lymphatic stem of the body (➤ Fig. 7.23).

7.8.5 Nerves of the peritoneal cavity

The abdominal viscera are innervated by the plexus of the autonomic nervous system, which lie anteriorly of the abdominal section of the aorta and in their entirety form the **Plexus aorticus abdominalis**. The plexus, which therefore lies in the retroperitoneum, contains **sympathetic** and **parasympathetic** nerve fibres. Their nerve fibres reach the target organs mainly as periarterial plexus, which run in the peritoneal duplicatures of the mesenteries and thus intraperitoneally.

In order to understand the organisation of the autonomic nerve plexus of the abdominal organs, it is important to look at the basic structure of the autonomic nervous system first.

The fundamental difference of autonomic efference compared to somatic efference is that 2 neurons are connected in series. The first **preganglionic** neuron, along with its nerve cell body (Pericaryon) sits in the central nervous system (CNS) and sends its axon as a nerve fibre into the peripheral nervous system (PNS), where the second **postganglionic** neurons sit in their nodular-shaped structures **(ganglia)**. The switch from preganglionic to postganglionic neurons sitting in the ganglion happens via synaptic switching (➤ Fig. 7.51).

The preganglionic neurons of the **sympathetic nervous system** are located in the lateral horns of the thoracic and lumbar sections of the spinal cord (**C8–L3**), whereas the **parasympathetic neurons**, are in the nuclei of the **cranial nerves III, VII, IX and X**, as well as

in the sacral part of the spinal cord (**S2–4**), which is why the parasympathetic nervous system as a **craniosacral** part of the autonomic nervous system is in opposition to the **thoracolumbar** sympathetic nervous system.

Sympathetic nervous system

The preganglionic neurons of the sympathetic nervous system engage with the **anterior root of the spinal cord** and go through the Rr. communicantes albi of the spinal nerves to the **sympathetic trunk** (Truncus sympathicus), which forms a chain of ganglia both sides of the vertebral column (paravertebral) (➤ Fig. 7.51); however, the nerve fibres for the abdominal cavity are **not** switched in these ganglia of the sympathetic trunk; instead they run through them and run with the two visceral nerves (**N. splanchnicus major**, T5–9, and **N. splanchnicus minor**, T10–11) through the diaphragm to the ganglia on the abdominal section of the Aorta (prevertebral), where they are finally switched on the postganglionic neurones. In addition, the prevertebral ganglia also receive nerve fibres from the lumbar spinal cord segments, which reach the nerve plexus around the aorta via the abdominal part of the sympathetic trunk with its visceral nerves (Nn. splanchnici lumbales).

Parasympathetic nervous system

The preganglionic neurons of the parasympathetic nerves run with the **N. vagus [X]** from the base of the skull through the chest cavity and finally pass through the diaphragm as Trunci vagales anterior and posterior with the oesophagus. The **Truncus vagalis anterior** as a result of intestinal rotation, arises mainly from the left N. vagus, the **Truncus vagalis posterior** accordingly from the right N. vagus. In particular, branches (Rr. coeliaci) from the Truncus vagalis posterior extend to the Plexus coeliacus and further to the Plexus mesentericus superior, which ventrally surrounds the abdominal Aorta.

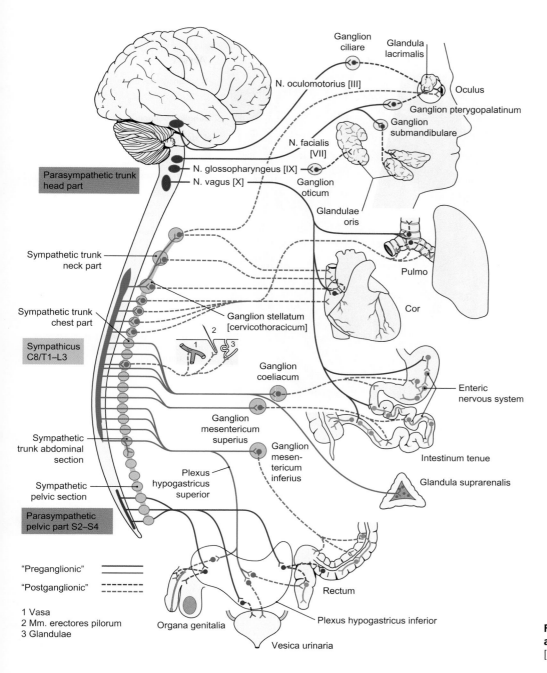

Fig. 7.51 Organisation of the autonomic nervous system. [L106]

Plexus aorticus abdominalis

The organisation of the autonomic nerve plexus of the abdominal Aorta (Plexus aorticus abdominalis) is easy to understand when you factor in that each plexus lies at the exit of the arterial branch of the same name and reaches the arterial target organs with the blood vessels (➤ Fig. 7.52, ➤ Fig. 8.64). Therefore, the arterial and nervous supply areas are similar.

While the sympathetic neurons descend from the Plexus coeliacus to the Plexus mesentericus superior from cranial to caudal and for the Plexus mesentericus inferior receives additional nerve fibres from the Nn. splanchnici lumbales, the innervation and supply area of the N. vagus (cranial parasympathetic nervous system) ends on the left colic flexure and, therefore, with the Plexus mesentericus superior (traditionally known as CANNON's point).

The left-sided sections of the large intestine receive their nerve fibres, as do all the pelvic organs, from the sacral parasympathetic trunk (S2–4), where they leave as the **Nn. splanchnici pelvici**, and then in the **Plexus hypogastricus inferior** in the vicinity of the rectum are switched to postganglionic neurons (➤ Fig. 7.52). The postganglionic nerve fibres ascend only to a small part of the Plexus mesentericus inferior and predominantly reach the Colon descendens and Colon sigmoideum as well as the proximal rectum as direct branches (➤ Fig. 7.52).

NOTE

The **plexus** of the abdominal aorta contains **sympathetic and parasympathetic** neurons. The **ganglia** of the arteries of the same name, however, are purely **sympathetic nerves.** The result is that the perivascular nerve plexus around the visceral arteries contain postganglionic sympathetic and preganglionic parasympathetic nerve fibres.

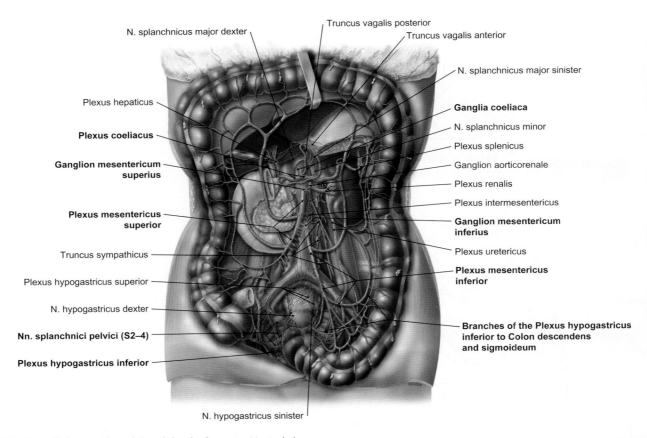

N. splanchnicus major dexter

Truncus vagalis posterior

Truncus vagalis anterior

N. splanchnicus major sinister

Plexus hepaticus

Plexus coeliacus

Ganglion mesentericum superius

Plexus mesentericus superior

Truncus sympathicus

Plexus hypogastricus superior

N. hypogastricus dexter

Nn. splanchnici pelvici (S2–4)

Plexus hypogastricus inferior

Ganglia coeliaca

N. splanchnicus minor

Plexus splenicus

Ganglion aorticorenale

Plexus renalis

Plexus intermesentericus

Ganglion mesentericum inferius

Plexus uretericus

Plexus mesentericus inferior

Branches of the Plexus hypogastricus inferior to Colon descendens and sigmoideum

N. hypogastricus sinister

Fig. 7.52 Autonomic innervation of the abdominal organs. Ventral view.

8 Pelvic viscera

Jens Waschke

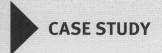
Prostate cancer

Medical history

A 72-year-old man reports to his GP that he has been suffering from increasing pain in the pelvic area and his back for some months, and recently also in his chest. He also says he is constantly tired and worn out, which is unusual for him.

Examination results

His pelvis, lumbar and thoracic spine and also his ribs are tender. All other physical examination findings are normal. As part of a routine cancer screening, which the patient has never undergone before, the GP carries out a rectal examination, in which the right lobe of the prostate exhibits a very dense node.

Diagnosis

On the basis of the physical findings the GP orders that the prostate-specific antigen (PSA) be tested in a previously taken blood sample and refers the patient to a urologist. In order to exclude coronary artery disease (CAD), which can also cause tightness in the chest with pain (angina pectoris), an ECG is carried out, which is normal. To check for oesophagitis, which is associated with retrosternal pain (heartburn) and could at least explain the discomfort in the chest area, the GP also arranges an appointment with a gastroenterologist in private practice for a gastroscopy.

The physical rectal findings are a strong indication for prostate cancer, which constitutes the most common malignant tumour in men over 70 years old. The urologist first confirms the diagnosis by means of a transrectal biopsy, in which parts of a prostate carcinoma are detected by a pathologist. Corresponding to the diagnosis, the PSA level is far beyond the age-appropriate normal range. Since the bone pain in this diagnosis can be seen as an indication of extensive bone metastasis, a nuclear medicine physician carries out a bone scintigraphy, which confirms metastases in pelvis, spine, ribs and sternum.

Treatment

Due to the extensive metastasis and the poor prognosis, surgical removal of the prostate is not meaningful. Because growth of prostate cancer is hormone-dependent, drug therapy is started, which restricts the distribution and effect of testosterone. In addition, pain medication is given.

Further developments

After 3 years the patient dies of the consequences of advanced stage tumour.

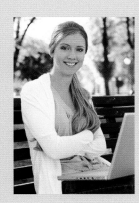

Your first day of a mandatory placement with a GP. You were present at the appointment with the patient. Now, the GP asks you to write a short letter for the urologist.
For this purpose, you make these bullet points:

First day – first doctor's letter...

Hx.: 72-year-old patient, with pain in pelvis, back and chest, worsening over last few months

Patient very tired and worn out, otherwise ⊠ known illnesses.

CE: pressure pain in pelvis, thoracic spine and lumbar spine and ribs; rough nodes in right prostate lobes palpable

DD.: BE for PSA control carried out, result pending, ECG (for the exclusion of AP) nothing evident, appt. for gastroscopy agreed (above all gastroesophageal reflux disease)

Palpation and CE are **highly suspect for metast. prostate cancer**

→ **request for biopsy to confirm diagnosis**

PSA value will be sent as soon as available, with confirmation of the suspected diagnosis: skeletal Scinti for metastases search

8.1 Kidneys

8.1.1 Overview

The kidney, ren, or nephros is a parenchymatous organ with a reddish-brown colour, which, together with the efferent tracts, forms (➤ Chap. 8.3) the **urinary system** (➤ Fig. 8.1). It is located in close proximity to the adrenal glands (➤ Chap. 8.2), an endocrine organ, in the **retroperitoneal space** of the upper abdomen.
The kidneys and efferent urinary tracts are of particular importance for the specialist field of urology.

8.1.2 Functions of the kidneys

The kidneys have a wide range of functions. Together with the liver it is the essential excretion organ of the body. Due to its regulation

of fluid and electrolyte balance, it is an absolutely **indispensable** organ. Its functions are:
- Excretion of urine, the body's own and foreign substances
- Regulation of fluid, electrolytes and acid-base balance
- Endocrine function (erythropoietin, renin, calcitriol)

The kidneys filter the blood and in the process form 170 litres of **primary urine** a day, which contains most of the bodily substances to be excreted (e.g. urine) and also foreign substances (e.g. medicines). From this primary urine the kidneys resorb over 90% of the liquid as well as the majority of electrolytes and nutrients, whilst other substances are excreted in a targeted way so that approximately 1.7 litres of **urine** a day is passed into the efferent urinary tracts. This principle enables a very effective elimination on the one hand and on the other hand, a delicately regulated recovery of valuable substances which is controlled by hormones and thus can be adapted to each respective metabolic state. Because of this excretion function the kidneys control not only fluid and electrolyte balance in the body, but also the pH level of the blood (acid-base homeostasis); however, the kidneys also have **endocrine functions:** erythropoietin, which is required by bone marrow for the production of red blood cells, as well as calcitriol, which regulates the calcium levels, are produced in the kidneys. Renin, which itself is not a hormone but an enzyme causes the formation of hormones, which are of critical importance for fluid balance.

8.1.3 Development of the kidneys

The kidneys develop, as do the genitalia, from the **intermediate mesoderm,** which in the *4th week* forms the **urogenital ridge,** the

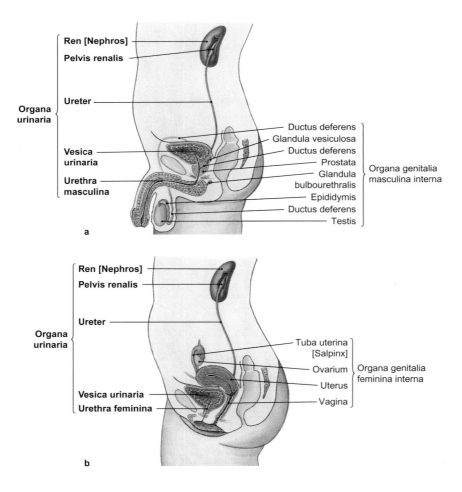

Fig. 8.1 Structure of the urinary system. Lateral view left. **a** Male urinary system. **b** Female urinary system.

lateral part of which is referred to as the **nephrogenic cord**. Between the *4th and 9th weeks* **3 generations of kidneys** (> Fig. 8.2) form one after the other from cranial to caudal:

- **Pronephros**
- **Mesonephros**
- **Metanephros**

Whilst the pronephros remains functionless and completely degenerates, the mesonephros is different and functions temporarily before it also largely degenerates. The primitive ureter of the mesonephros remains (**Ductus mesonephricus, WOLFFIAN duct**) in existence and enters into the caudal part of the hindgut (**cloaca**) (> Fig. 8.2). In men parts of the ductules system between testis and epididymis (Ductuli efferentes) also emerge from the mesonephros. From the WOLFFIAN duct the **ureteric bud** develops as a protrusion and forms the efferent urinary tracts and in the *5th week* induces the differentiation of the metanephros. The ureteric bud becomes (> Fig. 8.3):

- The ureter
- The renal pelvis (Pelvis renalis) with renal calyces (Calices renales)
- Collection ducts of the renal parenchyma

The definitive kidneys are thus formed from 2 parts, both of which come from the mesoderm:

- **Metanephros:** it forms the nephrons and the glomeruli become embedded in their renal corpuscles.
- **Ureteric bud:** it forms the collection ducts, which are connected to the nephrons.

The kidneys are thereby first divided into lobes, the boundaries of which can be seen as furrows on the surface anatomy.

The metanephroses first differentiate at the level of the future pelvis and ascend due to the strong growth of the lower half of the em-

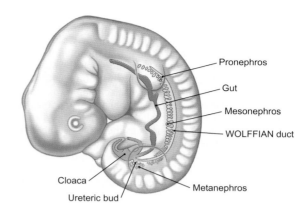

Fig. 8.2 Development of the kidneys in the 5th week of development.

bryonic body **up until** *the 9th week* (**ascent**), until they reach their final position (> Fig. 8.4). In the process they remain in a retroperitoneal location, but they rotate the hilum where blood vessels and the ureter enter and exit by 90°, so that they are no longer aligned ventrally, but medially. During their ascent, several generations of **renal arteries** develop one after the other, which first emerge from the pelvic artery (A. iliaca communis) and later from the abdominal aorta. These vessels usually degenerate, but may persist in some cases as accessory renal arteries.

N O T E

During development the kidneys rise out of the pelvis **(ascent)** and in the process do not take the supplying vessels and nerves along with them.

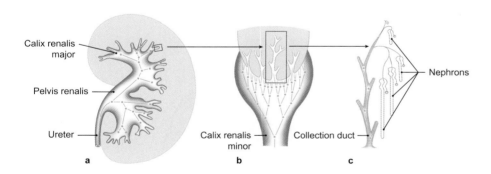

Fig. 8.3 Development of the kidneys from the ureteric bud. a Renal pelvis. **b** Renal calix. **c** Collecting duct. [L126]

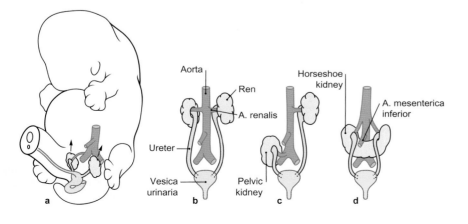

Fig. 8.4 Ascent of the kidneys with deformities. a Original position of the kidneys. **b** Normal final location of the kidneys. **c** Pelvic kidney, right. **d** Horseshoe kidney.

If ascent does not occur, this gives rise to a **pelvic kidney** (➤ Fig. 8.4c). What can also occur is that the inferior renal poles merge and form a **horseshoe kidney** (➤ Fig. 8.4d). Since this is hindered in its ascent by the unpaired A. mesenterica inferior, the horseshoe kidney also remains displaced caudally. Pelvic kidneys (1:2500 births) and also horseshoe kidneys (1:400 births) are usually accidental findings and have no clinical relevance so long as the course of the ureter is not affected in the process. Displacement of the ureter can cause urinary stasis, which can lead to kidney damage caused by increased pressure and by ascending infections. Similarly, **malrotations**, where the hilum points to ventral or dorsal, are usually clinically insignificant.

8.1.4 Projection and structure of the kidney

The kidneys are a 10–12 cm long, 5–6 cm wide and 4 cm thick parenchymatous organ with a weight of 120–200 g (averaging 150 g). They have a **superior and inferior pole** (Polus superior and Polus inferior), an **anterior and posterior surface** (Facies anterior and Facies posterior) and a **medial and lateral border** (Margo medialis and Margo lateralis). At the medial border is the **Hilum renale**, where the vessels and nerves and the ureter enter and exit (➤ Fig. 8.6). The kidneys are therefore kidney-shaped (!). They project (➤ Fig. 8.5)

* with the superior pole onto the XIIth thoracic vertebra and the XIth rib;
* with the hilum onto the IInd lumbar vertebra and
* with the inferior pole onto the IIIrd lumbar vertebra.

These specifications only apply to the left kidney. Due to the size of the liver the right kidney sits approximately half a vertebra deeper. The superior pole is thus positioned to the right just below the XIth rib.

Due to its proximity to the diaphragm, the location of the kidneys depends on breathing so that both kidneys can sink by up to 3 cm during inhalation.

In the **clinical examination** the kidneys are first examined using pain sensitivity as a rough guide, whereby finely-tuned fist punches are applied to the lumbar region at the level of the kidneys, i.e. on the posterior side just below the ribs; however, the patient must not be warned beforehand because the back muscles would otherwise be tensed and thus dampen the impact too much. In the case of an inflammation of the renal pelvis (pyelonephritis) the patient will, for example, not only wince in surprise but will also complain of experiencing significant pain. In its correct execution this diagnostic measure also always constitutes a certain stress test for the doctor–patient relationship.

The kidneys are divided into the **cortex** (Cortex renalis) and **medulla** (Medulla renalis) (➤ Fig. 8.7). The medulla is divided into different sections, which, corresponding to their shape are designated **renal pyramids** (Pyramides renales). Between the pyramids are renal columns (Columnae renales). A pyramid with its adjoining cortex segments is called a **renal lobe** (Lobus renalis). The border between the usually ca. 14 lobes is not usually visible on the surface anatomy in adults. The tips of the pyramids (Papillae renales) flow into the **renal calyces** (Calices renales majores and minores), where urine is released into the **renal pelvis** (Pelvis renalis). The renal pelvis is located together with adipose tissue and vascular, lymphatic and nervous systems in a recess of the kidney parenchyma (**Sinus renalis**), which is connected to the **Hilum renale**. Located in the hilum are the:

* V. renalis (anterior)
* A. renalis (in the middle)
* Renal pelvis (posterior)

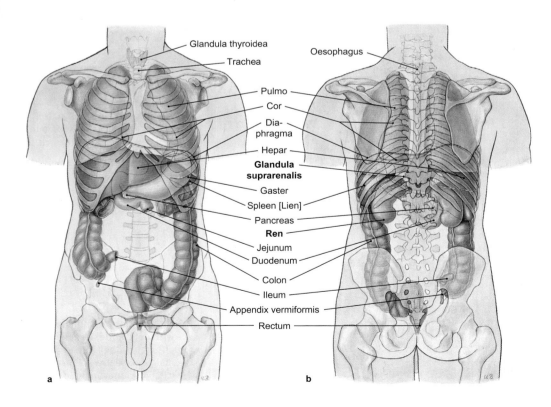

Glandula thyroidea
Trachea
Oesophagus
Pulmo
Cor
Diaphragma
Hepar
Glandula suprarenalis
Gaster
Spleen [Lien]
Pancreas
Ren
Jejunum
Duodenum
Colon
Ileum
Appendix vermiformis
Rectum

a   b

Fig. 8.5 Projection of inner organs onto the surface of the body. a Ventral view. **b** Dorsal view.

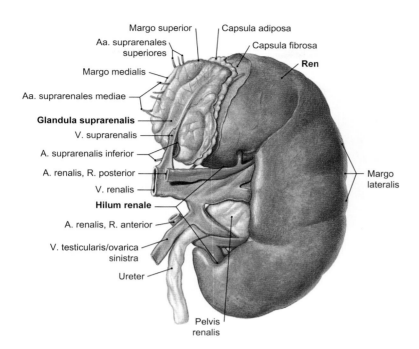

Margo superior
Aa. suprarenales superiores
Margo medialis
Aa. suprarenales mediae
Glandula suprarenalis
V. suprarenalis
A. suprarenalis inferior
A. renalis, R. posterior
V. renalis
Hilum renale
A. renalis, R. anterior
V. testicularis/ovarica sinistra
Ureter
Pelvis renalis
Capsula adiposa
Capsula fibrosa
Ren
Margo lateralis

Fig. 8.6 Kidney (Ren, Nephros) and adrenal gland (Glandula suprarenalis), left. Ventral view.

The kidney parenchyma consists of nephrons and collection ducts (➤ Fig. 8.12), in which urine is altered by filtration out of the blood with subsequent reabsorption and secretion. Finally, at the top of the papillae the collection ducts release the urine into the renal pelvis.

8.1.5 Fascial system of the kidney

The kidneys have a **3-fold fascial system** (➤ Fig. 8.8):
- **Capsula fibrosa:** organ capsule of dense connective tissue directly on the surface anatomy of the parenchyma
- **Capsula adiposa:** fat capsule that surrounds the kidney and adrenal gland
- **Fascia renalis:** fascial sac that is open in the inferior medial aspect for the passage of vessels and nerves and ureter. The anteri-

or layer of the renal fascia is referred to clinically as **GEROTA's fascia**. The posterior layer merges into the muscular fascia of the M. psoas major and M. quadratus lumborum.

Clinical remarks

The fascial systems and the topographical relationships of the kidneys are of clinical importance. The fat capsule secures the kidneys during breathing. If the capsule, e.g. during anorexia, is greatly reduced then the kidneys may sink **(nephroptosis)** or rotate, in which case the ureter bends down and the kidneys can be damaged by urinary backflow. In a **nephrectomy** due to malignant tumours of the kidneys, the kidneys and adrenal glands, including GEROTA's fascia, are removed.

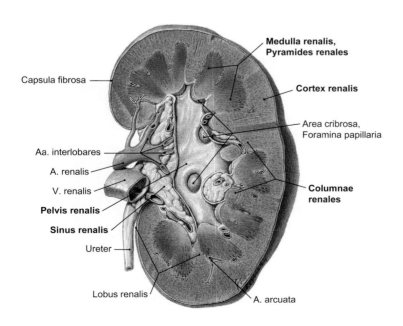

Capsula fibrosa
Aa. interlobares
A. renalis
V. renalis
Pelvis renalis
Sinus renalis
Ureter
Lobus renalis
A. arcuata
Medulla renalis, Pyramides renales
Cortex renalis
Area cribrosa, Foramina papillaria
Columnae renales

Fig. 8.7 Kidney (Ren, Nephros), left. Ventral view; after vertical dissection with exposed and opened renal pelvis.

355

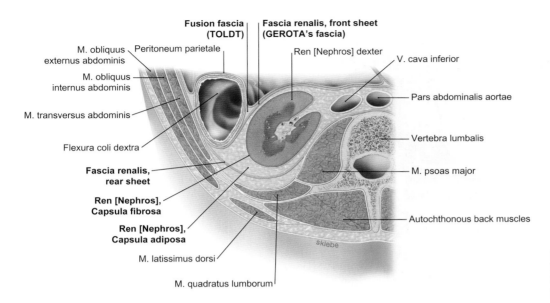

M. obliquus externus abdominis
M. obliquus internus abdominis
M. transversus abdominis
Flexura coli dextra
Fascia renalis, rear sheet
Ren [Nephros], Capsula fibrosa
Ren [Nephros], Capsula adiposa
M. latissimus dorsi
M. quadratus lumborum

Peritoneum parietale
Fusion fascia (TOLDT)
Fascia renalis, front sheet (GEROTA's fascia)
Ren [Nephros] dexter
V. cava inferior
Pars abdominalis aortae
Vertebra lumbalis
M. psoas major
Autochthonous back muscles

Fig. 8.8 Fascial systems of the kidneys; horizontal incision at the level of the III lumbar vertebra. Caudal view. [L238]

8.1.6 Topography

The kidneys are located **in the retroperitoneal space** of the upper abdomen and both **adrenal glands** sit above them (➤ Fig. 8.5). To the **anterior** they are separated from other organs by their 3-fold fascial system but nevertheless have a close topographical relationship on both sides to various viscera.

- The **right kidney** has broad surface contact with the Facies visceralis of the liver as well as contact to medial with the Pars descendens of the duodenum, and at its inferior pole to the jejunum and right colic flexure (➤ Fig. 7.19a).
- At its upper pole, the **left kidney** has contact with the posterior side of the stomach and at its lateral border it has contact with the Facies visceralis of the spleen. In front at the level of the hilum is the tail part of the pancreas. At the inferior pole there is contact with the Ileum and Colon descendens (➤ Fig. 7.19b, c).

Kidneys and adrenal glands are located **dorsally** in the retroperitoneal space directly against the posterior abdominal wall and thus ventrally of the M. psoas major and the M. quadratus lumborum.

Various **nerves of the Plexus lumbalis** are located directly at the renal fascia between the kidney and abdominal wall in the area of the inferior renal pole. (➤ Fig. 8.9):

- N. iliohypogastricus and N. ilioinguinalis which, among other things, provide sensory innervation to the inguinal region
- N. genitofemoralis, which courses further to caudal and therefore has no contact with the kidneys but only with the ureter.
- 11th and 12th intercostal nerves (12th intercostal nerve = N. subcostalis), which are located slightly further to cranial and therefore below both of the two lowest ribs.

Clinical remarks

The close proximity of the kidneys to the N. iliohypogastricus and N. ilioinguinalis explains why diseases of the kidneys, such as inflammation of the renal pelvis (pyelonephritis) or trapped kidney stones in the pelvis (nephrolithiasis) can cause **radiating pain up into the inguinal region**.

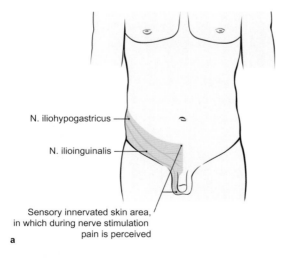

N. iliohypogastricus
N. ilioinguinalis
Sensory innervated skin area, in which during nerve stimulation pain is perceived

a

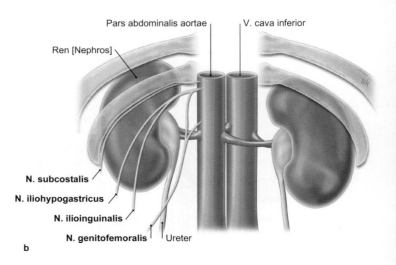

Pars abdominalis aortae
V. cava inferior
Ren [Nephros]
N. subcostalis
N. iliohypogastricus
N. ilioinguinalis
N. genitofemoralis
Ureter

b

Fig. 8.9 Proximity of the kidneys to nerves of the Plexus lumbalis. a Radiating pain into the inguinal region. **b** Course of the nerves of the Plexus lumbalis in relation to the kidneys. a[L126]; b[L238]

8.1.7 Vessels and nerves of the kidney

Arterial and venous supply

The **Aa. renales** (➤ Fig. 8.10a) originate in pairs from the abdominal section of the aorta and run dorsal to the veins to the hilum of the kidney, whereby the right A. renalis runs along behind the V. cava inferior. With 3–5 cm, the right A. renalis is considerably longer than the left (2–3 cm). In front of the hilum the A. suprarenalis inferior goes to the adrenal gland as well as thin branches to the ureter. The branches of the A. renalis divide the kidneys with their supply areas into **5 segments,** whereby the A. renalis branches at the hilum firstly into an **R. anterior,** which with various branches supplies the inferior, both anterior and the inferior segment of the kidney, and a **R. posterior** for the posterior segment (➤ Fig. 8.11, also ➤ Fig. 8.6). Alternatively, the lower segment can also receive an independent branch.

The renal capsule is reached by small branches from the A. renalis or the A. testicularis/ovarica or the Aa. lumbales.

The **Vv. renales** correspond with their branches to the arteries; they run ventrally of these and flow on both sides into the V. cava inferior (➤ Fig. 8.10b). Since the inferior vena cava lies to the right of the Aorta, the left V. renalis is, at 7.5 cm long, three times as long as the vessel on the right side (1–2.5 cm).

On the **left side,** the V. renalis takes up 3 veins; the corresponding veins flow to the right independently into the V. cava inferior:

- V. suprarenalis sinistra
- V. testicularis/ovarica sinistra
- V. phrenica inferior sinistra

Intrarenal blood vessels

The segmental branches of the A. renalis and V. renalis divide within the hilum and ascend as the **A. and V. interlobaris** at the edge of the pyramids, and then run at the cortex-medulla border as the **A. and V. arcuata** in an arch shape around the pyramids and leave them at their bases as the **A. and V. corticalis radiata,** which ascend to the capsule. From these, the fine vessels go to the capillary loops in the nephrons (➤ Fig. 8.12).

Clinical remarks

In contrast to the veins, the intrarenal arteries do not form closed vessel arches, i.e. they are terminal arteries. Thus, in the case of arterial occlusion, e.g. due to a transported blood clot (embolism), **renal infarction occurs.** Its extent corresponds to the segmental borders; however, the branching patterns are highly variable.

Accessory renal arteries (30%) are evolutionary relics and must be protected during operations in order to avoid haemorrhages. Up to 5 arteries can occur. **Aberrant arteries** enter into the parenchyma outside of the hilum. **Capsular vessels** can also cause haemorrhages during operations.

Because **kidney carcinoma** often grows into the Vv. renales, a tumour on the left hand side in men can cause backflow into the V. testicularis with a tangled ball-like expansion of the veins in the scrotum **(varicocele).** Therefore, in the case of a left-sided varicocele, a kidney tumour must always also be excluded (➤ Fig. 8.43)!

Lymphatic pathways

The regional lymph nodes of the kidneys are the **Nodi lymphoidei lumbales** around the Aorta and V. cava inferior (➤ Fig. 8.63). From there, the lymph on both sides goes into the **Trunci lumbales.**

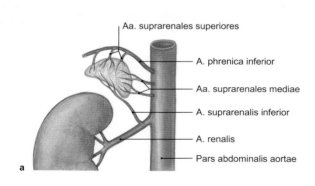

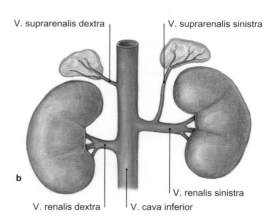

Fig. 8.10 Vascular supply of kidneys and adrenal glands. Ventral view. **a** Arteries. **b** Veins.

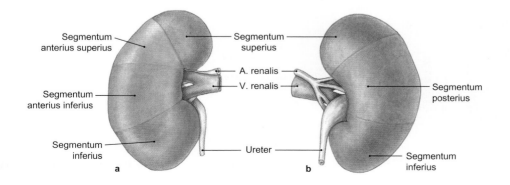

Fig. 8.11 Renal segments, Segmenta renalia, right. a Ventral view. **b** Dorsal view.

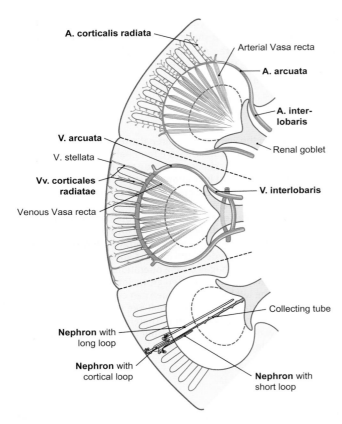

Fig. 8.12 Course of arteries, veins and nephrons in the renal parenchyma; schematic illustration. (according to [S010-1-16])

Innervation

The **autonomic innervation** of the kidneys is overwhelmingly sympathetic (➤ Fig. 8.13) and effects vasoconstriction and thus a reduction of blood flow as well as the secretion of renin. The postganglionic sympathetic nerve fibres from the Ganglion aorticorenale form the Plexus renalis around the A. renalis.

For the general organisation of the autonomic nervous system in the abdomen see ➤ Chap. 7.8.5 and on the autonomic ganglia in the retroperitoneum see ➤ Chap. 8.8.5.

8.2 Adrenal gland

Skills

After working through this chapter, you should be able to:
- explain the vital function of the adrenal glands and the diverse evolutionary origins of their parts
- show on a specimen the location of the adrenal glands with attachment to the different vessels and nerves on both sides of the body

8.2.1 Overview

The adrenal gland, Glandula suprarenalis, is an endocrine organ of gold-yellow colour, which rests on the upper pole of the kidney within the **retroperitoneal space**. In both diagnosis as well as in medical and surgical treatment, it is particularly important for specialists such as endocrinologists and highly experienced visceral surgeons.

8.2.2 Functions of the adrenal gland and development

The adrenal glands are an absolutely essential **endocrine gland. Cortex** and **medulla** have different evolutionary origins and form hormones, which are particularly necessary for managing stress and in emergency situations and they have a regulating effect on metabolism and the circulation (➤ Table 8.1).

Table 8.1 Hormones of the adrenal glands.

Hormones of the cortex (steroid hormones)	Hormones of the medulla
• Glucocorticoids (cortisol) • Mineralocorticoids (aldosterone) • Androgens (DHEA)	• Catecholamines (adrenaline, noradrenaline)

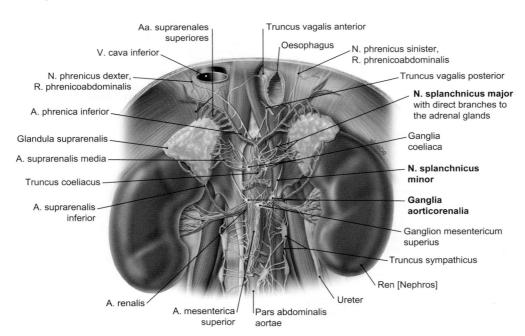

Fig. 8.13 Innervation of kidney and adrenal gland. [L238]

The cortex develops in the *6th week* from the **mesoderm** in the wall of the abdominal cavity (coelomic epithelium); the medulla, however, originates from the **neural crest (neuroectoderm)** and thus corresponds to a 'modified' sympathetic ganglion. Until birth, the adrenal glands are 10–20 times larger than in adults relative to body weight and then shrink in the first *2 years of life.*

Clinical remarks

If both adrenal glands are removed due to disease, mineralocorticoids and glucocorticoids must be replaced by medication because otherwise **life-threatening shock conditions** can ensue due to low blood sugar (hypoglycaemia) and low blood pressure (hypotension). This can also be the case with adrenal gland insufficiency (ADDISON's disease).

8.2.3 Structure, projection and topography of the adrenal glands

The adrenal glands are 5 cm long and 2–3 cm wide with a weight of 4 g. A distinction is made between **anterior, posterior and inferior surfaces** (Facies anterior, posterior and renalis) as well as a **medial (Margo medialis)** and a **superior border (Margo superior)** (➤ Fig. 8.6). At the medial border is the **hilum,** where the vascular, lymphatic and nervous systems enter and exit. The adrenal glands project onto the neck of the XIth and XIIth ribs. In the **retroperitoneum** they lie directly below the diaphragm and in the process rest upon the upper pole of the kidneys (➤ Fig. 8.6) and are embedded with these in a common fat capsule (**Capsula adiposa**), which are encased by the renal fascia (Fascia renalis, GEROTA's fascia). Hereby, they have the following topographical relationships:

* **Facies anterior:** Facies visceralis of the liver and Pars descendens of the duodenum as well as the V. cava inferior (right), posterior surface of the stomach (left, separated by the Bursa omentalis)
* **Facies posterior:** diaphragm
* **Facies renalis:** rests on the superior renal pole

8.2.4 Vessels and nerves of the adrenal glands

Arterial and venous supply

Usually there are **3 adrenal arteries** (➤ Fig. 8.10a):
* A. suprarenalis superior: usually several small vessels, originating from the A. phrenica inferior
* A. suprarenalis media: directly from the Aorta
* A. suprarenalis inferior: branch of the A. renalis

This 'luxury perfusion' prevents the occurrence of organ infarction that could jeopardise the vital organ; however, all 3 adrenal arteries are formed only in one third of cases, otherwise usually the middle or inferior artery is missing.

In contrast, for each adrenal gland there is only **one adrenal vein,** which collects blood and conducts it right into the V. cava inferior or left into the V. renalis (➤ Fig. 8.10b).

Lymphatic pathways

The regional lymph nodes of the adrenal gland are the **Nodi lymphoidei lumbales** around the Aorta and V. cava inferior (➤ Fig. 8.63). From there, the lymph on both sides goes in the **Trunci lumbales.**

Innervation

Autonomic innervation is carried out by preganglionic (!) sympathetic nerve fibres from the Nn. splanchnici from the **Plexus suprarenalis** medially of the gland. In the adrenal medulla they effect the release of catecholamines (the adrenal medulla corresponds to a modified sympathetic ganglion) (➤ Fig. 8.13).

For general organisation of the autonomic nervous system in the abdomen, see ➤ Chap. 7.8.5.

8.3 Efferent urinary tracts

Skills

After working through this chapter, you should be able to:
* explain the structure of the efferent urinary tracts with their development
* show sections and the precise course of the ureter on a specimen and pinpoint its constriction
* know the position and closure mechanisms of the urinary bladder as well as basic processes during micturition
* understand sections and differences of the urethra in both sexes and their clinical significance
* demonstrate the vessels and nerves of the efferent urinary tracts

8.3.1 Overview and function

The **efferent urinary tracts** include:
* Renal pelvis (Pelvis renalis)
* Ureter
* Urinary bladder (Vesica urinaria)
* Urethra

The efferent urinary tracts together with the kidneys (➤ Chap. 8.1) form the **urinary system** (➤ Fig. 8.1). They range from the renal pelvis in the **retroperitoneal space** of the upper abdomen via the ureters to the urinary bladder in the **subperitoneal space** of the pelvis and there facilitate the excretion of urine via the urethra (**micturition**).

With the exception of the urethra, the urinary system is identically formed in both sexes. In men, the urethra in the penis is a urine-semen duct, as it is also used to transport the ejaculate and thus is also part of the external male genitalia.

8.3.2 Development of the efferent urinary tracts

The efferent urinary tracts originate from 2 parts (➤ Fig. 8.14):
* **Ureteric bud:** forms ureters, renal pelvis and the collection duct of the kidney parenchyma
* **Sinus urogenitalis:** becomes the urinary bladder and urethra

Ureteric bud

The ureteric bud develops in the *5th week* as a protrusion from the primitive ureters of the mesonephros (**Ductus mesonephricus, WOLFFIAN duct**) and therefore emerges from the **mesoderm**. The ureter later includes attachment to the caudal part of the hindgut (**cloaca**), which differentiates from the **ectoderm** (➤ Chap. 8.1.3). The cloaca is then divided by the **urorectal septum** in the *7th week* into the anterior Sinus urogenitalis and the posterior rectum (➤ Chap 7.2.3) (➤ Fig. 8.14a–c).

Sinus urogenitalis

The upper part of the sinus urogenitalis develops into the **epithelium** of the **urinary bladder**, in that the inferior sections of the mesonephric ducts up to and including the ureteric buds are incorporated so that the **ureters** are now connected directly to the urinary bladder (➤ Fig. 8.14b, c). **Connective tissue** and **smooth muscles** emerge from the surrounding **mesoderm**. The apex of the urinary bladder continues into the **allantoic duct**, which ends as a blind sac within the body stalk . The allantoic duct degenerates into a connective tissue cord (**Urachus**) (➤ Fig. 8.14e, f), which after birth runs as the **Lig. umbilicale medianum** on the inside of the abdominal wall up to the navel.

The **Urethra** also originates from the Sinus urogenitalis (➤ Fig. 8.14e, f), whereby the middle section in a female embryo forms the epithelium of the whole of the urethra; however, in a male embryo it only forms the Pars intramuralis and prostate gland. In the inferior section of the Sinus urogenitalis its boundary invaginates into the amniotic cavity (**urogenital membrane**) between 2 folds (**urethral folds**) and tears in the *7th week* (➤ Fig. 8.31, ➤ Fig. 8.49). In this opening the **entoderm** of the Sinus urogenitalis forms the **urethral groove.** In a male embryo the urethral folds close over the urethral

groove and form the Pars membranacea and Pars spongiosa of the urethra, which are surrounded by the Pars spongiosa of the penis (Corpus spongiosum) (➤ Fig. 8.31). Only the distal part in the area of the glans of the penis originates from a depression of the **ectoderm**. In a female embryo the urethral groove does not close, but becomes the vestibule of the vagina (Vestibulum vaginae) (➤ Fig. 8.49).

Clinical remarks

Various **double formations** of the ureter can occur. The **ureter fissus** is usually an incidental finding and has no clinical relevance; however, where there is **ureteral duplication**, it often causes incorrect confluence into the urinary bladder, which can lead to vesicoureteral reflux or incontinence. Both ureters usually cross each other (MEYER-WEIGERT rule): the ureter originating from the more cranially located renal pelvis enters more into the urinary bladder or distally into the urethra, which can result in urinary incontinence; however, the ureter with a more cranially located urinary opening which usually originates from the lower renal pelvis, has a shorter Pars intramuralis in the urinary bladder wall, so that in this case it can lead to vesicoureteral reflux.

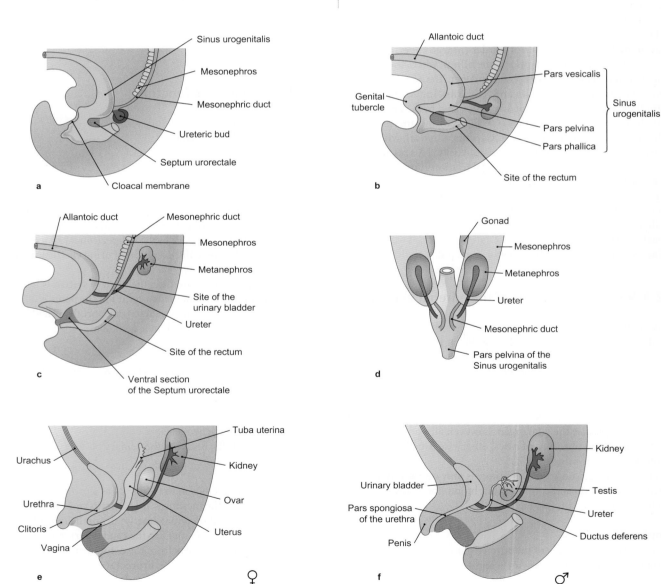

Fig. 8.14 Development of the efferent urinary ducts between the 5th **(a)** and 12th **(e, f)** weeks of development; view from left. [E347-09]

Reflux favours ascending infections, which can lead to permanent damage of the kidneys.
If the Urachus does not completely obliterate, then **urachus cysts** can remain and become infected. In the case of **urachus fistulas** a duct remains, which can still be connected to the urinary bladder, so that in newborns urine drains out of the naval.

8.3.3 Renal pelvis and ureter

The **renal pelvis** (Pelvis renalis) is surrounded by adipose tissue in the Sinus renalis of the kidneys (➤ Fig. 8.7). On the papillae of the medullary pyramids the renal pelvis is extended to the **renal calyces (Calices renales)** whereby the protrusions that emerge directly from the renal pelvis are referred to as the major calyces (Calices majores). These then divide into the minor calyces (Calices minores) that surround the papillae of the medullary pyramids. According to the width and length of the calyx, a distinction is made between **dendritic** and **ampullary** types of renal pelvis.

The **ureter** is 25–30 cm long and has a diameter of approximately 5 mm (➤ Fig. 8.15). It transports urine by regularly occurring peristaltic waves and is divided into **3 sections:**

- Pars abdominalis: in the retroperitoneal space
- Pars pelvica: in the lesser pelvis
- Pars intramuralis: traverses the urinary bladder wall

The ureter leaves the renal pelvis in an inferior medial direction and firstly crosses the inferior renal pole.

- The **Pars abdominalis** firstly *crosses* over the N. genitofemoralis and *crosses* below the A./V. testicularis/ovarica. On the **right side** it is covered by the duodenum, the A. colica dextra and the mesenteric root, and on the **left** by the A./V. mesenterica inferior or the A. colica sinistra. When entering the lesser pelvis the ureter *crosses* over the A./V. iliaca communis.
- The **Pars pelvica** in men passes *under* the Ductus deferens, and in women *behind* the ovary and in the vicinity of the uterus *under* the A. uterina.
- The **Pars intramuralis** runs 1.5–2 cm through the musculature of the urinary bladder wall and confluences with its two slot-shaped apertures (Ostia uteris) into the Trigonum vesicae of the urinary bladder. The valve-like openings are closed when no urine passes through the ureter in order to avoid a reflux of urine, which can damage the kidneys by ascending infections.

> **N O T E**
>
> **The over-under-over-under rule** for the course of the ureter: the ureter first runs *over* the N. genitofemoralis, crosses *under* the A. and V. testicularis/ovarica, crosses *over* the A. and V. iliaca and then crosses *under* the Ductus deferens in men and under the A. uterina in women.

The ureter has **3 constrictions** (➤ Fig. 8.15):
- at the outflow of the renal pelvis
- at the intersection of the A. iliaca communis or externa
- at the passageway through the wall of the urinary bladder (most narrow part)

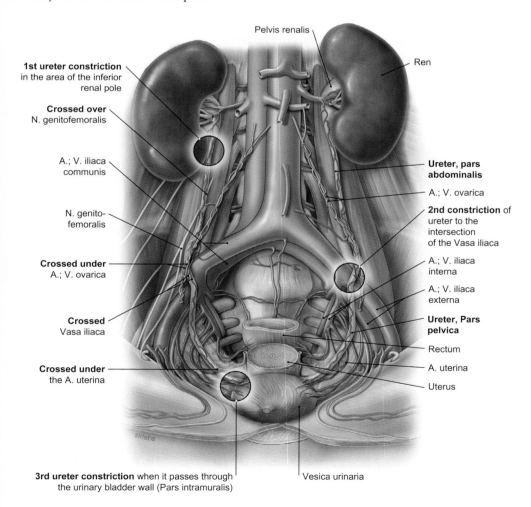

Pelvis renalis

Ren

1st ureter constriction in the area of the inferior renal pole

Crossed over N. genitofemoralis

A.; V. iliaca communis

N. genito-femoralis

Crossed under A.; V. ovarica

Crossed Vasa iliaca

Crossed under the A. uterina

Ureter, pars abdominalis

A.; V. ovarica

2nd constriction of ureter to the intersection of the Vasa iliaca

A.; V. iliaca interna

A.; V. iliaca externa

Ureter, Pars pelvica

Rectum

A. uterina

Uterus

3rd ureter constriction when it passes through the urinary bladder wall (Pars intramuralis)

Vesica urinaria

Fig. 8.15 Sections of the ureter with constrictions. [L238]

Kidney stones coming loose can remain stuck at the constrictions and then cause very strong wave-like radiating pain (renal colic). The proximity of the ureter to the A. uterina must be taken into consideration in **removal of the uterus** (hysterectomy) so that the ureter is not ligated with the artery. A urine blockage may lead to irreversible damage to the kidneys.

8.3.4 Urinary bladder

The **urinary bladder** (Vesica urinaria) lies **subperitoneally** and is covered on its superior side by the Peritoneum parietale of the pelvic cavity. It is divided into a **body** (Corpus vesicae), which tapers off above to the **apex** (Apex vesicae) and in a posterior inferior direction has a **bladder base** (Fundus vesicae) (➤ Fig. 8.16). In an anterior inferior direction the urinary bladder narrows into the **neck of bladder** (Cervix vesicae), which merges into the urethra. The wall of the urinary bladder has a thick layer of muscle, which is activated **parasympathetically** and is referred to as the **M. detrusor vesicae.**

At the fundus the exit of the urethra (Ostium urethrae internum) forms, together with the confluence found on both sides of the ureter (Ostium ureteris), the **trigone of the bladder** (Trigonum vesicae). The urinary bladder has a capacity of 500–1500 ml.

In **men** the prostate gland, which is crossed by the urethra, is located directly under the fundus of the bladder and there gives rise to the Uvula vesicae.

In pairs abutting the urinary bladder on the posterior side from **medial to lateral** are:
- Extended section of the Ductus deferens (Ampulla ductus deferentis)
- Seminal glands (Glandula vesiculosa)
- Ureter

The bladder is surrounded by paravesical adipose tissue and is secured by various **ligaments**:
- **Lig. umbilicale medianum** (contains the urachus = relic of the allantoic duct): runs from the apex of the urinary bladder to the navel
- **Lig. pubovesicale** (➤ Fig. 8.58), traverses the Spatium retropubicum and in women is anchored on both sides of the neck of the bladder on the posterior side of the pubic bone
- **Lig. puboprostaticum** (➤ Fig. 8.57), corresponding ligament in men

Behind the urinary bladder the peritoneal cavity in both sexes is extended caudally to a recess: the **Excavatio vesicouterina** and the **Excavatio rectovesicalis** separate the urinary bladder from the uterus and rectum in both women and men.

When full the urinary bladder protrudes over the pubic bone and can be punctured in the case of urinary retention, without opening the peritoneal cavity **(suprapubic catheter)**.

8.3.5 Urethra

The **urethra** is formed very variably in both sexes.
- The **female** urethra is 6 mm wide and, at 3–5 cm, very short and enters directly **ventral** of the vagina into the vestibule of the vagina (Vestibulum vaginae) (➤ Fig. 8.46).
- The **male** urethra, however, is relatively long at 20 cm and is divided into different sections (➤ Fig. 8.16):
  - **Pars intramuralis** (1 cm): in the urinary bladder wall, its begins at the Ostium urethrae internum
  - **Pars prostatica** (3.5 cm): traverses the prostate; here, the Ductus ejaculatorii (common exit duct of Ductus deferens

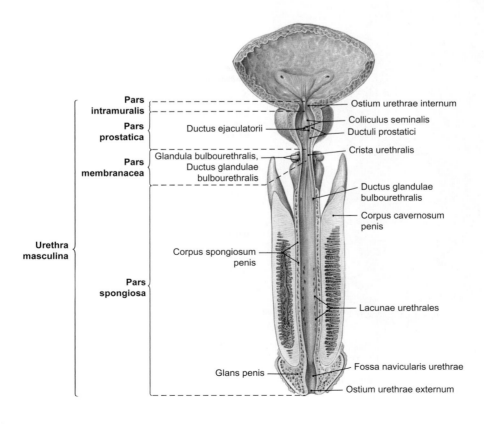

Pars intramuralis
Pars prostatica
Ductus ejaculatorii
Pars membranacea
Glandula bulbourethralis, Ductus glandulae bulbourethralis
Urethra masculina
Corpus spongiosum penis
Pars spongiosa
Glans penis

Ostium urethrae internum
Colliculus seminalis
Ductuli prostatici
Crista urethralis
Ductus glandulae bulbourethralis
Corpus cavernosum penis
Lacunae urethrales
Fossa navicularis urethrae
Ostium urethrae externum

Fig. 8.16 Urinary bladder and urethra. Ventral view; urinary bladder and urethra opened ventrally.

and seminal vesicle) confluences with the Colliculus seminalis and the prostate glands bilaterally
- **Pars membranacea** (1–2 cm): at the passage through the pelvic floor
- **Pars spongiosa** (15 cm): runs within the Corpus spongiosum of the penis up to the external orifice (Ostium urethrae externum). Here COWPER's glands (Glandulae bulbourethrales) and the LITTRÉ's glands (Glandulae urethrales) flow into each other. The proximal section is extended to the Fossa navicularis. The proximal section is also somewhat wider and is, therefore, sometimes referred to as the 'Ampulla urethrae'.

In this course, the male urethra has 2 **curvatures** (➤ Fig. 8.57) – at the transition from the Pars membranacea to the Pars spongiosa and in the middle section of the Pars spongiosa – and the following **constrictions** (➤ Fig. 8.16):
- Ostium urethrae internum
- Pars membranacea
- Ostium urethrae externum (narrowest point, diameter: 6 mm)

In contrast, the Pars spongiosa (especially proximally = 'Ampulla urethrae') and the Fossa navicularis are particularly wide.

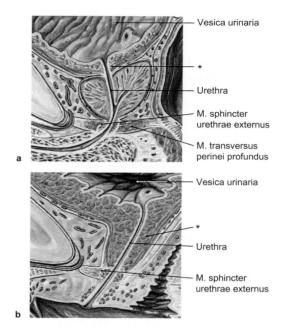

Fig. 8.17 labels: Vesica urinaria / * / Urethra / M. sphincter urethrae externus / M. transversus perinei profundus / a; Vesica urinaria / * / Urethra / M. sphincter urethrae externus / b

Fig. 8.17 Closure mechanisms of the urinary bladder and the urethra; median incision; view from left; * smooth muscles of the urethra. **a** Male view. **b** Female view.

Clinical remarks

Because the female urethra is much shorter than the male one, ascending infections of the urinary bladder **(cystitis)** are more common in women than in men.

Due to the stretched course of the female urethra the placing of a **urinary catheter** is much easier in women; however, care must be taken that the urethral orifice in the vestibule is located *in front of* the opening to the vagina. In men, however, the curvatures of the urethra must be offset by aligning the penis in order to prevent perforations especially in the tissue of the prostate, which are painful and can bleed severely. Firstly, the urethra is inserted with the catheter after stretching the penis in order to compensate for the bend in the Pars spongiosa. Resistance means the second curvature before the construction of the Pars membranacea has been reached. To compensate more easily for this second curvature, the penis is placed downwards between the legs of the patient.

Although the urinary bladder has a capacity of 500–1500 ml, the urge to urinate already starts from 250 ml. Via stretching receptors, an autonomic **reflex arc in the sacral portion of the parasympathetic nervous system (S2–4)** in the spinal cord is activated, which increases the tone of the smooth muscles of the urinary bladder wall (M. detrusor vesicae). Micturition is set in motion via a **micturition centre in the Pons** of the brain stem: firstly, the pelvic floor weakens so that the urinary bladder descends and then the tone of the smooth and striated closure muscles relaxes:
- via parasympathetic reflex arcs (S2–4):
  - reflex contraction of the M. detrusor vesicae (parasympathetic, S2–4)
- regulates via micturition centre in the brain stem (Pons):
  - atony of the pelvic floor → descent of the bladder
  - atony of the circular muscles of the urethra (inhibition of the sympathetic nervous system)
  - atony of the M. sphincter urethrae externus

Clinical remarks

If the closure mechanisms fail, **incontinence** ensues, which in older age is especially common in women, if the pelvic floor is weakened after pregnancy (pelvic floor weakness). Treatment consists of training the pelvic floor muscles and, if necessary, surgical tightening of the pelvic floor. In men, surgical removal of the prostate often leads to incontinence caused by damage to the smooth muscles of the proximal urethra.

8.3.6 Closure mechanisms of the urinary bladder and the urethra

Contributing to the closure mechanisms are both muscle tension from **smooth muscles** in the wall of the urethra and **striated muscles** in the perineal area (➤ Fig. 8.17):
- **Smooth muscles** of the annular muscle layer of the **urethra** ('M. sphincter urethrae internus'). This muscle layer is activated **sympathetically**. A true sphincter is not morphologically definable. In men, the muscles prevent retrograde ejaculation into the urinary bladder; however, their contribution to urinary continence is unclear.
- **M. sphincter urethrae externus:** in men this muscle is a division of the M. transversus perinei profundus, which does not form an independent muscle in women. This striated muscle, which is U-shaped and incomplete to the back towards the rectum, is innervated by the N. pudendus and facilitates arbitrary closure of the urinary tract.

In addition, the shape and **function of the pelvic floor** (Diaphragma pelvis) are also crucial for continence because the pelvic floor supports the urinary bladder.

8.3.7 Vessels and nerves of the efferent urinary tracts

Arterial blood supply

Only the urinary bladder has its own arteries; all other sections of the efferent urinary tracts are supplied from vessels in the surrounding.

- **Renal pelvis:** is concomitantly supplied by the A. renalis
- **Ureter:** due to its long course various arteries are involved (➤ Fig. 8.15)
  - Pars abdominalis: A. renalis, A. testicularis/ovarica, Pars abdominalis of the aorta, A. iliaca communis
  - Pars pelvica and intramuralis: A. iliaca interna with Aa. vesicales superior and inferior as well as the A. uterina
- **Urinary bladder:**
  - upper main part (around two thirds): A. vesicalis superior (from the A. umbilicalis of the A. iliaca interna)
  - fundus and neck of the bladder (approximately one third): A. vesicalis inferior; in women, the A. vaginalis often replaces the A. vesicalis inferior
- **Urethra:** A. vesicalis inferior or A. vaginalis; in men the Pars spongiosa is supplied by its own A. urethralis, which is the terminal branch of the A. bulbi penis (from the A. pudenda interna)

Venous drainage
The veins correspond to the respective arteries. In the pelvis the veins form extended plexi around the individual organs, which extensively communicate with each other. The **Plexus venosus vesicalis** drains via the **Vv. vesicales** into the V. iliaca interna.

Lymphatic pathways
The regional lymph nodes for the proximal ureter are the **Nodi lymphoidei lumbales** around the aorta and V. cava inferior (➤ Fig. 8.63). In the pelvis, corresponding to various lymph nodes in the immediate surroundings of the urinary bladder, the **Nodi lymphoidei iliaci interni and externi** are the central lymph node stations for the distal ureter, urinary bladder and urethra. From both groups, the lymph on both sides goes into the **Trunci lumbales.** Only the lymphatic pathways from the Pars spongiosa of the male urethra, like those of the penis, have a connection to the inguinal lymph nodes (**Nodi lymphoidei inguinales**).

Innervation
The efferent urinary tracts are both **sympathetically** and **parasympathetically** innervated:
- The **sympathetic nervous system** inhibits peristalsis of the M. detrusor vesicae and the smooth muscle of the ureter, but activates the smooth muscles of the urethra at the exit of the bladder.
- The **parasympathetic nervous system** in contrast, facilitates peristalsis and activates the micturition reflex.

Preganglionic **sympathetic** nerve fibres from the sympathetic chain (T11–L2) reach the Plexus aorticus abdominalis via the Nn. splanchnici lumbales and sacrales. The neurons for the proximal ureter are switched in the Ganglia aorticorenalia and reach the ureter via the **Plexus renalis and Plexus testicularis** along the respective arteries. The sympathetic neurons for the distal ureter, urinary bladder and urethra descend via the Plexus hypogastricus superior to the **Plexus hypogastricus inferior** in the pelvis, where they are connected to postganglionic neurons and reach the target organs via the **Plexus vesicalis**.

Preganglionic **parasympathetic** nerve fibres pass from the sacral spinal cord (S2–4) via the **Nn. pelvici splanchnici** to the Plexus hypogastricus inferior, where they are also switched and reach the Plexus vesicalis.

In the ureter and in the urinary bladder there can also be **afferent nerve fibres** that trigger the micturition reflex, but as nociceptors also detect hyperextension (e.g. in the case of descending kidney

stones). The Pars spongiosa of the male urethra, like the penis, receives sensory innervation via the N. pudendus and is thus highly sensitive to pain.

For the general organisation of the autonomic nervous system in the abdomen, see ➤ Chap. 7.8.5 and on the autonomic ganglia in the retroperitoneum, see ➤ Chap. 8.8.5.

8.4 Rectum and anal canal
Jens Waschke, Friedrich Paulsen

Skills

After working through this chapter, you should be able to:
- show the sections of the rectum and anal canal on a specimen and explain their evolutionary origins
- describe the topographical relationships of the rectum and anal canal and understand the mesorectum in its expansion and delineation
- explain the continence organ with the functions of its different parts and describe the key processes in defecation
- show on a specimen the boundaries of supply areas of the vascular, lymphatic and nervous systems of the rectum and anal canal and know their clinical relevance

8.4.1 Overview and function

Rectum and **anal canal (Canalis analis)** are the last segments of the large intestine (➤ Chap. 7.2) and serve the purpose of temporary storage and the controlled excretion of the faeces. They form a functional unit.

Due to various idiosyncrasies in topography, structure and vascular, lymphatic and nervous systems, both these sections are dealt with in the pelvic organs. For development, see ➤ Chap. 7.2.3.

8.4.2 Classification, projection and structure of rectum and anal canal

The rectum is joined to the Colon sigmoideum and begins at the level of the II or III sacral vertebra (➤ Fig. 8.5). It is located in the pelvic cavity and has a length of 12 cm. In passing through the pelvic floor the rectum continues into the anal canal, which is surrounded along its length of 3–4 cm by the two sphincters and ends at the anus. The anal canal is shorter in women. The anorectal transition projects onto the apex of the coccyx.

In the sagittal plane, the rectum exhibits 2 curvatures:
- the dorsally directed convex **Flexura sacralis** and
- the ventrally directed convex **Flexura perinealis**

Below the Flexura perinealis, which is induced by the pull of a muscle sling (M. puborectalis) of the M. levator ani, (➤ Fig. 8.22), is where the anal canal begins. The superior, proximal part of the rectum (⅔) up to the Flexura sacralis lies **in a secondary retroperitoneal** position, the inferior, distal part (⅓) and the anal canal are located in the **subperitoneal space**.

The rectum and anal canal just as the vermiform appendix differ from the other sections of the large intestine (➤ Fig. 8.18), so that the transition of the Colon sigmoideum into the rectum, e.g. during operations, can be seen with the naked eye:

- **no taenia** but a closed longitudinal muscle layer. On the anterior and posterior sides, the taenia first form 2 wide muscle strands, which then fuse into a continuous layer that surrounds the entire rectum
- **no haustra**
- **Folds:** the rectum has 3 (only visible from the inside) irregular transverse folds (Plicae transversae recti, ➤ Fig. 8.21); in contrast, in the anal canal there are longitudinal folds (Columnae anales)
- **no Appendices epiploicae.**

The transverse folds of the rectum cause in addition to the two curvatures in the sagittal plane, up to three curvatures (**Flexurae laterales**) in the frontal plane, which, however, are very irregular and usually difficult to discern. One of the folds is relatively consistently palpable 6–9 cm above the Linea anocutanea (**Plica transversa recti = KOHLRAUSCH's folds**). Under this fold the rectum is extended to the **Ampulla recti** (➤ Fig. 8.18). The **Linea anorectalis** forms the transition area to the anal canal, which is recognisable due to the change from the transverse folds of the rectum to the longitudinal folds of the anal canal.

Clinical remarks

From a clinical perspective, the anal canal usually begins in the area of the radiating in of the M. puborectalis ('rectally palpable anorectal ring') at the level of the Linea pectinata (➤ Fig. 8.18). Anatomically this boundary runs along the Linea anorectalis. Due to its position between the two lines (Linea anorectalis and Linea pectinata), the cavernous body in the anal canal is assigned either to the rectum ('Corpus cavernosum recti') or to the anal canal ('Corpus cavernosum ani'). In the following section, the Corpus cavernosum ani is discussed.

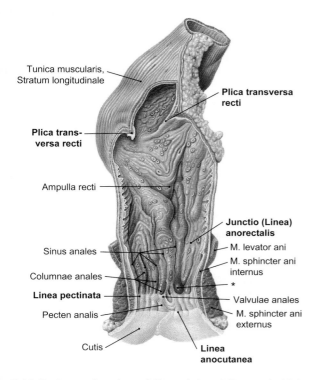

Tunica muscularis, Stratum longitudinale

Plica transversa recti

Plica transversa recti

Ampulla recti

Sinus anales

Columnae anales

Linea pectinata

Pecten analis

Cutis

Junctio (Linea) anorectalis

M. levator ani

M. sphincter ani internus

*

Valvulae anales

M. sphincter ani externus

Linea anocutanea

Fig. 8.18 Rectum and anal canal. Ventral view; * Haemorrhoidal nodes.

The **anal canal** is divided into **3 sections** (➤ Fig. 8.18, ➤ Fig. 8.20):

- **Zona columnaris:** it extends from the Linea anorectalis to the Linea pectinata and contains 6–10 longitudinal folds (**Columnae anales = MORGAGNI's columns**), which are elevated by a cavernous body ('**Corpus cavernosum ani**'). The longitudinal folds are delineated to the inferior by the **Valvulae anales**, which continue caudally into short pockets (Sinus anales), in whose depths the **anal glands (Glandulae anales,** Proctodeal glands,
- **Zona alba (anoderm enter) or Pecten analis (HILTON's zone):** the approximately 1 cm long section ranges from the **Linea pectinata (clinical term: Linea dentata),** runs jaggedly because here the Valvulae anales from above and the whitish squamous epithelium that tapers off on the longitudinal folds from below. Due to the multi-layered non-keratinised squamous epithelium, the mucosa has a whitish colour and is referred to synonymously as the '**Zona alba**'. The epithelium is firmly bound to the lower third of the M. spincter ani internus; a shift up or down is not possible, but there is a strong elasticity in the horizontal plane, as it is important for the passage of the faecal column.
- **Zona cutanea:** this starts at the blurred Linea anocutanea (HILTON's line) and forms the transitional zone to the outer skin. The skin is highly puckered, pigmented and hairless. Finally, somewhat distant from the anus, is the perianal region with hair, sebaceous glands and sweat glands (➤ Fig. 8.21). Located at the border between the Zona cutanea and perianal region is the subepithelial Plexus venosus subcutaneus.

Clinical remarks

As the rectum has transverse folds (Plicae transversae recti), whilst the anal canal, in contrast has longitudinal folds (Columnae anales), if there is a protrusion of intestinal sections out of the anus (prolapse) it can be seen with the naked eye, whether it is a case of **rectal prolapse** or **anal prolapse**. In the case of an anal prolapse there are longitudinally running mucosal folds and in a rectal prolapse the mucosal folds run circularly. Both can be associated with incontinence.

Because the supply areas of the vessels and nerves change here, the Linea pectinata is an important orientation line in the **diagnosis and treatment of cancer of the anal canal (see below).**

The proctodeal glands can penetrate the sphincter and in the case of inflammation can lead to the formation of **fistulas and abscesses,** which can spread into the Fossa ischioanalis.

8.4.3 Mesorectum

The topography of the rectum is of great clinical significance (➤ Fig. 8.19). The bony pelvis is covered on its inner side by a **parietal fascia (Fascia pelvis parietalis).** The section on the anterior side of the Os sacrum is referred to as the **Fascia presacralis** (clinically: **WALDEYER's fascia**). In addition, every single organ is surrounded by connective tissue that in its entirety constitutes the **visceral fascia (Fascia pelvis visceralis)**. Because these fascia are not disectable on a fixed specimen they were neglected for a long time in anatomy. The section of the visceral fascia around the rectum (clinically: **mesorectal fascia**) is of particular importance. It surrounds a space filled with fat and connective tissue, which contains the vascular, lymphatic and nervous systems of the rectum and the regional lymph nodes. This space within the 'mesorectal fascia' is, therefore, referred to clinically as the '**mesorectum**'.

Embedded in the 'mesorectum', in men the anterior wall of the rectum is firstly positioned from behind the urinary bladder (Vesica urinaria) and the seminal vesicles (Glandulae vesiculosae) and then further caudally the prostate gland. In the process, the rectum is separated from the prostate only by the thin **Fascia rectoprostatica** (clinically: **DENONVILLIER's fascia**) (➤ Fig. 8.19), which continues cranially into the **Septum rectovesicale**. In women, the rectum has a close topographical relationship to the posterior side of the vagina and is divided by this only by the **Fascia rectovaginalis (= Septum rectovaginale)** (➤ Fig. 8.58).

The mesorectal fascia thus separates the rectum with its vascular, lymphatic and nervous systems from the Plexus hypogastricus inferior, which represents the large autonomic nerve plexus of the pelvis and thus is responsible for the innervation of all pelvic viscera (➤ Chap. 8.8.5).

Clinical remarks

The mesorectal fascia is an important boundary structure in coloproctological surgery. In the case of **rectal cancer** it enables a bloodless removal of the rectum with its regional lymph nodes **(total mesorectal excision, TME)**. In the case of a TME, the Plexus hypogastricus inferior can be preserved, which is important for urinary and faecal continence, as well as erection and ejaculation in men, and among others the function of the cavernous body and BARTHOLIN's glands in women. In this way, incontinence and disorders of sexual functions can mostly be avoided.

Since in men the rectum is separated by just the thin Fascia rectoprostatica (DENONVILLIER's fascia) from the prostate, the **prostate is diagnostically accessible in a rectal examination**. Due to the high incidence of benign prostatic adenomata (prostatic hyperplasia) and malignant prostate carcinoma, digital rectal examination forms part of a complete physical examination in men over 50 years old.

8.4.4 Continence organ

Continence is the ability to hold back intestinal contents/faeces reflexively at will and to induce its emptying reflexively and at a desired point in time at will. For this, the anal canal has a locally and central nervous system-controlled **continence organ** (➤ Fig. 8.20, ➤ Fig. 8.21).

Components

The continence organ is composed of:
- **Ampulla recti:** the expansion of the ampulla on filling is registered by autonomous afferents (Nn. splanchnici pelvici) and perceived by central pathways as an impulse to defecate. Via spinal reflex arches it causes short-term atony of the M. sphincter ani internus (see below, **anorectal relaxation reflex**) with resulting contraction of all sphincters.
- **M. levator ani** (striated muscle, innervated arbitrarily by the N. pudendus and directly by the Plexus sacralis): the puborectal section of the M. levator ani (levator sling = M. puborectalis, ➤ Fig. 8.22) encompasses the distal section of the rectum at the transition to the anal canal (M. sphincter recti). The muscle is in a state of **permanent contraction**, which is only countermanded temporarily during defecation. The pubococcygeal section (M. pubococcygeus) of the M. levator ani is also involved in continence activity.
- **M. sphincter ani externus** (striated muscle, arbitrarily innervated by the N. pudendus): the muscle has 3 sections: Pars profunda, Pars superficialis and Pars subcutanea (➤ Fig. 8.20). The Pars profunda is functionally closely linked with the M. puborectalis, M. pubococcygeus and the retrorectal connective tissue. Via short-term atony of the M. sphincter ani internus (see below), an expansion of the ampulla causes the contents of the rectum to come into contact with the intermediate zone (Anoderm). This results in a reflexive contraction of the M. sphincter

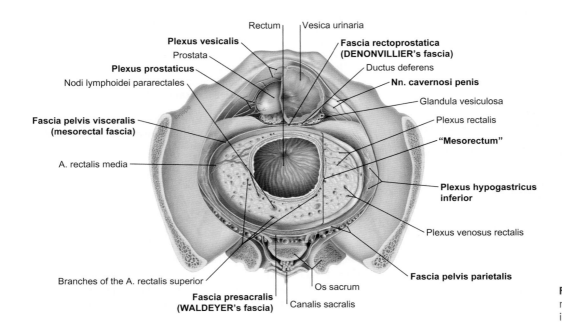

Rectum | Vesica urinaria
Plexus vesicalis
Prostata
Plexus prostaticus
Nodi lymphoidei pararectales
Fascia pelvis visceralis (mesorectal fascia)
A. rectalis media
Branches of the A. rectalis superior
Fascia presacralis (WALDEYER's fascia)
Fascia rectoprostatica (DENONVILLIER's fascia)
Ductus deferens
Nn. cavernosi penis
Glandula vesiculosa
Plexus rectalis
"Mesorectum"
Plexus hypogastricus inferior
Plexus venosus rectalis
Fascia pelvis parietalis
Os sacrum
Canalis sacralis

Fig. 8.19 Mesorectum; schematic diagram of a transversal incision, cranial view. [L238]

ani externus. If the muscle is now voluntarily contracted further, the M. sphincter ani internus also contracts again and excretion is suppressed. If the 'externus' is not voluntarily contracted, then excretion ensues. (➤ Fig. 8.21). Thus, with respect to defecation, the M. sphincter ani externus performs a **regulating function**.

• **M. sphincter ani internus** (70% of continence function at rest, protracted contraction, smooth muscles, involuntary, sympathet-

ically activated): the muscle forms the **centre of the continence organ**. It continues the circular layer of the intestinal wall and is, to a certain extent 'inserted' into the M. sphincter ani externus (between which is only connective tissue ➤ Fig. 8.21). Cranially it is connected to the M. puborectalis. The longitudinal layer runs on the outside of the circular layer as the so-called **M. corrugator ani** and terminates later with elastic tendons in the perianal skin.

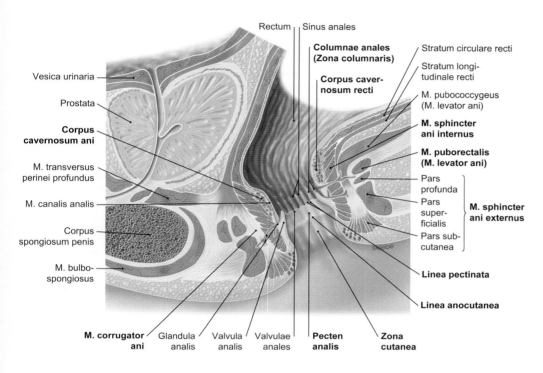

Fig. 8.20 Rectum and anal canal in men with presentation of the continence organ; median incision; view from left (according to [S010-1-16])

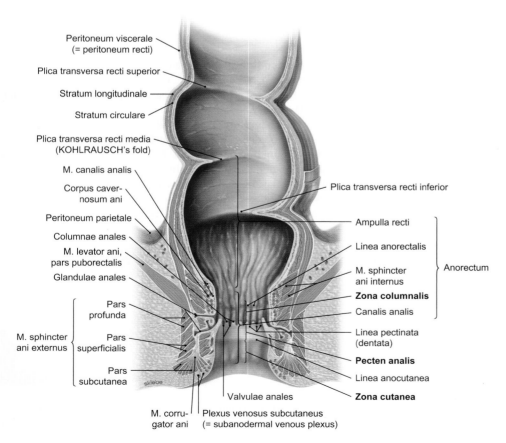

Fig. 8.21 Frontal incision through the pelvis with Ampulla recti and Canalis analis. [L238]

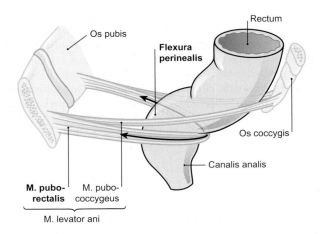

Os pubis
Rectum
Flexura perinealis
Os coccygis
Canalis analis
M. pubo- rectalis   M. pubo- coccygeus
M. levator ani

Fig. 8.22 Course of the M. puborectalis; schematic diagram. [L126]

A contraction of the M. corrugator ani causes a puckering of the anal skin and a 'drawing in' of the perianal skin into the outer anal canal with sealing of the anal edge. In defecation the M. corrugator ani contracts and leads to shortening of the anal canal. The circular layer increases in diameter caudally in the area of the M. sphincter ani internus (in comparison to the rest of the intestinal tract) = true sphincter. The smooth muscles of the 'internus' differ in their physiological behaviour from the rest of the intestinal muscles as there is no peristalsis and they are continually contracted. Only in defecation does a short-term, reflexively induced atony of the muscles occur.

- **M. canalis analis** (smooth musculature) and **Corpus cavernosum ani:** The sphincters alone are not in a position to seal the anal canal. Even at maximum contraction an opening of several millimetres remains. It is sealed by the M. canalis analis and the Corpus cavernosum ani that sits upon it.
  - The muscle originates from the M. sphincter internus ani and the longitudinal muscle layer of the rectum and radiates in a fan shape into the epithelium above the Corpus cavernosum, which it penetrates in the process. In this way, it creates a connection between the muscular, contractile part of the sealing mechanism with the vessels (**angiomuscular sealing mechanism**). Due to the fan-shaped course, variably long muscle fibres develop; the shortest terminate at the level of the Linea dentata. Due to radiation into the mucosa, the Linea dentata is kept taut and the Corpus cavernosum is fixed into its position above this line (➤ Fig. 8.21).
  - The Corpus cavernosum ani (approx. 10% of continence function) is fed arterially and consists of arteriovenous anastomoses with specialised vessels. It enables gas-tight, water-tight and faecal-tight sealing (**finely tuned continence**) of the anal canal. If the M. sphincter ani internus is contracted (during perpetuation of continence at rest), venous outflow is restricted, whilst arterial inflow is maintained. The cavernous body tissue fills with blood, becomes enlarged and effectively seals the lumen of the anal canal. In the process the vessel cushions interlock in a star shape. The A. rectalis superior divides at the level of the IIIrd sacral vertebra (corresponds to the KOHLRAUSCH's fold) into 2 main branches; the right branch divides again (➤ Fig. 8.24). In this way, 3 main arteries at 3, 7 and 11 o'clock reach the intestinal wall at the level of the Linea anorectalis and feed, among other things, the Corpus cavernosum ani (➤ Fig. 8.21).
- **Anal skin (Anoderm):** above the Linea anocutanea (HILTON's line) the skin has very good sensory innervation and contains

sebaceous glands. At approximately 1 cm wide, it is inseparably fixed with the M. sphincter ani internus at the latter's posterior edge: Pecten analis (HILTON's zone). The highly sensitive skin is of critical importance for the anorectal reflex. It controls volume, consistency (liquid, solid, gaseous) and position. This sensory detection is also the stimulus for voluntary termination of defecation. Here, the M. sphincter ani externus and M. puborectalis contract. After a slight delay, the M. sphincter ani internus also contracts again.

Clinical remarks

Haemorrhoids are pathologic extensions of the Corpus cavernosum ani and are a common occurrence. The causes are unclear, but appear to be associated with dietary habits in industrialised nations (too much fat, too little dietary fibre). The location of the haemorrhoidal nodes is given in terms of a clock face (in a 'lithotomy position'. Due to the branching pattern of the main branches of the A. rectalis superior on entering the Corpus cavernosum ani, the so-called main nodes typically form at 3, 7 and 11 o'clock. In addition, 'accessory nodes' may occur (corresponding to the accessory branches that emerge from the main branches), e.g. at 1 o'clock in ➤ Fig. 8.23.
Haemorrhoids can be divided into different **stages**:
- Stage I: only visible endoscopically
- Stage II: when pressed, they will emerge through the anal canal to the outside, but will return spontaneously back into the anal canal
- Stage III: emerge spontaneously, but can be repositioned with the finger
- Stage IV: emerge from the anal canal and cannot be repositioned
From stage II onwards treatment should be undertaken according to the stage and form: either using sclerotherapy or rubber band ligation (stage II) or surgery: fixation or removal (stages III and IV).

Defaecation (bowel movement)

Via stretching receptors in the Ampulla recti, an autonomic **reflex arc in the sacral portion of the parasympathetic nervous system (S2–4)** is activated in the spinal cord (defaecation reflex) (➤ Fig. 8.26), which increases the peristaltic activity of the muscles of the Colon sigmoideum and rectum and reduces the tone of the M. sphincter ani internus (➤ Table 8.2). Through voluntarily induced relaxation of the puborectal sling and the M. sphincter ani externus the anorectal angle is counteracted and the anal canal is widened. The blood-filled Corpus cavernosum ani is slowly 'squeezed' by the column of stool passing through. The flatly-oriented portions of

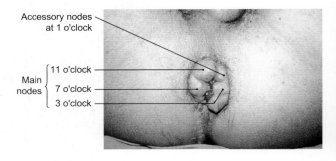

Accessory nodes at 1 o'clock
Main nodes { 11 o'clock / 7 o'clock / 3 o'clock

Fig. 8.23 Haemorrhoids stage IV; caudal view in the 'lithotomy position', when the patient is lying on his back and the examiner is looking at the bowel. [R234]

Table 8.2 Processes during bowel movement (defaecation).

Via parasympathetic reflex arc (S2–4, brain stem)	Arbitrary (thalamus and cerebrum)
• Reflex muscle contraction of the Colon sigmoideum and rectum (parasympathetic, S2–4) • Atony of the M. spincter ani internus (inhibition of the sympathetic nervous system)	• Weakness of the M. puborectalis and of the pelvic floor → spreading of the Flexura perinealis and raising of the rectum • Atony of the M. sphincter ani externus

the M. levator ani tense and thereby counteract the rising intra-abdominal pressure. The increase in pressure is based on the simultaneous contraction of the muscles of the diaphragm and abdominal wall and closure of the glottis. A squatting position facilitates defaecation. The column of stool passing along the anoderm is registered via somatic afferents of the N. pudendus. After the stool has passed through, defaecation is completed by contraction of both anal sphincters and the puborectal sling.

Clinical remarks

For a smooth course of **defaecation** several factors must work together: stool consistency must be such that
• intrarectal pressure is increased, so that the M. sphincter ani internus slackens;
• the Corpus cavernosum ani is compressed and emptied during the passage;
• the stool can be clearly perceived in the area of the anoderm in order to finish defaecation in a targeted manner.
If the stool is too soft (**diarrhoea**) or too hard (**constipation**), then this is not the case.

8.4.5 Arteries of the rectum and anal canal

The rectum and anal canal are supplied by **3 arteries (Aa. rectales superior, media and inferior)**. The innervation areas of the arteries correspond to their evolutionary origin. Since the whole rectum

and the upper part of the anal canal originates from the hind gut, but the lower sections of the anal canal from the proctodeum, it is understandable why anastomoses of vessels are located in the area of the Linea pectinata (clinically 'Linea dentata'). The arteries of the rectum and anal canal are (➤ Fig. 8.24):

• **A. rectalis superior** (unpaired): from the A. mesenterica inferior, supplies the majority of the rectum and the M. sphincter ani internus as well as the mucosa of the anal canal *above* the Linea pectinata and thus also the cavernous body ('Corpus cavernosum ani'). Its branches anastomose with the A. rectalis inferior.
• **A. rectalis media** (paired): outflow from the A. iliaca interna above the pelvic floor (M. levator ani); however, this artery is rarely formed on both sides and can even be missing on both sides. If present, it supports blood flow in the lower third of the rectum.
• **A. rectalis inferior** (paired): outflow from the A. pudenda interna *beneath* the pelvic floor. From the outside it supplies the anal canal and its sphincters up to the bottom third of the rectum as well as the mucosa of the anal canal *underneath* the Linea pectinata.

Between the various arteries numerous anastomoses are formed. The A. rectalis superior is the last branch of the A. mesenterica inferior. It gives off one branch, which anostomoses with the Aa. sigmoideae. From this point on (clinically: **SUDECK's point** [*]) it is a terminal artery.

Clinical remarks

The cavernous body of the anal canal ('Corpus cavernosum ani') is fed predominantly by the A. rectalis superior. Therefore, **bleeding from haemorrhoids**, which constitute the expanded caverns of the cavernous body, is arterial bleeding that is conspicuous due to its bright red colour.

8.4.6 Veins of the rectum and anal canal

As with all pelvic organs the veins of the rectum form an extensive plexus in the mesorectum (**Plexus venosus rectalis**). The blood

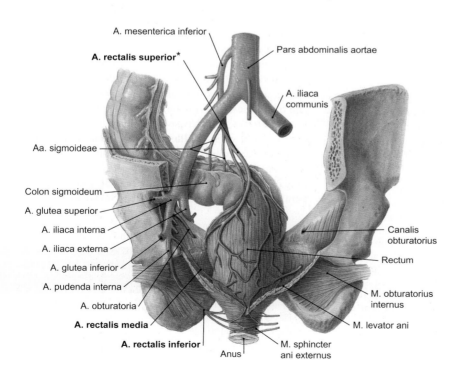

Fig. 8.24 Arteries of the rectum, Aa. rectales. Dorsal view. After the SUDECK's point (*) the A. rectalis superior is a terminal artery.

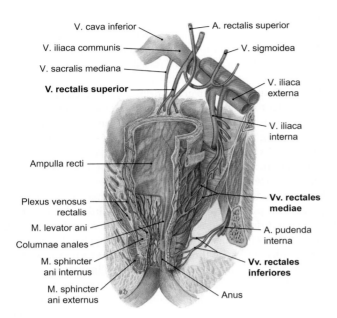

V. cava inferior
V. iliaca communis
V. sacralis mediana
V. rectalis superior
A. rectalis superior
V. sigmoidea
V. iliaca externa
V. iliaca interna
Ampulla recti
Plexus venosus rectalis
M. levator ani
Columnae anales
M. sphincter ani internus
M. sphincter ani externus
Vv. rectales mediae
A. pudenda interna
Vv. rectales inferiores
Anus

Fig. 8.25 Venous supply of rectum and anal canal, Canalis analis. Ventral view. Tributaries to the V. portae hepatis (purple) and to the V. cava inferior (blue).

flows out of this plexus according to the arteries of the rectum and anal canal via **3 veins** (➤ Fig. 8.25):

- **V. rectalis superior** (unpaired): connection via the V. mesenterica inferior to the portal vein (V. portae hepatis)
- **V. rectalis media** (paired, but very variable): connection via the V. iliaca interna to the V. cava inferior
- **V. rectalis inferior** (paired): connection via the V. pudenda interna and the V. iliaca interna to the V. cava inferior

The boundary between the drainage area of the V. portae hepatis and the V. cava inferior is located in the area of the **Linea pectinata**; however, here there are numerous links.

8.4.7 Lymphatic vessels of the rectum and anal canal

Lymph drainage follows the course of the arterial blood vessels. The regional lymph nodes are the **Nodi lymphoidei anorectales/pararectales**, which lie directly on the intestine, and the **Nodi lymphoidei rectales superiores**, which are also located in the mesorectum (➤ Fig. 8.19).

From the **proximal rectum**, the lymph passes into the **Nodi lymphoidei mesenterici inferiores** at the outflow of the A. mesenterica inferior and from there into the para-aortic lymph nodes (**Nodi lymphoidei lumbales**) located in the retroperitoneum and into the **Trunci lumbales** (➤ Fig. 7.23).

The **distal rectum** and the **anal canal** including the M. sphincter ani internus also have a connection to the drainage area of the Trunci lumbales. The first lymph node stations are the **Nodi lymphoidei iliaci interni** (or for the end section of the anal canal below the **Linea pectinata** and for the M. sphincter ani externus, the **Nodi lymphoidei inguinales superficiales**) in the groin (➤ Fig. 7.23).

8.4.8 Innervation of the rectum and anal canal

The **Plexus rectalis** is a part of the Plexus hypogastricus inferior and correspondingly contains sympathetic and parasympathetic nerve fibres (➤ Table 8.3, ➤ Fig. 8.26):

- The **sympathetic** fibres activate the M. sphincter ani internus and thereby ensure continence.
- The **parasympathetic** nerve fibres facilitate peristalsis and inhibit the sphincter.

The preganglionic **sympathetic nerve fibres** (T10–L3) reach the rectum via the **Plexus mesentericus inferior** or descend from the Plexus aorticus abdominalis via the Plexus hypogastricus superior and out of the sacral ganglia of the sympathetic trunk (Truncus sympathicus) via the Nn. splanchnici sacrales. They are predominantly converted in the **Plexus hypogastricus inferior** into postganglionic neurons (Ganglia pelvica). These reach the rectum with the branches of the Aa. rectales superiores and media.

Preganglionic **parasympathetic nerve fibres** pass out of the sacral parasympathetic nervous system (S2–S4) via the Nn. splanchnici

Table 8.3 Innervation of the rectum and anal canal.

Innervation of the rectum and anal canal above the Linea pectinata	Innervation of the anal canal below the Linea pectinata
• Sympathetically (T10–L3) via the Plexus mesenterius inferior and the Plexus hypogastricus inferior • Parasympathetically (S2–4) via the Plexus hypogastricus inferior	• Somatically via the N. pudendus

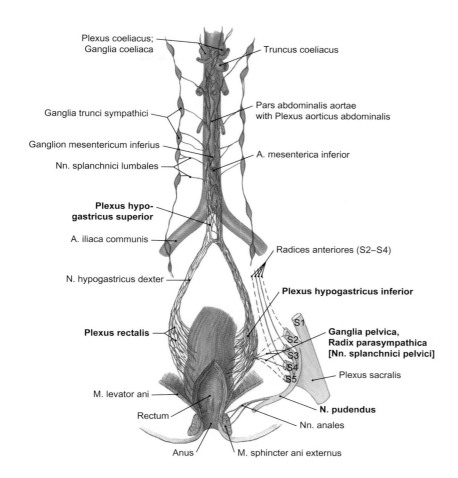

Plexus coeliacus; Ganglia coeliaca

Truncus coeliacus

Ganglia trunci sympathici

Pars abdominalis aortae with Plexus aorticus abdominalis

Ganglion mesentericum inferius

A. mesenterica inferior

Nn. splanchnici lumbales

Plexus hypogastricus superior

A. iliaca communis

Radices anteriores (S2–S4)

N. hypogastricus dexter

Plexus hypogastricus inferior

Plexus rectalis

S1
S2
S3
S4
S5

Ganglia pelvica, Radix parasympathica [Nn. splanchnici pelvici]

Plexus sacralis

M. levator ani

Rectum

N. pudendus

Nn. anales

Anus

M. sphincter ani externus

Fig. 8.26 Innervation of the rectum and anal canal. Ventral view; schematic diagram. The Plexus rectalis contains sympathetic (green) and parasympathetic (purple) nerve fibres.

pelvici into the ganglia of the **Plexus hypogastricus inferior.** They are converted either here or in the vicinity of the intestine into postganglionic fibres (Ganglia pelvica), which enter the mesorectum and there ascend, either independently or along the A. rectalis superior.

The autonomic innervation ends roughly in the area of the **Linea pectinata.** The inferior section of the anal canal has somatic innervation from the **N. pudendus** with sensory fibres. In addition, the N. pudendus activates the M. sphincter ani externus and the M. puborectalis with motor fibres and thus makes voluntary closure of the anus possible.

For general organisation of the autonomic nervous system in the pelvis, see ➤ Chap. 8.8.5.

N O T E

Evolutionarily, (such as at the left colic flexure) at the **Linea pectinata** there occurs a change of the innervation areas **of all vascular, lymphatic and nervous systems:**
- **Arteries:** A. mesenterica inferior ↔ A. iliaca interna
- **Veins:** V. portae hepatis ↔ V. iliaca interna
- **Lymph nodes:** Nodi lymphoidei iliaci interni ↔ Nodi lymphoidei inguinales
- **Innervation:** autonomic innervation (Plexus mesentericus inferior and Plexus hypogastricus inferior) ↔ somatic innervation (N. pudendus)

8.5 Male genitalia

Clinical remarks

Since the innervation areas of the vascular, lymphatic and nervous systems change there, the Linea pectinata is an important orientation line regarding **clinical and surgical treatment of carcinoma of the rectum and the anal canal:**
- Tumours situated proximally of the Linea pectinata metastasise into the pelvic lymph nodes and via venous blood to the liver. Proximal tumours are usually painless.
- Distal tumours metastasise firstly into the pelvic lymph nodes of the groin and into the lungs. Particularly because of their somatic innervation by the N. pudendus, distal tumours can be extremely painful.

Nevertheless, classification of rectal cancer tumours currently depends on the distance between the tumours and the Linea anocutanea.

Skills

After working through this chapter, you should be able to:
- explain the sections of the internal and external male genitalia and their function
- explain the development of the male genitalia, describe differences from the development of female genitalia, and understand possible deformities
- explain the structure and organisation of the penis and scrotum on a specimen
- show on a specimen the position, structure and fascia of the testes and epididymis, as well as the sections and course of the Vas deferens
- retrace fascia and content of the spermatic cord on a specimen
- explain the function and efferent ducts of the accessory sex glands

- explain the zonal classification of the prostate and topographical relationship to the rectum with its clinical relevance
- show arteries of the individual sexual organs and deduce their different origins from the development
- characterise drainage areas of veins and lymphatic pathways with their clinical importance
- understand the exact course of the arteries and veins of the penis with their importance for erection
- explain the autonomic and somatic innervation of the genital organs with their importance for the sexual functions

8.5.1 Overview

The male genitalia are divided into the internal and the external male genitalia (➤ Fig. 8.27). Whilst the external genitalia are located outside the body in the perineal region (➤ Chapter 8.9.3), the internal genitalia are found in the pelvic cavity or have been shifted according to their development from the abdominal cavity into the scrotum. Male genitalia are treated in medicine by the specialist field of urology.

The **external genitalia** include:
- Penis
- Urethra (Urethra masculina)
- Scrotum

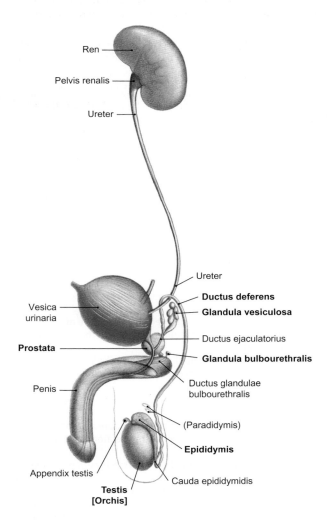

Fig. 8.27 Male urinary and reproductive organs. View from right

Labels (top to bottom, left side):
Ren
Pelvis renalis
Ureter
Vesica urinaria
Prostata
Penis
Appendix testis
Testis [Orchis]

Labels (right side):
Ureter
Ductus deferens
Glandula vesiculosa
Ductus ejaculatorius
Glandula bulbourethralis
Ductus glandulae bulbourethralis
(Paradidymis)
Epididymis
Cauda epididymidis

The urethra is described with the efferent urinary tracts (➤ Chap. 8.3).

The **internal male genitalia** include:
- Testis
- Epididymis
- Vas deferens (Ductus deferens)
- Spermatic cord (Funiculus spermaticus)
- Accessory sex glands:
  - Prostate gland
  - Seminal gland (Glandula vesiculosa), paired
  - COWPER's gland (Glandula bulbourethralis) paired

8.5.2 Function of the male genitalia

The **external genitalia** are sexual organs. The penis is used for sexual intercourse. The scrotum encases testis, epididymis, the first section of the Vas deferens as well as their vessels and nerves, and due to the storage of the testis outside the body, enables lowering of the surrounding temperature, which is necessary for the formation of sperm (spermatogenesis).

The **internal genitalia** are reproductive organs with different functions:
- Testis: formation of sperm cells and sex hormones (testosterone)
- Epididymis and spermatic duct: storage and transport of sperm cells
- Spermatic cord: guidance of spermatic duct and vessels and nerves of the testis
- Accessory sex glands: secretion of the ejaculate and lubricants

The sperm cells (spermatozoa) are formed in the testis and conveyed to the epididymis, where they are stored. During orgasm spermatozoa are transported via the spermatic duct into the urethra (**emission**), where they are mixed with secretions from the prostate and seminal glands into an ejaculate (volume: 3ml), before it is then released via the penis (**ejaculation**). The secretions of the ejaculate are important for the nourishment of spermatozoa and support fertilisation. COWPER's gland already issues secretion during the arousal phase, which moistens the woman's vagina as a lubricant. The testis, in addition to forming sperm cells, also has the important task of forming the male sex hormone testosterone. Because testis and epididymis have been shifted into the scrotum, the vessels and nerves arise according to their site of origin in the retroperitoneal space at the level of the kidneys and run in the inguinal canal together with the spermatic duct in the spermatic cord.

8.5.3 Development of the male genitalia

The internal and external genitalia in both sexes develop equally up to the *7th week* (sexually indifferent stage). Only afterwards do the genitalia differentiate specifically according to the genetic sex of the embryo.

Development of the internal genitalia (sexually indifferent stage)

The genitalia develop out of the **intermediate mesoderm**, which in the *4th week* forms the **urogenital ridge**. The medial section appears in the *5th week* as the **gonadal ridge** and thus a week later than the laterally located renal unit, which at this point in time is found at the stage of the mesonephros (➤ Fig. 8.28, ➤ Fig. 8.29). The **connective tissue** of the gonadal ridge is covered by a serous membrane (Tunica serosa), which emerges from the **coelomic epi-**

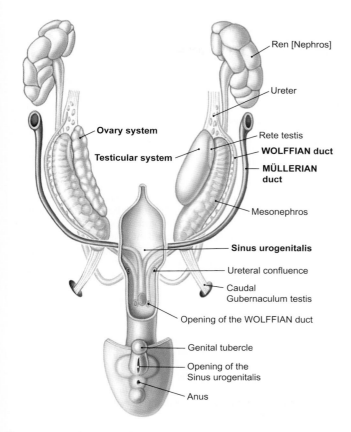

Ren [Nephros]

Ureter

Ovary system

Rete testis

Testicular system

WOLFFIAN duct

MÜLLERIAN duct

Mesonephros

Sinus urogenitalis

Ureteral confluence

Caudal Gubernaculum testis

Opening of the WOLFFIAN duct

Genital tubercle

Opening of the Sinus urogenitalis

Anus

Fig. 8.28 Development of the urinary organs and early development of the internal genitalia in both sexes in the 8th week of development. (according to [S010-1-16])

thelium of the abdominal cavity. In the *6th week* the **primary germ cords** form when the **primordial germ cells** migrate into the gonadal ridges (➤ Fig. 8.29). In the process, these take a complicated route: after they have already become differentiated in the *2nd week*

in the area of the primitive ridge, in the *4th week* they pass firstly with the yolk sac into the epithelium of the hindgut, which they leave again in order to migrate via its mesenterium into the gonadal ridge.

Laterally from these **sexually indifferent gonads** 2 pairs of ducts running in parallel develop one after the other: initially, in the *5th week* on both sides the mesonephric duct (Ductus mesonephricus) or **WOLFFIAN duct,** a primitive ureter of the mesonephros, is present, which enters the caudal part of the hindgut, from which the Sinus urogenitalis later emerges as a precursor of the urinary bladder (➤ Fig. 8.28). The sinus induces in the *7th week* the formation of the similarly paired **MÜLLERIAN duct** (Ductus paramesonephricus), which, therefore, sinks out of the coelomic epithelium of the gonadal ridge and remains in open connection with the abdominal cavity (➤ Fig. 8.28, ➤ Fig. 8.29). In contrast to the WOLFFIAN duct, the distal ends of the MÜLLERIAN duct fuse prior to entering the Sinus urogenitalis and form the uterovaginal canal.

Development of the internal male genitalia

At the end of the *7th week* in men, the gonad system develops into the testis. Responsible for the formation of the testis is a certain transcription factor (TDF, 'testis-determining factor'), which is expressed by a gene on the Y chromosome (SRY, 'Sex determining Region of the Y chromosome') of male embryos. The germinal cords now form the **testicular cords,** which become the **seminiferous tubules** (Tubuli seminiferi) (➤ Fig. 8.29). In their walls are the **SERTOLI cells**, the **spermatogonia**, which are incorporated into the epithelium as descendants of the primordial germ cells. Between the seminiferous tubules connective tissue cells differentiate into the **LEYDIG cells**. The testis has thus formed as the male gonad. If the TDF is missing, then an ovary forms.

The testis was generated in the lumbar region at the level of the mesonephros, which also prepares several ductules (Ductuli efferentes) as a connection to the later epididymis. In the process, the testis bulges out into the peritoneal cavity and is anchored dorsally by a

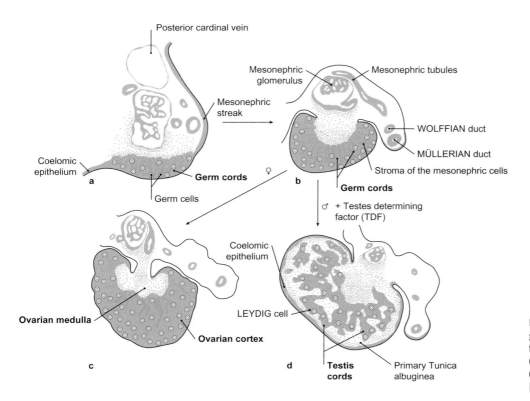

Posterior cardinal vein

Mesonephric glomerulus

Mesonephric tubules

Mesonephric streak

WOLFFIAN duct

MÜLLERIAN duct

Coelomic epithelium

Stroma of the mesonephric cells

Germ cords ♀

Germ cords

Germ cells

♂ + Testes determining factor (TDF)

Coelomic epithelium

Ovarian medulla

LEYDIG cell

Ovarian cortex

Testis cords

Primary Tunica albuginea

Fig. 8.29 Development of the gonads from the sexually indifferent gonad from the 6th week (a, b) into ovary (c) and testis (d). (according to [S010-1-16]) [L126]

peritoneal duplicature (**Mesorchium**), in which the coelomic epithelium runs over the surface of the testis. This peritoneal fold forms the upper and lower **gonadal ligaments** (➤ Fig. 8.28) cranially and caudally of the testis. In the course of the body's growth the testis is then shifted to caudal (**Descensus testis**), whereby it brings along its vascular and nerval supply as the spermatic cord. In the process, along the inferior gonad ligament, which becomes the **Gubernaculum testis**, a peritoneal protrusion first forms (**Proc. vaginalis peritonei**) up to the area of the later scrotum, where the testis descends until birth (➤ Fig. 8.30). As the Proc. vaginalis peritonei pushes the layers of the ventral wall apart from each other in front of it, these form the walls of the **inguinal canal**. Around birth the Proc. vaginalis peritonei closes in the area of the spermatic cord. The distal part of the Proc. vaginalis remains and forms the **Tunica vaginalis testis** as part of the testicular coatings.

The formation of the genital ducts depends on hormones, both of which are formed only in the testis:

- **Testosterone** (from the LEYDIG cells): promotes the differentiation of the WOLFFIAN ducts
- **AMH** (anti-MÜLLERIAN hormone, from the SERTOLI cells): inhibits the development of the MÜLLERIAN ducts

Testosterone causes the differentiation of the **WOLFFIAN duct** into:

- **Epididymis**
- **Vas deferens** (Ductus deferens)
- **Seminal glands** (Glandulae vesiculosae)

as well as the formation of the other accessory sex glands (**prostate, COWPER's glands**) from the **entoderm** of the **Sinus urogenitalis**, which has developed in this section into the urethra. In the process, only the epithelial parts of the organs are formed by the WOLFFIAN duct or the Sinus urogenitalis. Connective tissue, and smooth muscles emerge from the surrounding mesoderm.

Clinical remarks

The testes descend into the scrotum in 97% of all neonates, but only in 70% of premature babies. In the remaining cases cryptorchidism is present, whereby one or both testes are usually located in the inguinal canal (inguinal testis). Most of these testes spontaneously descend into the scrotum in the first half year of life but then no further so that surgical anchoring in the scrotum must be carried out due to the threat of infertility and because of an increased risk of testicular cancer. Small processes are present on the testes and epididymis as evolutionary relics (➤ Fig. 8.35), which are morbidly relevant in spite of their small size (see below). The Appendix testis at the upper testicular pole is a remnant of the MÜLLERIAN duct; in contrast the Appendix epididymidis at the head of the epididymis originates from the WOLFFIAN duct.

If the Proc. vaginalis peritonei fails to close completely, then fluid from the peritoneal cavity can cause a swelling of the scrotum (hydrocele). If the opening remains so wide that intestinal loops can shift into the inguinal canal, then a congenital inguinal hernia ensues.

Development of the external male genitalia

The external genitalia develop from the caudal part of the **Sinus urogenitalis**. In addition, the **ectoderm** with its inferiorly located connective tissue is also involved. In both sexes the external genitalia develop identically between the *4th and 7th week* (sexually in-

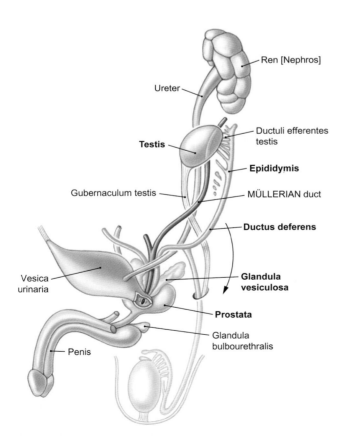

Fig. 8.30 Development of the internal male genitalia, Organa genitalia masculina interna. (according to [S010-1-16])

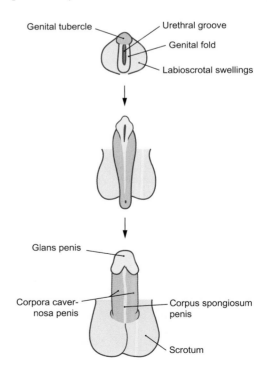

Fig. 8.31 Development of the external male genitalia, Organa genitalia masculina externa.

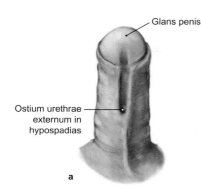

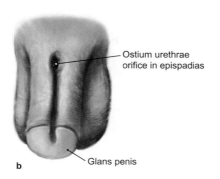

Fig. 8.32 Hypospadias and epispadias. The outer opening of the urethra is not located at the end of the glans penis, but, in the case of hypospadias, on the under side of the penis (**a**) and in epispadias (**b**) it is found dorsally at the penile shaft. [L266]

different stage). At the same time, the anterior wall of the Sinus urogenitalis sinks firstly to the **urethral groove** which is delineated on both sides by the **urethral folds**. Lateral to them are the **labioscrotal swellings** and at the anterior edge of the groove is the **genital tubercle** (➤ Fig. 8.31).

Afterwards in the male embryo under the influence of testosterone produced by the testis:

- the genital tubercle develops into the **penis (Corpora cavernosa)**
- the urethral folds develop into the **Corpus spongiosum** and into the **glans penis**
- the labioscrotal swellings develop into the **scrotum**

Due to the closure of the urethral folds over the urethral ridge the Pars spongiosa of the **urethra** is created at the same time.

Clinical remarks

When the closure of the urethral ridge is incomplete, the opening of the urethra is not located at the glans penis, but lies further proximally (➤ Fig. 8.32). In **hypospadias** (most common deformity of the penis) the urethra exits on the inferior side of the penis between the scrotum and the glans. In **epispadias** (rare) the urethra exits in a groove on the dorsal side of the penis. In addition to problems with urination, this condition can also cause a distorted curvature of the penis requiring surgical correction within the first years of life.

8.5.4 Penis and scrotum

The penis, in a flaccid state, is usually about 10 cm long and is divided into the **shaft (Corpus penis)** and the **root (Radix penis)** (➤ Fig. 8.33). The vascular, lymphatic and nervous systems of the penis lie on the dorsal side (Dorsum penis). The root of the penis is attached to the anterior abdominal wall by 2 ligaments:

- The superficial **Lig. fundiforme penis** emerges from the Linea alba and encompasses the penis on both sides as its fibre bundles form a loop.
- Lying underneath, the **Lig. suspensorium penis** is attached to the symphysis (➤ Fig. 8.34).

The distal end of the penis is thickened into the **glans penis**, which has a ridge (Corona glandis) at the base. When the penis is flaccid, the glans is covered by the foreskin (Preputium penis), which is secured to the inferior side of the penis by a ridge (Frenulum preputii).

The penis is constructed from the paired cavernous bodies of penis **(Corpora cavernosa penis)**, which are surrounded by a tough sheath (Tunica albuginea) and are separated by a Septum penis, as

well as from the cavernous body of the urethra (**Corpus spongiosum penis**), which surrounds the urethra. The Corpora cavernosa are fixed with the proximal ends (Crura penis) to the inferior pubic bones and are stabilised by the Mm. ischiocavernosi. The Corpus spongiosum is extended proximally to the Bulbus penis, which is covered by the M. bulbospongiosus, and forms the Glans penis distally. Externally, all the cavernous bodies are encased together by penile fascia (**Fascia penis**), which has superficial and deep fibres.

Clinical remarks

If the foreskin is too tight (**phimosis**) and cannot be retracted, problems with urination and infections can occur. Then the foreskin must be removed by circumcision.
Injuries to the suspensory ligaments can lead to curved deformities of the penis.

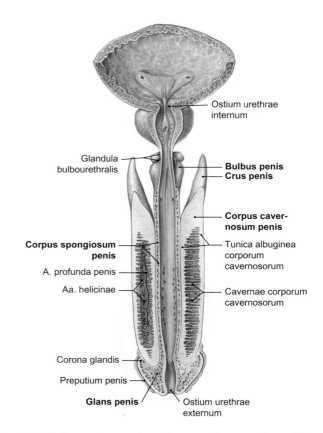

Fig. 8.33 Male member, penis, with exposed spongy tissue. Ventral view; urinary bladder and urethra opened, penile fascia removed.

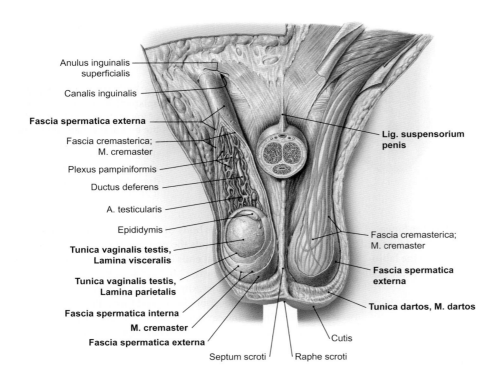

Anulus inguinalis superficialis
Canalis inguinalis
Fascia spermatica externa
Fascia cremasterica; M. cremaster
Plexus pampiniformis
Ductus deferens
A. testicularis
Epididymis
Tunica vaginalis testis, Lamina visceralis
Tunica vaginalis testis, Lamina parietalis
Fascia spermatica interna
M. cremaster
Fascia spermatica externa
Septum scroti
Raphe scroti
Cutis
Lig. suspensorium penis
Fascia cremasterica; M. cremaster
Fascia spermatica externa
Tunica dartos, M. dartos

Fig. 8.34 Scrotum and spermatic cord (Funiculus spermaticus). Ventral view; scrotum opened and penis frontally severed.

The **scrotum** is divided into two halves: externally in the median plane by a membranous raphe (Raphe scroti), and internally by a connective tissue separation layer (Septum scroti) (➤ Fig. 8.34). The wall of the scrotum consists of relatively strongly pigmented skin (Cutis), under which is a fat-free subcutis with much smooth musculature (Tunica dartos), which contributes to temperature regulation by its involuntary movement. Underneath, following as further layers, as with the spermatic cord, are the Fascia spermatica externa, the Fascia cremasterica and the Fascia spermatica interna (➤ Chap. 8.5.5).

8.5.5 Testis and epididymis

The **testis (Orchis)** is egg-shaped (➤ Fig. 8.35) and 4 × 3 cm in size (10–15 g). It has a **superior** and an **inferior pole** (Extremitas

superior and Extremitas inferior). The anterior and posterior borders (Margines anterior and posterior) are not clearly set and therefore indistinctly subdivide a **medial and a lateral surface** (Facies medialis and lateralis).

The **epididymis** sits above and distally to the testis and is secured by a superior and an inferior ligament (Ligg. epididymidis superius and inferius) (➤ Fig. 8.35). The epididymis is divided into the head (Caput), body (Corpus) and tail (Cauda).

The testis contains delicate ductules, which transport the spermatozoa formed in their walls to the epididymis. The epididymis consists of a single 6 m long coiled duct (Ductus epididymidis), which continues into the spermatic duct.

Between the wall of the scrotum and the testis is a further sheath, the **Tunica vaginalis testis** (➤ Fig. 8.34). It consists of an outer Lamina parietalis (Periorchium) on the inner side of the scrotum and an inner Lamina visceralis (Epiorchium) on the surface of the testis, which are connected to one another by the Mesorchium. Between these two layers is the '**Cavitas serosa scroti**', which corresponds to one of protrusions of the peritoneal cavity that arises in the course of the descent of the testes.

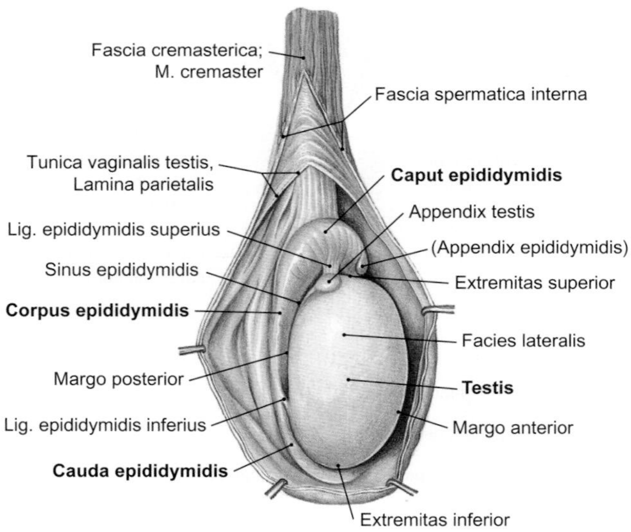

Fascia cremasterica; M. cremaster
Fascia spermatica interna
Tunica vaginalis testis, Lamina parietalis
Caput epididymidis
Lig. epididymidis superius
Appendix testis
(Appendix epididymidis)
Sinus epididymidis
Extremitas superior
Corpus epididymidis
Facies lateralis
Margo posterior
Testis
Lig. epididymidis inferius
Margo anterior
Cauda epididymidis
Extremitas inferior

Fig. 8.35 Testis (Orchis) and epididymis. View from right

Clinical remarks

Diseases of the testis, which often occur during childhood and adolescence, can to some extent be fulminant and associated with acute pain **(acute scrotum)**. The most common is **testicular torsion,** where the testis revolves around its longitudinal axis and, due to torsion of the spermatic cord and of the A. testicularis lying within, restricts blood flow, which can result in irreversible damage after just a few hours. Torsion usually occurs spontaneously or during exercise. After the blood flow disturbance has been established by a duplex ultrasonogram, surgery must take place immediately: the affected testis is turned back and both testes are fixed in the scrotum.

From a differential diagnostic point of view, there are torsions of the Appendix testis and the Appendix epididymis **(torsion of the hydatids)**, which, however, are treated conservatively with painkillers (➤ Chap. 8.5.3); there are also bacterial and viral (mumps) **infections**, where the testes or epididymis become inflamed and swollen.

In adults, asymptomatic testicular enlargements are always to be evaluated as an indication of a possible **testicular tumour**, which if necessary, should be excluded by a biopsy (see below).

8.5.6 Vas deferens and spermatic cord

The **Vas deferens (Ductus deferens)** is 35–40 cm long and 3 mm thick and runs with a scrotal, funicular, inguinal and pelvic section (➤ Fig. 8.36) via the spermatic cord and the inguinal canal. In the pelvis it crosses *over* the ureter, before it is attached to the dorsal side of the urinary bladder, where it expands (Ampulla ductus deferens) and, together with the efferent duct of the seminal gland, connects to the **Ductus ejaculatorius** (➤ Fig. 8.27), which finally flows into the Pars prostatica ➤ Fig. 8.16). In the spermatic cord, the Ductus deferens can clearly be felt due to its strong muscle wall!

The **spermatic cord (Funiculus spermaticus)** forms a fascia system in the scrotum and in the inguinal canal around the spermatic cord and the vascular, lymphatic and nervous systems of the testis.

The **coverings of the spermatic cord** are connected to the abdominal wall and therefore, like the latter, also form multiple layers (➤ Fig. 8.34, ➤ Fig. 8.37):

- Scrotal skin (Cutis)
- Tunica dartos: subcutis of scrotum with smooth musculature
- Fascia spermatica externa: continuation of the superficial abdominal fascia (Fascia abdominis superficialis)

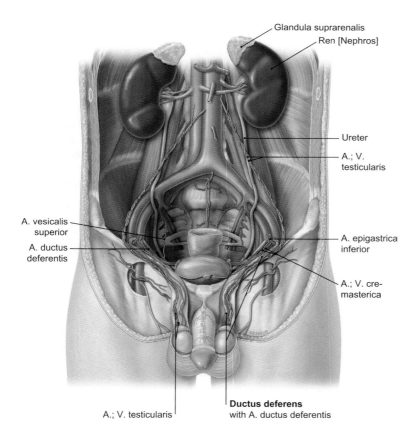

Fig. 8.36 Sections and course of the Ductus deferens. Ventral view. [L238]

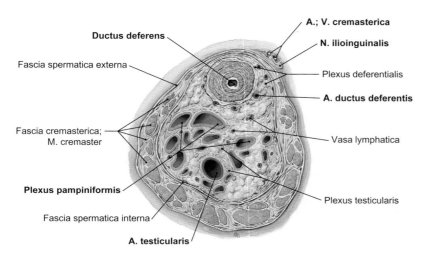

Fig. 8.37 Fascia and content of the spermatic cord, left. Frontal incision; ventral view. [S010-17]

- M. cremaster with Fascia cremasterica
- Fascia spermatica interna: continuation of the Fascia transversalis
- Tunica vaginalis testis

The **content of the spermatic cord** consist of the vas deferens and the different vessels and nerves of the testis as well as of the coverings (➤ Fig. 8.37):

- Vas deferens (Ductus deferens) with the A. ductus deferentis (from the A. umbilicalis)
- A. testicularis from the abdominal aorta and as venous accessory vessels of the Plexus pampiniformis
- N. genitofemoralis, R. genitalis (innervation of the M. cremaster)
- Lymph vessels (Vasa lymphatica) to the lumbar lymph nodes
- Autonomic nerve fibres (Plexus testicularis) from the plexus around the aorta

Attached **externally** to the spermatic cord are:

- N. ilioinguinalis
- A. and V. cremasterica (from A./V. epigastrica inferior)

Clinical remarks

During surgery **on an inguinal hernia** in men, care must be taken so that the inguinal canal is not narrowed too much, because otherwise the A. testicularis is compressed and infertility can ensue.

Since the spermatic cord is easily accessible before its entry into the inguinal canal, it can be cut on both sides for sterilisation **(vasectomy)**.

8.5.7 Accessory sex glands

The accessory sex glands include the unpaired prostate as well as the two seminal glands (Glandulae vesiculosae) and the two COWPER's glands (Glandulae bulbourethrales).

Prostate gland

The unpaired gland is $4 \times 3 \times 2$ cm in size (20 g) and is located below the fundus of the bladder. The prostate has a superior base and an inferior apex as well as an anterior and a posterior surface (Facies anterior and Facies posterior). It is divided into a right lobe and left lobe **(Lobus dexter and Lobus sinister)**, which are separated by a flat groove and also divided into a **Lobus medius** (➤ Fig. 8.38). Internally, the prostate is traversed by the urethra (Pars prostatica), into which its 30–50 individual glands each issue secretions via their own efferent ducts *on both sides* of the Colliculus seminalis. It forms 15–30% of the liquid volume of the ejaculate.

Internally, the prostate is divided into different **zones**, which are of the highest clinical relevance (➤ Fig. 8.39):

- **Central zone or internal zone** (25% of the glandular tissue): wedge-shaped segment between the Ductus ejaculatorii up to its confluence and the urethra
- **Peripheral zone or outer zone** (70% of the glandular tissue): surrounds the inner zone on the dorsal side like a mantle
- **Anterior zone:** gland-free area ventral of the urethra
- **Periurethral zone:** narrow strip of tissue immediately around the proximal urethra
- **Transition zone** (5% of the glandular tissue): both sides lateral of the periurethral zone

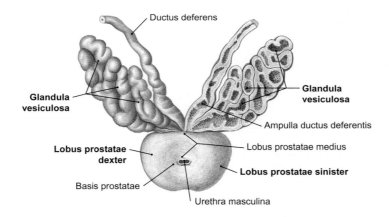

Fig. 8.38 Prostate and seminal vesicles. Cranial view.

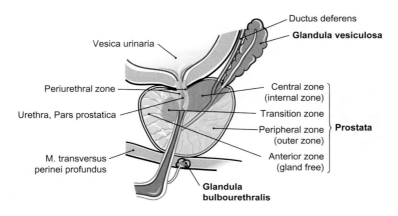

Fig. 8.39 Zones of the prostate. View from left; median incision.

Seminal gland (Glandula vesiculosa)

The paired gland rests on the dorsal side of the urinary bladder (➤ Fig. 8.38). The seminal glands are elongated oval glands (5 × 1 × 1 cm) and each consist of an individual raised gland of 15 cm in length. Its efferent duct combines with the Vas deferens to the Ductus ejaculatorius and ends in the Pars prostatica of the Urethra *on* the Colliculus seminalis (➤ Fig. 8.16). It secretions form 50–80 % of the ejaculate.

COWPER's glands (Glandulae bulbourethrales)

Embedded into the perineal muscles (M. transversus perinei profundus) are the COWPER's glands on both sides (➤ Fig. 8.16). The individual glands have a diameter of approximately 1 cm and flow on both sides with their 3 cm long efferent ducts proximally into the Pars spongiosa of the urethra (2.5 cm below the Membrana perinei).

Topography

The **prostate** sits in a **subperitoneal** position directly below the fundus of the urinary bladder. Its base, therefore, borders *above* onto the smooth muscles at the exit of the urethra ('M. sphincter urethrae internus'). The apex sits *inferior* of the perineal muscles and has contact with the external urethral sphincter (➤ Fig. 8.57). To the *anterior* the prostate is connected via the Ligg. puboprostatica to the posterior surface of the superior pubic bone branch; to the *posterior* it is separated from the rectum only by the Fascia rectoprostatica (DENONVILLIER's fascia). *Laterally* the parasympathetic Nn. cavernosi penis run from the Plexus hypogastricus inferior along the gland and reach the cavernous body of the penis via the perineal muscles (➤ Fig. 8.19).
The **seminal glands** lie in a directly **subperitoneal** position between the dorsal side of the urinary bladder and the anterior side of the Rectum.
The **COWPER's glands** are embedded below the pelvic floor (**extrapelvic**) into the perineal muscles of the deep perineal space.

> **NOTE**
> All accessory sex glands are important for the formation of ejaculate secretions or for moistening of the female genitalia. In contrast, the prostate with its different zones is of the greatest clinical importance! A malignant **prostate tumour** usually originates in the outer zone; a benign **prostate adenoma** in contrast, arises from the transition zone laterally of the central zone.

8.5.8 Vessels and nerves of the external and internal male genitalia

Arterial blood supply and venous drainage
External genitalia

The blood vessels of the penis are complicated. Their position in relation to the penile fascia is of great functional importance for erection of the penis (➤ Fig. 8.42).
The penis is supplied by **3 paired arteries** from the A. pudenda interna:

- **A. dorsalis penis:** runs *sub*fascially between the V. dorsalis profunda penis (medial) and the N. dorsalis penis (lateral), supplies the skin and glans of the penis
- **A. profunda penis:** lies in the Corpora cavernosa, and is responsible for their filling via their Aa. helicinae
- **A. bulbi penis:** penetrates into the Bulbus penis, supplies the Glandula bulbourethralis and, as the A. urethralis, supplies the urethra and Corpus spongiosum

Blood is taken up by **3 venous systems**:

- **V. dorsalis superficialis penis:** paired or unpaired; lies *epi*fascially in the subcutis and conducts blood from the penile skin to the V. pudenda externa
- **V. dorsalis profunda penis:** unpaired; runs *sub*fascially and drains the cavernous bodies via the Cv. cavernosae to the Plexus venosus prostaticus
- **V. bulbi penis:** paired; it brings blood from the Bulbus penis to the V. dorsalis profunda penis

During **penile erection** a dilation of the A. profunda penis occurs, activated parasympathetically, which causes filling of the Corpora cavernosa. These compress the V. dorsalis profunda penis under the stiff penile fascia so that blood cannot flow away. Erection occurs under additional contraction of the Mm. ischiocavernosi (innervated by the N. pudendus).

The **scrotum** is supplied by the A. pudenda interna (Rr. scrotales posteriores) and the Aa. pudendae externae (Rr. scrotales anteriores) as well as the A. cremasterica. The veins correspond to the arteries.

Internal genitalia

Testis and epididymis, Vas deferens and spermatic cord have their own respective arteries (➤ Fig. 8.36, ➤ Table 8.4). In contrast, the

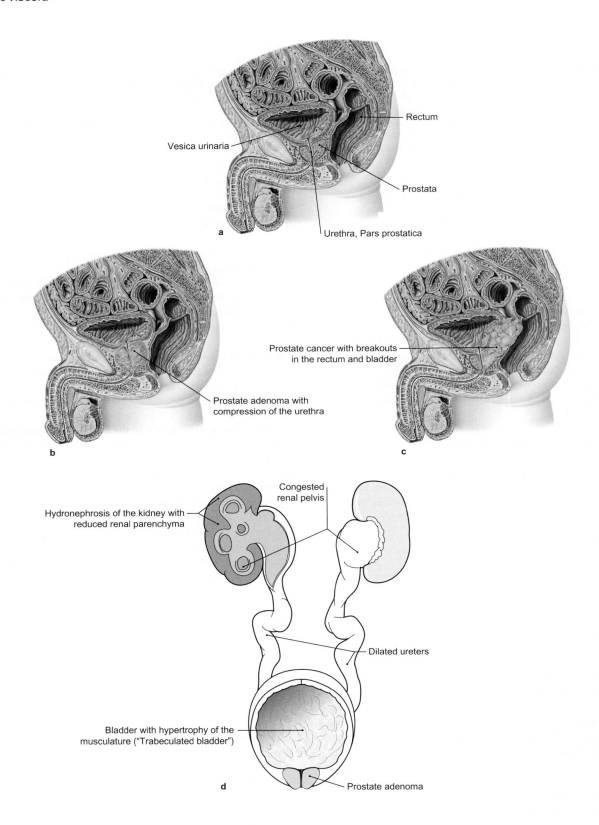

Fig. 8.40 Tumours of the prostate with clinical presentation. a–c Sagittal incision through a male pelvis. **a** Normal prostate. **b** Prostate adenoma. The adenoma emanates from the transition zone inside the gland and compresses the urethra, so that micturition is affected at an early stage. Enlargement of the prostate is palpable during a rectal examination. **c** Prostate cancer. In contrast to the adenoma, the carcinoma emanates from the peripheral zone of the prostate, so discomfort when urinating is rare. A rectal palpation finding of a hard nodular mass can, therefore, be the first clinical sign. **d** Due to backing-up of urine in the case of a prolonged narrowing of the urethra caused by a prostate adenoma, the muscles of the urinary bladder (trabeculated bladder) hypertrophy, the ureters and renal pelvis dilate and hydronephrosis ensues. [L266]

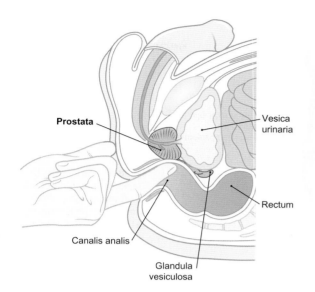

Fig. 8.41 Palpation of the prostate. [L126]

Prostata
Vesica urinaria
Rectum
Canalis analis
Glandula vesiculosa

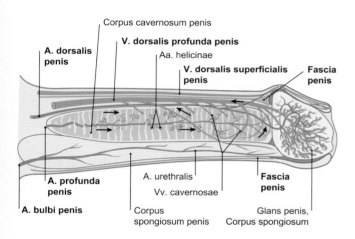

Fig. 8.42 Arteries and veins of the penis. [L126]

Corpus cavernosum penis
A. dorsalis penis
V. dorsalis profunda penis
Aa. helicinae
V. dorsalis superficialis penis
Fascia penis
A. profunda penis
A. urethralis
Vv. cavernosae
Fascia penis
A. bulbi penis
Corpus spongiosum penis
Glans penis, Corpus spongiosum

accessory glands are supplied by the visceral branches of the A. iliaca interna (➤ Fig. 8.61, ➤ Table 8.4).

The **A. testicularis** supplies the testis and epididymis. It originates from the abdominal section of the Aorta just below the renal arteries, and then descends in the retroperitoneal space, whereupon it crosses *over* the N. genitofemoralis, the ureter and the A. iliaca externa running, before entering into the inguinal canal, within the spermatic cord into the scrotum.

The **A. ductus deferentis** is a thin vessel that usually originates from the A. vesicalis superior or the A. vesicalis inferior and is attached to the pelvic section of the Vas deferens and accompanies it until its transition into the epididymis.

The fascia of the spermatic cord are supplied by the **A. cremasterica**, which originates shortly after its exit from the A. epigastrica inferior and is attached externally to the spermatic cord.

The accessory sex glands are supplied by the visceral branches of the A. iliaca interna in their vicinity. The prostate and seminal glands receive blood from the **A. vesicalis inferior** and **A. rectalis media** (➤ Fig. 8.61); the Glandulae bulbourethrales are supplied by the **A. pudenda interna** during its course in the deep perineal space.

Table 8.4 Blood vessels of the internal genitalia.

	Organ	Blood vessels
Arteries	Testis and epididymis	A. testicularis (from the Pars abdominalis of the Aorta)
	Ductus deferens	A. ductus deferentis (mostly from the A. umbilicalis)
	Spermatic cord (M. cremaster)	A. cremasterica (from the A. epigastrica inferior)
	Accessory sex glands:	A. vesicalis inferior, A. rectalis medialis and A. pudenda interna (all from the A. iliaca interna)
Veins	Testes, epididymis, Ductus deferens and spermatic cord	Plexus pampiniformis: venous plexus, the branches of which join to the V. testicularis, which flows to the right into the V. cava inferior and to the left into the V. renalis sinistra
	Accessory sex glands:	Plexus venosi vesicalis and prostaticus with connection to the V. iliaca interna

The blood from the testes, epididymis and Vas deferens accumulates firstly in a venous plexus, the **Plexus pampiniformis,** the branches of which unite proximally in the spermatic cord into the V. testicularis (➤ Fig. 8.36). The vein runs through the inguinal canal, ascends under the peritoneum of the pelvic cavity into the retroperitoneal space and flows to the right into the V. cava inferior, but to the left into the left V. renalis.

From the accessory sex glands, blood in the pelvis runs into the venous plexi in the vicinity of the prostate and urinary bladder (**Plexus venosi prostaticus and vesicalis**) and then drains via the **Vv. vesicales** into the V. iliaca interna (➤ Fig. 8.61).

The V. cremasterica accompanies the eponymous artery and flows into the V. epigastrica inferior.

Clinical remarks

An extension of the veins of the Plexus pampiniformis **(varicocele)** (➤ Fig. 8.43) can cause infertility due to backflow of blood.

Lymphatic pathways of the external and internal genitalia

The external and internal genitalia in men have completely **separated lymphatic drainage pathways** (➤ Fig. 8.44)!

- For the **external genitalia (penis and scrotum)** the lymph nodes of the groin (**Nodi lymphoidei inguinales superficiales**) represent the first lymph node stations.
- The regional lymph nodes of **the testis and epididymis** are the **Nodi lymphoidei lumbales** at the level of the kidneys, from which the lymph runs into the Trunci lumbales.
- In contrast, lymph from the **Vas deferens, spermatic cord and accessory sex glands** drains firstly into the lymph nodes of the pelvic cavity (**Nodi lymphoidei iliaci interni/externi and nodi lymphoidei sacrales**).

NOTE

The external and internal genitalia in men have completely separate lymphatic drainage pathways! Due to the descent of the testis during its development, the lymphatic pathways of the testis and epididymis ascend up to the Nodi lymphoidei lumbales at the level of the kidneys. In contrast, the regional lymph nodes of the external genitalia are the inguinal lymph nodes.

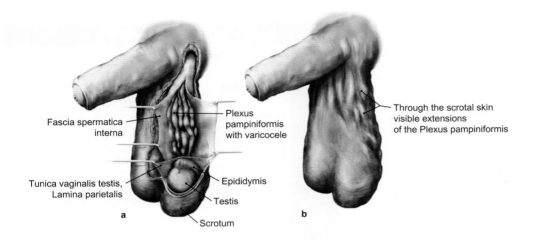

Fascia spermatica interna

Plexus pampiniformis with varicocele

Tunica vaginalis testis, Lamina parietalis

Epididymis

Testis

Scrotum

a

b

Through the scrotal skin visible extensions of the Plexus pampiniformis

Fig. 8.43 Varicocele. Due to backing-up of blood in the V. renalis sinistra, dilation of the Plexus pampiniformis can occur (**a**), which is visible through the skin of the scrotum (**b**). [L266]

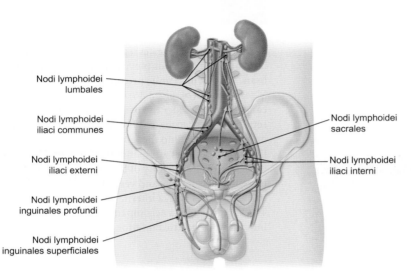

Nodi lymphoidei lumbales

Nodi lymphoidei iliaci communes

Nodi lymphoidei iliaci externi

Nodi lymphoidei inguinales profundi

Nodi lymphoidei inguinales superficiales

Nodi lymphoidei sacrales

Nodi lymphoidei iliaci interni

Fig. 8.44 Lymphatic drainage pathways of the external and internal male genitalia. Ventral view.

Clinical remarks

Due to the different lymphatic drainage pathways the first **lymph node metastases** in penile cancer are found in the groin; however, in the case of testicular cancer, they are found in the retroperitoneal space. Since the lymphatic drainage pathways of the internal and external genitalia do not communicate with each other, if a **testicular tumour is suspected, a transscrotal biopsy** must not be carried out, because tumour cells could be displaced into the lymphatic pathways to the inguinal lymph nodes. In this case, the biopsy must always be made via the inguinal canal.

Innervation of the external and internal genitalia

The external male genitalia have both **autonomic as well as somatic** innervation (➤ Fig. 8.45):

- The predominantly **parasympathetic innervation** increases blood flow to the cavernous body of the penis and thereby induces penile erection.
- The **somatic innervation** is sensory and for the purpose of sexual arousal.
- The **motor innervation** of the perineal muscles (M. bulbospongiosus and M. ischiocavernosus) supports ejaculation of the sperm out of the urethra.

In contrast, innervation of the internal genitalia is **purely autonomic:**

- The predominantly **sympathetic innervation** reduces the blood flow of the testis and epididymis and by means of contraction of

the smooth muscles of the Vas deferens, produces emission of sperm into the urethra and issue of secretions by the accessory glands. At the same time, the circular muscles of the urethra at the exit of the bladder prevent retrograde ejaculation into the urinary bladder.

- Individual **parasympathetic fibres** promote the formation of secretions during arousal.

The preganglionic **sympathetic nerve fibres** (T10–L2) descend from the Plexus aorticus abdominalis via the Plexus hypogastricus superior and from the sacral ganglia of the sympathetic chain (Truncus sympathicus) via the Nn. splanchnici sacrales and are synaptically converted mainly in the Plexus hypogastricus inferior into postganglionic neurons (➤ Fig. 8.45). These postganglionic fibres reach the pelvic organs and thus also the accessory sex glands and the Ductus deferens (Plexus deferentialis). Some fibres also join the Nn. cavernosi penis, which penetrate the pelvic floor and supply the cavernous bodies of the penis. The (mostly) postganglionic sympathetic fibres for the testis and epididymis run within the Plexus testicularis along the A. testicularis, after they have already been converted within either the Ganglia aorticorenalia or the Plexus hypogastricus superior (➤ Table 8.5).

The preganglionic **parasympathetic nerve fibres** pass from the sacral parasympathetic nervous system (S2–S4) via the Nn. splanchnici pelvici into the ganglia of the Plexus hypogastricus inferior (➤ Fig. 8.45). They are converted either here or in the vicinity of the organs into postganglionic fibres, which then reach the accessory sex glands. The **Nn. cavernosi penis** penetrate the pelvic

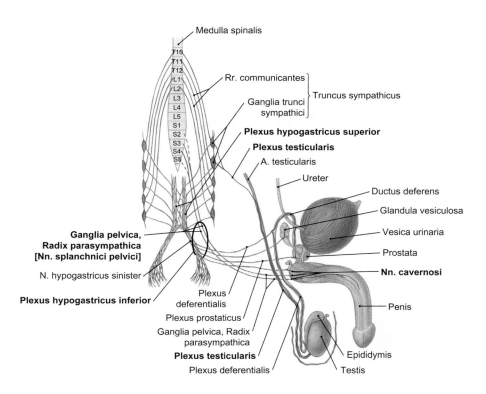

Medulla spinalis

Rr. communicantes

Truncus sympathicus

Ganglia trunci sympathici

Plexus hypogastricus superior

Plexus testicularis

A. testicularis

Ureter

Ductus deferens

Glandula vesiculosa

Vesica urinaria

Prostata

Nn. cavernosi

Penis

Ganglia pelvica, Radix parasympathica [Nn. splanchnici pelvici]

N. hypogastricus sinister

Plexus hypogastricus inferior

Plexus deferentialis

Plexus prostaticus

Ganglia pelvica, Radix parasympathica

Plexus testicularis

Plexus deferentialis

Epididymis

Testis

Fig. 8.45 Innervation of the male reproductive organs. Ventral and lateral views; schematic diagram. The Plexus hypogastricus inferior contains sympathetic (green) and parasympathetic (purple) nerve fibres.

Table 8.5 Innervation of the male genitalia.

Innervation	Target structures
Sympathetic innervation (T10–L2)	• Ductus deferens and accessory sex glands (Plexus hypogastricus inferior) • Testis and epididymis (Plexus testicularis)
Parasympathetic innervation (S2–4)	• Accessory sex glands (Plexus hypogastricus inferior) • Cavernous bodies of the penis (Nn. cavernosi penis)
Somatic innervation	• Sensory: mainly N. pudendus to penis and scrotum • Motor: N. pudendus to the perineal muscles

floor and run (partly below the attachment to the N. dorsalis penis) into the cavernous bodies, where they trigger erection (➤ Fig. 8.65, ➤ Table 8.5).

The somatic innervation via the **N. pudendus** sensorily innervates the penis via the N. dorsalis penis (➤ Fig. 8.45). The scrotum is also mostly sensorily innervated by the N. pudendus (Rr. scrotales posteriores) and only to a small extent by the N. cutaneus femoris posterior (Rr. perineales), N. ilioinguinalis (Rr. scrotales anteriores) and N. genitofemoralis (R. genitalis). Motor fibres run to the perineal muscles (M. bulbospongiosus and M. ischiocavernosus, ➤ Table 8.5).

N O T E

The **parasympathetic nervous system** induces the erection; the **sympathetic nervous system** effects emission and the **N. pudendus** effects ejaculation.

Clinical remarks

In surgical removal of the para-aortic lymph nodes, e.g. in the case of testicular cancer or cancer of the descending colon or during surgery to the abdominal Aorta and the large pelvic arteries, the **sympathetic nervous system** can be damaged. Disorders in emission and thereby ejaculation of sperm lead to infertility **(Impotentia generandi)**.

In surgical removal of the Rectum or prostate, e.g. due to rectal cancer or prostate cancer or pronounced prostatic hyperplasia of the prostate, the **parasympathetic** fibres to the penis can be separated so that an erection is no longer possible **(Impotentia coeundi)**.

For general organisation of the autonomic nervous system in the abdomen, see ➤ Chap. 7.8.5 and on the autonomic ganglia in the retroperitoneum, see ➤ Chap. 8.5.5.

8.6 Female genitalia

Skills

After working through this chapter, you should be able to:
• explain the sections of the internal and external female genitalia and their function
• explain the development of the female genitalia and demonstrate differences from the development of the male genitalia
• identify parts of the vulva on a specimen
• know the structure, sections and topographical relationships of the internal female genitalia
• understand changes of the uterus in overview with structure and function of the placenta
• explain all peritoneal duplicatures and ligaments of the internal genitalia with course and contents
• show arteries of the individual sexual organs and derive their different origins from the development
• characterise drainage areas of veins and lymphatic pathways with their clinical importance and demonstrate characterisation differences from the male genitalia
• explain the autonomic and somatic innervation of the genital organs with their importance for the sexual functions

8.6.1 Overview

In the female sex organs a distinction is made between **external genitalia** outside the pelvis in the perineal region and **internal genitalia** within the pelvic cavity. As well as diagnostics, the specialist field of gynaecology also focuses on with both conservative and surgical treatment of the female genitalia.

The **external genitalia** are collectively called the **vulva** (➤ Fig. 8.46). Parts include:

- Mons pubis
- Labia majora pudendi
- Labia minora pudendi
- Clitoris
- Vestibule of the vagina (Vestibulum vaginae)
- Greater vestibular glands (Glandulae vestibulares majores (BARTHOLINI's and minores)

The vestibule of the vagina extends to the hymen, which delineates the entrance of the vagina (Ostium vaginae). The vagina itself is part of the internal genitalia.

The **internal genitalia** include (➤ Fig. 8.47):

- Vagina
- Uterus
- Fallopian tube (Tuba uterina)
- Ovary (Ovar)

The fallopian tubes and ovaries are located as pairs and are collectively known as **adnexa** (attachments).

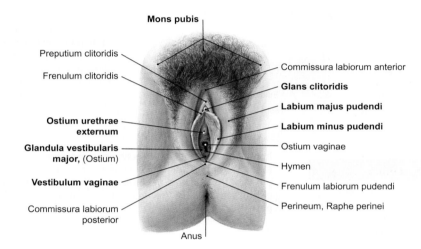

Fig. 8.46 External female genitalia. Caudal view.

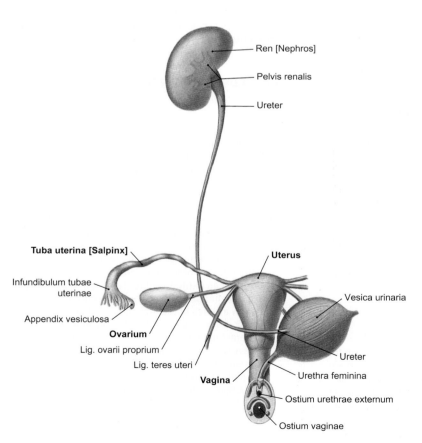

Fig. 8.47 Internal female genitalia and urinary organs. Ventral view.

8.6.2 Function of the female genitalia

The external genitalia are the **sexual organs** and serve the purpose of intercourse. Also flowing into the vestibule of the vagina is the external opening of the urethra (Ostium urethrae externum), which is located ventrally to the entrance into the vagina. Female internal genitalia are both **reproductive** as well as **sexual organs:**

- **Ovaries:** formation of oocytes and sex hormones (oestrogen)
- **Fallopian tubes:** uptake of the ovum and the site of fertilisation
- **Uterus:** development of the child
- **Vagina:** cohabitation organ and birth canal

8.6.3 Development of the external and internal female genitalia

Development of the internal female genitalia

The internal and external genitalia in both sexes develop ambiguously (indifferent stage, ➤ Chap. 8.5.3, ➤ Fig. 8.28, ➤ Fig. 8.29) up to the *7th week*. Only afterwards do the genitalia differentiate specifically according to the genetic sex of the embryo.
As no TDF is formed in the female sex ('**t**estis-**d**etermining **f**actor'), which is expressed by a gene onto the Y chromosome, from the *10th week* an ovary develops on each side out of the ambiguous gonadal units (➤ Fig. 8.28, ➤ Fig. 8.29). The primary germ cords now form the **cortex of the ovary**, in which the **ova** that emerge from the primordial germ cells are surrounded by **epithelial cells** and in the process up to the *17th week* they form **follicles**. Similar to the testes, the ovary protrudes into the abdominal cavity and receives the **Mesovarium** as a peritoneal duplicature for the purpose of attachment to the dorsal abdominal wall with a superior and an inferior enveloping fold **(superior and inferior gonadal ligaments);** however, in the case of the ovary the coelomic epithelium remains on the surface (superficial epithelium) so that it maintains its **intraperitoneal** location.
Similar to the testes, the ovary is also located in the lumbar region at the level of the Mesonephros. (➤ Fig. 8.28, ➤ Fig. 8.29). As the body grows, the ovary is shifted, but only to the level of the lesser pelvis **(descent)** and does not leave the peritoneal cavity (➤ Fig. 8.48). The upper gonadal ligament becomes the **Lig. suspensorium ovarii,** in which the vessels and nerves run, which the ovary has taken with it in its descensus. The superior part of the inferior gonadal ligament, which originates directly at the ovary, becomes the **Lig. ovarii proprium** and later connects the ovary with the uterus. From there the inferior section, which corresponds to the Gubernaculum testis, runs into the inguinal canal and becomes the **Lig. ovarii proprium**, which later anchors the uterus within the connective tissue of the Labia majora. Without the suppressing effect of the anti-MÜLLERIAN hormone from the testes the MÜLLERIAN ducts develop into female genital tracts.

- **Fallopian tube** (Tuba uterina)
- **Uterus**
- **Vagina**

The WOLFFIAN ducts, however, degenerate as there is no testosterone. The cranial, un-fused sections of the MÜLLERIAN ducts develop from the *12th week* into the fallopian tubes, while the uterus and the distal part of the vagina emerge from the distally fused parts to the uterovaginal canal (➤ Fig. 8.28, ➤ Fig. 8.48). The **inferior part of the vagina**, the majority of its epithelium and also the **BARTHOLIN's glands** originate from the Sinus **urogenitalis.** Here, the MÜLLERIAN ducts and the Sinus urogenitalis only form the epithelium of various organs, whilst connective tissue and smooth muscles emerge from the surrounding mesoderm. The

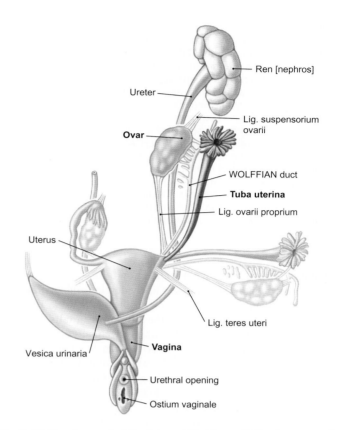

Fig. 8.48 Development of the internal female genitalia, Organa genitalia feminina interna. (according to [S010-1-16])

peritoneal duplicatures of the MÜLLERIAN ducts, which protrude into the peritoneal cavity, later form the peritoneal folds of the fallopian tube **(Mesosalpinx)** and of the Uterus **(Lig. latum uteri)**, which divide the caudal part of the peritoneal cavity into the dorsally located **Excavatio rectouterina (DOUGLAS pouch)** and the ventral **Excavatio vesicouterina.**
There, where the uterovaginal canal flows into the Sinus urogenitalis, it bulges out as the **sinus mount**. Developing in this area from the ectoderm of the Sinus urogenitalis is the **vaginal plate**, the lumen of which only forms subsequently. The sinus mount remains preserved as the **hymen** and demarcates the vagina downwards from the vestibule of the vagina (Vestibulum vaginae). The hymen usually ruptures after birth and remains as a remnant at the dorsal edge of the vaginal orifice.

NOTE

If hormones formed in the testis (testosterone, anti-MÜLLERIAN hormone) are missing, an ovary is formed and the MÜLLERIAN ducts differentiate into the Tuba uterina, uterus and vagina. Similarly to the male embryo, the internal female genitalia originates from 3 sources:
- Gonadal ridge with migrated germ cells → ovary
- MÜLLERIAN duct → Tuba uterina, uterus, vagina (superior section)
- Sinus urogenitalis → vagina (inferior section)

Clinical remarks

If the MÜLLERIAN ducts do not fuse with each other, **septation** of the uterine lumen (Uterus septus or subseptus) or even double formation (**Uterus duplex**) can ensue. In the case of a Uterus bicornis only the superior part is separated. If the uterovaginal canal does not form a vaginal plate together with the Sinus urogentialis, then **uterus and vagina are absent** (MAYER-ROKITANSKY-KÜSTER-HAUSER syndrome). If the vaginal plate does not form a lumen, the vagina remains closed in the superior part **(vaginal atresia)**. In **hymenal atresia** the inferior part of the vagina is not opened, so that the hymen does not tear after birth and impedes menstruation at puberty. **Relics** of the various systems can be clinically remarkable in rare cases if they form cysts, which can appear as tumours or inflammation: remnants of the WOLFFIAN ducts can remain extant as the Appendix vesiculosa in the vicinity of the ovary or as GARTNER's duct in the Lig. latum uteri and in the vaginal wall. The cranial end of the MÜLLERIAN duct can form a vesicle at the fallopian tube (hydatid of MORGAGNI). Relics of the mesonephric tubercles can remain as the epoophoron within the Mesovarium or the paroophoron within the Lig. latum uteri.

Development of the external female genitalia

The external genitalia in both sexes firstly develop ambiguously (sexually ambiguous stage) between the *4th and 7th week*. They are formed from the caudal section of the **Sinus urogenitalis**. At the same time, the anterior wall of the Sinus urogenitalis descends firstly to the **urethral groove** which is delineated on both sides by **genital folds**. Lateral to these are the **labioscrotal swellings** and at the posterior edge of the groove is the **genital tubercle** (➤ Fig. 8.49). Subsequently, in females, the following develop under the influence of the ovary and female sex hormones (oestrogen):
- the genital tubercle develops into the **clitoris** (Corpora cavernosa)
- the genital folds develop into the **Labia minora**
- the labioscrotal swellings develop into the **Labia majora** and into the **Mons pubis**

Unlike in men, the genital folds do not close and the labioscrotal swelling only close anterior and posterior at the unification points of the Labia majora (Commissura labiorum anterior and posterior). The **BARTHOLIN's glands** develop from the **Sinus urogenitalis**.

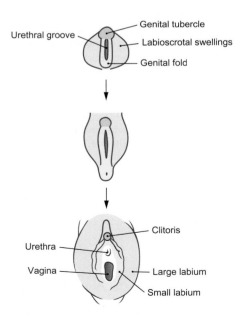

Fig. 8.49 Development of the external female genitalia, Organa genitalia feminina externa.

Labels:
Urethral groove — Genital tubercle — Labioscrotal swellings — Genital fold
Urethra — Clitoris
Vagina — Large labium — Small labium

The common features with the development of the external male genitalia explain why, in the case of disorders which involve excessive production of male sex hormones **(adrenogenital syndrome)**, penis-like hyperplasia of the clitoris can occur.

8.6.4 Vulva

The **Mons pubis**, which is covered by pubic hair after puberty, runs down into the **Labia majora pudendi**, which unite ventrally and dorsally (Commissura labiorum anterior and posterior). The approximately 3 cm long **cavernous bodies of the vestibule** are embedded on both sides into the Labia majora (Bulbus vestibuli) and behind these into the **vestibular glands** (Glandulae vestibulares majores BARTHOLINI and minores, clinical term: **BARTHOLIN's glands**). The BARTHOLIN's glands have a 2 cm long efferent duct corresponding to the COWPER's glands in men and moisten the vestibule of the vagina during sexual arousal.
Located between the Labia majora are the **Labia minora** (Labia minora pudendi), which encompass the **vestibule of the vagina** Vestibulum vaginae). In front the Labia minora run with a ridge of tissue (Frenulum clitoridis) to the glans of the clitoris as well as its prepuce (➤ Fig. 8.50). Flowing into the vulvar vestibule are:
- the vagina (dorsal)
- the urethra (ventral), approximately 2.5 cm below the clitoris
- the efferent ducts of the BARTHOLIN's glands (lateral)

Inflammation of BARTHOLIN'S glands can cause painful swellings of the Labia majora **(BARTHOLIN's abscess)**. A cause is a obstruction of the efferent ducts of the glands.
The topography of vaginal and urethral orifices in the vestibule of the vagina is important when **inserting a urinary catheter** in order to prevent the catheter being placed in the vagina (➤ Chap. 8.3.5).

The **clitoris** is the sensory organ for sexual arousal and 3–4 cm long. Evolutionarily there exist some common features between the construction of the clitoris and the penis. Therefore, the mechanisms for filling the cavernous bodies and for erection are comparable in both sexes. The clitoris consists of the two **cavernous bodies (Corpora cavernosa clitoridis)**, which are sheathed by a **fascia (Fascia clitoridis)** and merge ventrally into a short **body (Corpus clitoridis)**, in which, however, they remain separated by the Septum corporum cavernosorum (➤ Fig. 8.50). Caudally adjoining is the **Glans clitoridis**, which is covered by a **prepuce (Preputium clitoridis)**. The Corpora cavernosa gives way dorsally of the body to the crus of the clitoris (Crura clitoridis), which are anchored to the inferior branches of the pubic bone. The crura are surrounded by the Mm. ischiocavernosi. The M. bulbospongiosus stabilises the Bulbus vestibuli, which thus, as a cavernous body, corresponds to the Corpus spongiosum of the penis. Similarly to the penis, the clitoris is also anchored via 2 suspensory ligaments with the superficial **Lig. fundiforme clitoridis** and the more deeply located **Lig. fundiforme clitoridis,** which is attached to the symphysis (➤ Fig. 8.50).

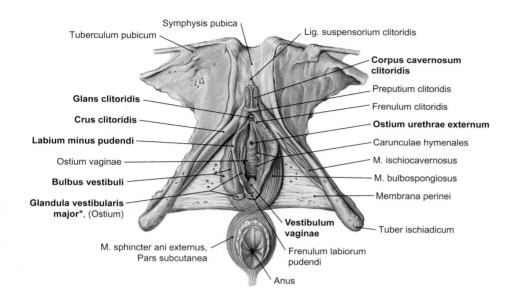

Fig. 8.50 **External female genitalia.** Caudal view, after removal of the superficial fascia and the vascular, lymphatic and nervous systems.

8.6.5 Ovary and fallopian tubes

The ovary and fallopian tubes are referred to as **adnexa**. They are covered by the peritoneum and lie, therefore, in an **intraperitoneal** position in the pelvic cavity (➤ Fig. 8.51).

Ovary

In a female of child-bearing age, the ovary (Ovar) is 4 × 2 × 3 cm large, 7–14 g in weight and oval (➤ Fig. 8.51). In pregnancy it doubles in size and after the menopause the ovary shrinks significantly. A distinction is made between a superior pole (Extremitas tubaria) and an inferior pole (Extremitas uterina) as well as a medial and lateral surface (Facies medialis and lateralis). Secured to the anterior border as a peritoneal duplication is the **Mesovarium** (Margo mesovaricus); while the posterior border remains free (Margo liber). The vessels and nerves enter and exit at the hilum of the ovary.

The ovary is secured by 2 suspensory ligaments:

- **Lig. ovarii proprium:** is attached to the Extremitas uterina and connects the ovary and the uterus

- **Lig. suspensorium ovarii** (clinically: Lig. infundibulopelvicum): connects the ovary from the Extremitas tubaria outwards with the lateral pelvic wall. It guides the A. and V. ovarica.

Dorsally, the ovary has contact with the ureter and the N. obturatorius as well as on the right side with the vermiform appendix (Appendix vermiformis) of the large intestine if it is suspended in the lesser pelvis (descending type). To the left the Colon sigmoideum traverses the superior pole of the ovary. Running **caudally** are the A. umbilicalis and the A. obturatoria (both branches of the A. iliaca interna, ➤ Fig. 8.62).

Fallopian tube

The fallopian tube (Tuba uterina [Salpinx]) connects the ovary and uterus (➤ Fig. 8.51). It is 10–14 cm long and has various sections:

- **Infundibulum** (Infundibulum tubae uterinae) : 1–2 cm long, has an aperture to the abdominal cavity (Ostium abdominale tubae uterinae) and fringe-like processes (Fimbriae tubae uterinae) for receiving the ovum during ovulation
- **Ampulla** (Ampulla tubae uterinae): 7–8 cm, runs in an arch shape around the ovary

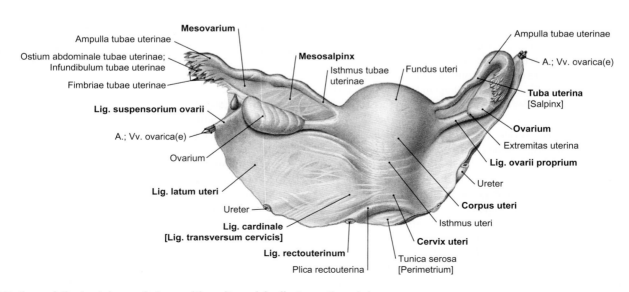

Fig. 8.51 Ovary, fallopian tubes and uterus with peritoneal duplicatures. Dorsal view.

- **Isthmus** (Isthmus tubae uterinae): 3–6 cm, constriction at the passageway to the uterus
- **Intramural section** (Pars uterina), 1 cm long, runs into the uterus (Ostium uterinum)

Comparable to the Mesovarium, the fallopian tube with the **Mesosalpinx** has a peritoneal duplicature, which runs to the Lig. latum uteri.

> **NOTE**
>
> **The ovary** and **Tuba uterina,** which are grouped as adnexa, are located in the same way as the body of the **Uterus intraperitoneal** and are, therefore, covered on their surface anatomy by peritoneum. In contrast, there are no intraperitoneal genitalia in men.

Clinical remarks

The intraperitoneal location of the adnexa is clinically significant:
- A large proportion of malignant tumours of the ovary **(ovarian cancer)** do not arise from the organ itself, but from the peritoneal epithelium on its surface.
- The open connection of the fallopian tube to the abdominal cavity means that an **ectopic pregnancy** can occur, in which the fertilised ovum does not implant in the uterus, but rather in the peritoneum in the vicinity of the ovary. This can cause life-threatening haemorrhaging due to erosion of blood vessels.

After ascending bacterial infections of the fallopian tube **(salpingitis)** its walls can stick together, so the fallopian tube is no longer accessible and fertilisation becomes impossible. In **sterilisation** the tube is ligated or separated in a targeted manner. The close topographical relationship of the adnexa (ovary and Tuba uterina) to the vermiform appendix (Appendix vermiformis) of the large intestine explains why an inflammation of the vermiform appendix **(appendicitis)** as well as an inflammation of the fallopian tubes **(salpingitis)** can be associated with similar pain in the right lower abdomen.

8.6.6 Uterus

Structure and location

The uterus (Metra) is 8 cm long, 5 cm wide and 2–3 cm thick. It has a variable weight of between 30–120 g (on average 50 g), which reaches up to 1 kg in pregnancy, and greatly diminishes with age. The uterus is divided into an intraperitoneally located **body (Corpus uteri)** with an anteriorly directed base (Fundus uteri) and a subperitoneally anchored **cervix (Cervix uteri)** of approximately 2.5 cm in length, which are set apart from each other by a constriction (Isthmus uteri) (➤ Fig. 8.51). The fallopian tubes (Tuba uterina) are attached on both sides to the body of the uterus as a connection to the ovaries (Ovar).

The uterus has an anterior surface (Facies anterior or vesicalis), which points to the urinary bladder, and a posterior surface (Facies posterior or intestinalis) which has contact with the rectum. The anterior of the peritoneal cavity sinks into the depths between these as the **Excavatio vesicouterina** and posteriorly as the **Excavatio rectouterina (DOUGLAS pouch)**.

In the normal position the uterus is curved forwards towards the **vagina (anteversion)** and the body is bent backwards towards the cervix **(anteflexion)** (➤ Fig. 8.52). This position has a protective purpose and prevents the uterus from being everted out of the vagina in the case of an increase in intra-abdominal pressure (sneezing, coughing).

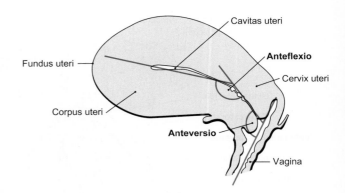

Fig. 8.52 Location of the uterus and vagina. View from right.

The space inside the **uterus** is divided into the **Cavitas uteri** in the body of the uterus and into the **cervical canal (Canalis cervicis uteri)** in the cervix. The cervix runs with its posterior section via the **external uterine orifice** (Ostium uteri) into the vagina, which is thus referred to as the **Portio vaginalis cervicis**. The superior section, which begins at the isthmus with the **internal uterine orifice** (Ostium anatomicum uteri internum) is the **Portio supravaginalis cervicis**.

Clinical remarks

Inspection and smear tests of the cervix are included in gynaecology as part of routine diagnostics in Germany and are remunerated by health insurances for women from the 20th year of age as a **preventative screening**. Screening should be carried out at least once a year for early recognition of any changes, such as precursors of a malignant tumour **(cervical cancer)** so as to remove them. Cervical cancer is one of the most frequent malignant cancers in women under the age of 40 years.

The **wall of the uterus** consists internally of the endometrium, which is followed by the strong muscular layer (myometrium) made of smooth muscles as well as externally by the peritoneal lining (perimetrium).

> **NOTE**
>
> **Endometrium:** mucosal membrane of the uterus
> **Myometrium:** smooth muscles of the uterus
> **Perimetrium:** peritoneal lining of the uterus
> **Parametrium** (= Lig. cardinale): connective tissue anchoring of the cervix in the pelvis
> **Mesometrium** (= Lig. latum): anteriorly placed peritoneal duplicature

Suspensory ligaments

The two sections of the uterus have various suspensory ligaments, which have clinical relevance in gynaecological operations:
- Corpus uteri:
  - **Lig. latum uteri** (= Mesometrium): forms together with the peritoneal duplicatures of the adnexa (Mesosalpinx, Mesovarium) an anteriorly positioned fold in the lesser pelvis, which covers the body of the uterus (➤ Fig. 8.51) → uterus, fallopian tube and ovary thus lie in an intraperitoneal position
  - **Lig. teres uteri** (clinical term: Lig. rotundum): connective tissue cord, which runs from the angle of the uterine tubes anteriorly to the lateral pelvic wall and through the inguinal canal to the Labia majora, where it inserts into the skin and adipose tissue; its purpose is to stabilise position of the uterus

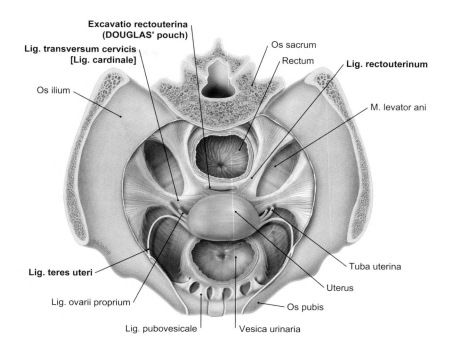

Excavatio rectouterina
(DOUGLAS' pouch)

Lig. transversum cervicis
[Lig. cardinale]

Os ilium

Lig. teres uteri

Lig. ovarii proprium

Lig. pubovesicale

Os sacrum

Rectum

Lig. rectouterinum

M. levator ani

Tuba uterina

Uterus

Os pubis

Vesica urinaria

Fig. 8.53 Anchoring ligaments of the uterus and connective tissue spaces of the pelvis. Transverse incision at the level of the Cervix uteri; cranial view; partial schematic diagram. [L238]

- Cervix uteri (> Fig. 8.53):
  - **Lig. cardinale** (Lig. transversum cervicis): connective tissue strands from the cervix laterally to the pelvic wall (also referred to as the Parametrium)
  - **Lig. rectouterinum** (clinical term: Lig. sacrouterinum): connective tissue strands from the cervix dorsally around the rectum and up to the sacrum
  - **Lig. pubocervicale:** secures the cervix ventrally at the pubic bone

The **Lig. rectouterinum** is also delineated in gynaecological operations in order to be able to protect the nerve fibres of the Plexus hypogastricus inferior, which run inferiorly in this connective tissue. Cranially, the connective tissue raises a peritoneal fold (**Plica rectouterina**), which constitutes on both sides the lateral border of the Excavatio rectouterina (DOUGLAS pouch).

Changes in the uterus during pregnancy

The child develops in the uterus. After the ovum is fertilised by spermatozoa in the fallopian tube, it is transported into the uterus, where it implants in the endometrium. The **placenta** develops in the endometrium from maternal and neonatal tissue . The placenta is differentiated in the *4th month* and at birth has a diameter of 20 cm and a weight of 350–700 g. Simplified, the disc-shaped structure of the placenta can be imagined as a shallow pot with a lid. The bottom of the pot corresponds to the **basal plate**, which is embedded into the endometrium of the uterus. The lid is the **chorionic plate**, from which the blood vessels originate and run via the **umbilical cord** to the child. In the umbilical cord, the two arteries (Aa. umbilicales) are twined in a spiral around a vein (V. umbilicalis). The **V. umbilicalis** brings blood, which has been *oxygen-enriched* in the placenta to the child and connects to the inferior vena cava whilst circumventing the liver (> Chap. 6.1.4). The two **Aa. umbilicales** branch from the internal iliac arteries (Aa. iliacae internae) and conduct the *deoxygenated* blood to the placenta. Between the basal plate and chorionic plate is a cavity filled with maternal blood, which is referred to as the **intervillous space**, since the **placental villi** hang into it from the chorionic plate for enlargement of the surface area. Located in the villi are the fetal blood ves-

sels, which take up respiratory gases and nutrients and merge in the chorionic plate into the umbilical cord vessels.

Functions of the placenta are:
- Exchange of respiratory gases and nutrients between maternal and fetal blood
- Hormone production (amongst others to maintain the placenta)
- Immune tolerance (to prevent rejection of the child)

8.6.7 Vagina

The **vagina** is a hollow muscular organ with a length of 10 cm and lies in a subperitoneal position. A distinction is made between the anterior and posterior walls (Paries anterior and Paries posterior), which both point towards the transverse folds on the inner surface (Rugae vaginales). Bordering onto the Portio vaginalis of the cervix is the **vaginal vault (Fornix vaginae)**, which is divided into anterior, lateral and posterior sections (> Fig. 8.58).

Because the uterus is tipped forwards (anteversion), the posterior wall is longer than the anterior wall and the posterior vaginal fornix is correspondingly higher than the anterior section (> Fig. 8.52). Caudally, the vagina opens dorsal to the urethra into the **vestibule of the vagina (Vestibulum vaginae)**, which is counted among the external genitalia. Before the first occurrence of sexual intercourse, this connection is closed by the remnants of the **hymen**.

To the posterior, the vagina borders on the rectum and is only separated from the latter by the **Fascia rectovaginalis (= Septum rectovaginale)** (> Fig. 8.58). The connective tissue in front towards the urinary bladder is also referred to clinically as the **Septum vesicovaginale.**

Clinical remarks

From the posterior vaginal vault outwards the **Excavatio rectouterina** (DOUGLAS pouch) can be aspirated in order to investigate free fluid.

8.6.8 Vessels and nerves of the external and internal female genitalia

From a developmental point of view, the supply of the female genitalia has many common features with the vessels and nerves of the male genitalia (➤ Chap. 8.5.8).

Arterial supply and venous drainage of the external genitalia

The external genitalia are supplied by the terminal branches of the **A. pudenda interna** and the **Aa. pudendae externae** (➤ Table 8.6). The blood vessels of the vulva thus correspond to those of the penis and scrotum. Accordingly, the mechanisms for filling the cavernous bodies, which are important for sexual sensation, are comparable (➤ Chap. 8.5.8). The Labia majora, which correspond developmentally to the **scrotum**, are supplied by the A. pudenda interna (Rr. labiales posteriores) and the A. pudenda externa (Rr. labiales anteriores). The veins correspond to the arteries.

Arterial supply and venous drainage of the internal genitalia

The internal female genitalia are supplied by three arteries, which originate from the abdominal section of the Aorta and the A. iliaca interna (➤ Fig. 8.54, ➤ Fig. 8.62).
The **A. ovarica** supplies the ovary and adjacent sections of the Tuba uterina. It originates from the abdominal section of the Aorta just below the renal arteries and then descends into the retroperitoneal space, whereupon it crosses *over* the N. genitofemoralis, the ureter and A. iliaca externa, before approaching the ovary in the Lig. suspensorium ovarii.
The **A. uterina** is a visceral branch of the A. illiaca interna. In the Lig. latum uteri the artery crosses over the ureter and branches into its terminal branches, with which it is involved in blood supply to all internal genitalia (➤ Fig. 8.54):

- **Rr. helicini,** wind along the uterus, which they supply and can adapt to the massive growth of the uterus during pregnancy
- **R. tubarius,** supplies the ampulla of the Tuba uterina

Table 8.6 Vessels of the clitoris and Bulbus vestibuli.

Arteries	Veins
• **A. dorsalis clitoridis:** supplies the Glans clitoridis • **A. profunda clitoridis:** penetrates into the Crura clitoridis and supplies the Corpora cavernosa clitoridis • **A. bulbi vestibuli:** supplies the Bulbus vestibuli	• **V. dorsalis superficialis clitoridis:** conducts blood from the Glans to the V. pudenda externa • **V. dorsalis profunda clitoridis:** drains blood from the Corpora cavernosa to the Plexus venosus vesicalis • **V. bulbi vestibuli:** paired, brings blood from the Bulbus vestibuli to the V. dorsalis profunda clitoridis

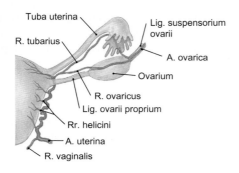

Fig. 8.54 Arterial blood supply of the internal female genitalia. Dorsal view.

- **R. ovaricus,** in addition to the A. ovarica it is involved in blood flow of the ovary
- **Rr. vaginales,** descend at the superior section of the vagina, which they supply in addition to the A. vaginalis

The vagina is predominantly supplied by the **A. vaginalis** from the A. iliaca interna.
Blood from the ovary and Tuba uterina is drained via the **V. ovarica**. The vein ascends in the Lig. suspensorium ovarii to the pelvic wall and flows to the right into the V. cava inferior (➤ Fig. 8.62); but on the left side it flows into the left V. renalis. Blood from the uterus, tube and vagina accumulates within the pelvis in the venous plexus in the vicinity of the organs (**Plexus venosi uterinus and vaginalis**) and then drains via the **Vv. uterinae** into the V. iliaca interna (➤ Fig. 8.62).

> **Clinical remarks**
>
> In the case of **endometrial cancer** or benign tumors **(fibroids)** of the Myometrium, which can bleed heavily, surgical removal of the uterus **(hysterectomy)** is necessary, which is often carried out transvaginally. Here, there is the danger that the ureter can be accidentally ligated with the Aa. uterina. The resulting urinary backflow can lead to kidney loss and, therefore, requires surgical correction.

Lymphatic pathways of the external and internal genitalia

In contrast to men, the external and internal genitalia in women do *not* have completely separated lymphatic drainage pathways, since the female reproductive organs have a connection to the inguinal lymph nodes (➤ Fig. 8.55)!
For the **external genitalia (vulva)**, just like in men, the lymph nodes of the groin (**Nodi lymphoidei inguinales superficiales**) are the first lymph node station.
The regional lymph nodes of the **ovary**, which correspond developmentally to the testis, of the Tuba uterina and of the adjacent uterus ('tube angle') are the **Nodi lymphoidei lumbales** at the level of the kidneys, from which the lymph runs into the Trunci lumbales. The lymphatic pathways ascend within the Lig. suspensorium ovarii.
Lymph is drained from the **uterus, Tuba uterina and vagina** firstly into the lymph nodes of the pelvic cavity (**Nodi lymphoidei iliaci interni/externi and Nodi lymphoidei sacrales**).
Specific to the lymphatic drainage of the internal female genitalia is that both the **uterus**, at the origin of the **Lig. teres uteri** ('tube angle') via the lymphatic pathways along this ligament, and the **inferior sections of the vagina** have a connection to the lymph nodes of the groin (**Nodi lymphoidei inguinales superficiales and profundi**) (➤ Fig. 8.55).

> **Clinical remarks**
>
> Due to the different lymphatic drainage pathways, the first **lymph node metastases** in the case of vulval cancer are found in the groin; in the case of endometrial cancer of the uterus and cervical cancer the metastases are found in the lesser pelvis, and in the retroperitoneal space in the case of ovarian tumours.

Innervation of the external and internal genitalia

The internal and external genitalia have both autonomic and somatic innervation (➤ Fig. 8.56, ➤ Table 8.7).

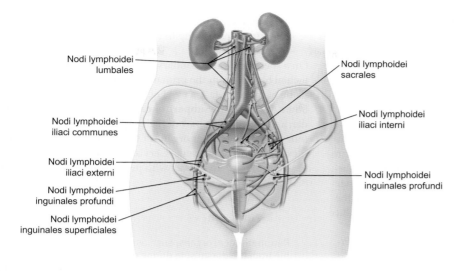

Fig. 8.55 Lymphatic drainage pathways of the external and internal female genitalia. Ventral view.

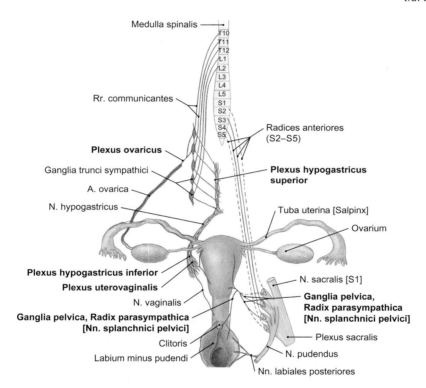

Fig. 8.56 Innervation of the female genitalia. Ventral view; schematic diagram. The Plexus hypogastricus inferior and the Plexus uterovaginalis contain sympathetic (green) and parasympathetic (purple) nerve fibres.

The mostly **parasympathetic innervation of the vulva** increases blood flow in the cavernous bodies and thus supports sexual arousal, which is perceived by somatic innervation.

Depending on hormone status, the autonomic innervation of the **internal genitalia** modulates the tone of the uterine muscles, tubal motility and the secretion of the glands. The **sympathetic innervation** reduces the blood flow of the organs and causes a contraction of the muscles of the uterus. In contrast, the **parasympathetic nervous system** has a dilating effect on the vessels of the uterus and reduces the tone of the uterine muscles. It fosters secretion formation of the vagina (transudate from the blood vessels as there are no glands!) as well as secretions of the BARTHOLIN's glands during arousal. The inferior sections of the vagina have somatic innervation, which promotes **sexual arousal**.

Preganglionic **sympathetic nerve fibres** (T10–L2) descend from the Plexus aorticus abdominalis via the Plexus hypogastricus supe-

rior and out of the sacral ganglia of the sympathetic chain (Truncus sympathicus) via the Nn. splanchnici sacrales and are mostly in the Plexus hypogastricus inferior converted synaptically into postganglionic neurons (➤ Fig. 8.56). Their axons reach the pelvic organs

Table 8.7 Innervation of the female genitalia.

Autonomic innervation	Somatic innervation
Sympathetic (T10–L2) and parasympathetic (S2–4): • Uterus, Tuba uterina, vagina (Plexus hypogastricus inferior) • Ovary (Plexus ovaricus) • Cavernous bodies of the clitoris and BARTHOLIN's glands (Nn. cavernosi clitoridis)	• Sensory: mainly N. pudendus to the clitoris, labia and vagina (lower section) • Motor: N. pudendus to the perineal muscles

and continue into the **Plexus uterovaginalis** (FRANKENHÄUS-ER's plexus), which innervates the uterus, Tuba uterina and vagina. The predominantly postganglionic sympathetic nerve fibres for the ovary run in the Plexus ovaricus along the A. ovarica, after they have already been converted in the Ganglia aorticorenalia or in the Plexus hypogastricus superior.

The preganglionic **parasympathetic nerve fibres** pass from the sacral parasympathetic nervous system (S2–S4) via the Nn. splanchnici pelvici into the ganglia of the Plexus hypogastricus inferior (➤ Fig. 8.56). They are converted either here or in the vicinity of the organs into postganglionic neurons, which innervate the uterus, Tuba uterina and vagina. The **Nn. cavernosi clitoridis** penetrate the pelvic floor and run (partly below the attachment to the N. dorsalis clitoridis) into the cavernous bodies, where they induce filling (erection), and to the BARTHOLIN's glands.

Somatic innervation by the **N. pudendus** provides sensory innervation to the inferior part of the vagina as well as to the posterior two thirds of the labia via the Rr. labiales posteriores nerves and to the clitoris via the N. dorsalis clitoridis (➤ Fig. 8.56). The anterior third of the labia receives sensory innervation from the N. ilioinguinalis (Rr. labiales anteriores) and the lateral sections receive additional innervation from the N. cutaneus femoris posterior (Rr. perineales) and the N. genitofemoralis (R. genitalis).

For the general organisation of the autonomic nervous system in the abdomen, see ➤ Chap. 7.8.5 and on the autonomic ganglia in the retroperitoneum, see ➤ Chap. 8.8.5 .

8.7 Retroperitoneal space and pelvic cavity

Skills

After working through this chapter, you should be able to:
• understand the structure of the retroperitoneum and pelvic cavity
• describe the topographical relationships of individual organs on a specimen

8.7.1 Overview

The **abdominal cavity** (Cavitas abdominalis) and the **pelvic cavity** (Cavitas pelvis) are predominantly lined with peritoneum and together form the **peritoneal cavity** (Cavitas peritonealis) (➤ Chap. 7.7). Behind and below the peritoneal cavity is the **extraperitoneal space** (Spatium extraperitoneale), which dorsally as the **retroperitoneum** (Spatium retroperitoneale), ➤ Chap. 8.7.2) is lined predominantly with adipose tissue between the organs and the vascular, lymphatic and nervous systems; this continues caudally into the pelvic cavity into the **subperitoneal space** (Spatium extraperitoneale pelvis, ➤ Chap. 8.7.3).

The organs of the **retroperitoneal space** are usually only covered on their anterior side by Peritoneum parietale (➤ Fig. 7.47). These organs are either
• already located outside the abdominal cavity (primary retroperitoneal organs)
  – Kidneys
  – Adrenal glands
• or have been shifted to the dorsal abdominal wall only during development (secondary retroperitoneal organs, ➤ Chap. 7):
  – Duodenum (apart from the Pars superior)
  – Colon ascendens

– Colon descendens
– Proximal rectum (up to the Flexura sacralis)
– Pancreas

On a specimen, the secondary retroperitoneal organs can be detached bluntly from the primary retroperitoneal organs in the plane of the tolot-fascia (➤ Fig. 8.8).

Some organs in the **subperitoneal space**, such as the urinary bladder, are covered on a part of their superior side with parietal peritoneum, whereas other organs of the pelvis (distal rectum from the Flexura sacralis, anal canal, Cervix uteri, vagina, prostata, Glandula vesiculosa) have no contact with peritoneum (➤ Fig. 8.57, ➤ Fig. 8.58).

N O T E

Extraperitoneal organs:
• Located outside of the peritoneal cavity in the retroperitoneal space of the abdominal cavity (Spatium retroperitoneale) or in the subperitoneal space of the pelvis (Spatium extraperitoneale pelvis)
• Not or only partially covered by Peritoneum parietale

8.7.2 Retroperitoneal space

The Retroperitoneum (Spatium retroperitoneale) is a slit-shaped space dorsal to the peritoneal cavity, which is delineated ventrally by the Peritoneum parietale and dorsally by the muscles of the posterior abdominal wall (M. psoas major and M. quadratus lumborum). Located in this space are the kidneys, the adrenal glands and the ureter, which together are surrounded by a fascia system (➤ Chap. 8.1, ➤ Chap. 8.2). Located between the two kidneys run the vessels and nerves of the retroperitoneal space (➤ Chap. 8.8).

8.7.3 Subperitoneal space

Caudal to the pelvic section of the peritoneal cavity (Cavitas peritonealis pelvis) the extraperitoneal space is extended to the subperitoneal space (Spatium extraperitoneale pelvis), in which connective tissue surrounds the individual organs with their vascular, lymphatic and nervous systems. The connective tissue is partially thickened to so-called fasciae, which surround the individual organs and subdivide individual compartments, such as the 'Mesorectum', which constitutes a clinically very relevant space around the rectum (➤ Chap. 8.4.3). The space behind the pubic symphysis is referred to as the **Spatium retropubicum** (clinically: RETZIUS' space) (➤ Fig. 8.57, ➤ Fig. 8.58).

The fasciae in the pelvis are divided into:
• **Fascia pelvis parietalis:** covers the bony pelvis on the inside; the section ventrally of the sacrum is referred to as the **Fascia presacralis (WALDEYER's fascia).**
• **Fascia pelvis visceralis:** encases the individual organs with their vascular, lymphatic and nervous systems, e.g. the 'mesorectal fascia' around the rectum with its 'Mesorectum'; in addition,

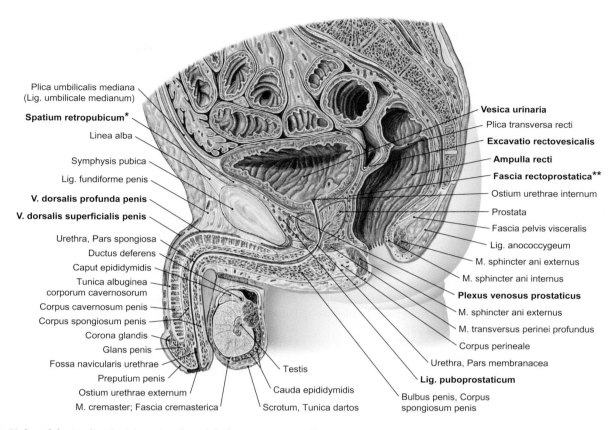

Plica umbilicalis mediana
(Lig. umbilicale medianum)

Spatium retropubicum*

Linea alba

Symphysis pubica

Lig. fundiforme penis

V. dorsalis profunda penis

V. dorsalis superficialis penis

Urethra, Pars spongiosa

Ductus deferens

Caput epididymidis

Tunica albuginea
corporum cavernosorum

Corpus cavernosum penis

Corpus spongiosum penis

Corona glandis

Glans penis

Fossa navicularis urethrae

Preputium penis

Ostium urethrae externum

M. cremaster; Fascia cremasterica

Testis

Cauda epididymidis

Scrotum, Tunica dartos

Bulbus penis, Corpus
spongiosum penis

Lig. puboprostaticum

Urethra, Pars membranacea

Corpus perineale

M. transversus perinei profundus

M. sphincter ani externus

Plexus venosus prostaticus

M. sphincter ani internus

M. sphincter ani externus

Lig. anococcygeum

Fascia pelvis visceralis

Prostata

Ostium urethrae internum

Fascia rectoprostatica**

Ampulla recti

Excavatio rectovesicalis

Plica transversa recti

Vesica urinaria

Fig. 8.57 Male pelvis. Median incision; view from left; *RETZIUS' space ** clinically: DENONVILLIER's fascia.

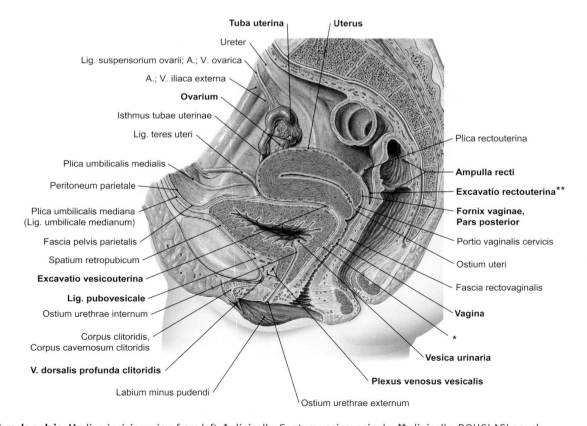

Tuba uterina

Uterus

Ureter

Lig. suspensorium ovarii; A.; V. ovarica

A.; V. iliaca externa

Ovarium

Isthmus tubae uterinae

Lig. teres uteri

Plica umbilicalis medialis

Peritoneum parietale

Plica umbilicalis mediana
(Lig. umbilicale medianum)

Fascia pelvis parietalis

Spatium retropubicum

Excavatio vesicouterina

Lig. pubovesicale

Ostium urethrae internum

Corpus clitoridis,
Corpus cavernosum clitoridis

V. dorsalis profunda clitoridis

Labium minus pudendi

Ostium urethrae externum

Plica rectouterina

Ampulla recti

Excavatio rectouterina**

**Fornix vaginae,
Pars posterior**

Portio vaginalis cervicis

Ostium uteri

Fascia rectovaginalis

Vagina

*

Vesica urinaria

Plexus venosus vesicalis

Fig. 8.58 Female pelvis. Median incision; view from left; * clinically: Septum vesicovaginale, ** clinically: DOUGLAS' pouch.

there are sheets of connective tissue, which separate individual organs from each other, such as in men the **Fascia rectoprostatica (= Septum rectoprostaticum**, clinically DENONVILLIER's fascia) and in women the **Fascia rectovaginalis (= Septum rectovaginale)**.

Further thickenings of the connective tissue are referred to as ligaments (Ligamenta) and serve the purpose of securing the individual organs to the bony pelvis. Even the remaining loose connective tissue, which continuously merges into connective tissue fascia or walls of the organs, have their own clinical terms:

- **Parametrium:** fibre strands from the cervix to the lateral pelvic wall (Lig. cardinale)
- **Paraproctium:** connective tissue around the rectum
- **Paracystium:** connective tissue around the urinary bladder
- **Paracolpium:** connective tissue around the vagina

The pelvic cavity is thereby divided into a total of **3 levels**. The pelvic organs lie in the clinically designated as the **'lesser pelvis'** caudal section below the Linea terminalis, which is composed of the anterior Pecten ossis pubis and the posterior Linea arcuata. The levels of the pelvic cavity (from cranial to caudal) are:

- **Pelvic section of the peritoneal cavity** (Cavitas peritonealis pelvis), caudally delineated by the Peritoneum parietale
- **Subperitoneal space**, which reaches caudally up to the pelvic floor (➤ Chap. 8.9)
- **Perineal region** (Regio perinealis), which lies underneath the pelvic floor and divides on both sides ventrally into the two perineal spaces and dorsally in the Fossa ischioanalis (➤ Chap. 8.9)

The peritoneal cavity runs with various recesses (Recessus), which are lined with Peritoneum parietale, into the subperitoneal space. In men the **Excavatio rectovesicalis** forms the deepest space of the abdominal cavity; in women this is the **Excavatio rectouterina (DOUGLAS' pouch)**, which runs still further caudally than the ventrally lying **Excavatio vesicouterina**.

⌐ Clinical remarks

In an **upright position**, in the deepest recesses of the peritoneal cavity, the **Excavatio rectovesicalis** in men, and the **Excavatio vesicouterina** (pouch of DOUGLAS) in women, may accumulate inflammatory exudate or pus if there is inflammation in the hypogastrium, which can be detected by sonography as free liquid. The pouch of DOUGLAS extends to the posterior vaginal vault and can be aspirated from there in order to investigate the free fluid.

8.8 Vessels and nerves of the extraperitoneal space and pelvic cavity

⌐ Skills

After working through this chapter, you should be able to:
- understand the basic structure of the vessels and nerves of the retroperitoneum, so that you can retrace the origin of the vascular and neural supply in the individual organs
- show on a specimen branches of the abdominal aorta and tributaries of V. cava inferior
- explain on a specimen branches of the Aa. iliacae externa and interna with course and supply areas
- know the venous plexuses of the pelvis with their connections and understand their clinical relevance
- identify lymph nodes and systems of lymphatic pathways with formation of the Ductus thoracicus
- explain the organisation of the autonomic nervous system with plexi and ganglia in the retroperitoneum and pelvis

8.8.1 Overview

The major arterial, venous and lymphatic vascular branches of the body in the **Retroperitoneum** continue caudally in the pelvic cavity into the **subperitoneal space** as well as from cranially into the **posterior mediastinum of the thoracic cavity** (➤ Chap. 6.6). In the process, the vessels supply both the dorsal abdominal wall (parietal vessels) as well as the viscera (visceral vessels) of the abdominal and pelvic cavities and continue as vessels of the lower extremities.

The **abdominal section of the Aorta (Pars abdominalis aortae)** enters through the diaphragm from the thoracic cavity into the retroperitoneal space. Their terminal branches are the iliac arteries (Aa. iliacae communes), which divide in the pelvis into the A. iliaca interna (to supply the pelvic wall and organs) and the A. iliaca externa (which merges under the inguinal ligament into the A. femoralis).

The **inferior vena cava (V. cava inferior)** with its tributaries extensively corresponds to the Aorta. After its passage through the diaphragm it flows directly into the right atrium of the heart.

In the Retroperitoneum, lymph trunks from the abdominal and pelvic cavities merge into the **thoracic duct (Ductus thoracicus)**, the largest lymph trunk of the body, which continues on to the left venous angle though the diaphragm into the posterior mediastinum. The retroperitoneal and subperitoneal spaces also contain sections of the somatic and autonomic nervous system. The **Plexus lumbosacralis** is a somatic nerve plexus, which is formed by the anterior branches of the spinal nerves and located between portions of the M. psoas major. Its nerves largely serve the purpose of innervating the lower extremities (➤ Chap. 5.6.1), but also of innervating the anal canal and external genitalia.

On the aorta, the nerve fibres of the **sympathetic and parasympathetic nervous systems** form an autonomic nerve plexus (**Plexus aorticus abdominalis**), the individual parts of which reach the individual organs with their respective arterial vessels. The autonomic nerve plexus continues via the Plexus hypogastricus superior into the pelvic cavity, where it innervates various organs as the **Plexus hypogastricus inferior**.

8.8.2 Arteries of the retroperitoneum and pelvic cavity

The **abdominal section of the Aorta (Pars abdominalis aortae)** passes at the level of the XIIth thoracic vertebra through the Hiatus aorticus of the diaphragm and afterwards descends to the left ventrally of the spinal column (➤ Fig. 8.59). On its way there **parietal branches** emerge for the abdominal wall and **visceral branches** for the viscera of the peritoneal cavity and retroperitoneal and subperitoneal spaces ➤ Table. 8.8). While the paired visceral branches supply organs in the retroperitoneum and pelvic cavity, the abdominal viscera receive blood from **3 unpaired arterial branches**:

- Truncus coeliacus
- A. mesenterica superior
- A. mesenterica inferior

At the level of the IVth lumbar vertebra the Aorta divides into its **terminal branches**. The Aa. iliacae communes pass over on both sides

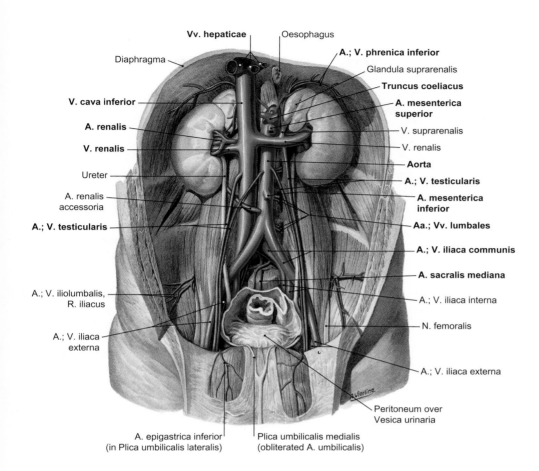

Vv. hepaticae
Oesophagus
Diaphragma
A.; V. phrenica inferior
Glandula suprarenalis
V. cava inferior
Truncus coeliacus
A. mesenterica superior
A. renalis
V. suprarenalis
V. renalis
V. renalis
Ureter
Aorta
A. renalis accessoria
A.; V. testicularis
A. mesenterica inferior
A.; V. testicularis
Aa.; Vv. lumbales
A.; V. iliaca communis
A. sacralis mediana
A.; V. iliolumbalis, R. iliacus
A.; V. iliaca interna
N. femoralis
A.; V. iliaca externa
A.; V. iliaca externa
Peritoneum over Vesica urinaria
A. epigastrica inferior (in Plica umbilicalis lateralis)
Plica umbilicalis medialis (obliterated A. umbilicalis)

Fig. 8.59 Abdominal Aorta and inferior vena cava. Retrositus. [S010-2-16]

into the pelvic cavity, where they branch. The thin A. sacralis mediana continues its course on the sacrum (➤ Fig. 8.59).
Before the sacroiliac joint the A. iliaca communis divides into the **A. iliaca externa**, which continues under the inguinal ligament into the A. femoralis (➤ Chap. 5.7.2), and into the **A. iliaca interna** in order to supply the pelvis and its viscera (➤ Fig. 8.60). The A. iliaca interna usually splits (in 60% of cases) into an anterior and a posterior main branch. Since the branch sequence is relatively variable, it is worthwhile instead to group the branches according to their supply areas into **parietal branches** for the pelvic wall and the external genitalia and into **visceral branches** for the pelvic viscera.

Table. 8.8 Branches of the Pars abdominalis aortae

Parietal branches to the thoracic wall	• A. phrenica inferior: on the underside of the diaphragm, gives off the A. suprarenalis superior to the adrenal gland • Aa. lumbales: 4 pairs directly from the Aorta, the 5th pair originates from the A. sacralis mediana
Visceral branches for the viscera	• Truncus coeliacus: unpaired, originates directly beneath the Hiatus aorticus and supplies the organs of the upper abdomen (➤ Fig. 7.48) • A. suprarenalis media supplies the adrenal glands • A. renalis: to the kidneys, also gives off the A. suprarenalis inferior to the adrenal glands • A. mesenterica superior: unpaired, supplies parts of the pancreas, the entire small intestine and the colon up to the left colonic flexure (➤ Fig. 7.49) • A. testicularis/ovarica: supplies the testis and epididymis in men and the ovaries in women • A. mesenterica inferior: unpaired, supplies the Colon descendens and upper rectum (➤ Fig. 7.50)
Terminal branches	• A. iliaca communis: for the pelvis and leg • A. sacralis mediana: descends onto the sacrum

The parietal branches are formed identically in both sexes ➤ Fig. 8.60:
- **A. iliolumbalis:** it supplies the Fossa iliaca and lumbar region and also gives off a branch to the spinal canal.
- **Aa. sacrales laterales:** these arteries enter into the sacral canal and supply the spinal meninx.
- **A. obturatoria:** it runs with the N. obturatorius through the Canalis obturatorius to the thigh. The **R. pubicus** anastomoses with an eponymous branch from the A. epigastrica inferior: in up to 20% of cases the entire A. obturatoria originates from this vessel. In the Canalis obturatorius the A. obturatoria divides into the **R. anterior**, which supplies the adductors of the thigh and anastomoses there with the A. circumflexa femoris medialis. The **R. posterior** runs to the gluteal muscles. The **R. acetabularis** runs via the Lig. capitis femoris to the head of the femur and is essential in children for nutrition of the proximal femoral epiphysis.
- **A. glutea superior:** it runs through the Foramen suprapiriforme into the gluteal region and supplies the gluteal muscles.
- **A. glutea inferior:** it passes through the Foramen infrapiriforme and similarly supplies the gluteal muscles.

Clinical remarks

If the anastomosis between the A. obturatoria and the A. epigastrica inferior is broad, this is traditionally called the **Corona mortis**, because in past times during operations in the inguinal region, e.g. due to inguinal hernias, there was a risk of life-threatening haemorrhaging. Nowadays, this clinical reference plays a minor role due to improved operative techniques and haemostatic capabilities.
If the R. acetabularis in children, due to trauma (e.g. hip dislocation) or because of unknown causes, such as in PERTHES

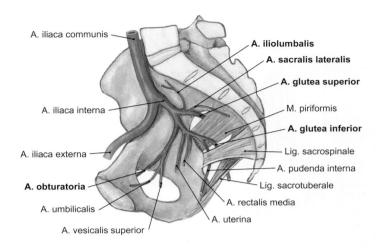

A. iliaca communis

A. iliolumbalis

A. sacralis lateralis

A. glutea superior

A. iliaca interna

M. piriformis

A. glutea inferior

A. iliaca externa

Lig. sacrospinale

A. pudenda interna

A. obturatoria

Lig. sacrotuberale

A. umbilicalis

A. rectalis media

A. vesicalis superior

A. uterina

Fig. 8.60 Parietal branches of the A. iliaca interna.

disease cannot ensure blood supply of the femoral head, then **bone necrosis occurs,** which can damage motion and stability of the hip joint.

In contrast, the **visceral branches** are somewhat different in men and women (➤ Fig. 8.61, ➤ Fig. 8.62):

- **A. umbilicalis:** it gives off the **A. vesicalis superior** to the urinary bladder, which in men usually gives rise to the **A. ductus deferentis** to the Vas deferens before it is closed (= Lig. umbilicale mediale) and gives rise to the Plica umbilicalis medialis.

- **A. vesicalis inferior:** it runs to the urinary bladder in men to the prostate and seminal vesicle and sometimes gives off here the A. ductus deferentis. In women, it also supplies the vagina, but can also be missing and is then replaced by the A. vaginalis.

- **A. uterina** *(only in women):* before its entrance into the Lig. latum uteri, the artery crosses *over* the ureter, before it branches and supplies the uterus, Tuba uterina, ovary and vagina with its respective branches.

- **A. vaginalis** *(only in women):* it supplies the majority of the vagina and sometimes replaces the A. vesicalis inferior.

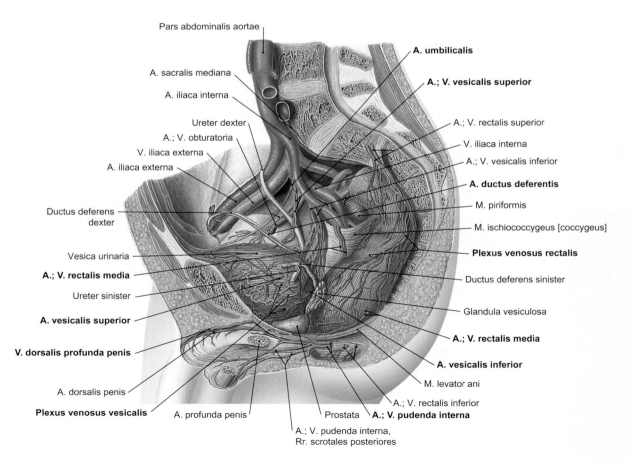

Pars abdominalis aortae

A. umbilicalis

A. sacralis mediana

A.; V. vesicalis superior

A. iliaca interna

A.; V. rectalis superior

Ureter dexter

V. iliaca interna

A.; V. obturatoria

A.; V. vesicalis inferior

V. iliaca externa

A. ductus deferentis

A. iliaca externa

M. piriformis

Ductus deferens dexter

M. ischiococcygeus [coccygeus]

Vesica urinaria

Plexus venosus rectalis

A.; V. rectalis media

Ductus deferens sinister

Ureter sinister

Glandula vesiculosa

A. vesicalis superior

A.; V. rectalis media

V. dorsalis profunda penis

A. vesicalis inferior

M. levator ani

A.; V. rectalis inferior

A. dorsalis penis

Plexus venosus vesicalis

A. profunda penis

Prostata

A.; V. pudenda interna

A.; V. pudenda interna, Rr. scrotales posteriores

Fig. 8.61 Blood supply of the male pelvic viscera. View from left.

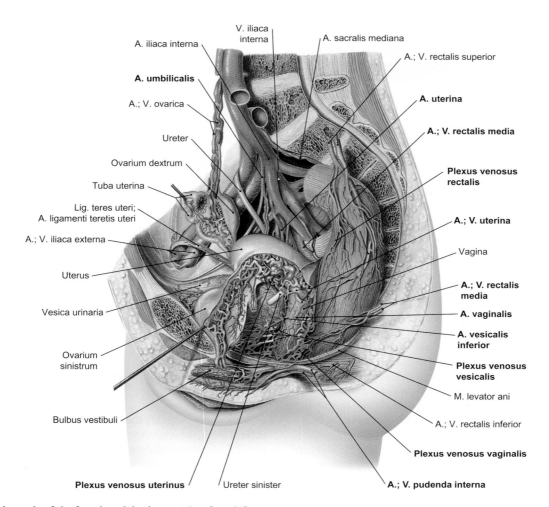

Fig. 8.62 Blood supply of the female pelvic viscera. View from left.

- **A. rectalis media:** it runs above the pelvic floor to the rectum. The vessel is rarely formed on both sides and can even be missing completely.
- **A. pudenda interna:** it passes through the Foramen infrapiriforme and then through the Foramen ischiadicum minus into the lateral wall of the Fossa ischioanalis (Canalis pudendalis, ALCOCK's canal) Here, it gives off the A. rectalis inferior for the inferior anal canal and then divides gender-specifically into its superficial and deep terminal branches in order to supply the external genitalia:
  - In men, the superficial **A. rectalis inferior** supplies the intestine and gives off the Rr. scrotales posteriores to the scrotum. The **deep branches** supply the penis with its cavernous bodies (A. bulbi penis, A. dorsalis penis, A. profunda penis).
  - In women, the superficial **A. perinealis** runs to the intestine and gives off the Rr. labiales posteriores to the labia. The **deep branches** supply the clitoris with its cavernous bodies and the vulval cavernous body in the Labia majora (A. bulbi vestibuli, A. dorsalis clitoridis, A. profunda clitoridis).

8.8.3 Veins of the retroperitoneum and pelvic cavity

The **inferior vena cava (V. cava inferior)** forms to the right of the aorta at the level of the lumbar vertebra vein through unification of the two Vv. iliacae communes. Via the **Vv. iliacae communes** these conduct blood out of the lower limbs and via the **V. iliaca interna**

from the pelvic viscera. A peculiarity in the pelvic cavity is that the veins in the vicinity of the individual organs form **plexus (Plexus venosi)**, all of which communicate with each other and also establish via the **cavocaval anastomoses** connections to the superior vena cava (V. cava superior). The inferior vena cava ascends to the right in front of the spinal column and passes in the Foramen v. cavae through the diaphragm. The **vein plexus of the pelvis** are (➤ Fig. 8.61, ➤ Fig. 8.62):

- **Plexus venosus rectalis:** this plexus of the rectum is located within the 'Mesorectum' and is in contact via the V. rectalis superior with the portal artery circulation and via the Vv. rectales media and inferior with the drainage area of the V. cava inferior (portocaval anastomosis).
- **Plexus venosus vesicalis:** the venous plexus at the fundus of the bladder collects blood from the urinary bladder and in men from the accessory sex glands. In women it also collects blood from the cavernous bodies (V. dorsalis profunda clitoridis).
- **Plexus venosus prostaticus:** in men, in addition to the blood of the prostate, it also takes up blood from the cavernous bodies of the penis (V. dorsalis profunda penis).
- **Plexus venosi uterinus and vaginalis:** the plexus around the uterus and vagina collect the blood of both organs.

From these plexus the Vv. rectales mediae , Vv. vesicales and Vv. uterinae flow outwards into the V. iliaca interna. Included among them are the veins which correspond predominantly to the parietal branches of the A. iliaca interna (Vv. gluteae superiores and inferiores, Vv. obturatoriae and Vv. sacrales laterales).

Table 8.9 Tributaries from the V. renalis sinistra and the V. cava inferior.

Tributaries of the V. renalis sinistra	Tributaries of the V. cava inferior
• V. phrenica inferior (sinistra) • V. testicularis/ ovarica (sinistra) • V. suprarenalis (sinistra)	• Vv. iliacae communes • V. sacralis mediana • Vv. lumbales • V. phrenica inferior dextra, entering left into the V. renalis • V. testicularis/ovarica dextra, entering left into the V. renalis • V. suprarenalis dextra, entering left into the V. renalis • Vv. renales dextra and sinistra • 3 Vv. hepaticae (Vv. hepaticae dextra, intermedia and sinistra)

The **V. cava inferior** corresponds extensively in its tributaries to the corresponding branches of the abdominal aorta (➤ Table 8.9); however, there are no veins which correspond to the three unpaired visceral arteries (Truncus coeliacus, A. mesenterica superior, A. mesenterica inferior), since blood from the unpaired abdominal organs is firstly siphoned via the portal vein (V. portae hepatis) through the liver. Instead, therefore, the **3 Vv. hepaticae** flow into the inferior vena cava, which conducts all of the blood of the intraperitoneal abdominal organs. The second difference is found in an asymmetry in the outlet relationship of individual vessels. Whilst on the right-hand side all tributaries flow directly into the inferior vena cava, on the left 3 vessels merge with the V. renalis (➤ Table 8.9).

The superior and inferior vena cava flow directly into the right atrium of the heart, so they do not communicate directly with each other. There are, however, bypass circulations (collaterals) that connect the two vessels indirectly (**cavocaval anastomoses**) and if there is occlusion or compression of one of the two venae cavae the blood can be redirected accordingly (➤ Chap. 6.6.3).

Clinical remarks

The asymmetrical confluence of the left V. testicularis into the left V. renalis can, in the case of a **malignant renal carcinoma**, be diagnostically relevant in men. As renal carcinomas tend to spread from the kidneys outwards continuously within the venous system, inflow congestion of the V. testicularis can occur with an extension of the Plexus pampiniformis in the scrotum, which is referred to as a **varicocele** (➤ Fig. 8.43). Therefore, in the case of a left hand varicocele, steps should always be taken to exclude cancer of the kidneys.

The connections of the Plexus prostaticus to the venous plexus of the spinal column (cavocaval anastomoses) explain to some extent why, in the case of **prostate cancer, spinal metastases** often occur, which extend up into the neck area; via spinal fractures these can cause injuries to the spinal cord with paraplegia.

8.8.4 Lymphatic vessels of the retroperitoneum and pelvic cavity

Located in the pelvis are the **Nodi lymphoidei iliaci interni and externi** along the respective blood vessels and the **Nodi lymphoidei sacrales** on the anterior surface of the sacrum (➤ Fig. 8.63). Due to their close topographical relationships, it is not possi-

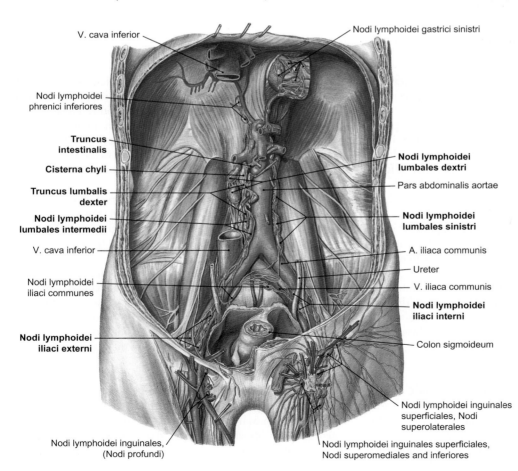

Fig. 8.63 Lymphatic vessels and lymph nodes of the retroperitoneal space. Ventral view.

ble to strictly differentiate between parietal lymph nodes for the abdominal wall and visceral lymph nodes for the organs. Thus, the pelvic viscera (rectum, urinary bladder, internal genitalia) are connected to all of the lymph node groups.

Via the **Nodi lymphoidei iliaci communes** the lymph runs out of the pelvis into the parietal lymph nodes of the retroperitoneal space, which are grouped as the **Nodi lymphoidei lumbales**. These are positioned in 3 chains as the Nodi lymphoidei lumbales sinistri around the aorta, as the Nodi lymphoidei lumbales dextri to both

sides of the V. cava inferior, and as the Nodi lymphoidei lumbales intermedi between both vessels. The lumbar lymph nodes are the collection lymph nodes for:

- the lower extremities
- the entire pelvic viscera
- the left side of the large intestine (Colon descendens, Colon sigmoideum, rectum, anal canal)
- kidneys and adrenal glands
- testicles/ovaries

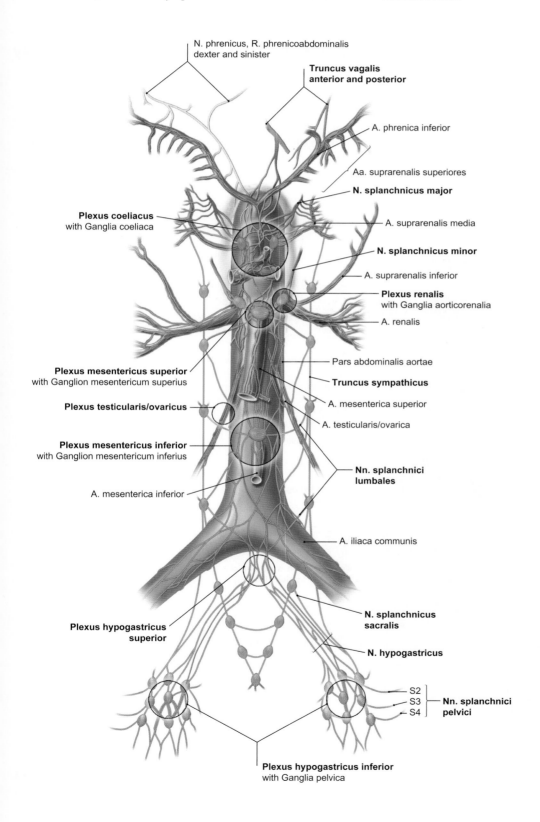

N. phrenicus, R. phrenicoabdominalis dexter and sinister

Truncus vagalis anterior and posterior

A. phrenica inferior

Aa. suprarenalis superiores

N. splanchnicus major

A. suprarenalis media

Plexus coeliacus with Ganglia coeliaca

N. splanchnicus minor

A. suprarenalis inferior

Plexus renalis with Ganglia aorticorenalia

A. renalis

Pars abdominalis aortae

Plexus mesentericus superior with Ganglion mesentericum superius

Truncus sympathicus

A. mesenterica superior

Plexus testicularis/ovaricus

A. testicularis/ovarica

Plexus mesentericus inferior with Ganglion mesentericum inferius

Nn. splanchnici lumbales

A. mesenterica inferior

A. iliaca communis

Plexus hypogastricus superior

N. splanchnicus sacralis

N. hypogastricus

S2
S3   **Nn. splanchnici pelvici**
S4

Plexus hypogastricus inferior with Ganglia pelvica

Fig. 8.64 Plexus aorticus abdominalis with sympathetic ganglia. [L238]

The lymphatic pathways of the individual organs and their regional lymph nodes are explained together with the individual organs of the abdominal and pelvic cavities.

Emerging on both sides from the efferent lymphatic pathways of the lumbar lymph nodes are the **Trunci lumbales**, which merge to the right of the aorta within the retroperitoneum beneath the diaphragm with the **Trunci intestinales** (they collect the lymph of the visceral lymph nodes from the abdominal cavity) into the **Ductus thoracicus**. The merging point is often dilated to the Cisterna chyli (➤ Fig. 8.63), which, however, is formed very variably. Thus, the Ductus thoracicus, as the main lymphatic trunk of the body beneath the diaphragm guides all of the lymph from the lower half of the body. It runs dorsal to the aorta at the level of the XII thoracic vertebra to the right, through the Hiatus aorticus of the diaphragm, ascends in the posterior mediastinum and finally enters into the left venous angle, which is located behind the sternoclavicular joint.

Clinical remarks

The systematics of major lymphatic trunks explain why malignant tumours of the abdominal organs (e.g. gastric cancer) or pelvic viscera (e.g. ovarian cancer) can also cause lymph node metastasis in the area of the left venous angle. These lymph node swellings in the *left* supraclavicular fossa are referred to as **VIRCHOW's nodes** after the first person to describe them and a doctor must always check for tumours in the abdominal and pelvic cavities.

8.8.5 Nerves of the retroperitoneum and pelvic cavity

For the basic structure of the autonomic nervous system, see ➤ Chap. 7.8.5.

To the anterior in the retroperitoneal space on the abdominal section of the aorta is a plexus of the autonomic nervous system (**Plexus aorticus abdominalis**), which innervates the abdominal viscera (➤ Fig. 8.64, ➤ Fig. 8.65). The aortic plexus at the outlets

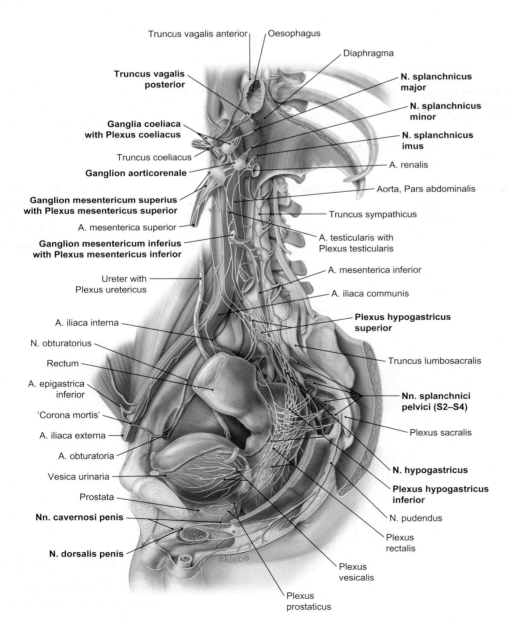

Truncus vagalis anterior
Oesophagus
Diaphragma
Truncus vagalis posterior
N. splanchnicus major
N. splanchnicus minor
Ganglia coeliaca with Plexus coeliacus
N. splanchnicus imus
Truncus coeliacus
A. renalis
Ganglion aorticorenale
Aorta, Pars abdominalis
Ganglion mesentericum superius with Plexus mesentericus superior
Truncus sympathicus
A. mesenterica superior
A. testicularis with Plexus testicularis
Ganglion mesentericum inferius with Plexus mesentericus inferior
A. mesenterica inferior
Ureter with Plexus uretericus
A. iliaca communis
A. iliaca interna
Plexus hypogastricus superior
N. obturatorius
Rectum
Truncus lumbosacralis
A. epigastrica inferior
'Corona mortis'
Nn. splanchnici pelvici (S2–S4)
A. iliaca externa
Plexus sacralis
A. obturatoria
Vesica urinaria
N. hypogastricus
Prostata
Plexus hypogastricus inferior
Nn. cavernosi penis
N. pudendus
N. dorsalis penis
Plexus rectalis
Plexus vesicalis
Plexus prostaticus

Fig. 8.65 Plexus hypogastricus inferior. [L238]

of the visceral vascular branches is further divided into eponymous sections:

- Plexus coeliacus
- Plexus mesentericus superior
- Plexus mesentericus inferior
- Plexus renalis
- Plexus testicularis/ovaricus

These autonomic plexus contain sympathetic and parasympathetic nerve fibres. The **sympathetic nerve fibres** originate mainly from the thoracic section of the sympathetic trunk (Truncus sympathicus) and as the Nn. splanchnici major and minor pass through the diaphragm (➤ Fig. 8.64, ➤ Fig. 8.65). In addition, from the abdominal section of the sympathetic trunk neurons run as the Nn. splanchnici lumbales up to the plexus on the Aorta. The **parasympathetic neurons** run as the Trunci vagales together with the oesophagus through the diaphragm and are the terminal branches of the Nn. vagi.

From the Plexus aorticus abdominalis outwards the nerve fibres in the abdominal cavity reach their target organs mainly as **periarterial plexus**, which each form an organ-specific plexus at the respective organs. As in all sections of the autonomic nervous system, the visceral efferent to the effector organ consists of 2 neurons, whereby the preganglionic neuron originates in the central nervous system and is converted synaptically within a ganglion into the so-called postganglionic neuron. Whilst the parasympathetic neurons are first converted in close vicinity to the organs and thus pervade the plexus of the Plexus aorticus abdominalis as preganglionic neurons, the sympathetic neurons are converted into ganglia away from the organs and are located at the eponymous vascular outlets of the abdominal aorta. The ganglia of the Plexus aorticus abdominalis are (➤ Fig. 8.64, ➤ Fig. 8.65):

- Ganglia coeliaca
- Ganglion mesentericum superius
- Ganglion mesentericum inferius
- Ganglia aorticorenalia

In the pelvis, the Plexus aorticus abdominalis continues as the **Plexus iliacus** on the A. iliaca communis and as the **Plexus hypogastrici superior and inferior** to supply the pelvic organs (➤ Fig. 8.65). Whilst the sympathetic neurons to some extent continue from the abdomen and derive additionally as the Nn. splanchnici sacrales from the pelvic section of the sympathetic trunk, all parasympathetic nervous originate as **Nn. splanchnici pelvici** from the sacral spinal cord (S2–4).

The sympathetic and parasympathetic neurons are converted (Ganglia pelvica) in the ganglia of the Plexus hypogastricus inferior and reach the pelvic organs largely autonomously and thus independently of the blood vessels.

The Plexus hypogastricus inferior is embedded on both sides between the Fascia pelvis visceralis, which surrounds the 'Mesorectum', and the Fascia pelvis parietalis on the bony pelvis in the connective tissue of the subperitoneal space (➤ Fig. 8.65; also ➤ Fig. 8.19). In women, the plexus is thus located in the Lig. rectouterinum between the Cervix uteri and rectum, which raises a peritoneal fold, which, as the **Plica rectouterina** marks the entrance to the Excavatio rectouterina (DOUGLAS' pouch).

NOTE

- The autonomous **plexus on the abdominal aorta** contain sympathetic and parasympathetic nerve fibres. In contrast, only sympathetic fibres are located in the **ganglia,** which are converted synaptically from preganglionic to postganglionic neurons.
- The **Plexus hypogastricus inferior** in the pelvis, in contrast, has both sympathetic and parasympathetic ganglia, in which the nerve fibres are converted close to the organs.

8.9 Pelvic floor and perineal region

8.9.1 Overview

The pelvic cavity (➤ Chap. 8.7) is delineated caudally by the muscular **pelvic floor (Diaphragma pelvis)**. Included in it is the **perineal region (Regio perinealis)** in the posterior section of which on both sides the **Fossa ischioanalis** is located, whilst the anterior section with the **superficial (Spatium superficiale perinei)** and the **deep perineal spaces (Spatium profundum perinei)** is divided into 2 levels, which contain the perineal muscles to support the pelvic floor. The anatomy of the pelvic floor is particularly relevant in gynaecology, since the pelvic floor and muscles of the perineal region can be damaged during pregnancy and childbirth. Since these muscles are of central importance for faecal continence, their topographical relationships are also important for visceral surgeons.

8.9.2 Pelvic floor

The pelvic floor (Diaphragma pelvis) is a plate of striated muscles, which complete the pelvic cavity caudally. The pelvic floor has the same construction in both sexes.

Function: the pelvic floor stabilises the position of the pelvic organs and thus ensures urinary and faecal continence.

The **muscles** of the pelvic floor are (➤ Fig. 8.66, ➤ Table 8.10):
- **M. levator ani,** which comprises the M. pubococcygeus, M. iliococcygeus and M. puborectalis.
- **M. ischiococcygeus**

In contrast to the M. pubococcygeus and the M. ischiococcygeus, the M. iliococcygeus does not originate from the hip bone but from the **Arcus tendineus musculi levatoris ani**, which constitutes a reinforcement of the fascia of the M. obturator internus on its superior surface.

Individual muscle fibres of the M. pubococcygeus run to the anal canal and to the prostate or the vagina and are therefore correspondingly referred to as the M. puboanalis, M. prostaticus, M. vaginalis or collectively as the 'M. pubovisceralis'.

On its anterior surface, the pelvic floor has contact with the urinary bladder, rectum, prostate or vagina.

The pelvic floor muscles of both sides leave a space ('**Hiatus levatorius**') between them, which is divided by the connective tissue of the **Corpus perineale (Centrum perinei)** into a **Hiatus urogenitalis** (anterior) as a passageway for the urethra and in women for the vagina, as well as into a '**Hiatus analis**' (posterior) for the rectum. The M. puborectalis forms a loop around the rectum and due its tone induces the development of the Flexura perinealis, which thus constitutes part of the continence organ (➤ Chap. 8.4.4).

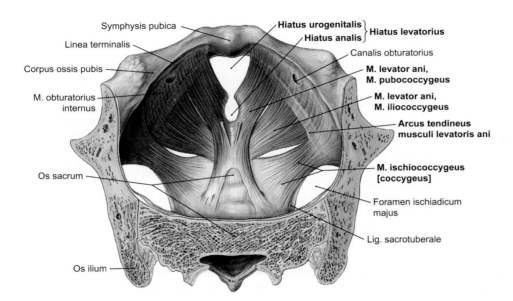

Fig. 8.66 Pelvic floor, diaphragma pelvis, female. Cranial view.

Table 8.10 Muscles of the pelvic floor (Diaphragma pelvis).

Innervation	Origin	Attachment	Function
M. levator ani			
Plexus sacralis (S3–S4)	• M. pubococcygeus: inner surface of the Os pubis near the symphysis • M. iliococcygeus: Arcus tendineus musculi levatoris ani	• Centrum tendineum perinei, Os coccygis, Os sacrum • Loop formation with fibres of the opposite side behind the anus (M. puborectalis)	Stabilises the pelvic organs, hence facilitates urinary and faecal continence, encompasses the rectum from behind, hence distal rectal occlusion (M. puborectalis)
M. ischiococcygeus			
Plexus sacralis (S3–S4)	Spina ischiadica, Lig. sacrospinale	Os coccygis, Os sacrum	Same as the M. levator ani

The pelvic floor is innervated by direct branches from the **Plexus sacralis (S3–S4)**. Only the M. puborectalis is also supplied by the N. pudendus. Blood comes from various branches of the **A. iliaca interna** (A. glutea inferior, A. vesicalis inferior and A. pudenda interna).

N O T E
• **Perineal region (Regio perinalis):** whole area between the pubic symphysis and coccyx
• **Perineum:** narrow section between the posterior margin of the Labia majora/root of penis and the anus

Clinical remarks

In women, weakness of the pelvic floor **(pelvic floor insufficiency)** is much more common than in men, because the pelvic floor is strained during pregnancy and childbirth, during which the levator is greatly stretched. As a result, there can ensue a **drop** (descent) or a **prolapse** of the uterus and vagina. Since the uterus is connected to the posterior wall of the urinary bladder and the vagina is connected to the anterior surface of the rectum, this is often associated with a prolapse of the urinary bladder (cystocele) and the rectum (rectocele) and thus **urinary** and **faecal incontinence** (➤ Fig. 8.67).

Clinical remarks

During childbirth uncontrolled tearing of the skin and muscles of the perineum up to the sphincters of the anus **(perineal fissures) can occur,** which in some cases can be prevented by targeted incisions laterally or in the median plane (perineal incision) **(episiotomy).**

The perineal region can be divided into an **anterior Regio urogenitalis** with sexual organs and urethra and a **posterior Regio analis** around the anus (➤ Fig. 8.68, ➤ Fig. 8.69). Both areas include spaces:
• Regio analis:
  – Fossa ischioanalis
• Regio urogenitalis
  – Superficial perineal space (Spatium superficiale perinei)
  – Deep perineal space (Spatium profundum perinei)

Fossa ischioanalis
The Fossa ischioanalis is a pyramid-shaped space filled with fat on both sides of the anus, which is very similarly formed in both sexes (➤ Fig. 8.68, ➤ Fig. 8.69). Its boundaries are set out in ➤ Table 8.11. Located in the lateral wall within a fascial duplicature on

8.9.3 Perineal region

Located underneath the pelvic floor is the **perineal region (Regio perinealis)**, which stretches from the pubic symphysis (Symphysis pubica) to posterior up to the apex of the coccyx , (➤ Fig. 8.68, ➤ Fig. 8.69). In contrast, the term **perineum** describes only the narrow connective tissue bridge between the posterior margin of the Labia majora (in women) or the root of penis (in men) and the anus. The taut connective tissue between the anus and coccyx is referred to as the Lig. anococcygeum.

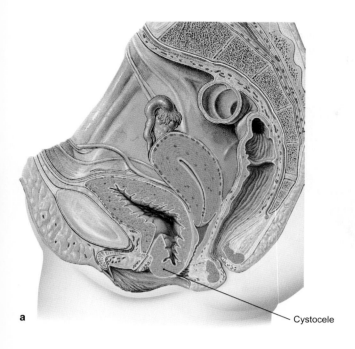

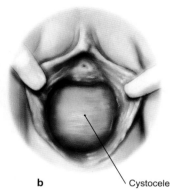

a   Cystocele   b   Cystocele

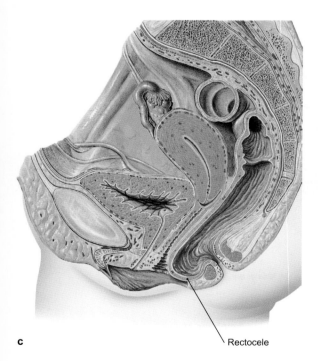

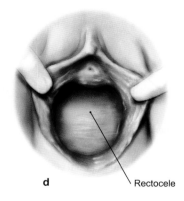

c   Rectocele   d   Rectocele

Fig. 8.67 Pelvic floor weakness.
When the stabilising function of the pelvic floor fails, the posterior wall of the urinary bladder or the anterior wall of the rectum can prolapse. **a, b** Prolapse of the urinary bladder wall with cystocele and incontinence. The cystocele is visible vaginally, by which the dorsal shadow should indicate that it concerns the urinary bladder wall. **c, d** Protrusion of the anterior wall of the rectum with rectocele and faecal incontinence. The rectocele is visible vaginally, the shadow is shown here ventrally. [L266]

the inferior side of the M. obturatorius internus is the Canalis pudendalis (ALCOCK's canal). The Fossa ischioanalis contains:
* A. and V. pudenda interna
* N. pudendus

Table 8.11 Delineation of the Fossa ischioanalis.

Delineation	Structures
Medial and cranial	M. sphincter ani externus and M. levator ani
Lateral	M. obturator internus
Dorsal	M. gluteus maximus and Lig. sacrotuberale
Ventral	Posterior border of the superficial and the deep perineal space, extensions stretch up to the symphysis
Caudal	Fascia and skin of the perineum

The vessels and nerves run through the Foramen ischiadicum minus out of the Regio glutealis via ALCOCK's canal into the Fossa ischioanalis.

Clinical remarks

The Fossa ischioanalis has significant clinical relevance because of its expansion on both sides of the anus. **Abscesses**, e.g. in the case of fistulas from the anal canal, can expand in the whole Fossa ischioanalis right up to anterior to the pubic symphysis. Besides non-specific symptoms of inflammation, these kinds of abscesses are only detected due to intense pressure pain in the perineal region.

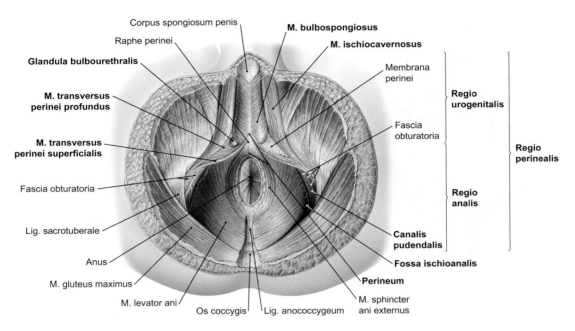

Fig. 8.68 Perineal region, Regio perinealis, male. Caudal view; after removal of all vascular, lymphatic and nervous systems.

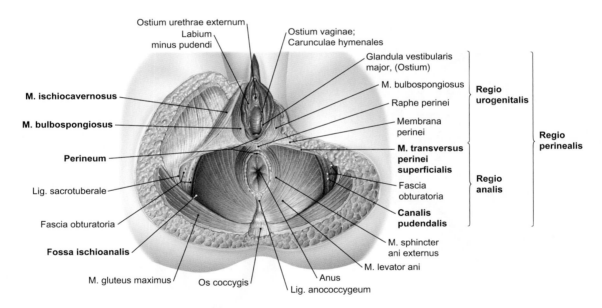

Fig. 8.69 Perineal region, Regio perinealis, female. Caudal view; after removal of all vascular, lymphatic and nervous systems.

Deep and superficial perineal space

Ventrally of the Fossa ischioanalis the **perineal spaces** form 2 levels, which differ in structure and contents in both sexes (➤ Table 8.12):

- The **deep perineal space** (Spatium profundum perinei) is delineated caudally by the Membrana perinei (reinforced fascia of the M. transversus perinei profundus) and contains the M. transversus perinei profundus, which is distinctly formed in men, but only weakly in women, and the M. sphincter urethrae externus.

- Located in the **superficial perineal space** (Spatium superficiale perinei), which is delineated cranially by the Membrana perinei and caudally by perineal fascia (Fascia perinei) are the M. transversus perinei superficialis, the M. bulbospongiosus and the M. ischiocavernosus, which in men stabilise the cavernous bodies of the root of the penis and support erection and ejaculation. In women they cover the cavernous bodies of the vulva and clitoris.

Perineal spaces in men

In men, the Hiatus urogenitalis between the two levator muscles on bothsides, is closed largely by the underlying perineal muscles, so that only the passageway of the urethra remains free.

In men, the perineal muscles consist of a relatively strong **M. transversus perinei profundus**, at the posterior edge of which is located the thin **M. transversus perinei profundus** (➤ Fig. 8.70, ➤ Table 8.13). Since these muscles form a kind of muscle plate, they used to be compared with the term 'Diaphragma urogenitale' to the Diaghragma pelvis of the pelvic floor; however, since there is no real diaphragm and a comparable muscle plate in women is not usually present, the term ceased to be used in anatomy; however, it continues to be used in clinical language.

On its superior and inferior surfaces the M. transversus perinei profundus is covered by a fascia. It is reinforced on the underside and is referred to here as the **Membrana perinei**.

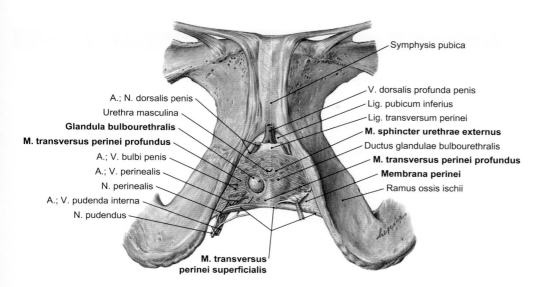

A.; N. dorsalis penis
Urethra masculina
Glandula bulbourethralis
M. transversus perinei profundus
A.; V. bulbi penis
A.; V. perinealis
N. perinealis
A.; V. pudenda interna
N. pudendus

Symphysis pubica
V. dorsalis profunda penis
Lig. pubicum inferius
Lig. transversum perinei
M. sphincter urethrae externus
Ductus glandulae bulbourethralis
M. transversus perinei profundus
Membrana perinei
Ramus ossis ischii

M. transversus perinei superficialis

Fig. 8.70 Perineal muscles, male. Caudal view; after removal of all other muscles.

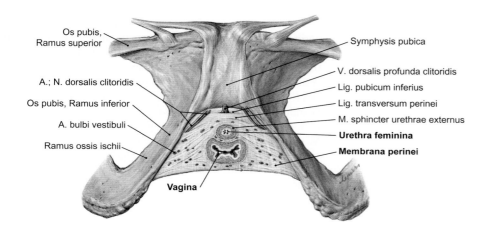

Os pubis, Ramus superior
A.; N. dorsalis clitoridis
Os pubis, Ramus inferior
A. bulbi vestibuli
Ramus ossis ischii

Symphysis pubica
V. dorsalis profunda clitoridis
Lig. pubicum inferius
Lig. transversum perinei
M. sphincter urethrae externus
Urethra feminina
Membrana perinei

Vagina

Fig. 8.71 Perineal muscles, female. Caudal view; after removal of all other muscles.

Table 8.12 Content of the Perineum.

Shared content	Content, male	Content, female
Spatium profundum perinei		
• Deep terminal branches of the A./V. pudenda interna and N. pudendus	• M. transversus perinei profundus and M. sphincter urethrae externus	• M. sphincter urethrovaginalis (M. transversus perinei profundus)
	• Urethra	• Vagina with confluence of the urethra
	• Nn. cavernosi penis	• Nn. cavernosi clitoridis (parasympathetic fibres to the erectile tissue)
	• Glandulae bulboure-thrales (COWPER)	
Spatium superficiale perinei		
• Superficial terminal branches of the A./V. pudenda interna and N. pudendus	• Crura penis	• Crura clitoridis
	• Bulbus penis	• Bulbus vestibuli
• M. transversus perinei superficial-is, M. bulbospon-giosus, M. ischio-cavernosus		• Glandulae vestibulares majores (BARTHOLIN)

The space between the two fascia, which is almost completely filled by the M. transversus perinei profundus, is the **deep perineal space**. In men, in addition to the urethra, this contains COWPER's glands (Glandulae bulbourethrales) and is traversed by the deep branches of the N. pudenus and the A. and V. pudenda interna on its way to the root of the penis (➤ Table 8.12). The Nn. cavernosi penis penetrate the deep perineal space and enter into the cavernous bodies of the penis. The **superficial perineal space** attaches caudally to the Membrana perinei and contains the superficial perineal muscles (M. transversus perinei superficialis, M. ischio-cavernosus, M. bulbospongiosus) as well as the superficial vessels and nerves.

Perineal spaces in women
In women the **deep perineal space** is filled predominantly by connective tissue and by individual muscle fibres of the M. transversus perinei profundus (➤ Fig. 8.71, ➤ Table 8.13). Although the muscle is usually not highly developed, the **Membrana perinei** is present as a dense connective tissue layer and allows demarcation of the two perineal spaces. The deep perineal space contains the passageway of the vagina and urethra. As in men, it is pervaded by the N. pudendus and by the deep branches of the A. and V. pudenda interna (➤ Table 8.12). The Nn. cavernosi clitoridis reach the cavernous bodies of the clitoris.

Table 8.13 Perineal muscles

Innervation	Origin	Attachment	Function
M. transversus perinei profundus			
N. pudendus (plexus sacralis)	Ramus inferior ossis pubis	Centrum tendineum perinei	Secures the levator hiatus
M. sphincter urethrae externus (part of the M. transversus perinei profundus)			
N. pudendus (Plexus sacralis)	Annular muscle, fibres from the M. transversus perinei profundus	• Connective tissue around the urethra (Pars membranacea) • Vaginal wall (M. sphincter urethrovaginalis)	• Closure of the urethra • Closure of the urinary bladder during ejaculation
M. transversus perinei superficialis (inconstant muscle)			
N. pudendus (Plexus sacralis)	Ramus ossis ischii	Centrum tendineum perinei	Supports the M. transversus perinei profundus
M. ischiocavernosus			
N. pudendus (Plexus sacralis)	Ramus ossis ischii	Crus penis/clitoridis	Stabilisation of cavernous body, ejaculation
M. bulbospongiosus			
N. pudendus (Plexus sacralis)	• Centrum tendineum perinei • In men, additionally at the Raphe penis	Encompasses the Bulbus penis and the Bulbus vestibuli	Stabilisation of cavernous body, ejaculation

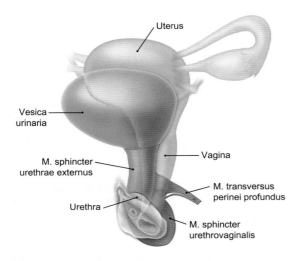

Uterus

Vesica urinaria

M. sphincter urethrae externus

Urethra

Vagina

M. transversus perinei profundus

M. sphincter urethrovaginalis

Fig. 8.72 Voluntary sphincters of the urinary bladder.

The **superficial perineal space** stretches between the Membrana perinei and the perineal fascia (Fascia perinei). In addition to the M. transversus perinei superficialis, it also contains the flanks of the cavernous bodies of the clitoris and the cavernous body of the vestibule of the vagina (Bulbus vestibuli) with its enveloping muscles (M. ischiocavernosus or M. bulbospongiosus) as well as the Glandulae vestibulares majores (BARTHOLIN's glands).

In both sexes, the M. transversus perinei profundus also forms the **M. sphincter urethrae externus**, which constitutes the voluntary sphincter of the urinary bladder (➤ Fig. 8.70, ➤ Fig. 8.71, ➤ Table 8.13). As the **M. urethrovaginalis** in women it also encompasses the vagina (➤ Fig. 8.72).

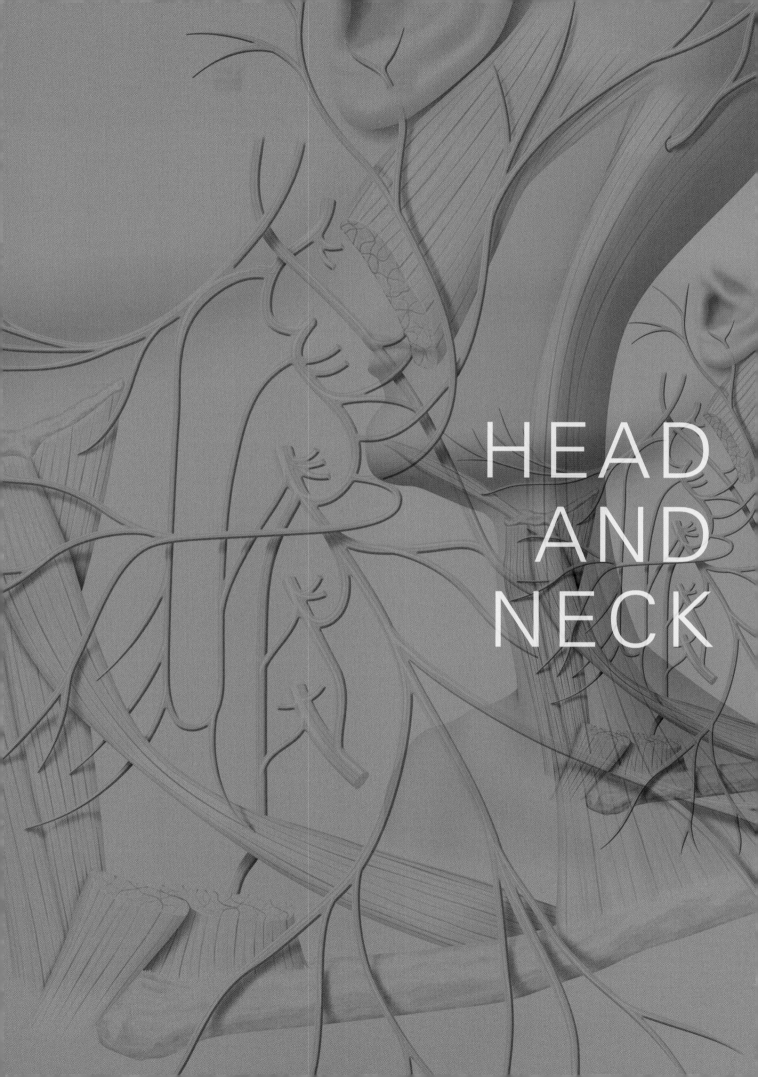

HEAD
AND
NECK

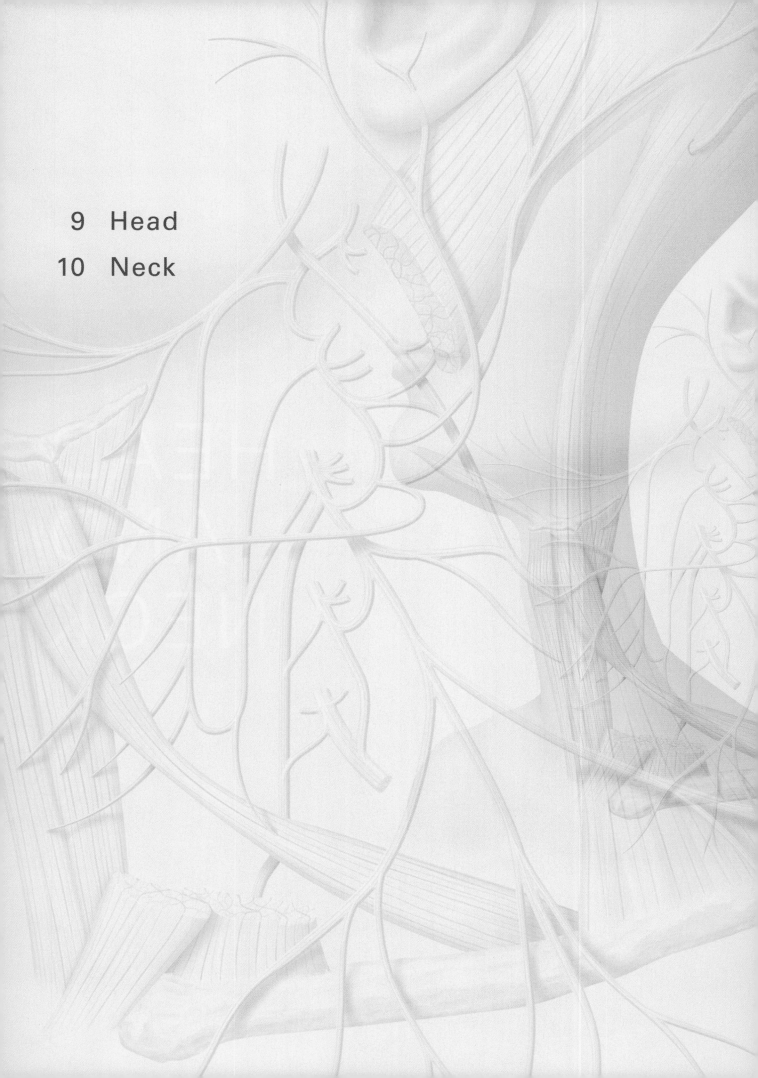

9 Head

Epidural haematoma

Accident

A 23-year-old male student is cycling to university without wearing a safety helmet. At an intersection, shortly before reaching the auditorium, he is hit by a car. He hits the front windscreen of the car with the side of his head. After a brief loss of consciousness of less than 20 seconds, he regains consciousness, reacts to speech and has no impairments except for pain in his leg and a haematoma on the left temple: he can stand up, does not want an ambulance and opts for a short recovery pause on a bench in front of the auditorium building; however, within the next half an hour he becomes extremely sleepy and is no longer responsive. Other students call an ambulance which brings him as fast as possible to the nearby emergency department of the university hospital.

Diagnosis

In the emergency room the student's respiration suddenly severely deteriorates, necessitating an emergency intubation. The doctors immediately arrange a head CT scan, on which the radiologist determines an intracranial lens-shaped (biconvex) area in the left half of the head. Based on the findings, the radiologist diagnoses an epidural haematoma, width approx. 3 cm, with midline shift.

Pathogenesis

On impact with the front windscreen of the car the patient has suffered a fracture in the area of the pterion, fracturing the inner hard bone layer of the calvaria (Lamina vitrea) creating sharp-edged fracture elements: the outer skull bone, on the other hand, is not fractured. Through the jagged bone fragments, the A. meningea media (between the dura mater and cranial bone) was injured, which resulted in arterial bleeding. Due to the pressure of the bleeding the dura mater has slowly become detached in a circumscribed area from the cranial bone, which in turn has led to an intracranial space-occupying lesion. The symptom-free interval, which caused the patient to waive an ambulance, is typical for this type of injury.

Treatment

The student is immediately brought into the operating room and the skull is opened (trepanation). Then the treating trauma surgeon (neurosurgeon) clears out the haematoma, seals off the source of bleeding and reinserts the removed bone fragment. The patient remains in the ICU after surgery for 2 days, followed by 1 week in the hospital for observation. After 2 weeks all cerebral deficits, which were caused by the lesion, have receded. He can continue studying, but has decided to wear a helmet when riding his bicycle from now on.

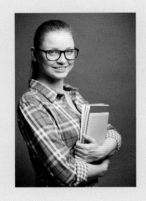

You're in your 3rd year at university and as a fellow student, you have witnessed the accident. In hindsight, you wonder if the bleeding could have been detected faster on the basis of the symptoms. You are under the impression that it is not so easy to tell the characteristics of a cerebral haemorrhage apart and therefore you draw an overview map of the topic.

Cerebral haemorrhages and how I recognise them	
Epidural haematoma	
Fracture of the skull bone → injury to vessels of the dura:	
Often A. meningea media	
Typical: (symptom-) **free interval**	
In CT: hyperdense, (Bi)convex expansion	
Subdural haematoma	
Acute:	Chronic: **after a mild trauma**
usually tear of Bridging veins	trauma, often can't remember,
Within 72 h after trauma	even weeks after
Symptoms very variable, rapid	promotion of anticoagulation
Vigilance reduction possible.	Headache, change in character
CT: hyperdense, crescent-shaped,	Memory impairment, etc.
Extra-cerebral expansion	CT: sickle-shaped, hypodense

characteristics:
epidural: arterial bleeding
subdural: venous bleeding

The **head (Caput)** encloses organs with very different functions. The bony basis is the skull, which surrounds the brain and the large remote sensory organs:

- Visual organ
- Hearing organ
- Vestibular organ
- Olfactory organ
- Gustatory sense

The respiratory and the digestive tracts begin in the head. Together with the nose paranasal sinuses, the mouth, throat and masticatory apparatus make a significant contribution to the shape of our face. Humans additionally use the oral cavity and its organs for articulation, speech and singing. The head is movable and sits on the cervical spine. The Protuberantia occipitalis externa (see below) on the back of the skull, the base of the ears and the mandible mark the boundary between the head and the neck.

9.1 Skull
Lars Bräuer

Skills

After working through this chapter, you should be able to:
- outline the development of the skull and its bones
- name sutures and fontanelles (closure times)
- outline the principal structure of the skull and of the facial bones, as well as their connections to each other
- know the structure of the neurocranium, viscerocranium, base of the skull, calvaria and Fossae cranii
- name the major points of penetration, foramina, fissures, impressions of the inner and outer surfaces of the skull base
---

9.1.1 Neurocranium and viscerocranium

The bony skull (Cranium) with the exception of the 3 auditory ossicles and the mandible is composed by of 22 single bones, which are connected to one another by sutures. The mandible (Mandibula) articulates with the remaining skull in the paired temporomandibular joint (Articulatio temporomandibularis) and can thus be moved against the skull. Embryologically and functionally, the skull is divided into two portions:

- Skull (neurocranium):
  - **Temporal bone (Os temporale),** paired
  - **Hammer (Malleus), anvil (Incus)** and **stirrup (Stapes)** = auditory ossicles
  - **Parietal bone (Os parietale),** paired
  - Parts of the **frontal bone (Os frontale),** unpaired
  - **Sphenoid bone (Os sphenoidale),** unpaired
  - **Ethmoid bone (Os ethmoidale),** unpaired
  - **Occipital bone (Os occipitale),** unpaired
- Facial skeleton (viscerocranium or splanchnocranium):
  - the orbital parts of the **frontal bone (Os frontale),** unpaired
  - **Zygomatic bone (Os zygomaticum),** paired
  - **Upper jaw (Maxilla),** paired
  - **Lacrimal bone (Os lacrimale),** paired
  - **Nasal bone (Os nasale),** paired
  - **Palantine bone (Os palatinum),** paired
  - **Vomer,** unpaired
  - **Inferior nasal concha (Concha nasalis inferior),** paired
  - **Lower jaw (Mandibula),** unpaired

On the **neurocranium** the skull roof **(Calvaria)** can be morphologically differentiated from the skull base **(Basis cranii).** The skull is used to hold and protect the brain and also includes parts of the outer ear, the middle ear and the inner ear (➤ Chap. 9.1.6).

The **viscerocranium** forms the basis for the face (➤ Chap. 9.1.5). Strictly speaking the incisive bone of the Maxilla (Os incisivum) should be listed with the abovementioned bones; however, it merges *in utero* with the Maxilla.

9.1.2 Skull development – Embryology

Desmocranium and chondrocranium

When the skull is being divided functionally into neurocranium and viscerocranium, a distinction can be made embryologically according to the ossification mode of the individual bones between a **desmocranium** and a **chondrocranium:**

- In the case of desmal ossification bones emerge directly from an embryonal connective tisue precursor.
- In contrast, in chondral ossification bones initially develop via the intermediate stage of a cartilage scaffold, which is later converted to bone and mineralised by differentiation processes.

The construction material is, however, the same for both forms of ossification, namely the **cranial mesenchyme,** which comes from the the paraxial cranial mesoderm, the prechordal mesoderm, occipital somites and the neural crest. The auditory ossicles hammer (Malleus) and anvil (Incus) are created as a continuation of **MECKEL's cartilage** (1st pharyngeal arch) and the stirrup (Stapes) from **REICHERT's cartilage** (2nd pharyngeal arch) – this is a purely chondral ossification mode. The Concha nasalis inferior and the Os ethmoidale are also created purely chondrally (➤ Table 9.1). The Maxilla, Os zygomaticum, Os palatinum, Os nasale, Vomer, Os lacrimale, Os frontale and Os parietale are created from desmal ossification (➤ Table 9.1). Mixtures of both ossification modi can be found in the Os sphenoidale, Os temporale and Os occipitale (➤ Table 9.2).

Table 9.1 Ossification forms of the skull bones

Bones	Ossification mode
Maxilla	Desmal
Mandibula	Desmal (except Proc. condylaris)
Os zygomaticum	Desmal
Os palatinum	Desmal
Os nasale	Desmal
Vomer	Desmal
Os lacrimale	Desmal
Os frontale	Desmal
Os parietale	Desmal
Os ethmoidale	Chondral
Concha nasalis inferior	Chondral
Os temporale	Chondral (except Pars squamosa and Proc. styloideus)
Os sphenoidale	Chondral (except Lamina medialis)
Os occipitale	Chondral (except Pars squamosa)
Malleus (hammer)	Chondral from MECKEL's cartilage
Incus (anvil)	Chondral from MECKEL's cartilage
Stapes (stirrup)	Chondral from REICHERT's cartilage

Table 9.2 Mixtures of ossification modi

Bones	Parts
Os sphenoidale	Lamina medialis: desmal, remaining parts: chondral
Os temporale	Partes petrosa and tympanica: chondral, Pars squamosa: desmal, Proc. styloideus: of 2nd pharyngeal arch
Os occipitale	Pars squamosa: desmal, Partes laterales and Pars basilaris: chondral

The Mandibula is initially created as a cartilaginous continuation of the 1st pharangeal arch (MECKEL's cartilage), this then recedes and the Mandibula is created from desmal ossification up to the Proc. condylaris (chondral) (➤ Table 9.1).

> **NOTE**
> The main part of the skull base develops from chondral ossification, the main part of the calvaria and facial skeleton by desmal ossification.

Fontanelles

At the time of birth and also a certain amount of time afterwards, the roof bones of the calvaria are separated from each other within the sutures by connective tissue – these ossify over the course of life through desmal ossification (➤ Chap. 9.1.3). If more than 2

Table 9.3 Fontanelles.

Fontanelle	Number	Closure	Location
Fonticulus anterior (front, large fontanelle)	Unpaired	24th–36th month	Between the two frontal and parietal bones, at the interface between Sutura coronalis and sagittalis (➤ Fig. 9.1a)
Fonticulus posterior (posterior, small fontanelle)	Unpaired	2nd–3rd month	Between the two parietal bones and the occipital bone, at the interfaces of the Suturae sagittalis and lambdoidea (➤ Fig. 9.1b)
Fonticulus sphenoidalis (sphenoidal fontanelle)	Paired	5th–7th month	Laterally between the frontal and parietal bones, as well as the large sphenoidal bone wings (➤ Fig. 9.1b)
Fonticulus mastoideus (posterolateral fontanelle)	Paired	17th–20th month	Laterally between parietal, temporal and occipital bones and the Proc. mastoideus (➤ Fig. 9.1b)

bone edges come together, the sutures are expanded to fontanelles (Fonticuli) and filled with connective tissue (➤ Table 9.3, ➤ Fig. 9.1). A distinction is made between 2 unpaired main fontanelles and 2 paired, smaller fontanelles that allow a slight deformation of the skull during parturition.

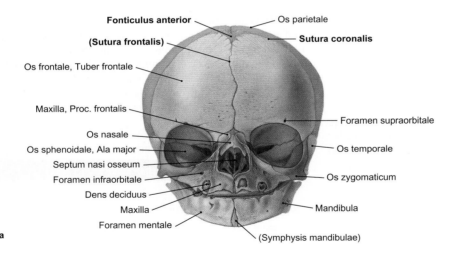

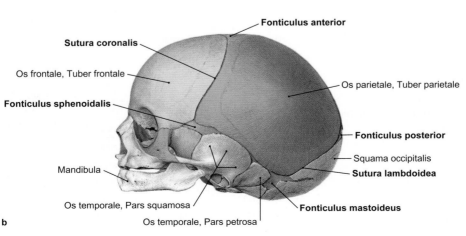

Fig. 9.1 Skull of a neonate with fontanelles. The viscerocranium is still much smaller than the neurocranium; during the development to an adult skull these proportions will balance out or be reversed due to the rapid growth of the viscerocranium. **a** Frontal view. **b** Lateral view.

9.1.3 Calvaria

The roof of the skull (Dome, calvaria) includes:
- both **Ossa parietalia**
- **Squama ossis frontalis**
- **Os occipitale**
- **Pars squamosa** of the **Os temporale**

Bone layers

The bones of the skull have a typical stratification from outside to inside:
- **Lamina externa** (corresponds to the outwardly directed compact bone)
- **Diploë** (corresponds to the spongiosa)
- **Lamina interna** (or Lamina vitrea, corresponds to the inward facing compact bone)

On the outside the periosteum forms the **pericranium;** the periosteal sheet (**Stratum periostale**) lies on the inside of the skull directly on the **dura mater** (hard meninx). The latter is, with the exception of the areas of venous sinus firmly fused with the meningeal sheet (**Stratum meningeale**) of the dura (SHARPEY's fibres). This also means that under physiological conditions there is no epidural space (space between Lamina interna and dura mater). In contrast the epidural space lies in the spinal canal between the periosteum of the vertebral body and the dura mater, which is filled with adipose tissue and the vertebral venous plexus. Therefore, a distinction is made between the Dura mater encephali and Dura mater spinalis.

bone plates. Often only the Lamina interna splinters. It can lead to injury of the meninges and the brain. If the trauma affects a wider area of the skull, there are generally **burst fractures** (e.g. after falling on the head).

Sutures

The bones of the skull are fused together with sutures (cranial seams, loose connective tissue seams, are among the syndesmoses, false joints), which are particularly easy to determine on the bony (macerated) skull in the area of the calvaria (➤ Fig. 9.2, also ➤ Fig. 9.9). The **sagittal suture** runs in the median line in which the two parts of the parietal bone are connected (Sutura sagittalis), which is connected frontal vertically with the **coronal suture** (Sutura coronalis) and occipitally with the **lambda suture** (Sutura lambdoidea). The point of contact between the coronal suture and the sagittal suture is referred to as the bregma and the contact point between the sagittal suture and the lambdoid suture as the lambda (➤ Fig. 9.2). An anatomical variant is the **interparietal bone** (inca bone, Os incae, **Os interparietale**). This is an accessory bone (sutural bone) in the area of the lambdoid suture, which has no clinical relevance but in the radiological findings should be known as a variant. In a number of vertebrates, the Os interparietale occurs regularly. The **squamous suture** (Sutura squamosa) connects the two Ossa temporalia with the Ossa parietalia in the form of an arch. The sutures of the skull ossify at different times well after the birth (➤ Table 9.4).

Sulci, foveolae

If one looks at the inner relief of the skull-cap, impressions of meningeal arteries are apparent, **Sulci arteriosi,** (in addition to the sutures), which develop from the arterial pulse of the Aa. meningeae. Also the venous Sinus sagittalis superior leaves a wide depression (Sulcus sinus sagittalis superioris) medially on the inside of the

Table 9.4 Sutures.

Suture	Ossification	Localisation
Sutura lambdoidea (lambdoid suture)	40th–50th year of life	Between Ossa parietalia and Squama occipitalis
Sutura frontalis (frontal suture)	1st–2nd year of life	Between the Ossa frontalia
Sutura sagittalis (sagittal suture)	20th–30th year of life	Between Ossa parietalia
Sutura coronalis (coronal suture)	30th–40th year of life	Between the Os frontale and Os parietale

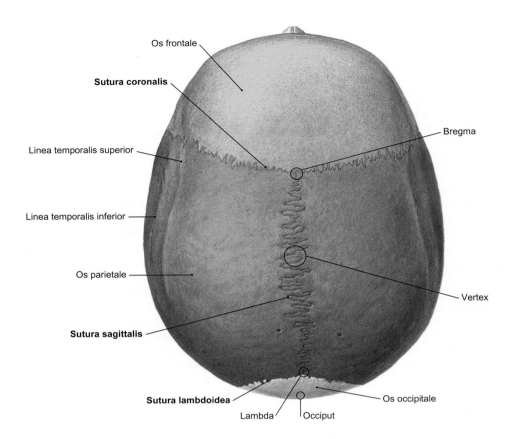

Fig. 9.2 Cranial bones with sutures. Superior view. The Sutura sagittalis (sagittal suture) connects the Ossa parietalia (vertex), the Sutura coronalis (coronal suture) connects the Os frontale with the two Ossa parietalia and the Sutura lambdoidea (lambdoid suture) connects the Ossa parietalia with the Os occipitale.

skull bone. At the very front it is raised into a crest (Crista frontalis), which functions as an attachment point of the **Falx cerebri** (a dural duplicature, which separates both hemispheres of the brain). Lateral of the Sulcus sinus sagittalis superioris small depressions are distributed irregularly but over the entire path of the Sulcus (**Foveolae granulares**). In these dimples there are the Granulationes arachnoideae (PACCHIONI granulations) in living persons, through which the cerebral fluid (Liquor cerebrospinalis) is reabsorbed. At some points openings can be seen, which penetrate all three layers of the calvaria and can also be found on the surface anatomy of the skull. These are points of penetration for emissary veins (emissary veins, **Vv. emissariae**), venous shortcuts between the superficial skull veins, the diploë veins and the blood-conducting sinus of the brain.

9.1.4 Base of the skull

At the base of the skull (Basis cranii) an inner base of the skull (**Basis cranii interna**) can be distinguished from a outer base of the skull (**Basis cranii externa**). The inner and outer bases of the skull are interspersed by a large number of passageways, fissures and apertures, through which the vascular, lymphatic and nervous systems pass. A large part of the bone of the skull base is pneumatised (filled with air), reducing the weight of the skull.

Inner surface of skull base

The inner surface of the skull base (Basis cranii interna, ➤ Fig. 9.3) is divided into 3 separate areas that together form the base of the skull and serve as a contact surface for the brain:
- The anterior cranial fossa (Fossa cranii anterior)
- The middle cranial fossa (Fossa cranii media)
- The posterior cranial fossa (Fossa cranii posterior)

Fossa cranii anterior

The anterior cranial fossa (Fossa cranii anterior) is formed from the following bones:
- **Os frontale** (Partes orbitales), forms the front and side parts
- **Os ethmoidale** (Lamina cribrosa), forms the base of the anterior cranial fossa
- **Os sphenoidale** (Rostrum, Jugum and Alae minores), forms the border to the middle base of the skull

The frontal lobe of the brain lie on the surface of the anterior cranial fossa, which leaves corresponding impressiones gyrorum in the thin bony lamellae. In the anterior portion medially there is the Lamina cribrosa of the Os ethmoidale, through the foramina of which the Fila olfactoria of the N. olfactorius [I] penetrate to connect with the Bulbus of the cranial nerve of the same name (➤ Fig. 9.4, ➤ Table 9.5). Between the right and left Lamina cribrosa a crest-shaped bone protrusion (Crista galli) is elevated, which serves as an attachment point for the Falx cerebri (a loose connective tissue dural duplicature, which separates both cerebral hemispheres). At the rostral end of the Crista galli, directly on the transition to the Crista frontalis, the Foramen caecum is located, which in children hosts an emissary vein for connection with the nasal cavity (in adults this Foramen is closed).

> NOTE
> The anterior cranial fossa forms the roof of the nasal cavity (Cavitas nasi) and the eye orbit (Orbita).

Fossa cranii media

The middle cranial fossa (Fossa cranii media) is formed by the following bones:
- **Os sphenoidale** (Alae majores), forms the front part of the floor
- **Os temporale** (Pars squamosa), together with the Alae majores forms the floor in the middle part

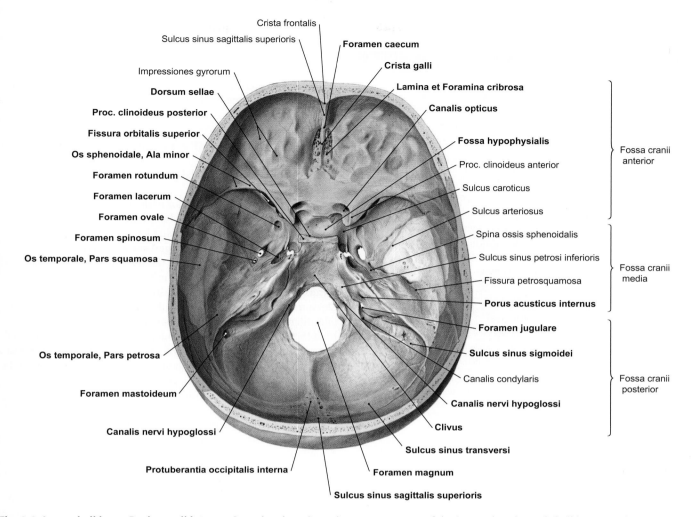

Fig. 9.3 Inner skull base, Basis cranii interna. Superior view. Conspicuous structures of the internal surface of skull base are the Foramen magnum (e.g. entry point of the extended spinal cord) within the Os occipitale, the Fossa hypophysialis (site of the pituitary within a dura duplicature) as well as the ethmoid bone (Lamina cribrosa of the Os ethmoidale) through which the nerve fibres of the N. olfactorius [I] extend. In particular in the area of the anterior cranial fossa one can also determine impressions of the gyri of the frontal lobe (Impressiones gyrorum lobus frontalis).

- **Os temporale** (Facies anterior of the Pars petrosa), forms the border to the posterior cranial fossa

The Corpus ossis sphenoidalis with the **Sella turcica** divides the Fossa cranii media in two halves. In this area there are the Fossa hypophysialis, which includes the Hypophysis cerebri (pituitary gland), the Dorsum sellae with the Procc. clinoidei posteriores, and in front of them is the Tuberculum sellae of the Sulcus prechias-maticus (Chiasma opticum) and the Procc. clinoidei anteriores. It is also the site of several openings (➤ Fig. 9.3):

- **Canalis opticus** (N. opticus and A. ophthalmica)
- **Fissura orbitalis superior** (Nn. oculomotorius [III], trochlearis [IV], ophthalmicus [V/1], lacrimalis, frontalis, nasociliaris and abducens [VI] as well as V. ophthalmica)
- **Foramen rotundum** (N. maxillaris [V/2])
- **Foramen ovale** (N. mandibularis [V/3])
- **Foramen spinosum** (R. meningeus of the N. mandibularis [V/3] and A. meningea media)

Medial of the Foramen ovale lies the Foramen lacerum, which is closed *in vivo* by connective tissue, but is traversed by various structures (➤ Fig. 9.4):

- **N. petrosus major**
- **A. canalis pterygoidei**
- **R. meningeus** (from the A. pharyngea ascendens)

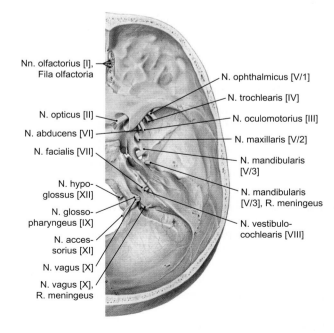

Fig. 9.4 Points of penetration of the inner skull base. Superior view.

Table 9.5 Points of penetration of the inner skull base and their contents.

Point of penetration	Content
Foramina cribrosa	• Nn. olfactorii [I] • A. ethmoidalis anterior (A. ophthalmica)
Canalis opticus	• N. opticus [II] • A. ophthalmica (A. carotis interna) • Meninges; Vaginae nervi optici

Fissura orbitalis superior	Medial area:
	• N. nasociliaris (N. ophthalmicus [V/1])
	• N. oculomotorius [III]
	• N. abducens [VI]
	Lateral area:
	• N. trochlearis [IV]
	• Joint stem of:
	  – N. frontalis (N. ophthalmicus [V/1])
	  – N. lacrimalis (N. ophthalmicus [V/1])
	• R. orbitalis (A. meningea media)
	• V. ophthalmica superior

Foramen rotundum	• N. maxillaris [V/2]
Foramen ovale	• N. mandibularis [V/3] • Plexus venosus foraminis ovalis
Foramen spinosum	• R. meningeus (N. mandibularis [V/3]) • A. meningea media (A. maxillaris)
Fissura sphenopetrosa, Foramen lacerum	• N. petrosus minor (N. glossopharyngeus [IX]) • N. petrosus major (N. facialis [VII]) • N. petrosus profundus (Plexus caroticus internus)
Apertura interna canalis carotici and Canalis caroticus	• A. carotis interna, Pars petrosa • Plexus venosus caroticus internus • Plexus caroticus internus (Truncus sympathicus, Ganglion cervicale superius)
Porus and Meatus acusticus internus	• N. facialis [VII] • N. vestibulocochlearis [VIII] • A. labyrinthi (A. basilaris) • Vv. labyrinthi
Foramen jugulare	Frontal area: • Sinus petrosus inferior • N. glossopharyngeus [IX] Posterior area: • A. meningea posterior (A. pharyngea ascendens) • Sinus sigmoideus (Bulbus superior venae jugularis) • N. vagus [X] • N. accessorius [XI] • R. meningeus (N. vagus [X])
Canalis nervi hypoglossi	• N. hypoglossus [XII] • Plexus venosus canalis nervi hypoglossi
Canalis condylaris	• V. emissaria condylaris
Foramen magnum	• Meninges • Plexus venosus vertebralis internus (Sinus marginalis) • Aa. vertebrales (Aa. subclaviae) • A. spinalis anterior (Aa. vertebrales) • Medulla oblongata/Medulla spinalis • Radices spinales (N. accessorius [XI])

Above the Foramen lacerum at the Sella turcica is the **Sulcus caroticus,** in which the A. carotis interna courses. On the medial Facies anterior of the Pars petrosa of the Os temporale there are points of penetration of the N. petrosus major (Hiatus canalis nervi petrosi majoris) as well as the N. petrosus minor (Hiatus canalis nervi petrosi minoris). With the N. petrosus minor the A. tympanica superior (from A. meningea media) penetrates the Hiatus canalis nervi petrosi minoris. The N. petrosus major leaves the middle cranial fossa via the Foramen lacerum; the N. petrosus minor pen-

etrates variably through the Fissura sphenopetrosa, Foramen lacerum or occasionally the Foramen ovale.

NOTE
The middle cranial fossa forms the bony basis for the two temporal lobes of the brain and for the pituitary gland.

Fossa cranii posterior
The posterior cranial fossa (Fossa cranii posterior) is formed by the following bones:
• **Os sphenoidale** (sphenoidal part of the clivus), forms the front part
• **Os temporale** (Facies posterior of the Pars petrosa), forms the anterolateral border to the middle cranial fossa
• **Os occipitale** (Partes basilaris and lateralis), forms the floor

The **Foramen magnum** as the largest site of penetration of the skull represents the connection to the vertebral canal (Canalis vertebralis). At its edge in close proximity to the **Condyli occipitales** is the Canalis nervi hypoglossi. Rostrally the **clivus** rises up to the Dorsum sellae of the Os sphenoidale. Occipitally the Crista occipitalis interna extends to the Protuberantia occipitalis interna. Behind the Foramen magnum the Sulcus sinus sigmoidei and the Sulcus sinus transversi limit the Fossa cerebellaris laterally. The Fossa cranii posterior includes other points of penetration apart from the Foramen magnum (➤ Fig. 9.3, ➤ Fig. 9.4):
• **Foramen magnum** – Medulla oblongata, Radix spinalis of the N. accessorius [XI], Aa. vertebrales, A. spinalis anterior, Aa. spinales posteriores, meninges and venous connections between Plexus basilaris and vertebralis internus
• **Canalis nervi hypoglossi** – N. hypoglossus [XII]
• **Foramen jugulare** – Nn. glossopharyngeus [IX], vagus [X], accessorius [XI], A. meningea posterior, V. jugularis interna
• **Porus acusticus internus** – Nn. facialis, intermedius, vestibulocochlearis, A. and V. labyrinthi

NOTE
The bony portions of the posterior cranial fossa form the floor for the cerebellum (Cerebellum), the bridge (Pons) and the extended medulla (Medulla oblongata).

Outer skull base
Similar to the inner skull base the outer skull base (Basis cranii externa, ➤ Fig. 9.5) is also subdivided into an anterior, middle and rear section.

Frontal section
The point of contact between Os incisivum and Maxilla is the Fossa incisiva with the rostrally lying Foramen incisivum and the Canalis incisivus. The N. nasopalatinus (N. maxillaris[V/2]) (➤ Fig. 9.6, ➤ Table 9.6) penetrates through this. At the point of contact between the Maxilla and the Os palatinum is the Foramen palatinum majus, as well as the Foramina palatina minora, through which the N. palatinus major and the A. palatina major or the Nn. palatini minores and Aa. palatini minores pass. The hard palate (Palatum durum) ends dorsal to the Choanae, which mark the entry into the nasal cavity.

NOTE
The front section of the outer skull base is actually part of the viscerocranium and forms the floor of the nasal cavity, as well as the hard palate (Proc. palatinus of the Maxilla, Os incisivum and Lamina horizontalis of the Os palatinum) and therefore the roof of the oral cavity.

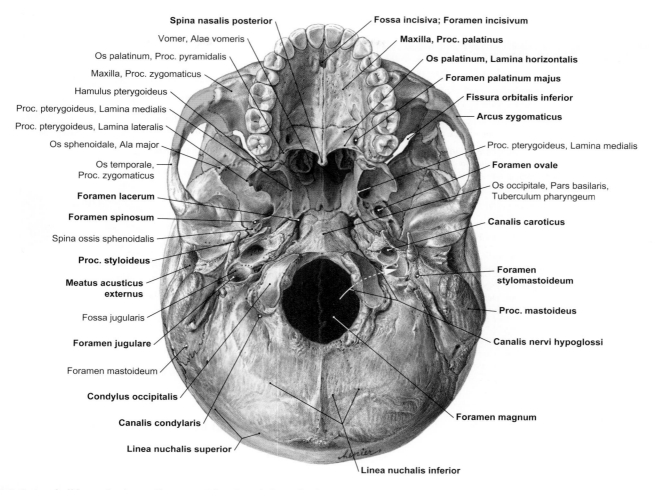

Fig. 9.5 Outer skull base, Basis cranii externa. View from below. The front part includes the palate with the maxillary teeth, the middle part extends from the posterior border of the hard palate to the anterior margin of the Foramen magnum and the rear part accordingly from the anterior margin of the Foramen magnum to the Linea nuchalis superior. The outer skull base includes, in particular, the points of penetration of the cranial nerves and vessels, as well as numerous attachment points for muscles and ligaments (e.g. Proc. styloideus or Proc. mastoideus). Lateral on both sides of the Foramen magnum are the joint surfaces (Condyli occipitales) for the two upper cranial joints (Articulationes atlantooccipitales).

Middle section

The middle section is mainly formed from the Os sphenoidale and the lower surface of the Os temporale. Prominent structures are the Proc. pterygoideus belonging to the Os sphenoidale and the Fossa pterygoidea. Lateral above the Proc. pterygoideus lies the Fossa pterygopalatina (pterygopalatine fossa) which hosts one of the parasympathetic cranial ganglia (Ganglion pterygopalatinum). The middle section also provides points of penetration for multiple structures. In the following, only structures and points of penetration are named which are different from the Basis cranii interna (➤ Fig. 9.5, ➤ Fig. 9.6):

- **Fissura orbitalis inferior** – Nn. infraorbitalis and zygomaticus [V/2], A. infraorbitalis, V. ophthalmica inferior
- **Canalis pterygoideus** – N. canalis pterygoidei
- **Fissura sphenopetrosa** – Chorda tympani, A. tympanica major (some authors are of the opinion that the Chorda tympani and the A. tympanica major run through the Fissura petrotympanica [GLASER's fissure])
- **Canaliculus mastoideus** – R. auricularis of the N. vagus [X]
- **Canaliculus tympanicus** – N. tympanicus [from IX]
- **Foramen stylomastoideum** – N. facialis [VII], A. stylomastoidea
- **Canalis musculotubarius** – M. tensor tympani, Tuba auditiva

Lateral and belonging to the surface of the Os temporale are the basis of the Pars petrosa, the Proc. mastoideus (mastoid process) as well as the Proc. styloideus (styloid process); in addition, at the side of it lie the Pars squamosa and the Pars tympanica.

Medial of the Proc. styloideus are the Foramen jugulare and the Foramen stylomastoideum. Rostral and thus in front of the Proc. mastoideus, the Porus acusticus externus opens (opening of the bony part of the external acoustic meatus) and in front of it the Fossa mandibularis, which takes up the joint head of the mandible and is limited at the front by the Tuberculum articulare.

Rear section

The main part of the posterior section is formed by the Os occipitale with the Pars basilaris and both Partes laterales; it extends to the rear via the Squama occipitalis through to the Protuberantia occipitalis externa (Inion). The Os occipitale is penetrated by the Foramen magnum, which is accompanied on both sides by the Condyli occipitales. The Canalis condylaris containing the **V. emissaria condylaris** runs through this structure. Behind the Proc. mastoideus lies the Foramen mastoideum, through which an emissary vein passes (V. emissaria mastoidea).

Table 9.6 Points of penetration of the outer skull base and their contents.

Point of penetration	Content
Foramen incisivum	• N. nasopalatinus (N. maxillaris [V/2])
Foramen palatinum majus	• N. palatinus major (N. maxillaris [V/2]) • A. palatina major (A. palatina descendens)
Foramina palatina minora	• Nn. palatini minores (N. maxillaris [V/2]) • Aa. palatinae minores (A. palatina descendens)
Fissura orbitalis inferior	• A. infraorbitalis (A. maxillaris) • V. ophthalmica inferior • N. infraorbitalis (N. maxillaris [V/2]) • N. zygomaticus (N. maxillaris [V/2])
Foramen rotundum	• N. maxillaris [V/2]
Foramen ovale	• N. mandibularis [V/3] • Plexus venosus foraminis ovalis
Foramen spinosum	• R. meningeus (N. mandibularis [V/3]) • A. meningea media (A. maxillaris)
Fissura sphenopetrosa, Foramen lacerum	• N. petrosus minor (N. glossopharyngeus [IX]) • N. petrosus major (N. facialis [VII]) • N. petrosus profundus (Plexus caroticus internus)
Apertura externa canalis carotici and Canalis caroticus	• A. carotis interna, Pars petrosa • Plexus venosus caroticus internus • Plexus caroticus internus (Truncus sympathicus, Ganglion cervicale superius)
Foramen stylomastoideum	• N. facialis [VII]
Foramen jugulare	Anterior area: • Sinus petrosus inferior • N. glossopharyngeus [IX] Posterior area: • A. meningea posterior (A. pharyngea ascendens) • Sinus sigmoideus (Bulbus superior venae jugularis) • N. vagus [X] • R. meningeus (N. vagus [X]) • N. accessorius [XI]
Canaliculus mastoideus	• R. auricularis nervi vagi (N. vagus [X])
Canalis nervi hypoglossi	• N. hypoglossus [XII] • Plexus venosus canalis nervi hypoglossi
Canalis condylaris	• V. emissaria condylaris
Foramen magnum	• Meninges • Plexus venosus vertebralis internus (Sinus marginalis) • Aa. vertebrales (Aa. subclaviae) • A. spinalis anterior (Aa. vertebrales) • Medulla oblongata/Medulla spinalis • Radices spinales (N. accessorius [XI])

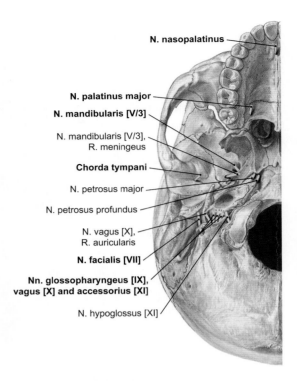

Fig. 9.6 Points of penetration on the outer skull base. View from below.

9.1.5 Individual bones of the viscerocranium

Mandibula

The unpaired **Mandibula (mandible),** the largest bone of the viscerocranium consists of 1 Corpus and 2 Rami, which merge together at the Angulus mandibulae. With the exception of the auditory ossicles the Mandibula is the only movable bone of the skull. Both Rami mandibulae have a Proc. coronoideus and at its free end a Proc. condylaris, which articulates via its Caput mandibulae with the Fossa mandibularis of the Os temporale and as such forms the mandibular joint (**Articulatio temporomandibularis,** see below). The Corpus consists of a base and a Pars alveolaris, which also bears the teeth of the lower jaw (➤ Fig. 9.7). The Pars alveolaris and basis are separated from each other by the Linea obliqua, which descends rostrally from the Proc. coronoideus. The indentation between the Proc. condylaris and Proc. coronoideus is referred to as the Incisura mandibulae. The most rostrally lying point of the Mandibula is the **Protuberantia mentalis,** which joins laterally on both sides of the Tubercula mentalia (mental tubercle) and gives the chin its characteristic shape. Between the Pars alveolaris and the Tubercula mentalia are the paired **Foramina mentalia,** through each of which the N. mentalis [V/3] runs and sensitively innervates large areas of the lower jaw.

Clinical remarks

As a result of violent force to the skull (especially sudden, blunt force violence, such as in a traffic accident) the bones of the skull base can fracture. This can affect the front, middle or posterior cranial fossa. Weakest points are the many openings in the middle area of the skull base. The fracture lines run through these when there is a **skull base fracture.** Often the penetrating structures are injured, resulting in bleeding and/or leakage of cerebrospinal fluid (liquorrhoea) from the nose or the external ear canal and nerve failures may occur.

Clinical remarks

If, in the case of **tooth loss** of permanent teeth no replacement is made, the Pars alveolaris mandibulae recedes in the area of the missing teeth. If left untreated, this progresses so far that the Foramen mentale comes to rest directly on the upper edge of the lower jaw. Pain, neuralgia and sensory disturbances in the supply area of the N. mentalis can be the result and those affected are very severely restricted and food intake becomes more difficult. Adaption of a dental prosthesis is very difficult in these cases and often only succeeds after reconstructing the bone structure.

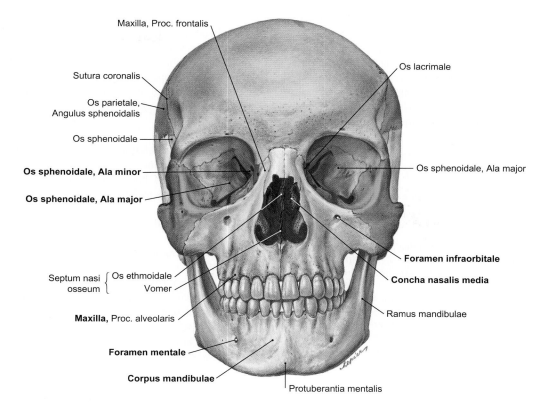

Maxilla, Proc. frontalis

Sutura coronalis

Os parietale,
Angulus sphenoidalis

Os sphenoidale

Os sphenoidale, Ala minor

Os sphenoidale, Ala major

Septum nasi { Os ethmoidale
osseum { Vomer

Maxilla, Proc. alveolaris

Foramen mentale

Corpus mandibulae

Os lacrimale

Os sphenoidale, Ala major

Foramen infraorbitale

Concha nasalis media

Ramus mandibulae

Protuberantia mentalis

Fig. 9.7 Cranial bones, Ossa cranii. Rostral view. The front part of the Os frontale, Os nasale, Os zygomaticum, Maxilla and Mandibula have the largest share in the formation of the facial structure. Maxilla, Os frontale, Os zygomaticum, Os sphenoidale, Os lacrimale and a small part of the Os palatinum form the Orbita. The Foramen supraorbitale (Os frontale), Foramen infraorbitale (Maxilla) and Foramen mentale (Mandibula) represent the penetration portals for the sensory parts of the N. trigeminus [V] and are used in the physical examination of a patient as trigeminal pressure points. The lower rim of the Maxilla is formed by the Proc. alveolaris, in which the teeth of the Maxilla are located. The Mandibula consists of a Corpus and both Rami mandibulae, both of which converge at the Angulus mandibulae. The Mandibula also has a Pars alveolaris, in which the teeth are anchored. Below this is the Basis mandibulae, which protrudes in the midline to the Protuberantia mentalis.

The paired Foramen mandibulae, which lead to the **Canalis mandibulae** are located at the inside of the Ramus mandibulae. The N. alveolaris inferior passes through the bony canal [from V/3], which emits sensory branches for innervation of the lower jaw. The **Lingula mandibulae**, is located in front of the Foramen manibulae which serves the Lig. sphenomandibulare as an attachment and presents a dental guiding structure for block anaesthesia. The **Sulcus mylohyoideus**, which runs rostally, emerges at the Foramen mandibulae. Further rostrally, the Linea mylohyoidea runs in tiers, which serves the M. mylohyoideus as attachment and originates from the level of the floor of the mouth. In 10–15% of all Mandibulae a **Foramen retromolare** can be found in the Fossa retromolaris immediately behind the last molar (Dens serotinus, wisdom tooth) which is connected via its own canal (Canalis retromolaris) with the Canalis mandibulae. Variable branches of the N. alveolaris inferior and the A. alveolaris inferior run through the foramen, which occurs mainly unilaterally. The knowledge of this variant is significant in dental surgery and conductive anaesthesia in this region.

NOTE

The Articulatio temporomandibularis is also known as the **secondary temperomandibular joint.** From an evolutionary perspective, the joint between the 1st and 2nd auditory ossicles (hammer and anvil) are referred to as **primary mandibular joint**. This emerges from the 1st pharyngeal arch.

Clinical remarks

The second most common fracture of the viscerocranium is the **mandibular fracture.** Due to the exposed location and U-shape, the lower jaw is often affected by fractures; particularly in the area of the Mentum (incisors) and of the Corpus (3rd molar). Fracture-related injuries of blood vessels (often A. alveolaris inferior) lead to small surface bleeding in the area of the floor of the mouth (ecchymoses) that are characteristic for a fracture. The Os nasale is most commonly affected by fractures.

Maxilla

The paired **Maxilla (upper jaw bone)** is connected to the upper jaw (➤ Fig. 9.8) via the Sutura palatina mediana, which is connected to every other bone of the viscerocranium (exception: Mandibula). The upper jaw bone is shaped like a pyramid and forms part of the orbital floor and includes as Os pneumaticum the **Sinus maxillaris (maxillary sinus).** A total of 4 surfaces (Facies orbitalis, anterior, nasalis and infratemporalis) and 4 processes (Procc. frontalis, zygomaticus, palatinus and alveolaris) can be differentiated. The Sulcus infraorbitalis runs within the Facies orbitalis, it converges to the Canalis infraorbitalis and, ultimately, to the Foramen infraorbitale, which has its outlet aperture (for N. and A. infraorbitalis) immediately below the bony lower orbital rim. The Facies nasalis forms the shape of the lateral nasal wall and is penetrated by the Hiatus maxillaris. The Proc. alveolaris bears the teeth of the Maxilla, comparable to the Mandibula. Above the Proc. alveolaris is is the Crista zygomaticoalveolaris, which represents a limit to the Proc. zygomaticus. The front two thirds of the hard palate are formed from the Proc. palatinus of the Maxilla. The Proc. frontalis of the Maxilla is connected to the Os frontale via the Sutura fronto-maxillaris, the Sutura zygomaticomaxillaris represents the corresponding connection to the Os zygomaticum. The **Os incisivum** is a self-contained bone within the Maxilla, which is fused with it in the area of the incisors (already in utero) and forms the Foramen incisivum and the Canalis incisivus.

Os palatinum

The paired L-shaped **Os palatinum (palatine bone)** forms the posterior third of the hard palatine through its Lamina horizontalis and is connected via the Sutura palatina transversa with the Proc. palatinus maxillae (Maxilla) (➤ Fig. 9.8). The palatine bone also consists of a Lamina perpendicularis with a Proc. sphenoidalis and a Proc. orbitalis through which the Os palatinum is connected with the Os sphenoidale. It is interrupted in this area by the Incisura sphenopalatine, which is simultaneously involved in the formation of the Foramen sphenopalatinum (point of penetration of N. naso-palatinus, A. sphenopalatina). On its cranial side the Lamina horizontalis forms the floor of the nasal cavity via the Facies nasalis and with the Facies palatina forms the bony roof of the oral cavity.

Os zygomaticum

The paired **Os zygomaticum (zygomatic bone)** consists of 3 processes and 3 surfaces and is largely responsible for the contour of the cheek (➤ Fig. 9.9). It is connected via
- the Proc. maxillaris with the Maxilla (Sutura zygomaticomaxillaris),
- via the Proc. frontalis with the Os frontale (Sutura zygomaticofrontalis) and
- via the Proc. temporalis with the Os temporale (Sutura zygomaticotemporalis)

Its facies orbitalis forms part of the orbital floor, the Facies temporalis is penetrated by the Foramen zygomaticotemporale (R. zygomaticotemporalis) and the Facies lateralis by the Foramen zygomaticofaciale (R. zygomaticofacialis). The Proc. temporalis, together with the Proc. zygomaticus of the Os temporale forms the Arcus zygomaticus (zygomatic arch).

> **N O T E**
> The Os zygomaticum, Os palatinum, Maxilla and Mandibula together with the Os hyoideum, which does not belong to the skull, form the jaw skeleton .

Os lacrimale

The paired **Os lacrimale (lacrimal bone)** is the smallest single bone of the viscerocranium and is involved to a minor degree in

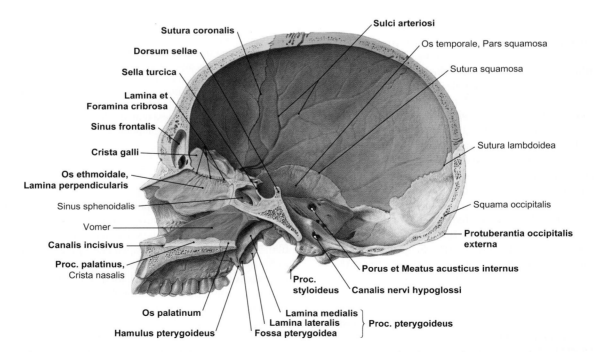

Fig. 9.8 Skull bones (right), Ossa cranii. Medial view. In this mediosagittal section through the skull the bony parts of the nasal skeleton (Lamina perpendicularis of the Os ethmoidale, vomer and Os nasale) can be recognised as well as the parts of the hard palate (Maxilla lamina horizontalis of the Os palatinum). In addition, in the section the pneumatic parts of the Os frontale (Sinus frontalis) and of the Os sphenoidale (Sinus sphenoidalis) become visible. The impressions of the meningeal vessels (Sulci arteriosi) between the hard meninges (Dura mater) and the skull bone are conspicuous.

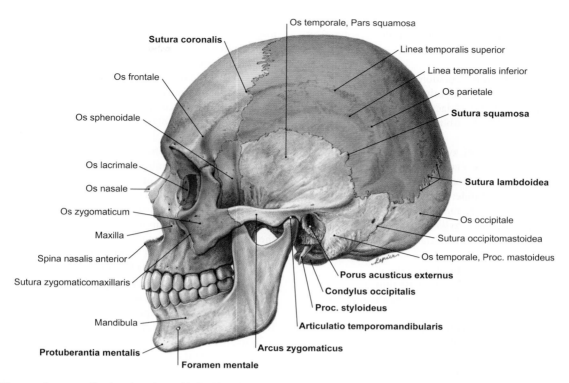

Fig. 9.9 Skull bones, Ossa cranii. View from lateral left side. The main part of the lateral relief of the skull is formed from both Ossa parietalia and temporalia (mainly Pars squamosa) which count as part of the neurocranium. The Os zygomaticum is adjacent to the Arcus zygomaticus (zygomatic arch) of the Os temporale and forms the contours of the cheek. At the leading edge to the Proc. mastoideus is the Porus acusticus externus which is part of the outer ear. Within the temporomandibular joint the Caput mandibulae (head of mandible) articulates with the Fossa mandibularis (Os temporale) in the Articulatio temporomandibularis.

the structure of the Orbita (➤ Fig. 9.7). The medial part forms the **Sulcus lacrimalis** (for the Ductus nasolacrimalis) which continues cranially to the **Fossa sacci lacrimalis** (for the inclusion of the Saccus lacrimalis). The rear edge of the Fossa sacci lacrimalis continues into the Crista lacrimalis posterior and downwards into the Hamulus lacrimalis.

Concha nasalis inferior
The paired **Concha nasalis inferior (inferior nasal concha)** is a self-contained bone and is located beneath the Concha nasalis media of the Os ethmoidale. It is connected on the lateral nasal wall with the Os palatinum and via the Proc. maxillaris with the Maxilla. Below the Concha nasalis inferior is the lower nasal passage (Meatus nasi inferior), into which the Canalis nasolacrimalis opens.

Vomer
The unpaired **Vomer** has the shape of a classical plough (➤ Fig. 9.8). It forms the lower and also largest part of the bony nasal septum and is connected at the top with the Lamina perpendicularis of the Os ethmoidale, as well as with the Os sphenoidale. The Sulcus vomeris runs on its outer side on which the cartilaginous part of the nasal septum is anchored. It also forms the medial wall of each posterior nasal aperture.

Os ethmoidale
The unpaired **Os ethmoidale (ethmoid bone)** is an irregular, porous bone, which belongs to the Ossa pneumatica (➤ Fig. 9.8). It is a component of the nasal cavity and includes the anterior and posterior cells of the ethmoidal sinusess **(Cellulae ethmoidales anteriores and posteriores)**. Its cranial part, the **Lamina cribrosa,** is permeated right and left by a large number of holes (Foramina

cribrosa) (like a sieve), which enable the passage of the Fila olfactoria (N. olfactorius [I]) from the anterior cranial fossa into the roof of the nasal cavity. In the midline of the Lamina cribrosa the **Crista galli** (like a cock's comb) protrudes into the Fossa cranii anterior and divides the Lamina cribrosa into two halves.

Os nasale
The paired **Os nasale (nasal bone)** is connected laterally to the Maxilla and via the Sutura frontonasalis to the Os frontale (➤ Fig. 9.8). The two Ossa nasalia are connected in the midline via the Sutura internasalis. The Os nasale forms only a small proportion of the nasal scaffold.

Clinical remarks

Fractures of the nasal bone belong to the **fractures of the nasal scaffold.** They are the most common fractures of the viscerocranium. Nasal scaffold fractures typically occur in martial arts, violent assaults and traffic accidents.

NOTE

The nasal skeleton is the bony basis of the nose and together with the nose cartilage forms the nasal scaffold. The Os nasale, Os ethmoidale, Concha nasalis inferior, Vomer, Os frontale, Os lacrimale and Maxilla are involved in the construction of the nasal skeleton.

Orbita
The orbit (Orbita) is a deep, pyramid-shaped pit with its tip facing occipitally. The penetration portals for nerves and blood vessels are located in the Orbita:

- Roof
  - **Incisura frontalis** or **Foramen supraorbitale:** N. supraorbitalis (N. ophthalmicus [V/1]), R. medialis
- Lateral wall
  - **Fissura orbitalis superior:** N. oculomotorius [III], N. trochlearis [IV], N. nasociliaris (N. ophthalmicus [V/1]), N. frontalis (N. ophthalmicus [V/1]), N. lacrimalis (N. ophthalmicus [V/1]), N. abducens [VI], R. orbitalis (A. meningea media), V. ophthalmica superior
  - **Fissura orbitalis inferior:** N. zygomaticus (N. maxillaris [V/2]), N. infraorbitalis (N. maxillaris [V/2]), A. infraorbitalis (A. maxillaris), V. ophthalmica inferior
  - **Foramen zygomaticoorbitale:** N. zygomaticus divided into R. zygomaticotemporalis (N. maxillaris [V/2]) (via Foramen zygomaticotemporale) and R. zygomaticofacialis (N. maxillaris [V/2]) (via Foramen zygomaticofacialis)
- Medial wall
  - **Canalis nasolacrimalis:** Ductus nasolacrimalis
  - **Canalis opticus:** N. opticus [II], A. ophthalmica
  - **Foramen ethmoidale anterius:** A. ethmoidalis anterior, N. ethmoidalis anterior (N. ophthalmicus [V/1])
  - **Foramen ethmoidale posterius:** A. ethmoidalis posterior, N. ethmoidalis posterior (N. ophthalmicus [V/1])
- Floor
  - **Canalis infraorbitalis** and **Foramen infraorbitale:** N. infraorbitalis (N. maxillaris [V/2]), A. infraorbitalis
- Bones of the Orbita
  - **Os frontale** (roof, in part)
  - **Os zygomaticum** (lateral wall)
  - **Os sphenoidale, Ala major** (lateral wall)
  - **Os sphenoidale, Ala minor** (medial wall)
  - **Maxilla, Proc. frontalis** (medial wall)
  - **Os ethmoidale** (medial wall)
  - **Os lacrimale** (medial wall)
  - **Os frontale** (medial wall)
  - **Maxilla** (floor)
  - **Os zygomaticum** (floor)
  - **Os palatinum** (floor)

Clinical remarks

Fractures of the orbital floor are referred to as **blow-out fractures.** They are created by frontal point force on the Bulbus oculi (e.g. tennis ball). This results in the fracture of the Orbita floor. In the process, structures within the eye socket (Mm. recti inferiores and obliquus inferior) can become clamped in the fracture gap or even pushed all the way into the Sinus maxillaris (**orbital hernia**) in extreme cases. Symptoms may be ghosting (by limitation of eyeball mobility), enophthalmus (retraction of the eyeball into the viscerocranium/facial skeleton) or conjugate paralysis upwards. If the N. infraorbitalis running in the orbital floor is also affected, **sensory disturbances** in the area of the facial skin of the Maxilla occur. The selective application of force can also lead to fracture of the Lamina papyracea of the Os ethmoidale (medial orbital wall, with involvement of the Cellulae ethmoidales).

9.1.6 Individual bones of the neurocranium

Os frontale

The anterior part of the skull is formed by the Squama frontalis of the **Os frontalis** (frontal bone) which also provides the shape of the roof of the Orbita (➤ Fig. 9.7) and the floor of the anterior cranial fossa (➤ Fig. 9.3). Therefore the Os frontale forms the transition between the viscerocranium and the neurocranium. The paired Sinus frontalis (frontal sinus) is located above the Orbita on both sides within the Squama frontalis, which protrudes forward in a bulge as the Arcus superciliaris (the eyebrows are here) (➤ Fig. 9.8). The Arcus superciliaris is more intensely formed in men than in women. Between the two Arcus superciliares lies the **glabella** (area between the eyebrows). In the view from below, the Foveolae ethmoidales are found below the glabella on both sides, which mark both the entrance to the frontal sinus and at the same time are part of the roof of the ethmoidal cells. The front edge of the bilateral orbital roof is formed by the **Margines supraorbitales** which show an Incisura frontalis or a Foramen frontale (point of penetration of the N. supraorbitalis). The Os frontale extends to the **Sutura coronalis** and is connected by this to the Os parietale. Caudally, it borders on the Os ethmoidale and forms a part of the medial orbital wall with the Foramina ethmoidalia anterius and posterius, which enable the passage of the vessels and nerves of the same name. The Facies orbitalis, which also forms the roof of the Orbita, is temporally deepened to the Fossa glandulae lacrimalis (location of the lacrimal gland). Above the Sutura frontosphenoidalis the frontal bone borders on the sphenoid bone. Inside the skull, starting at the Foramen caecum, the Crista frontalis runs medially, which continues into the Sulcus sinus sagittalis superioris. As already described, on the inner side of the bone Sulci arteriosi (location of the A. meningea anterior) and Foveolae granulares (PACCHIONI). can be recognised.

Os temporale

The paired **Os temporale** (temporal bone) partly belongs to the viscerocranium and partly to the neurocranium (➤ Fig. 9.9). In addition, it is involved in the formation of the **temporomandibular joint** (Fossa mandibularis), the outer wall of the skull (➤ Fig. 9.8) and the skull base (➤ Fig. 9.3). The temporal bone articulates with the lower jaw in the **Articulatio temporomandibularis** (temperomandibular joint, ➤ Fig. 9.9) via the Fossa mandibularis and the Tuberculum articulare lying in front of it. Dorsal of the Fossa mandibularis is the **Meatus acusticus externus** (outer ear canal), which joins the **Proc. mastoideus** (mastoid process) and in adults is filled with air (**Cellulae mastoideae**). The Os temporale is divided into:

- **Pars petrosa** (petrous part of the temporal bone, petrous pyramid): it borders at the back on the Ossa parietale and occipitale, its central external opening is the Meatus acusticus externus. At the back and below, it joins the Proc. mastoideus. The Pars petrosa accomodates the middle and the inner ear. Openings/spaces are the internal auditory canal (Meatus acusticus internus) with passage of the N. facialis [VII], N. intermedius [VII], N. vestibulocochlearis [VIII] and A. labyrinthi and the Foramen stylomastoideum with passage of the N. facialis [VII] and Canalis musculotubarius (passage of the Tuba auditiva [EUSTACHII] and position of the M. tensor tympani). In addition, it forms the Apertura externa canalis carotici for the A. carotis interna and together with the eardrum forms the side wall of the tympanic cavity (Cavitas tympani).
- **Pars tympanica:** it limits the bony wall of the external auditory canal from the front, bottom and rear, extends to the eardrum and lies annularly on the Partes squamosa and petrosa.
- **Pars squamosa** (squamous = scale): it occupies the largest part according to area and borders the Os parietale via the Margo parietalis. It forms the front and top part of the temple. At the front and above the Meatus, the Proc. zygomaticus bulges and stretch-

es forward as part of the zygomatic arch. It is connected to the Os occipitale via the Sutura occipitomastoidea and to the Os sphenoidale via the Sutura sphenosquamosa.

Os sphenoidale

The butterfly-shaped unpaired **Os sphenoidale** (sphenoid bone) is, like the Os frontale and the Os temporale part of the neurocranium and the viscerocranium (➤ Fig. 9.3). It is located in the middle of the skull base, contains points of penetration for numerous vessels and nerves and is the interface to all other bones of the internal surface of the skull base. The Os sphenoidale articulates at the front with the Os frontale and to a minor extent with the Os ethmoidale. Laterally it is adjacent to the two Ossa temporalia and at the back it is connected with the clivus of the Os occipitale. It is also involved in the structure of the Orbita. In the centre of the sphenoid bone is the **Turkish saddle** (Sella turcica, ➤ Fig. 9.8) and in its **Fossa hypophysialis** lies the pituary gland (Glandula pituitaria). A distinction is made between 2 lower, large wings(Alae majores) and 2 upper, small wings (Alae minores), which exit from the **Corpus sphenoidale**. The sphenoidal body is pneumatised and includes the Sinus sphenoidales (sphenoidal bone cavities) which belong to the paranasal sinuses. From its lateral edges access to the Orbita can be attained through the Ala minor via the Canalis opticus. Between the two **sphenoidal wings** the Fissura orbitalis superior also leads into the Orbita. The Alae majores are penetrated on both sides by the Foramina rotundum, ovale, spinosum. Caudal from the Corpus the Procc. pterygoidei (pterygoid processes) rise on both sides; these are divided into the smaller Lamina medialis and larger Lamina lateralis.

Os parietale

The paired **Os parietale** (parietal bone) constitutes the major part of the lateral skull and of the skull roof (➤ Fig. 9.9, ➤ Fig. 9.10). It is convex and has 4 edges, through which it is connected to the adjacent bones:

- Anterior via the Sutura coronalis with the Os frontale
- Lateral via the Sutura squamosa with the Os temporale (and to a minor degree with the Os sphenoidale)
- Below via the Sutura lambdoidea with the Os occipitale
- Medial to the respective contralateral Os parietale

The inner relief of the Os parietale is characterised by the impressions of the Aa. meningeae media and anterior (**Sulci arteriosi,** ➤ Fig. 9.8) as well as the Sinus durae matris (Sulcus sinus sigmoidei). On the outer wall a Linea temporalis superior and a Linea temporalis inferior can be recognized (➤ Fig. 9.9).

Os occipitale

The unpaired **Os occipitale** (occipital bone) forms the main part of the skull base and consists of 4 bone parts (➤ Fig. 9.10) that together make up the Foramen magnum (passage of the Medulla oblongata):

- **Pars squamosa**
- **Pars basilaris**
- **Partes laterales**
- **Planum occipitale**

The 4 bone parts fuse in the *4th year of life,* so that in infants 4 individual bones can be distinguished. Similar to the Ossa parietalia, to which it is connected via the Sutura lambdoidea, on the inside to both the right and left impressions of the Sinus durae matris can be seen: the **Sulcus sinus sigmoidei, Sulcus sinus petrosi inferioris, Sulcus sinus occipitalis** as well as the **Sulcus transversus** and **Sulcus sinus sagittalis superioris** (➤ Fig. 9.8). The latter merge at the Protuberantia occipitalis interna (Confluens sinuum). This is connected to the Crista occipitalis interna. Futhermore, on the inside within the respective Squama occipitalis the Fossa cerebellarisa can be seen, in which the cerebellum is located. Externally the Linea nuchalis inferior and the above lying Linea nuchalis superior are raised up (in some bony skulls a Linea nuchalis suprema can also be found). The Condyli occipitales are located on the surface of the Partes laterales, through which the skull articulates with the first cervical vertebra (Atlas). Above the condyles, on the lateral edges of the Foramen magnum, lies the **Canalis nervi hypoglossi** (point of penetration of the N. hypoglossus [XII]).

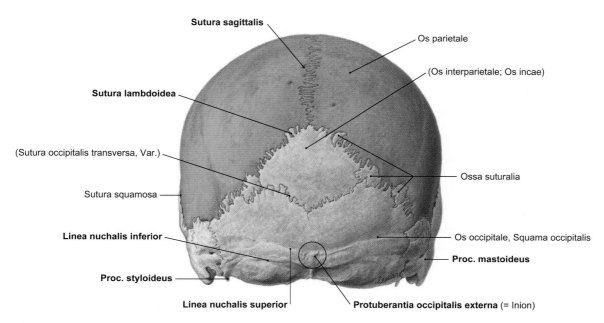

Fig. 9.10 Skull bones, Ossa cranii. Dorsal view. The majority of the occiput is formed by the Os occipitale and its central structure is the Squama occipitalis. The most protruding point of the occiput is the well palpable Protuberantia occipitalis externa (Inion), which continues on both sides into the Linea nuchalis superior (attachment point for muscles of the autochthonous back muscles).

The **stylohyoid syndrome** or also **EAGLE syndrome** is a bunch of symptoms, which is triggered by a Proc. styloideus that is too long. The Proc. styloideus can not only be too long, but in extreme cases also makes flexible joint-like contact with the Os hyoideum. The Proc. styloideus which is too long sometimes touches the pharyngeal wall and leads to foreign body sensation, swallowing problems (dysphagia) and unclear sore throat.

9.2 Soft tissue covering
Lars Bräuer, Friedrich Paulsen

Skills

After working through this chapter, you should be able to:
- describe the mimic musculature with attachment, origin, function and innervation
- be orientated in the face and the lateral facial region and systematically assign the areas
- name the structure, blood supply, innervation and lymphatic drainage as well as the function of the scalp
- describe the topographic course of blood vessels, nerves and lymph vessels in the various facial regions
- name important topographical clinical correlations of the lateral facial region
- envisage the three-dimensional anatomical structures which are lying deep in the lateral facial region and are not visible from the outside

9.2.1 Overview
Friedrich Paulsen

The skull is externally covered by soft tissues, which are divided into different regions (**Regiones capitis**) (➤ Table 9.7, ➤ Fig. 9.11) as in the throat area and torso:
- **Regio frontalis**
- **Regio nasalis***
- **Regio orbitalis***
- **Regio infraorbitalis***

- **Regio zygomatica***
- **Regio buccalis**
- **Regio oralis***
- **Regio mentalis***
- **Regio parotideomasseterica**
- **Regio temporalis***
- **Regio parietalis***
- **Regio occipitalis***

*The regions marked with an asterisk together form the Regio facialis.

The soft tissue includes skin, subcutaneous fat and facial muscles that form a functional unit with respect to facial expression and physiognomy. The facial muscles originate at the skull bone and radiate via elastic tendons into the dermis of the skin.

N O T E

The face-to-face encounter is an important aspect of the **contact** between two individuals. Facial expression plays a major role for the expression of emotions and a doctor can obtain valuable information about the emotional and health status of the patients. Understanding the facial structures is therefore of great relevance for practical medical activities.
With increasing age, the **elasticity** of the elastic tendons of the facial muscles that radiate into the skin becomes reduced. The result is the formation of wrinkles.

The facial muscles are used in addition to facial expression and physiognomy for the protection of sensory organs and food intake. The masticatory muscles also have a great influence on the form of the facial region. The muscles from the shoulder girdle (M. sternocleidomastoideus) and from the vertebral column (neck muscles) which extend onto the head are involved in head movements in relation to the spine.

Table 9.7 Facial regions (Regiones faciales).

Regio facialis anterior	Regio facialis lateralis superficialis	Regio facialis lateralis profunda
• Regio orbitalis • Regio nasalis • Regio infraorbitalis • Regio zygomatica • Regio oralis • Regio mentalis	• Regio buccalis • Regio parotideomasseterica	• Fossa infratemporalis • Fossa pterygopalatina

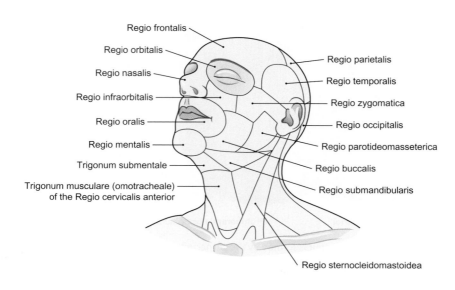

Fig. 9.11 Regions of the head.
[L126]

Regio frontalis
Regio orbitalis
Regio nasalis
Regio infraorbitalis
Regio oralis
Regio mentalis
Trigonum submentale
Trigonum musculare (omotracheale) of the Regio cervicalis anterior
Regio parietalis
Regio temporalis
Regio zygomatica
Regio occipitalis
Regio parotideomasseterica
Regio buccalis
Regio submandibularis
Regio sternocleidomastoidea

The soft tissues of the head can be divided into 3 parts due to structural features and regional affiorigin:
- **SCALP** (scalp)
- **Frontal facial region**
- **Lateral facial region**
  - Superficial lateral facial region
  - Deep lateral facial region

9.2.2 Scalp
Friedrich Paulsen

The soft tissues of the Calvaria (scalp) extend from the Arcus superciliaris to the Protuberantia occipitalis and the Linea nuchalis superior, as well as laterally to the Arcus zygomaticus.

Layers
The functional unit of skin, subcutis and tendon hub (Galea aponeurotica), which lies above the roof of the skull (Calvaria) (total thickness approx. 5 mm), is referred to as the **scalp**. It consists of several layers that can easily be remembered using the term SCALP. (➤ Fig. 9.12):
- **S** = Skin (Cutis)
- **C** = Connective tissue (Subcutis)
- **A** = Aponeurosis (Aponeurosis epicranialis, Galea aponeurotica with M. epicranius)
- **L** = Loose connective tissue (subgaleal movable layer)
- **P** = Pericranium (periosteum of the outer surface of the skull bones)

The loose subaponeurotic connective tissue connects the Galea aponeurotica with the pericranium, thus allowing the free movement of the scalp on the Calvaria.

Cutis
The cutis forms the outer layer of the scalp. It is structurally designed like the skin of the body surface but is coarse at the hairy head surface and contains a particularly large number of hair shafts, sebaceous glands and sweat glands. On the forehead there are only few hairs and no terminal hairs.

Subcutis
The subcutis contains hair papillae, hair follicles and hair roots in the area of the hairy scalp. The subcutis consists for the most part of **dense connective tissue,** which anchors the skin to the underlying Galea aponeurotica (see below). Arteries, veins and nerves for blood supply and innervation of the scalp also run here. In bald areas the subcutis is thinner.

Aponeurosis
The base of the scalp is the **Galea aponeurotica,** a widespread tendon, which radiates into the front, back and side muscles:
- At the front it is the Venter frontalis of the **M. epicranius** (M. occipitofrontalis), its paired muscle bellies originate between the Arcus superciliares from the subcutaneous connective tissue of the eyebrows and the Glabella and pass in a V-shape to the back.
- At the back it is also the paired Venter occipitalis of the M. epicranius, which originates at the Linea nuchalis suprema and radiates at the level of the middle of the auricle into the aponeurosis.
- Laterally it is the variably occurring **M. temporoparietalis.** The part facing the skull is also referred to as the M. auricularis superior. It belongs to a rudimentary sphincter system that moves the ear and can close the auditory canal.

The Galea aponeurotica is firmly fused with the subcutis due to its strong connective tissue trabecula (retinacula). On contraction the muscles allow a small shift movement of the scalp on the skull. The Venter frontalis of the M. epicranius can pull the forehead into wrinkles (frowning).

Subgaleal layer
The lower side of the Galea aponeurotica is attached to the periosteum of the skull (pericranium) via loose connective tissue. It forms the supraperiostal space and for functional reasons is referred to as the **subgaleal (subgaleatic) layer.**

Pericranium
The periosteum of the Calvaria is firmly fused with the Lamina externa of the skull bones and the connective tissue of the cranial sutures.

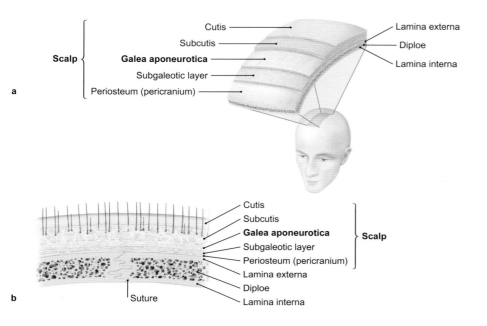

Fig. 9.12 Structure of the scalp.
a SCALP. **b** Layers of the scalp.
[L127]

Due to the taut connective tissue in the subcutis, the arteries are often kept open after injury of the entire scalp. This can create strong arterial **bleeding**. If only the skin and subcutis are injured there is only little bleeding. Venous bleeding is in contrast mostly pronounced, as the vessels in the taut connective tissue can practically not retract.

Scalping, as known from Indian stories, involves the scalp being pulled from the skull, whereby the periosteum can be relatively easily detached from the bone. This can be taken advantage of when practising procedures on the brain by moving the scalp using a temple cut (from one ear to the other) forwards and backwards from the periosteum, repositioning it after the operation and suturing the skin incision. Injuries **(scalping injuries)** are also possible in this way. If long hairs get caught up in a rotating machine, the entire scalp can be torn off. For this reason, occupational health and safety dictates that a hat should be worn when working with such machines.

During birth, a bloody serous oedema in the subcutis of the child can occur (particularly in the occiput and parietal bone area), which appears as a **head bulge (Caput succedaneum)**. Subperiostal bleeding is also possible during birth. Subperiostal bleeding therefore remains limited to individual bones of the Calvaria **(cephalhaematoma)** since the periosteum is very strongly fused in the area of the cranial sutures.

Vascular, lymphatic and nervous systems

The vascular, lymphatic and nervous systems reach the scalp from a frontal, temporal and occipital direction. Here, the vessels, with the exception of the forehead, lie in the subcutis. In the forehead the blood vessels run in the subgaleal layer. Vascular, lymphatic and nervous systems are:

* Frontal
  - A., V. and N. supraorbitalis
  - A. and V. supratrochlearis
* Temporal
  - A. and V. temporalis superficialis
  - N. auriculotemporalis (from [V/2])
  - R. zygomaticotemporalis nervi zygomatici (from [V/2])
* Occipital
  - A. and V. occipitalis
  - A. and V. auricularis posterior
  - N. occipitalis major
  - N. occipitalis minor
  - N. auricularis magnus

Arteries

The scalp is supplied with blood from branches of the A. ophthalmica or branches of the A. carotis externa.

Branches of the A. ophthalmica

The front and upper sections of the scalp in the forehead are supplied by:
* **A. supratrochlearis**
* **A. supraorbitalis**

They branch off in the Orbita from the A. ophthalmica, pass through the Orbita rostrally and penetrate with veins and nerves of the same name through the Septum orbitale and the A. supratrochlearis through the Incisura or the Foramen supratrochleare. Together with the nerves and veins the arteries run over the forehead upwards and provide the scalp roughly up to the vertex with blood.

Branches of the A. carotis externa

The largest part of the scalp is supplied with blood from 3 branches of the A. carotis externa (➤ Fig. 9.13).
* **A. auricularis posterior:** it is the smallest branch, exits backwards in the area of the Fossa retromandibularis from the A. carotis externa and then passes below and behind the auricle to the surface, to supply the area of the scalp.

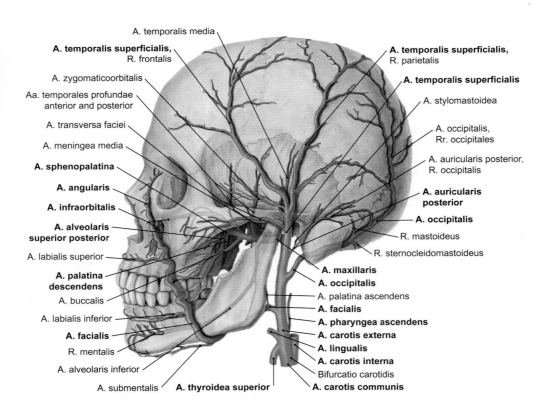

A. temporalis media
A. temporalis superficialis, R. frontalis
A. zygomaticoorbitalis
Aa. temporales profundae anterior and posterior
A. transversa faciei
A. meningea media
A. sphenopalatina
A. angularis
A. infraorbitalis
A. alveolaris superior posterior
A. labialis superior
A. palatina descendens
A. buccalis
A. labialis inferior
A. facialis
R. mentalis
A. alveolaris inferior
A. submentalis
A. thyroidea superior

A. temporalis superficialis, R. parietalis
A. temporalis superficialis
A. stylomastoidea
A. occipitalis, Rr. occipitales
A. auricularis posterior, R. occipitalis
A. auricularis posterior
A. occipitalis
R. mastoideus
R. sternocleidomastoideus
A. maxillaris
A. occipitalis
A. palatina ascendens
A. facialis
A. pharyngea ascendens
A. carotis externa
A. lingualis
A. carotis interna
Bifurcatio carotidis
A. carotis communis

Fig. 9.13 Branches of the A. carotis externa.

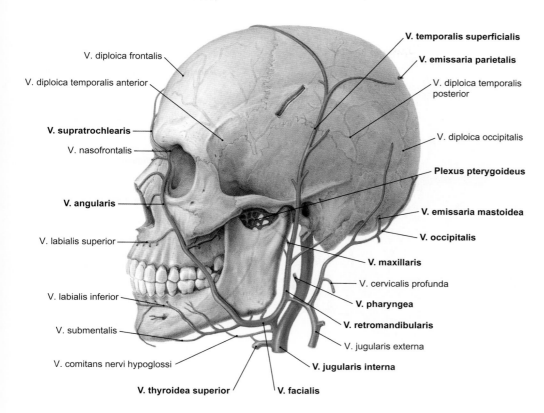

V. temporalis superficialis
V. emissaria parietalis
V. diploica temporalis posterior
V. diploica frontalis
V. diploica temporalis anterior
V. diploica occipitalis
V. supratrochlearis
V. nasofrontalis
Plexus pterygoideus
V. angularis
V. emissaria mastoidea
V. occipitalis
V. labialis superior
V. maxillaris
V. cervicalis profunda
V. pharyngea
V. labialis inferior
V. retromandibularis
V. submentalis
V. jugularis externa
V. comitans nervi hypoglossi
V. jugularis interna
V. thyroidea superior
V. facialis

Fig. 9.14 Tributaries Contributing vessels of the V. jugularis interna.

- **A. temporalis superficialis:** it is a terminal branch of the A. carotis externa, which runs cranially directly in front of the auricle and divides on the Os temporale into anterior and posterior branches.
- **A. occipitalis:** it exits from the A. carotis externa a little further down, passes further to the back and rises, sloping through the neck muscles on the surface anatomy to supply the scalp at the occiput and back of the head.

Veins
The veins, which drain the blood from the scalp, run with the respective arteries (➤ Fig. 9.14):
- **V. supratrochlearis** and **V. supraorbitalis:** they collect the blood from the front scalp from the vertex to the Arcus supraciliaris, enter the Orbita with the arteries of the same name and drain into the V. ophthalmica superior. There are anastomoses in front of the entrance into the Orbita to the V. angularis (branch of the V. facialis) in the nasal angle of the eyelid.
- **V. auricularis posterior:** it collects blood behind and below the auricle and drains into the V. retromandibularis.
- **V. temporalis superficialis:** it collects blood from the entire lateral scalp above the auricles and also drains also into the V. retromandibularis.
- **V. occipitalis:** it drains the rear section of the scalp between the Protuberantia occipitalis externa and the Linea nuchalis superior to the vertex. Below the Linea nuchalis superior it runs through the neck muscles into the depth in the dorsal section of the throat area. Here, the strong vein is involved in the drainage of the neck region and flows variably into the V. vertebralis, V. jugularis externa or V. jugularis interna. In addition, it is connected to the V. diploica occipitalis.

Lymph vessels
The lymph drainage from the scalp also essentially follows the catchment area of the arteries. A total of 4 drainage areas are differ-

entiated (➤ Fig. 9.15), whereby the temporal, parietal and occipital regions always have lymph nodes in the head, while the frontal region drains variably to lymph nodes in the head or throat area:
- Frontal – **Nodi lymphoidei preauriculares, Nodi lymphoidei submandibulares** (variable Nodi lymphoidei faciales)
- Temporal – **Nodi lymphoidei parotidei**
- Parietal – **Nodi lymphoidei infraauriculares**
- Occipital – **Nodi lymphoidei occipitales, Nodi lymphoidei mastoidei** (Nodi lymphoidei retroauriculares, Nodi lymphoidei auriculares posteriores)

Finally, from these primary lymph node stations, the lymph reaches the deep cervical lymph nodes.

Innervation
The scalp is sensitively innervated (➤ Fig. 9.16) via the cranial nerves and the Plexus cervicalis. The vertex can be considered as the limit. The M. occipitofrontalis and the M. temporoparietalis are, like all facial muscles, innervated by branches of the **N. facialis [VII]**.

Rostral from the vertex
The area in front of the vertex and in front of the auricle is innervated by branches of the **N. trigeminus [V]**:
- **N. supraorbitalis** (branch of the N. frontalis from [V/1]): it leaves the Orbita with a **R. lateralis** (enters through the Foramen supraorbitale/Incisura supraorbitalis) and a **R. medialis** (enters through the Incisura frontalis). Both branches penetrate the Venter frontalis of the M. occipitofrontalis and sensitively innervate the frontal area up to the vertex region.
- **N. supratrochlearis** (branch of the N. frontalis from [V/1]): after leaving the Orbita slightly above the nasal angle of the eyelid its branches innervate the lower middle forehead region.
- **R. zygomaticotemporalis nervi zygomatici** (branch from [V/2]): its branches innervate a small area of the temporal scalp.
- **N. auriculotemporalis** (branch from [V/3]): it extends with the Vasa temporalia superficialia in front of the ear on the surface

427

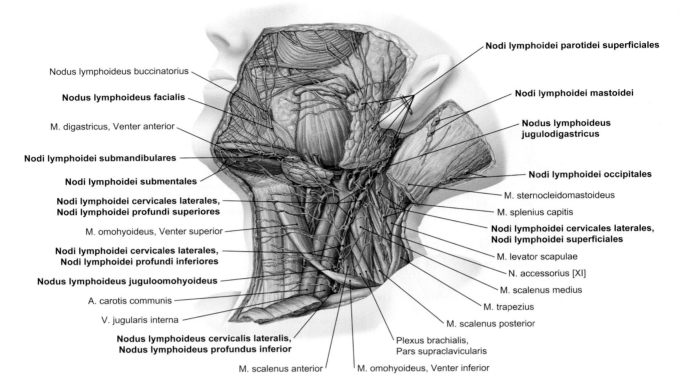

Fig. 9.15 Superficial lymph nodes of the face.

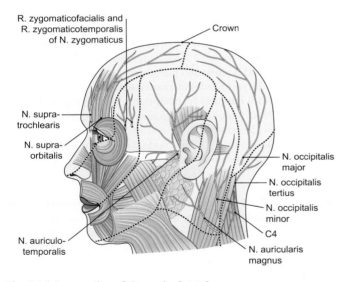

Fig. 9.16 Innervation of the scalp. [L126]

and innervates the usually hairy part of the temporal region and the scalp with its **Rr. temporales superficiales.**

Occipital from the vertex
Behind the auricle and the vertex, the scalp is sensitively innervated by branches of the Plexus cervicalis (➤ Fig. 9.16).

- **N. auricularis magnus** (from the Punctum nervosum [ERB's point], Rr. anteriores of C2 and C3): the powerful nerve innervates the skin behind the auricle with its branches. The branches also reach skin areas in the throat area underneath the auricle.
- **N. occipitalis minor** (from the Punctum nervosum [ERB's point], R. anterior of c2): It runs along the rear edge of the M. sternocleidomastoideus up via the attachment area of the muscle

into the lateral occipital region, from where it directs sensory information of the scalp.

- **N. occipitalis major** (R. posterior of C2): it arises below the M. obliquus capitis inferior (➤ Chap. 3.2.2) from the depth of the Trigonum vertebrale upwards, penetrates the Mm. semispinalis capitis and trapezius and then runs with its branches from the occipital region to the vertex, to sensitively innervate the largest part of the scalp.
- **N. occipitalis tertius** (R. posterior of C3): like the N. occipitalis major, it initially penetrates the Mm. semispinalis and trapezius. In doing so, it runs on the centre line and then innervates a small area at the rear of the scalp close to the midline.

9.2.3 Face and facial soft tissue
Lars Bräuer, Friedrich Paulsen

Surface anatomy
Friedrich Paulsen
The face extends from the nose root and the eyebrows up to the ears, including the auricles, as well as to the rear edge of the Mandibula and comprises the Regiones orbitalis, nasalis, infraorbitalis, zygomatica, oralis and mentalis (➤ Fig. 9.11).
From a clinical perspective the face is divided into:
- A middle (frontal) area (**Regio facialis medialis**)
- A paired lateral area (**Regio facialis lateralis**)
The lateral area is divided into:
- Superficial (**Regio facialis lateralis superficialis**) and
- Deep (**Regio facialis lateralis profunda**)
Anatomically, the frontal region (**Regio facialis,** ➤ Fig. 9.11) belongs to the Calvaria due to its relationship with the cranial cavity; however, in general usage the face extends up to the hairline and therefore includes the forehead. Characteristics of the face (Facies) are the eyes, nose and mouth. If the eyes and mouth are taken as

the horizontal limits, the face can be divided into an upper, a middle and a lower section.

The foundations of the face are the skull skeleton and cartilaginous skeleton from the external nose and auricle. They are covered with a relatively thin soft tissue coat, which includes the skin, the subcutaneous connective and fatty tissues and the mimic muscles. Prominent points of the face are the eyebrow bulges (Arcus supraciliares), the outer nose, the zygomatic arch (Arcus zygomatici), the auricles and the chin (Mentum).

The fatty material of the cheek is involved in the formation of the lateral facial region as well as (Corpus adiposum buccae, BICHAT'S fat-pad), the M. masseter and the Glandula parotidea.

Eye area, Regio orbitalis

The Regio orbitalis (➤ Fig. 9.11) is determined by the eyelids (Palpebrae) and by the shape, density and position of the eyebrows (**Supercilii**). An upper (**Palpebra superior**) and a lower (**Palpebra inferior**) eyelid limit the palpebral fissure (**Rima palpebrarum**) and cover the front part of the eyeball when the eyes are closed. On the side the eyelids merge at the nasal and temporal palpebral angle (**Angulus oculi medialis** and **Angulus oculi lateralis**) (➤ Fig. 9.11).

Nasal region, Regio nasalis

The Regio nasalis (➤ Fig. 9.11) is determined by the external scaffold of the nose. The foundations are the root of the nose (**Radix nasi**), the the nasal bridge (**Dorsum nasi**), the paired nose wings (**Alae nasi**), the tip of the nose (**Apex nasi**), the nostrils (**Nares**) and the interjacent nasal septum (**Septum nasi**). The nasal orifices form the entrance to the respiratory tract. The nasolabial folds descend laterally on the nasal wings (**Sulcus nasolabialis**) to the corners of the mouth (➤ Fig. 9.11). It is only weakly formed in young people and emerges more prominently from the 4th decade of life.

Oral region, Regio oralis

The Regio oralis (➤ Fig. 9.11) is limited by the upper lip (**Labium superius**) and bottom lip (**Labium inferius**), which merge on the corners of the mouth (**Angulus oris**) (**Commissura labiorum**). A small bump is formed in the midline on the upper lip (**Tubercle labii superioris**), and the border of the vermilion to the facial skin describes a double arch (Cupid's bow). From here a 8-10 mm wide groove runs, narrowing from the bottom upwards (**Philtrum**) to the nose root (in ancient times, the Philtrum was considered as one of the erogenous zones of the body, therefore Cupid's bow) (➤ Fig. 9.11).

Chin area, Regio mentalis

The Regio mentalis (➤ Fig. 9.11) is limited from the Regio oralis by the transverse chin-lip furrow (**Sulcus mentolabialis**) (➤ Fig. 9.11). The different protrusion at the chin is mainly based on the amount of subcutaneous fat and less on the bony chin protrusion (**Protuberantia mentalis**). In some people the M. mentalis (➤ Table 9.8), which radiates into the skin, causes an intense dimple in the skin of the chin.

Facial skin

The nature and properties of the skin and subcutis show large regional differences. Above the nasal wings, the cheeks and the chin the skin is comparatively thick, in contrast it is relatively thin above the eyelids. The distribution of sweat and sebaceous glands also show extreme variation on a regional level. On the eyelids and on the auricle there is a lack of subcutaneous fat tissue; in contrast it is strongly developed on the cheeks and chin. The vessels and nerves run in the subcutis.

Clinical remarks

Due to the loose subcutaneous connective tissue on the eyelids, severe swelling may occur, which make it impossible to open the eyelids (**lid oedema**). The incision during surgical interventions on the face always follow the **tension lines of the skin** (RSTL, 'relaxed skin tension lines') in order to avoid visible scars to a large extent.

Mimic muscles (Mm. faciei)
Lars Bräuer

The Mm. faciei are muscles, which are decisively responsible for the expression of the face and the formation of an individual face expression (**physiognomy**). They are also important for food intake and speech development (muscles in the area of the mouth). Moreover, they have protective functions (muscles of the eye, corneal reflexes). On an evolutionary level the facial muscles, which are arranged around the eyes, ears, nose and mouth, have a protective function because they can close the corresponding body opening; however, some of these muscles in humans are only in rudimentary form (around the ear).

The paired M. orbicularis oculi, the unpaired M. orbicularis oris and unpaired M. occipitofrontalis form the largest area of the facial muscles (➤ Fig. 9.17). The small facial muscles are highly individually distinct and enable delicate and unique facial expressions (e.g. M. risorius, M. corrugator supercilii).

The facial muscles are directly connected with the dermis above the superficial muscular aponeurotic system (SMAS, see below), so that by corresponding contraction or relaxation they stretch or compress and therefore enable the facial expressions. The exception is the M. buccinator, which has a **muscle fascia**. The facial muscles originate mostly from bony or cartilaginous structures of the skull skeleton and are attached to elastic tendons in the skin. Circularly routed muscles around the ocular and oral cavities resemble a sphincter, which facilitates the closing of the mouth and eye cavities. The facial muscles (including the Platysma) develop as a unit of the 2nd pharyngeal arch with the nerve (N. facialis [VII]), which innervates them. In the following the two larger and circular muscles running around the eye and mouth openings are described in detail. All facial muscles are summarised in ➤ Table 9.8.

M. orbicularis oris

The M. orbicularis oris is an annular muscle around the mouth opening (➤ Fig. 9.17). It forms the muscular basis for the lips and is motorically innervated by 3 branches of the N. facialis:
- Upper lip – Rr. zygomatici
- Corner of the mouth – Rr. buccales
- Lower lip – R. marginalis mandibulae

The arch-shaped muscle fibres can be divided according to their location and their course into 2 large parts:
- **Pars marginalis** – around the oral fissure
- **Pars labialis** – the largest part of the muscle, extends from the upper lip to the nasal septum and from the lower lip to the chin

A further part known as the M. rectus labii, is formed from the individual radially running muscle fibres. If the peripheral parts of the muscle (Pars labialis) are contracted, the lips become pointed (pouting, whistling).

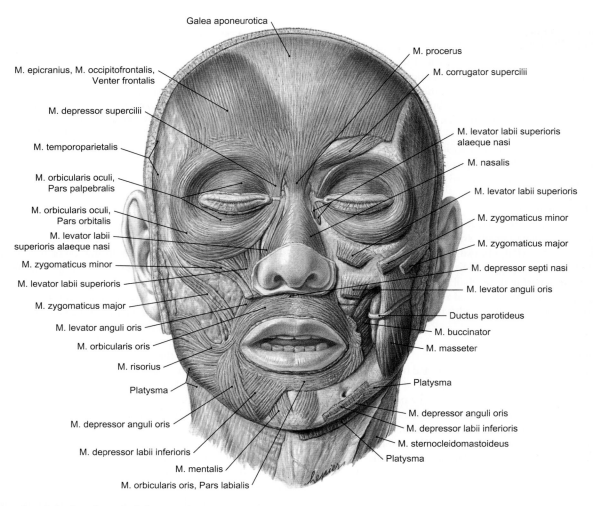

Galea aponeurotica

M. procerus

M. corrugator supercilii

M. epicranius, M. occipitofrontalis,
Venter frontalis

M. depressor supercilii

M. levator labii superioris
alaeque nasi

M. temporoparietalis

M. nasalis

M. orbicularis oculi,
Pars palpebralis

M. levator labii superioris

M. orbicularis oculi,
Pars orbitalis

M. zygomaticus minor

M. levator labii
superioris alaeque nasi

M. zygomaticus major

M. zygomaticus minor

M. depressor septi nasi

M. levator labii superioris

M. levator anguli oris

M. zygomaticus major

Ductus parotideus

M. levator anguli oris

M. buccinator

M. orbicularis oris

M. masseter

M. risorius

Platysma

Platysma

M. depressor anguli oris

M. depressor anguli oris

M. depressor labii inferioris

M. depressor labii inferioris

M. sternocleidomastoideus

M. mentalis

Platysma

M. orbicularis oris, Pars labialis

Fig. 9.17 Muscles of the face (Mm. faciei). Rostral view.

Clinical remarks

The **Orbicularis oris reflex** (moustache reflex) is for checking and excluding disorders of the upper motor neuron of the N. facialis [VII] or the nerve tracts between the pons and cortex. By tapping the face above the corner of the mouth affected patients contract the M. orbicularis oris as a reflex and the point of their lips. Healthy people and patients with damage of the lower motor neuron do not show this reflex. The N. trigeminus [V] is an afferent leg of the reflex, the facial nerve [VII] is the efferent leg.

The highly toxic exotoxins of the bacterial species *Clostridium botulinum* and *Clostridium butyricum* have been increasingly applied in recent years very highly diluted in clinical and plastic/cosmetic treatment. As such **Botox** has achieved record sales worldwide as a drug and wrinkle treatment. This involves low concentrations of the botulinus toxin being injected subcutaneously or intramuscularly, depending on the indications.

M. orbicularis oculi

The M. orbicularis oculi is the only muscle which can close the eye (➤ Fig. 9.17). It has a similar arch-shaped course as the M. orbicularis oris. Its fibres run around the bony edge of the Orbita and are used for the tight closure of the eye by the eyelids. The muscle, which is also innervated by the N. facialis [VII] (upper lid – Rr. temporales, lower eyelid – Rr. zygomatici) is divided into the following three parts:

- **Pars orbitalis:** the Pars orbitalis lies completely externally, runs above and below the bony orbital rim, and overlaps the Venter frontalis of the M. occipitofrontalis at the top. The Pars orbitalis emits fibres to the eyebrows, which lowers them (M. depressor supercilii). The lower part of the Pars orbitalis borders on the M. zygomaticus minor.
- **Pars palpebralis:** the Pars palpebralis forms the foundation for the eyelids and lies between subcutis and tarsus or Septum orbitale. The muscle fibres originate at the Lig. palpebrale mediale and run when the lid is closed to the Lig. palpebrale laterale. On the edge of the eyelid muscle fibres radiate from the Pars palpebralis into the tarsus and entwine the excretory ducts of the Glandulae tarsales located in the tarsus. These muscle fibres are referred to as Fasciculi ciliares or RIOLAN's muscles.
- **Pars lacrimalis:** the part also designated as HORNER's muscle is covered by the other two muscle units. It runs from the Saccus lacrimalis to the Pars palpebralis and entwines on the way the Canaliculi lacrimales superior and inferior. It is essential for the tear transport when the eyelids are closed.

The M. orbicularis oculi is integrated into the reflex arch to be able to quickly close the eye if required (e.g. opticofacial reflex, corneal and conjunctival reflex).

Table 9.8 Mimic muscles. The facial nerve [VII] is responsible for innervation.

Origins	Attachment	Function
Forehead, vertex, temples		
M. occipitofrontalis		
• Venter frontalis: skin of the forehead (➤ Fig. 9.17) • Venter occipitalis: Linea nuchalis suprema (➤ Fig. 9.18)	Galea aponeurotica	*Forehead:* • Venter frontalis: frowning (amazement) • Venter occipitalis: smooths forehead wrinkles
M. temporoparietalis (➤ Fig. 9.18)		
Skin of the temple, Fascia temporalis	Galea aponeurotica	Moves the scalp downwards
M. occipitofrontalis and M. temporoparietalis are referred to together as the M. epicranius		
Auricle		
M. auricularis anterior (➤ Fig. 9.18)		
Fascia temporalis	Front of the auricle	Moves the auricle upwards to the front
M. auricularis superior (➤ Fig. 9.18)		
Galea aponeurotica	Top of the auricle	Moves the auricle upwards to the back
M. auricularis posterior (➤ Fig. 9.18)		
Proc. mastoideus	At the back of the auricle	Moves the auricle backwards
Eyelids		
M. orbicularis oculi (surrounds the Aditus orbitalis like a sphincter), ➤ Fig. 9.17)		
• Pars orbitalis: Pars nasalis of the Os frontale, Proc. frontalis of the Maxilla, Os lacrimale, Lig. palpebrale mediale • Pars palpebralis: Lig. palpebrale mediale, Saccus lacrimalis • Pars lacrimalis: crista lacrimalis posterior of the Os lacrimale, Saccus lacrimalis	• Pars orbitalis: Lig. palpebrale laterale • Pars palpebralis: Lig. palpebrale laterale • Pars lacrimalis: lacrimal canaliculus, eyelid margins	Closes the eyelids (tight closure) Eyelid closure Extends the lacrimal sac
M. depressor supercilii (separation of the Pars orbitalis from the M. orbicularis oculi, ➤ Fig. 9.17)		
Pars nasalis of the Os frontale, bridge of the nose	Medial third of the skin of the eyebrows	Lowers the skin of the eyebrows
M. corrugator supercilii (➤ Fig. 9.17)		
Pars nasalis of the Os frontale	Middle third of the skin of the eyebrows	Pulls the skin of the forehead and eyebrows towards the root of the nose, creates a vertical fold above the root of the nose (anger, thinking)
M. procerus (➤ Fig. 9.17)		
Os nasale	Skin of the glabella	Horizontal folding of the bridge of the nose (frowning)
Nose		
M. nasalis (➤ Fig. 9.17)		
• Pars alaris: Maxilla at the level of the lateral incisor tooth • Pars transversa: Maxilla at the level of the canine tooth	• Pars alaris: nasal wings, edge of the nostrils • Pars transversa: tendon plate of the bridge of the nose	Moves the nostrils and thus the nose • Pars alaris: expands the nostrils • Pars transversa: narrows the nostrils
M. depressor septi nasi (➤ Fig. 9.17)		
Maxilla at the level of the medial incisor tooth	Cartilago septi nasi	Moves the nose downwards
Mouth		
M. orbicularis oris (➤ Fig. 9.17)		
Pars marginalis and Pars labialis: lateral of the Angulus oris	Skin of the lips	Closes the lips, tips of the mouth
M. buccinator (➤ Fig. 9.17)		
Maxilla, Raphe pterygomandibularis, Mandibula	Angulus oris	Tenses the lips, results in an increase of the internal pressure of the oral cavity, e.g. when blowing or chewing
M. levator labii superioris (➤ Fig. 9.17)		
Maxilla via Foramen infraorbitale	Upper lip	Pulls the upper lip laterally upwards
M. depressor labii inferioris (➤ Fig. 9.17)		
Mandibula below the Foramen mentale	Bottom lip	Pulls the lower lip laterally downwards
M. mentalis (➤ Fig. 9.17)		
Mandibula at the level of the lower lateral incisor tooth	Skin of the chin	Creates chin dimples, pushes the lower lip forwards (together with the M. orbicularis oris; 'pout')

Table 9.8 Mimic muscles. The facial nerve [VII] is responsible for innervation *(continued)*

Origins	Attachment	Function
M. transversus menti		
Transverse separation from the M. mentalis	Skin of chin bulge	Moves the chin skin
M. depressor anguli oris (➤ Fig. 9.17)		
Lower rim of the Mandibula	Angulus oris	Pulls the mouth downwards
M. risorius (➤ Fig. 9.17, ➤ Fig. 9.18)		
Fascia parotidea, Fascia masseterica	Angulus oris	Broadens the mouth (grin), creates dimples
M. levator anguli oris (➤ Fig. 9.17)		
Fossa canina of the Maxilla	Angulus oris	Pulls the mouth angle medially upwards
M. zygomaticus major (➤ Fig. 9.17)		
Os zygomaticum	Angulus oris	Pulls the mouth angle laterally upwards
M. zygomaticus minor (➤ Fig. 9.17)		
Os zygomaticum	Angulus oris	Pulls the mouth angle laterally upwards
M. levator labii superioris alaeque nasi (➤ Fig. 9.18)		
Proc. frontalis of the Maxilla (medial Orbita wall)	Nasal wings, upper lip	Lifts the lips and the nasal wing
Throat		
Platysma (➤ Fig. 9.17, ➤ Fig. 9.18)		
Basis mandibulae, Fascia parotidea	Skin underneath the Clavicula, Fascia pectoralis	Tenses the skin of the neck, generates longitudinal folds

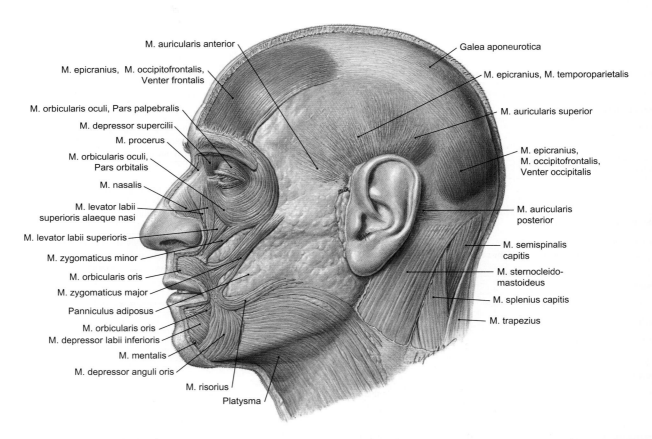

Fig. 9.18 Facial muscles (Mm. faciei) left. Lateral view. The M. occipitofrontalis is connected by a connective tissue plate (Galea aponeurotica) and is divided into a front (Venter frontalis) and posterior part (Venter occipitalis). The Platysma is in scope and size highly variable, developed more strongly in men than in women and ranges from the base of the Mandibula to above the Clavicula (sometimes even up to the Fascia pectoralis).

Vascular, lymphatic and nervous systems
Friedrich Paulsen

In the Regio facialis anterior the arteries, veins and nerves run largely independently of each other to supply the soft tissue coating.

Arteries

The arterial blood supply is mostly undertaken by branches of the A. carotis externa (➤ Fig. 9.13, ➤ Fig. 9.19, ➤ Fig. 9.20) and to a minor degree by a branch of the A. carotis interna.

A. carotis externa

The **A. facialis** is the most important arterial vessel of the middle facial region. It originates in the throat area in the Fossa retromandibularis from the A. carotis externa and passes diagonally towards the upper front . It runs on the inside of the Angulus mandibulae runs up to the posterior margin of the Glandula submandibularis to the front and turns at the Corpus mandibulae from the outside over the bones. From here it continues in a diagonal course past

the M. masseter (where it is strongly coiled [reserve stretching apparatus]), laterally at the corner of the mouth and past the nose towards the nasal corner of the eye. It enters here as the A. angularis into the Orbita. It its course the artery is located
- below the Platysma, M. risorius, M. zygomaticus major, M. zygomaticus minor
- above the M. masseter, M. buccinator, M. levator anguli oris
- above the M. levator labii superioris or penetrates it

Branches of the A. facialis are:
- **A. labialis inferior:** supplies the upper lip with blood
- **A. labialis superior:** supplies the upper lip and with an **A. septi nasi** anterior parts of the nasal septum with blood
- **A. nasalis lateralis:** serves the blood supply of nasal wing and the bridge of the nose

The terminal branch of the A. facialis is the **A. angularis.** It anastomoses with the A. dorsalis nasi (see below).

> **NOTE**
>
> The Aa. labiales inferiores and the Aa. labiales superiores on both sides anastomose with each other and form a vascular ring around the mouth.

The **A. maxillaris** (➤ Fig. 9.20) emits several branches for the supply of the face:
- **A. infraorbitalis:** enters through the Foramen infraorbitale and supplies the Regio infraorbitalis with blood

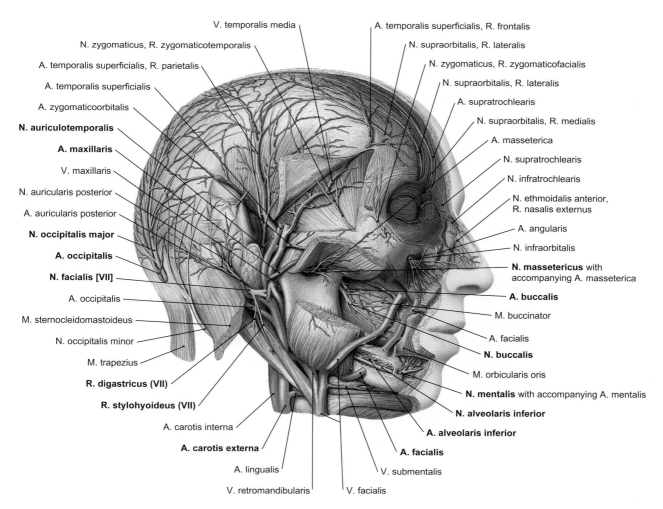

Fig. 9.19 Vessels and nerves in the Fossa retromandibularis.

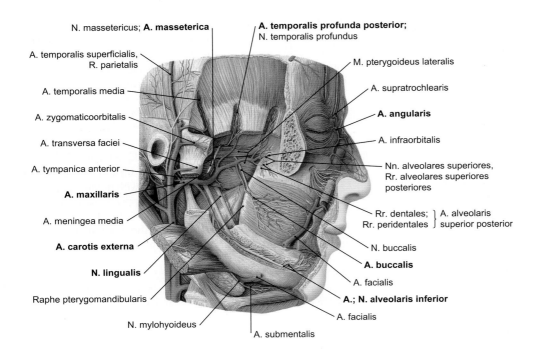

Fig. 9.20 Arteries and nerves of the deep facial regions.

- **A. alveolaris inferior, R. mentalis:** passes through the Foramen mentale to the chin and supplies a small area of the chin with blood
- **A. buccalis:** arrives at the outside of the M. buccinator to the face and supplies a border area of the mid-facial region

The **A. temporalis superficialis** ascends in the lateral facial region in front of the ear to the temporal region and emits branches in the direction of the mid-facial region:

- **A. transversa faciei:** arrives at the front edge of the Glandula parotidea in the lateral facial region and reaches the Regio infraorbitalis with its branches
- **A. zygomaticoorbitalis:** passes above the Arcus zygomaticus to the lateral corner of the eye

A. carotis interna

The **A. ophthalmica** lies in the Orbita and emits smaller branches for the blood supply of the face:

- **A. dorsalis nasi:** terminal branch of the A. ophthalmica, exits mostly at the nasal corner of the eyelid and supplies the bridge of the nose
- **R. nasalis externus of the A. ethmoidalis:** passes at the cartilage-bone demarcation of the bridge of the nose to the surface and contributes to the blood supply to the external nose
- **A. zygomaticofacialis:** branch of the A. lacrimalis, passes through the Foramen zygomaticofaciale into the face and sup-

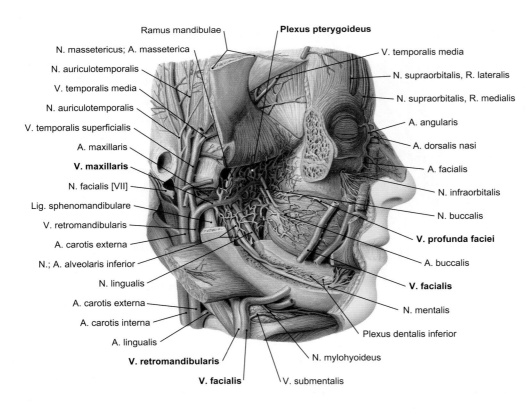

Fig. 9.21 Veins and nerves of the lateral deeper facial region.

plies the area above the Arcus zygomaticus to above the lateral area of the upper eyelid
- **Aa. palpebrales laterales:** branches of the A. lacrimalis, which pass through the Foramen zygomaticotemporale or Foramen zygomaticofaciale to the Regio zygomatica and to the Fossa temporalis; are involved in the formation of the Arcus palpebrales in the upper and the lower eyelids
- **Aa. palpebrales mediales:** branches of the A. supratrochlearis and are involved in the formation of the Arcus palbebrales of the upper and the lower eyelids

Veins
The main vessel of the middle facial region is the **V. facialis,** which originates as **V. angularis** in the nasal corner of the eye (➤ Fig. 9.14). First, the vein runs behind the artery, then passes more dorsally below the Mm. zygomatici major and minor in front of the M. masseter over the M. buccalis. At the Corpus mandibulae, the V. and A. facialis lie next to each other again, the artery crosses the Mandibula in front of the vein before both vessels reach the Glandula submandibularis. The V. angularis is connected via the Orbita to the V. ophthalmica superior and via this with the Sinus cavernosus. There are connections from the V. facialis via the **V. transversa faciei** to the V. temporalis superficialis. The V. facialis combines with the V. retromandibularis and flows into the V. jugularis interna (➤ Fig. 9.21). In addition, all of the abovementioned arteries of the middle facial region are accompanied by veins, which connect to the larger vein stems. They are named the same as the arteries. The course of the veins varies greatly in the facial area.

Lymph vessels
The lymph of the middle facial region (➤ Fig. 9.15) is drained to the:
- **Nodi lymphoidei submentales**
- **Nodi lymphoidei submandibulares**
- Nodi lymphoidei faciales buccales (inconstant)
- **Nodi lymphoidei parotidei**

Innervation
Sensory
Sensory information from the middle facial region passes via the branches of the **N. trigeminus [V]** and a branch from the **Plexus cervicalis** to the CNS (➤ Fig. 9.19, ➤ Fig. 9.20, ➤ Fig. 9.21). Innervation by the
- **N. ophthalmicus [V/1]** of the upper part of the face, including the forehead to the vertex, the upper eyelids, the nasal corner of the eyelid and bridge of the nose
- **N. maxillaris [V/2]** of the middle face from the lower eyelids up to the corners of the mouth including the upper lip and the nostrils
- **N. mandibularis [V/3]** of the lower part of the face with lower lip and chin up to the lower rim of the Mandibula
- **N. auricularis magnus** (Rr. anteriores of C2 and C3) of a small area in front of and below the ear lobes and the mandibular angle

Detailed information on sensoy innervation is summarised in ➤ Table 9.9.

Motor
The facial muscles, the mimic muscles around the auricle and those inserted on the scalp emerge from the 2nd pharyngeal arch. The nerve of the 2nd pharangeal arch is the **N. facialis [VII],** which innervates all the facial muscles(➤ Fig. 9.22). After leaving via the Foramen stylomastoideum on the external skull base, the nerve turns forward and enters the Glandula parotidea, where it forms the *Plexus parotideus*. Its main stem often divides into an upper *R. temporofacialis* and a lower *R. cervicofacialis*. Between the two

Table 9.9 Sensory innervation of the face.

Branch	Innervation area	Point of penetration
N. ophthalmicus [V/1]		
• N. lacrimalis	Lateral area of the upper lid	
• N. frontalis		
• R. medialis of the N. supraorbitalis	Middle portions of the forehead to the vertex	Incisura frontalis
• R. lateralis of the N. supraorbitalis	Lateral portions of the forehead to the vertex	Incisura supraorbitalis (Foramen supraorbitale)
• N. supratrochlearis	Medial area of the upper and the lower eyelids	From the Orbita
• N. nasociliaris		
• N. infratrochlearis	Skin at the nasal corner of the eyes	From the Orbita
• Rr. nasales externi from N. ethmoidalis anterior	Skin of the bridge of the nose	
N. maxillaris [V/2]		
• N. infraorbitalis		Foramen infraorbitale
• Rr. palpebrales inferiores	Lower eyelids, particularly lateral area	
• Rr. nasales externi and interni	Outer nose and Vestibulum nasi	
• Rr. labiales superiores	Upper lip	
• N. zygomaticus		
• R. zygomaticofacialis	Skin above the Os zygomaticum	Foramen zygomaticofaciale
• R. zygomatico-temporalis	Frontal area of the temple	Foramen zygomaticotemporale
N. mandibularis [V/3]		
• N. auriculotemporalis		
• Rr. temporales superficiales	Temporal region in front and above the auricle	
• Nn. auriculares anteriores	The front part of the auricle surface	
• N. buccalis	Skin of the cheek	
• N. mentalis from N. alveolaris inferior	Skin of the chin and the lower lip	
Plexus cervicalis		
• N. auricularis magnus	Jaw angle and ear lobes	From Punctum nervosum (ERB's point)

branches a number of fibres are exchanged (hence Plexus parotideus) within the parotid gland in the procedure. At the top, front and lower rim of the Glandula parotidea, 5 terminal branch groups emerge from the plexus parotideus: **Rr. temporales, Rr. zygomatici, Rr. buccales, R. marginalis mandibulae and R. colli.** In principle, the distribution pattern is variable, but basically the 5 terminal branch groups, which according to ➤ Table 9.10 innervate the facial muscles, can be distinguished. Shortly after leaving the Foramen stylomastoideum, the **N. auricularis posterior** runs back to innervate the mimic muscles behind and above the ear and the Venter posterior of the M. occipitofrontalis (➤ Table 9.10).

Vegetative
Postganglionic **parasympathetic nerve fibres** for the innervation of blood vessels and skin glands of the middle facial region originate from the Ganglion pterygopalatinum and the Ganglion oticum.

435

Table 9.10 Motor branches of the N. facialis [VII] for innervation of the facial muscles.

Muscle	Branch
Venter frontalis of the M. occipitofrontalis	Rr. temporales
M. corrugator supercilii	Rr. temporales
M. orbicularis oculi (above the eyelids)	Rr. temporales
M. procerus	Rr. temporales and/or Rr. zygomatici
M. depressor supercilii	Rr. temporales and/or Rr. zygomatici
M. orbicularis oculi (below the eyelids)	Rr. zygomatici
M. levator labii superioris alaeque nasi	Rr. zygomatici
M. zygomaticus major	Rr. zygomatici
M. zygomaticus minor	Rr. zygomatici
M. levator labii superioris	Rr. zygomatici
M. nasalis	Rr. zygomatici and/or Rr. buccales
M. depressor septi nasi	Rr. zygomatici and/or Rr. buccales
M. buccinator	Rr. zygomatici and/or Rr. buccales
M. levator anguli oris	Rr. zygomatici and/or Rr. buccales
M. orbicularis oris	Rr. buccales
M. depressor anguli oris	Rr. buccales
M. transversus menti	Rr. buccales
M. risorius	Rr. buccales
M. depressor labii inferioris	R. marginalis mandibulae
M. mentalis	R. marginalis mandibulae
Platysma	R. colli
Venter occipitalis of the M. occipitofrontalis	N. auricularis posterior
M. temporoparietalis	R. auricularis of the N. auricularis posterior
M. auricularis inferior	R. auricularis of the N. auricularis posterior
M. auricularis anterior	R. auricularis of the N. auricularis posterior
M. auricularis superior	R. auricularis of the N. auricularis posterior

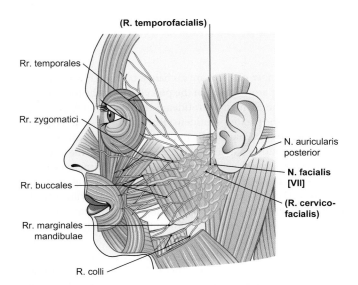

Fig. 9.22 Terminal branches of the N. facialis [VII]. [E402]

Sympathetic nerve fibres are derived from postganglionic neurons of the Ganglion cervicale superius, which run as periarterial plexusi with the branches of the A. carotis externa (Plexus caroticus externus) or the A. carotis interna (Plexus caroticus internus) and e.g. innervate blood vessels, sweat glands and hair. Some nerve fibres connect in the area of the Ganglion trigeminale to the branches of the N. trigeminus [V] and reach their target areas of the face in this way.

9.2.4 Superficial lateral facial region
Friedrich Paulsen

Limits of the Regio facialis lateralis superficialis are the Sulcus nasolabialis, the external ear to the Proc. mastoideus, the Arcus zygomaticus and the lower margin of the Corpus mandibulae. It is divided into
- **Regio buccalis** and
- **Regio parotideomasseterica.**

Surface anatomy
Regio buccalis
The central element of the Regio buccalis is the **M. buccinator** (➤ Fig. 9.19, ➤ Fig. 9.20), which forms the basis of the cheek. It is the only mimic muscle with a fascia (Fascia buccopharyngea). Its front muscle fibres radiate into the corner of the mouth, where they end in muscular nodes (Modiolus anguli oris). Here all muscles extending to the corners of the mouth interlace. Mucous membrane of the oral vestibule in this area is fused with the underlying musculature and is immovable. At the level of the second upper molar the **Ductus parotideus** (STENSEN's duct) penetrates the muscle. To the rear, the M. buccinator passes into the **Raphe pterygomandibularis**, which originates at the Proc. pterygoideus and runs to the Ramus mandibulae. It is not only the attachment point for the M. buccinator, but also for the M. constrictor pharyngis superior and forms the border to the Regio parotideomasseterica. Between the Raphe pterygomandibularis and the M. pterygoideus medialis running on the inside of the Ramus mandibulae there is a gap. It is filled by a **fatty body (Corpus adiposum buccae, BICHAT's fat-pad)** (➤ Fig. 9.23), the front part of which bulges out into the Regio buccalis over the rear end of the M. buccinator. The fatty body consists of structural fat.

On the bottom edge of the fatty body, the Ductus parotideus extends into the depth and penetrates the M. buccinator. The juxtaoral organ (CHIEVITZ's organ) lies on the M. buccinator near to the site where the Ductus parotideus penetrates (➤ Fig. 9.23). The M. zygomaticus major, the M. risorius and the upper part of the Platysma run in the Regio buccalis.

Clinical remarks

In the case of severe emaciation (e.g. due to cancer cachexia [wasting]) existing cheek fat made from structural fat can be broken down. The cheeks then appear sunken. the same is true for the structural fat in the Orbita, the eyes 'fall back into the eyeball'. The BICHAT's fat-pad therefore gives the cheek its contour.

N O T E

The **juxtaoral organ (CHIEVITZ's organ)** is a small, approximately 8×3 mm epithelial organ in the cheek, which is embedded in connective tissue rich in nerves and cells, and surrounded by a tight perineural sheath. A branch of the N. buccalis reaches the organ,

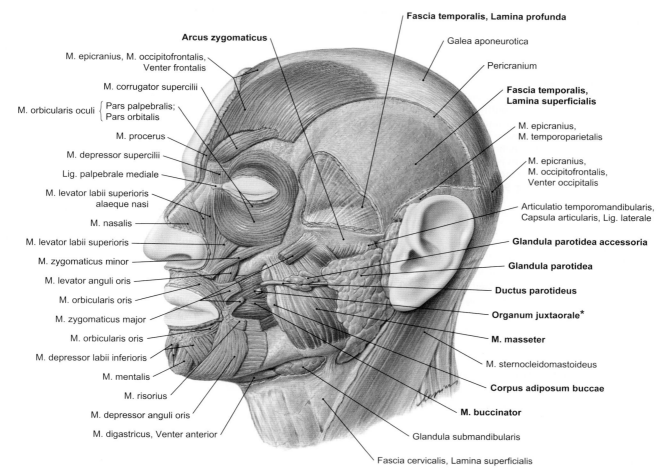

Fig. 9.23 Facial muscles, Mm. faciei, masticatory muscles and juxtaoral organ CHIEVITZ's organ.

providing blood supply from the Fossa infratemporalis (see below) via the A. buccalis. The function of the juxtaoral organ has not been conclusively clarified. It is assumed to have a receptor function, which recognises dynamic changes in chewing, swallowing and speaking and, among other things, helps to ensure that one does not bite the cheeks when chewing.

Clinical remarks

In the past due to a lack of knowledge the juxtaoral organ was frequently confused with a malignant **tumour,** which resulted in extensive and partially disfiguring operations.

Regio parotideomasseterica

The Regio parotideomasseterica extends from the anterior margin of the M. masseter upwards to the Arcus zygomaticus and downwards to the front edge of the upper part of the M. sternocleidomastoideus. Between the rear edge of the Ramus mandibulae and the anterior border of the M. sternocleidomastoideus or Proc. mastoideus is the **retromandibular space (Fossa retromandibularis),** which is filled mainly from the deep part of the **Glandula parotidea** (➤ Chap. 9.7.9). The superficial part of the gland partially overlaps the M. masseter. The glandular tissue extends upwards variably until the tragus and extends caudally to close to the Glandula submandibularis (➤ Fig. 9.23). The parotid gland is covered on the surface by a single fascia (Fascia parotidea, see below). Through the fascia and the Fossa retromandibularis, a compartment is created **(parotid gland compartment).** On the front of the

superficial part of the Glandula parotidea the ductus parotideus (STENSEN's duct) leaves the gland and passes in a horizontal course through the fascia of the M. masseter up to its front edge. Here it bends into the depths and penetrates the M. buccinator (see above). In its course, it is accompanied in variable shape by the salivary gland tissue (Glandulae parotideae accessoriae).

Fascia of the superficial lateral facial region

The M. masseter and M. temporalis have their own fascia. The **Fascia masseterica** covers the M. masseter and divides into a superficial and a deep layer that includes as a fascia compartment the Mm. pterygoidei lateralis and medialis as well as the M. masseter. The superficial layer is connected to the fascia sheet that covers the Glandula parotidea (**Fascia parotidea**). Both leaves together form the **Fascia parotideomasseterica.** The deep layer includes the Mm. pterygoidei. The **Fascia temporalis** also consists of a superficial and a deep layer. The strong Fascia temporalis originates along the Linea temporalis superficialis. It is the original field for the superficial parts of the M. temporalis. It therefore covers the M. temporalis and splits approximately 1–1.5 cm above the zygomatic arch into a superficial and a deep layer. The superficial layer inserts at the outer edge of the zygomatic arch, the deep layer extends to the inner edge of the zygomatic arch. Therefore, a fat-filled osteofibrous space is created between both sheets.

The M. buccinator, as the only mimic muscle, is enveloped by a fascia (**Fascia buccopharyngea**). In addition, the Glandula parotidea is enclosed by a fascia (Fascia parotidea). The Fascia masseterica and Fascia parotidea are part of the superficial throat fascia layer (**Fascia cervicalis superficialis**).

In conjunction with loose subcutis connective tissue of the facial skin and with the facial muscles in the face, the fasciae form a thin, but surprisingly resistant layer, which is referred to in its entirety as **the superficial muscular aponeurotic system (SMAS)**. It extends to the scalp. The SMAS plays the decisive role in plastic surgery for **facelifting**: the SMAS can be dissected in the direction of the face and released from the base by means of an arc-shaped incision in front of the ear. A part of the dissected tissue is then removed and the cut edge with all pertaining hanging structures is moved in the direction of the ear and firmly sutured. The facial skin is practically tautened in the process (➤ Fig. 9.24).

Vascular, lymphatic and nervous systems

The vascular, lymphatic and nervous systems of the superficial lateral facial region are divided according to their course:
- Vascular, lymphatic and nervous systems in the parotid gland compartment (either for the innervation of the gland or as a transit route)
- Vascular, lymphatic and nervous systems outside the parotid gland compartment

Vascular, lymphatic and nervous systems of the parotid gland compartment

These include the A. carotis externa, the V. retromandibularis, the N. facialis [VII] and the N. auriculotemporalis (from [V/3]).
The **A. carotis externa** reaches the Fossa retromandibularis from medial below the throat area, where it still runs in the carotid artery sheath, Glandula parotidea and rises in a cranial direction. It then divides usually at the level of the Collum mandibulae into the A. maxillaris and the A. temporalis superficialis (➤ Fig. 9.19). The **A. maxillaris** remains in the depth of the Fossa retromandibularis and generally extends behind the Ramus mandibulae into the lateral deep facial regions (see below). The **A. temporalis superficialis** rises upwards through the gland parenchyma and reaches the surface at the upper edge of the Glandula parotidea together with the V. temporalis superficialis. Both vessels run from the outer ear via the zygomatic arch further cranially into the Regio temporalis and branch out. The **A. transversa faciei** is a branch of the A. temporalis superficialis and supplies a part of the superficial lateral facial

region with blood. It generally branches in the gland parenchyma of the Glandula parotidea almost at right angles from the Aa. temporalis superficialis and then runs in a horizontal, slightly descending direction over the upper part of the M. masseter through the lateral facial region forwards to the Regio infraorbitalis. Anastomoses with branches of the A. facialis are possible.
The **V. retromandibularis** (➤ Fig. 9.19) forms the continuation of the V. temporalis superficialis caudally and drains its blood. Its largest portion runs within the Glandula parotidea. Here it incorporates the Vv. maxillares and usually runs superficially to the A. carotis externa. At the lower gland pole it leaves the gland and flows after a short course into the V. facialis.
The **N. facialis [VII]** after leaving the Foramen stylomastoideum from dorsal extends into the Glandula parotidea. It divides here superficially to the abovementioned vessels usually within the glandular tissue into an upper and a lower branch (➤ Fig. 9.22). Both branches exchange numerous fibres *(Plexus intraparotideus)*, continue to branch out and eventually form 5 terminal branch groups (➤ Chap. 9.2.3):
- Rr. temporales
- Rr. zygomatici
- Rr. buccales
- R. marginalis mandibulae
- R. colli

Operations within the Glandula parotidea (e.g. in the case of parotid gland tumours) are extremely challenging due to the close topographic relationship between the gland and the N. facialis [VII], since all nerve branches have to be retained to avoid triggering a partial paralysis of the facial muscles (peripheral damage of the N. facialis [VII]). Since the Fascia parotidea does not stretch **swelling caused by inflammation** (e.g. in the case of Parotitis epidemica = mumps) is extremely painful.

The **N. auriculotemporalis** (from [V/3]) extends behind the Collum mandibulae into the Fossa retromandibularis (➤ Fig. 9.20). In doing so, it often envelops the A. meningea media in a loop form. Shortly after its entry into the Glandula parotidea, it divides into several branches:
- The main trunk runs cranially in front of the outer ear and merges with the A. temporalis superficialis (**Rr. temporales superficiales**).
- The other branches within the Glandula parotidea extend
  - to the mandibular joint capsule (**R. capsularis articulationis temporomandibularis**)
  - to the front surface of the auricle (**Nn. auriculares anteriores**)
  - to the external auditory canal (**N. meatus acustici externi**)
  - to the tympanic membrane (**Rr. membranae tympani**)
  - directly to the Glandula parotidea (**Rr. parotidei**)
  - indirectly via the branches of the N. facialis (**Rr. communicantes cum nervo faciali**)

The **Rr. parotidei** and the **Rr. communicantes cum nervo faciali** lead postganglionic parasympathetic fibres for the innervation of the parotid gland. The cell body of the preganglionic fibres originate from the Nucleus salivatorius inferior and extend via the N. glossopharyngeus via the N. tympanicus (JACOBSON's plexus), Plexus tympanicus and N. petrosus minor to the Ganglion oticum where the switch to postganglionic is made. From here, the post-gangionic fibres initially extend to the N. mandibularis [V/3] and then into the N. auriculotemporalis. Recent research suggests

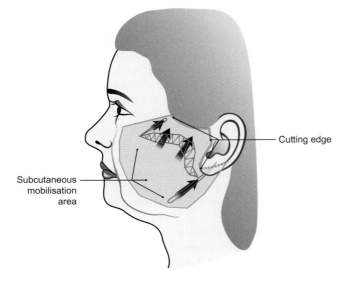

Subcutaneous mobilisation area

Cutting edge

Fig. 9.24 Facelifting. [L126]

that the parasympathetic fibres reach the Glandula parotidea only via Rr. parotidei of the N. auriculotemporalis and not via Rr. communicantes cum nervo faciale; however, this has not yet been conclusively clarified.

Vascular, lymphatic and nervous systems outside the parotid gland compartment

These include (➤ Fig. 9.19, ➤ Fig. 9.20) the A. and V facialis, the A. transversa faciei, the A. and V. buccalis and the N. buccalis.

The **A. facialis** and **V. facialis** usually run separately via the front portion of the M. buccinator and in front of the M. masseter. The artery runs in a coiled path and lies mostly in front of the vein – its pulse can be felt above the Corpus mandibula. In the Regio buccalis anastomoses with the **A. transversa faciei** (from A. temporalis superficialis) and the A. buccalis (a branch of the A. maxillaris) are common. The vein extends via the Angulus mandibulae caudally and to the rear and merges below the Angulus mandibulae with the V. retromandibularis to flow into the V. jugularis interna.

The **A. buccalis** and **V. buccalis** reach the lateral facial region from the rear (➤ Fig. 9.20). They extend between the M. pterygoideus medialis and M. buccinator to the surface and branch out onto the M. buccinator to supply blood to the muscle. Anastomoses often occur to the A. and V. facialis.

The **N. buccalis** reaches the cheek together with the Vasa buccalia via the Fossa infratemporalis (see below) (➤ Fig. 9.20). It is responsible for the sensory innervation of the skin above the cheek and the buccal and vestibular gingiva in the area of the molar teeth; however, the innervation can extend to the canine teeth.

9.2.5 Deep lateral facial region
Friedrich Paulsen

Fossa infratemporalis

The temporal fossa (Fossa temporalis) continues below the Arcus zygomaticus caudally into the **infratemporal fossa (Fossa infratemporalis)**. As such the latter belongs to the deep part of the lateral facial region (Regio facialis lateralis profunda) and stretches into the depth of the external skull base. Its limitations and relationships are summarised in ➤ Table 9.11 (➤ Fig. 9.5).

The contents of the Fossa infratemporalis are muscles and vascular, lymphatic and nervous systems. Muscles are (➤ Fig. 9.25):

- **M. pterygoideus medialis:** its attachment to the mandibula forms the caudal limit to the Fossa infratemporalis. The slit-like pterygomandibular space (Spatium pterygomandibulare) lies between the muscle and the mandibula.
- **M. pterygoideus lateralis**

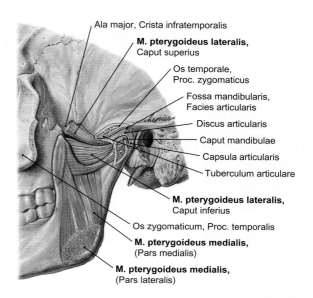

Fig. 9.25 Location of the Mm. pterygoidei in the Fossa infratemporalis.

- **M. buccinator:** only a small rear part of the muscle with the transition to the M. constrictor pharyngis superior lies in the Fossa infratemporalis and is covered by the M. pterygoideus medialis. The front portion is part of the superficial lateral facial region (see above).

Vascular, lymphatic and nervous systems

Vascular, lymphatic and nervous systems of the Fossa infratemporalis are the intermuscular part of the A. maxillaris (Pars pterygoidea), of the venous Plexus pterygoideus the branching of the N. mandibularis [V/3], the Ganglion oticum and the Chorda tympani.

The **A. maxillaris** is one of the two terminal branches of the A. carotis externa. It moves at a right angle behind the mandibular ramus into the Fossa infratemporalis (➤ Fig. 9.20). It therefore runs in front of the Lig. sphenomandibulare. It penetrates the Fossa infratemporalis mostly lateral to the M. pterygoideus lateralis and less often it penetrates the muscle medially. Its end section extends into the Fossa pterygopalatina. The artery has numerous vessel exits and is divided into three sections (➤ Table 9.12).

The **Plexus venosus pterygoideus** is a distinctive venous plexus between M. temporalis, M. pterygoideus lateralis and M. pterygoideus medialis (➤ Fig. 9.21). Its inflows and outflows are summarised in ➤ Table 9.13. In addition to the drainage of blood it also has a function within the scope of temperature regulation of the brain.

Table 9.11 Bony margins and relationships of the Fossa infratemporalis.

Direction	Limitation	Connection/neighbourhood relationships
Cranial	Facies infratemporalis of the Ala major ossis sphenoidalis, lower front part of the Os temporale	Foramen ovale (N. mandibularis [V/3]), Foramen spinosum (A. meningea media, R. meningeus from [V/3]) with the middle cranial fossa, under the zygomatic arch with the Fossa temporalis
Medial	Lamina lateralis of the Proc. pterygoideus ossis sphenoidalis	Opens into the Fossa pterygopalatina
Rostral	Facies infratemporalis and Proc. alveolaris maxillae, Facies temporalis ossis zygomatici	Fissura orbitalis inferior with the orbit, Regio buccalis, Foramina alveolaria to the Tuber maxillae
Lateral	Ramus mandibulae with Proc. coronoideus (and the attachment of the M. temporalis), Arcus zygomaticus	Foramen mandibulae with the mandibula
Occipital	Arcus zygomaticus ossis temporalis	Fossa retromandibularis (parotid gland compartment), peripharyngeal space (Spatium peripharyngeum)

Table 9.12 Sections and branches of the A. maxillaris.

Section	Branch	Blood supply
Pars mandibularis (Fossa retromandibularis)	A. auricularis profunda	Temporomandibular joint, auditory canal, tympanic membrane
	A. tympanica anterior	Middle ear
	A. alveolaris inferior • Rr. dentales • Rr. peridentales • R. mentalis • R. mylohyoideus	Lower teeth, chin, floor of the mouth
	A. meningea media	Meninges
	(A. pterygomeningea [A. meningea accessoria]) (not regularly formed)	M. pterygoideus lateralis, M. pterygoideus medialis, M. tensor veli palatini, Tuba auditiva, Meninges
Pars pterygoidea (Fossa infratemporalis)	A. masseterica	M. masseter
	A. temporalis profunda anterior	M. temporalis
	A. temporalis profunda posterior	M. temporalis
	Rr. pterygoidei	M. pterygoideus lateralis, M. pterygoideus medialis
	A. buccalis	M. buccinator
Pars pterygopalatina (Fossa pterygopalatina)	A. alveolaris superior posterior • Rr. dentales • Rr. peridentales	Maxilla, upper teeth, upper jaw gums, Sinus maxillaris

	A. infraorbitalis
	• Aa. alveolares superiores anteriores
	  – Rr. dentales
	  – Rr. peridentales
		Adjacent extra-ocular muscles, upper part of the efferent lacrimal ducts, upper teeth, Sinus maxillaris, upper part of the front face half under the Orbita

	A. canalis pterygoidei	Nasopharynx, Tuba auditiva
	A. palatina descendens • A. palatina major • Aa. palatinae minores	Palate
	A. sphenopalatina	Large parts of the nose and paranasal sinuses, KIESSELBACH's area

Table 9.13 Inflows and outflows of the Plexus venosus pterygoideus.

Inflows	Outflows
• V. sphenopalatina • V. ophthalmica inferior • V. alveolaris inferior • Vv. temporales profundae • Vv. meningeae mediae	• V. maxillaris • V. retromandibularis • V. profunda faciei • V. facialis • Sinus cavernosus

The **N. mandibularis [V/3]** reaches the Fossa infratemporalis via the *Foramen ovale*. Here, it divides into its branches, whose courses within the sub-temporal fossa are summarised in ➤ Table 9.14 (➤ Fig. 9.26, ➤ Fig. 9.35).

Clinical remarks

Due to the connection of the valveless veins of the Plexus venosus pterygoideus to the Sinus cavernosus pathogen transmission with subsequent thrombosis of the Sinus cavernosus can occur in bacterial infections of the face **(Sinus cavernosus thrombosis)** (➤ Chap. 11.5.8).

The **Chorda tympani** (➤ Fig. 9.37) lies on the N. lingualis medial of the M. pterygoideus medialis. It reaches the Fossa infratemporalis after passing through the *Fissura sphenopetrosa* (medial and dorsal of the mandibular joint) in the skull base (the Fissura petrotympanica [GLASER's fissure] lies in close proximity laterally from the Fissura sphenopetrosa); however, contrary to popular

Table 9.14 Branches and courses of the N. mandibularis [V/3] in the Fossa infratemporalis; innervation areas.

Branch	Course	Innervation
R. meningeus	Backflow through the Foramen spinosum into the middle cranial fossa	Parts of the meninges
N. massetericus	From medial through the Incisura mandibulae to the	M. masseter
Nn. temporales profundi	From medial to the	M. temporalis
N. pterygoideus lateralis	From medial to the	M. pterygoideus lateralis
N. pterygoideus medialis	From medial to the	M. pterygoideus medialis
N. musculi tensoris veli palatini	To the	M. tensor veli palatini
N. musculi tensoris tympani	To the	M. tensor tympani
N. buccalis	Between Caput superius and Caput inferius of the M. pterygoideus lateralis to the	Skin and mucosa of the cheek and gingiva of the lower jaw

Table 9.14 Branches and courses of the N. mandibularis [V/3] in the Fossa infratemporalis; innervation areas. *(continued)*

Branch	Course	Innervation
N. auriculotemporalis	Includes in a loop-shape the A. meningea media and then flexes between the mandibular joint and the external ear canal cranial to the temporal region	Postganglionic fibres from the Ganglion oticum to the parotid gland, external ear canal, tympanic membrane, skin of the auricle, skin of the rear part of the temporal region
N. lingualis	Picks up the Chorda tympani and passes between Mm. pterygoidei lateral from N. alveoaris inferior, below rostrally to the tongue	Skin of the soft palate, mucous membrane of the floor of the mouth, sensory innervation and palate fibres of the anterior two thirds of the tongue, preganglionic parasympathetic fibres to the Ganglion submandibulare
N. alveolaris inferior	Passes behind and to the side of the N. lingualis under the M. pterygoideus lateralis caudally, penetrates through the Foramen mandibulae into the mandibula	Teeth and gingiva of the lower jaw, M. mylohyoideus and Venter anterior of the M. digastricus, skin of the chin

opinion it is not the usual point of penetration for the Chorda tympani through the skull base.

The parasympathetic **Ganglion oticum** (➤ Fig. 9.39) is located close below the Foramen ovale on the medial side of the N. mandibularis [V/3]. Via the Rr. ganglionares it is in contact with the N. mandibularis [V/3].

Fossa pterygopalatina

The funnel-shaped **pterygopalatine fossa (Fossa pterygopalatina)**, which tapers from cranial to caudal, forms the medial continuation of the Fossa infratemporalis. Like the Fossa infratemporalis it belongs to the deep part of the lateral facial region (Regio facialis lateralis profunda) and stretches even further into the depths of the external skull base. The Maxilla, Os palatinum and Os sphenoidale are involved in the bony border of the more or less triangular space (➤ Fig. 9.27). Together the bones form the *Fissura pterygomaxillaris* as the boundary to the Fossa infratemporalis. The limits and relationships of the Fossa pterygopalatina are summarised in ➤ Table 9.15. Functionally, the Fossa pterygopalatina forms a central junction or distribution point for vessels and nerves of the Regio facialis lateralis profunda.

Vascular, lymphatic and nervous systems

Vascular, lymphatic and nervous systems of the Fossa pterygopalatina are the Pars pterygopalatina of the A. maxillaris (➤ Fig. 9.28), accompanying veins of the arterial branches of the Pars pterygopalatina (Vv. infraorbitalis, sphenopalatina, palatina descendens, Vv. canalis pterygoidei), the branches of the N. maxillaris [V/2] and the Ganglion pterygopalatinum.

The end section of the **A. maxillaris** extends into the Fossa pterygopalatina (Pars pterygopalatina). The vessel exits are summarized in ➤ Table 9.12.

The **veins** of the same name accompany the arterial branches of the Pars pterygopalatina and can be taken from ➤ Table 9.16. They are also connected to the Plexus pterygoideus, the V. facialis and the V. ophthalmica inferior.

The **N. maxillaris [V/2]** passes through the Foramen rotundum into the skull base to the Fossa pterygoidea and divides into its

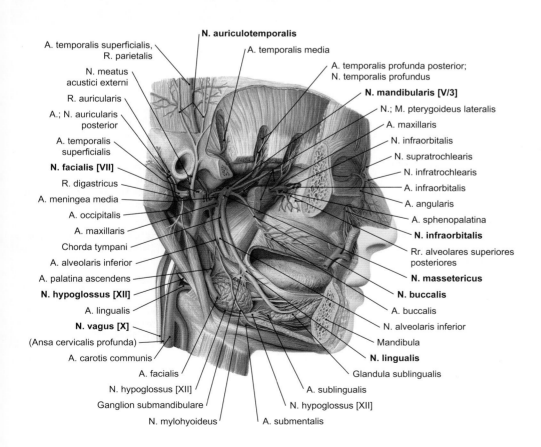

Fig. 9.26 Arteries and nerves in the deep lateral facial region.

Table 9.15 Limits and relationships of the Fossa pterygopalatina.

Direction	Limit	Connection/neighbourhood relationship
Cranial	Corpus ossis sphenoidalis, Radix alae majoris of the Os sphenoidale	
Medial	Lamina perpendicularis ossis palatini (at the same time, it forms the lateral wall of the nasal cavity in the area of the choane)	Foramen sphenopalatinum with the nasal cavity
Rostral	Tuber maxillae, Proc. orbitalis ossis palatini	Fissura orbitalis inferior with the Orbita, Foramina alveolaria posteriora to the Tuber maxillae
Lateral	Fossa infratemporalis	Fissura pterygomaxillaris
Occipital	Facies maxillaris of the Ala major ossis sphenoidalis, front edge of the Proc. pterygoideus ossis sphenoidalis	Foramen rotundum to the middle cranial fossa, Canalis pterygoideus (VIDIANUS canal) with the external skull base
Caudal	Oral cavity	Canalis palatinus major, Canales palatini minores with the palate

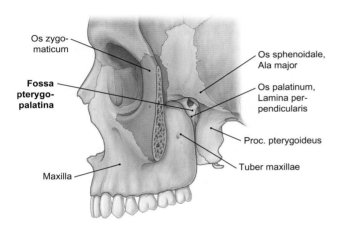

Fig. 9.27 Bony margins of the Fossa pterygopalatina. [E402]

Os zygomaticum
Fossa pterygopalatina
Maxilla
Os sphenoidale, Ala major
Os palatinum, Lamina perpendicularis
Proc. pterygoideus
Tuber maxillae

branches which leave the fossa again via different exit points (➤ Table 9.16, ➤ Fig. 9.29).

The parasympathetic **Ganglion pterygopalatinum** lies at the level of the Foramen sphenopalatinum. It is located medially and below the N. maxillaris [V/2] (➤ Fig. 9.30). Cranially there are fibre connections to the N. maxillaris [V/2]. From the rear the N. canalis pterygoidei reaches the ganglion from the Canalis pterygoideus. It carries preganglionic parasympathetic fibres that can be switched in the ganglion to postganglionic. The sympathetic fibres from the N. canalis pterygoidei (via N. petrosus profundus) are already postganglionic and pass through the ganglion without switching. The sensitive Rr. ganglionares emerging from the Orbita, nose and throat pass the Ganglion pterygopalatinum to the N. maxillaris.

Table 9.16 Connections and relationships of the Fossa pterygopalatina to neighbouring regions, and penetrating structures.

Connection via	Connection to	Pathway
Fissura orbitalis inferior	Orbita	A. infraorbitalis, V. infraorbitalis, N. infraorbitalis (from [V/2]), N. zygomaticus (from [V/2]), Rr. orbitales (from [V/2])
Foramen rotundum	Middle cranial fossa	N. maxillaris [V/2] (with small accompanying arteries)
Canalis pterygoideus (VIDIANUS canal)	External skull base	A. canalis pterygoidei, Vv. canalis pterygoidei, N. canalis pterygoidei (fibres from N. petrosus major – parasympathetic and N. petrosus profundus – sympathetic)
Foramen sphenopalatinum	Nasal cavity	A. sphenopalatina (Aa. nasales posteriores laterales and Rr. septales posteriores), V. sphenopalatina, Rr. nasales posteriores superiores mediales and laterales (from [V/2])
Canalis palatinus major, Canales palatini minores	Palate	A. palatina descendens, A. palatina major, Aa. palatinae minores, V. palatina descendens, N. palatinus major (from [V/2]), Nn. palatini minores (from [V/2])
Fissura pterygomaxillaris	Fissura infratemporalis	A. maxillaris, Plexus pterygoideus
	Foramina alveolaria at the Tuber maxillae	Aa. alveolares superiores posteriores (with accompanying veins), N. alveolaris superioris posterioris (from [V/2])

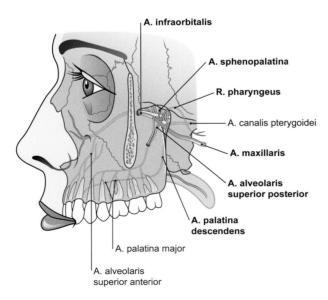

Fig. 9.28 A. maxillaris in the Fossa pterygopalatina. [E402]

A. infraorbitalis
A. sphenopalatina
R. pharyngeus
A. canalis pterygoidei
A. maxillaris
A. alveolaris superior posterior
A. palatina descendens
A. palatina major
A. alveolaris superior anterior

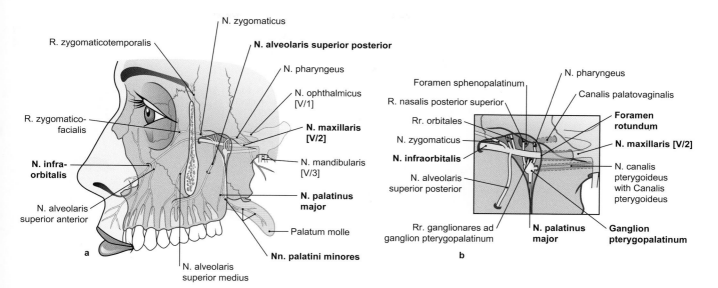

Fig. 9.29 N. maxillaris in the fossa pterygopalatina. a Terminal branches; **b** spatial relationship with the Ganglion pterygopalatinum. [E402]

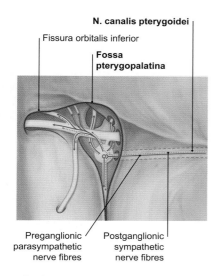

Fig. 9.30 Sympathetic and parasympathetic fibres in the Fossa pterygopalatina. [E402]

9.3 Cranial nerves
Lars Bräuer

Skills

After processing this chapter, you should be able to:
• describe the basic anatomical aspects of origin, course, fibre quality and innervation areas of the 12 cranial nerves

Clinical case

Prolactinoma

Case study
A 32-year-old patient consults her gynaecologist because of amenorrhoea. She also states that there is an enlargement of the breasts, with sporadically occurring milk flow (galactorrhoea).

Diagnostics
The gynaecologist initially suspects a pregnancy, but this is not confirmed. A subsequent mammography (x-ray of the chest) shows no pathological changes of the glandular tissue. Breast cancer can be ruled out. The patient casually reports that she has sometimes noticed blind spots in her field of vision. The gynaecologist takes a sample of the patient's blood to determine her hormonal status, and refers her to an ophthalmologist in the same house for clarification of the ocular symptoms. The ophthalmologist inspects the blind spots more closely and describes the symptoms as 'sporadic bitemporal hemianopsia'. Because this indicates a possible process at the Chiasma opticum (visual nerve intersection), the ophthalmologist immediately arranges for magnetic resonance imaging (MRI) in a radiological practice. The MRI images show a large tumour (macroadenoma) of the pituitary gland (Sella turcica) which is already pressing on the Chiasma opticum from below.
The examination of the blood values by the gynaecologist, shows prolactin levels of 240 ng/ml (reference: < 20 ng/ml), which explain the gynaecological symptoms. The doctors diagnose a prolactinoma (most frequent pituitary tumour).

Treatment
An immediately initiated drug therapy with bromocriptine (dopamine antagonist) causes the tumour to shrink, thus reducing the visual field defects and also the gynaecological complaints recede and after some time disappear completely.

Long-term follow-up
However, after 3 years the patient suffers from the symptoms again and it is concluded that the tumour has grown again (relapse). This time the patient is advised to have it surgically removed through a procedure in which a neurosurgeon gains transnasal and transphenoidal access. After the operation the patient is without complaints.

Note: the cranial nerves are also presented in ➤ Chap. 12.5. The human brain has **12 pairs of cranial nerves,** which are numbered using Roman numerals and have their exit and entry points on the brain and brain stem (➤ Fig. 9.31). All nerves, with the exception of the N. vagus [X] have their supply area in the head and throat area where they innervate all structures, such as glands but also muscles (both striated, as well as smooth). By definition the cranial nerves, with the exception of the N. olfactorius [I] and the N. opticus

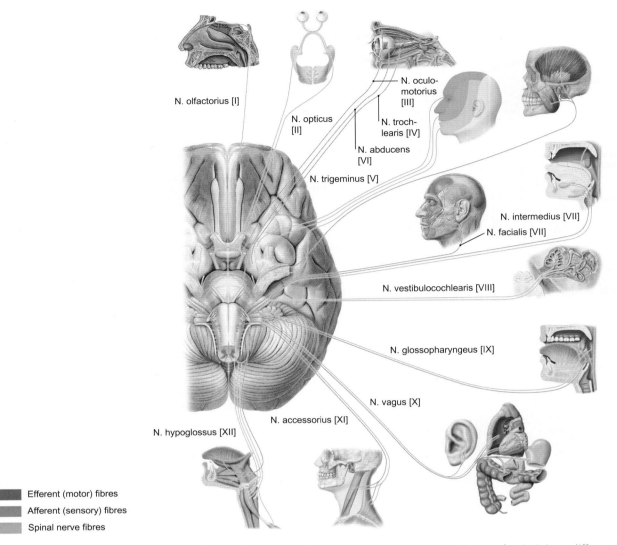

N. olfactorius [I]

N. opticus [II]

N. oculo-motorius [III]

N. troch-learis [IV]

N. abducens [VI]

N. trigeminus [V]

N. intermedius [VII]

N. facialis [VII]

N. vestibulocochlearis [VIII]

N. glossopharyngeus [IX]

N. vagus [X]

N. accessorius [XI]

N. hypoglossus [XII]

■ Efferent (motor) fibres
■ Afferent (sensory) fibres
■ Spinal nerve fibres

Fig. 9.31 Cranial nerves, overview. At the base of the brain there are 12 pairs of cranial nerves exiting (entering), which have different fibre qualities and are numbered from frontal to occipital with Roman numerals from I-XII.

[II] are peripheral nerves. The N. olfactorius [I] and N. opticus [II], however, are an extension of the telencephalon [I] or of the diencephalon [II] and thus belong to the central nervous system. Although the cranial nerves III – XII belong to the peripheral nerves, they differ significantly from them (and from spinal nerves): they are not segmentally arranged have no separate roots for afferent or efferent fibres and also differ significantly with respect to their function and fibre quality. The cranial nerves V, VII, IX, X and XI are derived from the site of the pharyngeal arches (branchial arches) and are therefore also referred to as **branchial nerves**. The following elaborates on the individual nerves, innervation areas and the corresponding ganglia.

9.3.1 N. olfactorius [I]

The N. olfactorius (olfactory nerve), which has special somatoafferent (SSA) fibres, consists of the **Fila olfactoria.** These thin axons that are less myelinated correspond to primary sensory cells originating in the Regio olfactoria (olfactory mucosa) at the roof of the nose (➤ Fig. 9.32). From there they extend through the foramina of the Lamina cribrosa of the Os ethmoidale (ethmoid bone) into the anterior cranial fossa to be switched within the **Bulbus olfacto-**

rius to the 2nd neuron. They then run as **Tractus olfactorius** to the corresponding primary and secondary olfactory areas (e.g. Corpus amygdaloideum) (➤ Chap. 13.6.2). A special feature of the N. olfactorius [I] is that fibres without prior interpretation (extrathalamic) pass directly to the primary and secondary olfactory areas. Smells are therefore of very special significance within the context of the long-term memory. The Fila olfactoria only have a limited life span (about 60 days) and must therefore be constantly renewed from corresponding stem cells.

> **Clinical remarks**
>
> In the context of **basal skull fractures** the Fila olfactoria can become detached at the point of penetration at the Lamina cribrosa. This results in a generally irreversible inability to smell **(anosmia).** If not all Fila olfactoria are damaged, there is an olfactory reduction **(hyposmia).** In this instance, those affected can generally no longer perceive aromatic substances, 'irritating' inorganic compounds, on the other hand (e.g. ammoniac) are perceived via the N. trigeminus [V] and felt as pain (nociception). Very often the patients also suffer from impaired taste sensation as no flavours but only isolated sweet, sour, salty, bitter and umami can be perceived.

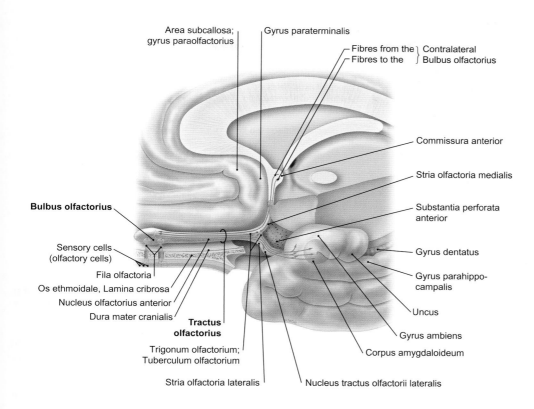

Area subcallosa;
gyrus paraolfactorius

Gyrus paraterminalis

Fibres from the ⎱ Contralateral
Fibres to the ⎰ Bulbus olfactorius

Commissura anterior

Stria olfactoria medialis

Substantia perforata
anterior

Bulbus olfactorius

Gyrus dentatus

Sensory cells
(olfactory cells)

Gyrus parahippo-
campalis

Fila olfactoria

Os ethmoidale, Lamina cribrosa

Uncus

Nucleus olfactorius anterior

Dura mater cranialis

Tractus
olfactorius

Gyrus ambiens

Corpus amygdaloideum

Trigonum olfactorium;
Tuberculum olfactorium

Stria olfactoria lateralis

Nucleus tractus olfactorii lateralis

Fig. 9.32 N. olfactorius with Fila olfactoria. In the roof of the nasal cavity lies the Regio olfactoria with its olfactory sensory cells (primary, bipolar sensory cells = olfactory neurons).

9.3.2 N. opticus [II]

The N. opticus [II] (optic nerve) also has specific somatoafferent (SSA) fibre qualities. During ocular development, it forms as a diverticulum of the diencephalon and is thus an integral part of the brain. The optic tract (➤ Chap. 13.3.1) starts within the retina

- for *colour vision (photopic)* with the first three projection neurons (1. cone cells, 2. cone bipolars, 3. ganglion cells) and interneurons (horizontal cells, amacrine cells)
- for *light-dark vision (scotopic)* containing up to 40 rod cells (1st neuron) which transmit their signal to a bipolar rod (2nd neuron) and then transmit the signal by an indirect way while relaying amacrine cells (3rd neuron) to a ganglia cell (4th neuron)

The approximately 1 million axons are non-myelinated and run to the **Papilla nervi optici** (blind spot) and leave the eyeball there. From the Lamina cribrosa scleri the specific somatoafferent fibres are myelinated by oligodendrocytes. In the physiological ageing processes everyone loses approximately 5,000 axons/year. The N. opticus [II] is surrounded by meninges (Pia mater, Arachnoidea, Dura mater). It leaves the Orbita through the **Canalis opticus,** in order to shortly afterwards unite with its contralateral part in the **Chiasma opticum**. From this point it is no longer referred to as N. opticus, but as Tractus opticus. In the Chiasma opticum the nasal retinal fibres (depiction of the temporal fields of vision) cross to the contralateral side but the temporal retinal fibres (depiction of nasal fields of vision) do not. The largest part of the fibres then proceeds as the Tractus opticus to the **Corpus geniculatum laterale** (thalamus). After switching it continues to the Area striata within the occipital cortex at the Sulcus calcarinus. The course of the N. opticus [II] and Tractus opticus from the Bulbus opticus up to the Sulcus calcarinus within the Lobus occipitalis is presented in ➤ Fig. 9.33. About 10 % of the fibres run extrageniculary to the Colliculi superiores (Lamina quadrigemina) and are responsible for **optical reflexes** by way of the corresponding interneurons (e.g. corneal reflex).

Clinical remarks

The optic tract can be damaged at several points in its course. If the **N. opticus [II]** is affected before the Chiasma opticum, in particular in the Canalis opticus, e.g. after traumatic brain injury, this can lead to blindness of the affected eye. If the **damage is in the area of the Chiasma opticum,** e.g. in the case of pituitary tumours (most frequent tumour: prolactinoma) a bitemporal hemianopsia is generally the result: both temporal visual fields fail (see tunnel vision), while the nasal visual fields are still intact, as the cells and projecting neurons in the Chiasma opticum located in the temporal retina run at the edge and are not initially affected by the tumour. Lesions of the **Tractus opticus** (e.g. bleeding) lead to failure of the temporal visual field of the contralateral eye and nasal visual field of the ipsilateral eye (homonymous hemianopia). If the **visual radiation** running at the front in the temporal lobes is damaged (e.g. by ischemia), the result is an upper quadrant anopsia. Lesions of the entire visual radiation (e.g. from mass bleeding), such as lesions of the Tractus opticus lead to a homonymous hemianopsia.

9.3.3 N. oculomotorius [III]

The N. oculomotorius [III] (➤ Fig. 9.34) innervates the outer optic muscles with the exception of the M. obliquus superior (N. trochlearis [IV]) and the M. rectus lateralis (N. abducens [VI]). It is a mixed nerve with general somatoefferent and visceroefferent qualities (GSE, GVE), with preganglionic parasympathetic neurons in the **Nucleus accessorius nervi oculomotorii EDINGER-WESTPHAL** (Mesencephalon). Its somatomotoric neurons, on the other hand, are in the **Nucleus nervi oculomotorii.** The N. oculomotorius [III] exits at the front edge of the bridge within the Fossa interpeduncularis and runs between A. cerebri posterior and A. superior cerebelli, to extend medially from the Tentorium cerebelli to-

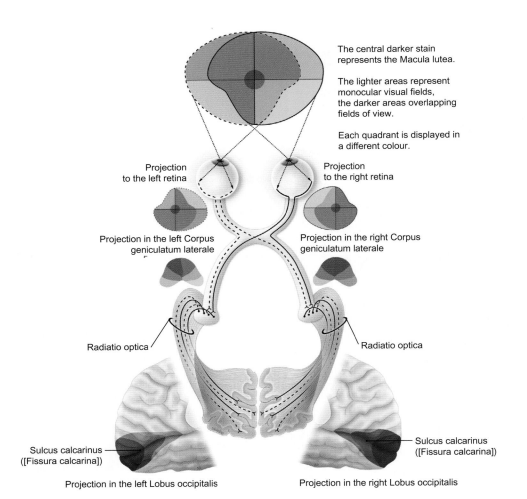

The central darker stain represents the Macula lutea.

The lighter areas represent monocular visual fields, the darker areas overlapping fields of view.

Each quadrant is displayed in a different colour.

Projection to the left retina

Projection to the right retina

Projection in the left Corpus geniculatum laterale

Projection in the right Corpus geniculatum laterale

Radiatio optica

Radiatio optica

Sulcus calcarinus ([Fissura calcarina])

Sulcus calcarinus ([Fissura calcarina])

Projection in the left Lobus occipitalis

Projection in the right Lobus occipitalis

Fig. 9.33 N. opticus and configuration in retina and optic tract (simplified). The first three neurons (colour vision) or 4 neurons (light-dark vision) of the visual tract lie within the retina. They leave the Bulbus oculi as the N. opticus [II] and later after partial fibre crossing over in the Chiasma opticum as the Tractus opticus. They run to a large extent to the Corpus geniculatum laterale and after switching run as the Radiatio optica to the Sulcus calcarinus in the area of the Lobus occipitalis.

wards the Sinus cavernosus. From there, it runs via the Fissura orbitalis superior into the Orbita and divides into a **R. superior,** an **R. inferior** and a **branch to the Ganglion ciliare** (➤ Chap. 12.5.6). The R. superior innervates the Mm. levator palpebrae superioris and rectus superior; the R. inferior supplies the M. rectus medialis, the M. rectus inferior and the M. obliquus inferior. The parasympathetic fibres coming from the EDINGER - WESTPHAL core extend to the **Ganglion ciliare,** are switched from preganglionic to postganglionic and run as **Nn. ciliares breves** to the **M. ciliaris** and to the **M. sphincter pupillae,** which they innervate. By innervation of the corresponding eye muscles the N. oculomotorius [III] is responsible for raising the eyelid (M. levator palpebrae superioris) and for the eyeball movement upwards laterally, upper medially, medially and lower medially. The M. tarsais, which consists of smooth muscle and is responsible for tightening of the eyelids is also positioned in the eyelids. It is innervated by the sympathetic system, so that in the event of failure of the N. oculomotorius III] it is still possible to slightly open the eyelids. The parasympathetic fibres mediate via the M. ciliaris the accommodation of the lens and regulate via the **M. sphincter pupillae** the narrowing of the pupils.

Clinical remarks

Damage to the N. oculomotorius [III] leads to ptosis (drooping of the affected eyelid), mydriasis (widening of the pupil), as well as the inability for accommodation. In addition, patients display an abducted and downward facing eyeball.

Ganglion ciliare

The Ganglion ciliare lies within the Orbita, lateral of the N. opticus and approximately 1.5 cm behind the Bulbus oculi (➤ Fig. 9.34). In the ganglion, the **parasympathetic fibres** of the N. oculomotorius [III] are switched from preganglionic and then innervate the inner eye muscles. The sympathetic and sensitive fibres that also run through the ganglion are not switched here. The ganglion gets its afferents from 3 different roots:

* From a parasympathetic root (**Radix parasympatica**) of the N. oculomotorius which is responsible for the innervation of the inner eye muscles (M. sphincter pupillae and M. ciliaris)
* From a sympathetic root (**Radix sympatica**) with fibres from the cervical sympathetic trunk for the innervation of the M. dilator pupillae (inner eye muscle which governs the width of the pupil)
* From a sensory root (**Radix sensoria**) with fibres from the N. nasociliaris for sensory innervation of the cornea and conjunctiva

Both the sensory as well as the sympathetic fibres run through the Ganglion ciliare without switching. The **Nn. ciliares breves** leave the Ganglion ciliare as postganglionic efferents, to pass through the sclera to the inner eye muscles.

9.3.4 N. trochlearis [IV]

The **N. trochlearis [IV]** is a purely motor nerve (general somatoefferent, GSE), which innervates the M. obliquus superior that belongs to the external ocular muscles. Its original neurons are locat-

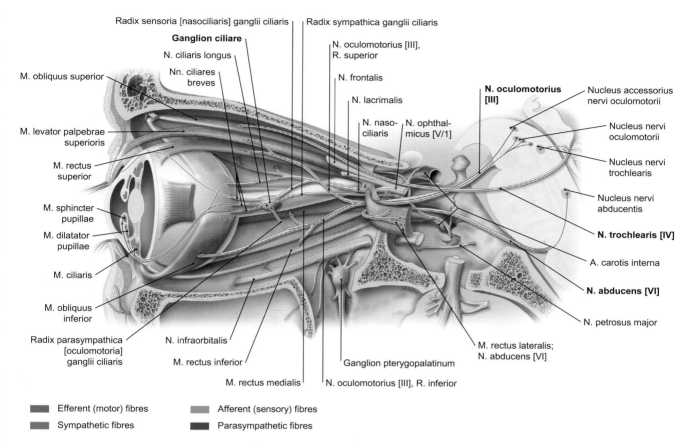

Fig. 9.34 Motor eye nerves and core areas, Nn. oculomotorius, trochlearis and abducens. Lateral view, opened Orbita, retrobulbar adipose tissue is removed, M. rectus lateralis resection.

ed in the **Nucleus nervi trochlearis** of the mesencephalon (➤ Fig. 9.34). Its fibres leave the brain at the back of the brainstem at the lower part of the **Lamina quadrigemina** (quadrigeminal plate) as a thin nerve. From there, it passes lateral of the two brain halves to the Tentorium cerebelli to enter into the Dura mater. Together with the N. oculomotorius [III] and the N. ophthalmicus [V/1] it passes through the Fissura orbitalis superior into the Orbita and runs outside the Anulus tendineus communis (annulus of ZINN) to the **M. obliquus superior,** for motor innervation. The contraction of the M. superior oblique, which is deflected via a connective tissue loop (trochlea, giving the name of the nerve) functioning as a hypomochlion leads to the medial rotation of the eyeball with simultaneous movement to lateral below. If the Bulbus is already in an adducted position, the M. obliquus superior lowers the Bulbus laterally downwards.

Clinical remarks

A **lesion of the N. trochlearis [IV]** is associated with double vision in patients. This is evoked by a **strabismus** (squinting) in a nasal direction and upwards. Affected patients try to compensate for the misalignment of the eyeball with corresponding head movements, which can be seen in a tilting of the head. The patients also report difficulty in climbing stairs, as a glance downwards through the eyeball is no longer possible.

9.3.5 N. trigeminus [V]

The N. trigeminus [V] is the strongest of the 12 cranial nerves and, at the same time, also the *first pharyngeal arch nerve (mandibular arch)*. It carries both motor and sensory fibres (SVE, GSA), which respectively originate from different core areas. Three cores are generally somatosensory and range from the brain stem to the upper cervical medulla (➤ Fig. 9.35):

- **Nucleus mesencephalicus nervi trigemini** (GSA, proprioception)
- **Nucleus pontinus nervi trigemini** (GSA, mechanoreception)
- **Nucleus spinalis nervi trigemini** (GSA, nociception, thermoception and mechanoreception)

The special visceroefferent (SVE) core of the N. trigeminus, the **Nucleus motorius nervi trigemini,** is located within the pons. All nerve fibres are bundled in the area of the pons, to leave the brain at its lateral border and to run as a common nerve (Radix sensoria and Radix motoria) rostrally via the Pars petrosa of the Os temporale. There, the nerve enters at the level of the Foramen lacerum into a Dura duplicature (Cavum trigeminale = MECKEL). At this point the perikaryon of sensory fibres forms the Ganglion trigeminale (Ganglion semilunare, GASSER's ganglion) which divides into 3 large main branches (hence the name triplet nerve):

- The **N. ophthalmicus [V/1]** (GSA, purely sensory, ➤ Table 9.17) passes through the Fissura orbitalis superior into the Orbita and then into the upper facial region. It innervates the eye (in particular cornea and conjunctiva), the skin of the upper eyelid, forehead, back of the nose and the mucous membranes of the nasal cavities and sinuses. It also stores vegetative fibres for the innervation of the lacrimal gland within the Orbita.

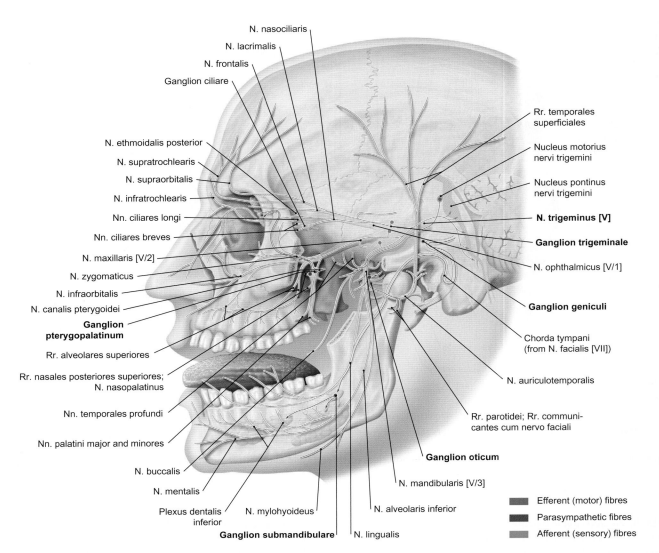

Fig. 9.35 N. trigeminus [V], core areas and fibre qualities. Lateral view, Arcus zygomaticus and Proc. coronoideus removed. The N. trigeminus [V] is divided into 3 parts and penetrates with each branch through another opening of the skull base.

- The **N. maxillaris [V/2]** (GSA, purely sensory, ➤ Table 9.19) leaves the skull through the Foramen rotundum. It innervates the skin of the anterior temporal region, the upper part of the cheek, the lower eyelid and underlying skin. It is also responsible for the sensory innervation of the palate, teeth of the upper jaw, the corresponding gingiva, and the mucosa of the Sinus maxillaris.
- The **N. mandibularis [V/3]** (GSA, SVE, sensory and motoric, ➤ Table 9.20) enters through the Foramen ovale and sensory innervates the skin of the posterior temporal region, the lower part of the cheek, the chin, as well as the teeth of the lower jaw

and the pertaining gums. It motorically innervates the masticatory muscles, two muscles at the floor of the mouth (M. mylohyoideus, Venter anterior of the M. digastricus), as well as the M. tensor veli palatini and the M. tensor tympani. Similar to the N. ophthalmicus [V/1] it stores vegetative fibres for the innervation of several glands (Glandulae linguales, sublingualis, submandibularis), as well as additional fibres for sensors (taste) of the anterior two thirds of the tongue (**Chorda tympani**).

The course of the N. trigeminus and its branches is summarised in ➤ Table 9.17- ➤ Table 9.20.

Table 9.17 Branches of the N. ophthalmicus [V/1] (purely somatoafferent).

Branch	Sub-branches	Innervation area
R. meningeus recurrens (R. tentorius)		Parts of the meninges
N. frontalis	N. supraorbitalis	Skin of forehead and mucosa of the frontal sinus
	N. supratrochlearis	Skin and conjunctiva at the nasal corner of the eye
N. lacrimalis		Lacrimal gland (for secretary innervation postganglionic parasympathetic fibres are attached to the N. zygomaticus), skin and conjunctiva of the temporal corner of the eye
N. nasociliaris	➤ Table 9.18	Nasal sinuses, anterior part of the nasal cavity and iris, Corpus ciliare, cornea of the eye (➤ Table 9.18)

Table 9.18 Branches of the N. nasociliaris [from V/1].

Branch	Course	Innervation area
Radix sensoria ganglii ciliarii (R. communicans cum ganglio ciliarii)	Controls the sensory component for the Ganglion ciliare, from which the Nn. ciliares breves emerge	Eyeball and conjunctiva (together with the Nn. ciliares longi)
Nn. ciliares longi	Attached to the N. opticus [II] and extend with the Nn. ciliares breves from the Ganglion ciliare to the Bulbus oculi; also joined by sympathetic fibres from the Plexus caroticus	Eyeball (Bulbus oculi) and its conjunctiva; the sympathetic fibres innervate the M. dilatator pupillae
N. ethmoidalis posterior	Runs through the identically named foramen to the posterior ethmoidal sinuses and the sphenoidal sinus	Mucosa of the posterior ethmoidal cells and the sphenoidal sinus
N. ethmoidalis anterior	Runs through the identically named foramen back into the anterior cranial fossa, courses through the Lamina cribrosa into the nasal cavity; it ends with the Rr. nasales externi in the skin of the dorsum of the nose	Mucosa of the anterior nasal cavity and the anterior ethmoidal cells; skin of the dorsum of the nose
N. infratrochlearis	Extends below the trochlea to the nasal corner of the eye	Skin at the nasal corner of the eye

NOTE

The exit points from the sensory facial branches (Foramen supraorbitale, Foramen infraorbitale and Foramen mentale) are referred to as **trigeminal pressure points** and are of practical clinical significance for the examining doctor (➤ Chap. 12.5.8).

Clinical remarks

Trigeminal neuralgia **(tic douloureux)** is a complex and sensory disorder of the trigeminal root, which leads to severe pain and sometimes even to skin irritation in the face. The pathogenesis has not yet been fully elucidated. It is thought that disorders or stenoses of the supplying vessels, especially in the area of the **Ganglion trigeminale** and the cerebellopontine angle, lead to a reduction in supply to nerve cells. The patients suffer from acute and sudden severe pain that reaches maximum values on a subjective pain scale. Even the lightest touch or even wind can trigger the pain, mainly in the supply areas of the N. mandibularis [V/3] and of the N. maxillaris [V/2]. Pain medication or anaesthesia can bring symptomatic relief. The patients often turn to suicide as a way to escape the pain. Trigeminal neuralgia can also occur as a result of infection with the varicella zoster virus **(postherpetic neuralgia)**. Since the N. ophthalmicus [I] is used as a transport route for the virus (axonal transport), there are restrictions in its innervation area. The involvement of the surface of the eye is particularly feared, which is not only associated with very severe pain, but in extreme cases can lead to a loss of sight **(Zoster ophthalmicus)**.

9.3.6 N. abducens [VI]

The N. abducens [VI] is comparable to the N. trochlearis [IV] a general somatoefferent nerve (GSE), which only innervates one muscle, the **M. rectus lateralis**. Muscle contraction of this external ocular muscle leads to the abduction of the eyeball and thus to gaze in a temporal direction (abducens = abduction). The neurons are in the **Nucleus nervi abducentis** within the pons. The abducens core is dorsally encircled by the fibres of the N. facialis [VII] that still runs in the pons **(internal genu of the facial nerve)**. The N.

abducens [VI] exits within the **Sulcus bulbopontinus** between pons and medulla and runs parallel to the A. basilaris in the direction of the clivus, to enter into the Dura mater. Within the Dura mater it runs together with the Nn. oculomotorius [III] and trochlearis [IV] to the **Sinus cavernosus**, where it does not run as a single cranial nerve in the lateral wall but through the middle right of the venous plexus. From here it passes through the Fissura orbitalis superior into the Orbita, enters through the Anulus tendineus communis (common tendinous ring) and innervates the M. rectus lateralis. The course and the fibre quality of the N. abducens [VI] is presented in ➤ Fig. 9.34 (together with the Nn. oculomotorius [III] and trochlearis [IV]).

Clinical remarks

Due to its long extradural course and its passage through the Sinus cavernosus the N. abducens is particularly susceptible to damage **(abducens palsy)**. If the patient is asked to move the affected eye to the temporal side, the eyeball remains pointing straight ahead, since the M. rectus lateralis is paralysed. It is comparable to trochlearis palsy and patients often suffer from the development of **double vision** (diplopia).

9.3.7 N. facialis [VII]

The N. facialis [VII] is the second pharyngeal arch nerve. Its main function is the special visceroefferent (SVE) innervation of the facial muscles. It consists of two major parts (**N. facialis [VII]** and **N. intermedius**) with different fibre qualities. According to its conducting qualities the parts of the N. facialis [VII] have 3 different origin cores:

- The **special visceromotor (SVE) Nucleus nervi facialis** that lies within the pons consists of an upper cell group (innervation of the forehead and eyelid muscles, controlled by the Gyrus precentralis of ipsilateral and contralateral sides) and a lower cell group (innervation of the remaining [lower] facial muscles, controlled by the Gyrus precentralis of the contralateral side). The upper nuclear portion therefore receives double innervation from both

Table 9.19 Branches of the N. maxillaris [V/2] (purely somatoafferent).

Branch	Sub-branches	Innervation area
R. meningeus		Meninges of the middle cranial fossa
N. zygomaticus	R. zygomaticotemporalis	Skin in the area of the temple
	R. zygomaticofacialis	Skin in the upper cheek region; for secretory innervation of the lacrimal gland postganglionic parasympathetic fibres run with the N. zygomaticus, which it emits to the N. lacrimalis (R. communicans cum nervo zygomatico)
Rr. ganglionares to ganglion pterygopalatinum		Control sensitive fibres for the Ganglion pterygopalatinum, innervation of the palate and nose, it connects to the sympathetic and parasympathetic fibres for the Glandulae nasales and palatinae (especially visceroefferent) as well with the taste fibres
N. infraorbitalis (terminal branch of the N. maxillaris)	Nn. alveolares superiores with Rr. alveolares superiores posteriores, medii and anteriores (Plexus dentalis superior)	Mucosa of the maxillary sinus, teeth of the upper jaw and corresponding gingiva
	Rr. palpebrales inferiores, Rr. nasales externi et interni and Rr. labiales superiores	Skin and conjunctiva of the lower eyelid, lateral skin area of the nasal wings, skin of upper lip and lateral cheek region between lower eyelid and upper lip
N. palatinus major	Runs via the Canalis palatinus major through the Foramen palatinum majus	Mucosa of the hard palate, Glandulae palatinae, palatine taste buds
Nn. palatini minores	Leave the Canalis palatinus major through the Foramina palatina minora	Mucosa of the soft palate, Tonsilla palatina, Glandulae palatinae, palatine taste buds
Rr. nasales posteriores superiores laterales and mediales	Pass through the Foramen sphenopalatinum into the nasal cavity and emit the N. nasopalatinus which reaches the hard palate through the Canalis incisivus	Mucosa of the nasal conchae, nasal septum, mucosa of the anterior part of the hard palate, upper incisors and gingiva, Glandulae nasales

Table 9.20 Branches of the N. mandibularis [V/3] (somatofferent and visceroafferent).

Branch	Sub-branches	Innervation area
R. meningeus		Parts of the meninges
N. massetericus		M. masseter
Nn. temporales profundi		M. temporalis
N. pterygoideus lateralis		M. pterygoideus lateralis
N. pterygoideus medialis		M. pterygoideus medialis
N. musculi tensoris veli palatini		M. tensor veli palatini
N. musculi tensoris tympani		M. tensor tympani
N. buccalis		Skin and mucosa of the cheek and gingiva of the lower jaw
N. auriculotemporalis	Rr. parotidei	Postganglionic parasympathetic fibres from the Ganglion oticum join and innervate the parotid gland
	Rr. communicantes cum nervo faciali	Postganglionic parasympathetic fibres from the Ganglion oticum join and innervate the parotid gland (controversial)
	N. meatus acustici externi	External ear canal, tympanic membrane
	Nn. auriculares anteriores	Skin of the external ear
	Rr. temporales superficiales	Skin of the posterotemporal region
N. lingualis	Rr. isthmi faucium	Skin of the soft palate
	N. sublingualis	Mucosa of the floor of the mouth
		Sensory innervation of the anterior two thirds of the tongue, taste fibres of the anterior two thirds of the tongue, association with preganglionic parasympathetic fibres from the Chorda tympani and transfer to the Ganglion submandibulare
N. alveolaris inferior	Plexus dentalis inferior	Teeth and gingiva of the lower jaw
	N. mylohyoideus	M. mylohyoideus and Venter anterior of the M. digastricus
	N. mentalis	Skin of the chin

hemispheres. The lower part is only reached by corticonuclear fibres of the contralateral side.

- The **general visceroefferent (GVE)** (parasympathetic) **Nucleus salivatorius superior** also lies within the pons and is responsible for the autonomic innervation of the salivary glands (exception: Glandula parotidea) of the lacrimal gland and a part of the nasal glands.
- The **special visceroafferent (SVA)** (taste) **Nuclei tractus solitarii** (Pars superior) which extend from the pons to the Medulla oblongata, contain the original neurons for sensory innervation of the anterior two thirds of the tongue (taste).

Additionally, **general somatoafferent fibres (GSA)** from the auditory canal rear wall, the skin behind the ear, the outer ear and the eardrum also run with the N. facialis [VII]. The fibres run for a short distance with the N. vagus [X] (R. communicans nervi vagi) and dock in the Pars petrosa of the N. facialis [VII]. The cell bodies of neurons lie, just as the perikarya of taste fibres, in the Ganglion geniculi and project via the intermediate part of the N. facialis [VII] into the **Nucleus spinalis nervi trigemini.**

The two main parts (facial and intermediate parts) leave the brain at the **cerebellopontine angle,** Then, together with the N. vestibulocochlearis [VIII] enter into the **Porus and Meatus acusticus internus.** Shortly before reaching the inner ear the main part of the nerve bends almost at a right angle dorsally and downwards (➤ Fig. 9.36). This bending point is referred to as the **external genu of the facial nerve** (internal genu of the facial nerve: course of intrapontine fibres of the N. facialis [VII] around the Nucleus nervi abducentis). The exterior genu of the facial nerve is based in the **Ganglion geniculi,** which contains pseudo-unipolar perikarya for the sensory fibres (taste) of the anterior two thirds of the tongue and the sensory nerve fibres from the outer ear. During the course

through the **Canalis nervi facialis** in the petrous bone, the N. facialis [VII] emits 3 more branches:

- The **N. petrosus major** (parasympathetic) runs through the Hiatus canalis nervi petrosi majoris and then runs in the middle cranial fossa between dura and the Pars petrosa of the Os temporale to the Foramen lacerum (➤ Fig. 9.36). Sympathetic fibres connect to it, forming the N. petrosus profundus. After both nerves have penetrated through the Foramen lacerum the parasympathetic fibres of the N. petrosus major and the sympathetic fibres of the N. petrosus profundus merge to the N. canalis pterygoidei (VIDIANUS), which passes through the canal of the same name into the Fossa pterygopalatina to the Ganglion pterygopalatinum (see below).
- The **N. stapedius** (➤ Fig. 9.36) remains within the petrous bone and runs to the M. stapedius lying in the Proc. pyramidalis of the petrous bone, to innervate it motorically (muscle contraction leads to tilting of the stirrup base plate in the oval window with resulting stiffening of the auditory ossicles and reduced sound transmission).
- Shortly before the N. facialis [VII] exits from the bony Canalis nervi facialis through the Foramen stylomastoideum, the **Chorda tympani** branches off (➤ Fig. 9.36). After a short course through an independent canal in the temporal bone it comes into the tympanic cavity. Surrounded by middle ear mucosa, it runs through the tympanic cavity towards the ossicles, passes between Collum mallei (hammer neck) and the upper part of the Crus longum incudis (long limb of the incus) and then bends down to the **Fissura sphenopetrosa** and via which in most cases leaves the middle ear (much less frequently the Chorda tympani penetrates the skull base via the **Fissura petrotympanica** [GLASER's fissure]). The Chorda tympani runs to the

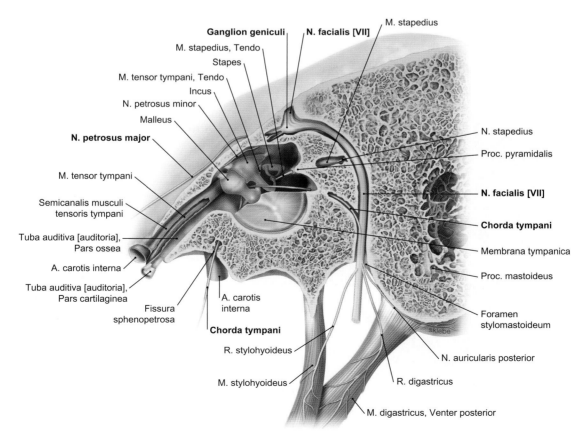

Fig. 9.36 Course of the N. facialis [VII]. Vertical section through the Canalis facialis, view from the left.

area behind or medial of the Fossa mandibularis via both fissures and runs medial from the Condylus and Ramus mandibulae downwards. About 1 cm below the Incisura mandibulae the Chorda tympani connects to the N. lingualis.

- From the **N. lingualis** the Chorda tympani takes up gustatory sensory fibres from the taste buds of the anterior two thirds of the tongue, which have their perikarya in the Ganglion geniculi of the N. facialis [VII] and project into the Nucleus spinalis nervi trigemini.
- **Parasympathetic fibres** run along with the Chorda tympani, the core area of which is the **Nucleus salivatorius superior**. They branch off from the N. lingualis and pass to the Ganglion submandibulare (see below).

The main part of the N. facialis [VII] leaves the skull base through the **Foramen stylomastoideum** of the Os temporale. Shortly after its exit, it emits motor branches:

- **N. auricularis posterior** for the innervation of the M. occipitofrontalis, Venter posterior
- **R. auricularis** (mostly as a branch of the N. auricularis posterior) for the innervation of the rudimentarily created facial Mm. auriculares
- A **direct branch** for the innervation of the M. digastricus, Venter posterior
- A **direct branch** for the innervation of the M. stylohyoideus

The main trunk then enters into the Glandula parotidea, where it branches to the **Plexus intraparotideus** (➤ Fig. 9.37). It usually divides into an upper R. temporofacialis and a lower R. cervicofacialis. Resulting terminal branches leave the parotid gland at the front and lower margins as **Rr. temporales** (also referred to clinically as the forehead branch), **Rr. zygomatici, Rr. buccales, R. marginalis mandibulae and R. colli** for the innervation of the mimic muscles (➤ Chap. 9.2.3) in the face.

Clinical remarks

In the case of space occupying processes in the cerebellopontine angle (usually a benign but displacingly growing acoustic neurinoma, see above next clinical box) both the N. vestibulocochlearis [VIII] (hearing and balance disturbances) as well as the N. facialis [VII] can be affected. Possible consequences of an **infranuclear lesion** (lesion below the facial core) are:

- Limited tear secretion (Result: dry eye)
- Failure of the N. stapedius (Result: hyperacousia)
- Failure of the Chorda tympani (Result: problems with sense of taste, limited production of saliva on one side)
- Failure of the motor branches (Result: **peripheral facial paresis** with lagophthalmus [inability to close the eye due to paralysis of the M. orbicularis oculi] and resulting detachment of the lacrimal film or signs of dehydration on the surface of the eye up to clouding and subsequent blindness on the affected side)

Supranuclear lesions describe damage in the area of corticonuclear fibres of the nerve. They are also referred to as **central facial palsy**. This is characterised by motor deficits of the contralateral lower facial muscles (so-called lower facial palsy). As the eye and forehead muscles are innervated by both halves of the brain, the upper half of the face is not affected in central facial palsy but the forehead can be wrinkled.

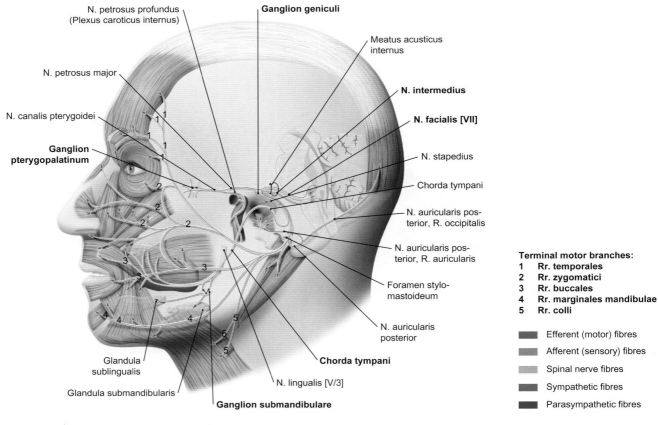

Fig. 9.37 N. facialis [VII], core and fibre qualities. View from the left.

Labels:
N. petrosus profundus (Plexus caroticus internus)
N. petrosus major
N. canalis pterygoidei
Ganglion pterygopalatinum
Ganglion geniculi
Meatus acusticus internus
N. intermedius
N. facialis [VII]
N. stapedius
Chorda tympani
N. auricularis posterior, R. occipitalis
N. auricularis posterior, R. auricularis
Foramen stylomastoideum
N. auricularis posterior
Chorda tympani
N. lingualis [V/3]
Ganglion submandibulare
Glandula submandibularis
Glandula sublingualis

Terminal motor branches:
1 Rr. temporales
2 Rr. zygomatici
3 Rr. buccales
4 Rr. marginales mandibulae
5 Rr. colli

Efferent (motor) fibres
Afferent (sensory) fibres
Spinal nerve fibres
Sympathetic fibres
Parasympathetic fibres

Ganglion pterygopalatinum

The N. petrosus major (preganglionic parasympathetic fibres) and the N. petrosus profundus (postganglionic sympathetic fibres) reach the Ganglion pterygopalatinum as the N. canalis pterygoidei (➤ Fig. 9.37). Furthermore, the ganglion is still used by sensory fibres of the palate, as a transit route on the way to the N. maxillaris [V/2]:

- A part of the parasympathetic fibres from the N. petrosus major connects after switching from preganglionic to postganglionic to the **N. zygomaticus** and extends together with it through the Fissura orbitalis inferior into the Orbita. These fibres pass via the connection to the **R. zygomaticotemporalis** and then to the **R. communicans cum nervo zygomatico** to the **N. lacrimalis,** to finally innervate the Glandula lacrimalis (lacrimal gland).
- A second part of the parasympathetic fibres extends from the Fossa pterygopalatina with the **N. nasalis posterior superior** through the Foramen sphenopalatinum into the nose. The fibres spread out into the nasal mucosa and innervate the Glandulae nasales.
- A third part of the parasympathetic fibres extends with the **N. palatinus major** and the **Nn. palatini minores** after passing the identically named foramina to the hard and soft palate and innervates the **Glandulae palatinae.**
- **Postganglionic sympathetic fibres** run with the named parasympathetic fibres from the N. petrosus profundus to the corresponding glands, which have already been switched from preganglionic to postganglionic in the Ganglion cervicale superius.
- **Sensory branches** from the soft palate run with the N. palatinus major and the Nn. palatini minores to the Ganglion pterygopalatinum, extend through this without switching and connect shortly before the Foramen rotundum to the N. maxillaris [V/2]. Their perikarya reside in the Ganglion trigeminale and project to the Nucleus pontinus nervi trigemini.

Ganglion submandibulare

The Ganglion submandibulare is located in the immediate vicinity (above) of the Glandula submandibularis and is responsible for their innervation and the innervation of the Glandula sublingualis and the Glandulae linguales (➤ Fig. 9.37). The parasympathetic fibres run with the **Chorda tympani,** , which connect to the N. lingualis. The fibres only run for a short distance with the N. lingualis [V/3], then subdivide and reach the **Ganglion submandibulare** lying medial of the Angulus mandibulae. Here, the fibres are switched from preganglionic to postganglionic, then part of the fibres passes directly into the neighbouring **Glandula submandibularis** and innervates this while the other part again docks at the N. lingualis and either passes with it into the tongue for innervation of the **Glandula lingualis anterior (Apicis linguae, BLANDIN-NUHN gland)** located in the tongue tip or leaves the N. lingualis [V/3] again after a short distance to innervate the **Glandula sublingualis**.

Similar to the Ganglion pterygopalatinum the parts of the Radix sympathica originate from the Plexus caroticus, which originate from the cervical Truncus sympathicus. Within the ganglion only the parasympathetic fibres are switched; the sympathetic fibres run through the ganglion unswitched.

9.3.8 N. vestibulocochlearis [VIII]

The N. vestibulocochlearis [VIII], which is also clinically referred to as N. statoacusticus, is a specially somatoafferent (SSA) nerve that also contains efferent fibres referred to as olivocochlear bundles (➤ Chap. 12.5.11). It is divided into two parts (➤ Fig. 9.38):
- The **cochlear part** relays information from the hearing organ (Cochlea) to the core areas in the brainstem.
- The **vestibular part** relays information of the balance organ (vestibular organ) to corresponding core areas in the brainstem.

The special somatoafferent nerve fibres of the **N. cochlearis** originate in the organ of CORTI of the cochlea. The perikarya of bipolar neurons lie within the cochlea in the **Ganglion spirale cochleae** within the modiolus. Here, the primary sensory cells of the organ of CORTI are switched to the peripheral N. cochlearis. This passes

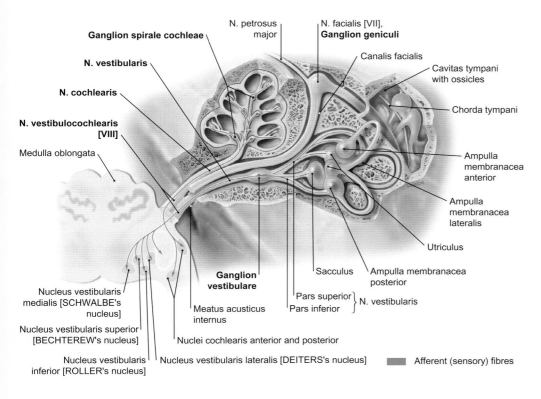

Ganglion spirale cochleae
N. vestibularis
N. cochlearis
N. vestibulocochlearis [VIII]
Medulla oblongata
N. petrosus major
N. facialis [VII], **Ganglion geniculi**
Canalis facialis
Cavitas tympani with ossicles
Chorda tympani
Ampulla membranacea anterior
Ampulla membranacea lateralis
Utriculus
Ampulla membranacea posterior
Sacculus
Nucleus vestibularis medialis [SCHWALBE's nucleus]
Nucleus vestibularis superior [BECHTEREW's nucleus]
Nucleus vestibularis inferior [ROLLER's nucleus]
Meatus acusticus internus
Ganglion vestibulare
Nuclei cochlearis anterior and posterior
Nucleus vestibularis lateralis [DEITERS's nucleus]
Pars superior
Pars inferior } N. vestibularis
Afferent (sensory) fibres

Fig. 9.38 N. vestibulocochlearis [VIII], cores and fibre qualities. View from above, Pars petrosa opened.

(with the N. vestibularis and the N. facialis) through the internal auditory canal and via the cerebellopontine angle into the brainstem to project to the **Nuclei cochleares anterior and posterior**. The central processes of the **1st neuron of the vestibular pathway** from Sacculus (vertical linear acceleration), Utriculus (horizontal linear acceleration) and the three semicircular canals (rotational acceleration) initially merge into 2 bundles, **Pars superior** and **Pars inferior,** which converge to the **N. vestibularis** and together with the N. cochlearis run through the internal auditory canal and enter the brainstem via the cerebellopontine angle. Their perikarya reside in the **Ganglion vestibulare** on the edge of the internal auditory canal. They project to the 4 **Nuclei vestibulares superior (BECHTEREW), inferior (ROLLER), medialis (SCHWALBE) and lateralis (DEITERS)** (➤ Fig. 9.38). Some fibres pass via the Pedunculus cerebellaris inferior to the cerebellum.

Clinical remarks

An **acoustic neurinoma** is a slow (years to decades), but suppressingly growing benign tumour which originates from SCHWANN cells of the nerve cell sheath of the N. vestibulocochlearis [VIII] (schwannoma). It usually develops in the area of the Porus acusticus internus. First symptoms are often a hearing loss (especially a high-frequency hearing loss) and/or tinnitus and as the third most common symptom dizziness (balance disorders). These 3 signs are already manifested when the acoustic neurinoma is still relatively small and is primarily or exclusively in the bony auditory canal (intrameatal). The N. facialis [VII] can be affected by the suppression of growth. Following diagnosis, the neurinoma is removed neurosurgically.

9.3.9 N. glossopharyngeus [IX]

The 3rd branchial nerve, the N. glossopharyngeus [IX], is a mixed nerve with general viscoefferent (GVE), special viscoefferent (SVE), general somatoafferent (GSA), as well as general visceroafferent (GVA) and special visceroafferent (SVA) units. It is therefore very similar to the N. vagus [X] (➤ Chap. 9.3.10). According to its different fibre qualities, it has a large innervation area: it innervates the Glandula parotidea, muscles and epithelium of the pharynx as well as sensory innervation to the rear third of the tongue. It also relays information from the **Glomus caroticum** and from the **Sinus caroticus** and is thus involved in blood pressure regulation. Its 4 core areas are in the Medulla oblongata:

- **Nucleus salivatorius inferior** (GVE), secretory core
- **Nucleus ambiguus** (SVE), motor core
- **Nucleus spinalis nervi trigemini** (ASA), core for surface sensitivity
- **Nucleus tractus solitarii** [Nucleus solitarius] (SVA, GVA), sensory core for taste fibres

The N. glossopharyngeus [IX] exits together with (and above) the N. vagus [X] (➤ Chap. 9.3.10) and the N. accessorius [XI] (➤ Chap. 9.3.11) from the Medulla oblongata in the **Sulcus retroolivaris** (➤ Fig. 9.39). It passes hidden from the cerebellum below the Flocculus cerebelli to the **Foramen jugulare,** through which it leaves the skull together with the N. vagus [X] and N. accessorius [XI]. At the level of the Foramen jugulare are its 2 sensory ganglia (**Ganglion superius** [inside the skull] and **Ganglion inferius** [outside the skull]), which are thrown up by pseudo-unipolar nerve cell bodies of sensory (Ganglia superius and inferius) and spinal (only Ganglion inferius) nerve fibres. After passing through the skull base, it runs between the A. carotis interna and V. jugu-

laris interna caudally to the **M. stylopharyngeus,** which serves as a guiding structure. Along the muscle it extends to the pharynx from behind and along the parapharyngeal space to the tongue. On its way, it emits the following branches:

- **N. tympanicus (JACOBSON)** (GVE and GSA): it branches at the level of the Ganglion inferius directly below the Foramen jugulare and reaches the tympanic cavity via a bony canal. Here its nerve fibres branch out into the mucosa of the tympanic cavity and form, together with sympathetic fibres from the Plexus caroticus, the **Plexus tympanicus** (➤ Fig. 9.39). The sensory nerve fibres innervate the middle ear mucosa, a part rejoins the **R. tubarius** and innervates the mucosa of the Tuba auditiva. The nerve cell bodies of the sensory fibres are located in the **Ganglion superius** and project into the **Nucleus and Tractus spinalis nervi trigemini**. Preganglionic parasympathetic fibres from the **Nucleus salivatorius inferior** run without switching with the N. tympanicus and the Plexus tympanicus through the middle ear and then merge with sympathetic fibres of the Plexus caroticus internus, which also runs in the middle ear mucosa to the **N. petrosus minor**. This enters through the **Hiatus canalis nervi petrosi minoris** into the middle cranial fossa and leaves it via the Foramen lacerum. From here the fibres run to the **Ganglion oticum** at the stem of the N. mandibularis [V/3] and the Foramen ovale. In the ganglion the switching of the parasympathetic fibres from preganglionic to postganglionic takes place, the sympathetic fibres are already postganglionic and continue unswitched. The postganglionic fibres attach onto the **N. auriculotemporalis** to the **Glandula parotidea** and within the parotid gland partially to the intraparotideal fibres of the **N. facialis [VII]** with which they pass into the parenchyma of the gland. The connection from the Nucleus salivatorius inferior to the parotid gland is referred to as **JACOBSON's plexus**. Some fibres continue and innervate the **Glandulae buccales** and **labiales**.
- **R. sinus carotici** (GVA): nerve fibres run within the R. sinus carotici which originate in the **Sinus caroticus** (pressoreceptors – blood pressure regulation) and in the **Glomus caroticum** (chemoreceptors O_2, CO_2 partial pressure) (➤ Fig. 9.39). Their nerve cell bodies are located in the Ganglion inferius of the N. glossopharyngeus and project into the **Tractus solitarius**.
- **Rr. pharyngei** (GVE, SVE, GSA, SVA): the branches have different fibre qualities (➤ Fig. 9.39):
  - Afferent (sensory) fibres (GSA) come from the pharyngeal wall. The nerve cell bodies reside in the Ganglion inferius and project to the Tractus spinalis nervi trigemini.
  - Motor fibres (SVE) derived from the Nucleus ambiguus innervate the pharyngeal muscles and the muscles of the soft palate in conjunction with motor fibres of the N. vagus [X] as Plexus pharyngeus.
  - Parasympathetic fibres (GVE) from the Nucleus salivatorius inferior reach the mucous Glandulae pharyngeales.
- **Rr. tonsillares and linguales** (GSA, SVA): they have 2 fibre qualities (➤ Fig. 9.39):
  - Afferent (sensory) fibres (GSA) originate in the base of the tongue and from the Isthmus faucium including the tonsils. The nerve cell bodies reside in the Ganglion inferius and project to the Tractus spinalis nervi trigemini.
  - Spinal nerve fibres (SVA) conduct taste sensations from the posterior third of the tongue and the neighbouring mucous membrane in the area of the Isthmus faucium to the Nucleus and Tractus solitarius. Its nerve cell bodies reside in the Ganglion inferius.
- **R. musculi stylopharyngei** (SVE): this branch of the Nucleus ambiguus innervates the M. stylopharyngeus (➤ Fig. 9.39).

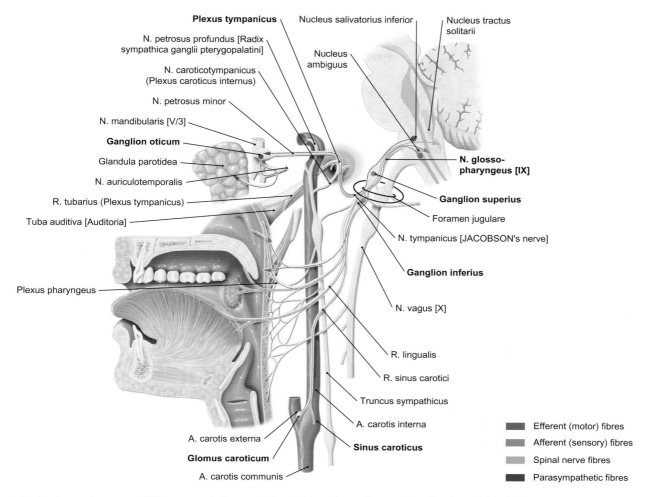

Fig. 9.39 N. glossopharyngeus [IX], cores and fibre qualities. Schematic median section, view from the left side.

Ganglion oticum

The Ganglion oticum is located at the stem of the N. mandibularis [V/3] near the Foramen ovale. In the ganglion parasympathetic fibres are switched from preganglionic to postganglionic. The nerve cell bodies of the fibres reside in the Nucleus salivatorius inferior and initially run with the N. glossopharyngeus [IX] via the above-mentioned JACOBSON's plexus to the Ganglion oticum. The postganglionic fibres pass via the N. auriculotemporalis [V/3] and partly with intraparotidal branches of the N. facialis [VII] into the parotid gland and innervate it parasympathetically. Further parasympathetic fibres extend from the Ganglion oticum to the base of the tongue and innervate the Glandulae linguales. Postganglionic parasympathetic fibres also pass through the Ganglion oticum without switching and reach the described target tissue with the parasympathetic fibres.

> **Clinical remarks**
>
> **Lesions of the N. glossopharyngeus [IX]** primarily cause swallowing difficulties, because the motor innervation of the M. constrictor pharyngis superior is disrupted. Other typical symptoms are a deviation of the uvula to the healthy side (also referred to as the backdrop phenomenon; paralysis of the Mm. levator veli palatini, palatoglossus, palatopharyngeus and uvulae), sensory disturbances in the upper pharynx (e.g. absence of gag reflex) and disorders of taste sensation at the base of the tongue.

9.3.10 N. vagus [X]

The N. vagus [X] (➤ Fig. 9.40) has the largest innervation area of all cranial nerves. It innervates up into the abdomen and is the main nerve of the cranial parasympathetic nervous system (autonomic nervous system). It has the same fibre qualities as the N. glossopharyngeus [IX] (GVE, SVE, GSA, GVA, SVA, ➤ Chap. 9.3.9) and for the most part uses the same core areas:

- **Nucleus ambiguus** (SVE), motor core
- **Nucleus tractus solitarii** [nucleus solitarius] (SVA, GVA), sensory core for taste fibres
- **Nucleus spinalis nervi trigemini** (GSA), core for surface sensitivity
- **Nucleus dorsalis nervi vagi** (GVE, GVA), parasympathetic core

The nerve exits as a relatively flat bundle between the N. glossopharyngeus [IX] (➤ Chap. 9.3.9) and the N. accessorius [XI] (➤ Chap. 9.3.11) in the **Sulcus retroolivaris** from the Medulla oblongata and passes together with the other two nerves to the Foramen jugulare. It also has 2 ganglia (Ganglion superius [Ganglion jugulare in the Foramen jugulare or inside the skull] and Ganglion inferius [Ganglion nodosum, outside of the skull]). It picks up 2 branches when still within the cranial cavity:

- **R. meningeus** (GSA): sensory fibres of the meninges of the posterior cranial fossa
- **R. auricularis** (GSA): sensory fibres from the external auditory canal

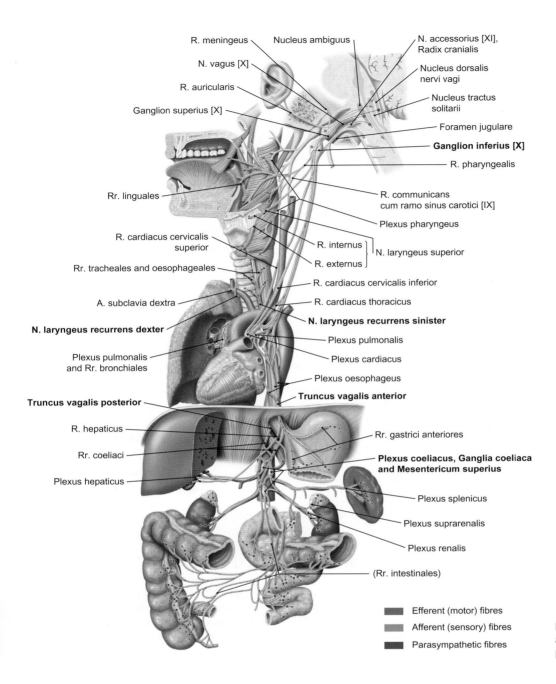

R. meningeus · Nucleus ambiguus
N. vagus [X]
R. auricularis
Ganglion superius [X]
Rr. linguales
R. cardiacus cervicalis superior
Rr. tracheales and oesophageales
A. subclavia dextra
N. laryngeus recurrens dexter
Plexus pulmonalis and Rr. bronchiales
Truncus vagalis posterior
R. hepaticus
Rr. coeliaci
Plexus hepaticus

N. accessorius [XI], Radix cranialis
Nucleus dorsalis nervi vagi
Nucleus tractus solitarii
Foramen jugulare
Ganglion inferius [X]
R. pharyngealis
R. communicans cum ramo sinus carotici [IX]
Plexus pharyngeus
R. internus ⎱ N. laryngeus superior
R. externus ⎰
R. cardiacus cervicalis inferior
R. cardiacus thoracicus
N. laryngeus recurrens sinister
Plexus pulmonalis
Plexus cardiacus
Plexus oesophageus
Truncus vagalis anterior
Rr. gastrici anteriores
Plexus coeliacus, Ganglia coeliaca and Mesentericum superius
Plexus splenicus
Plexus suprarenalis
Plexus renalis
(Rr. intestinales)

■ Efferent (motor) fibres
■ Afferent (sensory) fibres
■ Parasympathetic fibres

Fig. 9.40 N. vagus [X], cores and fibre qualities, highly simplified diagram.

Clinical remarks

Manipulation in the external auditory canal, e.g. when the ear nose and throat (ENT) doctor removes ear wax, irritation of the throat area is triggered via the sensory fibres of the N. vagus [X]. In excessive irritation of the throat, there may also be vomiting. Also, the stimulation of the R. meningeus, e.g. in the case of meningitis in the area of the posterior cranial fossa may trigger vomiting.

The main stem of the nerve runs together with the A. carotis interna and the V. jugularis interna within a common sheath (**Vagina carotica**) as a vascular nerve cord caudally through the throat area. On its way, it emits the following branches:

- **R. pharyngeus** (SVE, GSA): it forms together with the N. glossopharyngeus [IX] the **Plexus pharyngeus** and provides motor innervation to the pharyngeal muscles. Sensory information is relayed via Rr. linguales and the Plexus pharyngeus from the

mucosa of the throat area, Isthmus faucium, base of the tongue and entrance of the larynx to the Nucleus spinalis nervi trigemini. The nerve cell bodies reside in the Ganglion nodosum (inferius).

- **N. laryngeus superior** (SVE, GSA): the branch leaves the N. vagus [X] usually shortly after leaving the skull and passes between A. carotis interna and pharyngeal wall caudally to the level of the larynx. Here it branches into:
  - The **R. externus** innervates the M. cricothyroideus.
  - The **R. internus** provides sensory innervation of the larynx epithelium above the glottis.
- **Rr. cardiaci cervicales superiores and inferiores, Rr. cardiaci thoracici** (GVE, GVA): the branches leave the N. vagus already in the throat area and upper chest area and run to the heart. The N. vagus continues its course through the upper thoracic aperture. The Rr. cardiaci form the **Plexus cardiacus** at the heart. They are switched to the 2nd neuron and then innervate the atrium, the sinus nodes (right vagus part) and the AV nodes (left

vagus part) parasympathetically. The chambers of the heart are not innervated by the N. vagus.

- **N. laryngeus recurrens** (SVE, GSA): it passes on the left side from front to back around the aortic arch (and is wound around the Lig. arteriosum BOTALLI). On the right side, it extends from front to back around the A. subclavia and passes as on the left-hand side into the groove between trachea and oesophagus. On both sides, it emits **Rr. tracheales and oesophageales** (parasympathetic) and continues cranially to the larynx, which it reaches as the **N. laryngeus inferior**. Its fibres divide and innervate all other laryngeal muscles and the mucosa of the glottis and below the glottis (subglottis), with the exception of the M. cricothyroideus which has already been innervated by the N. laryngeus superior.
- In the thorax numerous fibres leave the N. vagus and form the **Rr. bronchiales**, the **Plexus pulmonalis** and the **Plexus oesophageus** for the parasympathetic innervation of the corresponding structures.
- Below the tracheal bifurcation the fibres which originally belonged to the left N. vagus [X] shift to the front and form the **Truncus vagalis anterior,** the fibres belonging to the right N. vagus [X] move dorsally and form the **Truncus vagalis posterior.** This shift is based on the gastric rotation during embryonic development. Both Trunci vagales pass together with the oesophagus through the Hiatus oesophageus of the diaphragm into the abdominal cavity and then branch out with the vessels as part of the enteric nervous system in: R. hepaticus (Omentum minus), Plexus hepaticus, Rr. gastrici anteriores, Plexus coeliacus, Ganglia coeliaca and Mesentericum superius, Plexus splenicus, Plexus suprarenalis, Plexus renalis and Rr. intestinales. They therefore parasympathetically innervate the viscera of the upper abdomen and gastrointestinal tract. The switch from preganglionic to postganglionic occurs directly at the respective organ.

The innervation area of the N. vagus [X] ends at the level of the colic flexure (**CANNON-BÖHM point**). From there, the parasympathetic innervation is guaranteed for all further distally located sections from the sacral medulla. The two autonomic nervous parts overlap extensively in this area, so that there can be no sharp border between the cranial (N. vagus [X]) and the sacral parasympathetic nervous system.

NOTE

The **course of the N. laryngeus recurrens** is different on both sides (left around the aortic arch, right around the A. subclavia). This can be explained from the development. A thicker myelin sheath on the left side ensures that despite the longer course both vocal folds can swing synchronously. In rare cases, the A. subclavia dextra originates as the last branch from the aortic arch (so-called **A. lusoria**) and runs behind or in front of the oesophagus or between the oesophagus and trachea on the right side of the body. In such a case, there is no N. laryngeus recurrens on the right side. The N. laryngeus inferior then originates either together or a few millimetres below the N. laryngeus superior from the N. vagus [X].

Clinical remarks

Damage to the N. vagus [X] is common in the context of skull fractures in the area of the Foramen jugulare; however, the nerve can also be damaged due to tumours of the cerebellopontine angle or iatrogenically (from medical procedures), e.g. biopsy incision of lymph nodes or a neck dissection (neck lymph node evacuation). Depending on the location of the damage, the following can be caused, difficulty in swallowing, sensory disturbances in the pharynx and the epiglottis (lack of gag reflex, taste disturbances), hoarseness (via Nn. laryngei), tachycardia, arrhythmia as well as respiratory and circulatory problems.

9.3.11 N. accessorius [XI]

By definition, the N. accessorius [XI] (SVE) is *not actually a cranial nerve* as its main section (**Radix spinalis**) does not originate from cerebral core areas, but from the anterior horn (**Nucleus nervi accessorii**) in the cervical spinal cord (up to C5). Hence the name 'accessorius' = additional. Only a smaller part (**Radix cranialis**) leaves the brainstem together with the N. glossopharyngeus [IX] (➤ Chap. 9.3.9) and the N. vagus [X] (➤ Chap. 9.3.10) in the Sulcus retroolivaris. The neurons are in the Nucleus ambiguus. Within the Foramen jugulare the two Radices merge to the N. accessorius [XI] (➤ Fig. 9.41). It is not conclusively clarified whether the fibres of the Radix cranialis pass over below the Foramen jugulare as **R. internus** to the N. vagus [X] or whether there is no connection to the N. vagus at all. The Radix cranialis participates in the innervation of the pharyngeal and laryngeal muscles and, strictly speaking, is not part of the N. accessorius [XI]. The fibres of the Radix spinalis, with their neurons in the Nucleus nervi accessorii, pass as **R. externus** via the M. levator scapulae caudally to the M. sternocleidomastoideus and innervate it. One part then continues through the lateral triangle of the neck to the anterior border of the M. trapezius, which it also innervates.

Clinical remarks

Since the N. accessorius [XI] runs very superficially in the throat area, it is at risk of injury (e.g. in the case of the removal of lymph nodes). In most cases the **damage** lies below the outlet for the M. sternocleidomastoideus in the lateral triangle of the neck, so that the innervation of the M. trapezius fails. The consequences are dropping of the shoulder and difficulties in raising the arm above the horizontal plane (distorted elevation). If the damage is above the outlet to the M. sternocleidomastoideus, it will also no longer be innervated and apart from the difficulties in raising the arm the patient can also no longer turn the head to the healthy side.

9.3.12 N. hypoglossus [XII]

The N. hypoglossus [XII] is a purely motor nerve with a quality (GSE). Its core area is the **Nucleus nervi hypoglossi.** It leaves the brain as the only cranial nerve with multiple small fibres in the **Sulcus anterolateralis** between olive and pyramid. After the merger of the fibres to the N. hypoglossus [XII] the nerve passes through the **Canalis nervi hypoglossi** at the side of the Foramen magnum through the skull base (➤ Fig. 9.42). Below this, fibres of the spinal nerves C1 and C2 (Plexus cervicalis) accumulate, which run to the Mm. geniohyoideus and thyrohyoideus and innervate them. After passing through the skull base, it passes into the **Spatium lateropharyngeum** between A. carotis interna and V. jugularis interna to the front in the direction of the floor of the mouth. In doing so, the fibres from C1 and C2 also runs with them as **Ansa cervicalis nervi hypoglossi**. It passes between M. mylohyoideus and M. hyoglossus laterally into the tongue and provides motor innervation to the internal muscles (Mm. longitudinales superior and inferior linguae,

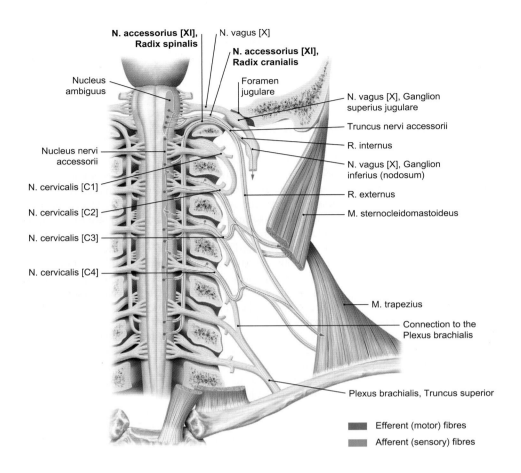

Fig. 9.41 N. accessorius[XI], cores and fibre qualities. Ventral view, vertebral canal and skull are opened.

Efferent (motor) fibres
Afferent (sensory) fibres

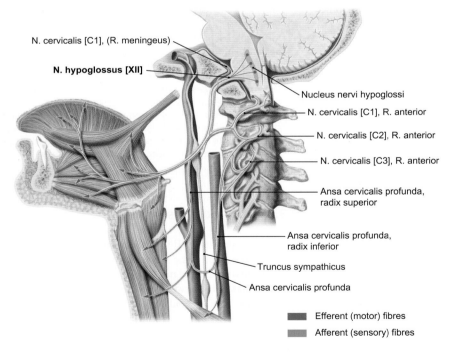

Fig. 9.42 N. hypoglossus [XII], cores and fibre qualities. Schematic median section, view from left.

Efferent (motor) fibres
Afferent (sensory) fibres

M. transversus linguae, M. verticalis linguae and the Mm. styloglossus, hyoglossus and genioglossus). It is the only motor muscle for the tongue and therefore vital for eating, drinking, swallowing and speaking.

Clinical remarks

Skull base fractures or infarcts in the flow area of the A. vertebralis may cause **damage to the N. hypoglossus [XII]**. Usually only one side is affected. The patients are conspicuous due to articulation disorders (dysarthria) and swallowing difficulties (dysphagia). When prompted to stick out the tongue, it deviates to the *diseased side,* as the muscles on the healthy side are predominant. If the lesion persists longer, the result is an atrophy of the tongue muscles on the affected side.

9.4 Eye
Michael Scholz

Skills

After processing this chapter, you should be able to:
- understand the embryological development of the eye and assess the resulting special features of the respective structures of the eye
- name the construction and the structures of the orbita
- differentiate the auxiliary structures of the Orbita and explain their functions
- describe and distinguish between the structure and function of the extraocular muscles, their blood supply and the innervation of the Bulbus oculi and the Orbita
- differentiate the components of the Bulbus oculi and assign their functions

Clinical case

Rupture of the N. opticus [II]
Accident
A 32-year-old man falls from his racing bike in a light descent and hits his right temple hard on the asphalt ground. Although the man is not wearing a helmet, he does not become unconscious as a result of the fall. He notes a coruscation for a few seconds in the right eye and by covering his left eye finds that he can see nothing through the right eye. Apart from minor abrasions a haematoma forms on the right temple.

Diagnosis
After admission to hospital an emergency computed tomography (CT) is conducted to evaluate possible fractures. A fracture cannot be detected, the optic nerve channel (Canalis opticus) is also intact. The alternating light exposure test which was also conducted to determine pupil reaction shows a complete afferent disruption of light perception in the right eye.

Treatment
The immediate intravenous administration of a megadose of the anti-inflammatory glucocorticoid prednisolone does not improve the vision loss on the right side.

Long-term diagnosis
After about 7 weeks an optical atrophy is detected. Due to the side impact of the unprotected head (helmet on when cycling!) on the road, there was a rupture of the Nn. opticus [II] and/or the relevant vessels in the Canalis opticus.

The eye (Organum visus) as the optical organ in humans consists functionally of the **eyeball (Bulbus oculi)** with the actual optical apparatus, the external **eye muscles (Mm. bulbi)**, numerous blood vessels and nerves and various auxiliary structures such as the **eyelids (Palpebrae)**, the **conjunctiva (Tunica conjunctiva)** and the **lacrimal apparatus (Apparatus lacrimalis).** With the exception of the eyelids, all auxiliary structures together with the eyeball and a filling **fat body (Corpus adiposum orbitae)**, which is developed around the Bulbus oculi as a **connective tissue capsule (Vagina bulbi; TENON's capsule)** are accommodated in the bony **orbit (Orbita)** (➤ Fig. 9.43).
- Each eye has an **upper (Palpebra superior)** and a **lower eyelid (Palpebra inferior).**
- The **lacrimal apparatus** is composed of the lacrimal gland (Glandula lacrimalis), the accessory lacrimal gland (Glandulae lacrimales accessoriae) and the MEIBOM's glands (Glandulae tarsales) in the eyelids, the upper and the lower tear ducts (Canaliculi lacrimales superior and inferior), the lacrimal sac (Saccus lacrimalis) and the nasolacrimal duct (Ductus nasolacrimalis).
- In the orbit there are **6 muscles that move the eyeball,** and the **(upper) lid elevator (M. levator palpebrae superioris).** Of the 6 muscles that move the eyeball, 4 run straight (M. rectus superior, M. rectus inferior, M. rectus medialis and M. rectus lateralis) and 2 have an oblique course (M. obliquus superior and M. obliquus inferior).
- The **eyeball (Bulbus oculi)** resembles an onion in its layered structure. On the outer optic membrane the layer looks like a husk (Tunica fibrosa bulbi), the middle eye membrane follows with sclera and cornea (Tunica vasculosa bulbi), which consists of the choroid, the ciliary body and the iris. The inner eye membrane (Tunica interna bulbi) is the retina. On the inside of the eyeball are the intraocular fluid, lens and vitreous body.

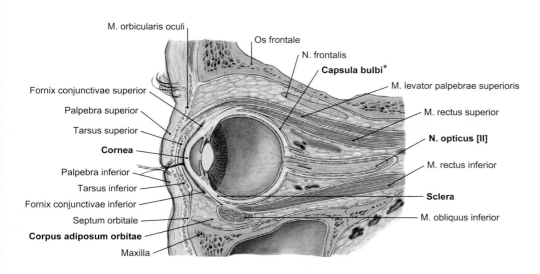

M. orbicularis oculi
Os frontale
N. frontalis
Capsula bulbi*
Fornix conjunctivae superior
M. levator palpebrae superioris
Palpebra superior
M. rectus superior
Tarsus superior
Cornea
N. opticus [II]
Palpebra inferior
M. rectus inferior
Tarsus inferior
Fornix conjunctivae inferior
Sclera
Septum orbitale
M. obliquus inferior
Corpus adiposum orbitae
Maxilla

Fig. 9.43 Vertical section through the middle area of the Orbita. Medial view. All structures within the Orbita are embedded in a fat body, which is similar to a filling or padding mass surrounding the content structures. *TENON's capsule

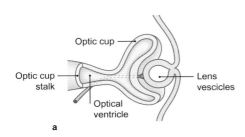
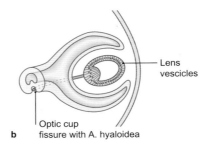

Fig. 9.44 Phases of ocular development In the 5th and 6th weeks (schematic diagram). **a** 5th week. **B** 6th week. [E838]

9.4.1 Embryology

Tissue of origin

The development of the organ of sight is principally controlled by a series of inductive signals, which initially take place within the neuroectoderm of the diencephalon (diencephalon) and later in mutual interaction between the respective portions of the eye system. In principle, the later eye tissue originates from 3 different areas during embryonic development (➤ Table 9.21):
- The neuroectoderm of the diencephalon
- The superficial ectoderm of the head
- The head mesenchyme

Development of the eye system

The development of the eye system is already visible at the beginning of the 4th week. First of all, a trough-shaped dent of the neuroectoderm is created on both sides (optical/farrow, Sulcus opticus). This creates eye vesicles by fusing the neural folds, which come into contact with the surface ectoderm during the further course of development. The surface ectoderm becomes thicker at the contact points and each develops a lens placode as a unit of the subsequent lens. The lens placodes then sink and merge finally to the spherical lens vesicles, which subsequently lose their connection to the surface ectoderm. The eye vesicles laterally surround the lens vesicles, so that the lens vesicles can emerge from the optic cups. Via the Sulcus opticus, the optic cup is still connected to the diencephalon. As an oblong indentation on the ventral side of the optic cup, the optic cup fissure (Fissura optica) develops along the optic cup stalk, through which mesenchymal cells can migrate along the entire length of the eye unit into the inside of the optic cup but not into the optic ventricle located between the two layers of the optic cup. This optic fissure forms blood vessels, which are partly surrounded by the first nerve fibres of the later N. opticus [II]. These blood vessels supply as A. and V. hyaloidea (vitreous body vessels), the inner layer of the optic cup, the lens vesicles as well as the optic cup mesenchyme. During the continuing development process the edges of the optic cup fissure finally begin to merge distally. Due to the proximal progressive extension of this merger zone, the vitreous

Table 9.21 Tissue of origin of the eye system with the parts of the eye developed during the course of the organ development.

Tissue of origin	Resulting components of the eye
Neuroectoderm (diencephalon)	• Retina • Inner layers of the ciliary body • Rear layers of the iris • N. opticus
Surface ectoderm (head)	• Ocular lens • Corneal epithelium
Head mesenchyme	• Sclera • Cornea • Choroidea

vessels are increasingly enclosed by the N. opticus [II] emerging in the optic cup stalk. The distal branches of the vitreous body vessels subsequently degenerate, while the proximal branches remain as a. and V. centralis retinae in the N. opticus (➤ Fig. 9.44).

Clinical remarks

Because the eye development is very complex, there may be a whole range of **congenital malformations of the eye**. Usually the malformations are caused by closure disorders of the optic cup fissure. Basically the type and severity of the respective anomalies depend on the embryonic stage of the developmental disorder. Apart from exogenous factors (e.g. environmental toxins) disturbances in the expression of important molecular factors may have an influence which plays an important role in the development of the eye (e.g. the transcription factor Pax6 or secreted signal molecules, such as Shh [sonic hedgehog]).

Development of the retina

The retina develops from the layers of the optic cup. The outer, thin layer of of the optic cup becomes a single-layered pigment epithelium, while the inner layer thickens during the invagination of the optic cup and develops to the actual neuroretina (➤ Fig. 9.45). The optic ventricle, which lies between the two units, disappears completely until birth due to the close approximation of both retinal layers; however, as a result no defined cell contacts are developed between the two layers, which means that the connection is not particularly resilient mechanically and clinically plays a key role e.g. in the development of age-related retinal detachment (Ablatio retinae).

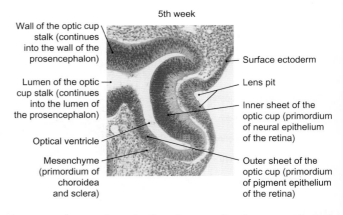

Fig. 9.45 Microscopic sagittal section; eye development; 5th week, 200x. The eye vesicle has already invaginated into the optic cup and has close contact to the lens placode. The inner and outer layers of the optic cup and the still existing optical ventricle can be clearly differentiated. [E581]

Development of the inner eye tissue

The exterior corneal epithelium develops from the surface ectoderm, while the stromal cells and the inner epithelium, which is known as the endothelium, develop from neural crest cells. The corneal curvature for normal visual acuity critical corneal curvature is formed in direct dependency on the intraocular pressure. The mesenchyme surrounding the optic cup (from the neural crest cells) is stimulated by the inducing effect of pigment epithelium to further differentiation and forms 2 layers: the internal, vessel-rich and later also pigmented layer, which is referred to as the choroid (Choroidea) and an external, connective tissue and initially vessel-poor layer, as the sclera. In the creation of the sclera the mesenchyme thickens and passes seamlessly in a transition zone (Limbus corneae) into the cornea. The Choroidea changes on the optic cup edge and forms the core of the ciliary body process which is covered by the double layered ciliated epithelium. The iris develops from the front edge (Pars caeca) of the optic cup, which bulges inwards and in this way partially covers the lens from the outside. In the same way as the layers of the optic cup, the iris displays a bilayered epithelium, which continuously procedes proximally into the epithelium of the ciliary body. Early in the development the pigmentation spreads in the iris up to the transition to the ciliary epithelium from the outside and to the inner layer of the optic cup, rendering the iris fully impermeable to light and justifying the subsequent function as a screen for the eye against incidental light.

Development of the eyelids and lacrimal glands

The eyelids develop during the 6th week from 2 skin folds growing successively over the cornea, which contain the cells of the head mesenchyme. Roughly from the beginning of the 10th week these wrinkles fully cover the cornea and connect to each other up to the 26th week. As long as the connection exists, the conjunctiva in front of the cornea, which has previously differentiated, forms a closed pouch. Through the keratinization of the epidermis system on the eyelid edges the epithelium connection dissolves approximately from the 7th month in this area and the eye can be opened. The systems of the two lacrimal glands develop as bud-like consolidations of the surface ectoderm. In adults the buds form branching in the mesenchyme, in which the duct system and gland end pieces differentiate. The lacrimal glands are not yet fully functional at the

time of birth, which is why newborns cannot form tears when crying.

9.4.2 Protective and auxiliary structures of the eye

The protective and auxiliary structures of the eye include the eyelids, the conjunctiva, the lacrimal apparatus and the extraocular muscles. They also include the orbital fat body and the vascular, lymphatic and nervous systems running in it.

Eyelids and conjunctiva

The **eyelids (Palpebrae)** can be described as movable soft tissue folds of the face, which in particular cover the cornea of the eyeball from the front and protect it against mechanical damage. At the same time, regular blinking (10–15 times per minute) ensures an even distribution of the tear fluid to the cornea and conjunctiva and protects the eye from drying out. The epidermis on the eyelids is relatively thin and fat free. Along the front edge of the eyelids are several dense rows of eyelashes (Cilia), which curve upwards and are usually longer than on the lower eyelid. The excretory ducts of the large sebaceous glands (glands of ZEIS; Glandulae sebaceae flow in the hair funnel of the eyelashes). On the hair roots there are apocrine sweat glands (MOLL's glands, Glandulae ciliares). In the upper eyelid there are small accessory lacrimal glands (KRAUSE's glands, WOLFRING glands) in the vicinity of the Fornix conjunctivae and on the top edge of the MEIBOM glands.

The eyelid (upper and lower eyelid are basically structured the same) is divided into an outer and inner layer (➤ Fig. 9.46):

- The **outer layer** of the eyelid contains the striated, facial **M. orbicularis oculi** with its **Pars palpebralis** as a sphincter of the palpebral fissure. The opening of the eyelids is especially the function of the **M. levator palpebrae superioris,** its tendon radiates into the upper edge of the fibrous eyelid plate of the upper lid (Tarsus). The section of the muscle near to the eyelid edge is known as the RIOLAN muscle (see below). Both in the upper and the lower eyelid the smooth muscle fibres of the **M. tarsalis** begin at the tarsal edge which is innervated sympathetically and ensures the retraction of the eyelids. Decreased activation of the muscle e.g. in the case of fatigue (parasympathetic nervous sys-

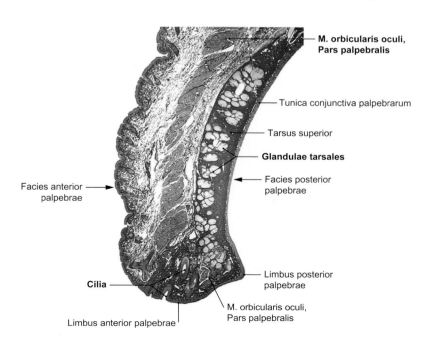

M. orbicularis oculi, Pars palpebralis

Tunica conjunctiva palpebrarum

Tarsus superior

Glandulae tarsales

Facies posterior palpebrae

Facies anterior palpebrae

Limbus posterior palpebrae

Cilia

M. orbicularis oculi, Pars palpebralis

Limbus anterior palpebrae

Fig. 9.46 Upper eyelid, Palpebrae superior. Photograph of a microscopic preparation; azan stain; sagittal section, magnified. [M375]

tem activation) causes in the truest sense of the word 'the eyes to fall closed'.

- The **internal layer** of the eyelid includes the **eyelid plate (Tarsus)** consisting of tough collagen connective tissue with the elongated MEIBOM glands (Glandulae tarsales) stored in it, 25-35 (upper eyelid) and 15-25 (lower eyelid), which as modified sebaceous glands flow on the rear edge of the eyelid (➤ Fig. 9.47). In the area of the eyelid edge there are muscle fibres of the M. orbicularis oculi (Pars palpebralis) grouped concentrically around the excretory ducts of the MEIBOM glands, which radiates into the Tarsus and are referred to as RIOLAN muscles or Fasciculi ciliares. Whether the muscle portion is for pressing out the oily secretion of the MEIBOM glands or the closure of the glands (e.g. during sleep), has not been clarified to date. The eyelid conjunctiva (Tunica conjunctiva palpebrarum) is the mucosa at the inner side of the eyelids.

The **conjunctiva (Tunica conjunctiva)** not only covers the inside of the eyelids. In its course in the direction of the eyeball it changes in the area of the orbital rim to the eyeball and thus forms reserve wrinkles, which are important for eye movements (Fornix conjunctivae superior/inferior). In the further course the conjunctiva covers - with the exception of the cornea – as eye connective tissue (Tunica conjunctiva bulbi) the entire front surface of the Bulbus oculi. Both units together form the conjunctival sac. This enables the movements of the eyelids and also provides protection for the eye. In the nasal eye angle there is a third, small and slightly curved mucosal fold (Plica semilunaris conjunctivae), which is considered in humans as rudiment of the nictitating membrane that is partially well developed in animals (Membrana nictitans). In the multi-layered epithelium of the conjunctiva cup cells are stored, their secretion

products are part of the lacrimal film. They also occur in the conjunctiva lymph follicle which belong to the conjunctiva-associated lymphatic tissue (CALT).

Clinical remarks

The **hailstone (chalazion)** is a pain-free swelling of the eyelid, mostly due to clogging of the excretory duct of a MEIBOM gland, with subsequent non-bacterial inflammation. It is differentiated from the painful infection of the eyelid edge glands (ZEIS or MOLL's glands), which is referred to as a **stye (Hordeolum externum)** and is mostly caused by bacteria *(Staphylococcus aureus)*. The **Hordeolum internum** is a bacterial inflammation of a MEIBOM gland. In both cases, the clinical picture shows a significant redness of the eyelid edge with oedematous swelling and possible pus formation.

Lacrimal apparatus
Lacrimal gland (Glandula lacrimalis)

Within the Orbita lies the **lacrimal gland (glandula lacrimalis)** immediately below the periorbita in the Fossa glandulae lacrimalis of the os frontale, lateral above the temporal eyelid angle (➤ Fig. 9.48). Its front edge extends to the Septum orbitale that closes the orbita to the outside with connective tissue. It is separated by the tendon of the M. levator palpebrae incompletely into a larger upper part (Pars orbitalis) and a smaller lower part (Pars palpebralis), which in turn is divided into 2–3 lobes. In the rear lateral part of the gland both parts are connected. The approximately 10 excretory ducts of this branched, tubuloalveolar gland ultimately flow into

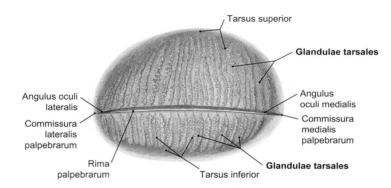

Fig. 9.47 Eyelids, Palpebrae, right. Rear view; glandular ducts of the Glandulae tarsales in a brightened preparation. Each eyelid contains approximately 20–30 individual glands with their own excretory duct opening into the rim of the eyelid.

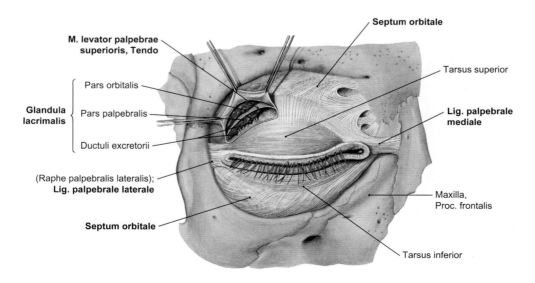

Fig. 9.48 Right orbital opening (Aditus orbitalis) with Septum orbitale and the underlying lacrimal gland (Septum orbitale opened in the temporal upper quadrant).

the upper fornix (Fornix conjunctivae superior) behind the eyelid. Their most important feature is the secretion of large parts of the aqueous component of the lacrimal film (➤ Table 9.22).

Lacrimal film

Corneal and conjunctival epithelium are moistened with a **lacrimal film** up to 40 μm thick. Its main component is the aqueous component derived from the lacrimal gland, an isotonic electrolyte solution, containing antimicrobial proteins and peptides and high molecular gel-forming mucins (main component of mucus) from the cup cells of the conjunctiva and from the lacrimal gland. The accessory lacrimal glands of the eyelids also make a small part of the aqueous component of the lacrimal film. The adhesion of the lacrimal film is made possible by microplicae on the superficial epithelial cells and membrane mucins in the apical cell membrane of the surface cells of the cornea and Tunica conjunctiva. Evaporation of the aqueous component is prevented by a superficial lipid layer that lies on the aqueous component and originates mainly from MEIBOM's glands of the eyelids (➤ Table 9.22). The lacrimal film protects and nourishes the ocular surface while forming the refractive anterior aspect of the visual system.

Table 9.22 Highly simplified division of the lacrimal film built in 3 physically different portions that continuously merge together.

Structure of the lacrimal film	Secreting glands/cells
Lipid layer Function: prevents a fast evaporation of the lacrimal film	Mainly MEIBOM's glands (Glandulae tarsales), with a small proportion of cell membrane lipids of desquamated epithelial cells
Aqueous component • Isotonic electrolyte solution • Gel-forming mucins and cleavage products of membrane-bound mucins • Antimicrobial substances (e.g. lysozyme, lactoferrin, lipocalin, defensins, surfactant proteins A and D) • IgA (by transcytosis) **Function:** irrigation fluid, equilibrates surface irregularities, antimicrobial protection	• Lacrimal gland (Glandula lacrimalis) • Cup cells of the conjunctiva (Tunica conjunctiva) • Accessory lacrimal gland (KRAUSE's glands, WOLFRING's glands)
Mucosal component • Membrane-bound mucins in the cell membrane of microplicae of the superficial epithelial cells of cornea and conjunctiva **Function:** part of the glycocalyx represents the connection between epithelium and aqueous component of the lacrimal film and thus serves adhesion of the lacrimal film	• Corneal epithelial cells • Conjunctiva (Tunica conjunctiva)

Vessel supply and innervation

The lacrimal gland is supplied with blood via the **A. lacrimalis** (branch of the A. ophthalmica) (➤ Fig. 9.49). The venous blood flows via the **V. ophthalmica superior** to the Sinus cavernosus. The parasympathetic nervous system increases tear secretion, the sympathetic nervous system inhibits it. Preganglionic fibres of the sympathetic nervous system are switched in the Ganglion cervicale superius of the sympathetic trunk to postganglionic fibres. These reach the lacrimal gland by following the Aa. carotis interna, ophthalmica and lacrimalis or they leave the plexus around the A. carotis interna as N. petrosus profundus, the parasympathetic fibres of which connect to its fibres in the Canalis pterygoideus as N. canalis pterygoidei, in order to reach the lacrimal gland. The preganglionic fibres of the parasympathetic nerve system (1st neuron in the Nucleus salivatorius superior) reach the Ganglion pterygopalatinum via the intermediate part of the N. facialis [VII] as N. petrosus major and then as N. canalis pterygoidei (in conjunction with sympathetic fibres from the N. petrosus profundus). Here, the switching of the parasympathetic fibres to postganglionic takes place, which then reach the N. lacrimalis and ultimately the lacrimal gland with the N. zygomaticus (branch of the N. maxillaris [V/2]) via the R. communicans cum nervo zygomatico (➤ Fig. 9.49).

Efferent lacrimal ducts
Michael Scholz, Friedrich Paulsen

The beat of the eyelid runs in a time-shifted manner from temporal to nasal (Pars palpebralis, M. orbicularis oculi) and wipes the tear fluid in the direction of nasal eye angle. The efferent lacrimal ducts begin here with the upper and lower Puncta lacrimalia (**Punctum lacrimale**), which are on the nasal eyelid edge of the upper or lower eyelid, respectively, near the medial angle of eye (➤ Fig. 9.50a). The Puncta lacrimalia submerge in the Lacus lacrimalis when the eyelid closes (**Lacus lacrimalis**). This is the 'old' used tear fluid that has collected at the eyelid angle at the nose. The lacrimal fluid reaches the upper and lower lacrimal canaliculi via the Puncta lacrimalia (**Canaliculi lacrimales superior and inferior**), which either flow individually or combined in a short common tract into the lacrimal sac (**Sac-**

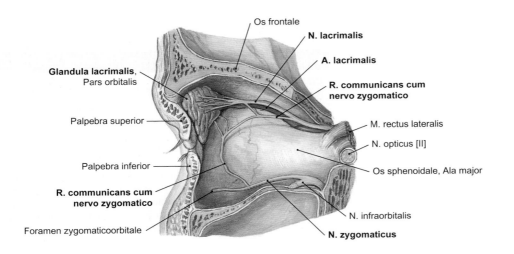

Os frontale
N. lacrimalis
A. lacrimalis
R. communicans cum nervo zygomatico
Glandula lacrimalis, Pars orbitalis
Palpebra superior
Palpebra inferior
M. rectus lateralis
N. opticus [II]
Os sphenoidale, Ala major
R. communicans cum nervo zygomatico
Foramen zygomaticoorbitale
N. infraorbitalis
N. zygomaticus

Fig. 9.49 Arterial blood supply and nervous innervation of the lacrimal gland. Medial view, schematic drawing.

cus lacrimalis) (➤ Fig. 9.50a, b). Around the lacrimal canaliculi the **Pars lacrimalis of the M. orbicularis oculi (HORNER's muscle)**, is arranged which is essential for the tear transport through the canaliculi. This so-called tear pump function of the Pars lacrimalis is not yet fully understood. The muscle fibres insert via small tendons on the Septum lacrimale of the lateral lacrimal sac wall.

The lacrimal sac, which lies in the Fossa lacrimalis and is separated lateral to the Orbita by the Septum lacrimale (➤ Fig. 9.51) extends cranially to the Fornix sacci lacrimalis and passes caudally in approx. 25 mm long **nasolacrimal ducts (Ductus nasolacrimalis)**. The Ductus nasolacrimalis is located in one of the bony canals formed by the

Maxilla and the Os lacrimale and has a dorsal topographic relationship to the maxillary sinus. Medially, an ethmoid bone cell (Agger nasi cell) can push between the wall of the bony canal and the lateral nasal wall. The Ductus nasolacrimalis continues downwards into the lower nasal duct (Meatus nasi inferior) below the lower nasal concha (Concha nasalis inferior). The outlet area in the nasal cavity is below the front portion of the inferior nasal concha and is very variably formed. In many cases there is a **mucosal fold (Plica lacrimalis, HASNER's valve)** at the outlet area. The lumen of the lacrimal sac and lacrimal nasal duct are surrounded by a strong vessel plexus, which is functionally comparable with a cavernous body. Around

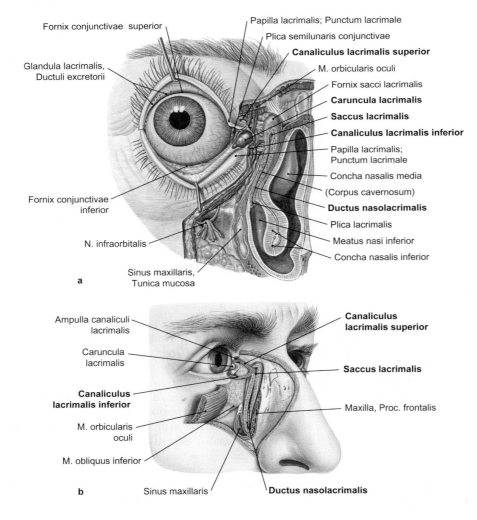

Fornix conjunctivae superior
Glandula lacrimalis, Ductuli excretorii
Fornix conjunctivae inferior
N. infraorbitalis
Sinus maxillaris, Tunica mucosa
Papilla lacrimalis; Punctum lacrimale
Plica semilunaris conjunctivae
Canaliculus lacrimalis superior
M. orbicularis oculi
Fornix sacci lacrimalis
Caruncula lacrimalis
Saccus lacrimalis
Canaliculus lacrimalis inferior
Papilla lacrimalis; Punctum lacrimale
Concha nasalis media
(Corpus cavernosum)
Ductus nasolacrimalis
Plica lacrimalis
Meatus nasi inferior
Concha nasalis inferior

a

Ampulla canaliculi lacrimalis
Caruncula lacrimalis
Canaliculus lacrimalis inferior
M. orbicularis oculi
M. obliquus inferior
Sinus maxillaris
Canaliculus lacrimalis superior
Saccus lacrimalis
Maxilla, Proc. frontalis
Ductus nasolacrimalis

b

Fig. 9.50 Structures of the lacrimal apparatus, Apparatus lacrimalis right. a View from the front lateral. Upper and lower canaliculi, lacrimal sac and lacrimal nasal passage. The lacrimal nasal passage is open before it flows into the Meatus nasi inferior (underneath the Concha nasalis inferior). **b** Horizontal section at the height of the lacrimal sac.

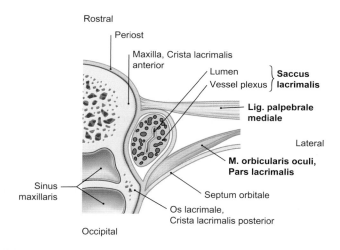

Fig. 9.51 Lacrimal apparatus, Apparatus lacrimalis, right side. Horizontal section at the height of the lacrimal sac (diagram). [E402]

and between the vessels of the cavernous body connective tissue fibres from the lacrimal sac run spirally to the lower nasal concha. Due to the attachment in the area of the inferior nasal concha and the spiral course of the connective tissue fibres, the lacrimal sac and lacrimal nasal duct are pulled cranially on contraction of the Pars lacrimalis of the M. orbicularis oculi; in the process the lacrimal system is wrung out like a towel and the tear liquid drained distally.

Clinical remarks

The most common pathological changes of the efferent lacrimal ducts include **inflammation (dacryocystitis), constriction (dacryostenosis)** and **stone formations (dacryolithiasis).** The symptoms are **epiphora** (Greek: 'downflow'), an overflow of the tear fluid through the eyelid margins. In the case of dacryostenosis it can also be a congenital defect, which e.g. can be attributed to **persistance of HASNER's valve,** a thin fibrous membrane at the transition to the lower nasal passage and prevents a normal lacrimal drainage. In most cases it ruptures shortly after birth. If it persists longer than a year, it must be therapeutically pierced.

NOTE

If the cavernous body tissue swells, the tear transport is reduced or no longer possible through the efferent lacrimal ducts. Then the tears flow down the cheeks and one 'cries.' Except for mechanical causes (foreign objects in the conjunctival sac; 'reflex tears') the blood vessels of the cavernous body may fill even with strong emotions (e.g. great pleasure, anxiety or grief) (at the same time the liquid lacrimal gland production considerably increases). **In the course of life a person cries up to 80 litres of tear fluid.** There are different theories and opinions to the cause for the development of 'emotional tears'. Without a doubt, crying has an important social function between people. While crying in infancy and small children is the only form of communication up to a certain degree, it is usually an expression of different emotions in adults. In the animal world the emotional tears of man are probably unique. Other mammals and reptiles can weep with a corresponding lacrimal apparatus, but the so-called **crocodile tears** are actually reflectory tears and are probably due to the fact that the reptiles open their mouth wide when eating and thus mechanically increase the pressure on the lacrimal gland. Nevertheless: animals demonstrably also experience the pain and grief sensation, even if there are no tears to accompany these feelings.

9.4.3 Orbita

The orbit (**Orbita**) is a bony limited, conically constructed space. 'It is formed by various bony parts of the neurocranium (skull) and the viscerocranium Viscerocranium/facial skeleton (➤ Fig. 9.52, also ➤ Fig. 9.7). The parts of the neurocranium consist of:

- the Facies orbitalis of the Os frontale (roof of the Orbita)
- the Lamina orbitalis of the Os ethmoidale (medial wall)
- the Ala major and minor of the Os sphenoidale (rear limitation of the Orbita)

The bony boundaries of the viscerocranium are formed by the

- Proc. orbitalis of the Os palatinum
- Facies orbitalis of the Maxilla (floor of the Orbita)
- Os lacrimale (medial wall)
- Fascies orbitalis of the Os zygomaticum (lateral wall)

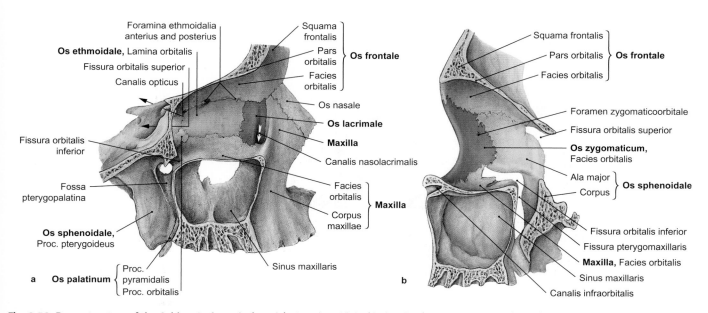

Fig. 9.52 Bony structure of the Orbita. Os frontale (purple), Os ethmoidale (dark yellow), Os sphenoidale (green), Os palatinum (blue), Maxilla (light yellow), Os lacrimale (dark red), Os zygomaticum (light red). **a** View of the medial wall of the Orbita. **b** View of the lateral wall of the Orbita.

The bony structure of the Orbita requires very close **topographic relationships** to the directly adjacent neighbouring regions that are clinically of great importance (➤ Fig. 9.53). The treatment of pathological changes within or in the area of the Orbita may require the interdisciplinary cooperation of different disciplines. Inflammatory processes or tumour events in the Orbita can, for example, spread very quickly to the neighbouring regions and usually make a multidisciplinary approach to treatment necessary. In such cases, in addition to the ophthalmologist, ENT doctors, radiologists, maxillofacial and brain surgeons or neurologists are involved in appropriate therapeutic management.

The frontal opening of the orbita bordered by a bone edge (Margo orbitalis) is called the **Aditus orbitalis**. The bony Orbita is lined by the periosteum which is known as the **Periorbita**. At the Canalis opticus and the Fissura orbitalis superior, the Periorbita is connected to the Dura mater of the brain and bridges as **Membrana orbitalis** the Fissura orbitalis inferior. The fibres of the **M. orbitalis** run in this membrane, a smooth muscle innervated sympathetically via the N. petrosus profundus, the tone of which regulates the flow of blood through the V. ophthalmica inferior. On the outside, the Orbita is closed according to the two eyelids by a thin connective tissue plate, the **Septum orbitale**, (➤ Fig. 9.54). The Septum orbitale is attached at the top and bottom in the area of the Margo orbitalis and passes close behind the M. orbicularis oculi of the eyelids to the outer edge of the tarsal plate.

The bony boundaries between Orbita and sinuses (Sinus maxillaris; Cellulae ethmoidales) are extremely thin. So they can be easily fractured by a trauma. **Inflammatory processes** can then easily spread from the physiologically pathogen populated mucous membranes of the sinuses into the 'sterile' Orbita (e.g. as orbital phlegmon).

Vessels and innervation of the Regio orbitalis

Above the Septum orbitale the Orbita is surrounded by a circular arterial plexus of vessels (➤ Fig. 9.54). In this region the **innervation areas of A. carotis interna** overlap with its branches (A. supraorbitalis, Aa. palpebrales laterales [from A. lacrimalis] and Aa. palpebrales mediales) with those of the **A. carotis externa** (A. facialis, A. angularis, A. infraorbitalis, A. temporalis superficialis and A. zygomaticoorbitalis). The veins of the same name accompany the arteries. The **N. supraorbitalis** leaves the Orbita variably as a branch of the N. ophthalmicus [V/1] via the Foramen supraorbitale or the Incisura supraorbitalis of the same name. The **N. infraorbitalis** passes as a branch of the N. maxillaris [V/2] below the Orbita through the Foramen infraorbitale into the superficial facial region. Both nerve exit points (N. supraorbitalis and N. infraorbitalis) are used as pressure points in the context of the physical examination of a patient to check the function of the top two nerve branches of the N. trigeminus [V] (trigeminal pressure points).

N O T E

The V. angularis connects the superficial facial region with the V. ophthalmica inferior, which in turn drains into the Sinus cavernosus. By infections in the face (e.g. after squeezing a spot on the cheek) pathogens can be relayed to the **Sinus cavernosus**. This may create a **thrombosis** that can be associated with intracranial complications (e.g. damage to the cranial nerves running through or on the edge of the Sinus cavernous with resulting deficits or meningitis).

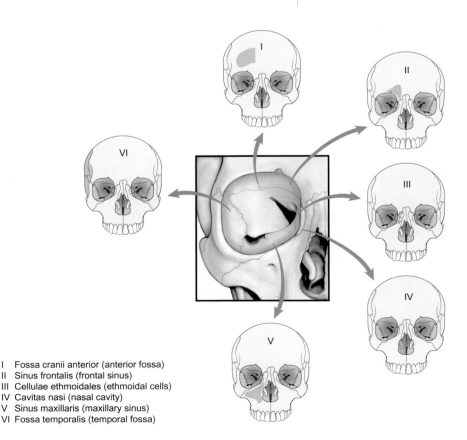

I   Fossa cranii anterior (anterior fossa)
II Sinus frontalis (frontal sinus)
III Cellulae ethmoidales (ethmoidal cells)
IV Cavitas nasi (nasal cavity)
V   Sinus maxillaris (maxillary sinus)
VI Fossa temporalis (temporal fossa)

Fig. 9.53 Localisation and presentation of the directly neighbouring regions of the Orbita.

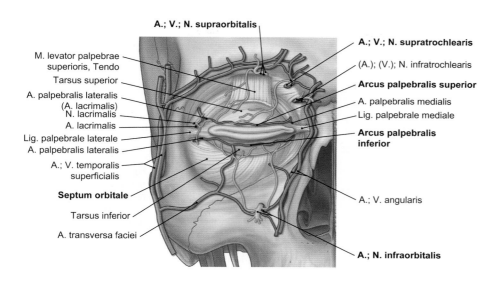

A.; V.; N. supraorbitalis

M. levator palpebrae
superioris, Tendo
Tarsus superior
A. palpebralis lateralis
(A. lacrimalis)
N. lacrimalis
A. lacrimalis
Lig. palpebrale laterale
A. palpebralis lateralis
A.; V. temporalis
superficialis
Septum orbitale
Tarsus inferior
A. transversa faciei

A.; V.; N. supratrochlearis
(A.); (V.); N. infratrochlearis
Arcus palpebralis superior
A. palpebralis medialis
Lig. palpebrale mediale
Arcus palpebralis
inferior
A.; V. angularis
A.; N. infraorbitalis

Fig. 9.54 Arteries, veins and nerves of the Regio orbitalis, on the right. Anterior view. [E460]

Content of the Orbita

In the Orbita embedded in the surrounding fat body (Corpus adiposum orbitae), the M. levator palpebrae and the 6 extraocular muscles are situated. Vessels and nerves enter and exit the Orbita through bony openings (➤ Table 9.23).

Extraocular muscles

At the tip of the orbital bowl a tendon ring begins formed by the Periorbita (**Anulus tendineus communis; anulus of ZINN**) which forms the origin of most extraocular muscles. The cranial nerves II (N. opticus), III (N. oculomotorius) and VI (N. abducens) run through its central opening and as a branch of the N. ophthalmicus [V/1], the N. nasociliaris and the A. ophthalmica (➤ Fig. 9.55).

Table 9.23 Overview of the points of penetration of the Orbita with the respective associated vascular, lymphatic and nervous systems.

Points of penetration of the Orbita	Vascular, lymphatic and nervous systems
Canalis opticus	• N. opticus [II] • A. ophthalmica • Meninges; Vaginae nervi optici
Fissura orbitalis superior (lateral section)	• N. frontalis (N. ophthalmicus [V/1]) • N. lacrimalis (N. ophthalmicus [V/1]) • N. trochlearis [IV] • R. orbitalis (A. meningea media) • V. ophthalmica superior *Irregular:* • Anastomoses between the A. meningea media and the A. lacrimalis
Fissura orbitalis superior (annular section)	• N. nasociliaris (N. ophthalmicus [V/1]) • N. oculomotorius [III] with R. superior and R. inferior • N. abducens [VI]
Fissura orbitalis superior (medial section)	• Rr. venae ophthalmicae inferioris through to the Sinus cavernosus
Fissura orbitalis inferior	• V. ophthalmica inferior • N. zygomaticus (N. maxillaris [V/2]) • A., V., N. infraorbitalis (N. maxillaris [V/2]) • M. orbitalis
Foramina ethmoidalia anterius/posterius	• A., N. ethmoidalis anterior/posterior (N. ophthalmicus [V/1])
Foramen zygomaticum	• N. zygomaticus (N. maxillaris [V/2]) with R. zygomaticotemporalis and R. zygomaticofacialis

Clinical remarks

The **orbital apex syndrome (TOLOSA-HUNT syndrome)** is a painful paralysis of the extraocular muscles (ophthalmoplegia). The causes are chronical inflammatory processes, rarely malignancies in the area of the orbit tip. For certain clarification of the findings appropriate diagnostic imaging is usually required.

The Bulbus oculi can move around all 3 axes of the eyeball, similar to the rotating movements of a ball joint. There are 3 pairs of antagonistically acting muscles responsible for this: the 4 straight Mm. recti and the 2 oblique Mm. obliqui. The M. levator palpebrae superioris serves to raise the eyelid and is not involved in the movement of the eyeball. The 4 straight ocular muscles (M. rectus superior, M. rectus inferior, M. rectus lateralis, M. rectus medialis) have their origin at the Anulus tendineus communis (ZINN's tendon ring) and attach before the equator of the Bulbus oculi at the sclera. The origin of the two oblique eye muscles is in contrast to the straight ocular muscles not at the Anulus tendineus communis. Its end tendons radiate as the straight extraocular muscles into the sclera of the Bulbus; however, behind the equator (➤ Fig. 9.56). Particularly worth mentioning here is the course of the attachment tendon of the M. obliquus superior, which passes during its forward-facing course

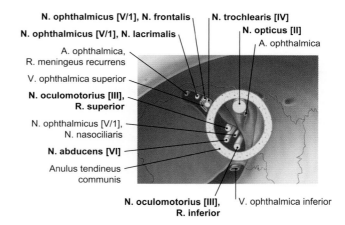

N. ophthalmicus [V/1], N. frontalis
N. ophthalmicus [V/1], N. lacrimalis
A. ophthalmica, R. meningeus recurrens
V. ophthalmica superior
N. oculomotorius [III], R. superior
N. ophthalmicus [V/1], N. nasociliaris
N. abducens [VI]
Anulus tendineus communis
N. trochlearis [IV]
N. opticus [II]
A. ophthalmica
N. oculomotorius [III], R. inferior
V. ophthalmica inferior

Fig. 9.55 Points of penetration of vascular, lymphatic and nervous systems into the Orbita through the Fissurae orbitales superior and inferior and within the Anulus tendineus communis (ZINN's tendon ring). [E460]

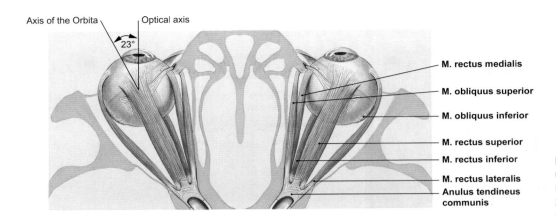

Axis of the Orbita   Optical axis

23°

M. rectus medialis
M. obliquus superior
M. obliquus inferior
M. rectus superior
M. rectus inferior
M. rectus lateralis
Anulus tendineus communis

Fig. 9.56 Course of the extraocular muscles and their position relative to the Bulbus oculi (diagram). The optical axis and the axis of the Orbita differ by 23°.

through a trochlea (fibrous connective tissue loop) serving as a hypomochlion, and is deflected back laterally to the rear before it radiates behind the equator of the bulbus into the sclera.

The axis of each Orbita is slightly laterally aligned viewed from the rear to the front. The Bulbus oculi with the optical axis is in contrast aligned exactly to the front (➤ Fig. 9.56). As a result, the interaction of the 6 extraocular muscles leads to various movements of the eyeball in a 3-dimensional space (➤ Table 9.24).

Clinical remarks

In the case of an outer **oculomotor paralysis** there is a highly complex impairment of eye movement, since the N. oculomotoris [III] innervates all extraocular muscles, with the exception of the Mm. rectus laterales (N. abducens [VI]) and the obliquus superior (N. trochlearis [IV]). Because of the preponderance of the two unaffected muscles the gaze of the eye

is directed downwards. If, at the same time, the innervation of the M. levator palpebrae superioris is affected, there is also ptosis, the drooping eyelid over the optical axis, so that the patient has no double vision, in spite of the deformity of the Bulbus. If the eyelid of the affected patient is manually pulled upwards, this will result in diplopia (double vision). In an internal oculomotor paralysis the parasympathetic innervation of the M. sphincter pupillae and M. ciliaris is stopped. This is characterised by a wide, light rigid pupil and a reduced ability of accommodation.

Vascular, lymphatic and nervous systems of the Orbita
Arteries

As a general rule, all structures within the Orbita including the Bulbus oculi are supplied with blood via the **A. ophthalmica**, the first branch from the Pars cerebralis of the A. carotis interna immediately after penetration through the dura mater (➤ Fig. 9.57). The

Table 9.24 Extraocular muscles of the eyeball with respective origin and attachment as well as function and innervation of the muscle.

Innervation	Origins	Attachment	Function
M. rectus superior			
N. oculomotorius [III], R. superior	Upper section of the Anulus tendineus communis	Above, ventral of the equator at the bulbus	Elevation of the optical axis, adduction and inward rotation of the eyeball
M. rectus inferior			
N. oculomotorius [III], R. inferior	Lower section of the Anulus tendineus communis	Below, ventral of the equator at the bulbus	Lowering of the optical axis, adduction and inward rotation of the bulbus
M. rectus lateralis			
N. abducens [VI]	Lateral section of the Anulus tendineus communis	Lateral, ventral of the equator at the bulbus	Abduction of the bulbus
M. rectus medialis			
N. oculomotorius [III], R. inferior	Medial section of the Anulus tendineus communis	Medial, ventral of the equator at the bulbus	Adduction of the bulbus
M. obliquus inferior			
N. oculomotorius [III], R. inferior	Medial section of the orbital base behind the orbital edge; on the Maxilla lateral of the Sulcus lacrimalis	Lateral rear quadrant of the Bulbus oculi	Elevation of the optical axis, adduction and outward rotation of the bulbus
M. obliquus superior			
N. trochlearis [IV]	Corpus ossis sphenoidalis, above and medial of the Canalis opticus	Lateral rear quadrant of the Bulbus oculi	Lowering of the optical axis, adduction and inward rotation of the bulbus
M. levator palpebrae superioris			
N. oculomotorius [III], R. superior	Ala minor ossis sphenoidalis, in front of the Canalis opticus	Front surface of the tarsus in the upper lid; fibres for skin and Fornix conjunctivae	Elevation of the upper eyelid

A. ophthalmica, enters the Orbita together with the N. opticus [II]. There, it divides into:

- The **A. lacrimalis** exits lateral of the N. opticus from the A. ophthalmica and runs temporally to supply the lacrimal gland, the extraocular muscles in this area, the Bulbus (as Aa. ciliares anteriores) and the lateral portion of the upper and lower eyelids (as A. palpebralis lateralis) with blood.
- The **A. centralis retinae** passes centrally in the N. opticus [II] up to the Papilla nervi optici and divides there into several branches. It is responsible within the Bulbus as a terminal artery (risk of blindness in closure of this vessel!) for the supply of the inner layers of the retina.
- The **Aa. ciliares posteriores longae and breves** emerge from dorsal through the sclera into the Bulbus and supply structures within the Bulbus.
- After the A. ophthalmica has crossed the N. opticus [II] in its course, it emits the **A. supraorbitalis**. It runs together with the N. supraorbitalis through the Foramen supraorbitale of the Os frontale and brings blood to the forehead and scalp.
- The **A. ethmoidalis anterior** runs through the Foramen ethmoidale anterius from the Orbita and on to the nasal cavity. Here it supplies the side wall of the nasal cavity, the upper section of the nasal septum and the Cellulae ethmoidales (➤ Chap. 9.6.5). Finally it flows into the Aa. dorsalis nasi that supplies the surface anatomy of the nose as one of the 2 terminal branches of the A. ophthalmica.
- The **A. ethmoidalis posterior** leaves the orbita through the Foramen ethmoidale posterius and provides the upper rear of the nasal cavity and also in part the Cellulae ethmoidales with blood (➤ Chap. 9.6.5).
- The second terminal branch of the A. ophthalmica is the **A. supratrochlearis,** which leaves the Orbita together with the N. supratrochlearis and in its course supplies parts of the forehead with arterial blood (➤ Fig. 9.57).

Veins

The venous blood leaves the Orbita via 2 large vessels, the **Vv. ophthalmicae superior and inferior** (➤ Fig. 9.58). Both Vv. ophthalmicae receive inflow from venous vessels of the superficial and deep facial regions: V. supraorbitalis, V. nasofrontalis, V. angularis

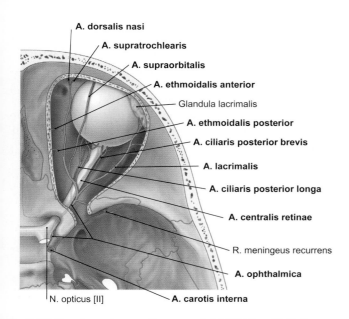

Fig. 9.57 View from above on the opened right Orbita with Bulbus oculi and the arterial vessel exit points from the A. carotis interna. [E460]

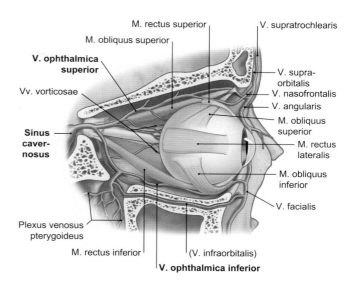

Fig. 9.58 Lateral view of the venous blood vessels of the Orbita in their course from rostral to occipital. The lateral wall of the Orbita has been removed. [E460]

(→ V. ophthalmica superior) and V. facialis (→ V. ophthalmica inferior). In principle, the V. ophthalmica superior runs through the upper part and the V. ophthalmica inferior through the lower part of the Orbita. Both veins receive corresponding inflows from the muscles and the veins that run in the respective part of the Orbita with the arteries. The V. ophthalmica superior leaves the Orbita dorsally via the Fissura orbitalis superior, and then flows into the Sinus cavernosus. The V. ophthalmic inferior combines in its dorsal section with the Vv. ophthalmica superior, but can also occur as an independent vessel through the Fissura orbitalis superior, to then flow as an independent vessel into the Sinus cavernous. A further dorsal vessel branch combines with the V. infraorbitalis, passes through the Fissura orbitalis inferior and drains into the Plexus pterygoideus which lies in the Fossa infratemporalis.

Innervation

The innervation of the eyeball as well as the orbital structures takes place via the cranial nerves II–VI and sympathetic fibres from the thoracic medulla. In ➤ Fig. 9.59 the view from the top of the opened orbital cavity is shown, after the dura mater, the roof of the Orbita and finally the Periorbita with parts of the Corpus adiposum orbitae have been removed. At the same time, the dura mater was removed above the Ganglion trigeminale (Ganglion semilunare, GASSER's ganglion).

N. opticus [II]

Within the retina of the eyeball are the first three projection neurons of the optic tract. The processes of the ganglion cells merge with the optic nerve papillae (Discus nervi optici) to the N. opticus [II] that leaves the Bulbus to the rear. The nerve runs through the retrobulbar adipose tissue towards the Anulus tendineus communis (ZINN's tendon ring), passes through it and continues via the Canalis opticus into the anterior cranial fossa (➤ Fig. 9.55; the A. ophthalmica runs in the opposite direction through the Canalis opticus and then through the Anulus tendineus communis to continue to branch in the Orbita). Within the Orbita the N. opticus [II] generally forms a slightly outwardly convex arch during dissection. This is the reserve length for the various eye movements. As a diverticulum of the diencephalon, the N. opticus [II] is not an actual cranial nerve, but is completely surrounded by the three meninges. At the Bulbus oculi the dura mater passes into the sclera;

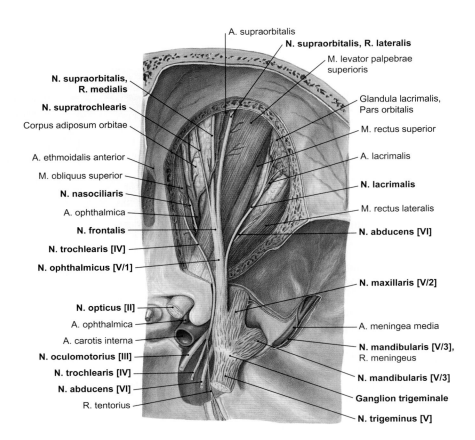

A. supraorbitalis

N. supraorbitalis, R. lateralis

M. levator palpebrae superioris

N. supraorbitalis, R. medialis

N. supratrochlearis

Corpus adiposum orbitae

A. ethmoidalis anterior

M. obliquus superior

N. nasociliaris

A. ophthalmica

N. frontalis

N. trochlearis [IV]

N. ophthalmicus [V/1]

N. opticus [II]

A. ophthalmica

A. carotis interna

N. oculomotorius [III]

N. trochlearis [IV]

N. abducens [VI]

R. tentorius

Glandula lacrimalis, Pars orbitalis

M. rectus superior

A. lacrimalis

N. lacrimalis

M. rectus lateralis

N. abducens [VI]

N. maxillaris [V/2]

A. meningea media

N. mandibularis [V/3], R. meningeus

N. mandibularis [V/3]

Ganglion trigeminale

N. trigeminus [V]

Fig. 9.59 Contents of the Orbita opened cranially with Ganglion trigeminale. The course of the N. ophthalmicus [V/1] and its branches can be determined through the opened Fissura orbitalis superior. In addition, the entries into the Orbita from the cranial nerves III, IV and VI, which innervate the extraocular muscles and the penetration of the N. opticus [II] are represented by the Canalis opticus.

portions of the soft meninges (leptomeninx) are continued by the Choroidea.

N. oculomotorius [III]

Shortly before or after passing through the Fissura orbitalis superior into the Orbita the N. oculomotorius [III] branches into an upper and a lower branch (➤ Fig. 9.60, ➤ Fig. 9.34) which pass through the Anulus tendineus communis when entering the Orbita (➤ Fig. 9.55). In the Orbita the **R. superior** runs lateral to the N. opticus [II] upwards and innervates the Mm. rectus superior and levator palpebrae superioris (➤ Fig. 9.60). The larger **R. inferior** in its course is divided into 3 other branches which supply the motor innervation to the Mm. rectus medialis, rectus inferior and obliquus inferior (➤ Fig. 9.61). On the way to the M. obliquus inferior the 3rd branch of the R. inferior emits another branch to the Ganglion ciliare (see below). These preganglionic fibres form the parasympathetic root of the Ganglion ciliare. After switching to postganglionic (within the Ganglion ciliare) the parasympathetic fibres pass via the Nn. ciliares breves into the bulbus and innervate the M. sphincter pupillae and the M. ciliaris.

Ganglion ciliare

The uppermost of the 4 parasympathetic cranial ganglia lies lateral to the N. opticus [II] (➤ Fig. 9.60, ➤ Fig. 9.61, ➤ Fig. 9.34). Here,

the preganglionic parasympathetic fibres from the R. inferior nervi oculomotorii (Radix oculomotoria) are switched. As with all cranial ganglia, there is also an additional sensory root in the Ganglion ciliare (**Radix sensoria**) of the N. trigeminus [V] (N. nasociliaris) and a sympathetic root (**Radix sympathica**) with postganglionic fibres from the Plexus caroticus internus. The fibres of the two latter roots pass unswitched through the Ganglion ciliare. The sensory fibres originate for the most part from the surface of the eye (cornea and conjunctiva). They leave the Bulbus via the Nn. ciliaris breves. The sympathetic fibres take the opposite way and pass within the Bulbus mainly to the M. dilatator pupillae (➤ Fig. 9.34).

N. trochlearis [IV]

The N. trochlearis [IV] runs like the N. oculomotorius [III] intradurally in the lateral wall of the Sinus cavernosus (➤ Fig. 9.59, ➤ Fig. 9.60). Shortly before it reaches the Orbita, it runs upwards, crosses the N. oculomotorius (➤ Fig. 9.60) and enters the Orbita above the Anulus tendineus communis (ZINN's tendon ring) through the Fissura orbitalis superior. In its relatively short intraorbital course, it runs medially over the M. levator palpebrae superioris and provides motor innervation radiating from above into the M. obliquus superior (➤ Fig. 9.34).

N. trigeminus [V]

N. ophthalmicus [V/1]

Also after an intradural course in the lateral wall of the Sinus cavernous, the N. ophthalmicus [V/1] enters the Orbita as the most cranial main branch of the N. trigeminus [V], through the Fissura orbitalis superior (➤ Fig. 9.59). Shortly before the purely sensory nerve divides into three branches:

- N. nasociliaris
- N. frontalis
- N. lacrimalis

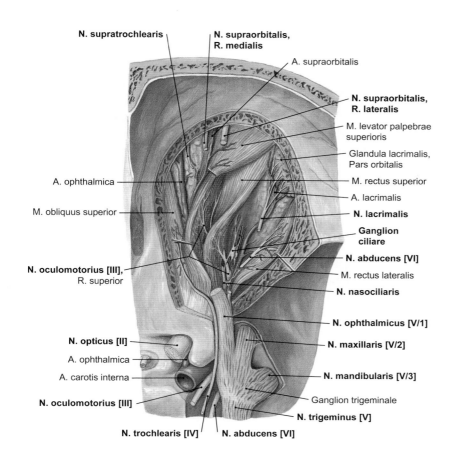

Fig. 9.60 Orbita from above after folding away the M. levator palpebrae superioris and the M. rectus superior. The nerve branches of the cranial nerves III, IV and VI can be clearly recognized in the respective muscles. After removing the orbital fat tissue, the approximately 2 mm in size Ganglion ciliare is visible, which is located approximately 2 cm behind the Bulbus oculi, lateral of the N. opticus [II].

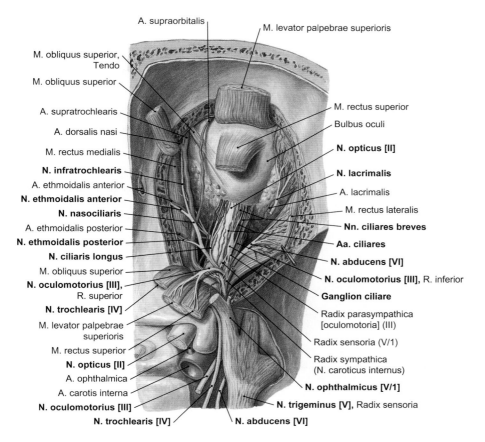

Fig. 9.61 View of the Orbita from above after separation and folding up of the Mm. levator palpebrae superioris, rectus superior and obliquus superior. In addition to the Ganglion ciliare and branches of the A. ophthalmica, the N. opticus [II] and the branches of the N. nasociliaris are visible.

The N. frontalis and N. lacrimalis run outside around the Anulus tendineus communis (ZINN's tendon ring), the N. nasociliaris usually penetrates through the ring.

The purely sensory **N. nasociliaris** is the most caudal in the Orbita. It crosses in its course the N. opticus [II] (➤ Fig. 9.61) and passes below the M. rectus superior medially. Its branches are listed in ➤ Table 9.18 .

The **N. frontalis** runs between the M. levator palpebrae superioris and periorbita ventrally after penetrating through the Fissura orbitalis superior. It divides in the centre of the Orbita into its 2 terminal branches:

- N. supraorbitalis
- N. supratrochlearis (➤ Fig. 9.60).

The thicker **N. supraorbitalis** leaves the Orbita via the Foramen supraorbitale or the Incisura supraorbitalis. Both nerves innervate the forehead and part of the scalp.

The **N. lacrimalis** runs ventrally as the smallest branch of the N. ophthalmicus [V/1] on the upper edge of the M. rectus lateralis. In its course it takes up fibres from the R. zygomaticotemporalis nervi zygomatici which contributes both parasympathetic postganglionic (Ganglion pterygopalatinum) as well as postganglionic sympathetic fibres (Ganglion cervicale superius) to the innervation of the lacrimal gland. In addition, the N. lacrimalis sensitively innervates parts of the conjunctiva as well as the lateral area of the upper eyelid.

N. maxillaris [V/2]

The **N. zygomaticus** is a branch of the N. maxillaris [V/2] and in its course separates in the fossa pterygopalatina from the N. maxillaris. After taking up postganglionic parasympathetic fibres from the Ganglion pterygopalatinum it runs through the Fissura orbitalis inferior into the Orbita and divides there into 2 sensory skin innervating branches:

- R. zygomaticofacialis
- R. zygomaticotemporalis

The parasympathetic (visceroefferent) fibres are conveyed by the R. communicans cum nervo zygomatico and the N. lacrimalis to the lacrimal gland and innervate it (➤ Fig. 9.62).

N. abducens [VI]

After leaving the brain stem The N. abducens [VI] runs through the Sinus cavernosus lateral of the A. carotis interna and then goes via the Fissura orbitalis superior through the Anulus tendineus communis (ZINN's tendon ring) into the Orbita (➤ Fig. 9.55, ➤ Fig. 9.34). There it runs laterally to the M. rectus lateralis and provides motor innervation.

Clinical remarks

In the case of damage to the N. trochlearis [IV] **(trochlear paresis)** the M. obliquus superior can no longer be moved. In these patients the optic axis is therefore displaced medially. Due to its central course through the Sinus cavernosus the N. abducens [VI] is particularly frequent in a thrombosis of the Sinus cavernosus and is often the first cranial nerve affected **(abducens palsy).** The patient can no longer abduct the affected eye laterally.

In order to find suitable surgical access the following **classification of the Orbita** is used according to various clinical aspects:

- Bulbar/retrobulbar section
- Central or intraconal part/peripheral or extraconal part
  - The intraconal part is the part of the Orbita which is bordered by the cone-shaped (conal) straight extraocular muscles
- Upper/middle/lower level of the Orbita
  - The upper level extends from the Orbita roof to the M. rectus superior and includes the M. levator palpebrae superioris, the Nn. frontalis, trochlearis [IV] and lacrimalis as well as the Aa. supraorbitalis, supratrochlearis, the A. and V. lacrimalis and the V. ophthalmica superior (➤ Fig. 9.43; ➤ Fig. 9.59)
  - The middle level is the same as with the above-mentioned intraconal space between the straight extraocular muscles and includes the Nn. opticus [II], oculomotorius [III], nasociliaris, abducens [VI] and zygomaticus, the Ganglion ciliare, the A. ophthalmica, the V. ophthalmica superior and the Aa. ciliares posteriores breves and longae (➤ Fig. 9.61)
  - The lower level extends from the M. rectus inferior to the Orbita floor and includes the N. infraorbitalis as well as the A. infraorbitalis and the V. ophthalmica inferior (➤ Fig. 9.43; ➤ Fig. 9.58).

9.4.4 Bulbus oculi

The **eyeball (Bulbus oculi)** is almost spherical and in adults has a diameter of about 2.5 cm. It weighs between 8 and 10 g and fills the

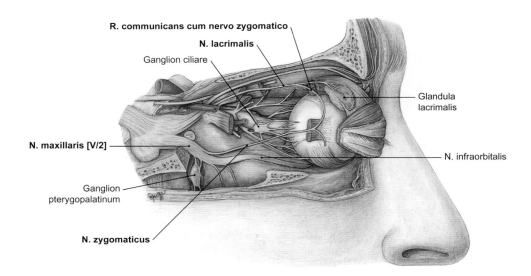

Fig. 9.62 Nerve pathways in the Orbita. Lateral view after removal of the temporal wall and the orbital fat body.

front section of the orbit. The largest part of the eyeball is surrounded by the **sclera**. It consists of strong connective tissue which contains collagen and elastic fibres. The **Vagina bulbi (TENON's capsule)** is a connective tissue sheath and covers the entire surface anatomy of the bulbus from the point of entry of the N. opticus [II] to the Limbus corneae where the sclera transforms into the cornea. Between the sclera and Vagina bulbi there is a thin gap (**Spatium episclerale**).

Penetrating the Vagina bulbi, the tendons of the external ocular muscles attach at the sclera. At the front, the round shape of the bulbus is interrupted by the swelling of the transparent **cornea** (➤ Fig. 9.63). It passes into the sclera and the conjunctiva covering it (Tunica conjunctiva) in the area of the Limbus corneae. The cornea has no vessels and remains so up to the transition into the vascularised Tunica conjunctiva, so that the superficial epithelial layers of the cornea have to be supplied with nutrients and oxygen via the tear fluid.

Clinical remarks

The **endocrine orbitopathy** is a disease that is one of the organ-specific autoimmune diseases and occurs mostly in the context of BASEDOW's disease. It is believed that the immune system forms faulty antibodies against specific tissue in the Orbita (e.g. eye muscles, fatty tissue) and leads to inflammatory reactions. Clinically, this type of disease is manifested as protruding of the eyes (exophthalmus), an enlargement of the palpebral fissure with eyelid retraction and movement disorders of the eye.

Inside the eyeball is hollow. The **anterior chamber of the eyeball** connects behind the cornea in the direction of the optic nerve that is stretched between the cornea and the front side of the iris. The anterior chamber of the eyeball is connected to the **posterior eye chamber** through the **pupil opening of the iris**. Here the aqueous humour circulates from the back of the eye chamber into the anterior chamber of the eye. The **aqueous humour (Humor aquosus)** is secreted by the ciliary epithelium of the **ciliary body (Pars plicata)** into the posterior eye chamber and flows between the lens and the

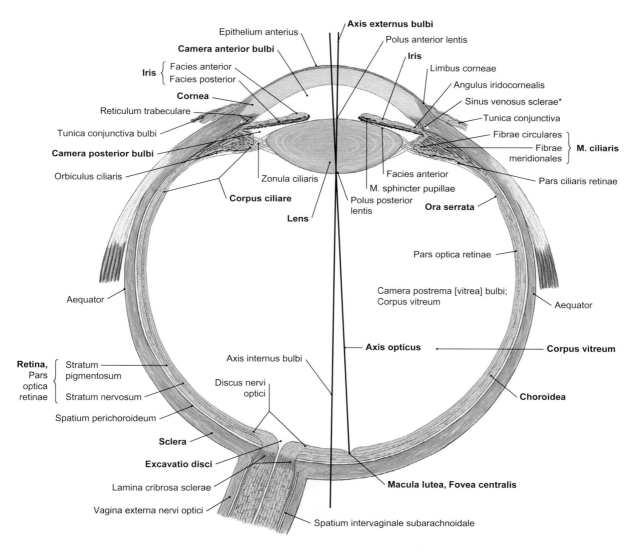

Fig. 9.63 Right Bulbus oculi in middle horizontal cut with section of the N. opticus [II] at the height of the pupil opening. Below the sclera is the uvea (vessel skin), which at the front area of the eye consists of the iris (Iris) and the ciliary body (Corpus ciliare) and at the rear area of the choroid (Choroidea). The Ora serrata marks the transition from the ciliary body into the choroid. This is important for the nutrition of the inner overlying retina but at the same time for the temperature regulation of the Bulbus oculi. The retina with its visual sense cells forms the innermost layer of the Bulbus oculi. In the front part of the eye the pigment epithelium of the ciliary body and the epithelium of the iris also belong to this layer.

back of the iris through the pupil into the anterior chamber of the eye. In the **iridocorneal angle (Angulus iridocornealis),** which is bordered by the iris root, the ciliary body and the cornea, lies the **trabecular meshwork (Trabeculum corneosclerale),** and the aqueous humour drains into the annular **Sinus venosus sclerae (SCHLEMM's canal)** through its connective tissue fissure spaces and is then diverted via the intrascleral and episcleral veins into the venous system (➤ Fig. 9.64). The continuous production and draining of the aqueous humour (approximately 6–7 ml per day) is important for the nutrition of the inner layers of the cornea and the lens and for maintaining the physiological intraocular pressure (normal range from 10 to 21 mmHg), which guarantees the stable spherical shape of the Bulbus oculi and the stable spacing of the optical media inside the eye to each other.

Clinical remarks

If draining of the aqueous humour is impaired, the result may be a **glaucoma ('green star').** The increased intraocular pressure often causes neuronal damage in the area of the retina and optic disc, as the sclera is constructed from connective tissue and is not very elastic. Glaucoma diseases are among the most common causes of blindness worldwide. The cause of a decreased outflow of aqueous humour is, for example, the shift of the iridocorneal angle by adhesion of the iris to the cornea (synechia), which may lead to closed-angle glaucoma. When the chamber angle is open the outflow of aqueous humour through the trabecular meshwork of SCHLEMM's canal can also be disrupted due to other causes (open-angle glaucoma). In the case of normal pressure glaucoma that can be seen as a special form of primary open-angle glaucoma, there is damage of the optic nerve, even though the intraocular pressure is not increased in these patients.

The posterior chamber borders on the back of the **eye lens.** This consists of a lens core (Nucleus lentis) and the lens cortex (Cortex lentis) and is surrounded by a dense fibre capsule (Capsula lentis). In the equator region new cells are formed below the lens capsule in a growth zone (Zona germinativa) for a lifetime. These then re-shape into long fibres, store transparent crystalline proteins and then lose their cell organelles. The transparent, biconvex formed resilient lens loses elasticity during the continuous growth process with increasing age, which at around the age of 40-45 years leads to presbyopia. The **ciliary zonules (Zonula ciliaris)** insert in the lens capsule, which emerge from the ciliary processes of the **ciliary body (Corpus ciliare)** (➤ Fig. 9.63). As a result of the contraction of the M. ciliaris the ciliary body moves towards the lens, which reduces the tension of the ciliary zonules. This rounds off the lens and the eye focuses on the close proximity (near accommodation). In the non-contracted condition of the ciliary muscle the tension of the ciliary zonules prevails and the lens flattens out. In this way the eye focuses on far-sightedness. Behind the lens and its holding apparatus the eye is filled up to the retina with the transparent **vitreous body (Corpus vitreum)**constructed from a gel-like substance, which consists almost to 98 % of water. It assumes almost four fifths of the total volume of the Bulbus (➤ Fig. 9.63). Cornea, aqueous humour in the eyes chambers, iris, lens and vitreous body form the optical apparatus of the eye.

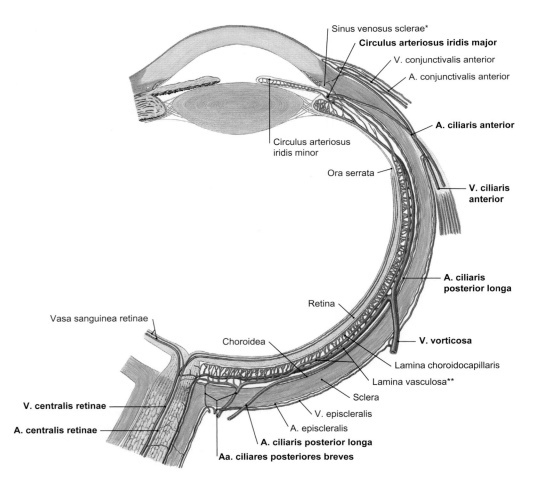

Fig. 9.64 **Blood vessels of the right Bulbus oculi** (diagram).
* clinically: SCHLEMM's canal
** clinically: uvea

Vessel supply

The eyeball is supplied with blood from different *arterial inflows*, all of which come from the A. ophthalmica (➤ Fig. 9.64):

- **A. centralis retinae:** it originates from the A. ophthalmica (➤ Fig. 9.50) and runs after its entry centrally in the N. opticus [II], enters into the Bulbus at the Discus nervi optici and supplies the innermost layer of the retina.
- **Aa. ciliares anteriores:** they supply all internal eye muscles and form anastomoses with the Aa. ciliares posteriores longae.
- **Aa. ciliares posteriores longae:** they penetrate the sclera medial and lateral of the N. opticus [II] and run forwards inside the choroid (Choroidea).
- **Aa. ciliares posteriores breves:** these branches penetrate the sclera immediately around the N. opticus [II] and pass into the Choroidea.

The *venous blood flow* from the Bulbus oculi takes place primarily via the vortex veins (**Vv. vorticosae**), 4 vessels which come from the Choroidea and run in one of the four quadrants of the rear bulbus through the sclera and then flow into the V. ophthalmica superior or the V. ophthalmica inferior. The venous blood of the inner retina is diverted through the **V. centralis retinae** which in its course flows into the V. ophthalmica superior or directly into the Sinus cavernosus.

Clinical remarks

Central venous thrombosis is a relatively frequent vascular disease of the V. centralis retinae. Patients initially perceive a painless deterioration of vision. Except for general risk factors for the development of thrombosis, the cause of a central venous thrombosis has not yet been sufficiently clarified.

Wall structure of the bulbus

The content of the Bulbus oculi is surrounded by a wall, which can be divided into three layers (➤ Table 9.25).

Tunica fibrosa bulbi

The Tunica fibrosa bulbi consists of 2 units, the sclera and cornea:
- The **sclera,** the so-called white of the eyes, forms the rear and side portion of the Bulbus and is traversed by numerous vessels.
- The **cornea** is constructed from 5 layers:
  - Epithelial layer,
  - BOWMAN's membrane (a thick basal membrane),
  - Stroma (makes up around 90 % of corneal thickness),
  - DESCEMET's membrane (a thick basal membrane) and
  - Endothelial layer (it is involved specifically in the metabolic control between aqueous humour and stroma)

Clinical remarks

After injury of the cornea regeneration is only limited. After untreated damage there is often scarring that can lead to severe vision loss. To restore the vision after scarring or a deterioration of the cornea, a **corneal transplantation (keratoplasty)** is usually necessary. This procedure is the most frequently carried out tissue transplantation in Germany. The healing tendency in this procedure is good to very good (clear healing of the graft is achieved in approximately 90 % of operations), since the cornea is an avascular tissue (it is one of the immune privileged organs). Rejection of the donor tissue is rare (<5 %); however, if vessels have already immigrated in the receptor cornea, the risk of rejection significantly increases

(high-risk keratoplasty). To minimise this risk, a tissue typing is conducted on the recipient using a blood sample (HLA typing) before the operation, to find suitable transplants conforming to the recipient's tissue type (via corneal banks).

Tunica vasculosa bulbi

In the Tunica vasculosa bulbi (Tunica media bulbi, Uvea) there are many blood and lymph vessels. It includes all the inner eye muscles, which are necessary for regulation of incident light in the eye and are necessary to control the lens shape and is responsible for the secretion of the aqueous humour. The iris, the ciliary body and the Choroidea belong to it (➤ Fig. 9.65).

Choroidea

The Choroidea forms the rear part of the Tunica vasculosa bulbi and makes up around two thirds of the entire vessel layer. Oxygen and nutrients reach the outer portions of the retina via its capillary system. The Choroidea is pigmented and internally firmly connected to the outer retina and on the exterior loosely connected to the sclera.

Corpus ciliare

The ciliary body (Corpus ciliare) is connected at the front to the Choroidea. It extends at the front to the transition of cornea and sclera and at the back up to the Ora serrata. It is formed mainly from the **M. ciliaris** which consists of smooth muscle fibres arranged in a circular, radial and longitudinal fashion. Thus the ciliary muscle protrudes into the inside of the eye and contraction leads to a loosening of the **ciliary zonules** of the holding apparatus of the lens and thus to close accommodation. The ciliary zonules originate from the Procc. ciliares of the ciliary body and are visible as lengthwise aligned folds on its inner surface (➤ Fig. 9.65). The totality of the connective tissue fibres is called the Lig. suspensorium lentis. The ciliary body is divided into an evenly running part (**Pars plana**) and into a folded part (**Pars plicata**). Approximately 70 **ciliary processes (Proc. ciliares),** originate from the Pars plicata from which the ciliary zonules of the lens holding apparatus radiate. The **ciliary epithelium** in the area of the Pars plicata also secretes the aqueous humour.

Table 9.25 Wall layers of the eyeball with their parts.

Tunica fibrosa bulbi	Tunica vasculosa bulbi	Tunica interna bulbi
• Sclera	• Choroidea	• Retina
• Cornea	• Corpus ciliare	– Pars caeca retinae
	• Iris	– Pars optica retinae

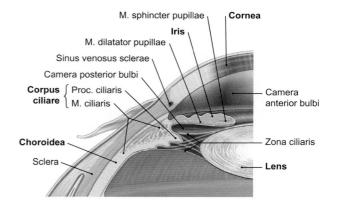

Fig. 9.65 Structures of the iridocorneal angle (diagram). [E460]

Iris

The Tunica vasculosa bulbi is closed at the front through the iris. The iris represents the adjustable aperture of the eye and is visible through the cornea as the coloured part of the eye. At the back it is covered by a pigment sheet (➤ Fig. 9.66). It has a central opening, the **pupil (Pupilla).** The size of the pupil opening (variable between approximately 1.5 and 8 mm) can be changed by smooth muscle fibre traction, which are positioned in the connective tissue of the iris stroma. Extending annularly around the pupil opening, muscle fibres form the **M. sphincter pupillae** and leads by contraction to a reduction in pupil diameter (miosis; ➤ Fig. 9.66). They are innervated by postganglionic parasympathetic nerve fibres from the Ganglion ciliare (Nn. ciliares breves). In the course fan-shaped and radially outwards extending smooth muscle fibres are attached, which form the **M. dilator pupillae.** On contraction this leads to a widening of the pupil opening (mydriasis). Its muscle fibres are located directly on the pigment sheet of the iris and are innervated by postganglionic sympathetic nerve fibres from the Ganglion cervicale superius, which also reach the Bulbus via the Ganglion ciliare but are not switched. The blood supply of the iris is via 2 arterial rings, the outer **Circulus arteriosus iridis major** and the incomplete inner **Circulus arteriosus iridis minor** (➤ Fig. 9.66). Both artery rings are connected to one another by anastomoses. The back of the iris has a radiating-like structure which is created by the serrated edge of the retina (Pars ciliaris retinae) and by the arrangement of the ciliary body processes (Plicae iridis).

Tunica interna bulbi

The Tunica interna bulbi (retina) consists of two portions:

- The **Pars caeca retinae** covers the inner surface of the Corpus ciliare (Pars ciliaris retinae) and the iris (Pars iridica retinae) by their two parts in front of the Ora serrata.
- Dorsally and laterally in the eye up to the Ora serrata there is the **Pars optica,** the actual light sensitive part of the retina. It consists of two layers:
  - The outer **retinal pigment epithelium (Stratum pigmentosum),** which is firmly connected to the Choroidea and continues to the front as a pigment layer in the area of the Pars caeca retinae,
  - The inner **neuronal retina (Stratum neuroepitheliale),** which is only directly connected with the Stratum pigmentosum around the N. opticus [II] and on the Ora serrata

The neuronal retina, in turn, is divided into several layers. The outer layer that rests directly on the pigment epithelium, contains the

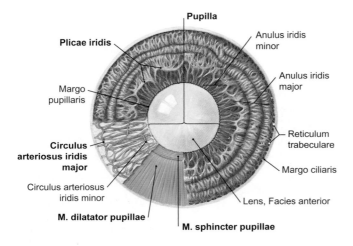

Fig. 9.66 Iris with lens from the front (diagram). [L127]

Labels:
Pupilla
Plicae iridis
Margo pupillaris
Circulus arteriosus iridis major
Circulus arteriosus iridis minor
M. dilatator pupillae
M. sphincter pupillae
Anulus iridis minor
Anulus iridis major
Reticulum trabeculare
Margo ciliaris
Lens, Facies anterior

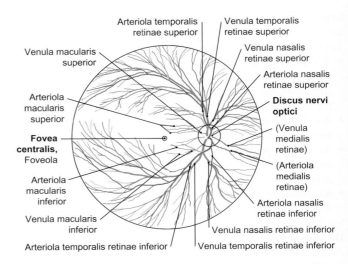

Fig. 9.67 Branching of the blood vessels of the retina with localization of the Discus nervi optici and the Fovea centralis (diagram).

Labels:
Arteriola temporalis retinae superior
Venula temporalis retinae superior
Venula macularis superior
Venula nasalis retinae superior
Arteriola macularis superior
Arteriola nasalis retinae superior
Discus nervi optici
Fovea centralis, Foveola
(Venula medialis retinae)
(Arteriola medialis retinae)
Arteriola macularis inferior
Arteriola nasalis retinae inferior
Venula macularis inferior
Venula nasalis retinae inferior
Arteriola temporalis retinae inferior
Venula temporalis retinae inferior

photo receptors (rods and cones), which are unevenly distributed over the retina and in which the signal transduction of a light stimulus (photon) takes place in a physiological nerve impulse (phototransduction). The photo receptors form synaptic connections to the inner retinal neurons **(bipolar cells, horizontal cells, amacrine cells),** which in turn are synaptically connected to the innermost retinal neurons, the **ganglion cells.** A photon must therefore first penetrate all retinal layers before it can come to a signal transduction in the outer segments of the photoreceptors. The ganglion cells are the only neurons of the retina which send visual sense stimuli to the brain via the joint course of their axons. The axons of the retinal ganglion cells converge for this in the **optic disc (Discus nervi optici)** and run as the N. opticus [II] and after the Chiasma opticum as Tractus opticus in the direction of the thalamus (Corpus geniculatum laterale) of the diencephalon (➤ Chap. 9.3.2). In the area of the papillae, except for the axons of the ganglion cells there are no retinal structures. For this reason, this area of the retina is referred to as the **blind spot.** This is where the A. centralis retinae enters into the inside of the eye and divides into various branches to supply blood to the inner retina (➤ Fig. 9.67). The corresponding vein (V. centralis retinae) leaves the eye above the optic disc. Lateral to the Discus nervi optici is the **yellow spot, the Macula lutea.** It is characterised by a depression (**Fovea centralis**) which represents both the thinnest part of the retina as well as the area of sharpest vision. Here the highest visual sensitivity within the retina is based on the large density of cone cells without the presence of rod cells. When directly focusing on an object the picture falls into this area of the retina and can thus be sharply seen.

Clinical remarks

Pathological changes of the retina in the area of the Macula lutea are referred to as **macular degeneration**. The most common form of this disease which gradually lead to a progressive vision loss is the **age-related or senile macular degeneration (AMD).** In industrialised countries it most often results in blindness for people over 50 years, followed by glaucoma diseases and diabetic retinopathy. Apart from a genetic predisposition the main risk factors for AMD are smoking and high blood pressure.

The retinal pigment epithelium supplies the outer parts of the retina. In the case of a **retinal detachment (Ablatio retinae)** the connection between the neuronal retina and pigment epithelium becomes detached for various reasons. If the photoreceptors are no longer sufficiently nourished due to the loss of contact, depending on the duration and location of the ablation a massive loss of function in the affected areas may occur. A retinal detachment is treated depending on the cause, location and extent. After repositioning of the retina a functional regeneration can be achieved.

9.5 Ear
Friedrich Paulsen

Skills

After processing this chapter, you should be able to:
- describe the anatomical construction of the auricle, middle ear and inner ear and name its content structure
- correctly describe the various regions of the ear, clearly define their limits and to place them into a topographical and clinical context with neighbouring structures
- describe the structure of the Tuba auditiva, the muscles involved in the tube function and the relationship to the middle ear
- describe the course of the vascular, lymphatic and nervous systems in the Pars petrosa and understand the arrangement of their different supply or innervation areas
- describe the embryological development of the auricle, the middle ear and the inner ear and explain the structure and function

Clinical case

Auricular haematoma

Case study
A young man consults the ENT doctor in charge late at night with a severely swollen auricle on the front. He is a kick boxer and states that he had received a kick to the head when train-

ing. The auricle hurt for a short period then the pain disappeared quickly; however, the auricle became swollen relatively quickly and the trainer sent him immediately to the ENT clinic.

Initial examination
The doctor examines the auricle, the external auditory canal and the eardrum in detail. The bluish swelling of the auricle is soft and fluctuating. The ENT doctor diagnoses an auricular haematoma, i.e. a serous bloody effusion between the perichondrium and cartilage. The box kick led to a tangential, shearing force impact on the auricle, causing the perichondrium to be pushed off the cartilage. A gap is formed, which has secondarily filled with liquid.

Treatment
The ENT doctor incises the swelling under sterile conditions in order to prevent an auricular perichondritis. A serous bloody secretion drains out in the process. In order to optimally reattach the perichondrium to the cartilage, he makes 2 mattress sutures. In addition, he prescribes an antibiotic. He then explains to the patient that this type of injury is quite frequent in boxing and advises him in the future to regularly wear head protection because in the long-term recurrent auricular haematoma can cause a 'cauliflower ear'. A connective tissue organisation of the haematoma occurs with restrictions of the nutrient supply of the ear cartilage and with loss of cartilage, which ultimately leads to deformity of the auricle.

The ear (Auris) includes the hearing organ and the equilibrium organ. It is divided into the **external ear, middle ear** and **internal ear**.(➤ Fig. 9.68):
- The **external ear** includes the auricle, the external auditory canal and the eardrum.
- The **middle ear** consists of the tympanic cavity, which lies centrally in the temporal bone (Pars petrosa of the Os temporale). It is separated from the external auditory canal through the tympanic membrane, accommodates 3 ossicles and is connected via the Eustachian tube with the nasopharynx as well as via the Antrum mastoideum with the mastoid process.
- Also referred to as the labyrinth the **internal ear** also lies in the temporal bone. It consists of various cavities, which border laterally on the middle ear and medially on the Meatus acusticus internus.

The hearing organ in the internal ear (Organum vestibulocochleare) converts the sounds and noises received via the auricle, which are forwarded and amplified by the middle ear as mechanical informa-

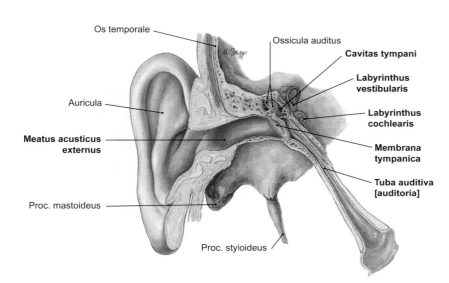

Fig. 9.68 Parts of the ear, Auris, right. Longitudinal section through ear canal, middle ear and Eustachian tube; frontal view.

tion, into electrical impulses in such as way that the information can be forwarded to the brain. In addition there are specialised receptor cells in the internal ear to determine movements and positions in space (organ of equilibrium).

9.5.1 Embryology

Development of the auricle
The auricle which has the function of receiving sound develops from the 1st pharyngeal groove, between the 1st and 2nd pharyngeal arches.

Development of the auricle from the six auricular hillocks
At the dorsocranial end of the 1st pharyngeal groove, at the beginning of the 6th week there are 2 rows each of 3 **auricular hillocks** that grow at different speeds and fuse quickly to the auricle. With the extension of the mandibular branch in the 1st pharyngeal arch, the auricles are indirectly shifted cranially and finally lie at the level of the eye.

Clinical remarks

Excessive or inadequate fusing of the auricular hillocks is not uncommon and spontaneous **(auricle malformations)**; auricles that are positioned too deep are often associated with chromosome-related malformations.

Development of the external acoustic meatus from the first pharyngeal groove
The external auditory canal develops from the ectoderm in the depth of the 1st pharyngeal cleft that grows inwards as a funnel-shaped tube until it reaches the entodermal lining of the tympanic cavity (Recessus tubotympanicus, from the 1st pharyngeal pouch) and at the start of the 9th week forms a solid auditory canal plate on the auditory canal floor.

Clinical remarks

If the auditory canal plate does not dissolve after the 7th month, **congenital deafness** occurs.

Middle ear development
The entodermal lining of the 1st pharyngeal pouch grows from the 5th week as a lateral bulge of the pharyngeal skin and becomes the **middle ear.** It meets with ectodermal tissue at the bottom of the 1st pharyngeal cleft. At the point of contact, only a thin membrane remains, the **tympanic membrane.** Now the distal portion of the 1st pharyngeal pouch extends, Recessus tubotympanicus, and becomes the primitive **tympanic cavity.** The proximal part remains narrow and becomes the **auditory tube** (Tuba auditiva [auditoria], EUSTACHIAN tube).

Development of the auditory ossicles
Also at the start of the 5th week the ossicles begin to differentiate in the mesenchyme of the 1st and 2nd pharyngeal arches :
- Hammer and anvil as derivatives of MECKEL's cartilage as well as the M. tensor tympani in the 1st pharyngeal arch (innervation therefore by the N. mandibularis [V/3], the 1st pharyngeal arch nerve)

- The stirrup as a derivative of REICHERT's cartilage and the M. stapedius in the 2nd pharyngeal arch (innervation therefore by the N. facialis [VII], the 2nd pharyngeal arch nerve)

Development of the internal ear
On approximately the 22nd day the **otic placode** forms in the **surface ectoderm** on both sides of the position of the rhombencephalon as a thickening of the epithelium; it soon bulges out to form an **auditory pit** and constricts the **ear vesicle.** Each vesicle is divided into a front **(rostral) part,** to form the Sacculus and Ductus cochlearis and in a rear **(occipital) part,** to form the Utriculus, semicircular canals and Ductus endolymphaticus; rostral and occipital parts remain connected through a narrow path and form, in total the **membranous labyrinth.**

9.5.2 External ear

The external ear is divided into the externally visible **auricle** (Auricula) as well as the **external auditory canal** (Meatus acusticus externus), which leads to the inside and the eardrum (Membrana tympanica). It is used for sound transmission and improvement of the directional location.

Auricle
The auricle (> Fig. 9.69) consists of a basic framework made up of elastic cartilage. The skin on the lateral surface is immovable and fixed to the perichondrium without folds; on the rear side the skin is movable. No subcutaneous fatty tissue. The **ear lobe** (Lobulus auriculae) has no cartilage, is variably formed and consists of subcutaneous adipose tissue with skin coating. The outer edge of the auricle, the **helix,** is rolled together, the **antihelix** is the inner auricular fold, **tragus** and **antitragus** are prominent cartilage parts that limit the central depression **(Cavitas conchae)** at the entrance of the auditory canal. The tragus continues in the cartilaginous part of the external auditory canal. Other names are commonly used for the auricle, but are negligible for understanding.

Muscles
On the auricle rudimentary muscles are often present, such as the Mm. auriculares anterior, superior and posterior or the M. tragicus (some people can waggle their ears but only in conjunction with the M. epicranius). These are mimic muscles (innervated by the N. auricularis posterior of the N. facialis [VII]) which belong to a rudimentary sphincter system (M. orbicularis conchae) that is still well pronounced in many animals. Hence horses, for example, can turn the outer ears towards the direction of sound. Hedgehogs and

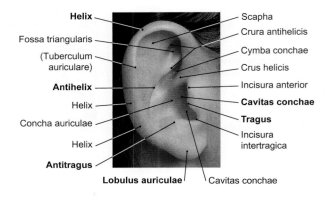

Fig. 9.69 Auricle, Auricula, right. Lateral view.

bears can close the external auditory canal so as not to be disturbed by noise during hibernation.

Vascular, lymphatic and nervous systems
Arteries
The auricle has an abundant blood supply by virtue of its exposed position (protection against cold, heat loss). The arteries are branches of the A. carotis externa. The **A. temporalis superficialis** with Rr. auriculares anteriores reaches the front of the auricle; Rr. auriculares of the **A. auricularis posterior** supply the back.

Veins
Corresponding **Vv. auriculares anteriores** drain into the **Plexus pterygoideus**; the V. auricularis posterior flows into the V. jugularis externa and the Vv. temporales superficiales into the V. jugularis interna.

Lymph vessels
Lymph is drained from the auricle forwards into the **Nodi lymphoidei parotidei** and backwards into the **Nodi lymphoidei mastoidei**, In some cases also into the upper **Nodi lymphoidei cervicales profundi**.

Innervation
Innervation of the auricle (➤ Fig. 9.70) takes place in front of the ear via the **N. auriculotemporalis** (from the N. mandibularis [V/3]), behind and below the ear from the Plexus cervicalis (**N. auricularis magnus, N. occipitalis minor**). The auricle itself is innervated via the N. facialis [VII] (which part of the **N. facialis [VII]** is exactly supplied, is not conclusively clarified) and at the entrance to the external auditory canal via the **N. vagus [X]**.

External auditory canal
The external auditory canal in adults is approximately 25-35 mm long and generally in the horizontal and vertical plane bent slightly forward in an S-shape (in neonates it is still straight) (➤ Fig. 9.71). It stretches from the depth of the Cavitas conchae to the tympanic membrane and consists of two parts:
- A longer cartilaginous (elastic cartilage) externally located **Pars fibrocartilaginea** (up to 20 mm)
- A bony **Pars ossea**

The Pars ossea belongs to the Pars tympanica of the Os temporale, which borders the Meatus acusticus externus from the front, below and behind. In its superior aspect, the bony ring is interrupted by the Incisura tympanica (attachment point for the Pars flaccida of the tympanic membrane, see below). The end of the external auditory canal is formed by the Sulcus tympanicus and the Incisura tympanica, the eardrum is attached here. Functionally the auditory canal is a sound funnel (approx. 8 mm diameter at the entrance, in the Pars ossea only 6–7 mm, narrowest point at the transition from cartilage into the bony part). The auditory canal cartilage is connected to the tragus of the auricle. The cartilaginous part is covered by skin on the inside on its entire course, which contains hair, specialised free sebaceous glands and apocrine tubulous olfactory glands (ceruminous glands, Glandulae ceruminosae). The secretion of the glands forms the earwax (cerumen), which contains shed epithelial cells, lipids and protein pigments (brown colour) as well as bitter substances (unpleasant for all types of insects).

Vascular, lymphatic and nervous systems
Arteries
The external auditory canal is arterially supplied by **Rr. auriculares anteriores** of the A. temporalis superficialis and the **R. auricularis posterior** of the A. carotis externa.

Veins
The venous drainage occurs via **Vv. auriculares anteriores** into the Vv. temporales superficiales and from here into the V. jugularis interna, as well as via the **V. auricularis posterior** in both the V. jugularis interna as well as the V. jugularis externa.

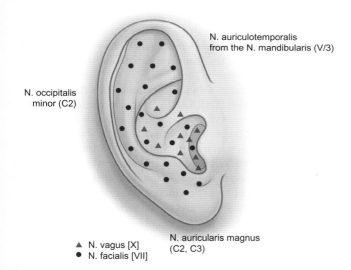

Fig. 9.70 Sensory innervation of the auricle, Auricula, right. Lateral view. [E402]

N. auriculotemporalis from the N. mandibularis (V/3)

N. occipitalis minor (C2)

▲ N. vagus [X]
● N. facialis [VII]

N. auricularis magnus (C2, C3)

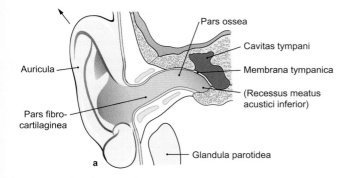

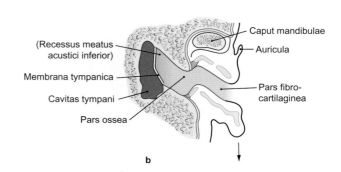

Pars ossea
Cavitas tympani
Membrana tympanica
(Recessus meatus acustici inferior)
Auricula
Pars fibro-cartilaginea
Glandula parotidea

a

Caput mandibulae
Auricula
(Recessus meatus acustici inferior)
Membrana tympanica
Cavitas tympani
Pars ossea
Pars fibro-cartilaginea

b

Fig. 9.71 External ear canal, Meatus acusticus externus, right (diagram). The arrows indicate the pulling direction of the examiner on the auricle, to stretch the ear canal in order gain a view of the tympanic membrane. **a** Frontal section. **b** Horizontal section.

Lymph vessels

Regional lymph node stations are the **Nodi lymphoidei parotidei superficiales** and **profundi** and **Nodi lymphoidei infraauriculares,** which drain into the **Nodi lymphoidei cervicales profundi.**

Innervation

The front and upper wall are innervated by the **N. meatus acustici externi** from the **N. auriculotemporalis** (from the N. mandibularis [V/3]); the posterior and partially the lower wall are reached by the R. auricularis of the **N. vagus [X].** The rear wall and the external side of the tympanic membrane are innervated by the Rr. auriculares of the **N. facialis [VII]** and of the **N. glossopharyngeus [IX].**

Topography

The external auditory canal is directly adjacent to the Glandula parotidea, to the Proc. mastoideus, the middle cranial fossa and the mandibular joint. When opening the mouth the head of the temporomandibular joint glides on the slope of the Tuberculum articulare ossis temporalis, which slightly extends the cartilaginous portion of the external auditory canal.

Clinical remarks

An inflammation of the elastic cartilage may occur **(auricular perichondritis)** as a result of injuries or insect bites to the auricle. The ear lobe is unaffected because it contains no cartilage.

Since the ear lobe is well supplied with blood, is very easily accessible and has no elastic cartilage, it is often used for taking a blood sample, e.g. in diabetic patients for the determination of blood glucose levels. Through the exposed location and the lack of a fat layer, frostbite and sunburn, however, are not unusual.

Abnormalities of the auricle often require plastic reconstructive surgery. Mechanical manipulation (e.g. cleaning the external auditory canal with a cotton bud) or damage often result in an inflammation of the auricle and the external auditory canal **(Otitis externa).**

Excessive formation of cerumen (ear wax) often results in a ceruminal plug that may close the external auditory canal **(Cerumen obturans)** and leads to **conductive hearing loss.**

Due to the sensory innervation of the external auditory canal through the N. vagus [X] during manipulations in the auditory canal (e.g. when removing earwax or when foreign bodies are trapped in the auditory canal) a **throat irritation** is almost always triggered. In a worst case scenario the manipulation can cause vomiting or collapse.

In order to be able to inspect the tympanic membrane with an ear mirror or a microscope **(otoscopy),** the auricle has to be pulled back and upwards. This stretches the cartilaginous portion of the auditory canal and the tympanic membrane can be seen (at least partially) (➤ Fig. 9.71).

Zoster oticus is the secondary manifestation of infection with varicella zoster virus in the area of the ear, resulting in blistering of the auricle and/or on the external auditory canal. Severe pain is typical for zoster. The infection can also spread to the internal ear and cause hearing loss up to deafness (N. cochlearis) or equilibrium disorders (N. vestibularis).

Tympanic membrane

Each medium has a distinctive sound wave resistance, which is referred to as the impedance. The impedance of air and one of the fluids (perilymph) located in the inner ear are so different that 98 % of the incident sound waves would be reflected in direct transmission from the air to the inner ear. The remaining 2 % would be too little to provide sufficient cortical perception. Tympanic membrane (Membrana tympanica) and auditory ossicles of the middle ear, however, serve as a kind of impedance converter and reduce the reflection of the noise, so that on average 60 % of the sound energy can be transferred to the oval window of the inner ear.

The **tympanic membrane** (➤ Fig. 9.72a, ➤ Fig. 9.73) forms the border between the external ear and the middle ear and closes both spaces against each other in an airtight closure (the middle ear is therefore solely ventilated by the Tuba auditiva in the case of an intact eardrum). The eardrum is grey, with a mother-of-pearl-like gloss, elliptically rounded in shape and has a diameter of approximately 9 mm with an area of 85 mm^2. Structures lying in the middle ear close behind the tympanic membrane shimmer through. A distinction is made between 2 areas:

- The very much smaller, thinner and slacker **Pars flaccida** located in the cranial section (SHRAPNELL's membrane, approx. 25 mm^2), which does not vibrate on sound (➤ Fig. 9.72a)
- The large, thicker (approx. 0.1 mm) and tighter **Pars tensa,** which is used for sound transmission to the hammer head.

The eardrum has a thickened edge (**Limbus membranae tympanicae**), which is attached in the area of the Pars tensa via a connective tissue ring (**Anulus fibrocartilagineus**) in the bony Sulcus tympanicus of the temporal bone and the Incisura tympanica, a recess of the Sulcus at the upper front. It sits obliquely to the auditory canal axis. The position of eardrums can be imagined if the outstretched palms of the hand are placed together like the bows of a ship so that only the tips of the 3rd–5th fingers touch: the backs of

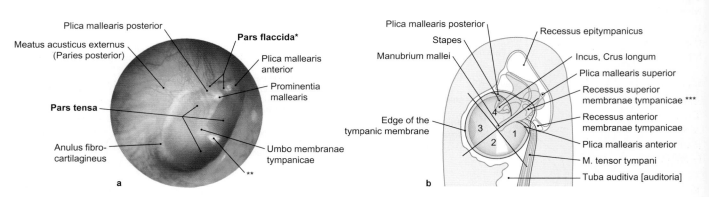

Fig. 9.72 Tympanic membrane, Membrana tympanica, right. Lateral view. **a** Mirror image of the ear. **b** Schematic representation with Recessus of the tympanic cavity, Cavitas tympani and division into 4 quadrants. * clinically: SHRAPNELL's membrane, ** typically positioned light reflex, *** clinically: PRUSSAK's space.

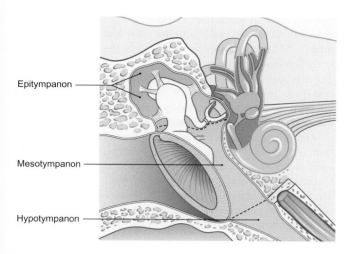

Epitympanon

Mesotympanon

Hypotympanon

Fig. 9.73 Levels of the tympanic cavity, Cavitas tympani, right. Anterior view. [L126]

hand point to the auditory canals, the palms in the direction of the cranial cavity. In the case of small children and infants the eardrum is even more inclined than in adults. The eardrum is drawn inside like a funnel. The eccentrically lying tip corresponds to the lowest point on the auditory canal side or Umbilicus of the tympanic membrane **(Umbo membranae tympanicae);** the tip of the hammer grip (Manubrium mallei) is attached at this point, on the middle ear side, which continues obliquely towards the upper front. At the most cranially located attachment point of the hammer the short hammer process protrudes (Proc. lateralis mallei) as the Prominentia mallearis in the direction of the auditory canal. From this bulge the Plicae malleares anterior and posterior run on the inner surface of the tympanic membrane and separate the Pars flaccida from the Pars tensa of the tympanic membrane.

If one creates an imaginary line through the Manubrium mallei and a line perpendicular to it that leads exactly through the Umbo, one can divide the eardrum into 4 quadrants:
- An anterior upper
- A posterior upper
- An anterior lower
- A posterior lower

The division into quadrants (➤ Fig. 9.72b) is of practical clinical significance. The auditory ossicles are located behind the upper quadrants. In addition, the Chorda tympani (branch of the N. facialis [VII]) and the attachment tendon of the M. tensor tympani (see below) run here. The basis of the tympanic membrane is a layer of connective tissue (Stratum fibrosum), which forms a network from radial and circular fibres and provides the stiffness of the tympanic membrane. On the auditory canal side, the connective tissue is covered by squamous epithelium, in the middle ear by a Stratum mucosum (single layered cuboidal epithelium).

Vascular, lymphatic and nervous systems
Arteries
The external side of the tympanic membrane is fed arterially by the **A. stylomastoidea** which comes via the A. auricularis profunda from the A. maxillaris; the internal side receives its blood supply from the **A. tympanica anterior,** a branch of the A. carotis externa.

Veins
The venous drainage occurs on the outside and the inside via the Vv. perforantes into the V. stylomastoidea and from here into the Plexus pterygoideus.

Lymph vessels
Regional lymph nodes are the **Nodi lymphoidei parotidei superficiales** and **profundi** and the **Nodi lymphoidei infraauriculares** and from here the **Nodi lymphoidei cervicales profundi.**

Innervation
The eardrum is extremely well sensory innervated. On the outside via the Rr. auriculares of the **N. vagus [X]** and the **N. auriculotemporalis** (from the N. mandibularis [V/3]); on the inside via the **Plexus tympanicus from fibres of the N. facialis [VII]** and the **N. glossopharyngeus [IX].**

> **Clinical remarks**
>
> In the anterior lower quadrant one can see when inspecting the eardrum through the otoscope a bright pyramid-shaped light reflex, which is referred to as a **mirror or tympanic membrane reflex.** It can be used to draw conclusions about the tension of the tympanic membrane. The base of the light reflex pyramid is directed to the Anulus fibrocartilagineus.
> The Pars flaccida of the eardrum is thinner than the Pars tensa and therefore in the case of **suppurating middle ear infections** (Otitis media) is the preferred location for a spontaneous perforation.
> Hydromyrinx can be seen and drained through the tympanic membrane. To ensure that the middle ear structures during a **paracentesis** are not put at risk (incision through the tympanic membrane) it is performed in the anterior lower or posterior lower quadrant. A **tympanostomy tube** can then be inserted through the incision for long-term aeration of the middle ear.

9.5.3 Middle ear

The middle ear (Auris media) includes the tympanic cavity (Cavitas tympani) with the 3 ossicles. Connections are present via the Antrum mastoideum with the air-containing cells of the mastoid process, as well as the Eustachian tube (Tuba auditiva [auditoria], 'tube', EUSTACHIAN tube) with the nasopharynx.

Tympanic cavity
The **tympanic cavity (Cavitas tympani)** is separated from the external auditory canal by the eardrum which is airtight and thus represents a closed space which must be ventilated. This ventilation of the tympanic cavity (and the air-containing cells of the mastoid process) only takes place during the swallowing process in which the tube, which is otherwise sealed, opens briefly and enables the air exchange between nasopharynx and middle ear.

The tympanic cavity is anatomically and clinically divided (➤ Fig. 9.73) into:
- The **Epitympanum** (dome recess, tympanic dome, attic) contains the suspension device and the largest part of the auditory ossicles and is connected to the mastoid cells (retrotympanal spaces) via the Antrum mastoideum. Below the Antrum the semicircular canals of the labyrinth bone bulge out. The area between Pars flaccida of the tympanic membrane (lateral) and hammer head and anvil body (medial) is the **Recessus epitympanicus.** An even smaller space between Pars flaccida and hammer neck is the Recessus superior membranae tympanicae (PRUSSAK's space).
- The **Mesotympanum** (tympanic space) includes the Manubrium mallei, the Proc. lenticularis of the anvil, and the tendon of the M. tensor tympani and lies directly behind the tympanic membrane.

- The **Hypotympanon** which merges into the Tuba auditiva (tympanic cellar, Recessus hypotympanicus) is the lowest point of the tympanic cavity and is located below the tympanic membrane level.

The distance between the Epitympanum and the Hypotympanum is 12–15 mm at a depth of 3–7 mm. The internal volume of the tympanic cavity is only about 1 cm³.

The tympanic cavity is lined by a single layer of isoprismatic epithelium; individual goblet cells and ciliated epithelium are also present. The auditory ossicles are covered by multilayered squamous epithelium. In the Lamina propria there are tubulous glands (Glandulae tympanicae), which are innervated by the Plexus tympanicus.

Delineations

The tympanic cavity has 6 walls (➤ Fig. 9.74, ➤ Table 9.26): a rear, a front, a roof, a floor and a medial and a lateral wall:

- A thin bony plate (Tegmen tympani, **Paries tegmentalis**) separates the Epitympanum above from the middle cranial fossa.
- The paper thin front wall of the Mesotympanum (**Paries caroticus**) has a connection to the A. carotis interna.
- The lateral wall (**Paries membranaceus**) is almost exclusively formed by the eardrum. At the top edge lies the Fissura spheno-

petrosa, through which the Chorda tympani, the A. tympanica anterior and the Lig. mallei anterior enter and exit. The auditory tube (Tuba auditiva [auditoria]) flows into the tympanic cavity in the lower wall section.

- The rear panel (**Paries mastoideus**) borders on the mastoid process (Proc. mastoideus, ➤ Fig. 9.75). At the upper rear there is a direct connection to the normally pneumatic spaces (**Cellulae mastoideae**) of the mastoid (Aditus ad antrum). In the upper part of the rear wall the Eminentia pyramidalis forms an elevation. At this point, the tendon of the M. stapedius exits. Just below flows the Canaliculus chordae tympani, through which the Chorda tympani enters the tympanic cavity.
- The lower wall of the tympanic cavity (**Paries jugularis**) is part of the Hypotympanum. It demarcates the tympanic cavity from the V. jugularis interna. The bone is very thin at this section (approx. 0.5 mm) and partially pneumatised. Here, the N. tympanicus together with the A. tympanica inferior enter through the Canaliculus tympanicus into the tympanic cavity.
- The medial wall (**Paries labyrinthicus**) separates the cochlea from the tympanic cavity and therefore forms the border to the inner ear (labyrinth). It has two openings (➤ Fig. 9.75): the **oval window** (Fenestra vestibuli), in which the stirrup foot plate lies, which is attached in the oval window via the Lig. anulare stape-

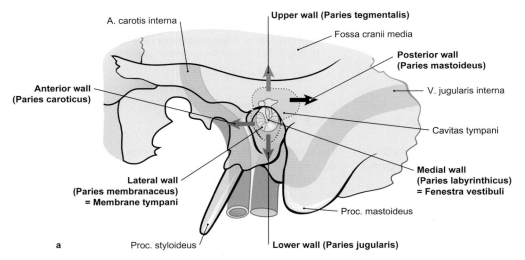

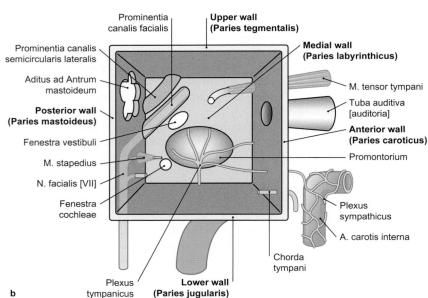

Fig. 9.74 Topographical relationships of the tympanic cavity, Cavitas tympani, to the adjacent structures. a Right side; lateral view exterior; schematic representation (➤ Table 9.26). **b** Right side; view from lateral into the tympanic cavity schematically shown as a box.

Table 9.26 Walls of the tympanic cavity.

Wall	Relationship	Openings/connections
Posterior, rear wall (Proc. mastoideus)	Mastoid wall (Paries mastoideus)	Aditus to Antrum mastoideum (transition to the mastoid cells); Eminentia pyramidalis (passage of the tendon of the M. stapedius); opening of the Canaliculus chordae tympani
Anterior, frontal wall (carotid canal)	A. carotis interna (Paries caroticus)	Canaliculi caroticotympanici (passage sympathetic nerve fibres); Semicanalis tubae auditivae (bony connection in the direction of the nasopharynx)
Superior, upper wall (middle cranial fossa)	Middle cranial fossa (Paries tegmentalis)	Opening of the Semicanalis musculi tensoris tympani and passage of its tendon; Fissura petrosquamosa (passage of the A. tympanica superior); Canaliculus nervi petrosi minoris (contains preganglionic parasympathetic fibres of the N. glossopharyngeus [IX], which run to the Ganglion oticum)
Inferior, lower wall (Fossa jugularis)	V. jugularis (Paries jugularis)	Canaliculus tympanicus (passage of N. tympanicus and A. tympanica inferior)
Medial, medial wall (labyrinth)	Oval window (Paries labyrinthicus)	Fenestra vestibuli (above the Promontorium, contains stirrup base plate); Fenestra cochleae (below and behind Promontorium; closed from Membrana tympanica secundaria)
Lateral, lateral wall (tympanic membrane)	Tympanic membrane (Paries membranaceus)	Fissura sphenopetrosa (passage of the Chorda tympani)

diale, and the **round window** (Fenestra cochleae) located further below which is closed by the Membrana tympanica secundaria. Between the oval and the round window, the medial tympanic cavity wall bulges out towards the **Promontorium** through the basal cochlear coil. Above the oval window, the medial wall protrudes outward through the lateral semicircular canal towards the **Prominentia canalis semicircularis lateralis**. The N. facialis [VII] runs through the medial wall in the **Canalis nervi facialis**. The canal bulges the medial wall towards the horizontally running **Prominentia canalis nervi facialis**.

The Tuba auditiva [auditoria] commences at the Ostium tympanicum tubae auditivae and is demarcated at the top by the Septum canalis musculotubarii from the Semicanalis musculi tensoris tympani.

Vascular, lymphatic and nervous systems
Arteries
The middle ear including the ossicles and the Cellulae mastoideae are supplied by 10 arteries (➤ Table 9.27). They are listed here for the sake of completeness but exact knowledge is superfluous infor-

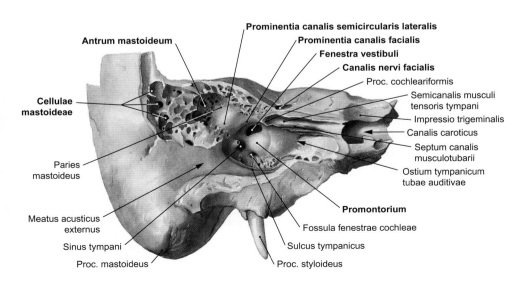

Fig. 9.75 Medial wall, Paries labyrinthicus, the tympanic cavity, Cavitas tympani, right. Vertical section in the longitudinal axis of the temporal bone; frontal lateral view.

Prominentia canalis semicircularis lateralis
Prominentia canalis facialis
Fenestra vestibuli
Canalis nervi facialis
Antrum mastoideum
Proc. cochleariformis
Semicanalis musculi tensoris tympani
Impressio trigeminalis
Canalis caroticus
Cellulae mastoideae
Septum canalis musculotubarii
Ostium tympanicum tubae auditivae
Paries mastoideus
Promontorium
Meatus acusticus externus
Fossula fenestrae cochleae
Sinus tympani
Sulcus tympanicus
Proc. mastoideus
Proc. styloideus

Table 9.27 Arteries of the tympanic cavity.

Artery (original vessel)	Entry site	Supply area
Aa. caroticotympanicae (A. carotis interna)	Canaliculi caroticotympanici	Promontorium
A. tympanica superior (A. meningea media)	Canalis nervi petrosi minoris	M. tensor tympani, Epitympanum, Stapes
R. petrosus (A. meningea media)	Hiatus canalis nervi petrosi minoris	N. facialis [VII], Stapes
A. tympanica anterior (A. maxillaris)	Fissura sphenopetrosa	Epitympanum, hammer, anvil, Antrum mastoideum, tympanic membrane
A. tympanica posterior (A. stylomastoidea)	Canaliculus chordae tympani	Chorda tympani, hammer, tympanic membrane
A. tympanica inferior (A. pharyngea ascendens)	Canaliculus tympanicus	Stapes, Promontorium, Hypotympanum, Pars cartilaginea of the Tuba auditiva
A. auricularis profunda (A. maxillaris)	Basis partis petrosae ossis temporalis	outer ear canal, tympanic membrane, Hypotympanum
A. stylomastoidea (A. auricularis posterior)	Canalis nervi facialis	Cellulae mastoideae, Antrum mastoideum, Paries mastoideus, Stapes, M. stapedius
R. mastoideus (A. occipitalis)	Foramen mastoideum	Cellulae mastoideae
A. subarcuata (A. labyrinthi)	Below the front semicircular canal	Cellulae mastoideae

mation and not necessary to understand the middle ear. If necessary it can be looked up. With the exception of the Aa. caroticotympanicae all vessels are branches of the A. carotis externa. Most of the arteries form an anastomosis system in the area of the Promontorium.

Veins

The veins of the same name drain into the Sinus petrosi superior and inferior, the Sinus sigmoideus, the Bulbus superior venae jugularis, the V. meningea media and the Plexus pharyngeus

Lymph vessels

Regional lymph nodes are the **Nodi lymphoidei parotidei profundi** and the **Nodi lymphoidei retropharyngeales,** which drain to the nodi lymphoidei cervicales profundi.

Innervation

The tympanic cavity, the ossicles and the Cellulae mastoideae are innervated sensitively from the **N. tympanicus of the N. glossopharyngeus[IX].** Preganglionic parasympathetic fibres of the N. facialis [VII] and the N. glossopharyngeus [IX] form the Plexus tympanicus below the tympanic cavity mucosa. A part of the fibres is switched here in small groups of multipolar ganglion cells to postganglionic neurons and innervates the tympanic cavity mucosa. The other part leaves the tympanic cavity and forms the **N. petrosus minor** (innervation of the Glandula parotidea, JACOBSON's anastomosis). Apart from parasympathetic fibres, sympathetic fibres also occur in the Plexus tympanicus (sometimes referred to as R. communicans cum plexu tympanico), which reach it as Nn. caroticotympanici (passage through the Paries caroticus) coming from the Plexus nervosus of the A. carotis interna.

Auditory ossicles

The 3 ossicles coated by mucous membranes (➤ Fig. 9.76), hammer (**Malleus**), anvil (**Incus**) and stirrup (**Stapes**) are suspended in

the tympanic cavity and form a movable chain from the eardrum to the oval window (Fenestra vestibuli):

- The **Malleus** consists of head (**Caput** mallei), neck (**Collum** mallei), handle of Malleus (**Manubrium** mallei), a long (**Proc. anterior**) and a short (**Proc. lateralis**) process. Manubrium mallei and Proc. lateralis are fused with the tympanic membrane. The tendon of the M. tensor tympani is also attached at the Manubrium mallei.
- The **anvil** consists of a body (**Corpus** incudis) and 2 legs (**Crus longum** and **Crus breve** incudis). On the front of the Corpus is the articular surface for articulation with the Malleus. The Crus longum runs parallel to the Manubrium mallei. At the end, there is the **Proc. lenticularis,** which bends at a right angle and bears the joint surface for articulation with the stirrup.
- The **stirrup** consists of a head (**Caput** stapedis), 2 legs (**Crus anterius** and **Crus posterior** stapedis) as well as the base of the stirrup (**Basis stapedis**). The base plate is movably fixed in the oval window via a connective tissue ring ligament (**Lig anulare stapediale**) and transmits the sound vibrations to the perilymph of the inner ear.

The 3 bones are connected in a series and linked by true joints (**Articulatio incudomallearis,** a saddle joint, and **Articulo incudostapedialis,** a ball joint). In the tympanic cavity the bones are fixed with ligaments:

- Ligg. mallei superius, anterius (remnants of the MECKEL's cartilage) and posterius (Ligg. mallei anterius and posterius together form the 'axis ligament', which acts as a lever of the hammer)
- Ligg. incudis superius and posterius

The ligaments are listed just for the sake of completeness.

NOTE

The auditory ossicles form a flexible chain for the transmission of sound waves conducted by the tympanic membrane to the perilymph of the inner ear. Low air impedance has to be transferred to the significantly higher inner ear fluid impedance. This requires the amplification of the sound waves (impedance matching), which is accomplished by the size difference between the tympanic membrane (55 mm²) and the oval window (3.2 mm²; 17 times) and the lever action of the auditory ossicles (1.3-times). This boosts acoustic pressure 22-fold.

Muscles

The sound transmission is influenced by 2 striated muscles (Mm. ossiculorum auditus) (➤ Fig. 9.77), the M. tensor tympani and the M. stapedius. Its contraction leads to a reduction of high sound intensities and the volume range is adjusted dynamically. They also weaken the transfer of one's own voice.

The **M. tensor tympani** originates in the Semicanalis musculi tensoris tympani of the temporal bone. Its tendon enters at the Proc.

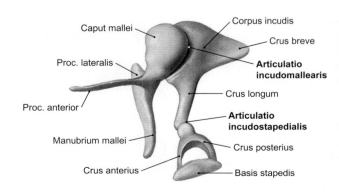

Fig. 9.76 Ossicles, Ossicula auditus, right. View from medial above.

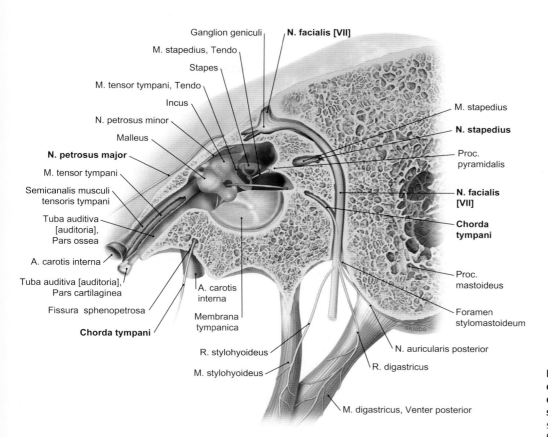

Ganglion geniculi
M. stapedius, Tendo
Stapes
M. tensor tympani, Tendo
Incus
N. petrosus minor
Malleus
N. petrosus major
M. tensor tympani
Semicanalis musculi tensoris tympani
Tuba auditiva [auditoria], Pars ossea
A. carotis interna
Tuba auditiva [auditoria], Pars cartilaginea
Fissura sphenopetrosa
Chorda tympani
A. carotis interna
Membrana tympanica
R. stylohyoideus
M. stylohyoideus

N. facialis [VII]
M. stapedius
N. stapedius
Proc. pyramidalis
N. facialis [VII]
Chorda tympani
Proc. mastoideus
Foramen stylomastoideum
N. auricularis posterior
R. digastricus
M. digastricus, Venter posterior

Fig. 9.77 Tympanic cavity with ossicles, ossicular muscles, course of the N. facialis [VII] and some of its branches. Vertical section through the Canalis facialis; view from the left side.

cochleariformis through the Paries tegmentalis into the tympanic cavity and is deflected almost at right angles. It inserts after a short course at the top edge of the hammer handle. The **A. tympanica superior** supplies it with blood, the **N. pterygoideus medialis** of the N. mandibularis [V/3] innervates the muscle. Functionally the M. tensor tympani tenses the eardrum by tension at the hammer handle and stiffening of the ossicular chain. It is used for a better transmission of high sound frequencies.

The **M. stapedius** originates in the Cavum musculi stapedii. Its tendon enters at the tip of the Proc. pyramidalis in the Paries mastoideus into the tympanic cavity and passes to the Caput stapedis. The **A. stylomastoidea** supplies it with blood, the **N. facialis [VII]** innervates the muscle. A contraction tips the stirrup foot plate in the oval window and reduces energy transfer. Very loud noises are thus weakened, the inner ear is protected.

Vascular, lymphatic and nervous systems

The blood supply for the tympanic cavity was already discussed above. The ossicles are sensitively innervated from the **N. mandibularis [V/3]**, vegetatively innervated via the **N. tympanicus and Nn. caroticotympanici,** exactly in the same way as the tympanic cavity mucosa.

Mastoid process

In neonates, only the tympanic cavity and the Antrum mastoideum are filled with air. First in young children (finishing approximately in the *6th year of life*) air-filled cells are formed in the mastoid process starting from the anvil. The degree of **pneumatisation** differs greatly according to the individual case. Zygomatic and temporal bone pyramids can be almost completely pneumatised (extensive pneumatisation); the pneumatisation can also be completely missing (compact mastoid bone) or only slightly formed (partially pneumatised). All pneumatised spaces (Cellulae mastoideae) are in contact with the tympanic cavity via the Antrum

mastoideum (➤ Fig. 9.75), are lined with mucous membrane and must be ventilated. Blood supply and innervation in the tympanic cavity were already discussed.

Clinical remarks

An inflammation of the Cellulae mastoideae **(mastoiditis)** is often an inflammation transferred from the tympanic cavity. It is one of the most common complications of a middle ear inflammation. The inflammation can spread from the mastoid to the soft tissue parts behind and in front of the ear, the M. sternocleidomastoideus, the inner ear, the Sinus sigmoideus, the meninges, the cerebellum and the N. facialis [VII].

Topography of the N. facialis [VII] and its branches
Course

The **N. facialis [VII]** runs in its peripheral section over a long distance through the Os temporale (➤ Fig. 9.77). It is composed of two branches, the actual N. facialis and the N. intermedius. Both branches combine in the depth of the facial canal (Canalis nervi facialis) to the N. intermediofacialis (generally referred to as N.facialis [VII]) (➤ Fig. 9.81). After it leaves the cerebellopontine angle, it passes together with the N. vestibulocochlearis [VIII] through the Meatus acusticus internus of the temporal pyramid **(meatal and labyrinthine distance)** up to the Ganglion geniculi (outer facial bend), flexes here to the rear and continues in the medial tympanic wall (Paries labyrinthicus) in a thin bony canal between Epitympanum and Mesotympanum **(tympanal distance).** Its bony channel bulges the bones above the oval window. Shortly afterwards, the N. facialis [VII] bends to caudal and passes through the front section of the mastoid **(mastoidal distance).** Between the mastoid and Proc. styloideus it leaves the skull base at the Foramen stylomastoideumi.

Branches

On the way through the petrous bone, the N. facialis [VII] emits the N. petrosi major and stapedius and the Chorda tympani (also ➤ Chap. 9.3.7).

At the Ganglion geniculi the first branch to be emitted is the **N. petrosus major** (➤ Fig. 9.77). It runs in the Os temporale to the front medially and exits at the Hiatus nervi petrosi majoris on the Facies anterior of the Pars petrosa ossis temporalis below the dura. The nerve carries preganglionic parasympathetic fibres to the Ganglion pterygopalatinum for the innervation of lacrimal, nasal, palatine and pharyngeal glands and taste fibres from the palate.

Since the N. facialis [VII] runs directly passed the Proc. pyramidalis ossis temporalis in whose cavity the M. stapedius lies, the **N. stapedius** is a very short nerve, which originates directly from the N. facialis [VII] (➤ Fig. 9.77).

The **Chorda tympani,** which exits shortly before the end of the Canalis nervi facialis and regresses through its own bone canal goes back into the tympanic cavity and runs embedded in mucosa, between hammer and Crus longum of the anvil right through the tympanic cavity, to leave the skull base via the Fissura sphenopetrosa (or Fissura petrotympanica) (➤ Fig. 9.77).

Clinical remarks

The **N. facialis [VII]** can be damaged due to fractures of the petrous bone and inflammation of the middle ear or mastoid process, as well as surgical interventions because of these conditions. For **facial diagnostics** (the amount of the damage) and the follow-up after facial paralysis, various test procedures are used: SCHIRMER's test (lacrimal gland function), Stapedius reflex test, taste test and sometimes a sialometry (test of the salivary gland function) for testing the Chorda tympani and electromyography (EMG) and electroneuronography (ENoG) to test the facial muscles; however, these methods are increasingly being replaced by modern high-resolution imaging methods.

The course of the Chorda tympani renders it susceptible to injury in surgery conducted on the middle ear. During middle ear infections there is often an isolated **functional loss of the Chorda tympani** with dry mouth and loss of taste sensation on the affected side.

If the N. stapedius is involved, and thus the M. stapedius is paralysed, the result is impaired hearing on the affected side. Loud sounds are perceived as uncomfortably loud **(hyperacusis),** because of insufficient attenuation (due to a tilting of the base of the stirrup foot plate in the oval window).

The N. facialis [VII] can be exposed surgically via the Proc. mastoideus to provide relief, for example, in the context of an inflammatory swelling of the nerve. In the process the bony canal is opened or removed from behind.

Auditory tube

The Eustachian tube (Tuba auditiva [auditoria], EUSTACHIAN tube, Tuba EUSTACHII) is about 3.5 cm long and runs obliquely from the rear lateral above to medial at the front below. It connects the tympanic cavity with the nasopharynx and its function is pressure compensation (➤ Fig. 9.78). The requirement for optimal transmission of sound waves is equal air pressure in both the tympanic cavity and the external auditory canal. If this is not the case, e.g. during the ascent or descent in an aeroplane or when diving, there is hearing loss.

The Tuba auditiva [auditoria] connects to the Hypotympanum and starts in the front wall of the tympanic cavity (Paries caroticus) with the Ostium tympanicum tubae auditivae. It converges at the Ostium pharyngeum tubae auditivae, which protrudes at the side to the rear in the nasopharynx (the Ostia of both sides protrude as Torus tubarius). In its mucosa lies the Tonsilla tubaria as part of the lymphatic tonsillar ring (WALDEYER's tonsillar ring). A distinction is made between a bony section (**Pars ossea**) and an almost twice as long cartilaginous section (**Pars cartilaginea**) (➤ Fig. 9.68, ➤ Fig. 9.78a). The latter consists of a groove made of flexible cartilage (Cartilago tubae auditivae). The upside-down cartilage groove is medially enclosed by connective tissue (Lamina membranacea) to form a slit-shaped canal. The Tuba auditiva [auditoria] is opened by the contraction of the Mm. tensor and levator veli palatini as part of the swallowing action (➤ Fig. 9.78b, c).

The bony section of the Tuba auditiva [auditoria] is inside a triangular bony canal (Semicanalis tubae auditivae of the Canalis musculotubarius) of the Pars petrosa ossis temporalis. Separated by a thin bony layer the M. tensor tympani lies in the **Semicanalis musculi tensoris tympani** of the **Canalis musculotubarius** (➤ Fig. 9.77).

Clinical remarks

The Tuba auditiva [auditoria] is lined by respiratory ciliated epithelium with goblet cells; mixed Glandulae tubariae occur in the subepithelium. The ciliary beat is aimed in the direction of the nasopharynx. Failure of the protective mechanism in the tube can lead to an ascending inflammation with formation of a **tube catarrh** up to otitis media. By injection of air via the nose, adhesions and closures inside the tubes can be dissolved (e.g. swallowing for pressure problems).

One of the most common causes of conductive hearing loss in childhood is the relocation of the tube opening (**tube occlusion**) due to tube catarrh or restricted nasal breathing due to enlarged pharyngeal tonsils (**adenoids**). If the tube function disorder persists over a longer period of time, restructuring of the middle ear mucosa takes place. As a result, an actively secreting epithelium develops, with fluid retention formation in the tympanic cavity (**secretory otitis media**).

Muscles

The opening of the Tuba auditiva and thus the pressure compensation between tympanic cavity and nasopharynx takes place using the Mm. tensor and levator veli palatini and the M. salpingopharyngeus (➤ Fig. 9.78, ➤ Table 9.28).

The swallowing action involves contraction of the Mm. tensor and the levator veli palatini. The **contraction of the M. tensor veli palatini** causes the tubal lumen to expand by pulling on the Pars membranacea and the upper edge of the tubal cartilage (➤ Fig. 9.78b, c). **Contraction of the M. levator veli palatini** causes the muscle to bulge out and this muscle belly pushes against the cartilaginous part of the tube from below. In the process, the groove is bent open and the tube lumen expanded. The M. salpingopharyngeus is involved in occluding the tube (➤ Fig. 9.78a).

Clinical remarks

Cleft palate is associated with a non-functioning Mm. tensor and levator veli palatini, because the Punctum fixum of the muscles is missing and they contract into a void. This renders the tubular function redundant. If left untreated, an **adhesive process** occurs in the middle ear due to the absence of middle ear ventilation. Such children are hard of hearing and often do not learn to speak.

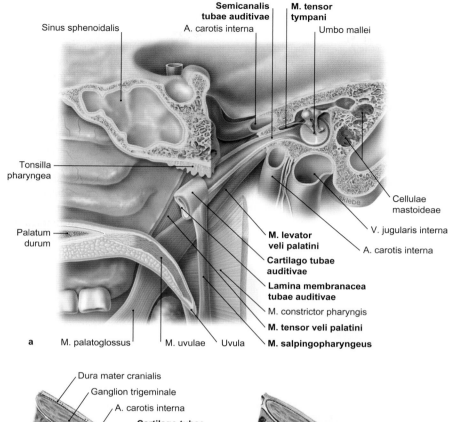

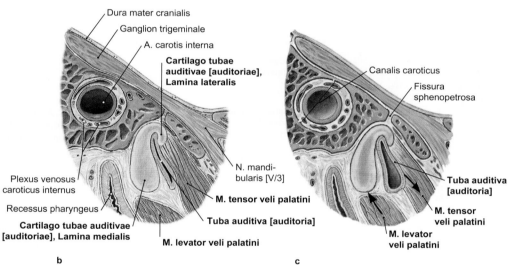

Fig. 9.78 Eustachian tube, Tuba auditiva [auditoria], right.
a Medial view, connection between the tympanic cavity and nasopharynx and location of muscles. [L238]
b, c Cross-sections at the level of the lateral portion of the Pars cartilaginea, closed (b) and open (c) tube, the effect of the muscles on the tube is illustrated by arrows.

Table 9.28 Muscles of the Eustachian tube.

Innervation	Origins	Attachment	Function
M. tensor veli palatini			
N. musculi tensoris veli palatini of the N. mandibularis [V/3]	Fossa scaphoidea at the Proc. pterygoideus, membrane part of the Tuba auditiva	Aponeurosis palatina	Extends the lumen of the Eustachian tube, tenses the soft palate
M. levator veli palatini			
Plexus pharyngeus from N. glossopharyngeus [IX] and N. vagus [X]	Lower surface of the Pars petrosa ossis temporalis, Cartilago tubae auditivae	Aponeurosis palatina	Extends the lumen of the Eustachian tube, elevates the soft palate
M. salpingopharyngeus			
Plexus pharyngeus mainly from the N. vagus [X]	Lower portion of tube cartilage in the area of the nasopharyngeal space	Cartilago thyroidea, side wall of the pharynx	Closes the tube, raises the pharynx

Vascular, lymphatic and nervous systems
Arteries
The Pars ossea receives blood from the **Aa. caroticotympanicae** (from the A. carotis interna); the Pars cartilaginea is fed via the **A. tympanica inferior** from the A. pharyngea ascendens (➤ Table 9.27).

Veins
The venous drainage occurs in the **Plexus pterygoideus.**

Lymph vessels
Regional lymph nodes are the **Nodi lymphoidei retropharyngeales,** which drain into the Nodi lymphoidei cervicales anteriores, as well as the **Nodi lymphoidei parotidei profundi,** which drain into the nodi lymphoidei jugulares interni.

Innervation
The Eustachian tube is sensitively innervated via the **Plexus (nervosus) tympanicus** of the R. tubarius from the **N. glossopharyngeus**

[IX]. Autonomic parasympathetic fibres also go through the Plexus tympanicus to the Pars ossea. The Pars cartilaginea is parasympathetically supplied by the **Plexus pharyngeus.** Sympathetic fibres originate in the nerve plexus around the A. carotis interna. The Ostium pharyngeum tubae auditivae is innervated with parasympathetic fibres of the R. tubarius from the N. glossopharyngeus [IX].

9.5.4 Internal ear

The internal ear (Auris interna) is a complex of bony canals and extensions inside the Pars petrosa of the Os temporale (**osseous labyrinth, Labyrinthus osseus,** ➤ Fig. 9.79). Inside is a system of membranous tubes and vesicles called the **membranous labyrinth (Labyrinthus membranaceus)** (➤ Fig. 9.80). It houses the organ for balance and hearing (Organum vestibulocochleare). The tip of the cochlea is pointed in an anterolateral direction. The semicircular canals (Canales semicirculares) are positioned at a 45° angle in

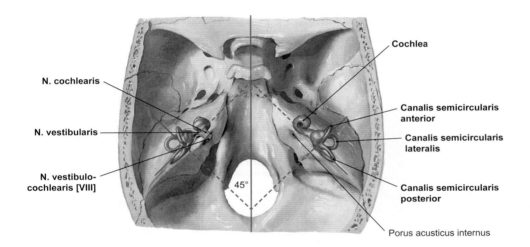

Fig. 9.79 Inner ear, Auris interna, and N. vestibulocochlearis [VIII]. View from above, internal ear projected in its natural position on the temporal bone.

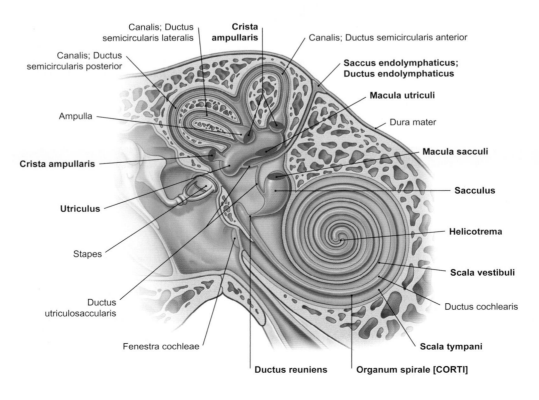

Fig. 9.80 Membranous labyrinth, Labyrinthus membranaceus, right. Longitudinal section through the temporal bone; frontal view, schematic drawing. [E402]

relation to the main planes of the skull (frontal, sagittal, and horizontal planes)(➤ Fig. 9.79).

Osseous labyrinth

The bony labyrinth consists of (➤ Fig. 9.80):
- Atrium (Vestibulum)
- 3 bony semicircular canals
- The bony cochlea
- The internal auditory canal (Meatus acusticus internus)

The **Vestibulum** is the starting point for the cochlea and semicircular canals. It is connected to the tympanic cavity via the oval window.

The **semicircular canals** (Canales semicirculares ossei) are divided into front/top (**Ductus semicircularis anterior**), rear (**Ductus semicircularis posterior**) and side (**Ductus semicircularis lateralis**) semicircular canals. They stretch from the Vestibulum in a posterosuperior direction. The canals account for approximately two thirds of a circle with one end each beginning at the vestibule and the other end extended to an Ampulla. Each canal is always perpendicular to the other two.

The **cochlea** consists of a canal (**Canalis spiralis cochleae**), which is wound in 2 ½ turns around the cochlear spindle (**Modiolus cochleae**). It is arranged so that its base (**Basis cochleae**) is aimed

posteromedial and its peak (**Apex cochleae**) anterolaterally. Thus, the base of the Modiolus lies near the Meatus acusticus internus. In the Canales spiralis and longitudinalis modioli sits the **Ganglion spirale cochleae** with the perikarya of bipolar nerve cells of the N. cochlearis (➤ Fig. 9.81). The Lamina spiralis ossea originates from the Modiolus into the cochlear canal. The **Ductus cochlearis** (part of the membranous labyrinth) winds around the Modiolus, which is attached to the Lamina spiralis and laterally on the outer wall of the cochlea. Through this arrangement 2 channels are created (one above, the Scala vestibuli and one below, the Scala tympani of the Ductus cochlearis), which pass through the entire cochlea and connect at the apex via the Helicotrema. The **Scala vestibuli** starts at the Vestibulum; the **Scala tympani** leads to the round window (Fenestra cochleae) and is separated by a connective tissue membrane from the middle ear. A small channel (Canaliculus cochleae) begins close to the round window, passes through the Os temporale and opens on the Facies posterior into the posterior cranial fossa. This is a link between the perilymphatic space and subarachnoid space (Spatium subarachnoideum).

The **internal auditory canal** starts at the **Porus acusticus internus** and continues laterally for around 1 cm. Here it ends in a perforated bony plate. In the 1 cm long segment the N. facialis [VII] and N. vestibulocochlearis [VIII] run (➤ Fig. 9.79).

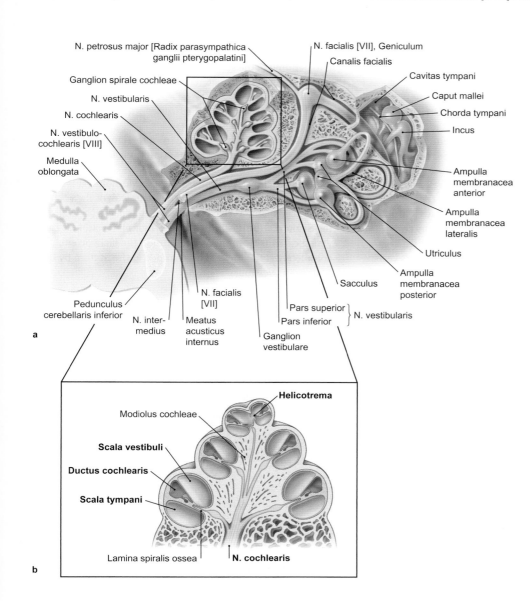

Fig. 9.81 labels:
- N. petrosus major [Radix parasympathica ganglii pterygopalatini]
- Ganglion spirale cochleae
- N. vestibularis
- N. cochlearis
- N. vestibulo-cochlearis [VIII]
- Medulla oblongata
- Pedunculus cerebellaris inferior
- N. inter-medius
- N. facialis [VII]
- Meatus acusticus internus
- Ganglion vestibulare
- Pars superior / Pars inferior } N. vestibularis
- Sacculus
- N. facialis [VII], Geniculum
- Canalis facialis
- Cavitas tympani
- Caput mallei
- Chorda tympani
- Incus
- Ampulla membranacea anterior
- Ampulla membranacea lateralis
- Utriculus
- Ampulla membranacea posterior

a

Inset labels:
- Helicotrema
- Modiolus cochleae
- Scala vestibuli
- Ductus cochlearis
- Scala tympani
- Lamina spiralis ossea
- N. cochlearis

b

Fig. 9.81 Cochlea. [E402]
a Cochlea together with organ of equilibrium, N. vestibulocochlearis [VIII] and N. facialis [VII], course into the Pars petrosa of the Os temporale; view from above; Pars petrosa opened. **b** Cross-section (diagram). [E402]

Membranous labyrinth

The membranous labyrinth is a coherent system of canals and bursae within the bony labyrinth and includes (➤ Fig. 9.80, ➤ Fig. 9.81):

- Ductus cochlearis
- Sacculus
- Utriculus
- 3 membranous semicircular canals (Ductus semicirculares)

The 3 **membranous semicircular canals** are in contact with the Utriculus. Each semicircular canal forms an extension at the crossing to the Utriculus (Ampulla membranenacea). The upper and posterior semicircular canals unite to form a common limb (Crus commune). Each ampulla contains sensory epithelium (**Crista ampullaris**, ➤ Fig. 9.82).

The membranous labyrinth is filled with sodium-poor and potassium-rich **endolymph**, (mainly formed in the Stria vascularis of the the Ductus cochlearis) and separated from the periosteum of the walls of the bony labyrinth by perilymph. It is not directly adjacent to the bony labyrinth, but is separated from it by the perilymphatic space filled with perilymph (Spatium perilymphaticum). It is thought that the perilymphatic space is formed by epithelial-like cells, which are adjacent to the bone and the membranous labyrinth. The **perilymph** originates as a exudate of perilymphatic capillaries and is probably reabsorbed in the region of postcapilliary venules of the perilymphatic space or reaches the Liquor cerebrospinalis (CSF) via the Aqueductus cochleae, a tube located in the bony Canaliculus cochleae. The membranous labyrinth is functionally divided into a vestibular and a cochlear section.

Organ of equilibrium
Structure

The **vestibular labyrinth** includes the Sacculus and Utriculus structures positioned in the Vestibulum, the Ductus utriculosaccularis, the three semicircular canals and the Ductus endolymphaticus (➤ Fig. 9.80). The **Utriculus** is larger than the Sacculus. It is located in the back of the upper part of the Vestibulum. All 3 semicircular canals lead into it with both their initial as well as their ampullar part. The **Sacculus** lies at the lower front in the Vestibulum. The Ductus cochlearis flows into it. The **Ductus utriculosaccularis** connects the Sacculus and Utriculus. The **Ductus endolymphaticus,** originates approximately in the middle which after a short course through the Vestibulum enters the Aqueductus vestibuli (part of the bony labyrinth), passes through the Os temporale to the Facies posterior of the Pars petrosa, and flows here with the Saccus endolymphaticus into the posterior cranial fossa.

> **NOTE**
> The Saccus endolymphaticus is an epidural enlargement located in the rear surface of the petrous bone, in which the endolymph drains into the lymph fissures of the hard meninges.

> **Clinical remarks**
>
> The triad of seizure-like dizziness attacks, unilateral hearing loss and unilateral tinnitus is referred to as **MENIÈRE's syndrome**. A reabsorption defect in the endolymph, with distension of the membranous labyrinth (Hydrops cochleae) is discussed as the cause. Pathological changes to the sensory cells are the result.

Sensory cells

The sensory cells of the vestibular labyrinth filled with endolymph sit as **Macula sacculi** in the Sacculus (registration of vertical linear acceleration), as **Macula utriculi** in the Utriculus (registration of horizontal linear acceleration) and as Cupulae in the Cristae ampullares of the three semicircular canals (registration of rotational acceleration) (➤ Fig. 9.80). The sensory cells of the vestibular organ each possess a long kinocilium and stereocilia which extend into a gelatinous substance (Cupula) (➤ Fig. 9.82). Movements of the Cupula lead to bending of the sensory cell processes. This stimulus leads to the synaptic activation of afferent fibres of the N. vestibularis.

Hearing organ
Structure

The **cochlear labyrinth** is formed from the Ductus cochlearis. The vestibular and cochlear labyrinths communicate via the **Ductus reuniens** (➤ Fig. 9.80).

The Ductus cochlearis winds around the Modiolus. It is attached to the Lamina spiralis and lateral to the outer wall of the cochlea and divides the Canalis spiralis cochleae into 3 spaces (➤ Fig. 9.81):

- the **Scala vestibuli** is filled with perilymph (vestibular canal), which extends from the Vestibulum to the Helicotrema, lies completely at the top and is separated at the bottom by the Membrana vestibularis from

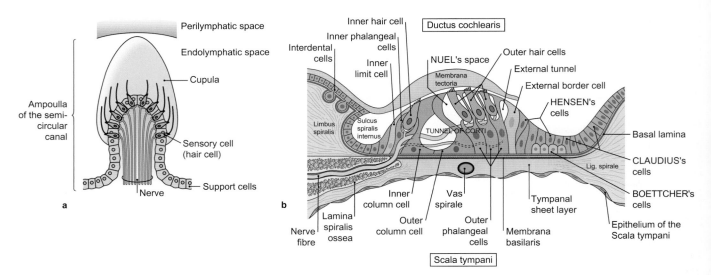

Fig. 9.82 Structure of the sensory cell-bearing organs (diagram). **a** Structure of the Crista ampullaris. **b** Structure of the Organum spirale (organ of CORTI). [L141]

- the **Ductus cochlearis,** filled with endolymph, which is delimited by the basilar membrane from
- the **Scala tympani** filled with perilymph (tympanic stairs), which extends from the Helicotrema to the round window in the medial wall of the tympanic cavity.

The Scala vestibuli and Scala tympani interconnect at the Helicotrema.

Sensory cells

The floor of the Ductus cochlearis is the basilar membrane (Lamina basilaris), which carries the auditory organ (Organum spirale, organ of CORTI). The **organ of CORTI** (➤ Fig. 9.82b) is the actual auditory organ. Auditory sensory cells (internal and external hair cells) are located here strictly organised together with supporting cells on the basilar membrane and are covered by a gelatinous membrane (Membrana tectoria). The organ of CORTI extends over the whole length of the Ductus cochlearis. The hair cells are very complexly innervated afferently and efferently.

Clinical remarks

Hair cell damage, e.g. if the music heard was too loud or after an explosion (acoustic shock), are very commonly associated with **tinnitus** . The term Tinnitus aurium (ringing of the ears) or tinnitus for short, refers to a symptom in which the affected person perceives sounds that have no perceptible external cause to other persons. In industrialised countries tinnitus is the most frequent common illness after obesity with 22 % affected in its acute form (up to 3 months) and with 4 % affected in its chronic form.

An **acute hearing loss** is a sudden hearing loss (up to deafness) with no identified cause. It is delimited from hearing disorders with an identifiable cause. The diagnosis is a **sensorineural hearing loss.** The course of the hearing loss is very variable, but a high spontaneous resolution rate is known. There are a number of therapies for conductive hearing loss; the most common is an infusion therapy.

Vascular, lymphatic and nervous systems
Arteries

The *bony labyrinth* is supplied via the **A. tympanica anterior** from the A. maxilliaris, the **A. stylomastoidea** from the A. auricularis posterior and the **R. petrosus** from the A. meningea media. The complete blood supply to the *membranous labyrinth* takes place from the branches of the **A. labyrinthi,** which divide into a R. cochlearis and 1 or 2 Rr. vestibulares; the Vv. labyrinthini drains the blood into the Sinus petrosus inferior or Sinus sigmoideus. The A. and V. inferior anterior cerebelli often project a few millimetres into the internal auditory duct and emit here the A. and Vv. labyrinthi supplying the labyrinth with blood (*Cave:* terminal artery). Rarely does the A. labyrinthini come directly from the A. basilaris.

Clinical remarks

Thrombotic closure of the A. labyrinthi or its afferent branches is associated with balance disorders and hearing loss, because the A. labyrinth is a terminal artery.

Innervation

The innervation takes place via the N. vestibulocochlearis [VIII] (often clinically referred to as N. statoacusticus) (➤ Fig. 9.81a). It bears sensory fibres for the ears (N. cochlearis) and the balance

(N. vestibularis). The **N. cochlearis** comes in a slightly curved course from the cochlea. The ganglion cells (Ganglion spirale) and fibres of the N. cochlearis lie in cavities of the bony Modiolus. They join at the base of the Modiolus to the N. cochlearis. The **N. vestibularis** consists of a Pars superior from the front and lateral semicircular canals as well as Sacculus and a Pars inferior from the Utriculus and rear semicircular canal. The perikarya of the neurons of both sections are combined into the **Ganglion vestibulare**. The N. vestibularis and N. cochlearis join together in the temporal bone. Before leaving the Porus acusticus internus, the N. facialis [VII] and its intermediate part lie on it. As N. vestibulocochlearis [VIII] they pass through the posterior cranial fossa and enter between Pons and Medulla oblongata into the lateral surface of the brain stem.

Clinical remarks

The **acoustic neurino** (Vestibularis schwannoma) is a benign tumour of the SCHWANN cells (➤ Chap. 9.3.8).

Sound conduction

Sound waves enter via the external ear (auricle and external acoustic canal) and are transmitted via the tympanic membrane and the auditory ossicular chain via the stirrup foot plate to the perilymph. This produces wave movements that migrate along the walls of the Ductus cochlearis (especially the basilar membrane) **(migrating waves).** This results in shearing movements of the organ of CONTI. The stereocilia of the inner hair cells are bent (deflexion). These biomechanical events are converted by the sensory cells into receptor potentials (mechanoelectrical transduction).

Clinical remarks

A **cholesteatoma** (syn.: pearl tumour in the ear; expanding growth of multi layered keratinizing squamous epithelium into the middle ear with chronic putrid inflammation of the middle ear), acute otitis media, mastoiditis, and trauma to the skull can result in a **labyrinthitis** with dizziness, stimulus or nystagmus (trembling of the eyes, uncontrolled rhythmic movements of the eyes). Entry ports for infectious agents are the round and oval windows, gaps in the bony labyrinth (after injury and bone erosion by infected pneumatic areas), or inflammation ascending via nerves and vessels, Canaliculus cochleae or Canaliculus vestibuli to the meninges. Consequences range from **sensorineural hearing loss** to deafness and destruction of the vestibular organ.

Stimulus processing

The stimulus processing is presented in ➤ Chap. 13.4.

9.6 Nose
Friedrich Paulsen

Skills

After processing this chapter, you should be able to:
- name the structures of the external nose, the bony and cartilaginous structure of the nasal skeleton, the boundaries of the nasal cavities and their distension

---

- name the location, bony limits, openings and topographic relation of the nasal sinuses to other structures
- know and be able to demonstrate the blood supply and innervation of the entire nose with respect to its clinical relevance
- describe the regional lymph flow
- describe the general development of the nose and nasal sinuses

---

Clinical case

Case study

A 22-year-old man is brought to the emergency surgery department of a large hospital at 3 o'clock in the morning by 5 passers-by. People say that they saw how the young man was beaten by 3 other men. In the process, he received a fist blow to the head. He was also allegedly kicked several times when on the ground. Only the shouts of the passers-by and their committed intervention caused the 3 men to leave him and flee. As the emergency department was nearby, they quickly linked arms with him and brought him in themselves.

Initial examination

The young man is in a state of shock and appears slightly disorientated when first questioned, but is responsive. His nose appears sunken and unnaturally broadened. The nose is somewhat askew. There is also dried blood under the nose and chin. His white t-shirt is stained with blood. On the right side the eye is severely swollen and protruding, the eyelids can no longer be closed properly and are under tension. The initial investigation shows a nasal fracture and a pronounced Protrusio bulbi on the right side. The patient can no longer properly close and open his eye on the affected side. In addition, the man displays abrasions on the right temple and has several bruises on the left arm and on the back.

Further diagnostics

An emergency so-called trauma spiral (a full-body CT) is conducted, which includes a CT scan of the head (CCT). With the exception of the bruising there are no injuries to the internal body or neck organs. The CCT shows a nasal framework fracture and air inclusions in the area of the orbita tip as well as bone fragments of the Lamina orbitalis in the cavities of two rear ethmoidal cells. Air is passing in this way from the ethmoidal cells into the orbita tip and has evoked the Protrusio bulbi. An injury of the dura mater is not detectable. The attending eye doctor establishes a significant vision reduction of 10 %.

Treatment

Following diagnosis, the patient is relocated in the same night to the ENT clinic. Due to the extensive Protrusio bulbi, the attending ENT doctor conducts a lateral canthotomy on the right eye edge with the patient under local anaesthesia. In doing so, all structures in the lateral eye angle (skin, Lig. palpebrale laterale, Septum orbitale) are cut with scissors (cantholysis) while protecting the eyeball. This results in a pressure relief in the posterior compartment of the Orbita, which relieves the structures (especially the N. opticus). In the same session, the nasal framework fracture is reconstructed. The patient is administered antibiotics intravenously and also receives a cortisone bolus.

Course

The next day the Protrusio bulbi begins to recede, the air pockets in the Orbita tip are rapidly rebsorbed over a short period of time (hours to days), the vision of the patient increases again and on day 3 after surgery reaches 100 %.

9.6.1 Overview

Respiratory organs

The respiratory tract serves as gas transport and exchange between the air and blood. It is divided into respiratory organs that conduct air and exchange air. The air conducting respiratory organs are divided into the upper respiratory tract (nose, throat) and lower respiratory tract (larynx, trachea, bronchial tree); the junction between the two is formed by the entrance to the larynx. The gas exchange (external breathing) is carried out in the lungs (Pulmones).

- Respiratory tract
- Air conducting respiratory organs
  - Upper respiratory tract
    - Nose (nose)
    - Throat (pharynx)
  - Lower respiratory tract
    - Larynx
    - Trachea
    - Bronchial tree (Bronchi)
- Gas exchange respiratory organs
  - Lungs (pulmones)

Upper respiratory tract

The upper respiratory tract includes the nose (Nasus) and throat (pharynx). The throat belongs to the aerodigestive tract, which means that it is used both for the transport of gas and food. Its upper section (nasopharynx) connects to the nose, transports respiratory gas, so it is purely an airway, the middle portion (oropharynx) has a dual function of gas and food transport. At the entrance to the larynx the respiratory and gastric tracts divide again. The air is fed to the lower respiratory tract, starting with the larynx, liquids and food components are forwarded in the lower section of the pharynx (laryngopharynx).

Nose

The nose is the entrance to the respiratory tract. It is divided into the externally visible **external nose** (Nasus externus) and the **nasal cavities** (internal nose, Cavitates nasi). The **two nasal cavities** are openly connected to the paranasal sinuses (Sinus paranasales) as well as the upper portion of the pharynx (nasopharynx).
Function of the nose is, apart from air conduction (aerodynamics) mechanical cleaning, warming and saturation (climatisation) of the respiratory air and the immune defence of pathogens. On the roof of the nose is the olfactory field, which controls the inhaled air (ability to smell). Nose-specific reflexes (e.g. sneezing) serve to protect the respiratory organs. In addition, the nasal cavities are involved in phonation as a resonance space and formation site for consonants.

9.6.2 Development

Nose

The nasal development belongs to the facial development and is closely associated with the palate and oral cavity development. Between the *4th and 5th embryonic weeks* the ectoderm consolidates on the supraorbital ridge near the Stomatodeum to the olfactory placodes. They submerge into the depth and become **olfactory pits** and **olfactory tubes,** from which the nasal cavities later form. The edges of the pits are raised to a medial and a lateral nasal bulge. The two **medial nasal bulges,** which are separated by the Area internasalis, grow out and down until they come in contact with the upper jaw bulge. Here they form the middle part of the upper lip, the philtrum, the membranous part of the nasal septum and the primary palate. The two **lateral nasal bulges** differentiate into the nasal wings. Right and left olfactory tubes grow on the roof of the primary oral cavity, stay for a short time separated by an epithelial plate (HOCHSTETTER's epithelial wall, epithelial choanal membrane, Membrana bucconasalis) and then gain connection by dissolution of the membrane in the *7th week* to the primary oral cavity. The two connections are referred to as **primary choanae**; the remaining area between external and internal openings are referred to as **primary palates**; however, it is not identical with the expansion of the later premaxillary segment. The further development of the nasal cavities is linked to the development of the secondary palate. On the roof of the primary oral cavity behind the primary palate the nasal septum is formed. It grows as a sagittal plate vertically downwards, and meets the two palatal processes in the transverse level from left and right from the side wall of the primary oral cavity growing to the centre line, with which it fuses forming a seam (Raphe palatini). The abutting palatal processes become **secondary palates.** At the point where the palatal processes and nasal septum meet on the V-shaped tapered primary palate, a canal (**Ductus nasopalatinus) forms.** The Canales incisivi and the Foramen incisivum result later in the upper jaw from the canal.

NOTE

The **primary palate** becomes a premaxilliary section of the definitive palate. The incisive bone (Os incisivum, 'GOETHE's bone') emerges from it with the incisors.

The development of the secondary palate leads to the separation of nasal and oral cavity; the development of the nasal septum separates the inner nose in 2 separate cavities, which run dorsally via a Meatus nasopharyngeus (secondary or definitive choane) into the nasopharynx.

Clinical remarks

Cleft formation of the palate, upper jaw and face can be attributed to inadequate mesenchymal proliferation and thus non-fusion of nose and jaw bulges and can be very differently pronounced. In the case of mild forms ('cleft lip') only the upper lip is affected on one or two sides. Severe forms continue occipitally as **cleft lip and palate** (frequency 1:2,500 births). Isolated cleft palates are the result of a non-fusion of the palatal process (rear cleft palate) or between palatal processes and primary palate (front cleft palate). Combinations are possible. The mildest form of a rear cleft palate is an uvula bifida (cleaved uvula). The causes of the palate, jaw and maxillofacial clefts are manifold.

The Vestibulum nasi emerges from the material of the **nasal tubes,** a part of the Cavitas nasi and the Regio olfactoria. The residual part originates from the material of the primary oral cavity. The mesenchyme that surrounds the secondary nasal cavity, differentiates to the cartilaginous nasal capsule. It ossifies partly enchondrially, partially desmally. The Cartilago septi nasi remain unossified with the Proc. posterior as well as the cartilage of the outer nose. While the nasal septum persists as a smooth wall, the surface of each lateral nasal wall increases by developing the **nasal conchae (Conchae nasi),** which protrude as epithelial bulges (Turbinalia) into the nasal cavity lumen. Usually 3 nasal conchae each differentiate, which are referred to as maxilloturbinal (Concha nasalis inferior, inferior nasal concha), ethmoturbinal I (Concha nasalis media, middle nasal concha) and ethmoturbinal II (Concha nasalis superior, upper nasal concha). As in the animal world the development of a 4th nasal

concha (Concha nasalis suprema) is also possible. Initially, the skeleton of the nasal conchae is still cartilageous and is replaced in the 5th fetal month by bone.

NOTE

In the context of nasal development a tube-like connection forms between the nasal septum and nasal floor, which sometimes appears as a blind sack, Ductus incisivus. This is the tube around the **vomeronasal organ** (JACOBSON's organ, Organum vomeronasale), which appears in humans as a rudimentary sensory organ. It belongs to the olfactory system in many animals and has key features, e.g. when looking for a partner, for food, for individual recognition or the identification of territorial markings. Pheromones play a crucial role in the function. Remnants of the vomeronasal organ are detectable in humans until after birth.

Paranasal sinuses

The paranasal sinuses grow as early as the foetal period as small epithelial buds of the nasal cavities in the mesenchyme of the surrounding cranial bone. They reach their full development only after completion of growth and can expand even further in the course of life. Their individual varying development is extremely closely linked to the development of the dentition and is associated with the formation of the face. An exception is the Sinus sphenoidalis. It develops as a detachment from the nasal cavity by creating a Concha sphenoidalis. Around the *4th year of age* the Sinus sphenoidalis grows into the sphenoidal body. The expansion is just as variable as for other sinuses.

9.6.3 External nose

On the **external nose** (Nasus externus, ➤ Fig. 9.83) a distinction is made between:
- The nasal root lying above the philtrum (Sulcus nasolabialis) (Radix nasi)
- The bridge of the nose (Dorsum nasi)
- The left and right ala of the nose (Alae nasi dextra and sinistra)

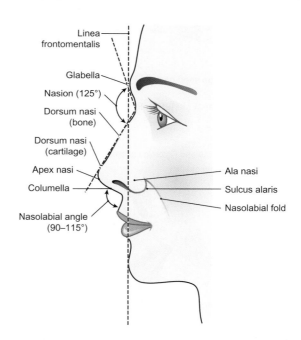

Linea frontomentalis
Glabella
Nasion (125°)
Dorsum nasi (bone)
Dorsum nasi (cartilage)
Apex nasi
Columella
Nasolabial angle (90–115°)
Ala nasi
Sulcus alaris
Nasolabial fold

Fig. 9.83 External nose with aesthetic nose angles and points of reference. [L126]

- The tip of nose (Apex nasi)
- The membranous portion of the nasal septum (Pars membranacea septi nasi, Columella, Pars mobilis septi)
- The nasal orifices (Nares)

The external nose has a great impact on the shape of the face.

Skeleton

Mechanical resilience is achieved through a skeletal system of hyaline cartilage and connective tissue, which is attached to the bony nose pyramid (nasal scaffold consisting of the Os frontale, Os nasale and Proc. frontalis of the Maxilla). The Ossa nasalia are connected via the Sutura internasalis and together form with the Incisura nasalis and the Proc. palatinus of the Maxilla, the outer bony nasal aperture (Apertura piriformis).

The movable cartilaginous proportion (➤ Fig. 9.84) consists on each side of:

- The triangular cartilage (Cartilago triangularis, Cartilago nasi lateralis, lateral cartilage)
- The nose tip cartilage (Cartilago alaris major, wing cartilage)
- Small cartilage plates (Cartilagines alares minores and Cartilagines nasi accessoriae)

The wing cartilage forms with a narrow Crus mediale (nose bridge) and a varyingly broad Crus laterale (nostrils) the shape of the nostril. The cartilaginous nasal septum begins between the wing cartilages (Cartilago septi nasi, ➤ Fig. 9.85). The cartilage-free areas are filled with solid connective tissue, which connects the cartilage to each other and to the bone.

Musculature

The external nose is moved by multiple facial muscles (➤ Table 9.30, ➤ Fig. 9.23), allowing for control of the width of the nose opening. For the innervation of the muscles ➤ Table 9.10, for the attachment ➤ Table 9.8.

Table 9.29 Descriptions in nasal plastic surgery.

Term	Explanation
Supra-tip area	The bridge of the nose just above the nose tip
Weak triangle	The region of the dorsum of the nose just above the nose tip is formed only by the nasal septum
Keystone area	Overlap of the lateral cartilage through the Os nasale
Soft triangle	Skin area at the top edge of the nostril, close to which the Crus mediale bends into the Crus laterale (the cartilage-free field consists only of a skin duplicature)
Columella	The front section of the nasal septum between nose tip and philtrum

Table 9.30 Muscles of the external nose.

Muscle	Function
M. nasalis, Pars alaris (M. dilatator)	Extends the nostrils
M. nasalis, Pars transversa (M. compressor)	Narrows the nostrils
M. depressor septi nasi	Moves the nose downwards
M. levator labii superioris alaeque nasi	Raises the nasal wing

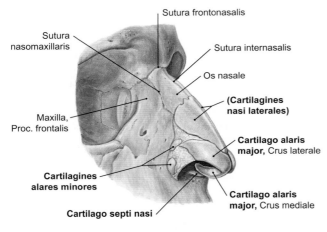

Fig. 9.84 External nasal skeleton. Right frontal view.

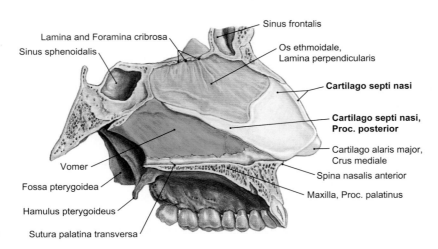

Fig. 9.85 Nasal septum (Septum nasi). View from the right

9.6.4 Nasal cavities

The **paired nasal cavities** with the pharynx belong to the upper respiratory tract and contain the olfactory fields. Each nasal cavity (Cavitas nasi) is a conical space, its base forms the nasal floor and its tip forms the nasal cavity roof. The front and narrower sections of each nasal cavity are enveloped by the skeleton of the outer nose, the wider, rear parts are located centrally in the skull. The inhalated air flows through the nasal orifices (Nares) into the nasal atrium (Vestibulum nasi). The border to the respective **nasal cavity** is the Limen nasi which is raised by the Crus laterale of the wing cartilage. The Limen nasi shapes together with the Crus mediale of the wing cartilage and a floor bar of the Maxilla, the inner nasal valve (narrowest point of the nose for the air flow). Here, the inhalated air is swirled and distributed in the respective nasal cavity – improving the contact between air and mucosa (diffusor effect). Each nasal cavity has 4 walls: a floor, roof and a medial and a lateral nasal cavity wall (➤ Fig. 9.85, ➤ Fig. 9.86, ➤ Fig. 9.87). The nasal cavities are separated:

- from the oral cavity by the hard palate
- from the base of the skull bones by parts of the Ossa frontalia, ethmoidalia and the Os sphenoidale
- each other by the nasal septum (Septum nasi)
- latteraly from the Orbitae and the paranasal sinuses

At the rear they continue via a choane into the nasopharynx (epipharynx).

Floor of the nasal cavity

The **nasal cavity floor** (➤ Fig. 9.85, ➤ Fig. 9.86, ➤ Fig. 9.87) is slightly concavely curved, smooth and much wider than the nasal cavity roof. It is created:

- at the front by the cartilaginous nasal skeleton of the outer nose
- from the surface anatomy of the Proc. palatinus of the Maxilla (including the Os incisivum [intermaxillary bone])
- the Lamina horizontalis of the Os palatinum

The nasal septum which lies in the midline at the base of the nose, is attached over the protruded Spina nasalis anterior and the Crista nasalis anterior. The nasal orifices open at the front on the floor.

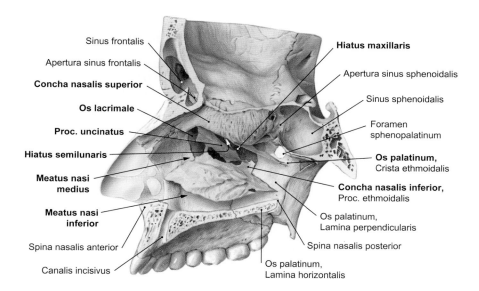

Fig. 9.86 Lateral nasal wall without middle nasal concha.

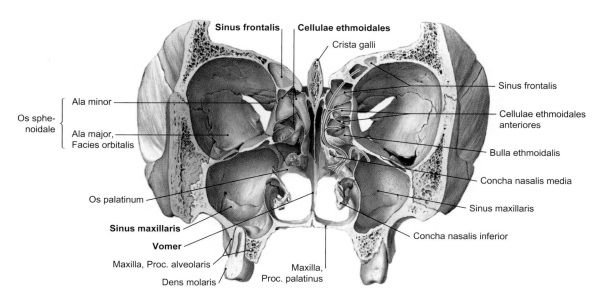

Fig. 9.87 Frontal section through the viscerocranium/facial skeleton. Right: representation of the bony topography, left: orifice of the paranasal sinuses: green = frontal sinus, purple = anterior ethmoidal sinuses, blue = maxillary sinus (arrows).

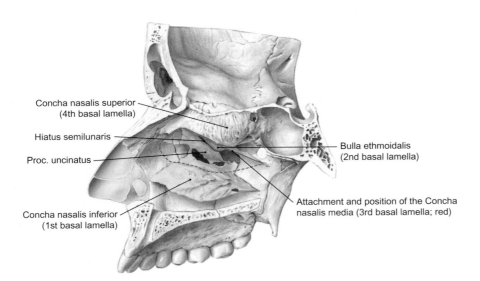

Concha nasalis superior
(4th basal lamella)

Hiatus semilunaris

Proc. uncinatus

Bulla ethmoidalis
(2nd basal lamella)

Attachment and position of the Concha
nasalis media (3rd basal lamella; red)

Concha nasalis inferior
(1st basal lamella)

Fig. 9.88 Lateral nasal wall with contour of the middle nasal concha (red).

The openings of the Canales incisivi are located near the nasal septum right behind the nasal atrium at the start of the nasal cavities. The Canales incisivi flow together in the unpaired Foramen incisivum in the oral cavity.

Roof of the nasal cavity

The **nasal cavity roof** (➤ Fig. 9.85, ➤ Fig. 9.86, ➤ Fig. 9.87) is narrow and stands in the centre, which is formed by the Lamina cribrosa of the Os ethmoidale at the highest point. In front of the Lamina cribrosa the roof drops off in the direction of the nasal orifices and is formed here from:

- the Spina nasalis of the Os frontale
- the Ossa nasalia
- the Procc. laterales of the Cartilago septi nasi
- the Cartilagines alares of the external nose

At the rear the roof lowers over the Recessus sphenoethmoidalis to the respective choane and is formed by the front surface of the Corpus ossis sphenoidalis. The olfactory fields lie directly below the Lamina cribrosa on the nasal cavity roof.

Medial nasal cavity wall

The basis of the **medial nasal cavity wall** is the **nasal septum** (Septum nasi) (➤ Fig. 9.85, ➤ Fig. 9.87), a Lamella standing vertically in the midsagittal plane made of connective tissue, cartilage and bone that separates the two nasal cavities from each other. The nasal septum consists of

- **Pars membranacea** – in the nasal atrium mainly of dense connective tissue (nose bridge, Columella)
- **Pars cartilaginea** – from the frontal Cartilago septi nasi and the variable Proc. posterior of the Cartilago septi nasi continuing from septum cartilage dorsally between Lamina perpendicularis ossis ethmoidalis and vomer, which slowly ossifies from dorsal to rostral with increasing age
- **Pars ossea** – from vomer and Lamina perpendicularis ossis ethmoidalis as well as a small part from the Ossa nasalia, the Spina nasalis superior ossis frontalis, the Spina nasalis anterior, the Crista incisiva maxillae, the Crista nasalis maxillae, the Crista nasalis ossis palatini and the Crista sphenoidalis

Clinical remarks

Slight variations of the nasal septum wall from the median occur regularly and are without functional importance. You can usually already tell whether the nasal septum is somewhat crooked by feeling the nasal bridge of the external nose. A more pronounced **nasal septum deviation** can hinder nasal breathing and restrict the ability to smell.

After traumatic effects on the external nose or in the case of coagulation disorders there may be a **nasal septum haematoma**, which requires immediate relief by puncture and, if necessary, incision and nasal packing, otherwise the septal cartilage is in danger of sinking.

Rhinitis (inflammation of the nose, nasal catarrh, rhinitis, coryza) is an acute or chronic nasal inflammation by infectious, allergic or vascular mechanisms. It is most common in the context of a common cold.

Lateral nasal cavity wall

The **lateral nasal cavity wall** of each nasal cavity is complexly structured (➤ Fig. 9.86, ➤ Fig. 9.87, ➤ Fig. 9.88). It consists, like the nasal septum of bone, of cartilage and connective tissue. Only the general structure is described here. Deviations are common. The bones involved in the development are:

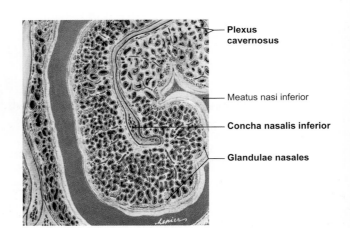

Plexus
cavernosus

Meatus nasi inferior

Concha nasalis inferior

Glandulae nasales

Fig. 9.89 Cavernous body tissue at the nasal septum (left) and on the lower nasal muscle (Concha nasalis inferior).

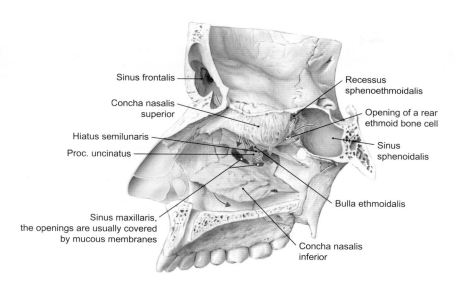

Fig. 9.90 Confluence of the paranasal sinuses and the Ductus nasolacrimalis at the lateral nasal wall. Brown = Ductus nasolacrimalis; green = frontal sinus; purple = anterior ethmoidal cells; blue = maxillary sinus; orange = posterior ethmoidal cells; red = sphenoid sinus (arrows).

- **At the front:**
  - The Os nasale
  - The Facies nasalis maxillae
  - The Os lacrimale
- **In the middle:**
  - The Corpus maxillae with its Hiatus maxillaris
  - The Os ethmoidale (with the thin Proc. uncinatus, the wall to the anterior and posterior ethmoidal cells [Cellulae ethmoidales anteriores and posteriores]) as well as the top and the middle nasal concha (Conchae nasales superior and media) protruding into the nasal cavity
  - The inferior nasal concha (Concha nasalis inferior) as an independent bone.
- **At the rear:**
  - The Lamina perpendicularis of the Os palatinum
  - The Lamina medialis of the Proc. pterygoideus ossis sphenoidalis

In the area of the outer nose, the lateral wall (Proc. lateralis of the cartilago septi nasi, Crus mediale of the ala major and Cartilagines minores) is formed from cartilage as well as from connective tissue. The **nasal conchae,** per nasal cavity a Concha nasalis superior, media and inferior, protrude from their attachment to the lateral nasal wall in the respective nasal cavity. They divide the nasal cavity into 4 air ducts. The upper canal is located directly below the olfactory field, the other 3 form the **nasal passages** (Meatus nasi superior, medius and inferior), which each run below the corresponding nasal concha. The bony parts of the nasal conchae are covered by a **cavernous body tissue** (> Fig. 9.89), which when swollen only leaves narrow spaces between themselves and the nasal septum (collectively referred to as the Meatus nasi communis). Depending on the particular state of swelling, approximately 35% of the nasal mucosa volume is composed of vascular plexus. The cavernous body tissue is most pronounced on the lower and middle nasal concha (as well as in the nasal septum at KIESSELBACH's area, see below). Between the vessels of the cavernous body tissue there are large quantities of serous glands, which moisten the respiratory ciliated epithelium covering the muscles. In approximately 80 % of people, there is a **nasal cycle,** i.e. the nasal mucosa of both nasal sides swells and subsides for 2-7 hours with alternating nasal resistance during breathing at a ratio of 1:3, but with the same overall resistance. The **inferior nasal concha** is the largest nasal concha. Its head lies approximately 1 cm behind the nasal valve and its tail ends approximately 1 cm in front of the entrance into the Tuba auditiva at the level of the corresponding choane. The **middle nasal**

concha lies above the lower nasal concha, the head is located approximately 1 cm further dorsal, the tail also ends at the level of the respective choane. The **upper nasal concha** is in relation to the middle and lower conchae significantly smaller. Its head begins approximately at the height of the middle area of the Lamina cribrosa. Its tail falls caudally before the bony front wall of the Sinus sphenoidalis and extends to the upper section of the respective choane. Above the choanae the inspired breath extends into the Meatus nasopharyngeus.

The most complex structure of the lateral nasal wall (**osteomeatal complex,** > Table 9.31) is the Hiatus maxillaris lying beneath the middle nasal concha (> Fig. 9.86, > Fig. 9.88, also > Fig. 9.91). It is only partially closed by 3 structures:

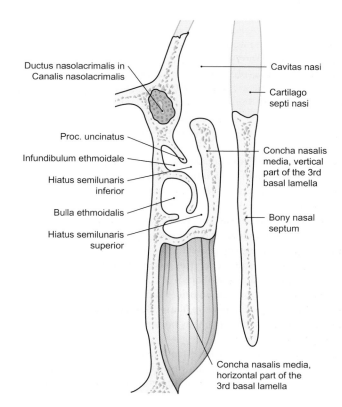

Fig. 9.91 Horizontal section through nasal septum and osteomeatal complex of the left side of the nose just above the inferior nasal concha. [L126]

Table 9.31 Clinical terminology of the lateral nasal cavity wall and the paranasal sinuses.

Term	Explanation
Agger nasi	An anterior ethmoidal cell in front of and above the attachment of the middle nasal concha with close topographical relationship to the Ductus nasolacrimalis
Atrium meatus medii	Region before the middle nasal passage above the head of the inferior nasal concha
Bulla ethmoidalis	Anterior ethmoidal cell above the Hiatus semilunaris, which very regularly develops, but can also be missing
Fontanelle	Accessory opening in the medial maxillary sinus wall that is covered by mucous membrane
Basal lamellae (➤ Fig. 9.88)	Lamellae, which pass through the ethmoid bone as embryological residues. Four basal lamellae (BL) can be distinguished: • BL 1: Proc. uncinatus • BL 2: Bulla ethmoidalis • BL 3: Concha nasalis media • BL 4: Concha nasalis superior
HALLER's cells	An ethmoidal cell that pneumatises the lower orbital wall (infraorbital cell)
Maxillary hiatus	A large opening of the Sinus maxillaris into the nasal cavity, which is partially closed by the Proc. uncinatus of the Os ethmoidale and mucous membranes
Hiatus semilunaris	A crescent-shaped and up to 3 cm wide cleft between the Bulla ethmoidalis and the upper free margin of the Proc. uncinatus; the Hiatus semilunaris provides access to the Infundibulum ethmoidale
Infundibulum ethmoidale	A deepening behind the Hiatus semilunaris, which lies between the Proc. uncinatus and the Bulla ethmoidalis
ÓNODI-GRÜNWALD cells	A posterior ethmoidal cell which bulges backwards over the Sinus sphenoidalis
Osteomeatal complex	Umbrella term for the complicated anatomy of the Hiatus semilunaris and its surroundings
Proc. uncinatus	A thin bone lamellar of the Os ethmoidale that forms part of the medial wall of the Sinus maxilaris by incomplete closure of the Hiatus maxillaris and confines the Hiatus semilunaris at its lower anterior aspect
Recessus frontalis	A gap that produces the connection between the nasofrontal sinus and nasal cavity (Ductus nasofrontalis, Canalis nasofrontalis)
Sulcus olfactorius	Channel between the anterior attachment of the Concha nasalis media at the skull base and the roof of the nose

- At the centre the **Proc. uncinatus** of the Os ethmoidale is inserted in the opening of the **Hiatus maxillaris**. At the top edge of the Proc. uncinatus a sickle-shaped smooth gap remains (**Hiatus semilunaris** ➤ Table 9.31). The front and cranial end of the Hiatus semilunaris form a depression, which is known as the Infundibulum ethmoidale. Behind and beneath the Proc. uncinatus further openings are present.
- The Os lacrimale and the inferior nasal concha border in front of and below the Hiatus maxillaris.
- From posterior above the anterior ethmoidal cells protrude into and in front of the Hiatus maxillaris (**Bulla ethmoidalis**, ➤ Table 9.31). At the same time, they border the Hiatus semilunaris to the back and above.

With the exception of the Hiatus semilunaris, all openings around the Proc. uncinatus which are not sealed by bone are normally covered with mucous membranes and therefore not visible (rear and front fontanelles, ➤ Table 9.31).

The lacrimal nasal passage and most of the sinuses confluence with their excretory ducts at the lateral nasal wall (➤ Table 9.32, ➤ Fig. 9.90, ➤ Fig. 9.87):

Table 9.32 Confluence points of the nasolacrimal ducts and of the paranasal sinuses.

	Lower nasal passage	Middle nasal passage	Upper nasal passage
Ductus nasolacrimalis	x		
Sinus frontalis		X	
Cellulae ethmoidales anteriores		X	
Cellulae ethmoidales posteriores			X
Sinus maxillaris		X	
Sinus sphenoidalis			x

- **Below the lower nasal concha:**
  - The lacrimal nasal passage (Ductus nasolacrimalis) confluences at the lateral nasal cavity wall of the Meatus nasi inferior via the Apertura ductus nasolacrimalis (HASNER's valve) under the front edge of the inferior nasal concha. In the mucosa of the lower nasal duct there is often a mucosal groove dorsally aligned from the aperture that corresponds to the flow of secretions. The Ductus nasolacrimalis is situated in a bony canal in the lateral nasal cavity wall formed by the Os lacrimale and the Maxilla, which runs from cranial to caudal in front of the head of the middle nasal concha and under the head of the inferior nasal concha. Dorsally the canal borders on the maxillary sinus.
- **Below the middle nasal concha:**
  - The frontal sinus (Sinus frontalis) directs its secretions via the Ductus nasofrontalis and the Infundibulum ethmoidale to the anterior, cranial area of the Hiatus semilunaris.
  - The anterior ethmoidal sinuses (Cellulae ethmoidales anteriores) also drain into the Ductus nasofrontalis or the Infundibulum ethmoidale of the Hiatus semilunaris. The Bulla ethmoidalis, which limits the Hiatus semilunaris at the upper rear and drains into it, belongs to the anterior ethmoidal cells. Other anterior ethmoidal sinuses will open on or just above the Bulla ethmoidalis and thus reach the Hiatus semilunaris.
  - The maxillary sinus (Sinus maxillaris) confluences in the lower section in the Hiatus semilunaris (Infundibulum maxillare), usually directly below the Bulla ethmoidalis.
- **Behind the upper nasal concha:**
  - The posterior ethmoidal sinuses (Cellulae ethmoidales posteriores) usually confluence on the lateral paranasal sinus wall of the meatus nasi superior.
  - The Sinus sphenoidalis flows as the only paranasal sinus not on the lateral paranasal sinus wall. Its Apertura sinus sphenoidalis is located on the rear wall of the nasal cavity and confluences in the Recessus sphenoethmoidalis (space above the Concha nasalis superior in the area of the nose roof at the transition between Lamina cribrosa and Corpus ossis sphenoidalis) behind the upper nasal concha in the Meatus nasi superior.

NOTE

Overall, the lateral nasal wall is individually constructed showing large differences in strength. The size of the upper nasal concha can vary greatly, even the confluence of the frontal sinus via the Hiatus semilunaris often differs from the manner described here.

Clinical remarks

The structures under the middle nasal concha summarised under the term **osteomeatal unit** are clinically not only extraordinarily important for ventilation, but also for the drainage of the paranasal sinuses. The area is used as a surgical access pathway in **endonasal surgery,** e.g. in the treatment of chronic sinusitis or Polyposis nasi.

In neonates, in the area of the confluence point of the Ductus nasolacrimalis in the lower nasal passage, there can be a thin connective tissue membrane (HASNER's valve) as an embryological relict or the Ductus nasolacrimalis finds no connection to the lower nasal passage. In these cases, the lacrimal drainage is hindered. The child suffers from a persistent epiphora (continuous tear production) on the affected side. The efferent lacrimal ducts mostly become inflamed above the membrane or occlusion **(Dacryocystitis neonatorum)** and there is pus discharge from the lacrimal points. If the HASNER's valve or the default canal remain, operative intervention is necessary to create the physiological flow to the nose.

9.6.5 Paranasal sinuses

A large part of the bones bordering directly on the paranasal sinuses are pneumatised in the first years of life up to an advanced age (Ossa pneumatica). This creates the **paranasal sinuses** (Sinus paranasales, ➤ Fig. 9.87, ➤ Fig. 9.90, ➤ Fig. 9.92), which are connected with the nasal cavities via ostias and are lined with mucous membrane. They are ventilated via the nasal cavities. It is assumed that this process functionally serves the lightweight construction of the skull. They do not have an importance as a resonance room. Through their topographic relationship with the adjacent structures the parasanal sinuses are of major clinical relevance.

Maxillary sinus

The paired maxillary sinus (**Sinus maxillaris,** ➤ Fig. 9.87, ➤ Fig. 9.90, ➤ Fig. 9.92) is usually the largest paranasal sinus. It often completely fills the Corpus maxillae and can be chambered by bony membranes (Recessus). The maxillary sinus floor bears a relationship to the alveolar process (alveolar recess). This applies in particular to the root tips of the 2nd premolars and the first two molars (15, 16, 17, 25, 26, 27; ➤ Chap. 9.7.2), which sometimes are only separated from the maxillary sinus by thin bony lamellae or by mucous membranes. If the Recessus alveolaris is extended, the 1st premolars, the Caninus and the Dens serotinus (see below) can be included in the maxillary sinus. The front wall is adjacent to the Sulcus lacrimalis on the efferent lacrimal ducts, the rear wall with the Tuber maxillae at the Fossa pterygopalatina. In the roof, which is also the floor of the Orbita, run the N. infraorbitalis and the Vasa infraorbitalia. The lateral wall borders on the Os zygomaticum, medial lies the Hiatus maxillaris with the osteomeatal complex (➤ Chap. 9.6.4). Here, the natural maxillary sinus ostium confluences close to the roof via the Infundibulum maxillare in the middle of the Infundibulum ethmoidale. In this way secretion products of the maxillary sinus mucosa and air can reach the Hiatus semilunaris and the respective nasal cavity. If the mucosa coating in the area of fontanelles below the Proc. uncinatus is missing, the maxillary sinus has in more than 10 % of the cases 1 or even 2 accessory ostia (open fontanelles).

Frontal sinus

The paired frontal sinus (**Sinus frontalis,** ➤ Fig. 9.87, ➤ Fig. 9.90, ➤ Fig. 9.92) is characterised by a particularly large variability in its expansion as well as between the two cavities. Both front cavities are usually separated by a bony wall (Septum frontalium), which is often not in a median position. A frontal sinus can extend over the median to the other side (and interfere with the expansion of the other cavity). The formation of the frontal sinus reaches the upper orbital edge around the *7th year of life*. It can then pneumatise the Squama frontalis, the Arcus superciliaris or the Pars orbitalis of the Os frontale. In the case of extensive pneumatisation it can extend up to close to the Canalis opticus. In cases of severe pneumatisation the bone to the anterior cranial fossa is usually only very thin. In approximately 5 % the frontal sinus can also be missing (frontal sinus aplasia). Usually the frontal sinus forms a funnel-shaped recess at its lowest point, in which the Ostium frontale forms the connection to the nasal cavity. As a rule, the typical confluence of the frontal sinus into the nasal cavity emerges in the form of the Ductus nasolacrimalis, which is formed by anterior ethmoidal sinuses that limit it and confluences in the Infundibulum ethmoidale which is followed by the Hiatus semilunaris. There are numerous deviations from the most common orifice shape of the frontal sinus described here.

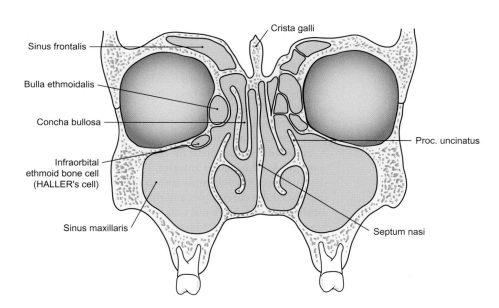

Fig. 9.92 Frontal section through the viscerocranium/ facial skeleton. Presentation of anatomic variants of the ethmoidal bone. [L126]

Labels on figure: Sinus frontalis · Bulla ethmoidalis · Concha bullosa · Infraorbital ethmoid bone cell (HALLER's cell) · Sinus maxillaris · Crista galli · Proc. uncinatus · Septum nasi

Ethmoidal cells

The ethmoidal cells (**Cellulae ethmoidales**, ➤ Fig. 9.87, ➤ Fig. 9.90, ➤ Fig. 9.92, ➤ Fig. 9.93) are also summarised under the terms ethmoidal cell complex or ethmoidal cell labyrinth (Labyrinthus ethmoidalis). According to their location in relation to the attachment of the middle nasal concha, they are divided from an embryological and clinical point of view into the front (**Cellulae ethmoidales anteriores**) and posterior (**Cellulae ethmoidales posteriores**) ethmoidal cells. Ultimately, all anterior ethmoidal sinuses drain into the Infundibulum ethmoidale and, therefore, in the same way as the maxillary sinus and the frontal sinus into the Hiatus semilunaris. In contrast, the posterior ethmoidal cells flow into the upper nasal passage. Size and shape of the ethmoidal sinuses and their relationship to each other are extremely variable; however, the cells are usually much smaller than the Sinus maxillares, frontales and sphenoidales and are therefore only referred to as cells. Since the ethmoidal sinuses often grow into bones outside of the Os ethmoidale, their walls can consist completely of Os frontale, Os maxillare, Os lacrimale, Os sphenoidale, Os palatinum or a combination of the individual bones. Examples of this are the Agger nasi cells, a Bulla frontalis, an infraorbital cell (HALLER's cell) and the Cellula sphenoethmoidalis (ÓNODI-GRÜNWALD cell) (➤ Table 9.31, ➤ Fig. 9.92, ➤ Fig. 9.93). The largest and most constant ethmoidal cell is the Bulla ethmoidalis that borders the Hiatus semilunaris from above. The ethmoid bone has a close topographic relationship to the Orbita. The bony walls between the ethmoidal cells and the Orbita are extremely thin. You can almost see through them on the bony skull (Lamina papyracea - paper thin). The bony walls of numerous ethmoidal cells form a part of the floor of the anterior cranial fossa in the area of the Crista galli. Here they form the Foveolae ethmoidales ossis frontalis.

Sphenoidal sinus

The paired sphenoidal sinus (**Sinus sphenoidalis**, ➤ Fig. 9.87, ➤ Fig. 9.90, ➤ Fig. 9.92) is located in the Corpus ossis sphenoidalis immediately below the Cella turcica. As with all other sinuses the pneumatisation of the sphenoidal bone is extremely variable and is laterally differently developed. A Septum sinuum sphenoidale separating both sphenoidal sinuses runs in most cases asymmetrically and can be partially or completely missing. Additional incomplete septa are possible. The sphenoidal sinus enters through the Apertura sinus sphenoidalis of the sphenoidal sinus front wall into the Recessus sphenoethmoidalis in the skull base. Close topographic relationships exist laterally to the Canalis opticus with the N. opticus (➤ Fig. 9.93), the A. carotis interna, the Sinus cavernosus and the N. trigeminus [V], as well as at the front to the rear ethmoidal cells and upper posterior to the pituitary gland. In the formation of an ÓNODI-GRÜNWALD cell (➤ Table 9.31, ➤ Fig. 9.93), the Sinus sphenoidalis lies partially below these sphenoidal cells. In the case of extensive pneumatisation the bony walls are usually only extremely thin.

Clinical remarks

Inflammation of the paranasal sinuses (sinusitis) is a common disease. In children the ethmoidal sinuses are particularly affected, in adults the maxillary sinus, but also frontal and sphenoidal sinuses can become inflamed. Unilateral Sinus maxillaris inflammation is often caused odontogenically **(odontogenic Sinusitis maxillaris)**. The inflammation usually originates at the 2nd premolar or the 1st molar (see above). Feared complications of ethmoiditis are the spreading to the Orbita via the thin Lamina papyracea (orbital phlegmon) and the spreading of the inflammation via the bony walls of the Canalis opticus to the N. opticus with risk of optic nerve damage if the posterior ethmoidal sinuses or the sphenoidal sinus are affected. If the Sinus frontalis is highly developed occipitally via the orbital roof (Recessus supraorbitalis), clinicians refer to a **dangerous frontal sinus**. A frontal sinus inflammation can lead via the thin bony walls of the anterior cranial fossa e.g. to meningitis, epidural abscesses or brain abscesses. **Malignant tumours** of the nose have become less frequent due to improved occupational health and safety measures. If they occur, they are extremely dangerous and difficult to treat due to their infiltrative growth into the neighbouring regions, such as the Orbita, skull base, palate and throat.

N O T E

Access to the nasal cavities

In the nasal skeleton there are various access points for nerves and blood vessels:
- Lamina cribrosa
- Foramen sphenopalatinum
- Canalis incisivus
- Nostrils

9.6.6 Vascular, lymphatic and nervous systems

Arteries

The blood supply to the nose and the paranasal sinuses (➤ Fig. 9.94) is provided by branches of the A. carotis externa and the A. carotis interna.

The A. ophthalmica originates from the A. carotis interna and passes through the Canalis opticus into the Orbita. It emits the **A. ethmoidalis posterior** at the medial orbital wall and further forward the **A. ethmoidalis anterior**. Both arteries penetrate through the corresponding Foramina ethmoidalia anterior and posterior into the ethmoidal complex and run through the Canales ethmoidales between the ethmoidal cells up into the nasal cavity. Here they branch out to the nasal septum and to the lateral nasal wall. The A. ethmoidalis anterior emits the Rr. nasales laterales anteriores and Rr. septales anteriores which anastomise with the other vessels supplying the nasal cavity. The A. ethmoidalis posterior perfuses a smaller area near the skull base.

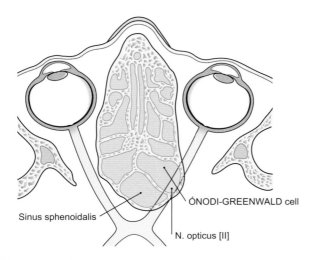

Sinus sphenoidalis

ÓNODI-GREENWALD cell

N. opticus [II]

Fig. 9.93 Horizontal section through the ethmoid bone at the level of the Canalis opticus. Relationships during formation of an ÓNODI-GRÜNWALD cell. [L126]

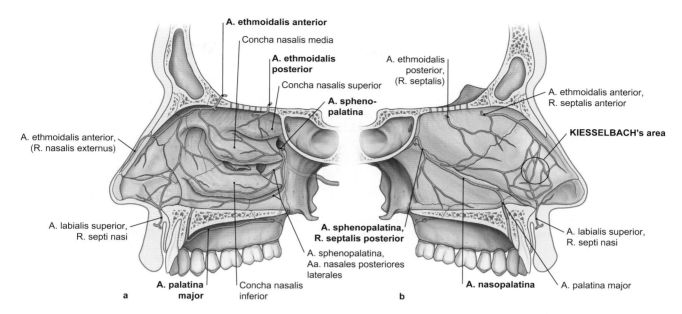

Fig. 9.94 Arterial blood supply to the nasal cavity. a Lateral wall of the right nasal cavity. **b** Nasal septum of the right nasal cavity. [E402]

The outer nose receives blood via the **A. dorsalis nasi,** which via the A. supratrochlearis is also a branch of the A. ophthalmica. Anastomoses exist to the A. angularis in the face. The Vestibulum nasi receives blood via the **R. septi nasi** from the A. labialis superior.

The main blood supply of the nasal cavity is carried out via the **A. sphenopalatina,** a terminal branch of the A. maxilliaris from the A. carotis externa. It passes via the Fossa pterygopalatina through the Foramen sphenopalatinum into the nose and splits into the Aa. nasales laterales posteriores and Rr. septales posteriores. Extensive anastomoses exist between the arteries and connections to the A. palatina descendens and to the A. palatina major (via Canalis incisivus). There is a vessel-rich region in the anterior lower area of the nasal septum with a thin mucous membrane (**KIESSELBACH's area**). It is supplied with blood mainly from the septal part of the A. ethmoidalis anterior with participation of the septal part of the A. sphenopalatina.

The arterial blood supply of the paranasal sinuses is carried out for:

- The maxillary sinus via a branch of the A. sphenopalatina, the A. infraorbitalis and the A. alveolaris superior posterior (all branches of the A. maxillaris)
- The ethmoidal cells via the Aa. ethmoidales
- The frontal sinus via the A. ethmoidalis anterior
- The sphenoidal sinus from above via branches of the dural arteries.

Veins

The external nose drains its blood via **Vv. nasales externae** in the V. facialis. The nasal cavities lead the blood into the Plexus cavernosi concharum and other venous networks of the nasal mucosa. From here, the blood is drained into **Vv. ethmoidales** to the V. ophthalmica superior, in **Vv. nasales internae** via Plexus pterygoideus, Vv. maxillares and V. retromandibularis in the V. jugularis interna and in the V. palatina major.

The paranasal sinuses drain their blood in different ways:

- The maxillary sinus in vascular networks of the dental roots to the Plexus pterygoideus
- The ethmoidal cells in Vv. ethmoidales to the orbital veins and from there to the Sinus cavernosus, into the cavernous body tissue of the efferent lacrimal ducts and from there to the orbital veins as well as in the Plexus pterygoideus

- The frontal sinus in the Sinus sagittalis superior and the Plexus pterygoideus
- The sphenoidal cavity in the Sinus cavernosus and the Plexus pterygoideus

The Plexus pterygoideus forms a central drainage station for all paranasal sinuses, which is of clinical significance due to its connections to the middle cranial fossa and the Sinus cavernosus.

Lymph vessels

The **Nodi lymphoidei submandibulares** are regional lymph nodes of the external nose and nasal atrium. The lymph of the nasal cavities and paranasal sinuses is drained largely in the direction of the throat to the Nodi lymphoidei retropharyngeales and from here to the **Nodi lymphoidei cervicales profundi** and to a lesser extent forward to the Nodi lymphoidei submandibulares.

Innervation

The nose and the paranasal sinuses are innervated sensitively by branches of the N. ophthalmicus [V/1] and the N. maxillaris [V/2] (➤ Fig. 9.95). The N. olfactorius [I] gives the sense of smell. The innervation of secretory active glands and of the blood vessels in the nose and paranasal sinus mucosa is provided via parasympathetic fibres of the N. facialis [VII], which rest primarily in the N. maxillaris [V/2] in the Fossa pterygopalatina, and via sympathetic fibres, which are switched in the Ganglion cervicale superius.

Sensory innervation:

- The N. ethmoidalis anterior (branch of the N. nasociliaris from V/3) divides into a R. nasalis externus for the innervation of the external nose and in Rr. nasales interni, which innervate as Rr. nasales laterales the front area of the lateral nasal wall and with Rr. nasales mediales innervate the nasal septum.
- The N. ethmoidalis posterior innervates the mucosa of the posterior ethmoidal cells and the sphenoidal sinus.
- Rr. nasales posteriores superiores laterales and mediales pass as branches of the N. maxillaris [V/2] through the Foramen sphenopalatinum into the nasal cavity and innervate the nasal mucosa at the back of the upper area of the nasal cavity (nasal septum, lateral and rear nasal cavity wall in the area of the Recessus sphenoethmoidalis).

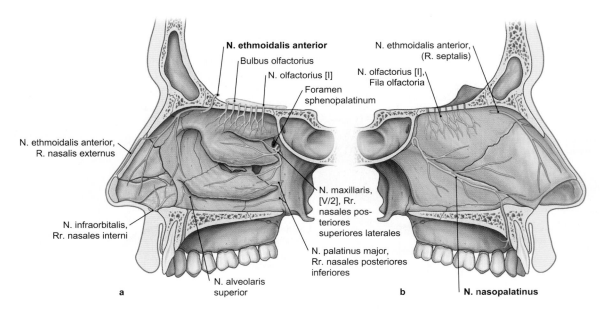

Fig. 9.95 Innervation of the nasal cavity. a Lateral wall of the right nasal cavity. **b** Nasal septum of the right nasal cavity. [E402]

- Rr. nasales posteriores inferiores emerge from the N. nasopalatinus and innervate in the area of the middle and lower nasal passage, including the lower nasal concha and the lower portion of the nasal septum.
- Sneezing reflex: the afferent arm of the triggered protective reflex in the nasal mucosa, which is associated with a reflectory closure of the glottis, runs across the N. maxillaris [V/2] to the Medulla oblongata.

Sense organ innervation:
- From the olfactory fields, the Fila olfactoria passes through the Lamina cribrosa of the skull base. After switching in the Bulbus olfactorius, the fibres continue via the Tractus olfactorius to the central core areas.

Parasympathetic innervation:
- The intermediate part of the N. facialis [VII] passes as N. petrosus major and in the further course as N. canalis pterygoidei to the Ganglion pterygopalatinum. After switching, the postganglionic fibres run together with the sensory fibres of the N. maxillaris [V/2] out of the Fossa pterygopalatina to the nasal mucosa. The fibres provide activation of the gland secretion, and vessel dilatation.

Sympathetic innervation:
- Postganglionic fibres from the Ganglion cervicale superius pass as N. petrosus profundus through the Canalis pterygoideus and reach the Fossa pterygopalatina and the Foramen sphenopalatinum via the nasal cavity. They are responsible for inhibiting gland secretion and for vasoconstriction.

Clinical remarks

A **hyposmia** (decreased olfactory sensation) or an **anosmia** (missing olfactory sensation) can be caused by viral infections, chronic sinusitis, obstructions due to relocation of the airways to the olfactory mucosa, e.g. in the case of allergies, drug side effects, brain tumours or brain trauma with injuries of the olfactory nerves when passing through the cribriform plate.

9.7 Oral cavity, masticatory apparatus, tongue, palate, floor of the mouth, salivary glands
Wolfgang H. Arnold

Skills

After working through this chapter, you should be able to:
- name all oral structures
- describe the nerve course in the oral cavity
- explain the vascular supply to the oral cavity
- explain the development of the teeth
- describe the detailed structure of the various teeth
- describe the structure and function of the Articulatio temporomandibularis, and the location and function of the masticatory muscles
- describe the construction, location and functions of the tongue and of the palate
- reproduce the location, structure and function of the salivary glands
- explain the construction of the floor of the mouth and its compartments
- name the blood supply, innervation and lymph drainage of the abovementioned structures and organs
- describe the topographical location and the neighbourhood relationships of the structures and organs to each other and to be able to classify the surrounding areas and describe their function
- explain the development of the oral cavity, masticatory apparatus, tongue, palate and salivary glands

Clinical case

Perimandibular abscess

Case study
A 50-year-old male patient, who underwent root canal treatment 1 year ago due to profound caries of tooth 46, presents with significantly reduced general health and an increased temperature of 38.5 °C. He states that he has pain in the right

cheek and throat area that radiates into the right ear so that he can no longer open his mouth properly and also has swallowing difficulties.

Initial examination
The pulse rate of the patient is increased, swallowing difficulties and limited mouth opening are clear. The patient has inadequate oral hygiene. The medical records show that in the preceding investigations the patient has had gingival recession (inflammation-free gum recession) and periodontal pocket depths up to 12 mm. The right cheek and the throat area at the right below the lower jaw are clearly swollen, whereby the swelling is only local and includes the submandibular soft tissue. The mandible is not palpable in this area. Submandibular lymph nodes are palpable. Clinically, this gives the impression of a spread of the swelling into the parapharyngeal area. With moderate spontaneous pain, there is severe pressure pain.

Diagnostics
From a differential diagnostic point of view the clinical findings indicate a perimandibular abscess on the right side, a salivary calculus in the Glandula submandibularis or a tumour of the Glandula submandibularis. In order to rule out a salivary calculus or tumour, an ultrasound examination is conducted. In addition, a panoramic x-ray and a dental CT are conducted to visualize a possible osteolytic process. The interpretation of the findings shows a diagnosis of a perimandibular abcess.

Treatment
The dentist opts for the intraoral opening of the abscess and the administration of an antibiotic. Penicillins are the preferred antibiotics for odontogenic infections. After opening the abscess, the dentist inserts a drainage, so pus and wound secretions can be drained away. The wound in the oral cavity heals completely within a short time. After healing the renovation of the root filling follows with apicoectomy in a second session. The dentist advises the patient to urgently improve his oral hygiene habits. In addition, he tells the patient to come every quarter year to check the periodontal condition with professional tooth cleaning.

9.7.1 Oral cavity

The oral cavity is the beginning of the digestive system and is divided into several sections (➤ Fig. 9.96): the **Vestibulum oris** forms the oral vestibule and is bordered outside by the lips and the cheeks and inside by the alveolar processes and the teeth. The **Cavitas oris propria** is the actual oral cavity. The **Isthmus faucium,** the oropharyngeal isthmus, borders the oral cavity dorsally. There the oral cavity passes to the Pars oralis of the pharynx (oropharynx). Between the tooth row of the lower jaw (Mandibula) there is the tongue body (Corpus linguae). In the oral cavity the excretory ducts of three large salivary glands emerge (Glandula parotidea, Glandula submandibularis and Glandula sublingualis), their secretions form the total saliva, which moistens the oral cavity. Overall, the oral cavity is lined with a cutaneous mucous membrane.

Development
In evolutionary terms, the development of the oral cavity originates from **2 germ leaves.** The rear section evolves from the **entodermal foregut,** the front section from the **ectodermal mouth recess.** Through the development of the front brain the **unpaired forehead bulge** grows forward and downwards, while the two paired **maxillary and mandibular bulges** grow forwards. Finally, all 5 face bulges include the **primary oral cavity (Stomatodeum).** The primary oral cavity is a uniform oral nasal space which is separated from the foregut by the pharangeal membrane (**Membrana buccopharyngea**). As early as the 3rd embryonic week the buccopharyngeal membrane tears, so that the Stomatodeum and the intestinal tube are connected to each other. Approximately in the 6th embryonic week the primary palate forms from the forehead bulge of the unpaired **primary palate;** from the two maxillary bulges the **palatinal processes** emerge laterally. These grow medially towards each other, where they fuse in the midline, so that oral and nasal cavity are completely separated from each other.

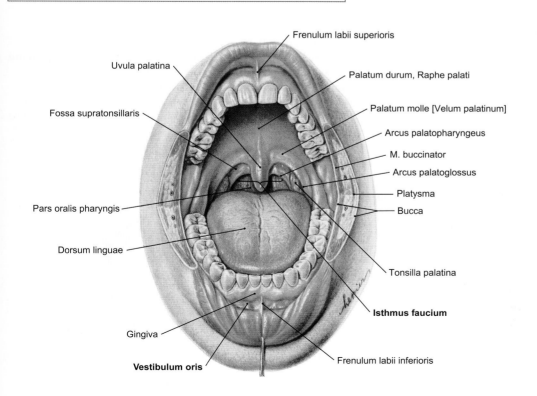

Fig. 9.96 Oral cavity, Cavitas oris. Frontal view, mouth open.

Labels:
- Frenulum labii superioris
- Uvula palatina
- Palatum durum, Raphe palati
- Fossa supratonsillaris
- Palatum molle [Velum palatinum]
- Arcus palatopharyngeus
- M. buccinator
- Arcus palatoglossus
- Platysma
- Pars oralis pharyngis
- Bucca
- Dorsum linguae
- Tonsilla palatina
- **Isthmus faucium**
- Gingiva
- **Vestibulum oris**
- Frenulum labii inferioris

Limitation of the oral cavity

The **oral opening (Rima oris)** represents the entrance to the **Cavitas oris.** Laterally, the oral cavity is restricted by the **cheeks** , the muscular base is the M. buccinator. The roof of the oral cavity forms the palate, which is divided into the **hard palate (Palatum durum)** and the **soft palate (Palatum molle).** The floor of the mouth is mainly formed by the **Corpus linguae.** Under the tongue is the Diaphragma oris, with the muscular base of the M. mylohyoideus. Dorsally the Cavitas oris opens through the Isthmus faucium into the oropharynx.

Orientation

Principally, the directional terms of the body also apply to the oral cavity: however, since the teeth are arranged in a ellipsoid dental arch, additional directional names are required. Dental surfaces, which face the Vestibulum oris are in the front tooth region in both the upper and lower jaw the **labial surfaces,** in the posterior region the **vestibular and buccal surfaces.** The surfaces facing the oral cavity are referred to in the lower jaw as **lingual,** in the upper jaw as **palatinal** surfaces. Together, one can also use the name: **oral.** Tooth surfaces that are in the direction of the throat, are referred to as **distal,** tooth surfaces in the direction of the Rima oris, as **mesial** surfaces. Together, the tooth surfaces of adjacent touching teeth are referred to as **approximal** surfaces (➤ Fig. 9.97).

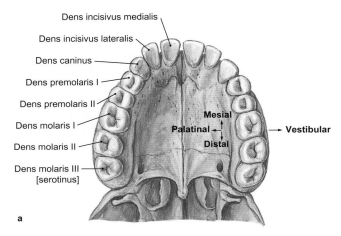

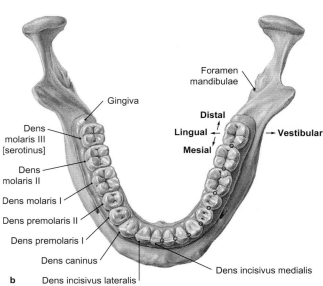

Fig. 9.97 Dental arches with presentation of the directional terms, as well as the individual types of tooth. a Upper jaw. **b** Lower jaw.

Oral mucosa
Classification

The **oral mucosa (Mucosa oralis)** is formed differently in the various regions of the oral cavity. In principle it is cutaneous mucosa, i.e., it is a multilayered epithelium that is mostly keratinised on the palate and on the back of the tongue, but is not keratinised on the cheeks and on the floor of the mouth. The **gums (Gingiva),** are located around the teeth, which are divided into different sections. Directly at the neck of the tooth one refers to the **Gingiva marginalis,** which is movable and forms the Sulcus gingivalis between the tooth neck and the Gingiva. The **Gingiva propria** that is firmly fused with the periosteum of the Proc. alveolaris connects to this and cannot be moved. Between the teeth there is the **Papilla interdentalis** (➤ Fig. 9.98). The upper lip is attached via the **Frenulum labii superioris,** which is situated between the first two incisors, to the Mucosa oralis and the Gingiva. The lower lip is attached via the **Frenulum labii inferioris,** which runs from the lower lip to the oral mucosa, usually between the canine and the first premolars on the right and left side.

Clinical remarks

Normally, the oral mucosa is coloured pink. Keratinisation disorders with cellular and epithelial atypia are often the cause of white mucosal changes **(leucoplakia).** If the mucosal changes cannot be wiped away, it is **precancerous,** and can be attributed to the premalignant diseases of the oral mucosa. They always require a histopathological evaluation, surgical removal and continuous observation. White deposits of the oral mucosa that can be wiped away are most commonly **fungal infections** *(Candida albicans),* which can be treated with medication.

In the context of analysing familial relationships (paternity test) or to detect criminal offences, a cytological **mouth swab** is taken for DNA analysis with which a genetic fingerprint is created. For this purpose, a few mucosal skin cells are taken with a sterile swab from the inside of the mouth cavity and the DNA is then extracted.

Vascular, lymphatic and nervous systems

The Gingiva and the oral mucosa are very well perfused. The **blood vessels** form a close capillary network directly under the epithelium. In the area of the Gingiva marginalis the capillaries are developed as vessel loops that are closely positioned (➤ Fig. 9.99). In the cheek and the base of the mouth there is a flatter network, lying under the epithelium.

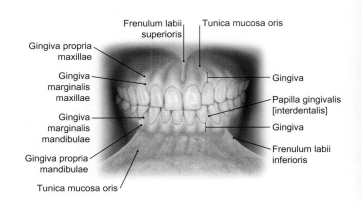

Fig. 9.98 Classification of the Gingiva and Mucosa oralis. [L127]

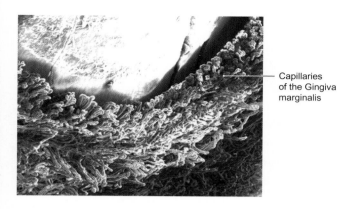

Capillaries of the Gingiva marginalis

Fig. 9.99 Scanning electron microscopy image of a corrosion preparation of capillary loops of the Gingiva marginalis. [T785]

Clinical remarks

Via the capillary network of the floor of the mouth and the cheek **medication** can be resorbed. This can be used in an emergency, e.g. in the treatment of angina pectoris seizures with nitroglycerin (nitrospray).

The oral mucosa is innervated via terminal branches of the N. trigeminus [V]. In the upper jaw area, it is the N. maxillaris [V/2], in the lower jaw area the N. mandibularis [V/3] (➤ Fig. 9.100, ➤ Table 9.33).

Table 9.33 Innervation of the oral mucosa.

Nerve	Innervation area	Course
N. maxillaris [V/2]	Upper jaw	• Foramen rotundum • Fossa pterygopalatina
• N. infraorbitalis	Vestibular gingiva of the upper front teeth	• Canalis infraorbitalis • Foramen infraorbitale
• N. nasopalatinus	Palatinal gingiva of the upper front teeth	• Septum nasi • Foramen incisivum
• N. palatinus major	Palatinal gingiva and mucosa of the Palatum durum	• Canalis palatinus major • Foramen palatinum major
• Nn. palatini minores	Mucosa of the Palatum molle	• Canaliculi palatini minores
N. mandibularis [V/3]	Lower jaw	• Foramen ovale • Fossa infratemporalis
• N. buccalis • N. lingualis	Buccal mucosa, front ⅔ of the tongue, floor of the oral mucosa, lingual gingiva	Under the M. pterygoideus medialis on the M. buccinator, on the inner side of the Ramus mandibulae under the M. pterygoideus medialis on the M. hyoglossus to the tongue
• N. alveolaris inferior	Lower jaw teeth, vestibular gingiva	• Foramen mandibulare • Canalis mandibulae • Foramen mentale

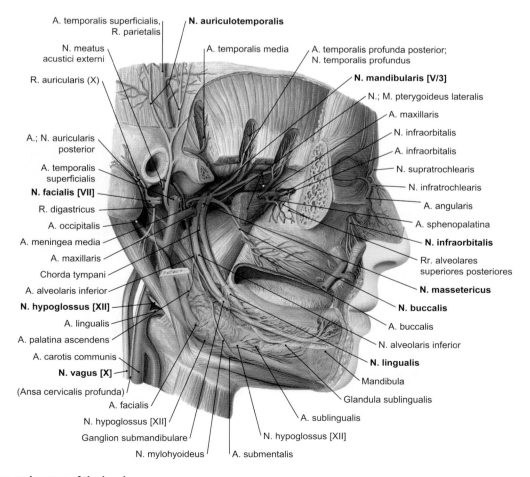

A. temporalis superficialis, R. parietalis
N. auriculotemporalis
N. meatus acustici externi
A. temporalis media
A. temporalis profunda posterior; N. temporalis profundus
R. auricularis (X)
N. mandibularis [V/3]
N.; M. pterygoideus lateralis
A. maxillaris
A.; N. auricularis posterior
N. infraorbitalis
A. infraorbitalis
A. temporalis superficialis
N. supratrochlearis
N. facialis [VII]
N. infratrochlearis
R. digastricus
A. angularis
A. occipitalis
A. sphenopalatina
A. meningea media
N. infraorbitalis
A. maxillaris
Rr. alveolares superiores posteriores
Chorda tympani
N. massetericus
A. alveolaris inferior
N. buccalis
N. hypoglossus [XII]
A. buccalis
A. lingualis
N. alveolaris inferior
A. palatina ascendens
N. lingualis
A. carotis communis
Mandibula
N. vagus [X]
Glandula sublingualis
(Ansa cervicalis profunda)
A. sublingualis
A. facialis
N. hypoglossus [XII]
N. hypoglossus [XII]
Ganglion submandibulare
N. mylohyoideus
A. submentalis

Fig. 9.100 Arteries and nerves of the head.

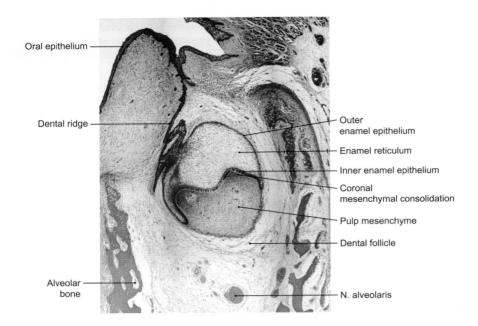

Oral epithelium

Dental ridge

Outer enamel epithelium

Enamel reticulum

Inner enamel epithelium

Coronal mesenchymal consolidation

Pulp mesenchyme

Dental follicle

Alveolar bone

N. alveolaris

Fig. 9.101 Dental development. Cap stage of the development of a molar in the lower jaw with enamel organ and pulp system. [T785]

9.7.2 Masticatory apparatus – teeth

Development

Dental development starts around the 40th day of embryonic development with the invagination of the oral cavity epithelium into the underlying mesenchyme. As a result, a U-shaped epithelial ridge is developed in each of the upper jaw and the lower jaw, the general **dental ridge**. The close relationship between the two different embryonic tissues triggers a complex cascade of genetic interactions that ultimately lead to the formation of the teeth (➤ Table 9.34). Reciprocally, in the epithelial cells (ectodermal origin) and in the mesenchymal connective tissue cells (cells from neural crest cells of the head) genes are activated that are responsible for the production of certain messengers (inductors). The inductors make another differentiation in neighbouring cells to highly specialised cells or the production of further differentiation factors.

The deeply proliferating epithelium of the dental ridge grows around the mesenchyme and leads to a consolidation of mesenchymal cells and thus to the formation of the *enamel bud*. The further proliferation of the epithelium is associated with the development of the enamel organ that consists of the **outer enamel epithelium,** the **enamel pulp** and the **inner enamel epithelium**. The cell density of the mesenchyme, in turn, has the consequence that the inner enamel epithelium is pushed in the direction of the outer enamel epithelium and as such can form the *enamel cap* (cap stage, ➤ Fig. 9.101). Due to continued growth of the enamel epithelium into the depths the dental cap enlarges to the **enamel bell** (bell stage). At this stage the mineralisation of hard dental substances begins. During the development of the enamel organ the determined dental mesenchyme compresses in the bell to dental papillae, into

which the blood vessels and nerves grow. In the immediate vicinity mesenchymal cells form an epithelial band due to factors from the inner enamel epithelium, which form the future dentine (**preodontoblasts**). The *tooth saccules,* which are the basis of the later dental holding apparatus, differentiates from the mesenchymal cells and fibres around the bell and the papilla. The preodontoblasts in the pulp form long processes (**odontoblast processes, TOMES' processes),** which begin with the secretion of organic basic substance (**predentine)** and are referred to as **odontoblasts** . After the first predentine is formed, the cells in the immediate vicinity of the predentine on the border between predentine and inner enamel epithelium begin to differentiate to **ameloblasts**, which in turn begins with the formation of the enamel matrix (➤ Fig. 9.102). As in the case of predentine the enamel matrix mineralises initially extracellularly.

Table 9.34 Germ layer, derivatives of teeth.

Germ layer	Embryonic tissue	Dental tissue
Ectoderm	Melting organ	Enamel
Mesenchyme (neural crest)	Tooth papilla	Dentine
		Odontoblasts
		Pulpar mesenchyme
	Dental sacules	Periodontium

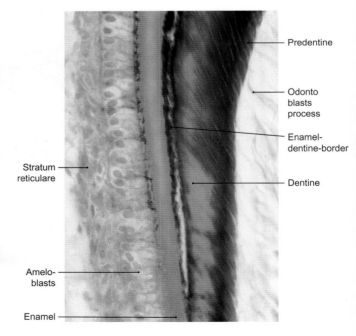

Predentine

Odonto blasts process

Enamel-dentine-border

Dentine

Stratum reticulare

Amelo-blasts

Enamel

Fig. 9.102 Dental development with incipient mineralisation of tooth enamel. [T785]

Unlike the odontoblasts the ameloblast processes are very short and only form pyramid-shaped protrusions of cells. The enamel matrix is resorbed again after the initiation of the mineralisation of the ameloblasts, so that the enamel is largely free of organic material. The structure of the enamel prisms comes from the arrangement of the ameloblasts. The result of the activity of the ameloblasts (secretion of the enamel matrix, initiation of mineralisation, absorption of the matrix proteins) is inorganic enamel prisms, which consist almost exclusively of hydroxyapatite. While the enamel is formed from the inside to the outside (centrifugal), this occurs in the case of dentine centripetal to the pulp. The predentine formed by the odontoblast processes consists mainly of collagen fibres, which are subsequently covered with hydroxyapatite and mineralised in this way. Dentine is therefore made of organic collagen fibres and inorganic hydroxyapatite. The odontoblast processsses remain in the cavities, the dentine canules, and continue to be able to produce predentine. The cell bodies of the odontoblasts remain lying at the inner wall of the pulp. With increasing dentine thickness the odontoblaste processes extend steadily. They are the cellular elements of the dentine, which are responsible for the reaction of the dentine to external stimuli.

Clinical remarks

With the odontoblast processes, nerve fibres pass into the dentine canules, so that dentine in contrast to enamel, is sensitive to pain. In the course of life, the pulp becomes smaller due to the constant dentine formation. Therefore, there is a **risk of opening of the pulp during caries removal** in children greater than in older people.

Due to further proliferation of enamel epithelium it extends like a tube into the depths, whereas the enamel reticulum always becomes narrower and ultimately touches the inner and outer enamel epithelium and the **epithelial root sheath** (HERTWIG's sheath). By touching the inner and outer enamel epithelium a further differentiation of the ameloblasts is prevented. On the inside of the root sheath odontoblasts continue to differentiate, which forms the **root dentine**. The cells of the epithelium of the HERTWIG's sheath die from apoptosis. Mesenchymal cells of the tooth saccule come into contact with the exposed root dentine, which differentiate to **cementoblasts** and deposit the **dental cement** onto the dentine as well as forming root skin (**desmodont**).

Tooth structure and components
Structure

Each tooth consists of a dental crown (Corona dentis), a tooth neck (Cervix dentis) and a tooth root (Radix dentis):
- The **dental crown (Corona dentis)** is covered cap-like by the **enamel (Enamelum)**. It protrudes from the gums (Gingiva).
- On the **tooth neck (Cervix dentis)** the coverage of the crown ends with enamel and passes into the dental cement.
- The dentine of the **tooth root (Radix dentis)** is covered by the **dental cement (Cementum)**. The lowest point of the tooth root is the **root tip (Apex radicis dentis)**. Here there is the **root papilla (Papilla dentis),** which is penetrated at the Foramen apicis dentis by the **root canal (Canalis radicis dentis)**. Through the Foramen apicis dentis, vessels and nerves enter the **pulp cavity (Cavitas dentis)**. The pulpa cavity is divided into the root pulp (Cavitas pulparis) and the crown pulp (Cavitas coronae). The pulp contains arteries and veins, lymph vessels and nerves and consists of loose connective tissue (➤ Fig. 9.103).

The root is attached by the **periodontal apparatus (periodontium)** In the upper and lower jaw. It is suspended from **SHARPEY's fibres** (Fibrae cementoalveolares, collagen fibres) of the root skin (syn.: Periodontium, periodontal or parodontal ligament, desmodentium alveolar dental membrane) in the dental alveola (Alveolus dentalis of the Proc. alveolaris of the Maxilla or the mandible). A distinction is made between the fibres of the periodontium:
- Dentoalveolar comb fibres which radiate from alveolar edge upward into the gingiva
- Horizontal fibres that run from the alveolar edge horizontal to the cement and complete the Sulcus dentalis
- Fibres, which run obliquely from the top exterior to the bottom

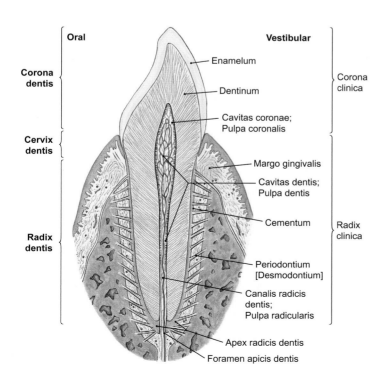

Fig. 9.103 Anatomical construction of a tooth with the Periodontium (incisor, Dens incisivus).

- Circular apical fibres in the area of the root tip
- Inter-radicular fibres in the bifurcation of the roots of multirooted teeth

Hard tooth tissue

Enamel, dentine and cement are the hard dental substances. In contrast to bones they have no blood vessels.

Enamel

Enamel (Enamelum, Substantia adamantina) is the hardest substance in the human body. Mature enamel consists almost entirely of hydroxylapatite crystals that are stored together to enamel prisms. The enamel prisms extend from the dentine enamel border to close under the enamel surface. As the enamel is cell-free, it can no longer be replaced after loss.

Dentine

Dentine (Dentinum, Substantia eburnea, dentine) is in contrast to enamel a living tissue and constitutes the major part of a tooth. It is traversed by dentine canules that run radially from the pulp cavity to the outside and in which the processes of the odontoblasts run for a lifetime as TOMES' fibres together with fine nerve fibre endings. In the dental crown the dentine is covered by enamel (crown dentine), at the root by cement (root dentine). The enamel-cement border above the dentine corresponds to the tooth neck. Dentine is after enamel the body's hardest substance.

Cement

Cement (Cementum) is relatively similar to bone, contains almost as much organic matrix, but a higher proportion of minerals and around only half the amount of water. Like the osteocytes in bone, the cementocytes lie in Lacunas of cement. The SHARPEY's fibres, which suspend the tooth in the alveola of the upper and lower jaw (see above) are fixed in the cement.

Characteristics of teeth

Since the teeth are not arranged in a circular arch, but are arranged in a parabolic arch, they have a different radius of curvature. They are also mirror imaged on both sides, so that they cannot be interchanged. The following characteristics are used for differentiation of individual teeth:

- **Curvature feature:** it describes the different curvature of the vestibular surface. The mesial area is more severely curved particularly in the posterior region than the distal area.
- **Angle feature:** the chewing edge of a crown forms a more acute angle with the mesial contact area than with the distal contact area.
- **Root feature:** it describes the deviation of the root course from the dental axis distally.

Permanent dentition (Dentes permanentes)

The permanent **adult dentition** consists of **32 teeth** with 16 upper and 16 lower jaw teeth. Each dental arch is divided into 2 symmetrical halves, making a total of 4 quadrants. The 4 quadrants are numbered in sequence from the top right to bottom right from 1 to 4, yielding a denture scheme each with 8 teeth. In each quadrant in turn 4 dental types are differentiated, 2 **front teeth (Dentes incisivi, incisors)**, 1 **canine (Dens caninus)**, 2 **premolars (Dentes premolares)** and 3 **molars (Dentes molares)** (➤ Fig. 9.104). The Fédération Dentaire International (FDI) (International Dental Federation) has developed a current globally valid dental scheme in which each tooth of a quadrant is numbered from 1 to 8, and the respective number of the quadrant is set before the tooth number. In the case of **deciduous dentition (20 teeth)**, the quadrants from 5 to 8 are counted according to the adult dentition.

Dental notation of the permanent dentition

18 17 16 15 14 13 12 11	21 22 23 24 25 26 27 28
48 47 46 45 44 43 42 41	31 32 33 34 35 36 37 38

Dental scheme in deciduous dentition

55 54 53 52 51	61 62 63 64 65
85 84 83 82 81	71 72 73 74 75

NOTE

The **incisors (Dentes incisivi)** are single root teeth with a cutting edge. The **canines (Dentes canini)** also have only one root, their crown resembles a sharp chisel. The **premolars (Dentes premolares)** are constructed differently: the first upper premolar is a double rooted tooth, whereby one root points in a palatinal and the other in a vestibular direction. The second premolar is like the two lower jaw premolars single rooted. The premolars have no cutting edge, but a chewing surface with a hump relief. The 3 **upper jaw**

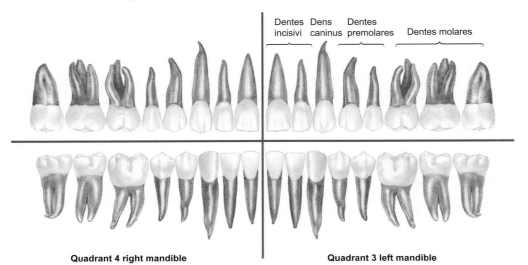

Quadrant 1 right maxilla   Quadrant 2 left maxilla

Dentes incisivi   Dens caninus   Dentes premolares   Dentes molares

Quadrant 4 right mandible   Quadrant 3 left mandible

Fig. 9.104 Permanent teeth, Dentes permanentes. Vestibular view.

molar teeth (Dentes molares) are three rooted teeth with 1 palatinal and 2 vestibular roots. The **lower jaw molars (Dentes molares)** each have 2 roots with a mesial and a distal root. All molars are characterised by a very differentiated hump relief in the occlusal surface that are used for food fragmentation.

Incisor teeth, Dentes incisivi

The incisors have chisel-shaped crowns and a root. The upper incisors are larger than those of the lower jaw.

Crowns

In the case of incisor crowns a distinction is made between a Facies vestibularis and a Facies lingualis. On the cutting edge of younger teeth there are several small edge tubercles. The Facies lingualis is characterised by marginal ridges (Cristae marginales), which run convex in a gingival direction and form the Tuberculum dentis in the cervical area of the tooth. Above the Tuberculum dentis of the upper incisors is the Foramen caecum, an enamel indentation in which caries often develops.

Roots

The incisors are single-rooted teeth, longitudinal ridges can often be found on their mesial and distal surfaces. The root tip is bent towards distal. The strongest and longest root is in the 1st upper incisor, the smallest root in the 1st lower.

Pulp

The Cavitas coronae of the incisors corresponds in their shape to the shape of the dental crown.

Root canal

The root canal (Canalis radicis dentis) is usually narrow and often interrupted by dentine bridges. The root canal often forms branches.

Canine teeth, Dentes canini

The canine teeth are the largest teeth in the frontal tooth area. They are important corner pillars between the incisors and the premolars and in prosthetic dentistry anchor teeth for bridges and brackets.

Crowns

The cutting edge runs obliquely in a slightly offset mesial tip so that the crown is more like a chisel. The mesial cutting edge is shorter and thinner than the distal. From the tip of the crown a flat, midline ridge runs cervically, which divides the vestibular area into a mesial and a distal facet. On the Facies lingualis there are 2 cervically merging marginal ridges. Also the lingual surface is divided by a medium edge into a mesial and distal facet. At the cervical end of the merging marginal ridges there is the Tuberculum dentis.

Roots

The canines are single-rooted teeth, whose roots are formed stronger vestibularly than lingually. The root of the upper jaw canine is the longest of all teeth.

Pulp

The Cavitas coronae of the canine is a narrow, long extended space which in the dental neck area runs continuously into the root canal.

Root canal

The Canalis radicis dentis of the upper canine tooth runs without branches and is relatively long. In the lower jaw the root canal is often split into 2 sub-branches.

Premolars, Dentes premolares

Crowns

The premolars have no cutting edge, but an **occlusal surface** (Facies occlusalis). The top premolars each have 2 humps, a vestibular and a palatal. The vestibular hump is greater than the lingual. Between the two humps a distinct side ridge runs on the mesial and distal side. A longitudinal fissure runs from mesial to distal, at its ends there is a mesial and a distal pit. In the lower premolars the humps are smaller and therefore the marginal ridges are less developed. The 1st molar has predominantly a double hump crown pattern, the 2nd lower premolar can also have 3 humps. The Facies occlusalis is similar in double hump premolars of the lower jaw to those of the upper premolars. Because the vestibular hump is larger than the lingual, the chewing surfaces incline inwards, which is referred to as a crown escapement. Consequently, the tip of the vestibular hump lies in the middle of the chewing surface and that of the lingual on the lingual crown edge. The triangular type of the Facies occlusalis, 2 lingual and 1 vestibular hump can be found. The two lingual humps are separated by a transverse fissure, so that a Y-shaped fissure pattern is created.

The **Facies vestibularis** of all premolars is similar to the canines. The occlusal crown section is moved to lingual, considerably reducing the crown escapement. The **Facies lingualis** is much narrower and smaller than the Facies vestibularis. The transverse arch of this surface passes directly into the approximal surface, the longitudinal arch is relatively flat, causing the lingual crown wall to stand perpendicular.

Roots

The upper 1st premolar usually has 2 roots, 1 stronger vestibular and 1 weaker palatinal. All other premolars have only 1 root, it is shaped like a canine tooth.

Pulp

The Cavitas coronae of premolars corresponds to the shape of the dental crowns.

Root canal

The single-rooted premolars very often have 2 root canals. Particularly often single-rooted first upper premolars have 2 root canals.

Molars, Dentes molares

The molars in permanent dentition are the biggest teeth. They have several humps in the masticatory surface that serve the disintegration of food. For this reason, they are referred to as the grinders. The molar teeth in the upper and the lower jaw differ greatly.

Upper jaw molars

Crowns

The Facies occlusalis usually has 4 humps, 2 vestibular and 2 lingual. Sometimes there are only 3 humps, sometimes a 5th hump occurs (Tuberculum CARABELLI see below). The mesial humps are higher than the distal ones. The largest is the mesiolingual hump which is connected by an enamel ridge (Crista transversalis) with the distovestibular hump. The smallest is the distolingual hump. The fissure system consists of a mesiovestibular and a distolingual fissure. Both fissures are connected to one another by a transvers fissure. The mesiovestibular fissure separates the two mesial humps and the mesiovestibular from the distovestibular hump. The distolingual fissure separates the two distal and lingual humps from each other. At the intersection points of the transverse fissure with the two other fissures there are small depressions, the Fovea mesialis and the Fovea distalis. In front of the edge between the mesiovestibular and mesiolingual or the distovestibular and distolingual humps is the Fovea triangularis. Mesially the Facies vestibulares and Facies lingualis are higher than distal. The crown of the upper wisdom tooth is similar to the crown of the 2nd molar; however, the crown shape of the upper wisdom tooth varies greatly.

Tuberculum CARABELLI

The Tuberculum CARABELLI (CARABELLI hump) is an additional hump in the mesial section of the lingual crown wall and can be most often found on the 1st molars.

Roots

The upper molars are three-rooted teeth with a Radix lingualis, a Radix vestibularis mesialis and a Radix vestibularis distalis. The Radix lingualis is the strongest of the three roots. It is projected between the two vestibular root origins. The roots are wide open, whereby the root tips are bent towards one another. The roots of the wisdom teeth show large form variability. The root tips of the upper jaw molars are in close contact to the base of the maxillary sinus. The bone lammelle between the alveoli and the maxillary sinus is often paper thin (➤ Fig. 9.105).

> ### Clinical remarks
>
> In the extraction of molars in the upper jaw, there is the **risk of opening the maxillary sinus.** A link between oral and maxillary sinus leads to the degeneration of the ciliated epithelium in the maxillary sinus with a chronic infection.

Mandibular molars
Crowns

The Facies occlusalis of the 1st molars very often has 5 humps, 2 vestibular, 2 lingual and 1 distal hump. In contrast, the 2nd lower molars has only 4 humps. The distal hump is not present. The biggest hump is the mesiovestibular hump. The smallest hump is the distal hump.

Fissures

At the first molars there is a mesiodistal longitudinal fissure and 3 transverse fissures. Through the mesiovestibular transverse fissure, the two vestibular humps are separated from each other, the two lingual humps by the lingual transverse fissure and the distal trans-

verse fissure separates the distal bump from the distovestibular. At the intersection points of the longitudinal and transverse fissures, smaller depressions are again present. The fissures pattern of the 2nd lower molars is formed by a transverse fissure which separates the hump into 2 vestibular and 2 lingual humps. The mesial humps are slightly larger than the distal.

The lower wisdom tooth shows a large number of size and shape variations. The chewing surface has often 4 or 5 humps which are separated from each other by the corresponding fissures.

Roots

The molar teeth in the lower jaw are double-rooted teeth with a mesial and distal root. The mesial root is flat and wide, the distal root round and relatively pointed. The Radix mesialis is bent forward; the Radix distalis runs quite straight. The roots of the 2nd molars are formed much more simply. They are not as far apart as the 1st molars. In the wisdom teeth the roots again show large shape variability.

Pulp and root canals

The shape and size of the Pulpa coronalis reflect the shape of the dental crown. In adolescents the crown pulp is larger than in older people. The **pulp of the upper molars** is relatively large and has 4 walls that bulge slightly into the pulp. They run cervically like a funnel, pulp horns can be found under the humps occlusally. The root canal of the lingual root is the widest; the two vestibular root canals are more closely constructed. The mesiovestibular root shows numerous variations, often the root canal is divided into 2 canals. The wisdom teeth have a very richly varying root canal system. The **pulp of the lower molars** corresponds to a cube with a smaller distal and a larger mesial wall. Under each hump there is usually a pulp horn. In the mesial root, especially in the 1st molars, there are often 2 root canals. The lower wisdom tooth also shows strong variability in the number and form of the root canals just as the upper wisdom tooth.

Milk dentition (Dentes decidui)

In contrast to the permanent dentition the **milk dentition (deciduous teeth)** contains only 20 teeth with 5 teeth in each quadrant (➤ Fig. 9.106).

> N O T E
>
> A distinction is made between milk incisors (Dentes incisivi deciduales), the milk canine (Dens caninus decidualis) and the milk molars (Dentes molares deciduales). The milk front and canine teeth are single-rooted teeth with chisel-shaped cutting edges in the crown. There are no premolars in milk teeth. The milk molars of the upper jaw are three-rooted with 1 palatal and 2 vestibular roots. The mandibular molars of the deciduous dentition each have 2 roots, of which one is mesial and the other distal oriented.

Milk incisors, Dentis incisivi deciduales

The crowns in the upper incisors are low and wide with a strongly protruding cervical enamel bulge, the **Cingulum.** The heads of the lower incisors have hardly any form differences. Sometimes the first incisor has 3 ridge tubercles in the masticatory edge.

Milk canines, Dentes canini deciduales

The upper milk canines have a wider crown than the first milk incisors. In addition, they have a wide Cingulum. The area on the lingual side is often divided by a ridge in the middle, on which a clear tubercle emerges cervically. The **lower canine** is narrower than the upper. The Cingulum is not as clearly pronounced.

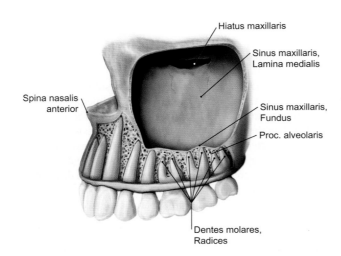

Hiatus maxillaris

Sinus maxillaris, Lamina medialis

Spina nasalis anterior

Sinus maxillaris, Fundus

Proc. alveolaris

Dentes molares, Radices

Fig. 9.105 Extent of the maxillary sinus with illustration of the relationship between the tooth roots to the maxillary sinus floor. [L266]

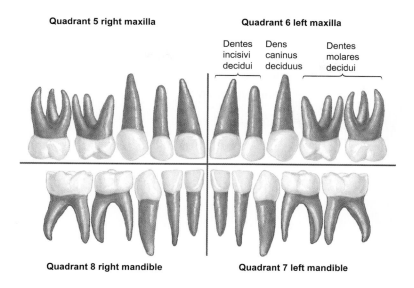

Quadrant 5 right maxilla

Quadrant 6 left maxilla

Dentes incisivi decidui

Dens caninus deciduus

Dentes molares decidui

Quadrant 8 right mandible

Quadrant 7 left mandible

Fig. 9.106 Milk teeth, Dentes decidui, approx. 3-year-old child. Vestibular view.

Milk molars, Dentes molares deciduales

The crown of the upper milk molars is similar to the crown shape of the permanent molars. On the Facies vestibularis the Tuberculum molare is located in the lower quadrant mesially. A Tuberculum CARABELLI can often be found on the Facies lingualis. The roots of the **upper milk molars** are spread far apart. The upper milk molar comes in two versions: as premolar type with 2 humps and as a molar type with 4 humps. The 4 hump variant shows an H-shaped fissure pattern, similar to the first permanent upper molar. At the **lower molars** there are 2 shape variants, the premolar and molar type. The chewing surface of the molar type has 4 or 5 humps. The lingual humps are long and pointed. Distally a 3rd hump can often be found. The roots are spread far apart and bend at the end together. The mesial root is wider and longer. The **lower 1st milk molar** has a significant crown escapement which is heightened by a projection of the Cingulum and a Tuberculum molare. The **lower 2nd milk molar** corresponds in its appearance to the first lower permanent molars. It has mostly 5 humps with an irregular fissure pattern. A Tuberculum molare is usually not present.

Tooth eruption and change of teeth

Roughly from the *6th month of life* the milk teeth erupt in a coordinated order into the oral cavity, the range of the eruption is, however, highly variable and can be less or exceed the times outlined in ➤ Table 9.35. The cutting teeth in the lower jaw come first, with the eruption of the 2nd milk molars up to the age of 2 ½ to 3 years, when the milk dentition is complete. The milk teeth are slightly smaller than the permanent teeth.

The **changing dentition period** starts roughly from the *6th year of life.* In the process, the tooth roots and the bony alveolar walls are resorbed. This loosens the milk tooth crown more and more, and it eventually falls out. The milk teeth are replaced by permanent teeth, which are referred to as **replacement teeth**. The additional teeth of the permanent dentition which do not replace milk teeth,

are the **additional teeth.** During the dental change the size of the Maxilla and mandible increases and reach their final size after all permanent teeth have erupted.

The dental changing period is in two phases:
- First, *(5th–9th year of life)* the additional teeth and the permanent incisors (replacement teeth) erupt.
- Then *(10th–12th year of life)*, the milk molars are replaced by the premolars (replacement teeth) and the milk canines by the permanent canines.

As a rule of thumb:
- the 1st molar is the 6-year molar,
- the 2nd molar is the 12-year molar and
- the 3rd molar is the wisdom tooth (Dens serotinus, Dens sapientiae, 17–25 years).

Innervation of the teeth
Upper jaw

The upper jaw teeth are all sensitively innervated by different individual branches of the **N. infraorbitalis,** a branch of the N. maxillaris [V/2], (➤ Table 9.36, ➤ Fig. 9.107). The result is that the teeth of the Maxilla are innervated individually. The entire nerve plexus, innervated by the upper jaw teeth, is referred to as **Plexus dentalis superior**.

Clinical remarks

Because of the individual innervation of the upper jaw teeth block anaesthesia is not possible. In the upper jaw **infiltration anaesthesia** of individual teeth is preferable. The upper jaw front teeth are innervated both from the vestibular as well as from the palatine side.

Table 9.36 Branches of the N. infraorbitalis and their innervation areas.

Nerve	Innervation area	Course
Rr. alveolares superiores	Molars	On the Tuber maxillae through the Foramina alveolaria to the lateral maxillary sinus mucosa
R. alveolaris superior medialis	Premolars	In the Canalis infraorbitalis to the maxillary sinus mucosa
Rr. alveolares superiores anteriores	Canine and incisors	From the Foramen infraorbitale on the Corpus maxillae to the front teeth

Table 9.35 Eruption times of milk teeth in months.

Dental type	1st incisor	2nd incisor	Canine	1st molar	2nd molar
Upper jaw ♂	9.1 ± 1.5	10.4 ± 2.4	18.9 ± 2.7	16.0 ± 2.3	27.6 ± 4.4
Upper jaw ♀	9.6 ± 2.0	11.9 ± 2.7	20.1 ± 3.2	15.7 ± 2.3	28.4 ± 4.3
Lower jaw ♂	7.3 ± 1.6	13.0 ± 2.8	19.3 ± 2.9	16.2 ± 1.9	25.9 ± 3.8
Lower jaw ♀	7.8 ± 2.1	13.8 ± 3.6	20.2 ± 3.4	15.6 ± 2.2	27.1 ± 4.2

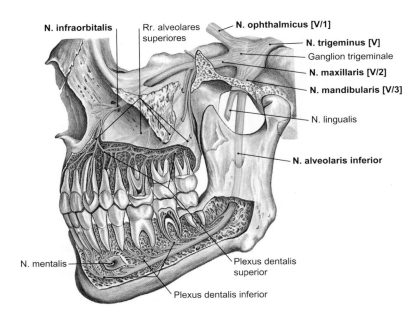

N. infraorbitalis
Rr. alveolares superiores
N. ophthalmicus [V/1]
N. trigeminus [V]
Ganglion trigeminale
N. maxillaris [V/2]
N. mandibularis [V/3]
N. lingualis
N. alveolaris inferior
N. mentalis
Plexus dentalis superior
Plexus dentalis inferior

Fig. 9.107 Innervation of the teeth.

Lower jaw

The lower jaw teeth are only sensitively supplied by a single nerve the **N. alveolaris inferior,** a branch of the N. mandibularis [V/3]. It passes through the Foramen mandibulae in the Canalis mandibulae, where it forms the **Plexus dentalis inferior**. Prior to entering the Canalis mandibulae the N. mylohyoideus leaves the nerve as a motor branch of the N. alveolaris inferior.

Clinical remarks

At the entrance of the N. alveolaris inferior in the Canalis mandibulae, all teeth of the lower jaw are simultaneously anaesthetised in a quadrant using **block anaesthesia**; however, due to the proximity, the N. lingualis and the N. mylohyoideus are are always anaesthetised with it, leading to taste and sensory failures of the tongue.

Periodontium

The **Periodontium** consists of 4 different elements (➤ Fig. 9.103):
• Gums (gingiva)
• Alveolar bone (Proc. alveolares maxillae and mandibulae)
• Root skin (periodontal ligament, desmodentium)
• Dental cement (Cementum)

The Periodontium is a tooth-dependent structure and reforms almost completely after loss of a tooth.

Clinical remarks

A **chronic parodontitis** leads to decomposition of the alveolar bone and degeneration of the periodontal ligaments with loss of SHARPEY's fibres (periodontosis). **Periodontitis** is the most common disease that leads to tooth loss in old age. The retraction of the alveolar bone can lead to problems in the insertion of implants for dental prostheses.

9.7.3 Masticatory apparatus – Masticatory muscles

The masticatory muscles are responsible for the movement of the lower jaw against the upper jaw. All 4 masticatory muscles (➤ Table 9.37) have their origin at the skull base and run to the mandible. They ensure that food can be bitten off and can be reduced to small pieces. The group of masticatory muscles is supported by further muscles of the head and throat area. These include mimic muscles, the suprahyoid and the infrahyoid muscles, the M. sternocleidomastoideus and neck muscles.

M. masseter

The **M. masseter** is attached on the outside of the Ramus mandibulae. The **Pars superficialis** runs obliquely from above downwards towards the lower front, the **Pars profunda** runs vertically. The rear edge of the muscle is covered by Glandula parotidea. The cheek fat globule lies at the front edge between the M. masseter and the M. buccinator (BICHAT's fat pad). It shapes the contour of the rear cheek area and forms a raphe at the rear edge of the Ramus mandibulae together with the M. pterygoideus medialis that originates at the inner side.

M. temporalis

The **M. temporalis** fills the Fossa temporalis and is covered on its front side by the Fascia temporalis, which passes from the Linea temporalis superior to the zygomatic arch. Just above the zygomatic arch the Fascia temporalisis forms a superficial and a deep layer that are attached on the outer and inner surface of the Arcus zygomaticus. The osteofibrous space created between is filled with structural fat. The attachment area at the Proc. coronoideus of the Mandibula is hidden by the zygomic bone and M. masseter. The M. temporalis is the largest and strongest masticatory muscle. It is often associated with the Mm. masseter (see above) and pterygoideus lateralis. At the bottom of the anterior border is the upper part of the cheek fat globule.

M. pterygoideus medialis

The **M. pterygoideus medialis** (➤ Fig. 9.108) and the M. masseter are usually connected to one another by a connective tissue raphe

Table 9.37 Masticatory musculature.

Innervation	Origins	Attachment	Function	Blood supply
M. masseter				
N. massetericus [from V/3]	• Pars superficialis: lower edge of the Os zygomaticum, anterior two thirds • Pars profunda: inner surface of the Os zygomaticum, rear third	• Pars superficialis: Tuberositas masseterica • Pars profunda: outer surface of the Proc. coronoideus	Adduction, protrusion in unilateral contraction, laterotrusion	A. masseterica (A. maxillaris), A. facialis, A. transversa faciei of the A. temporalis superficialis, A. buccalis (A. maxillaris)
M. temporalis				
Nn. temporales profundi [from V/3]	• Pars profunda: Planum temporale of the Os zygomaticum • Pars superficialis: Facies temporalis	Proc. coronoideus mandibulae	Adduction, retrusion	Aa. temporales profundae anterior and posterior (A. maxillaris), A. temporalis media (A. temporalis superficialis)
M. pterygoideus medialis				
N. pterygoideus medialis [from V/3]	• Pars medialis: Fossa pterygoidea • Pars lateralis: Lamina lateralis of the Proc. pterygoideus	Tuberositas pterygoidea mandibulae	Adduction, protrusion, mediotrusion	A. alveolaris superior, A. alveolaris inferior, A. buccalis (A. maxillaris)
M. pterygoideus lateralis				
N. pterygoideus lateralis [from V/3]	• Caput inferius: Lamina lateralis, Proc. pterygoidei • Caput superius: Facies and Crista infratemporalis	Fovea pterygoidea mandibulae, joint capsule and Discus articularis	Protrusion on bilateral contraction, mediotrusion and adduction in unilateral contraction	R. pterygoideus (A. maxillaris)

at the lower rim of the mandible, so that they encompass the Corpus mandibulae in the area of the Angulus mandibulae like stirrups. This way they can enforce maximum power and induce the mouth closure and the grinding movements for the disintegration of food. The M. pterygoideus medialis has 2 origins:

• The **Pars medialis** is bigger and comes from the Fossa pterygoidea.

• The **Pars lateralis** comes from the outside of the Lamina lateralis of the Proc. pterygoideus.

The Caput inferius of the M. pterygoideus lateralis slides between both parts.

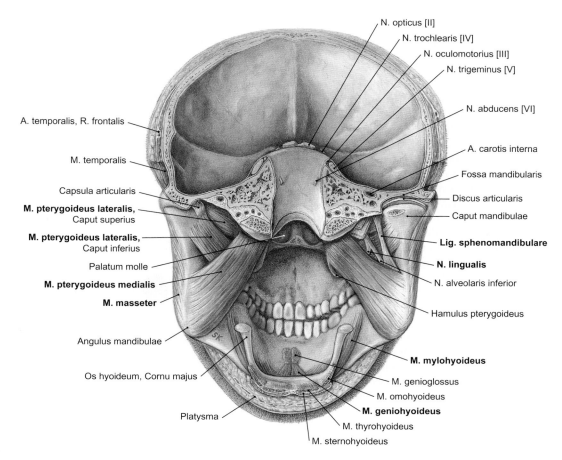

Fig. 9.108 Masticatory muscles. Dorsal view.

M. pterygoideus lateralis

The **M. pterygoideus lateralis** is essentially involved in the oral opening. It has a smaller upper head (**Caput superius**) and a larger lower head (**Caput inferius**). A part of the muscle fibres of the Caput superius inserts on the anterior ligament of the Discus articularis and on the joint capsule of the temporomandibular joint and attaches in bilateral activity the Caput mandibulae at the tuberculum slope during adduction of the lower jaw. Unilateral activity leads to the grinding movement on the working side and to stabilising the Caput mandibulae on the dormant side. The Caput inferius is the only masticatory muscle part which is involved in the jaw opening. It induces the oral opening and forces the further motion in the form of a combination of rotation and translation.

> N O T E
> The M. pterygoideus lateralis takes a key position for the kinematics of the temporomandibular joint.

9.7.4 Masticatory apparatus – temporomandibular joint

The paired temperomandibular joint is part of the masticatory apparatus. Functionally, the temporomandibular joints enable food intake and fragmentation, as well as articulation when speaking and singing. Both temporomandibular joints form a functional unit and thus work always at the same time.

Development

The temporomandibular joint is an **accumulation joint**. It is formed between the Mandibula and Os temporale from **secondary cartilage** with a growth zone. The joint form is connected to the development of the dentition and thus not only dependent on whether or not there are teeth, but also on the bite form.

Structure

The joint head (**Caput mandibulae**) of the temporomandibular joint forms the biconvex curved articular process of the lower jaw. It articulates with the front part of the **Fossa mandibularis** and the Tuberculum articulare of the Os temporale. The rear part of the Fossa mandibularis, which belongs to the Pars tympanica of the Os temporale, is not part of the temporomandibular joint and lies extracapsular. The **joint surfaces** are not covered with hyaline cartilage, but by a fibrous cartilage which indicates the biomechanical features of the temporomandibular joint. Between the joint surfaces there is a **Discus articularis,** which divides the joint cavity into 2 chambers (dithalamic joint). The axes of the joint heads are slanted and intersect in front of the Foramen magnum at an angle between 150° and 165°. The temporomandibular joint is completely enclosed by a rough joint capsule.

Caput mandibulae

It forms the upper end of the **Proc. articularis (Proc. condylaris, Condylus mandibulae)** and is roll-shaped. Its shape shows great individual variation. The joint heads are usually not bilaterally structured as a mirror image. The articular surfaces of the Caput mandibulae are covered by fibrous cartilage and are mainly on the front of the joint head.

Fossa mandibularis

The temporomandibular joint pit is located on the underside of the Os temporale and is two to three times larger than the articular surface of the Caput mandibulae. At the lowest point of the Fossa mandibularis the bone is paper thin and translucent at the skull. The articular surface passes forward to the vertex of the **joint tubercles (Tuberculum articulare)**. The Tuberculum articulare is located in front of the Fossa mandibularis and forms a slanting, downward angled articular surface, which is also called the **tubercular slope**. On the Tuberculum articulare the cartilage coating is especially thick, because here the power transfer takes place via the Discus articularis. Together with the Fossa mandibularis the Tuberculum articulare forms an S-shaped joint path.

Discus articularis

The Discus articularis sits like a cap on the joint head and divides the temporomandibular joint into an upper somewhat larger joint (Articulatio discotemporalis) and a lower joint (Articulatio discomandibularis). It has therefore 2 chambers (**dithalamic joint**). The discus is tightly frontally fused medially and laterally with the joint capsule. In the centre it is very thin and becomes thicker at the edges. It consists of connective tissue and fibrous cartilage and shows a regionally different structure (➤ Fig. 9.109) which is divided into 4 sections (from front to back):

* **Anterior ligament** (here the tendons of the muscle fibres of the Caput superius musculi pterygoidei lateralis radiate from the front into the Discus articularis)
* **Intermediate zone**
* **Posterior ligament**
* **Bilaminary zone** (connective tissue, which splits in front of the cartilaginous portion of the external auditory duct into 2 sheets, an upward and downward part)

The lower sheet of the bilaminary zone is attached at the Collum mandibulae with the joint capsule and thus forms the rear border of the lower joint fissure. It consists of taut collagen fibres and passes further to the rear into a highly vascularised connective tissue, the **Plexus retroarticularis.** The top layer consists mainly of elastic fibres, which are attached to the Fissura tympanosquamosa and the Fissura petrosquamosa. When the mouth is opened, the lower layer is stretched, while the top layer is relaxed. When closing it is vice versa. At the front the Discus articularis is connected medially and laterally to the joint capsule.

As the Caput mandibulae and the Fossa mandibularis (joint socket) do not fit together exactly, the Discus has the **function** of balancing this mismatch of articulating skeletal elements. When opening and

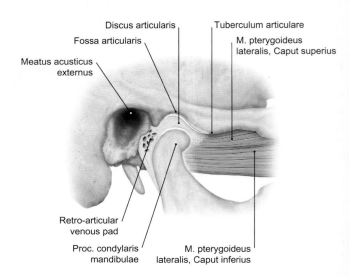

Fig. 9.109 Bony parts of the temporomandibular joint with Discus articularis and M. pterygoideus lateralis. [L127]

closing the mouth, the discus articularis is shifted (it slides on to the tubercular slope) and adapts to the changing size conditions.

NOTE

Even at maximum chewing force development on the occlusal surface, the temporomandibular joint in the Fossa mandibularis is barely loaded since the chewing pressure from the teeth is derived via the trajectories of the viscerocranium at the skull base and the cranium.

Clinical remarks

Occlusion disorders, dysgnathia or tooth loss may cause chronic biomechanical stress of the temporomandibular joint, which is often associated with degenerative changes of joint cartilage and the Discus articularis. **Degenerative changes (osteoarthritis)** are usually associated with defects in the lateral area of the Discus articularis **(perforation)**. As the jaw joints are true joints (diarthroses), they can be affected by all diseases, which also affect the large limb joints (e.g. diseases of the rheumatic type). Stronger violent impacts on the Mandibula can lead to fractures of the Collum mandibulae **(Collum fracture)**. with or without dislocation. Even without fracture, bleeding often occurs from the retroarticular venous plexus with difficulties to open the mouth. In older people, owing to strong atrophy of the bone in the Fossa mandibularis a central **fracture of the Fossa mandibularis** with an intrusion in the middle cranial fossa may occur after falls or knocks on the chin. The pain in all diseases of the temporomandibular joint is often projected into the external auditory canal. In this case the temporomandibular joint must always be taken into consideration.

Joint capsule

The thin joint capsule passes from the edge of the Fossa mandibularis around the Tuberculum articulare and attaches above the Fovea pterygoidea on the lower jaw. Because it is closely connected with the Discus, the Discus articularis separates the joint cavity into the Articulatio discotemporalis and discomandibularis. Both joint cavities typically have no connection to each other. The joint capsule is reinforced by ligaments (➤ Table 9.38).

Ligaments

The movements of the temporomandibular joint are influenced by ligaments of the joint capsule as well as through ligaments that are not associated with the joint capsule (➤ Table 9.38).

Biomechanics

The temporomandibular joint is a combination joint, which allows for movement in all three planes. Because of its shape, it is referred to as a **bicondylar joint (Articulatio bicondylaris)**. As both jaw joints are connected via the mandibular brace, independent movements of a joint is not possible (biomechanical coupling).

Clinical remarks

The shape of the articular surfaces, the shape and position of the teeth, the condition of the dentition, the occlusion, the muscles of mastication and their innervation form a common functional system (craniomandibular system; CMS) which affects the movements in the temporomandibular joint. Interference in this system, such as e.g. an incomplete dentition or occlusion disorders, lead to **disruptions of the movement process in the jaw joints.**

Table 9.38 Ligaments of the temporomandibular joint.

Ligament	Function	Relationship with the joint capsule	Connection
Lig. laterale (Lig. temporomandibulare)	Involved in the joint guidance, inhibits edge movements and stabilises the condylus on the working side	Reinforces the joint capsule on the outside	Arcus zygomaticus inclined towards the rear to the Collum mandibulae
Lig. mediale	Variably formed, reinforces the joint capsule, inhibits edge movements	Reinforces the joint capsule on the inside	Inner edge of the Fossa mandibularis to the Collum mandibulae
Lig. sphenomandibulare	Inhibits mouth opening near the end position	No relationships	Spina ossis sphenoidalis between Mm. pterygoidei to the Lingula mandibulae
Lig. stylomandibulare	Mostly weak, supports Lig. sphenomandibulare	No relationships	The lower margin of the Proc. styloideus to the posterior border of the Ramus mandibulae

Main movements of the jaw joints in the context of mastication are:
- **Abduction and adduction** (opening and closing, raising and lowering of the lower jaw): this is a combined gliding hinge movement that takes place bilaterally and symmetrically. The Discus articularis slides under the force of the M. pterygoideus lateralis on the Tuberculum articulare to forward below. In doing so, the Angulus mandibulae moves backwards. The axis of this hinge motion passes through the Foramen mandibularae, which is why the N. alveolaris inferior is not stretched in this movement.
- **Grinding movements:** These asymmetric movements are made up of combined translational and rotational motion:
  - **Protrusion and retrusion** (forward and backward movement) of the lower jaw: this movement takes place in the Articulatio discotemporalis and is guided through the rows of teeth. For this reason, deformities of the teeth and occlusion disorders can affect the movement in the jaw joints.
  - **Mediotrusion and laterotrusion** (medial or lateral translation): this movement is also guided by the rows of teeth. On one side the joint head turns around a vertical axis in the joint socket, while the other slides forward on the Tuberculum articulare and separates the teeth on this side.

The grinding movement takes place on the side of the rotation (working side, active side, laterotrusion side, rotation condyle, dormant condyle). The Mandibula is pushed against the upper jaw. The extent of the lateral transfer is the **BENNETT's angle,** and lies between 15° and 20° in healthy individuals. The contralateral side, which only responds to movement, is the balance side (mediotrusion side). This side is called the oscillating condyle or translational condyle.

Vascular, lymphatic and nervous systems
Arteries and veins
The temporomandibular joint is supplied with blood vessels via the following:
- A. temporalis superficialis
- A. transversa faciei
- A. auricularis profunda
- Rr. articulares (A. maxillaris)

The venous drainage occurs via corresponding veins, as well as the Plexus retroarticularis.

Innervation
The mandibular joint is sensory innervated by a multitude of nerve branches (➤ Table 9.39). In younger people, the Discus articularis is fully sensory innervated. In older people it should, however, only be innervated in areas where it is fused with the joint capsule. The Lig. laterale and the surrounding tissue are particularly finely innervated. This is the basis for the pain of the temporomandibular joint in the case of functional impairment.

Location positions of the Mandibula
In each position the Mandibula assumes a corresponding position relative to the Maxilla. The condyles are located in different positions in the joint cup:
- **Occlusion:** it describes the positional relationship between the upper and lower jaws and is the basis for functional analyses of the masticatory system. Different routes are taken into account:
  - Bite height (so-called vertical occlusion: describes the distance of the jaw position in a fully dentulous dentition in a vertical direction in the occlusion position
  - Lip closure line: describes the height of the masticatory level
  - Laughter line: corresponds to the course of the upper lip when laughing
  - Sagittal and horizontal occlusion: describes the positional relationship of upper and lower jaws in the sagittal and horizontal plane
- **Central relation:** at the central relation the lower jaw is in its most vital location relative to the skull. The joint heads are on both sides at the lowest point of the Fossa mandibularis.
- **Resting position:** in the resting position, the dental arches are unconsciously held a few millimetres apart at a distance. Both condyles and the Discus articularis lie at the rear wall of the Tuberculum articulare. The resting position is set by the tone of the masticatory muscles. If the muscles of mastication sag, e.g. during sleep, or in the case of loss of consciousness, the lower jaw drops down. The head position also affects the resting position.
- **Terminal occlusion location:** the final occlusion location (habitual intercuspidation) is the final position of the lower jaw, where the teeth are in their maximum tubercle-fossa-dentition position. The condyles are at the lowest point of the Fossa articularis. In the final occlusion location the roof of the socket is, however, only slightly loaded, because the chewing pressure is derived over the rows of teeth on the trajectories of the viscerocranium.
- **Ligament location:** in the ligament location (ligament position) the mouth is open to the maximum degree and the condyles lie behind the lowest point of the Tuberculum articulare. In doing

so, the ligaments and the joint capsule are at maximum tension, meaning that no further movements are possible.

> **Clinical remarks**
>
> The **bite height** (jaw occlusion) is of importance for the manufacture of prostheses in edentulous jaws.
> In a hyper-extension of the ligaments and the joint capsule or in the case of a flat tubercle the joint heads can slip in front of the Tuberculum articulare **(luxation)** and thus evoke a **jaw lock** (the lower jaw can no longer be adducted). A **jaw clamp** refers to a handicapped jaw opening, e.g. in the context of a retroarticular haematoma after falling or impact on the Mandibula or in the case of a parotid gland inflammation (parotitis).

9.7.5 Tongue

Overview
Functions
The tongue has a wide range of functions:
- **Transport, shaping and mechanical grinding:** during food grinding the food bolus is formed by the tongue, in that the tongue body pushes the food between the masticatory surfaces of the molars and then pushes the food bolus in the direction of the pharynx. In addition, softer food ingredients are pulverised by the pressure of the tongue against the hard palate.
- **Flavour:** in the epithelium of the dorsum of tongue, at the edge and the base of the tongue, there are numerous taste buds for taste sensation.
- **Feeling:** numerous sensitive tactile corpuscles of the tongue mucosal membrane make the tongue an extremely sensitive tactile organ, with which items in the oral cavity can be multiply enlarged in our perception.
- **Speech:** due to its very good mobility and formability thanks to the tongue muscles, the tongue significantly contributes to speech formation (phonation).

Structure of the tongue
The tongue is divided into **tongue body (Corpus linguae)** and **tongue root (Radix linguae).** Corpus linguae and Radix linguae are separated from each other by the V-shaped Sulcus terminalis, with the tip of the V in the middle of the tongue facing the Isthmus faucium. At the top of the V there is the **Foramen caecum** linguae, a rudimentary remnant of the Ductus thyroglossus (syn.: Ductus thyroglossalis), from which the Glandula thyroidea has developed. The front part of the tongue forms the tip of the tongue (**Apex linguae**). The tongue body passes seamlessly into the tip of the tongue.

Development
Roughly in der 4th embryonic week the development of the tongue unit begins in the 1st pharyngeal arch. First, 3 protrusions appear under the ectoderm of the Stomatodeum, 2 paired laterally, the Tubercula lingualia lateralia, and in the middle at the rear the Tuberculum impar. All 3 bulges merge with each other and later form the anterior two-thirds of the tongue. From the 2nd, 3rd and 4th pharyngeal arches another bulge develops behind the Tuberculum impar, the Copula, from which the tongue root emerges. The Sulcus terminalis marks the boundary between tongue body and tongue root. Between the Tuberculum impar and the Copula the Tuberculum impar is created in the middle, its epithelium constricted as a Ductus thyroglossus, grows in the neck area into the depth and

Table 9.39 Innervation of the temporomandibular joint.

Nerve	Innervation area
• N. auriculotemporalis • Rr. articulares • N. massetericus	Joint capsule lateral, dorsal, medial
• Nn. temporales profundi • N. pterygoideus lateralis, Rr. articulares	Joint capsule anterior
N. facialis [VII]	Lig. laterale
Ganglion oticum, Rr. articulares	Membrana synovialis, parasympathetic, secretory

forms the thyroid gland (Glandula thyroidea). The constriction point of the Ductus thyroglossus is marked by the Foramen caecum in adults. The tongue muscles develop in the areas of the occipital myotome of the N. hypoglossus [XII] and migrate from the dorsal side under the tongue epithelium. The development of the tongue from multiple pharyngeal arches and the occipital myotome explains the complex innervation of the tongue.

Tongue mucosa

The **tongue surface (Dorsum linguae)** passes on the **tongue margin (Margo linguae)** over to the **tongue lower surface (Facies inferior linguae)**. In the middle the tongue dorsum is divided by the **Sulcus medianus linguae** into a right and left half (➤ Fig. 9.110). The section of the dorsum of tongue in front of the **Sulcus terminalis** is referred to as Pars presulcalis (Pars anterior), the section behind the Sulcus terminalis as Pars postsulcalis (Pars posterior). The mucosa of the Dorsum linguae in the area of Pars presulcalis is covered with a variety of **tongue papillae (Papillae lingualis)**. A distinction is made between the following structures on the tongue surface:

- Mucosa
- Thread-shaped papillae, Papillae filiformes
- Mushroom-shaped papillae, Papillae fungiformes
- Leaf-shaped papillae, Papillae foliatae
- Valate papillae, Papillae vallatae

The papillae are distributed differently over the tongue. Papillae filiformes and fungiformes are mainly located on the back of the tongue. Papillae foliatae focus on the edge of the tongue, Papillae vallatae (only approx. 9-14) lie in front of the Sulcus terminalis (➤ Fig. 9.110).

Mucosa

The mucous membrane (Tunica mucosa linguae) is rough in the front section of the dorsum of the tongue and in front of the Sulcus terminalis a multilayered keratinized squamous epithelium with different degrees of keratinisation. The roughness comes from numerous small, partially macroscopically visible connective tissue papillae (Papillae linguae), which are for the touch and taste sensation. The papillae generally form a core (primary papilla), from the other small secondary pupillae. The mucosa is fixed on a rough plate of connective tissue **(Aponeurosis linguae)**, but a Tela submucosa is missing.

Tongue papillae

Papillae filiformes

The thread-shaped papillae (Papillae filiformes) are distributed over the entire dorsum of the tongue and are covered by a keratinized squamous epithelium. The tips are keratinized and point towards the throat. On the papillae there are free nerve ends, tactile corpuscles in the form of terminal clusters, non-myelinated nerve fibres and MEISSNER's tactile corpuscles which are for tactile, depth, temperature and pain perception. They enlarge felt items by a factor of 1.6 (stereognosis).

Papillae fungiformes

Mushroom papillae (Papillae fungiformes) are rare on the tongue and lie distributed between the Papillae filiformes. They can be recognised as bright red points between the Papillae filiformes. The Papillae fungiformes have a conical shaped connective tissue core from which superficial short secondary papillae radiate into the epithelium. In the periphery of the connective tissue core of the papillae there is a thick vascular plexus, which is responsible for the red colouring of the papillae. The Papillae fungiformes are covered by a multi-level keratinized squamous epithelium. In the epithelial surface a few taste buds are stored. There are also numerous mechanoreceptors and thermal receptors and free nerve endings in the connective tissue. Thus the fungal papillae are for taste perception as well as thermal and mechanoreceptors.

Papillae foliatae

Foliate papillae (Papillae foliatae) are located on the rear side of the tongue and run vertically from the tongue dorsum to the base of

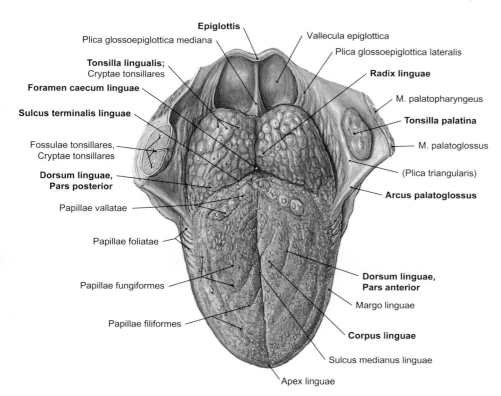

Fig. 9.110 Tongue, Lingua.
Superior view.

the tongue. They are covered by multilayered keratinized squamous epithelium; in their lateral folds there are taste buds. On the floor of the folds excretory ducts from serous VON-EBNER's glands confluence. The glands lie in the Lamina propria under the epithelium.

Papillae vallatae

On the front edge of the Sulcus terminalis there are approximately 9–14 valate papillae (Papillae vallatae). They consist of a wide papillary body that is surrounded by a deep circular walled trench. At the floor of the walled trench the excretory ducts of serous glands (Glandulae gustatoriae, VON-EBNER's glands) open. The papillary body is covered by a slightly keratinised squamous epithelium and is located on the level of the tongue surface. In the epithelium of the walls of the wall trench there are numerous taste buds on both sides.

NOTE
- Papillae filiformes: touch, depth, temperature and pain perception
- Fungiform papillae: taste sensation, thermal and mechanoreception
- Papillae foliatae: taste perception
- Papillae vallatae: taste perception

Taste buds

All **taste buds (Caliculi gustatorii)** together form the **taste organ (Organum gustus).** The taste buds are located in the epithelium of the Papillae vallatae, Papillae fungiformes and Papillae foliatae. In infants and children there are also taste buds on the laryngeal entrance and the oesophageal entrance, which slowly recede in the course of life. The taste buds consist of onion skin-like arranged sensory cells and support cells. The basal cell pole of sensory cells is attached to the basal membrane. The apical cell pole ends at the taste pore and has long microvilli. The basal section of the sensory cells is connected with the taste buds via synapses. It is assumed that the supporting cells are for the regeneration of the taste cells. Via the taste buds we perceive 5 taste qualities: **sweet, sour, salty, bitter** and **umami** (hearty). Recent findings assume that there is still another 6th taste quality **(greasy).**

Tongue inferior surface

The tongue inferior surface is covered by a smooth, multi-level non-keratinised, very thin squamous epithelium. The mucosa is located directly on the Lamina propria, a Tela submucosa is not present. In the midline is the mucosa to the tongue frenulum **(Frenulum linguae).** 2 serrated mucosal folds also run on the right and left from the tongue edge to the tip of the tongue **(Plicae fimbriatae).** Laterally on the underside of the tongue tip the excretory ducts of the Glandulae linguales anteriores empty (BLANDIN-NUHN glands). The two seromucous salivary glands lie between the muscles of the tongue tip. On both sides of the base of the fren-

ulum the joint excretory duct (Ductus submandibularis, WHARTON's duct) the Glandulae submandibularis and sublingualis confluence at the **Caruncula sublingualis.**

NOTE
Under the tongue there is a subepithelial vein network in the Lamina propria. Here, sublingually applied drugs are rapidly absorbed (e.g. nitroglycerin for angina pectoris).

Tongue root

Behind the Sulcus terminalis, lies the **tongue root (Radix linguae)** with the **tongue tonsil (Tonsilla lingualis),** which is part of WALDEYER's tonsillar ring. The base of the tongue is covered by multi-layered keratinised squamous epithelium and has in relation to the palatine tonsil (Tonsilla palatina) low, widely spaced crypts. In the crypts the excretory ducts of the mucous **Glandulae linguales** meet. On the tongue root the unpaired **Plica glossoepiglottica mediana** and the paired **Plicae glossoepiglotticae laterales** to the epiglottis originate and limit the intervening pits **(Valleculae epiglotticae).**

Clinical remarks

Tongue injuries are common from **scalding or chemical burns**. Especially in the case of pipe smoking, potential **precancerous** cells occur at the tongue base as hyperkeratoses or leucoplakias.
The term **glossitis** includes acute and chronic diseases or changes in the tongue surface and/or the tongue body, which could have very different causes, such as bacterial and viral infections, fungal infestation, toxic effects (smoking, alcohol), iron deficiency, and many more. If swallowed, **foreign bodies** can pass to the Valleculae epiglotticae at the base of the tongue and relocate the airway by pressure on the epiglottis. There is a danger of asphyxiation.

Tongue muscles

A difference is made between **intrinsic (own) muscles** and **extrinsic muscles,** which originate from the skeleton. Extrinsic muscles change the location, intrinsic muscles the shape of the tongue. A large part of the tongue muscles are anchored at the Aponeurosis linguae. In the midline the Septum linguae divides the tongue incompletely into two halves. The development of the tongue muscles is individually just as diverse as the movement options.

Intrinsic muscles

The intrinsic muscles have their origin and attachment in the tongue (➤ Table 9.40). They stand in the 3 planes perpendicular to each other and are interwoven. Functionally they enable chewing, talking, singing, sucking or whistling.

Table 9.40 Intrinsic muscles of the tongue.

Innervation	Origin	Attachment	Function
M. longitudinalis superior			
N. hypoglossus [XII]	Aponeurosis linguae	Aponeurosis linguae	Curvature of the tongue downwards
M. transversus linguae			
N. hypoglossus [XII]	Aponeurosis linguae of the tongue edge	Septum linguae	Tongue extension
M. verticalis linguae			
N. hypoglossus [XII]	Aponeurosis linguae of the superior surface of the tongue	Aponeurosis linguae of the inferior surface of the tongue	Flattening of the tongue and groove formation in the dorsum of the tongue

Table 9.41 Extrinsic tongue muscles.

Innervation	Origin	Attachment	Function
M. genioglossus			
N. hypoglossus [XII]	Spina mentalis	Corpus linguae	Management of the dorsum of tongue and the tongue base to the front, extension of the tongue
M. styloglossus			
N. hypoglossus [XII]	Proc. styloideus	Margo linguae to the Apex linguae	Withdrawal of the Corpus linguae
M. hyoglossus			
N. hypoglossus [XII]	• Os hyoideum, Cornu majus (M. ceratoglossus) • Os hyoideum, Cornu minus (M. chondroglossus)	Corpus linguae	Rotation of the tongue and flattening of the rear section of the tongue
M. palatoglossus			
N. glossopharyngeus [IX] and N. vagus [X]; R. pharyngeus	Rear section of the M. transversus linguae	Aponeurosis palatina	Closure of the Isthmus faucium, lowering of the velum

Table 9.42 Innervation of the tongue.

Nerve	Quality	Areas innervated
N. lingualis (branch from [V/3])	Sensible	Front ⅔ of the tongue
N. glossopharyngeus [IX]	Sensible Sensory	Posterior ⅓ of the tongue Papillae foliatae and vallatae
N. vagus [X] N. laryngeus superior (branch from [X])	Sensible Sensory	Transition to the epiglottis
Chorda tympani (branch of the intermedius part from [VII])	Sensory parasympathetic	• Papillae fungiformes • Glandula submandibularis, Glandula sublingualis, salivary glands of the oral mucosa
N. hypoglossus [XII]	Motor	All of the tongue muscles with the exception of the M. palatoglossus
Plexus pharyngeus (branches of [IX and X])	Motor	M. palatoglossus

Extrinsic tongue muscles

The extrinsic tongue muscles are all paired and radiate from outside into the tongue (➤ Table 9.41).

> ### Clinical remarks
>
> In deep unconsciousness the N. genioglossus sags and the tongue sinks back into the pharynx in the supine position and can relocate the airway. For this reason, unconscious people always have to be positioned in the stable **recovery position** as quickly as possible.

Vascular, lymphatic and nervous systems
Arteries and veins

The tongue is supplied with blood via the **A. lingualis** from the A. carotis externa. The A. lingualis passes via the rear edge of the Diaphragma oris medial to the N. hypoglossus and under the M. hyoglossus into the Corpus linguae and divides it into its terminal branches:

- **A. profunda linguae** (Main branch): runs to the tip of the tongue (Fig. 10.17)
- **Rr. dorsales linguae:** supply the base of the tongue and emit small branches to the Tonsilla palatina

- **A. sublingualis:** supplies the Glandula sublingualis and mucous membranes of the mouth floor

The arteries are accompanied by veins of the same name. The **V. lingualis** discharges the blood in the V. facialis to the V. jugularis interna.

Lymph vessels

The regional lymph nodes of the tongue are:
- **Nodi lymphoidei submandibulares**
- **Nodi lymphoidei submentales**
- **Nodus jugulodigastricus** (from the tongue root)

From here, the lymph is drained into the deep cervical lymph nodes (Nodi lymphoidei cervicales profundi) (also ➤ Chap. 9.7.8).

> ### Clinical remarks
>
> The A. sublingualis runs relatively superficially along the edge of the Corpus mandibulae. On surgical removal of molars or the preparation of the jaw crest for bone augmentation, care must be taken to ensure that the **A. sublingualis** is not injured when exposing the jaw.

Innervation of the tongue

The tongue has a complex innervation due to its development (➤ Table 9.42).

Sensible
- Anterior two thirds: the **N. lingualis** (branch from [V/3]) runs into the Spatium infratemporale and runs from dorsal to the M. constrictor pharyngis superior and the M. hyoglossus lying laterally in the tongue.
- Rear third: the **N. glossopharyngeus [IX]** lies on the M. stylopharyngeus and runs from dorsal under the M. hyoglossus into the base of the tongue. The mucosa at the transition to the epiglottis is innervated by the N. laryngeus superior (a branch of [X]).

Sensory

The **Chorda tympani** is responsible for sensory innervation of the anterior two thirds (branch from [VII]), the **N. glossopharyngeus [IX]** is responsible for the rear third. The Chorda tympani radiates from dorsal in the Spatium infratemporale into the N. lingualis and

519

continues with it to the tongue. The Papillae vallatae and foliatae of the tongue are sensory innervated via the N. glossopharyngeus [IX]. The branches of the taste buds in the transition area to the epiglottis partly join to the N. vagus.

Parasympathetic

The parasympathetic fibres for the Glandula submandibularis and the Glandula sublingualis run as preganglionic fibres with the **Chorda tympani** into the N. lingualis and branch from here to the **Ganglion submandibulare**, where they are switched to being postganglionic. The fibres then run with the terminal branches of the N. lingualis to the Glandula sublingualis or from the ganglion directly into the Glandula submandibular.

Motor

With the exception of the M. palatoglossus, all the tongue muscles are innervated by the **N. hypoglossus [XII]**. The M. palatoglossus gets its fibres from the Plexus pharyngeus (branches from [IX] and [X]).

Clinical remarks

Injuries of the N. hypoglossus [XII] lead to the tongue diverging to the affected side when extended; in the process, there is muscle atrophy on this side.

9.7.6 Palate

Development

From an evolutionary viewpoint, the palate is developed from 3 palatal processes. In the forehead bulge the unpaired primary palate emerges, which extends from horizontal to dorsal. In the maxillary bulges the two palatal bulges form on the left and right side, which initially grow around from cranial to caudal on the side edges of the tongue. Roughly in the *7th embryonic week* the floor of the mouth sinks, whereby the palatal processes rest on the tongue and reorientate in a horizontal direction. Then they grow as far medially until they touch in the midline and fuse with the vomer which is growing from top to bottom. The merger process begins between the primary palate and the palatal processes and continues gradually dorsally to the rear edge of the palate (➤ Fig. 9.111). It is completed approximately in the *12th week*. The epithelium wall lying between the palate processes (HOCHSTETTER's epithelial wall) recedes, so that a connective tissue bridge is formed and the closure of the palate is completed.

Clinical remarks

If the palatal processes do not fuse with each other, the result is a variety of cleft formations **(cleft lip and palate)**. A distinction is made between **cleft upper lip**, which is always created on the side and can be attributed to a lack of closure be-

tween the medial nasal process and maxillary bulge. It can also lead to the formation of **cleft jaw**, which occurs between the primary palatal processes and the palatal bulges and can be attributed to a non-fusion of the primary palate with the secondary palatal bulges. They run distally from the second upper incisors to the Foramen incisivum. Finally, **cleft palates** emerge in the middle of the palate, in which the secondary palatal plates do not fuse together and lead to a connection between the oral and nasal cavities either on both sides or only on one side. Between the different characteristics of the clefts, there are numerous combinations and degrees of severity. Lip, jaw and palate malformations are the most common developmental disorders in humans. The form known colloquially as a 'hare-lip' is a one or two-sided fissure formation on the upper lip. The mildest form is a split uvula. **(Uvula bifida.)** Not all clefts are of genetic origin, but can also be traced back to a folic acid deficiency of the mother during pregnancy.

Hard and soft palate

The palate forms the roof of the oral cavity and the floor of the nasal cavity. It is divided into the hard palate (**Palatum durum**) and the soft palate (**Palatum molle**). Functionally the hard palate contributes to the phonation of consonants and serves as an abutment for the tongue when crushing food. The soft palate blocks off the nasopharynx from the oropharynx during swallowing (➤ Chap. 10.7.6) by folding back onto the posterior pharyngeal wall.

Hard palate

The hard palate (Palatum durum) is a domed bony plate and consists of the Proc. palatinus of the Maxilla and the Lamina horizontalis of the Os palatinum. The bony plates meet in the middle in the **Sutura palatina mediana**. At the back the Lamina horizontalis is connected via the **Sutura palatina transversa** with the Proc. palatinus. The hard palate is penetrated at the front by the Foramen incisivum and at the back by the paired Foramen palatinum majus and the paired Foramina palatina minora.

Soft palate

The **soft palate (Palatum molle)** attaches onto the back of the hard palate and during the inspection of the oral cavity can be distinguished from the hard palate by the so-called A line. The basis of the Palatum molle is formed by a horizontal plate of connective tissue (**Aponeurosis palatina**), which radiates into the 5 muscles (➤ Table 9.43). The Aponeurosis goes back into the fibromuscular posterior edge of the soft palate, on which the uvula (Uvula palatina) sits. Laterally, 2 folds radiate into the uvula on each side, the front and the rear palatal arch (Arcus palatoglossus and Arcus palatopharyngeus).

Isthmus faucium

The **palatal arches (Arcus palati)** each enclose a pit (Fossa tonsillaris) in which the palatine tonsil (Tonsilla palatina) is located. There is a small triangular depression over the Tonsilla palatina (Fossa supratonsillaris).

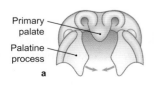
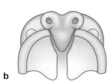
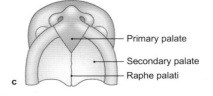

Fig. 9.111 Development of the palate, separation of the nose and throat area. a 7th week. **b** 8th week. **c** 10th week. [E838]

Primary palate · Palatine process · Primary palate · Secondary palate · Raphe palati

- The **anterior palatal arch (Arcus palatoglossus)** radiates into the lateral margin of the tongue. Its free medial border can easily cover the Tonsilla palatina. It is elevated by the M. palatoglossus.
- The **posterior palatal arch (Arcus palatopharyngeus)** radiates from behind into the pharyngeal wall. It is elevated by the M. palatopharyngeus.

The palatal arches together with the soft palate and the base of the tongue form the **pharyngeal isthmus (Isthmus faucium)** (> Fig. 9.112) and make the transition to the oropharynx.

Clinical remarks

About 60 % of men and 40 % of women over the age of 40 years snore on a regular basis. In children, it is only 10 %. **Snoring** (compensated snoring) is to a lesser extent normal and does not have any value as a disease. The soft palate generally flutters when it is relaxed during sleep. The clinicians call snoring **(ronchopathy)** a loud rattling noise, which is created in the upper respiratory system and leads to a reduced supply of oxygen and subsequently to sleep disorders. This is known as obstructive snoring.

If you touch the base of the tongue, the palatal arch or the rear wall of the pharynx, the **swallowing or gag reflex** is generally triggered. The muscles of the tongue, the throat, the larynx and the oesophagus are involved in the reflexes.

Allergic reactions can result in a life-threatening swelling of the mucosal lining of the soft palate.

Inflammation in the area of the soft palate is usually associated with severe difficulty in swallowing.

Circulatory disorders of the brain stem occur at an advanced age in many people. If they affect the catchment area of the A. vertebralis, they are often associated with paralysis of the palatal muscles on the affected side, the result is swallowing and tube ventilation disorders. This can lead to soft palate parese (damage to the core areas of the N. glossopharyngeus [IX] and N. vagus [X]). Due to paralysis of the M. levator veli palatini, the soft palate may hang down on the affected side and the uvula is shifted to the healthy side.

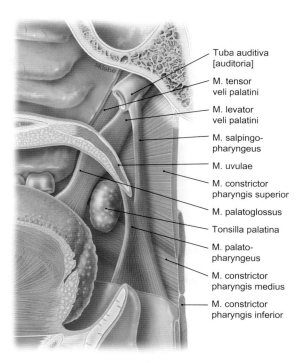

Fig. 9.112 **Muscular base of the Isthmus faucium and the muscles of the soft palate, as well as the pharynx.**

Palatal mucosa

The palatal mucosa consists of multilevel keratinised squamous epithelium. It cannot be moved on the hard palate, but can be moved on the soft palate. The hard palate is well perfused. Hundreds of **small salivary glands (Glandulae palatinae,** > Fig. 9.114) are located in the mucosa. Laterally, the mucous membrane runs to the front and side into the gingiva. In the midline, the mucosa is elevated to the **Raphe palati.** In the front part of the hard palate there are numerous transverse ridges (palatal graduations, Rugae palatinae) which serve the fixation and disintegration of food components. On the side facing the nose the soft palate is covered by

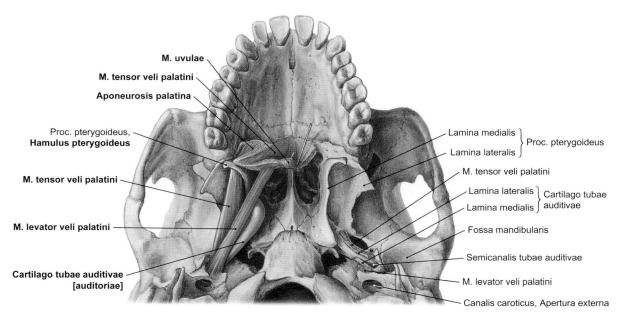

Fig. 9.113 **M. levator veli palatini, M. tensor veli palatini and cartilage of the pharyngotympanic tube, Cartilago tubae auditivae.**

multiple rows of ciliated epithelium, on the oral cavity side by multilayered squamous epithelium.

Palatal muscles

The Aponeurosis palatina forms the connective tissue anchor for 4 paired muscles and the unpaired M. uvulae (➤ Fig. 9.112, ➤ Fig. 9.113, ➤ Table 9.43).

The **M. tensor veli palatini** runs from the Lamina medialis of the Proc. pterygoideuss forwards below and then bends around the Hamulus pterygoideus, to horizontally radiate into the Aponeurosis palatina. The **M. levator veli palatini** crosses under the Tuba auditiva medially below on its way from the outside of the Os tem-

porale. On contraction it raises and opens the Ostium tubae auditivae.

Vascular, lymphatic and nervous systems

Arteries and veins

The arterial supply (➤ Fig. 9.114) is carried out by:

- **A. palatina descendens** (terminal branch of the A. maxillaris): it comes from the Fossa pterygopalatina via the Canalis palatinus major and the Foramen palatinum majus and reaches the mucosa at the transition from the hard to soft palate.
- **A. palatina major:** it originates from the A. palatina descendens and after penetrating the Foramen palatinum majus runs into

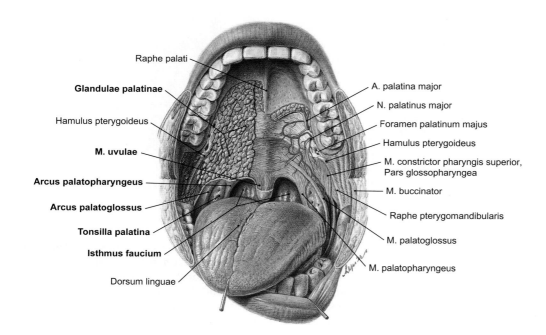

Fig. 9.114 Oral cavity, Cavitas oris, and palatal muscles, Mm. palati. Anterior view.

Table 9.43 Muscles of the soft palate.

Innervation	Origin	Attachment	Function
M. levator veli palatini			
Plexus pharyngeus (branches of [IX] and [X]), sometimes also the N. facialis [VII]	Facies inferior of the Pars petrosa of the Os temporale and Cartilago tubae auditivae	Aponeurosis palatina	Tenses and raises the soft palate, opens the Tuba auditiva and closes the nasopharyngeal space together with the M. constrictor pharyngis superior, bulges out the levator bulge of the pharyngeal wall
M. tensor veli palatini			
N. tensor veli palatini (from [V/3])	Lamina medialis of the Proc. pterygoideus, Ala major of the Os sphenoidale, Lamina membranacea of the Tuba auditiva, it bends horizontally around the Hamulus pterygoideus	Aponeurosis palatina	Tenses the soft palate, opens the Tuba auditiva and deforms the palate for articulation
M. palatopharyngeus			
Plexus pharyngeus (branches from [IX])	Aponeurosis palatina, Hamulus pterygoideus and Lamina medialis of the Proc. pterygoideus	Lateral pharyngeal wall and rear edge of the Cartilago thyroidea, base of Arcus palatoglossus	Elevates the pharynx, base of the Arcus palatopharyngeus
M. palatoglossus			
Plexus pharyngeus (branches from [IX] and [X])	Dorsal separation from M. transversus linguae	Aponeurosis palatina	Closes the Isthmus faucium, sinks the soft palate, base of the Arcus palatoglossus
M. uvulae			
Plexus pharyngeus (branches from [IX] and [X])	Aponeurosis palatina	Mucosa of the uvula	Shortens the uvula

the palatal mucosa forward to the Foramen incisivum, where it establishes contact with the A. nasopalatina of the A. sphenopalatina via the Canalis incisivus.

- **Aa. palatinae minores:** they originate from the A. palatina descendens and after passing through the Canalis palatinus and the Foramina palatina minora run to the back to the soft palate and to the adjacent structures.
- **A. palatina ascendens** (from the A. facialis) for the soft palate and the palatal arches.
- **A. pharyngea ascendens** (from the A. carotis externa) for the soft palate and the palatal arches.

The venous blood is transported in the **Plexus pterygoideus** in the Fossa infratemporalis.

Blood supply of the Tonsilla palatina

Together with the Tonsilla lingualis in the base of the tongue, the Tonsilla palatina belongs to WALDEYER's tonsillar ring (➤ Chap. 10.7.7). The Tonsilla palatina has a highly differentiated vascular supply (➤ Fig. 9.115, ➤ Table 9.44).

Clinical remarks

Tonsillitis is a highly painful inflammation of the Tonsillae palatinae. It is contagious and can be transmitted by aerosol infection. The main cause of acute tonsillitis are usually *Streptococci*. Tonsillitis is one of the 20 most common diseases in general medicine.

In the case of surgical removal of the Tonsilla palatina **(tonsillectomy)** the danger of postoperative bleeding is relatively large and feared due to the large number of arteries. If there is a so-called **dangerous carotid loop** (course variant of the Pars cervicalis of the A. carotis interna in relation to the rear pharyngeal wall), due to the close relationship of the A. carotis interna and the tonsil bed (location of the Tonsilla palatina at the posterior margin of the Isthmus faucium) within the framework of a tonsillectomy or when opening a peritonsillar abcess the A. carotis interna may be damaged and this may lead to a fatal bleeding.

Table 9.44 Vascular supply to the Tonsilla palatina.

Supplying artery	Terminal branch
A. lingualis	Rr. dorsales linguae
A. palatina ascendens	Rr. tonsillares
A. pharyngea ascendens	Rr. pharyngeales with Rr. tonsillares
A. palatina descendens	R. pharyngeus with Rr. tonsillares

Lymph vessels

The lymph enters regional **Nodi lymphoidei cervicales profundi** (also ➤ Chap. 9.7.8).

Innervation

It follows via (➤ Fig. 9.116):

- Terminal branches of the N. nasopalatinus: palatal mucosa and gingiva in the area of the front teeth (the N. nasopalatinus passes through the Foramen incisivum to the hard palate)
- N. palatinus major: gingiva and mucous membranes in the side tooth region (the N. palatinus major runs on both sides through the Foramen palatinum majus to the palate)
- Nn. palatini minores: mucosa of the soft palate (they pass through the Foramina palatina minora of the same name to the soft palate)

Clinical remarks

The N. palatinus major at the Foramen palatinum majus can be blocked by **conduction anaesthesia**. This attains freedom from pain in the palatal gingiva in the posterior region. Freedom from pain in the palatal gingiva of the front teeth is achieved by conduction anaesthesia of the N. nasopalatinus at the Foramen incisivum.

Innervation of the Tonsilla palatina

The innervation of the tonsil bed takes place via the Rr. tonsillares of the Nn. palatini minores and the N. glossopharyngeus [IX].

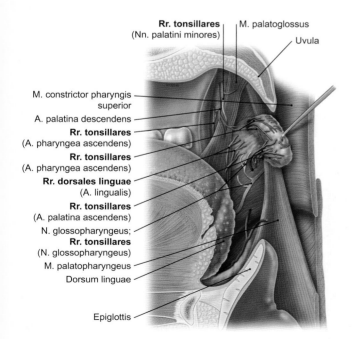

Fig. 9.115 Vascular supply to the Tonsilla palatina.

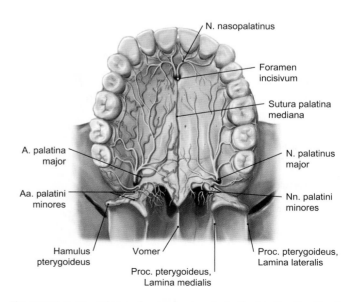

Fig. 9.116 Innervation and vascular supply to the hard and soft palate. [L266]

9.7.7 Floor of the mouth

The **floor of the mouth (Diaphragma oris)** consists of several muscles, which are stretched between the Corpus mandibulae and the Os hyoideum (➤ Fig. 9.117) (➤ Fig. 9.117–➤ Fig. 9.119). The central element of the Diaphragma oris are the two **Mm. mylohyoidei,** which are connected in the midline via the connective tissue Raphe mylohyoidea (➤ Fig. 9.118, ➤ Fig. 9.119). In addition the **Mm. geniohyoidei, digastrici and stylohyoidei** are involved in the formation of the floor of the mouth. All muscles are directly or indirectly connected with the hyoid bone (Os hyoideum, see ➤ Chap. 10.2.1) and are referred to as Mm. suprahyoidei or suprahyoid muscles (➤ Fig. 9.118, ➤ Fig. 9.119, ➤ Table 9.45). The floor of the mouth of the tongue functionally serves as an abutment.

Hyoid bone

The **hyoid bone (Os hyoideum)** is a U-shaped bone on the floor of the mouth (➤ Fig. 9.117). Since it is not connected with the rest of the skeleton, but is only suspended via muscles and ligaments, it is usually missing in the human skeletons used in training. Embryologically it consists of the cartilage of the 2nd and 3rd pharyngeal arches. 2 pairs of horns sit laterally on the body **(Corpus hyoidei).** The large horn **(Cornu majus)** is connected to the larynx via the Membrana thyrohyoidea and its reinforcements (➤ Chap. 10.2.1) and dorsally, the small horn **(Cornu minus)** is connected via the **Lig. stylohyoideum** with the Proc. styloideus of the temporal bone.

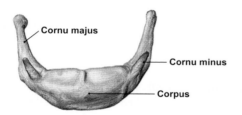

Fig. 9.117 Hyoid bone, Os hyoideum. Frontal view from above

Muscles of the floor of the mouth

The muscles of the floor of the mouth and the Venter posterior of the M. digastricus or the M. stylohyoideus (which do not belong to the muscles of the floor of the mouth) are presented in ➤ Table 9.45.

Compartments of the floor of the mouth

Between the muscles of the floor of the mouth, connective tissue gap spaces form, which are referred to as compartments of the floor of the mouth (➤ Fig. 9.120):

- The **Spatium parapharyngeum** continues between the M. genioglossus and the M. geniohyoideus in its **anterior part.** It contains the A. lingualis and the V. lingualis.
- The **Spatium sublinguale** extends between the M. geniohyoideus and the M. mylohyoideus. Medial to the Glandula sublingualis is the N. lingualis.
- Under the M. mylohyoideus covered by the platysma, is the **Spatium submandibulare** with the Glandula submandibularis.

Each of the three oral floor compartments is connected dorsally to the neurovascular cord of the neck.

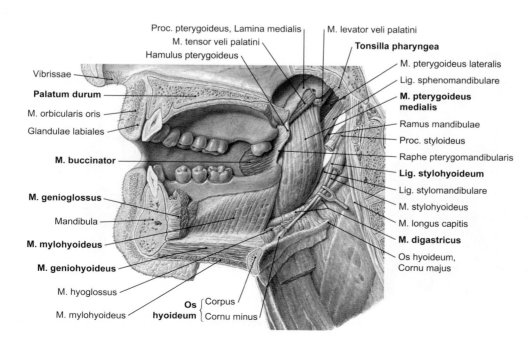

Proc. pterygoideus, Lamina medialis
M. tensor veli palatini
Hamulus pterygoideus
Vibrissae
Palatum durum
M. orbicularis oris
Glandulae labiales
M. buccinator
M. genioglossus
Mandibula
M. mylohyoideus
M. geniohyoideus
M. hyoglossus
M. mylohyoideus
Os hyoideum { Corpus / Cornu minus
M. levator veli palatini
Tonsilla pharyngea
M. pterygoideus lateralis
Lig. sphenomandibulare
M. pterygoideus medialis
Ramus mandibulae
Proc. styloideus
Raphe pterygomandibularis
Lig. stylohyoideum
Lig. stylomandibulare
M. stylohyoideus
M. longus capitis
M. digastricus
Os hyoideum, Cornu majus

Fig. 9.118 Oral cavity, Cavitas oris, with presentation of the Diaphragma oris.

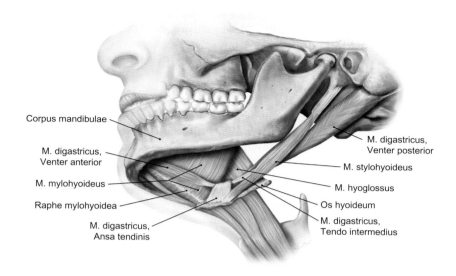

Corpus mandibulae

M. digastricus,
Venter anterior

M. mylohyoideus

Raphe mylohyoidea

M. digastricus,
Ansa tendinis

M. digastricus,
Venter posterior

M. stylohyoideus

M. hyoglossus

Os hyoideum

M. digastricus,
Tendo intermedius

Fig. 9.119 Muscles of the floor of the mouth. Lateral view from below.

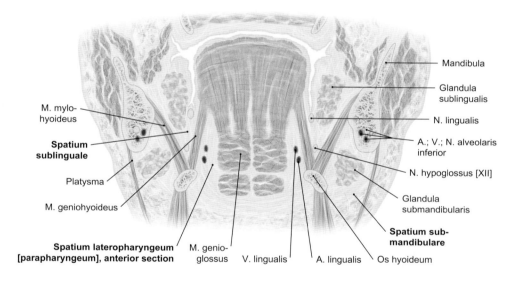

M. mylo-
hyoideus

**Spatium
sublinguale**

Platysma

M. geniohyoideus

**Spatium lateropharyngeum
[parapharyngeum], anterior section**

M. genio-
glossus

V. lingualis

A. lingualis

Os hyoideum

Mandibula

Glandula
sublingualis

N. lingualis

A.; V.; N. alveolaris
inferior

N. hypoglossus [XII]

Glandula
submandibularis

**Spatium sub-
mandibulare**

Fig. 9.120 Horizontal section through the musculature of the floor of the mouth in the area of the Os hyoideum with presentation of the compartments of the floor of the mouth. [L127]

Table 9.45 Suprahyoid muscles.

Innervation	Origin	Attachment	Function
M. mylohyoideus			
N. mylohyoideus (branch from [V/3])	Caudal to Linea mylohyoidea, medial to Raphe mylohyoidea	Hyoid bone and Raphe mylohyoidea	Elevation of the floor of the mouth during swallowing
M. geniohyoideus			
N. hypoglossus [XII], Plexus cervicalis (C1, C2)	Spina mentalis	Os hyoideum	In the case of fixation of the Os hyoideum by the Venter posterior of the M. digastricus and the M. stylohyoideus, opening of the mouth in fixation of the lower jaw by the masticatory muscles, lifting of the larynx
M. digastricus, Venter anterior			
N. mylohyoideus (branch from [V/3])	Fossa digastrica of the Mandibula	Intermediate tendon of the M. digastricus at the Os hyoideum	Elevation of the floor of the mouth during swallowing
M. digastricus, Venter posterior (not a muscle of the floor of the mouth)			
N. facialis [VII], R. digastricus	Incisura mastoidea medial of the mastoid process	Intermediate tendon at the Os hyoideum	Fixation of the hyoid bone, lifting the larynx
M. stylohyoideus (not a muscle of the floor of the mouth)			
N. facialis [VII], R. stylohyoideus	Proc. stylohyoideus	Corpus and Cornu majus of the Os hyoideum	Raises the hyoid bone upwards and backwards during swallowing

9.7.8 Lymphatic pathways of the oral cavity

The lymph from the oral cavity (➤ Fig. 9.121, ➤ Table 9.46) collects on both sides in the Truncus jugularis, which extends together with the A. carotis communis and the V. jugularis interna to the V. subclavia.

> **Clinical remarks**
>
> **Inflammatory processes** in the lower jaw area often lead to a swelling of the submental and submandibular lymph nodes. They are then palpable under the chin or in the Trigonum submandibulare. **Carcinomas of the floor of the mouth** metastasise in the submandibular lymph nodes, in contrast **carcinomas of the base of the tongue** metastasise to the Nodi lymphoidei cervicales profundi.

9.7.9 Salivary glands

The excretory ducts of the 3 paired large salivary glands as well as various small salivary glands flow into the oral cavity which, in their entirety, are summarised as Glandulae salivariae oris:

- **Major salivary glands:**
  - Parotid gland (Glandula parotidea, Parotis)
  - Saliva gland of the lower jaw (Glandula submandibularis, Submandibularis)
  - Sublingual gland (Glandula sublingualis, Sublingualis)
- **Minor salivary glands:**
  - Glandulae buccales (cheek)
  - Glandulae labiales (lips)
  - Glandulae palatinae (palate)
  - Glandulae linguales (tongue), this also includes the paired Glandula lingualis anterior (BLANDIN -NUHN gland)
  - Glandulae gingivales (gums)
  - Glandulae molares (area of the molar teeth)

The major salivary glands partly discharge via longer excretory ducts into the oral cavity.

Development

The salivary glands arise during the 6th–7th week as a solid epithelium sprouting of the ectodermal Stomatodeum.

Saliva

The oral cavity is continuously moistened by the **saliva** (daily approximately 1.5 l) which is produced in the three major and numerous minor salivary glands. The secretions of the Glandulae sublinguales and the minor salivary glands serve to moisten the mucosa of the oral cavity, the secretions of the Glandulae parotideae and submandibulares are in contrast excreted on stimulation. Saliva consists to 96 % of a liquid part and to 4 % of solid constituents. The liquid part consists of:

- Water
- Electrolytes
- Mucus components (mucines)
- Enzymes (α-amylase)
- Antimicrobial agents (e.g. IgA, lysozymes, defensins)

Solid components are sloughed epithelial cells and a number of bacteria that colonize inside the oral cavity as physiological flora. The saliva secretion is stimulated by mechanical, chemical, olfactory and psychological stimuli.

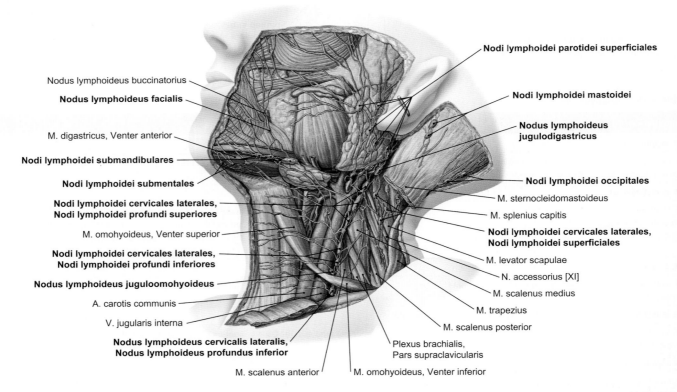

Fig. 9.121 Superficial lymph vessels, Vasa lymphatica superficialia and lymph nodes, Nodi lymphoidei of the head and throat. Lateral view.

Table 9.46 Regional lymph nodes of the oral cavity.

Lymph node group	Inflow	Outflow
Nodi lymphoidei occipitales lie on the origin of the M. trapezius at the level of the Linea nuchae	Occipital until the skull vertex, neck	Nodi lymphoidei cervicales profundi
Nodi lymphoidei retroauriculares lie on the attachment of the M. sternocleidomastoideus at the Proc. mastoideus	Back of the ear, skin at the occiput	Nodi lymphoidei cervicales profundi
Nodi lymphoidei parotidei lie on the Glandula parotidea in front of the outer ear canal	Forehead, temples, lateral part of the eyelids, nose root, outer ear, outer ear canal, tympanic membrane, Tuba auditiva, Glandula parotidea, nasopharyngeal space	Nodi lymphoidei cervicales profundi
Nodi lymphoidei submandibulares lie in the Spatium submandibulare	Split flow: • Superficial: middle of the forehead and eyelids, outer nose, upper lip and cheek • Deep: tip of the tongue, anterior palatal section and oral cavity, teeth, gingiva, Vestibulum nasi, Fossa infratemporalis In addition, they receive inflow from the Nodi lymphoidei faciales and submentales	Nodi lymphoidei cervicales superficiales and profundi
Nodi lymphoidei submentales lie laterally under the Mandibula in the Trigonum submentale	Chin and the middle of the lower lip, lower jaw incisors and gingiva, tongue tip and the floor of the mouth	• Nodi lymphoidei submandibulares • Nodi lymphoidei cervicales profundi and superficiales
Nodi lymphoidei buccales lie in the region of the cheek	Rear Cavitas nasi and oral cavity and tongue base – Fossa pterygoidea and infratemporal palate and pharynx	Nodi lymphoidei cervicales profundi

---

Clinical remarks

For the protection of the teeth they are covered by a largely bacteria-free, thin biofilm, the **pellicle,**. The pellicle consists of the organic components of the saliva and protects the enamel from abrasion and acids in food components; however, various bacteria can become attached and form the basis for the dental plaque (plaque, pathogenic bacterial biofilm). By brushing your teeth, the pellicle is removed and needs several minutes to form again from the saliva. Regular intake of food containing acids (e.g. apples) shortly before brushing can lead to damage to the enamel because brushing the teeth removes the pellicle, but not the entire acid of the saliva in the oral cavity, which then attacks the teeth. If minerals are deposited (calcium deposits) in the plaque, **calculus occurs.**

Parotid gland

The **Glandula parotidea** is situated in the Regio parotideomasseterica and is sheathed by a tough fascia (**Fascia parotidea**) which limits the parotid gland compartment. At the posterior margin of the Ramus mandibulae the Fascia masseterica divides into a superficial and a deep layer. The deep layer medially limits the Spatium parapharyngeum (➤ Fig. 9.122), the superficial layer lies close to the gland as the Fascia parotidea. At the front, the Glandula parotidea lies on the M. masseter, cranially it extends up to the Arcus zygomaticus, at the back it borders on the external auditory canal, the Tragus and the Proc. mastoideus, caudally it covers the upper part of the M. sternocleidomastoideus. The largest part of the gland lies behind the Ramus mandibulae and extends medially to the M. pterygoideus medialis and the Proc. styloideus (➤ Fig. 9.122). The excretory duct (**Ductus parotideus,** STENSEN's duct) runs over the M. masseter, penetrates the M. buccinator and flows into the **Papilla parotidea,** opposite the 2nd upper molars. Often, the Ductus parotideus is surrounded by widely dispersed glandular tissue. These glandular parts are referred to as **Glandulae parotideae accessoriae.**

The N. facialis [VII] radiates from the dorsal side into the gland and forms the Plexus parotideus within the gland. Through the Plexus parotideus, the gland is divided into a **Pars superficialis** and a **Pars profunda.** In the retromandibular section of the Glandula parotidea lie the A. carotis externa, the V. retromandibularis, the N. auriculotemporalis and the stem of the N. facialis [VII]. The A. transversa faciei and the Ductus parotideus, which leave the gland toward the anterior section.

Clinical remarks

On the outside, the parotid gland compartment is tightly bordered by the close-fitting Fascia parotidea, so inflammation and tumours can only spread with difficulty. **Inflammatory processes (parotitis)** spread medially into the Spatium parapharyngeum. On the other hand, infections of the tonsils can break through into the Spatium parapharyngeum. Above the A. carotis externa and the V. retromandibularis, there is a connection to the neurovascular cord of the neck to the mediastinum. **Suppurative processes in the parotid gland compartment** or the Spatium parapharyngeum can therefore spread to the mediastinum.

Parotid tumours often require operative treatment. In the process, sympathetic and parasympathetic nerve fibres within the glandular tissue are severed. In the context of the subsequent recovery parasympathetic fibres can connect to formerly sympathetically innervated sweat glands of the skin above the parotid gland and lead to **gustatory sweating (FREY's syndrome).** This is possible because the neurotransmitter on the postganglionic synapses of both sympathetic and parasympathetic nerves is acetylcholine. Each time when the parasympathetic system is now activated, e.g. when the affected person is hungry and sees something to eat, the sweat glands are activated with perspiration formation on the cheek.

Malignant **parotid gland tumours** can lead to peripheral facial palsy; benign tumours do not normally do this.

Mumps (Parotitis epidemica) is an acute systemic viral disease (mostly in childhood), which causes severe swelling of the gland within the parotid gland fascia. This is extremely painful for those affected.

SJÖGREN's syndrome is a chronic inflammation of the glands of the head and throat area region, but particularly the salivary glands. A distinction is made between primary and secondary SJÖGREN's syndrome. At the forefront of the disease is a Sicca symptomatic, including the dryness of oral (**xerostomia**) and eye surfaces (**xerophthalmia**). The salivary glands, in particular the Glandula parotidea, may be swollen.

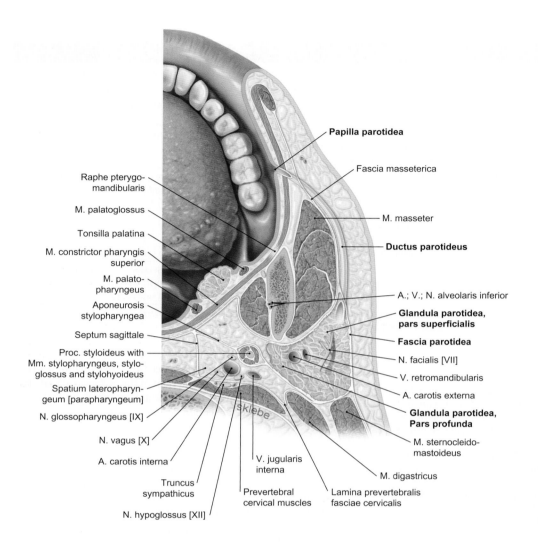

Papilla parotidea

Fascia masseterica

M. masseter

Ductus parotideus

Raphe pterygo-mandibularis

M. palatoglossus

Tonsilla palatina

M. constrictor pharyngis superior

M. palato-pharyngeus

Aponeurosis stylopharyngea

Septum sagittale

Proc. styloideus with Mm. stylopharyngeus, stylo-glossus and stylohyoideus

Spatium lateropharyn-geum [parapharyngeum]

N. glossopharyngeus [IX]

N. vagus [X]

A. carotis interna

Truncus sympathicus

N. hypoglossus [XII]

V. jugularis interna

Prevertebral cervical muscles

Lamina prevertebralis fasciae cervicalis

M. digastricus

A.; V.; N. alveolaris inferior

Glandula parotidea, pars superficialis

Fascia parotidea

N. facialis [VII]

V. retromandibularis

A. carotis externa

Glandula parotidea, Pars profunda

M. sternocleido-mastoideus

Fig. 9.122 Section preparation through the parotid gland compartment at the level of the Foramen mandibulae with presentation of the fascia of the parotid gland compartment. [L238]

Submandibular gland

The **Glandula submandibularis** lies in the **Trigonum submandibulare (Spatium submandibulare),** which is bordered laterally by the Corpus mandibulae lateral, the Venter anterior of the M. digastricus medial and the Venter posterior of the M. digastricus occipitally. The roof of the Trigonum submandibulare is formed by the M. mylohyoideus. The gland body bends together with the Ductus submandibularis in a hook shape around the rear edge of the M. mylohyoideus and connects the Trigonum submandibulare with the Spatium sublinguale (➤ Fig. 9.123). The Trigonum submandibulare and the Spatium sublinguale are connected at the rear to the neurovascular cord of the neck. The **Ductus submandibularis (WHARTON's duct)** is surrounded by glandular tissue and lies on the Diaphragma oris, where it passes medially beside the Glandula sublingualis to the Caruncula sublingualis. The gland excretory duct is accompanied by the N. lingualis and the A. and V. sublingualis. Initially, the A. lingualis is lateral of the glandular excretory duct, then crosses under it and finally enters medially into the tongue.

Sublingual gland

The **Glandula sublingualis** is located immediately below the mucosa of the floor of the mouth in the Spatium sublinguale on the M. mylohyoideus (➤ Fig. 9.123). The gland body forms the Plica sublingualis in the floor of the mouth, in which several small excretory ducts of the Glandula sublingualis flow (**Ductus sublinguales minores**) . The gland of the Mm. geniohyoideus, genioglossus and hyoglossus lies medially. At the rear the Glandula sublingualis borders on the Glandula submandibularis (➤ Fig. 9.123). Apart from the small excretory ducts the Glandula sublingualis has one large excretory duct (**Ductus sublingualis**), which merges with the Ductus submandibularis and flows into the Caruncula sublingualis.

Vascular, lymphatic and nervous systems
Glandula parotidea

The Glandula parotidea is supplied with blood via the **A. temporalis superficialis,** a branch of the A. carotis externa. The venous blood flows via the **Vv. parotideae,** which form the Plexus pterygoideus, in the V. facialis.

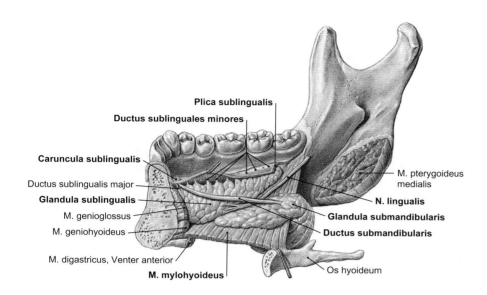

Plica sublingualis

Ductus sublinguales minores

Caruncula sublingualis

Ductus sublingualis major

Glandula sublingualis

M. genioglossus

M. geniohyoideus

M. digastricus, Venter anterior

M. mylohyoideus

M. pterygoideus medialis

N. lingualis

Glandula submandibularis

Ductus submandibularis

Os hyoideum

Fig. 9.123 Glandula subman-dibularis and Glandula sublin-gualis of the right side.

The **lymph** is transported away via Nodi lymphoidei parotidei superficiales and profundi in the Nodi lymphoidei cervicales superficiales.

The **parasympathetic innervation** takes place via **JACOBSON's anastomosis.** The nerve cell body lies in the Nucleus salivatorius inferior, the nerve fibres run with the **N. glossopharyngeus [IX]** via the N. tympanicus, Plexus tympanicus and N. petrosus minor to the Ganglion oticum.. The switched, postganglionic fibres join

the N. auriculotemporalis (branch from [V/3]), reach the parotid gland compartment via it and branch out as the Plexus parotideus in the gland parenchyma. They accompany the branches of the N. facialis [VII] in sections in the Glandula parotidea (➤ Fig. 9.124). The **sympathetic innervation** begins from the Ganglion cervicale superius. The postganglionic sympathetic fibres pass with the branches of the A. carotis externa into the gland.

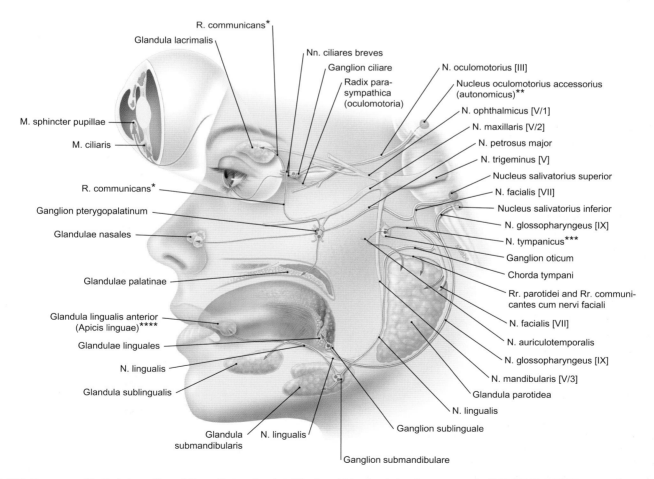

R. communicans*

Glandula lacrimalis

Nn. ciliares breves

Ganglion ciliare

Radix para-sympathica (oculomotoria)

N. oculomotorius [III]

Nucleus oculomotorius accessorius (autonomicus)**

N. ophthalmicus [V/1]

N. maxillaris [V/2]

N. petrosus major

N. trigeminus [V]

Nucleus salivatorius superior

N. facialis [VII]

Nucleus salivatorius inferior

N. glossopharyngeus [IX]

N. tympanicus***

Ganglion oticum

Chorda tympani

Rr. parotidei and Rr. communi-cantes cum nervi faciali

N. facialis [VII]

N. auriculotemporalis

N. glossopharyngeus [IX]

N. mandibularis [V/3]

Glandula parotidea

N. lingualis

Ganglion sublinguale

Ganglion submandibulare

M. sphincter pupillae

M. ciliaris

R. communicans*

Ganglion pterygopalatinum

Glandulae nasales

Glandulae palatinae

Glandula lingualis anterior (Apicis linguae)****

Glandulae linguales

N. lingualis

Glandula sublingualis

Glandula submandibularis

N. lingualis

Fig. 9.124 Parasympathetic innervation of the salivary glands of the head; * lacrimal gland anastomosis, ** EDINGER-WESTPHAL nucleus, *** JACOBSON'S nerve, **** BLANDIN-NUHN gland.

529

Glandula submandibularis

The Glandula submandibularis is supplied with blood via the **A. facialis** and the **A. lingualis** from the A. carotis externa. The venous blood flows via the **V. submentalis,** which discharges into the V. facialis. From here, the blood drains into the V. jugularis interna. The **lymph** is transported into the directly neighbouring Nodi lymphoidei submandibulares and from here to the Nodi lymphoidei cervicales superficiales and profundi.

The **parasympathetic secretory innervation** of the gland takes place from the Nucleus salivatorius superior via the N. intermedius of the N. facialis [VII]. This emits the Chorda tympani backwards in front of the Foramen stylomastoideum, which passes through the middle ear to the skull base, usually penetrates the Fissura sphenopetrosa and radiates behind the temporomandibular joint caudally in the N. lingualis. From the N. lingualis the Rr. ganglionares pass to the Ganglion submandibulare, in which the switch to postganglionic fibres is carried out (➤ Fig. 9.124). The **sympathetic innervation** takes place via the Ganglion cervicale superius. From here the postganglionic fibres pass together with the A. submandibularis into the gland.

Glandula sublingualis

The Glandula sublingualis is supplied with blood via the **A. lingualis,** from which the **A. sublingualis** leaves as a small branch. The A. lingualis originates from the A. carotis externa. The venous disposal takes place via the **V. sublingualis,** which flows into the V. lingualis. From here, the blood drains into the V. jugularis interna. As for the Glandula submandibularis, the **lymph** is transported in the directly neighbouring Nodi lymphoidei submandibulares and from here to the Nodi lymphoidei cervicales superficiales and profundi.

The **parasympathetic secretory innervation** corresponds to the innervation of the Glandula submandibularis and therefore follows the Chorda tympani, which passes with the N. lingualis to the Ganglion submandibulare. Postganglionic fibres join the N. lingualis again and reach the gland (➤ Fig. 9.124). The **sympathetic innervation** also corresponds to that of the Glandula submandibularis.

Clinical remarks

In the context of kidney disease, urea-containing substances are excreted via the salivary glands.
Radiation therapy for the treatment of tumours of the head and throat area region or radioactive irradiation can lead to **sicca syndrome (dry mouth)** with swallowing and speech difficulties.

---

10 Neck

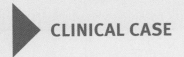
Branchial cleft cyst

Case study

A father comes with his 6-year-old daughter to the paediatrician. For some time now the daughter has been complaining of a recurrent swelling with pressure on the left side of the neck. Until now, the swelling always went away without medical treatment. For over a week now, however, the swelling has been permanently present with increasing pain, significant redness at the site and high temperature.

Further diagnostics and diagnosis

To determine the suspected diagnosis of a branchial cleft cyst, the paediatrician advises the girl to see an ear, nose and throat specialist, who carries out an ultrasound examination and magnetic resonance imaging (MRI) of the neck area. Here, a lateral neck cyst on the anterior margin of the left M. sternocleidomastoideus can be unequivocally seen and can be differentiated from any other possible swellings. Branchial cleft cysts (closed) or neck fistulae (perforating the skin) are created by congenital developmental abnormality of the neck structures. A differentiation is made between centrally located (median) branchial cysts and laterally located branchial cysts. A lateral neck cyst is the result of an incorrect degeneration of the embryonic pharyngeal arch system in this area (Sinus cervicalis). This means that in most cases lateral branchial cysts are found on the side of the neck area above the M. sternocleidomastoideus.

Treatment

Firstly the acute inflammation is treated with antibiotics, analgesics and fever-reducing medications; however, because the infection is likely to recur or a fistula may form, the neck cyst should be operatively removed. Typically, this operation is a relatively complication-free, routine procedure; however, great care should be taken to completely remove all of the cyst tissue, to ensure that there is no recurrence. When the parents decided on surgery, the girl was operated shortly after. She stayed overnight on a ward for observation and was discharged the next day. Since then, the wound has healed well and there are no further symptoms.

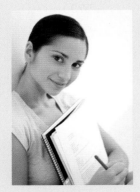

You are completing your paediatric rotational placement and are involved in examining a young patient with a suspected lateral cervical cyst. Since you find this case exciting and would like to use it for the patient presentation in the paediatric seminar, you make notes.

From the paediatrician to ENT
6 year-old female patient with recurrent swelling and feeling of pressure in the area of the left side of the neck, to date, the swelling has always disappeared by itself
Current: permanent swelling for more than 1 week, increasing level of pain, obvious redness, increased temperature.
Suspected diagnosis: lateral cervical cyst
CAVE! Difference median and lateral cervical cysts?!?
Further Proc: Transfer to ENT specialist (scan?)
Read at home: Etiology, pathology, clinical aspects, differential diagnosis, treatment!!!

The **neck (Collum, Cervix)** is the tubular, mobile connecting element between the head and the upper body. The cervical spine is the bony foundation on which the head sits. The arrangement and structure of the cranial joints permit the free rotation of the head in relation to the trunk by almost 90° on each side. In evolutionary development, this only became possible about 370 million years ago, at a time when the first amphibians conquered solid ground. In comparison, in fish the head and spine remain immobile in relation to each other even today; however, in phylogenetic terms, the neck area with its structures should not be thought of as a fundamentally new idea. In fact, this part of the body is expressed in the most understandable way as an almost protracted head–torso border area. Taken from this perspective, this also explains why, for example, the nerves of the head are also involved in the innervation of the shoulder muscles and why it is that the upper limbs are supplied by nerves exiting from the cervical spine. The neck is not just purely a connecting element; it also contains organs, such as the thyroid gland, parathyroid gland and the larynx.

Clinical remarks

Injuries to the neck region are generally regarded as very dangerous, since close to the cervical spine in the soft tissues there are many important structures, such as large blood vessels and nerves and the respiratory and digestive tracts.

10.1 Overview
Michael Scholz

Skills

After working through this chapter, you should be able to:
- name the specific structures of the neck and describe its anatomical structures
- describe the various regions of the neck in a topographically correct way and clearly define their limits

---

10.1.1 Surface anatomy of the neck

The shape and appearance of the throat area are primarily defined by the more or less strongly defined neck muscles, the size and shape of the thyroid gland (Glandula thyroidea) and larynx, as well as the distribution of subcutaneous fat. A cranial view reveals an elongated oval shape, while a caudal view shows a more transverse-oval cross-section of the neck. In men, the **thyroid cartilage (Cartilago thyroidea)** can be clearly recognised and palpated in the throat as the Adam's apple (**Prominentia laryngea**) (> Table 10.1). Conversely, in women and children this structure hardly stands out in relief from the throat area. The position of the hyoid bone (**Os hyoideum**) can be determined by a transverse skin fold above the larynx, which also represents the visible external border between the base of the mouth and neck.

The **bony limits** of the neck are cranially the lower jaw (Mandibula) and the occipital bone (Os occipitale), and caudally the collarbones (Claviculae) and the upper edge of the shoulder blades (Scapulae). Through the upper thoracic aperture, an interconnect-

Table 10.1 Easily palpable structures and bone points in the neck region.

Anatomical structure	Palpable section
Lower jaw (Mandibula)	• Lower edge
Os temporale	• Proc. mastoideus
Os occipitale	• Protuberantia occipitalis externa
Breast bone (Sternum)	• Upper edge
Clavicle (Clavicula)	• Upper edge
Shoulder blade (Scapula)	• Acromion
Os hyoideum	• Corpus • Cornu majus ossis hyoidei
Larynx	• Cartilago thyroidea • Cartilago cricothyroidea
Windpipe (Trachea)	• Cricoid cartilage
Jugular fossa (Fossa jugularis)	
VII Cervical vertebra; Vertebra prominens	• Proc. spinosus

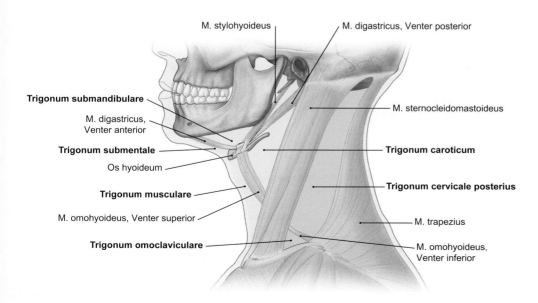

Fig. 10.1 Anterior (blue) and lateral (green) neck regions from left lateral (diagram). The 4 sections of the anterior neck triangle with the structures delimiting it are also shown. [E402]

ed bony ring made up of the breastbone (Sternum), the first pair of ribs and the first thoracic vertebra, the neck passes caudally by definition into the Mediastinum of the thorax. At the base of the anterior cervical region, just above the sternum as a clearly visible trough is the **jugular fossa (Fossa jugularis)**. By light pressure in this area, one can easily feel the upper cartilaginous braces of the windpipe (Trachea) just under the skin. To the dorsal side of the airway (larynx, trachea) in the throat area are the cervical sections of the gastrointestinal tract (pharynx, oesophagus) and behind them is the cervical spine.

10.1.2 Regions of the neck and neck triangles

In principle the neck can be divided into 4 large regions (➤ Fig. 11.2):
- Regio cervicalis anterior
- Regio sternocleidomastoidea
- Regio cervicalis lateralis
- Regio cervicalis posterior

In addition, several of the respective regions can be defined as single, subdividing neck triangles (Trigona cervicis) (➤ Fig. 10.1, ➤ Table 10.2). The **M. sternocleidomastoideus**, which is in the lateral neck area and represents a clear ridge under the skin, is the prominent structure for classifying the cervical regions. The muscle originates from the Manubrium sterni (Caput sternale) and at the sternal end of the clavicle (Caput claviculare) and runs cranially and to the back to the Proc. mastoideus of the Os temporale and the Linea nuchalis superior. The lateral neck region, which is defined by this muscle, is referred to as the **Regio sternocleidomastoidea**. Medial to the two Mm. sternocleidomastoidei is the **frontal triangle of the neck (Regio cervicalis anterior; Trigonum cervicale anterius)**. This region (➤ Fig. 10.1, blue) can be topographically divided, due to the deeper lying structures, into other smaller neck triangles (➤ Table 10.2). Lateral to the M. sternocleidomastoideus is the **lateral triangle of the neck (Regio cervicalis lateralis; Trigonum cervicale posterius)**, which is delimited posteriorly by the anterior border of the M. trapezius and caudally by the middle third of the clavicle. Here (➤ Fig. 10.1, green) the Venter inferior musculi omohyoidei runs in the lower part, creating another triangle, the **Trigonum omoclaviculare (Fossa supraclavicularis major)**, (➤ Fig. 10.1). The **posterior neck region (Regio cervicalis posterior)** is mainly characterised by compact, strongly built neck muscles.

Table 10.2 Subdivision of the Regio cervicalis anterior in its Trigona with its respective delimitations.

Subdivision	Delimitation
Trigonum submandibulare (paired)	• Lower rim of the mandibula • Venter anterior and Venter posterior of the M. digastricus
Trigonum submentale (unpaired)	• Venter anterior of the M. digastricus • Os hyoideum
Trigonum caroticum (paired)	• Venter posterior of the M. digastricus • M. stylohyoideus • Venter superior of the M. omohyoideus • Anterior border of the M. sternocleidomastoideus
Trigonum musculare (paired)	• Os hyoideum • Venter superior of the M. omohyoideus • Anterior border of the M. sternocleidomastoideus • Midline of the neck

10.2 Musculoskeletal system of the neck
Michael Scholz

In the neck, the parts of the musculoskeletal system can be divided up into passive and active elements.

10.2.1 Passive sections

The passive parts include the cervical spine and its skeletal joints, the intervertebral discs and ligaments (➤ Chap. 3.3.2) and the **hyoid bone (Os hyoideum)** with its ligament connections. The hyoid bone is a horseshoe-shaped, curved bone of approximately 3–5 cm in size, made up of a body (Corpus ossis hyoidei) and 2 greater horns (Cornua majora) and 2 lesser horns (Cornua minora) (➤ Fig. 10.2). The hyoid body and the Cornua majora can usually be easily palpated externally.

The medial constrictor muscles of the pharynx (**M. constrictor pharyngis medius**) are attached to this. The hyoid bone has no connection to other bony structures and is stretched between the muscles of the base of the mouth (suprahyal muscles) and the infrahyoid muscles. As a result it is hinged and mobile within this muscle sling. The **Lig. stylohyoideum** connects the hyoid bone with the base of the skull (Os temporale). The ligament stops the Os hyoideum from being pulled below the level of the IV cervical vertebra and can completely or partially ossify with age. Via the **Membrana thyrohyoidea**, the hyoid bone is connected with the thyroid cartilage (Cartilago thyroidea) of the larynx (➤ Fig. 10.3, also ➤ Chap. 10.6.3). The membrane is centrally reinforced by the **Lig. thyrohyoideum medianium** which runs from the Incisura thyroidea superior to the Corpus ossis hyoidei. The reinforced rear

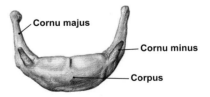

Fig. 10.2 Hyoid bone (Os hyoideum). View from upper front

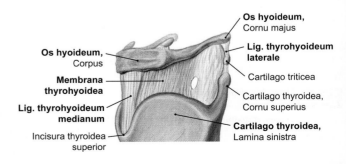

Fig. 10.3 Ligament connections between the hyoid bone (Os hyoideum) and the thyroid cartilage (Cartilago thyroidea) of the larynx.

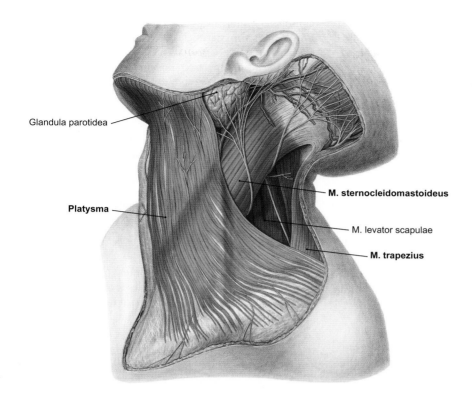

Glandula parotidea

Platysma

M. sternocleidomastoideus

M. levator scapulae

M. trapezius

Fig. 10.4 Superficial muscles of the neck in the anterior and lateral head and neck region. View from left, lateral.

edge of the Membrana thyrohyoidea is referred to as the **Lig. thyrohyoideum laterale** and in its course from the Cornu majus ossis hyoidei to the Cornu superius of the thyroid cartilage, it wraps around a small piece of elastic cartilage of just a few millimetres in size (**Cartilago triticea**).

> **Clinical remarks**
>
> In the case of a **fracture of the hyoid bone** by force (e.g. a chokehold) parts of the hyoid bone can drop down to the larynx and prevent swallowing (risk of aspiration).

10.2.2 Active sections – neck muscles

The active musculoskeletal system is formed by the throat and neck muscles. From a topographical viewpoint, the muscles of the nape of the neck as well as the M. trapezius are part of the throat area muscles; however, in functional terms the M. trapezius is part of the shoulder girdle muscles and the neck musculature is regarded as part of the autochthonous back muscles (M. erector spinae). The neck muscles can be divided into a superficial, medium and deep muscle layer (➤ Table 10.3).

Table 10.3 Stratifying structure of the neck muscles.

Superficial muscle layer	Middle muscle layer	Deep muscle layer
• Platysma • M. sternocleidomas-toideus	• Suprahyoid muscles • Infrahyoid muscles	• Mm. scaleni • Prevertebral muscles

Superficial layer of the cervical muscles

The superficial neck muscles include the platysma and the M. sternocleidomastoideus.

Platysma

The **platysma** is a thin, broad muscle plate located directly under the skin. It belongs to the facial muscles and has no fascia. It originates variably with its fibres in the skin below the Clavicula in the upper chest and inserts at the lower margin of the Mandibula. In its course it covers the superficial neck veins and a large part of the M. sternocleidomastoideus. Between the platysma and the M. sternocleidomastoideus is the lower pole of the parotid gland (Glandula parotidea) (➤ Fig. 10.4). There is a great variation in the extent of individual platysmas; in rare cases it extends only to the neck midline or is completely missing. The platysma is innervated by the **R. colli of the N. facialis [VII]**. This nerve branch generally arises from the branches of the N. facialis [VII] within the parotid gland and forms a nerve loop with the R. superior of the N. transversus

Table 10.4 M. sternocleidomastoideus.

Innervation	Origin	Attachment	Function
M. sternocleidomastoideus			
N. accessorius [XI])	• Caput sternale: upper edge of the Manubrium sterni • Caput claviculare: medial third of the Clavicula	Proc. mastoideus; Linea nuchalis superior	• With unilateral activity: lateral inclination of the head to the ipsilateral side and rotation to the contralateral side • Where there is bilateral activity: dorsiflexion of the head • Where the head is fixed: auxiliary respiratory muscle

colli (From the Punctum nervosum cervicis, ERB's point; Plexus cervicalis) (➤ Fig. 10.20). Using this connection, motor nerve fibres of the N. transversus colli reach the distant sections of the platysma. Due to its course, the platysma tenses the skin of the neck by contraction, so has an impact on facial expressions (threatening gestures).

N O T E

The N. transversus colli runs directly transversally via the M. sterno-cleidomastoideus and below the platysma.

M. sternocleidomastoideus

The **M. sternocleidomastoideus** (➤ Table 10.4) forms the border between the anterior (Regio cervicalis anterius) and lateral (Regio cervicalis lateralis) neck regions. It originates with a head for each muscle at the upper edge of the Manubrium sterni (**Caput sternale**) and at the sternal end of the Clavicula (**Caput claviculare**). Located between the two original heads is the **Fossa supraclavicularis minor** (➤ Fig. 10.5). The Caput sternale and the Caput claviculare join together in their course into a broad muscle belly, which rises obliquely from the chest to the head and is inserted with a strong tendon on the **Proc. mastoideus** and on the **Linea nuchalis superior**. Between the two sternal heads of the right and left muscles, the **Fossa jugularis** is easily visible on the surface (jugular fossa). The M. sternocleidomastoideus, together with the M. trapezius receives its motor innervation from the **N. accessorius [XI]** because at the embryo stage both muscles arose from a common system and are derived from former pharyngeal arch muscles. A unilateral contraction of the muscle causes a sideways tilting of the head to ipsilateral and a rotational movement to the

contralateral side ('head turning muscle'). Simultaneous contraction of both Mm. sternocleidomastoidei leads to the dorsiflexion of the head.

When the head is in a fixed position, the M. sternocleidomastoideus acts as an auxiliary respiratory muscle.

Clinical remarks

A unilateral shortening of the M. sternocleidomastoideus can lead to a **twisted neck muscle (Torticolis muscularis)**. The cause is usually a congenital malformation of the muscle; however, traumatic or inflammatory processes (myositis) may also lead to scarring and shortening of the muscle. Muscle contraction and the associated slanted position of the head can result in facial and cranial asymmetry.

Middle layer of the cervical muscles

The middle layer of the neck muscles form the suprahyoid and infrahyoid muscles (➤ Table 10.5). Both muscle groups are attached to the hyoid bone and their interaction determines the position of

Table 10.5 Suprahyoid and infrahyoid muscles.

Suprahyoid muscles	Infrahyoid muscles
• M. stylohyoideus	• M. sternohyoideus
• M. digastricus	• M. omohyoideus
– Venter anterior	– Venter superior
– Venter posterior	– Venter inferior
• M. mylohyoideus	• M. thyrohyoideus
• M. geniohyoideus	• M. sternothyroideus

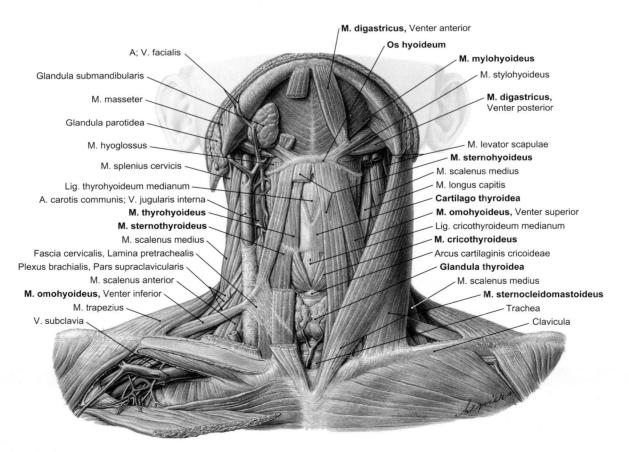

Fig. 10.5 **Various parts of the neck musculature and throat structures.** Ventral view.

the hyoid bone. They are functionally involved in swallowing and speech formation.

Suprahyoid muscles

The muscles summarised by the term suprahyoid have their origins in different embryonic structures:

- The **M. mylohyoideus** and the **Venter anterior of the M. digastricus** form from the 1st pharyngeal arch.
- The **Venter posterior of the M. digastricus** and the **M. stylohyoideus** arise from the 2nd pharyngeal arch.
- The **M. geniohyoideus** is part of the rectus system of the neck. It originates from the somites of the neck.

The varied origins of each individual superior hyoid bone muscles also explains why they are innervated by different nerves.

M. stylohyoideus

The M. stylohyoideus (➤ Table 10.5) originates with a thin tendon at the base of the Proc. stylohyoideus and runs ventrocaudally to the lateral wall of the Corpus ossis hyoidei. Immediately before its attachment to the hyoid bone it divides into 2 tendon strands and surrounds the intermediate tendon of the M. digastricus (Ansa tendinis), which it secures (➤ Fig. 10.6). During swallowing, it pulls the hyoid bone backwards and upwards. It is innervated by the N. facialis [VII].

M. digastricus

The M. digastricus (➤ Table 10.6) has 2 bellies, a shorter Venter anterior and a longer Venter posterior, which are connected together by a tendon. This, in turn, is held in place by a loose connective tissue loop (Ansa tendinis) at the Corpus ossis hyoidei (➤ Fig.

Table 10.6 Suprahyoid muscles.

Innervation	Origins	Attachment	Function
M. stylohyoideus			
R. stylohyoideus of the N. facialis [VII]	Proc. styloideus of the Os temporale	Corpus and Cornu majus ossis hyoidei	In bilateral activity pulls the hyoid bone backwards and upwards
M. digastricus, Venter anterior and Venter posterior			
• Venter anterior: N. mylohyoideus from [V/3] • Venter posterior: R. digastricus of the N. facialis [VII]	• Venter anterior: Fossa digastrica mandibulae • Venter posterior: Incisura mastoidea	Intermediate tendon via connective tissue at the Cornu majus of the hyoid bone	• Hyoid fixed and bilateral activity: sinking (abduction) of the Mandibula = mouth opening • Hyoid fixed and unilateral activity: grinding movement • Lower jaw fixed and bilateral activity: lifting of the hyoid bone during swallowing
M. mylohyoideus			
N. mylohyoideus of the N. mandibularis [V/3]	Linea mylohyoidea of the Mandibula	Raphe mylohyoidea, Corpus ossis hyoidei	• Raises the floor of the mouth, mouth opens (lowers the mandible with bilateral activity and fixed hyoid bone) • With unilateral activity and fixed hyoid bone: grinding movement • With bilateral activity and fixed lower jaw: lifts the hyoid bone during swallowing
M. geniohyoideus			
Muscular branches (C1, C2) which run with the N. hypoglossus [XII]	Spina mentalis of the Mandibula	Corpus ossis hyoidei	• Raises the floor of the mouth, mouth opens (lowers the mandible with bilateral activity and fixed hyoid bone) • With unilateral activity and fixed hyoid bone: grinding movement • With bilateral activity and fixed lower jaw: lifts the hyoid bone during swallowing

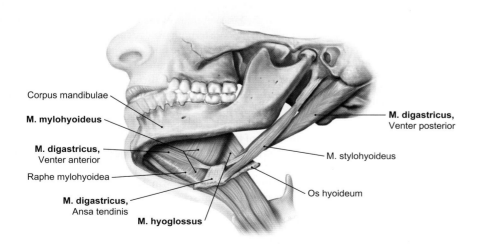

Corpus mandibulae
M. mylohyoideus
M. digastricus, Venter anterior
Raphe mylohyoidea
M. digastricus, Ansa tendinis
M. hyoglossus
M. digastricus, Venter posterior
M. stylohyoideus
Os hyoideum

Fig. 10.6 Mouth base region with suprahyoid muscles. View from the side below.

10.6). The **Venter anterior** originates in the Fossa digastrica on the inside of the Mandibula and is innervated as the superficial separation of the M. mylohyoideus in the same way as the one from the N. mylohyoideus (N. mandibularis [V/3]). The **Venter posterior** originates on the Incisura mastoidea at the medial side of the Proc. mastoideus (Os temporale). This arises from the same position as the M. stylohyoideus and is therefore also innervated by the N. facialis [VII] (R. digastricus). When the Mandibula is fixed, the M. digastricus raises the hyoid bone (swallowing); when the hyoid bone is fixed, it opens the mouth (lowering the Mandibula).

M. mylohyoideus

The M. mylohyoideus (➤ Table 10.6) originates at the Linea mylohyoidea of the Mandibula and is located above the Venter anterior of the M. digastricus. The wide muscle plates on both sides unite along the centre line in the approximately 4–5 cm long Raphe mylohyoidea. The posterior muscle fibres insert on the Corpus ossis hyoidei (➤ Fig. 10.5). The M. mylohyoideus is innervated by the N. mylohyoideus (N. mandibularis [V/3]) and supports and raises the floor of the mouth.

M. geniohyoideus

The M. geniohyoideus (➤ Table 10.6) lies cranially on the M. mylohyoideus and runs from the Spina mentalis of the Corpus mandibulae to the Corpus ossis hyoidei. It is a narrow, paired muscle, the medial sides of which are virtually touching in their course. The muscle arises from the rectus system of the neck and hence is innervated by a branch of the Plexus cervicalis (C1). When the Mandibula is fixed, it raises the hyoid bone and assists with opening the mouth when the Os hyoideum is fixed.

Infrahyoid muscles

The 4 flat muscle pairs of the infrahyoid muscles continue the rectus system of the trunk to cranial. All of these are within the Trigonum musculare of the Regio cervicalis anterius, and are stretched between the sternum, thyroid cartilage, hyoid bone and in their course cover the trachea, thyroid gland and a large part of the larynx. They are divided into 2 layers, with the upper layer formed from the **M. sternohyoideus** and the **M. omohyoideus**, and the lower layer from the **M. sternothyroideus** and the **M. thyrohyoideus** (➤ Fig. 10.5). All the infrahyoid muscles are innervated by nerve branches of the Plexus cervicalis (C1–C4), which clump to a nerve loop, the Ansa cervicalis (profunda). In conjunction with the suprahyoid muscles, the infrahyoid muscles determine the position of the hyoid bone and larynx, and therefore play an important role in swallowing and voice formation (phonation).

> **NOTE**
> The previously used terms Ansa cervicalis superficialis (anastomosis of the N. transversus colli with the R. colli of the N. facialis [VII]) and Ansa cervicalis profunda (motor innervation of the infrahyoid muscles) often led to confusion. Therefore, only **Ansa cervicalis** is still used, by which is meant the nerve loop around the V. jugularis interna, which serves to innervate the infrahyoid muscles; however, since no term for the former Ansa cervicalis superficialis has been proposed and the term is still familiar, the previous names are retained in the figures.

M. sternohyoideus

The M. sternohyoideus (➤ Table 10.7) is a long flat muscle arising from the dorsal side of the Manubrium sterni and the dorsal part of the Articulatio sternoclavicularis and runs to the lower margin of the Corpus ossis hyoidei. In its cranial course, the muscles of both sides increasingly converge up to the hyoid bone, with the Prominentia laryngea (Adam's apple) of the thyroid cartilage remaining uncovered (➤ Fig. 10.5). In the region of origin of the M. sternohyoideus an intermediate tendon can be individually present.

M. omohyoideus

The M. omohyoideus (➤ Table 10.7) originates from the upper border of the scapula in the area of the Lig. transversum scapulae and is attached to the hyoid bone (➤ Fig. 10.5). Its origin is also the reason for its name from the old anatomical term 'omoplata' for the shoulder blade. The muscle is divided by an intermediate tendon into 2 muscle bellies, a Venter superior and a Venter inferior. The **Venter inferior** originates medial of the Incisura suprascapularis on the Margo superior of the shoulder blade. In its course, it runs as an upper boundary of the Trigonum omoclaviculare (Fossa supraclavicularis major) through the lateral triangle of the neck to the front and continues with its intermediate tendon directly on the carotid sheath (Vagina carotica). The **Venter superior** has its origin at the intermediate tendon and runs upwards to the Corpus ossis hyoidei. Here it is located directly lateral to the attachment point of the M. sternohyoideus (➤ Fig. 10.5).

> **NOTE**
> The **intermediate tendon of the M. omohyoideus** is located behind the M. sternocleidomastoideus and crosses over the carotid sheath. At the intersection point, the intermediate tendon and the Vagina carotica merge together. Through the background tension of the M. omohyoideus, the carotid sheath is permanently under tension at this point. Therefore, the lumen of the V. jugularis interna is enlarged and the venous blood return to the heart is better than it would be without this tension. As a result the point of intersection at the level of the cricoid cartilage can also be used as a puncture point for intravenous access.

M. thyrohyoideus

The M. thyrohyoideus (➤ Table 10.7) runs from the Linea obliqua of the thyroid cartilage (Cartilago thyroidea) to the Cornu majus of the hyoid bone (➤ Fig. 10.7). In its course, it lies beneath the Venter superior of the M. omohyoideus and beneath the M. sternohyoideus (➤ Fig. 10.5). It lowers the hyoid and holds it in place. In the swallowing process, it raises the larynx.

M. sternothyroideus

The M. sternothyroideus runs in the caudal continuation of the M. thyrohyoideus and beneath the M. sternohyoideus (➤ Table 10.7). It has its origin at the rear surface of the Manubrium sterni and runs up to the Linea obliqua of the thyroid cartilage. Laterally the separation of the M. sternothyroideus and M. thyroideus is incomplete, since the lateral muscle fibres merge together and run to the hyoid bone. In its course, the muscle overlays the lateral lobes of the thyroid gland. The M. sternothyroideus pulls the larynx caudally and fixes the larynx through isometric contraction during phonation.

Deep layer of the neck musculature

Also included in the deep layer of the neck muscles are 2 muscle groups:

- The lateral, deep-running **Mm. scaleni**
- The **prevertebral muscles** passing in front of the cervical spine

The two muscle groups run to the cervical spine or ventrally to the skull base. They are antagonists of the neck muscles.

Mm. scaleni

The scalene muscles are the continuation of the intercostal muscles of the thorax in the neck region (> Fig. 10.7). There are usually three scalene muscles (> Table 10.8), all innervated by direct branches of the cervical spinal nerves (C3–C8). The strongest of these muscles is the M. scalenus medius and its origin can lie with some fibres on the atlas and the axis. Occasionally (in approximately one third of the population) a 4th scalene muscle (M. scalenus minimus) can also be present.

> **N O T E**
> The M. scalenus anterior and M. scalenus medius together with the upper edge of the 1st rib, form a triangle, the **scalene hiatus**, through which the A. subclavia and the Plexus brachialis pass. Some authors differentiate between a front and rear scalene hiatus; however, in this case the front scalene hiatus is not an actual gap but rather describes the course of the V. subclavia in front of the M. scalenus anterior over the 1st rib, whereas the rear scalene hiatus describes the topographical course shown above.

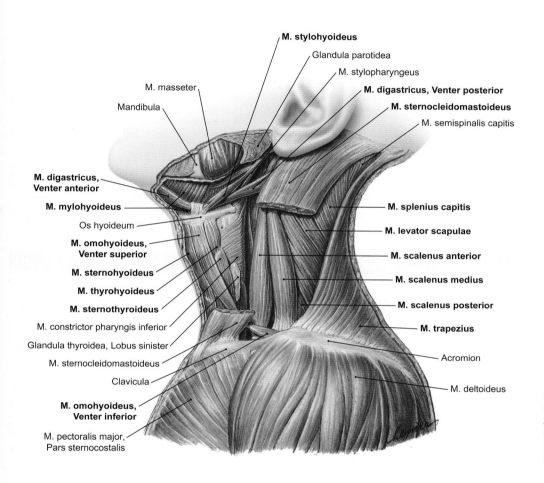

Fig. 10.7 Presentation of the neck musculature from lateral. All muscle fascia, the platysma and the median section of the M. sternocleidomastoideus are removed.

Table 10.7 Infrahyoid muscles.

Innervation	Origin	Attachment	Function
M. sternohyoideus			
Plexus cervicalis, Ansa cervicalis (profunda)	Inner surface of the Manubrium sterni	Corpus ossis hyoidei	Pulls the hyoid bone caudally, fixes the hyoid bone for opening the jaw and grinding movement
M. omohyoideus			
Plexus cervicalis, Ansa cervicalis (profunda)	Margo superior of the scapula	Venter superior of the Corpus ossis hyoidei	Draws the hyoid bone downwards, fixes the hyoid; tenses the middle neck fascia, promotes the venous backflow from the head and neck by holding the V. jugularis open
M. thyrohyoideus			
Plexus cervicalis, Ansa cervicalis (profunda)	Outer surface of the Lamina of the Cartilago thyroidea	Corpus ossis hyoidei	• Where the hyoid bone is fixed: raising the larynx for the act of swallowing • Where the larynx is fixed: lowering of the hyoid bone to influence phonation
M. sternothyroideus			
Plexus cervicalis, Ansa cervicalis (profunda)	Inner surface of the manubrium sterni	Lina obliqua of the Lamina of the Cartilago thyroidea	Pulls the larynx caudally, fixes the larynx during phonation

Table 10.8 Mm. scaleni.

Innervation	Origins	Attachment	Function
M. scalenus anterior			
Plexus cervicalis (Rr. anteriores of the Nn. cervicales IV–VII)	Cervical vertebrae III–VI (Tubercula anteriora)	1st rib (Tubercula musculi scaleni)	• Bilateral activity: forward tilt of the cervical spine • Unilateral activity: tilting sideways and rotating the cervical spine to the ipsilateral side • In the case of fixed cervical spine: lifting the 1st rib, support of inspiration
M. scalenus medius			
Plexus cervicalis (Rr. anteriores of the Nn. cervicales III–VIII)	Cervical vertebrae III–VII (Tubercula anteriora)	1st rib dorsolateral of the Sulcus arteriae subclaviae	• Bilateral activity: forward tilt of the cervical spine • Unilateral activity: tilting sideways and rotating the cervical spine to the ipsilateral side • In the case of fixed cervical spine: lifting 1st rib, support of inspiration
M. scalenus posterior			
Plexus cervicalis (Rr. anteriores of the Nn. cervicales VII–VIII)	Transverse processes cervical vertebrae V–VI (Tubercula posteriora)	2nd rib (outer surface), sometimes also 3rd rib	• Unilateral activity: tilting sideways and rotating the cervical spine to the ipsilateral side • In the fixed cervical spine: lifting of the 2nd rib, support of inspiration
M. scalenus minimus			
Plexus cervicalis (Rr. anteriores of the N. cervicalis VIII)	Cervical vertebra VII (Tuberculum anterius)	1st rib (posterior border, dorsal to the M. scalenus anterior)	• Unilateral activity: tilting sideways and rotating the cervical spine to the ipsilateral side • In the case of fixed cervical spine: lifting 1st rib, support of inspiration

Table 10.9 Prevertebral muscles

Innervation	Origins	Attachment	Function
M. rectus capitis anterior			
Plexus cervicalis (R. anterior of the N. cervicalis I)	Massa lateralis of the atlas	Pars basilaris of the Os occipitale	Fine adjustment of the head in the cranial joints, bending of the head to the front
M. rectus capitis lateralis			
Plexus cervicalis (R. anterior of the N. cervicalis I)	Proc. transversus of the atlas	Proc. jugularis of the Os occipitale	Fine adjustment of the head in the cranial joints, lateral bending of the head
M. longus capitis			
Plexus cervicalis (Rr. anteriores of the Nn. cervicales I–III)	Tubercula anteriora of the Procc. transversi of the IIIrd-VIth cervical vertebrae	Pars basilaris of the Os occipitale	• Bilateral activity: forward tilt of the head • Unilateral activity: sideways tilt of the head
M. longus colli			
Plexus cervicalis (Rr. anteriores of the Nn. cervicales II–IV)	Corpus of the Vth-VIIth cervical vertebrae and the Ist-IIIrd thoracic vertebrae; Tubercula anteriora of the Procc. transversi of the II–V cervical vertebrae	Procc. transversi of the Vth-VIth cervical vertebrae, Corpus of the IInd-IVth cervical vertebrae, Tuberculum anterius of the atlas	• Bilateral activity: assistance with the forward tilt of the cervical spine • Unilateral activity: tilting sideways and rotating the cervical spine to the ipsilateral side

---

Clinical remarks

Anatomical variations in the area of the scalene hiatus (cervical rib, narrowed scalene hiatus, accessory M. scalenus minimus, aberrant muscle fibres) can accompany a **scalenus anticus syndrome**. Here a compression of the Plexus brachialis and/or the A. subclavia commonly occurs with corresponding deficits.

Prevertebral muscles
The **prevertebral muscles** (➤ Fig. 10.8) are:
- **M. rectus capitis anterior**
- **M. rectus capitis lateralis**
- **M. longus capitis**
- **M. longus colli**

The muscles run on both sides between the transverse appendages (Proc. transversi) and the Corpora vertebrae of the cervical vertebrae and the upper 3 thoracic vertebrae. The muscle fibre cords of the M. longus capitis and M. longus colli are usually not clearly separated from each other, and form a muscle complex consisting of longitudinal and diagonal fibre cords. The prevertebral muscles are innervated by Rr. anteriores of the cervical spinal nerves.

M. rectus capitis anterior
The M. rectus capitis anterior (➤ Table 10.9) has its origin at the lateral mass of the atlas and runs to the Pars basilaris of the Os occipitale. Through its contraction, it assists with tilting the head forwards (inclination) and stabilises the Articulatio atlantooccipitalis.

M. rectus capitis lateralis
The M. rectus capitis lateralis (➤ Table 10.9) is a short flat muscle running from the Proc. transversus atlantis to the Proc. jugularis of

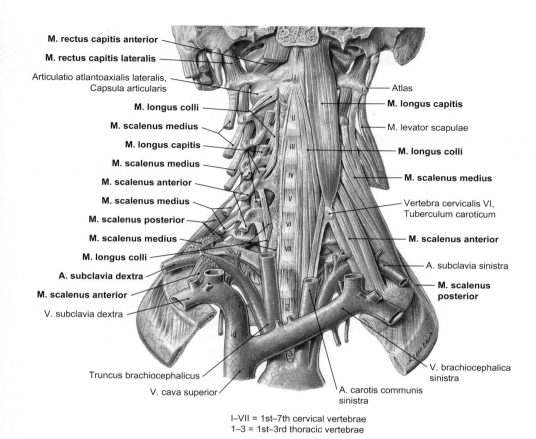

Fig. 10.8 Prevertebral muscles and M. longus capitis. Ventral view.

Labels (clockwise from upper left):
M. rectus capitis anterior
M. rectus capitis lateralis
Articulatio atlantoaxialis lateralis, Capsula articularis
M. longus colli
M. scalenus medius
M. longus capitis
M. scalenus medius
M. scalenus anterior
M. scalenus medius
M. scalenus posterior
M. scalenus medius
M. longus colli
A. subclavia dextra
M. scalenus anterior
V. subclavia dextra
Truncus brachiocephalicus
V. cava superior

Atlas
M. longus capitis
M. levator scapulae
M. longus colli
M. scalenus medius
Vertebra cervicalis VI, Tuberculum caroticum
M. scalenus anterior
A. subclavia sinistra
M. scalenus posterior
V. brachiocephalica sinistra
A. carotis communis sinistra

I–VII = 1st–7th cervical vertebrae
1–3 = 1st–3rd thoracic vertebrae

the Os occipitale (➤ Fig. 10.8). It supports the lateral flexion of the head.

M. longus capitis
The M. longus capitis (➤ Table 10.9) originates from the Tubercula anteriora of the transverse processes of cervical vertebrae III–VI and runs from caudal lateral to cranial medial to the Pars basilaris of the Os occipitale (➤ Fig. 10.8). A bilateral contraction of the M. longus capitis leads to a bending forward of the cervical spine and the head. A unilateral contraction of the muscle causes tilting and rotation of the head.

M. longus colli
The M. longus colli consists of 3 units, giving the muscle as a whole its characteristically triangular form (➤ Fig. 10.8). A **Pars obliqua superior**, running from the transverse processes of the upper cervical vertebrae III–V to the Tuberculum anterius of the atlas, a **Pars recta**, which originates from the anterior side of the lower cervical and upper thoracic vertebral bodies, and attaches at the front of cervical vertebrae II–IV, and a **Pars obliqua inferior** with its origin at the front of the thoracic vertebrae I–III, with the attachments at the Tubercula anteriora of the transverse processes of cervical vertebrae V–VII. A unilateral contraction leads to tilting and rotation of the head on the ipsilateral side. Bilateral contraction assists with the bending forwards of the cervical spine and the head.

10.3 Cervical fascia and connective tissue spaces
Michael Scholz

┌─ **Skills** ───────────────────────────────

After working through this chapter, you should be able to:
• name the various fasciae and anatomical spaces of the throat area and describe their boundaries

└──

The connective tissue of the cervical fascia (Fascia cervicalis) surrounds and connects the muscles, vascular, lymphatic and nervous systems and viscera of the neck with each other. Regionally it thickens into 3 different well-developed sheets. In their course, the respective fascial sheets delimit different transitional anatomical spaces from each other. These anatomical spaces, filled with loose connective tissue, surround the viscera and vascular, lymphatic and nervous systems, and ensure their ability to move against each other. This is necessary because the neck structures need to follow the natural movement of the cervical spine and the corresponding location changes during swallowing without any friction. The throat area structures themselves, like the vascular, lymphatic and nervous systems, are also surrounded by their own connective tissue sheaths.

N O T E

The anatomical spaces created by the fascia of the throat area run cranially and caudally to the skull base, and pass continually caudally into the mediastinum. Therefore, inflammatory processes or bleeding can spread virtually freely to the skull base and spread out into the mediastinum.

10.3.1 Neck fasciae

The cervical fascia is divided into a muscle fascia (Fascia cervicalis) with 3 sheets, a pathway fascia, a general organ fascia and special organ fasciae (➤ Fig. 10.9, ➤ Table 10.10).

Table 10.10 Neck fasciae.

Fascia	Enclosed/ensheathed structures
Muscle fascia (Fascia cervicalis)	
• Lamina superficialis (superficial layer)	• Complete throat area (also referred to as Fascia nuchae in the nape of the neck) • M. sternocleidomastoideus • M. trapezius
• Lamina pretrachealis (middle layer)	• Infrahyoid muscles
• Lamina prevertebralis (deep layer)	• Mm. scaleni • Prevertebral muscles • M. levator scapulae • Continues into the fascia of autochtonous back muscles • Truncus sympathicus, Pars cervicalis
Vascular, lymphatic and nervous systems fascia	
• Vagina carotica (carotid sheath)	• Aa. carotis communis, carotis interna and carotis externa • V. jugularis interna • N. vagus [X]
Organ fasciae	
• General organ fascia	All neck structures together (pharynx, larynx, thyroid gland, parathyroid gland, upper part of the trachea, Pars cervicalis of the oesophagus)
• Special organ fascia = organ capsule	Each individual neck organ, e.g. Fascia oesophagea

Muscle fascia

The non-uniformly structured **superficial sheet of the cervical fascia (Lamina superficialis)** in its course lies below the subcutaneous adipose tissue and under the platysma. The Lamina superficialis surrounds the entire circumference of the neck and encloses the Mm. sternocleidomastoidei and the upper parts of the Mm. trapezii (Partes descendentes) (➤ Fig. 10.10). Caudally, the superficial layer is attached both to the front surface of the Manubrium sterni and to the Clavicula, and continues into the Fascia pectoralis. Cranially the sheet is fixed to the lower margin of the Mandibu-

la and is attached laterally to the Fascia parotidea. In addition, the Lamina superficialis is fixed onto the hyoid bone (➤ Fig. 10.11). Above the hyoid bone, the Lamina superficialis covers the Trigonum submandibulare and the Glandula submandibularis which in turn is surrounded by its own capsule (specific organ fascia). The cutaneous branches of the cervical plexus and the superficial neck veins (Vv. jugulares externae and anteriores) run over the surface of the Lamina superficialis.

In comparison to the superficial cervical fascia, **the middle sheet of the cervical fascia (Lamina pretrachealis)** is a much coarser and hence more clearly defined structure. It is tensed bilaterally by the Mm. omohyoidei and lies protectively in front of the throat organs. All infrahyoid muscles are covered by it (➤ Fig. 10.9, ➤ Fig. 10.10); however, there is no direct connection to the trachea. The fascial sheet spans between the hyoid bone and the posterior side of the Manubrium sterni and of the Clavicula (➤ Fig. 10.11). At the point of intersection between the intermediate tendon of the M. omohyoideus and the carotid sheath, the Lamina pretrachealis and the Vagina carotica are fused.

The **deep sheet of the cervical fascia (Lamina prevertebralis)** is fixed on the Lig. longitudinale anterius along the medial cervical spine. It ensheathes the prevertebral muscles, the M. scaleni and the M. levator scapulae and merges into the fascia of the autochtonous back muscles at the nape of the neck (➤ Fig. 10.9). Cranially, the Lamina prevertebralis extends to the skull base and caudally it merges into the Fascia endothoracica. The Truncus sympathicus is enclosed in the lower neck section up to the C4 level of the Lamina prevertebralis. In addition, the Lamina prevertebralis covers the primary strands of the Plexus brachialis, the N. phrenicus and the A. subclavia.

Vascular, lymphatic and nervous systems fascia

The connective tissue enclosure of the vascular, lymphatic and nervous systems, which ensheathes the neurovascular strand lying to the side of the neck structures is the **Vagina carotica (carotid sheath; ➤** Fig. 10.10). It extends from the upper thoracic aperture to the skull base. Within it, running from caudal to cranial in the area of the Regio sternocleidomastoidea are initially the A. carotis communis, the V. jugularis interna with its adjacent deep lateral cervical lymph nodes and the N. vagus [X]. In the Trigonum caroticum the A. carotis communis splits into the A. carotis interna and the A. carotis externa, with the A. carotis interna continuing the course of the A. carotis communis and runs together with the V. jugularis interna and the N. vagus [X] within the Vagina carotica to the skull base.

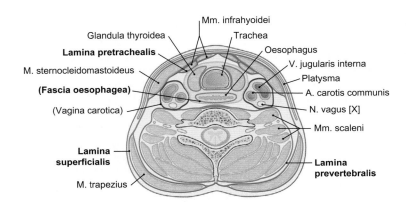

Fig. 10.9 Transverse section through the neck at the level of the thyroid gland (diagram). The respective courses of muscle fasciae, the pathway fascia and the visceral fascia are marked in colour with their respective content structures. Lamina superficialis (blue), Lamina pretrachealis (green), Lamina prevertebralis (red), carotid sheath (purple), general organ fascia (yellow), special organ fascia (brown). [E402]

Labels in figure:
Mm. infrahyoidei
Glandula thyroidea
Trachea
Lamina pretrachealis
Oesophagus
M. sternocleidomastoideus
V. jugularis interna
(Fascia oesophagea)
Platysma
A. carotis communis
(Vagina carotica)
N. vagus [X]
Mm. scaleni
Lamina superficialis
Lamina prevertebralis
M. trapezius

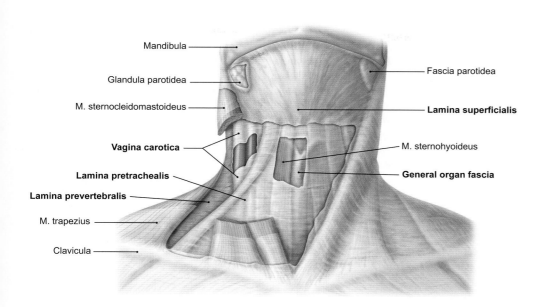

Fig. 10.10 Muscle fasciae of the neck. Ventral view. The platysma has been removed bilaterally. To the left, the superficial fascia sheet (Lamina superficialis) is intact and ensheathes the M. sternocleidomastoideus. To the right, the medial portion of the muscle and the majority of the Lamina superficialis is removed. As a result, the course of the middle and deep cervical fascia, as well as the carotid sheath, can be recognised. The medial fenestrated section makes it possible to view the thyroid cartilage of the larynx and the M. sternohyoideus, which would otherwise be covered by the lamina pretrachealis and the general organ fascia. Lamina superficialis (grey), Lamina pretrachealis (brown), Lamina prevertebralis (green), Vagina carotica (red).

NOTE

The **positional relationship between artery, vein and nerve** within the carotid sheath changes in its course from caudal to cranial. At the start in the Regio sternocleidomastoidea, the vein and nerve run lateral to the artery, then both migrate dorsally in their course to the skull base. In the Trigonum caroticum, the vein courses laterodorsally to the artery and the N. vagus [X] runs dorsally between the vessels.

Within the carotid bifurcation are the Glomus caroticum and the Sinus caroticus:

- The **Glomus caroticum** is a small knot-shaped paraganglion made up of an envelope and main cells. It has a diameter of approx. 3 mm. Apart from blood vessels, afferent nerve fibres leave the paraganglion, and these join onto the N. glossopharyngeus [IX] **(R. sinus carotici nervi glossopharyngei)**. The main cells are chemoreceptors that measure the partial pressures of oxygen and carbon dioxide and the pH of the blood.
- The **Sinus caroticus** contains pressure receptors (baroreceptors) in its wall that measure the blood pressure in the blood vessels and register changes of arterial pressure. Via the N. glossopharyngeus [IX] the information from both systems is sent to cardiovascular and respiratory centres in the Medulla oblongata. Respiratory rate and depth and heart rate are adjusted by reflexes. Other glomerulae and sinuses with a similar role are present e.g. in the wall of the aorta.

Organ fasciae

The organ fasciae are divided into a general and specific organ fasciae (➤ Fig. 10.9). The connective tissue of the general organ fascia encases all the neck organs, such as the pharynx, larynx, thyroid, parathyroid gland, the upper part of the trachea and the Pars cervicalis of the oesophagus; the special organ fasciae envelop each individual organ of the neck as a connective tissue organ capsule (e.g. Fascia oesophagea).

10.3.2 Connective tissue spaces of the neck

Due to the spatial structure of the individual fascial leaves of the Fascia cervicalis into a superficial, middle and deep sheet, movable connective tissue spaces are formed adjacent to each other. Apart

from their anatomical/physiological function to enable the freely movable nature of the structures of the throat area when swallowing, breathing and movements of the cervical spine, these spaces are also clinically relevant, since inflammatory processes can propagate along these anatomical spaces.

Spatium suprasternale

Between the Lamina superficialis and the Lamina pretrachealis there is the Spatium suprasternale, due to the different attachment points of these two sheets of the Fascia cervicalis to the Manubrium sterni and the Clavicula, (➤ Fig. 10.11). This movable space filled with adipose tissue is delimited caudally by the two sternoclavicular joints and by the Lig. interclaviculare which passes over the Manubrium sterni.

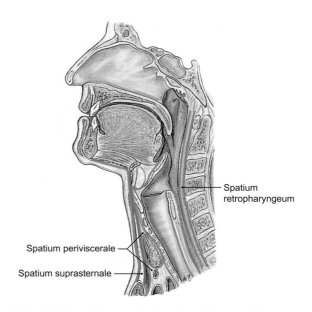

Fig. 10.11 Position of the cervical fascia and the resulting connective tissue spaces in sagittal section (diagram). Lamina superficialis (blue), Lamina pretrachealis (green), Lamina prevertebralis (red), general organ fascia (yellow), special organ fascia (brown).

543

Spatium periviscerale

The Spatium periviscerale (previscerale) can be defined as a movable space stretched between the Lamina pretrachealis and the general organ fascia (➤ Fig. 10.11). It extends from the Os hyoideum to the anterior mediastinum, where it ends at approximately the same level as the base of the heart.

Spatium peripharyngeum

The Spatium peripharyngeum dorsolaterally surrounds the throat (pharynx) and is divided into two parts:

* the **Spatium retropharyngeum (Spatium retroviscerale)**
* the **Spatium lateropharyngeum (Spatium parapharyngeum)**

Spatium retropharyngeum

The Spatium retropharyngeum (➤ Fig. 10.11) is the thin slit-like connective tissue space between the dorsal pharyngeal wall or the cervical part of the oesophagus and the deep layer of the cervical fascia (Lamina prevertebralis). The Spatium retropharyngeum starts at the skull base and continues caudally into the posterior mediastinum. The boundary with the adjacent Spatium lateropharyngeum is completed by a strong connective tissue plate (Septum sagittale) running from cranial to caudal.

Clinical remarks

Due to the connection of the Spatium retropharyngeum with the posterior mediastinum, there is here also the risk of transmission of inflammatory agents from within the neck to the thorax **(retropharyngeal abscess)**.

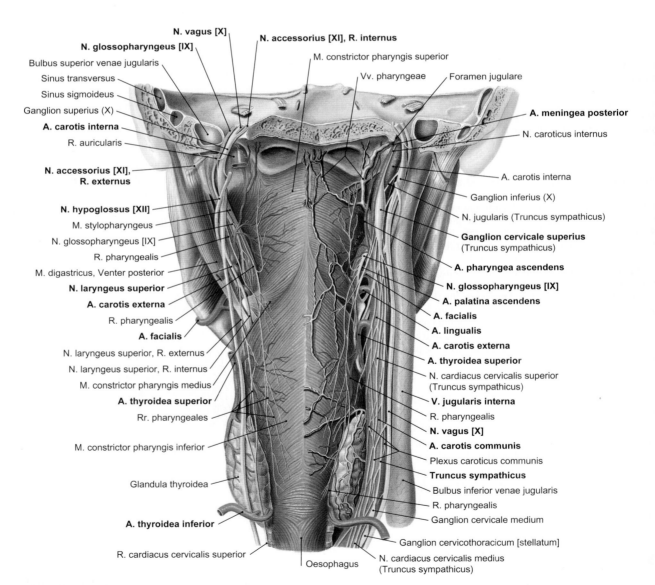

Fig. 10.12 Vessels and nerve pathways in the dorsal compartment of the Spatium lateropharyngeum, after removal of all connective tissue structures. Left side of image: course of the nerve routes following the removal of the major neck vessels with overlying nerve plexi; dorsal view.

Spatium lateropharyngeum

The Spatium lateropharyngeum like the Spatium retropharyngeum, reaches from the skull base into the mediastinum. It is divided into an anterior and posterior compartment by the course of the Fascia stylopharyngea, which runs from the Proc. styloideus to the lateral pharynx wall. The front section of the connective tissue space extends to the front into subcutis lying on the M. buccinator and only contains the vessels leading to the Tonsilla palatina (Rr. tonsilares of the A. and V. pharyngea ascendens). The section located dorsal of the Fascia stylopharyngea contains the large vascular, lymphatic and nervous systems of the neck, such as the A. carotis interna, the V. jugularis interna and the N. vagus [X], which are further caudally covered by the carotid sheath (Vagina carotica). The Truncus sympathicus, the N. glossopharyngeus [IX], the N. accessorius [XI] and the N. hypoglossus [XII] also run here (➤ Fig. 10.12).

10.4 Vascular, lymphatic and nervous systems of the neck
Michael Scholz

Skills

After working through this chapter, you should be able to:
- classify the course of the vascular, lymphatic and nervous systems of the throat area and structurally understand the different areas they innervate or supply

In the neck there are 2 large neurovascular pathways, which continue in their course to the upper extremities and the head (➤ Table 10.11). The cervical lymph is carried by superficial and deep lymph nodes (Nodi lymphodei cervicales) and is drained at the end of the Ductus lymphatic dexter and Ductus thoracicus into the respective venous angle. The innervation of the neck muscles and the muscles of the pharynx and larynx is carried out via the cervical spinal nerves (Plexus cervicalis and Plexus brachialis) and via the

Table 10.11 Structures within the two major neurovascular routes of the neck.

Vessels	Nerves	Lymph
Lateral cervical region		
• A. subclavia • V. subclavia	• Plexus brachialis	• Truncus subclavius
Dorsolateral cervical region		
• A. carotis communis • A. carotis externa • A. carotis interna • V. jugularis interna	• N. vagus • Truncus sympathicus	• Truncus jugularis

cranial nerves [V, VII, IX, X, XI]. The sensory innervation of the neck is provided by branches of the Plexus cervicalis and dorsal branches of the cervical spinal nerves. In addition, the N. hypoglossus [XII] and the N. phrenicus (C3–C5) run in their course to their respective innervation areas through different regions of the neck.

10.4.1 Arteries of the neck

There are 2 major arteries (A. subclavia and A. carotis communis) running through the neck, which in their course provide the blood supply via their junctions and branches to several areas of the throat area, the thoracic and abdominal walls and the head.

A. subclavia
The A. subclavia originates on the right side from the Truncus brachiocephalicus and on the left side as the last branch from the aortic arch. On both sides, the artery runs in the arch laterally over the pleural dome and, together with the primary strands of the Plexus brachialis, penetrates the scalene hiatus. In its further course it passes into the Sulcus arteriae subclaviae via the 1st rib and then subsequently continues on the lower edge of the 1st rib continuing by definition as the A. axillaris (➤ Fig. 10.13). Many branches exit

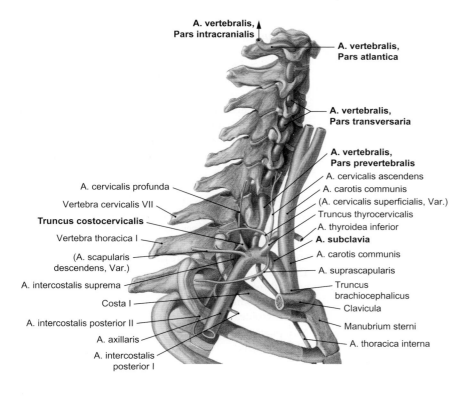

A. vertebralis, Pars intracranialis
A. vertebralis, Pars atlantica
A. vertebralis, Pars transversaria
A. vertebralis, Pars prevertebralis
A. cervicalis ascendens
A. carotis communis
(A. cervicalis superficialis, Var.)
Truncus thyrocervicalis
A. thyroidea inferior
A. subclavia
A. carotis communis
A. suprascapularis
Truncus brachiocephalicus
Clavicula
Manubrium sterni
A. thoracica interna

A. cervicalis profunda
Vertebra cervicalis VII
Truncus costocervicalis
Vertebra thoracica I
(A. scapularis descendens, Var.)
A. intercostalis suprema
Costa I
A. intercostalis posterior II
A. axillaris
A. intercostalis posterior I

Fig. 10.13 Branches of the A. subclavia with the Truncus thyrocervicalis and Truncus costocervicalis.

Table 10.12 Branches and junctions from the A. subclavia.

Arteries	Branches
A. vertebralis	
A. thoracica interna	
Truncus thyrocervicalis	• A. thyroidea inferior • A. cervicalis ascendens • A. suprascapularis • A. transversa cervicis (colli)
Truncus costocervicalis	• A. cervicalis profunda • A. intercostalis suprema

the A. subclavia, which apart from the A. thoracica interna and the A. intercostalis profunda are all involved in supplying blood to the neck (➤ Table 10.12).

Clinical remarks

The atypical outflow of an A. subclavia dextra, which originates as the last branch of the aortic arch instead of originating from the Truncus brachiocephalicus, is referred to as the **A. lusoria**. Here, the artery on its way to the right arm runs either behind the oesophagus or between the trachea and the oesophagus. This can affect the oesophageal function by creating difficulty in swallowing **(Dysphagia lusoria)** (also ➤ Chap. 10.6.6).

A high-grade stenosis in the region of the exit of the A. subclavia sinistra (less frequently of the A. subclavia dextra) can result in a retrograde flow into the A. vertebralis of the affected side during intense physical activity and load of the arm **(subclavian steal syndrome)**. This can lead to reduced perfusion of the brain resulting in dizziness and headaches.

A. vertebralis

The A. vertebralis originates as the first branch from the arc-shaped course in the first section of the A. subclavia. It runs almost vertically in a cranial direction and in 90% of cases (➤ Fig. 10.14) enters the Foramen transversale of the VIth cervical vertebra under the VIth cervical vertebra. From here it runs through the transverse processes of the cervical vertebra to the atlas. Together with the

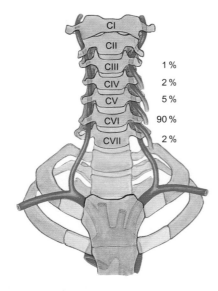

Fig. 10.14 Variations in the levels of entry of the A. vertebralis into the Foramina transversaria of the cervical spine.

A. carotis interna, as it runs cranially it supplies the brain and other structures of the CNS. As it runs through the neck, its small segmental branches supply the deep cervical musculature, the vertebral bodies, the spinal cord and the meninges of the medulla.

A. thoracica interna

The A. thoracica interna originates caudally from the A. subclavia and runs lateral to the sternum through the upper thoracic aperture. It runs parallel to the sternum caudally to the diaphragm.

Truncus thyrocervicalis

The Truncus thyrocervicalis originates at the medial margin of the M. scalenus anterior (➤ Fig. 10.15a). Usually 4 arteries arise from the short arterial trunk. Due to all these arteries having a high level of individual variability, they can also originate from the A. subclavia as stand-alone vessels (➤ Fig. 10.15b–g). The 4 vessels are:

- **A. thyroidea inferior:** it rises to the thyroid gland (Glandula thyroidea) and supplies the thyroid together with the A. thyroidea superior from the A. carotis externa. In addition, the A. thyroidea inferior during its course also supplies the parathyroid glands (Glandulae parathyroidae), the larynx, the pharynx, the oesophagus and the trachea.
- **A. cervicalis ascendens:** it runs slightly medial from the N. phrenicus on the M. scalenus anterior in a cranial direction and supplies the deep cervical muscles (➤ Fig. 10.16).
- **A. suprascapularis:** it runs on the dorsal side of the scapula and together with the A. axillaris circumflexa scapulae arising from the A. axillaris, forms the Rete scapulare.
- **A. transversa cervicis (colli):** as it courses through the lateral cervical region, it divides into 2 branches, the **R. superficialis** and the **R. profundis** (➤ Fig. 10.15a, ➤ Fig. 10.16). The R. superficialis runs together with the N. accessorius [XI] to the M. trapezius. The R. profundis goes deeper into the lateral cervical region together with the N. dorsalis scapulae to the Mm. rhomboidei and the M. latissimus dorsi.

A. carotis communis

The **A. carotis communis dextra** originates from the Truncus brachiocephalicus directly behind the right sternoclavicular joint. The **A. carotis communis sinistra** arises directly from the aortic arch and continues cranially behind the left sternoclavicular joint into the neck (➤ Fig. 10.8). The A. carotis communis courses on each side, together with the V. jugularis interna and the N. vagus [X] encased by the carotid sheath (Vagina carotica) and in its course through the neck, normally no other branches come off. In the Trigonum caroticum triangle, at the level of the upper edge of the Cartilago thyroidea, the A. carotis communis divides into its 2 terminal branches, the A. carotis externa and the A. carotis interna (➤ Fig. 10.17).

The **A. carotis interna** continues the course of the A. carotis communis directly without giving off other branches from the Trigonum caroticum through the parapharyngeal space in the direction of the skull base. It passes via the Canalis caroticus of the petrous bone (Pars petrosa ossis temporalis) into the inside of the skull in order to reach its supply areas.

The **A. carotis externa** provides branches for supplying the organs of the throat, tongue, face and scalp directly after leaving the A. carotis communis (➤ Fig. 10.17):

- A. thyroidea superior
- A. pharyngea ascendens
- A. lingualis
- A. facialis
- A. occipitalis

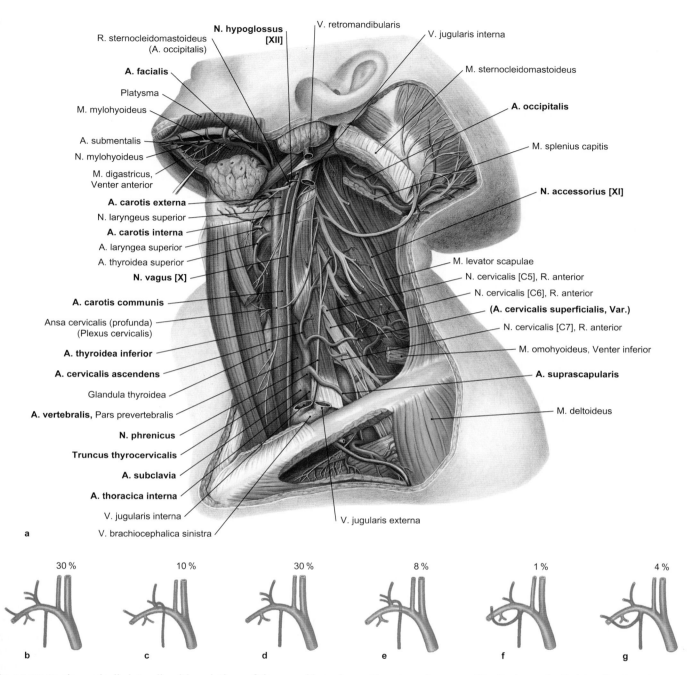

Fig. 10.15 Regio cervicalis lateralis with variations of the vessel branches. a Vessels and nerves of the Regio cervicalis lateralis, deep layer. Left lateral view after removal of the V. jugularis interna. **b–g** Variations of the vessel outflows from the A. subclavia and the Truncus thyrocervicalis.

- A. auricularis posterior
- A. temporalis superficialis
- A. maxillaris

A. thyroidea superior

The A. thyroidea superior arises as the first branch of the A. carotis externa on its anterior side just above the bifurcation of the carotid artery. It courses to the front caudally and supplies the right and left thyroid lobes. In its course to the thyroid gland, the A. thyroidea superior gives off the **A. laryngea superior** to the larynx. The thyroid gland is also supplied by the A. thyroidea inferior, a branch of the A. subclavia.

A. pharyngea ascendens

The A. pharyngea ascendens courses to the skull base as the second and smallest branch of the A. carotis externa in the posterior compartment of the lateropharyngeal space between the A. carotis interna and the pharynx. On its way it supplies the pharynx and the Tonsilla palatina and with its terminal branch reaches (**A. meningea posterior**) parts of the meninges.

A. lingualis

Directly above the outlet of the A. thyroidea superior, the A. lingualis courses at approximately the level of the hyoid bone to the front of the A. carotis externa (➤ Fig. 10.17). It passes behind the M. stylohyoideus and the Venter posterior of the M. digastricus into the Trigonum submandibulare, then continues into the Regio

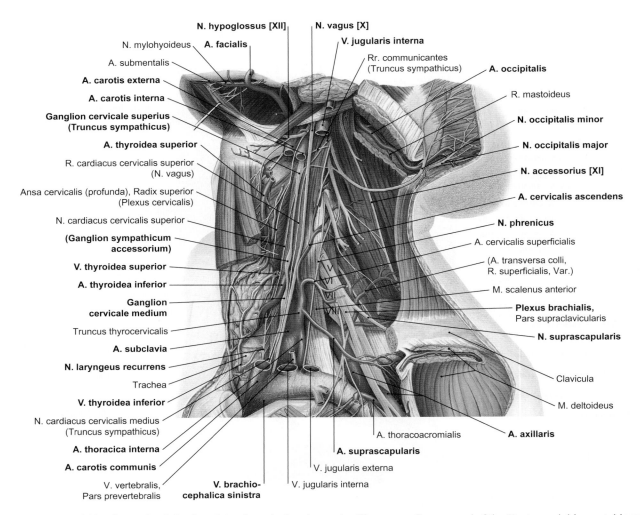

N. hypoglossus [XII]
N. mylohyoideus — **A. facialis**
A. submentalis
A. carotis externa
A. carotis interna
Ganglion cervicale superius
(Truncus sympathicus)
A. thyroidea superior
R. cardiacus cervicalis superior
(N. vagus)
Ansa cervicalis (profunda), Radix superior
(Plexus cervicalis)
N. cardiacus cervicalis superior
(Ganglion sympathicum
accessorium)
V. thyroidea superior
A. thyroidea inferior
Ganglion
cervicale medium
Truncus thyrocervicalis
A. subclavia
N. laryngeus recurrens
Trachea
V. thyroidea inferior
N. cardiacus cervicalis medius
(Truncus sympathicus)
A. thoracica interna
A. carotis communis
V. vertebralis,
Pars prevertebralis
V. brachio-
cephalica sinistra

N. vagus [X]
V. jugularis interna
Rr. communicantes
(Truncus sympathicus)
A. occipitalis
R. mastoideus
N. occipitalis minor
N. occipitalis major
N. accessorius [XI]
A. cervicalis ascendens
N. phrenicus
A. cervicalis superficialis
(A. transversa colli,
R. superficialis, Var.)
M. scalenus anterior
Plexus brachialis,
Pars supraclavicularis
N. suprascapularis
Clavicula
M. deltoideus
A. axillaris
A. thoracoacromialis
A. suprascapularis
V. jugularis externa
V. jugularis interna

Fig. 10.16 Nerves and blood vessels of the deep lateral cervical region and axillary area after removal of the M. sternocleidomastoideus, the major neck vessels and the anterior two thirds of the Clavicula. The Roman numerals V–VIII mark the corresponding cervical nerves.

sublingualis. It provides branches which supply blood to the tongue and other structures within the Regio sublingualis.

A. facialis

The A. facialis usually leaves the A. carotis externa directly above the outlet of the A. lingualis. As a variant, both blood vessels can also exit from a common trunk (Truncus linguofacialis) from the A. carotis externa. The A. facialis goes under the M. stylohyoideus and stretches along the Venter posterior of the M. digastricus, courses further between the Glandus submandibularis and the Mandibula, and at the front edge of the M. masseter it crosses the edge of the Mandibula, passing obliquely and forwards to the face (➤ Fig. 10.17). In its course in the Trigonum submandibulare, more branches are given off to supply the Tonsilla palatina (**R. tonsillaris of the A. palatina ascendens**), the area under the chin (**A. submentalis**) and various other small branches to supply the Glandula submandibularis (**Rr. glandulares**).

A. occipitalis

The A. occipitalis originates in the Trigonum submandibulare, often opposite the A. facialis. It courses dorsally to the Os. occipitale, where its branches form a dense vascular network.

A. auricularis posterior

The A. auricularis posterior is a small branch of the A. carotis externa, which also originates on the dorsal side and courses dorso-

cranially to the ear muscle, which is supplied by its smaller branches (**Rr. auriculares**). In addition it gives off branches to the middle and inner ear and to the dura mater.

A. temporalis superficialis and A. maxillaris

The A. temporalis superficialis and the A. maxillaris are the two terminal branches of the A. carotica externa. The **A. temporalis superficialis** starts dorsally to the Colum mandibulae, and runs between the rear edge of the Mandibula and cranially in front of the Porus acusticus externus to the temple. Here it divides into the **R. frontalis** and the **R. parietalis** to supply this region (➤ Fig. 10.17). The **A. maxillaris** normally courses as the larger of the two terminal branches dorsal of the Collum mandibulae into the Fossa infratemporalis, and there it branches out into its terminal branches (➤ Chap. 9.2.5).

10.4.2 Veins of the neck

Overview

The majority of the venous blood from the head and neck is drained through the **jugular system**, made up of the following paired veins:

- **V. jugularis interna**
- **V. jugularis externa**
- **V. jugularis anterior**

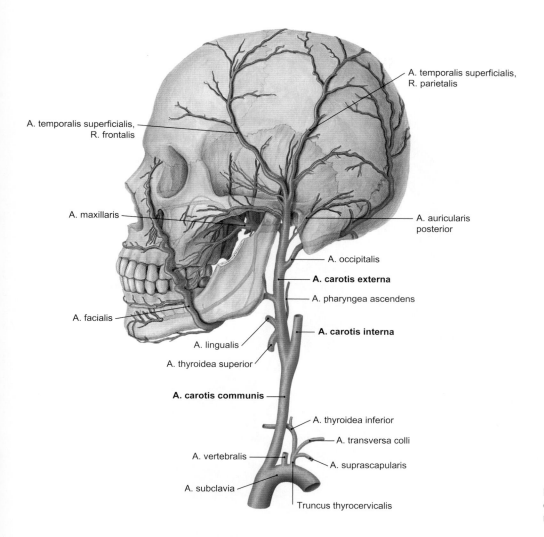

A. temporalis superficialis, R. parietalis

A. temporalis superficialis, R. frontalis

A. maxillaris

A. auricularis posterior

A. occipitalis

A. carotis externa

A. pharyngea ascendens

A. facialis

A. carotis interna

A. lingualis

A. thyroidea superior

A. carotis communis

A. thyroidea inferior

A. transversa colli

A. vertebralis

A. suprascapularis

A. subclavia

Truncus thyrocervicalis

Fig. 10.17 Course of the A. subclavia and the A. carotis communis. Lateral view.

To a lesser extent, the blood is also drained by the paired **V. subclavia**. The venous network of the throat area is individually extremely variable and the veins are connected with each other by various anastomoses.

The V. jugularis interna and the V. subclavia join together in the right and the left venous angle to the **V. brachiocephalica** (➤ Fig. 10.19). On both sides of the vein angle the major lymphatic trunks flow on both sides of the venous angle; on the right side of the **Ductus lymphaticus dexter** and on the left side of the **Ductus thoracicus**. The right and left V. brachiocephalica form the Vena cava superior (➤ Fig. 10.19), then flow into the right atrium of the heart.

Clinical remarks

The placing of an **intravenous access** is the most commonly used technique in preclinical emergency care. Where the veins are in poor conditions, an alternative access point using the V. jugularis externa can also provide a good alternative (cardiopulmonary resuscitation guidelines). For **central venous catheters (CVC)** thin plastic tubing is introduced under clinical conditions via a larger vein and advanced to the right atrium of the heart through the Vena cava superior or the Vena cava inferior. In this way it is possible to introduce drugs and highly concentrated nutritional solutions and to determine the **central venous pressure (CVP)**. To insert a CVC, access is preferably via the V. jugularis interna or the V. subclavia because they can be easily located anatomically and sonographically; however, access via other veins is also possible.

Course of the veins
V. jugularis interna

The paired V. jugularis interna starts at the Foramen jugulare at the skull base with the **Bulbus superior venae jugularis**, the extended continuation of the Sinus sigmoideus. Together with the N. glossopharyngeus [IX], the N. vagus [X] and the N. accessorius [XI] it passes through the Foramen jugularis and then runs within the carotid sheath together with the A. carotis interna and the N. vagus [X] caudally through the Spatium lateropharyngeum and the Trigonum caroticum. In the Regio sternocleidomastoidea it is accompanied by the A. carotis communis and the N. vagus [X]. The V. jugularis interna widens shortly before its junction with the V. subclavia into the **Bulbus inferior venae jugularis** (➤ Fig. 10.18, ➤ Fig. 10.19).

NOTE

The V. jugularis interna collects and drains the venous blood from the brain, scalp, facial region and thyroid gland.

V. jugularis externa

The paired V. jugularis externa is formed by the fusing of the **V. occipitalis** and the **V. auricularis posterior** and it runs epifascially on the M. sternocleidomastoideus to the V. subclavia (➤ Fig. 10.18, ➤ Fig. 10.20) in a caudal direction. It leads blood from the superficial head and ear areas.

549

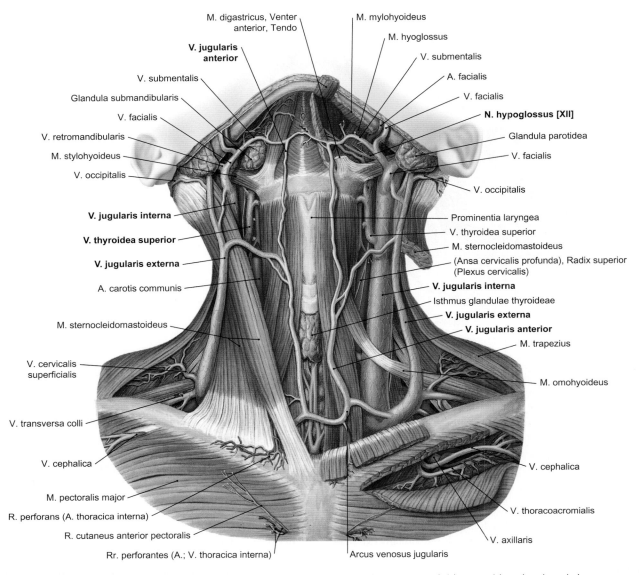

Fig. 10.18 Veins of the neck after removal of all cervical fasciae. On the left side, the M. sternocleidomastoideus has largely been removed. Ventral view.

V. jugularis anterior

The V. jugularis anterior is also paired and runs epifascially, beginning in the area of the hyoid bone and draining the venous blood of the floor of the mouth region and the front wall of the throat area. Shortly before the venous angle (Angulus venosus), it flows into the V. jugularis externa. In the Spatium suprasternale (➤ Fig. 10.11, ➤ Fig. 10.18), both Vv. jugulares anteriores are connected with each other by the **Arcus venosus jugularis**.

V. subclavia

The V. subclavia collects the venous blood from the cervical spine, arms and shoulder girdle, a part of the chest wall and the deep cervical muscles. The drainage area of the vein largely corresponds with the supply area of the artery (A. subclavia). The vein runs as a continuation of the **V. axillaris** between the 1st rib and the clavicle (Clavicula) and between the M. scalenus anterior and the clavicular origin of the M. sternocleidomastoideus. In this area it is covered by the Fascia pretrachealis and is connected with the surrounding structures by connective tissue. In the venous angle it combines with the V. jugularis interna to the V. brachiocephalica.

V. brachiocephalica

The V. brachiocephalica also receives direct inflows from the cervical region (➤ Fig. 10.19). The **V. thyroidea inferior** flows as a single vein or as the Plexus thyroideus impar into the V. brachiocephalica sinistra. The **V. vertebralis**, which previously still largely receives venous blood from the V. cervicalis profunda, also flows into the V. brachiocephalica.

10.4.3 Nerves of the neck

The innervation of the skin of the throat area is carried out by branches of the Plexus cervicalis (ventrolateral skin area) and by Rr. dorsales of spinal nerves C2–C8. Also involved in the motor innervation of the neck muscles are both cervical spinal nerves (Plexus cervicales; Plexus brachiales; Rr. dorsales C1–C8) and various cranial nerves (N. trigeminus [V], N. facialis [VII], N. glossopharyngeus [IX], N. vagus [X] and N. accessorius [XI]). Autonomic nerve fibres of the neck come from the sympathetic trunk of the neck, (Truncus sympathicus, Pars cervicalis) and the N. vagus [X].

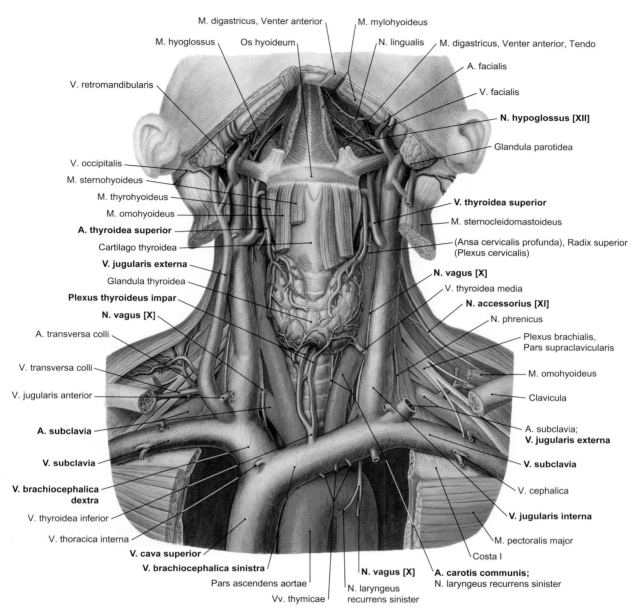

Fig. 10.19 Vessels and nerves of the neck and the upper thoracic aperture after removal of the sternum, parts of the clavicles and parts of the M. sternocleidomastoideus, and infrahyoid musculature. Ventral view.

The N. hypoglossus [XII] passes through the neck on its way to the tongue, for which it provides the motor innervation.

Cervical spinal nerves

Like all spinal nerves, the **spinal nerves of the neck** also include the **R. anterior** and **R. posterior** for the innervation of the different target areas:

- The Rr. anteriores combine to produce 2 large nerve plexi, the **Plexus cervicalis** and the **Plexus brachialis**. In the plexi nerve fibres from several spinal cord segments combine.
- By contrast, the Rr. dorsales (C2–C8) which are thinner than the Rr. anteriores, maintain their segmental course. Shortly after exiting from the cervical spinal nerves, they divide into a lateral (**R. lateralis**) and a medial (**R. medialis**) branch (➤ Table 10.13) and provide motor innervation of the neck muscles, parts of the autochthonous back muscles, the skin of the nape of the neck and the occipital region, which supply sensory innervation up to the transition of the supply area of the N. trigeminus [V] (➤ Fig. 10.21).

Table 10.13 Rr. posteriores of the spinal nerves of the neck with origins, fibre quality and innervation area.

Nerve	Origins	Quality	Supply areas
R. posterior (N. suboccipitalis)	C1	Motoric only	• Deep neck muscles • M. longus capitis • M. semispinalis capitis
R. posterior • Lateral branch • Medial branch (N. occipitalis major)	C2	Mixed	• M. semispinalis capitis • M. longissimus capitis • M. splenius capitis • Skin of the throat area up to the crown
R. posterior • Lateral branch • Medial branch (N. occipitalis tertius)	C3	Mixed	• Autochthonous back muscles • Innervation of the skin of the nape of the neck
Rr. posteriores • Lateral branch • Medial branch	C4–C8	Mixed	• Autochthonous back muscles • Overlying skin areas

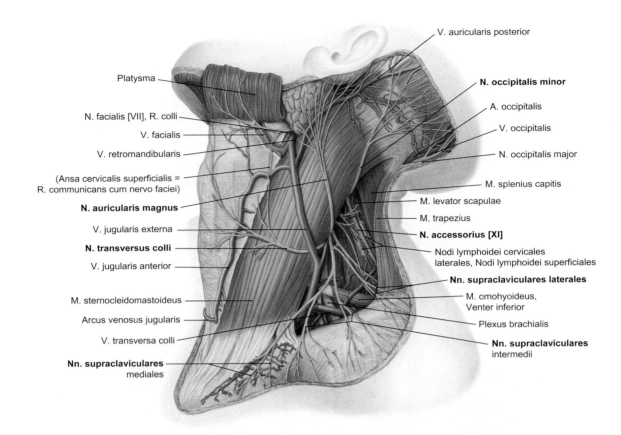

Fig. 10.20 Vessels and nerves of the lateral neck region after removal of the Lamina superficialis of the cervical fascia. The platysma is folded upwards. View from lateral left side.

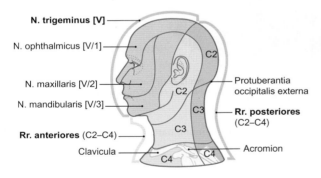

Fig. 10.21 Sensory innervation of the skin of the throat area and head with segmental arrangement of the skin areas (diagram). [E402]

Table 10.14 Sensory skin branches of the Plexus cervicalis from the Punctum nervosum (ERB's point) with their branches.

Nerve	Origins
N. occipitalis minor	C2–C3
N. auricularis magnus • R. anterior • R. posterior	C2–C3
N. transversus colli • Rr. superiores • Rr. inferiores	C2–C3
Nn. supraclaviculares • mediales • intermedii • laterales	C3–C4

Plexus cervicalis

The Plexus cervicalis is formed from the **Rr. anteriores of the spinal nerves C1–C4**. The nerves originating from this plexus innervate the skin in the front and side of the throat area, the infrahyoid muscles and the diaphragm and parts of the serosa skin, such as the Pleura parietalis, the pericardium in the thorax and the peritoneum in the abdomen. The branches from the Plexus cervicalis are surrounded by the Lamina pretrachealis, and are divided into **skin branches (Rr. cutanei)** and **muscle branches (Rr. musculares)**.

Rr. cutanei

The sensory skin branches of the Plexus cervicalis all penetrate at the posterior border of the M. sternocleidomastoideus, at about the halfway level of the course of the muscle, through the Lamina superficialis to the surface. The position is referred to as the **Punctum nervosum (ERB's point)** (➤ Table 10.14; ➤ Fig. 10.20). The **N. occipitalis minor** runs on the posterior border of the M. sternocleidomastoideus in a cranial direction and crosses over the N. accessorius [XI]. It supplies sensory innervation to the skin of the throat area and the head behind the outer ear (➤ Fig. 10.22). The **N. auricularis magnus** is usually the strongest branch from the Punctum nervosum. It runs from the posterior border of the M. sternocleidomastoideus diagonally upwards over the muscle to

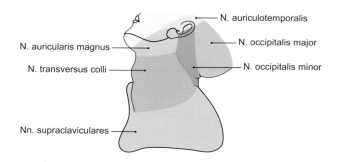

Fig. 10.22 Sensory innervation of the skin of the throat area and head via the nerves of the Plexus cervicalis and the Nn. occipitalis major and tertius.

the ear lobe. Its **R. anterior** supplies the sensory innervation to the front surface of the outer ear and to the jaw angle (➤ Fig. 10.22). The skin on the back of the outer ear is innervated by the **R. posterior**.

The **N. transversus colli** runs approximately level to the middle of the N. sternocleidomastoideus, horizontally across the muscle medially into the front throat area. It is covered by the platysma and is divided into the **Rr. superiores** (sensory innervation of the skin above the Os hyoideum) and the **Rr. inferiores** (skin of the throat area below the hyoid bone). One of the Rr. superiores, together with the R. colli of the N. facialis [VII], forms an anastomosis (formerly known as Ansa cervicalis superficialis) and therefore in a short section of the fibre course also leads motor fibres to the underside of the platysma (➤ Fig. 10.20).

The **Nn. supraclaviculares** are a group of cutaneous nerves radiating in a fan shape into the lateral triangle of the neck and only penetrate the Lamina superficialis and the platysma in the area of the

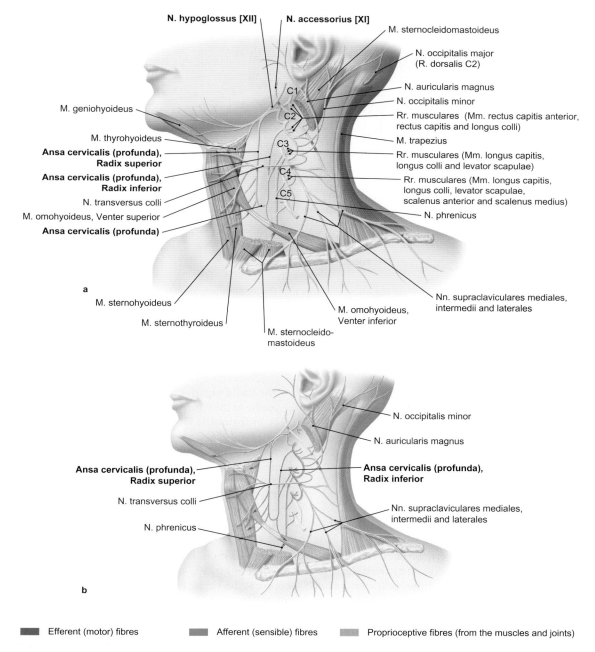

Efferent (motor) fibres   Afferent (sensible) fibres   Proprioceptive fibres (from the muscles and joints)

Fig. 10.23 Sensory and motor branches of the Plexus cervicalis (diagram). **a** Anatomical situation. **c** Functional distinction of the branches.

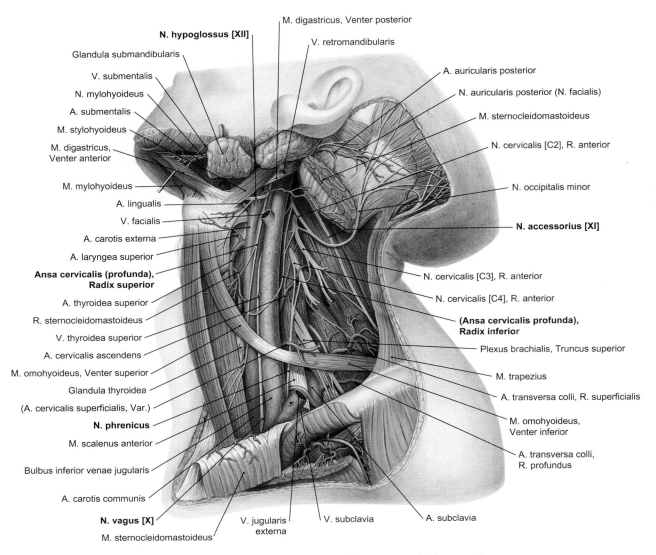

Fig. 10.24 Vessels and nerves of the lateral cervical region after removal of the M. sternocleidomastoideus.

Trigonum omoclaviculare. A distinction is made between (➤ Fig. 10.20, ➤ Fig. 10.22):

- **Nn. supraclaviculares mediales:** sensory innervation of the skin at the front of the Clavicula with bordering chest skin
- **Nn. supraclaviculares intermedii:** sensory innervation of the skin in the medial section of the Clavicula with chest skin to the 4th rib
- **Nn. supraclaviculares laterales:** sensory innervation of the skin over the acromion of the scapula and above the M. deltoideus

Rr. musculares

The Rr. musculares of the Plexus cervicalis innervate different muscle groups (➤ Fig. 10.23).

A main motor branch is the **N. phrenicus (C3–C5)**, which innervates the diaphragm (Diaphragma) and also sensorily supplies adjacent sections of the pericardium and peritoneum. It runs diagonally over the M. scalenus anterior caudally and between the A. and V. subclavia enters through the upper thoracic aperture into the mediastinum (➤ Fig. 10.16, ➤ Fig. 10.24). In its course on the M. scalenus anterior in the direction of the mediastinum, the N. phrenicus is crossed by 2 arteries, the A. transversa colli and the A. suprascapularis (➤ Fig. 10.16).

The **Ansa cervicalis** (formerly: Ansa cervicalis profunda) is a nerve loop of the cervical nerves C1–C3. It consists of a Radix superior (C1–C2) and a Radix inferior (C2–C3), which lies around the V. jugularis and is located in the carotid sheath (➤ Fig. 10.23):

- The **Radix superior** in its course is temporarily attached to the course of the Nn. hypoglossus [XII]. In the place where the N. hypoglossus [XII] crosses the Aa. carotides internae and externae, some of the nerve fibres leave it and pass downwards between the major vessels of the throat area. The Radix superior innervates the Venter superior of the M. omohyoideus and the upper portions of the M. sternohyoideus and M. sternothyroideus.
- The **Radix inferior** completes the nerve loop and, as a direct branch of the Plexus cervicalis, passes either medial or lateral of the V. jugularis interna in a caudal direction.

Both roots of the Ansa cervicalis come together individually at different levels ventral of the A. carotis communis and the V. jugularis interna (➤ Fig. 10.24). From here, branches of the Ansa cervicalis course to the Venter inferior of the M. omohyoideus and to the lower parts of the M. sternohyoideus and M. sternothyroideus.

Plexus brachialis

The Plexus brachialis is formed by the merging of the **Rr. anteriores of spinal nerves C5–C8**, as well as the **1st thoracic nerve**

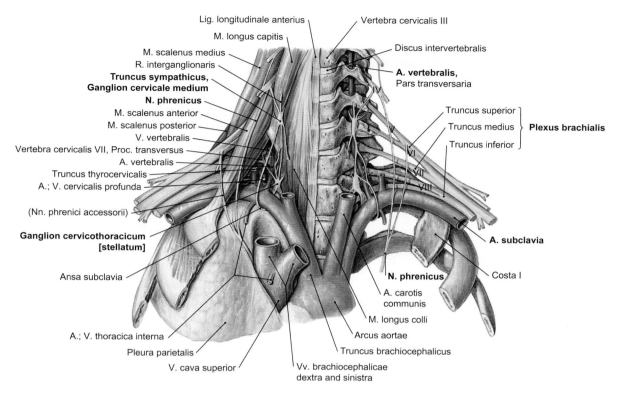

Lig. longitudinale anterius — Vertebra cervicalis III
M. longus capitis — Discus intervertebralis
M. scalenus medius
R. interganglionaris — **A. vertebralis,** Pars transversaria
Truncus sympathicus, Ganglion cervicale medium
N. phrenicus
M. scalenus anterior — Truncus superior
M. scalenus posterior — Truncus medius } **Plexus brachialis**
V. vertebralis — Truncus inferior
Vertebra cervicalis VII, Proc. transversus
Truncus thyrocervicalis
A. vertebralis
A.; V. cervicalis profunda
(Nn. phrenici accessorii)
Ganglion cervicothoracicum [stellatum]
Ansa subclavia
N. phrenicus — A. carotis communis — **A. subclavia** — Costa I
A.; V. thoracica interna
Pleura parietalis — M. longus colli
V. cava superior — Arcus aortae
Truncus brachiocephalicus
Vv. brachiocephalicae dextra and sinistra

Fig. 10.25 Vessels and nerves in the transition zone from the throat area and the thorax to the upper extremity (diagram).

(T1). The Rr. anteriores arise between the origins of the M. scalenus anterior and M. scalenus medius and are the roots of the Plexus brachialis. At the exit of the scalene hiatus, the Rr. anteriores attach to the 3 primary strands of the Plexus brachialis (Trunci) (➤ Table 10.15, ➤ Fig. 10.25).

Prior to entering into the axilla along the Aa. subclavia and axillaris, the 3 trunks (Trunci superior, medius and inferior), each divide into a ventral and a dorsal branch and then entwine again into 3 **secondary cords** (Fasciculi lateralis, medialis and posterior) (see also ➤ Chap. 4.6.2). The peripheral nerve for the innervation of the upper extremities and parts of the chest wall pass out of the cords. Due to the fibre exchange in the Plexus brachialis, they always have parts of at least 2 spinal nerves.

Clinical remarks

For local anaesthesia and analgesia in the arm, a clinical **block of the Plexus brachialis** (axillary block, axillary Plexus brachialis block, axillary Plexus anaesthesia) can be performed. It is a simple regional anaesthetic procedure with few side effects. A local anaesthetic is mostly injected at the C6 level into the perineural connective tissue between the M. scalenus anterior and M. scalenus medius. A disadvantage in contrast to the **infraclavicular Plexus block** is the partly insufficient deactivation of the innervation area of the N. radialis; however, there is no risk of a pneumothorax caused by breaching the immediately neighbouring dome of the pleura (➤ Fig. 10.25, right-hand side).

The **Pars supraclavicularis** of the Plexus brachialis surrounds the direct motor branches arising from the 3 Trunci. They all leave the Plexus brachialis in the lateral neck triangle. They include:

- **N. dorsalis scapulae** (C3–C5) that penetrates through the M. scalenus medius and runs to its target area, the M. levator scapulae and M. rhomboidei

- **N. thoracicus longus** (C5–C7), which further caudally penetrates the M. scalenus medius and courses over the 1st rib to the M. serratus anterior, which it innervates (➤ Fig. 10.16)
- **N. subclavius** (C5–C6), that courses to the M. subclavius and can additionally emit fibres to the N. phrenicus (Nn. phrenici accessorii)
- **N. suprascapularis** (C4–C6), that courses to the Scapula and runs beneath the Lig. transversum scapulae (in contrast to the A. suprascapulae, which typically runs above the ligament) passes through the Incisura suprascapulae to innervate the Mm. supraspinatus and infraspinatus (➤ Fig. 10.16)

Cranial nerves

Branches of the N. trigeminus [V], N. facialis [VII], N. glossopharyngeus [IX], N. vagus [X], N. accessorius [XI] , and N. hypoglossus [XII] run through the throat area (➤ Table 10.16). The cranial nerves IX–XI and the N. hypoglossus [XII], after exiting the internal surface of skull base, pass through the Spatium lateropharyngeum in close relationship to the A. carotis interna (➤ Fig. 10.12). As one of the terminal branches of the **N. mandibularis [V/3]** , the **N. mylohyoideus** runs forwards in the Sulcus mylohyoideus of the Mandibula into the Trigonum submandibulare and provides motor innervation to the M. mylohyoideus and Venter anterior of the M. digastricus (➤ Fig. 10.15a, ➤ Fig. 10.16). The Venter posterior of the M. digastricus and M. stylohyoidus are both innervated by branches of the **N. facialis [VII]**. At the lower edge of the Glandula

Table 10.15 Composition and origins of the primary strands of the Plexus brachialis.

Rr. anteriores from	Primary strand of the Plexus brachialis
C5–C6	Truncus superior
C7	Truncus medius
C8–T1	Truncus inferior

Table 10.16 Cranial nerves IX–XII with side branches and innervation areas through the course of the throat area.

Cranial nerves	Innervation areas
N. glossopharyngeus [IX] • R. musculi stylopharyngei • Rr. pharyngei • R. sinus carotici	• M. stylopharyngeus • Plexus pharyngeus • M. constrictor pharyngis superior • Wall of the Sinus caroticus/Glomus caroticum

N. vagus [X]
• R. pharyngeus
• N. laryngeus superior
  – R. externus
  – R. internus
• N. laryngeus recurrens
• Rr. cardiaci cervicales superiores/inferiores
	• Plexus pharyngeus
	• M. cricothyroideus
	• M. constrictor pharyngis inferior
	• Mucosa of the upper half of the larynx
	• Inner laryngeal muscles
	• Mucosa of the lower half of the larynx
	• Plexus cardiacus

N. accessorius [XI]	• M. sternocleidomastoideus • M. trapezius
N. hypoglossus [XII]	• Inner and outer tongue muscles

parotidea, the R. colli nervi facialis emerges from the glandular tissue and runs diagonally forwards and downwards to innervate the platysma (➤ Fig. 10.20).

The **N. glossopharyngeus [IX]** courses caudally, between the A. carotis interna and the V. jugularis interna through the Spatium lateropharyngeum. It is positioned dorsal of the M. stylopharyngeus, and continues to run between it and the M. styloglossus to the root of the tongue and its other innervation areas (➤ Table 10.16).

The **N. vagus [X]** is the main nerve of the parasympathetic nervous system and also contains visceromotor and viscerosensory fibres (➤ Chap. 9.3.10). In the throat area, it runs as part of the neurovascular bundle within the carotid sheath through the Spatium lateropharyngeum (➤ Fig. 10.12) in the direction of the mediastinum. From the throat area section of the N. vagus [X], nerve fibres go out to innervate the pharynx (Rr. pharyngei), larynx (N. laryngeus superior, N. laryngeus recurrens [the terminal branch of the N. laryngeus recurrens is also referred to as the N. laryngeus inferior]) and the heart (Rr. cardiaci cervicales superiores and inferiores) (➤ Table 10.16).

The **N. accessorius [XI]** also courses through the Spatium lateropharyngeus and enters in the top angle of the Trigonum caroticum,

usually in front of the V. jugularis interna, under the M. sternocleidomastoideus, and in order to supply this and then subsequently supply motor innervation to the M. trapezius (➤ Fig. 10.24).

The **N. hypoglossus [XII]** courses through the Spatium lateropharyngeum forward into the Trigonum carotis. Here it crosses over in an arch-like manner the A. carotis externa and the A. carotis interna and continues to run through the Trigonum submandibulare. From here, it passes between the M. hyoglossus and M. mylohyoideus to the tongue (➤ Fig. 10.26).

Clinical remarks

Damage to the N. hypoglossus [XII], e.g. due to tumour infiltration of a cervical lymph node metastasis can be easily diagnosed: when stretched out, the tongue deviates to the diseased side since the tongue muscles pushing out on the healthy side can carry out the motion, whereas it is not possible on the diseased side.

Truncus sympathicus (Pars cervicalis)

The sympathetic trunk (Truncus sympathicus) consists of two parallel nerve cords, running paravertebrally on each side. They extend from the cervical spine to the coccyx. Each of the two sympathetic trunks is characterised by the accumulation of neurons (ganglions) that thicken in segmental succession. A distinction is made between:

• Pars cervicalis
• Pars thoracica
• Pars lumbalis
• Pars sacralis

In its upper section, the Pars thoracica forms a ganglion located on the head of the rib, each of which is covered by the Fascia endothoracica. This first chest ganglion is usually fused with the lower cervical ganglion, forming the **Ganglion cervicothoracicum (stellatum)** with a length of up to 2 cm. It is located above the dome of the pleura behind the A. subclavia at the level where the A. vertebralis exits. The **Pars cervicalis trunci sympathici** continues from here embedded in the deep layer (Lamina profunda) of the Fascia cervicalis in front of the Mm. longus colli and capitis and behind

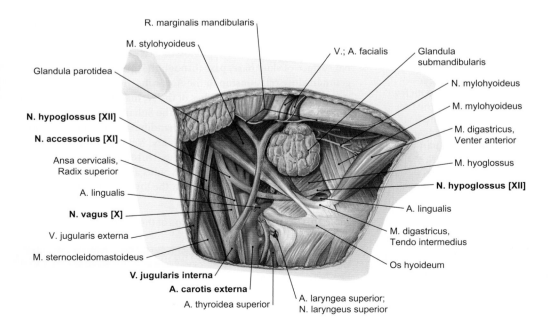

Fig. 10.26 Vessels and nerves in the upper region of the Trigonum caroticum and Trigonum submandibulare after removal of all fascia. View from right lateral below.

R. marginalis mandibularis
M. stylohyoideus
Glandula parotidea
N. hypoglossus [XII]
N. accessorius [XI]
Ansa cervicalis, Radix superior
A. lingualis
N. vagus [X]
V. jugularis externa
M. sternocleidomastoideus
V. jugularis interna
A. carotis externa
A. thyroidea superior
A. laryngea superior; N. laryngeus superior
V.; A. facialis
Glandula submandibularis
N. mylohyoideus
M. mylohyoideus
M. digastricus, Venter anterior
M. hyoglossus
N. hypoglossus [XII]
A. lingualis
M. digastricus, Tendo intermedius
Os hyoideum

the carotid sheath cranially (➤ Fig. 10.12, ➤ Fig. 10.16). Approximately at the level of the IV cervical vertebra the sympathetic trunk penetrates the deep sheet of the cervical fascia and now, resting behind the carotid sheath, runs towards cranial. At the level of the IIIrd cervical vertebra, the sympathetic trunk once again thickens on both sides, to the **Ganglion cervicale superius**. Between the Ganglion stellatum and the Ganglion cervicale superius, infrequently there is a **Ganglion cervicale mediale** (at the level of the VIth cervical vertebra). Connections between spinal nerves and the sympathetic trunk usually run via the Rr. communicantes albi to the sympathetic trunk and back to the respective spinal nerve via the Rr. communicantes grisei; however the Rr. communicantes albi only occur in the Pars thoracica and the Pars lumbalis. In the Pars cervicalis they are absent! In the ganglia, ascending preganglionic parasympathetic fibres are interlaced; these then continue as postganglionic fibres to a variety of target areas in the chest, throat area and head.

Ganglion cervicale superius

The Ganglion cervicale superius is positioned before the transverse processes of the IInd and IIIrd cervical vertebrae, and at about 3 cm in size, it is the largest sympathetic ganglion in the throat area. It is also the last switching station onto postganglionic parasympathetic fibres that go from here to their innervation areas in the head. The Rr. communicantes grisei run from the Ganglion cervicale superius to spinal nerves C1–C4. Additionally, the fibres form a Plexus around the Aa. carotis interna and externa, and its branches reach the parasympathetic cranial ganglia (Ganglia ciliare, pterygopalatinum, submandibulare, oticum), through which they pass to the end organs without being switched. Other fibres run down to the heart.

Ganglion cervicale medium

The Ganglion cervicale medium is frequently poorly developed and can be either entirely absent as an individual variability, it can be replaced by several smaller ganglia, or it can be fused with the Ganglion cervicale inferius. When present, it is found at the level of the VIth cervical vertebra, in close proximity to the A. thyroidea inferior. The Rr. communicantes grisei for the spinal nerves C5–C6 and branches to the thyroid gland, parathyroid gland and the heart come from the ganglion.

Ganglion cervicale inferius

The Ganglion cervicale inferius is usually fused together with the first chest ganglion of the Truncus sympathicus to the **Ganglion cervicothoracicum (Ganglion stellatum)**. The ganglion is located ventrally on the head of the 1st rib and in front of the Proc. transversus of the VIIth cervical vertebra (C7). The Rr. communicantes grisei run from the ganglion to spinal nerves C7–C8 and T1. Other branches course as the N. vertebralis and in the Ansa subclavia to the vessels, and as the Nn. cardiaci inferiores to the heart. Thus the fibres reach the oesophagus, larynx, trachea, bronchi, pharynx and the heart.

10.4.4 Lymph nodes of the neck

In the throat area there are approximately 200–300 lymph nodes, strung together like a chain, running mainly along the V. jugularis interna. This large number (approximately 30% of the lymph nodes of the entire body) is explained by the immediate proximity of the oral and nasal cavities, providing entry for potential pathogens and antigens. Running along a horizontal line from the chin via the mandibular edge to the Occiput is a series of lymph nodes which serve as

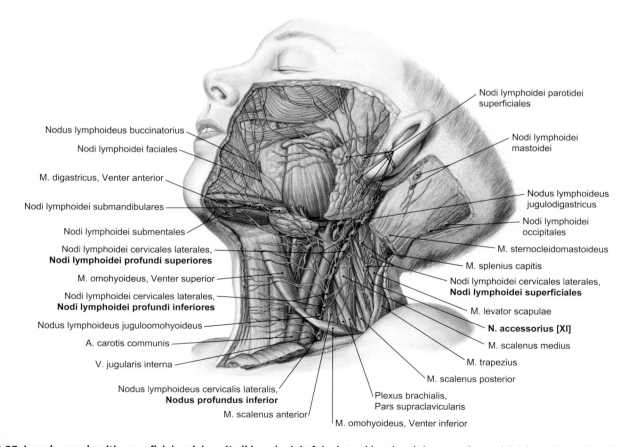

Fig. 10.27 Lymph vessels with superficial and deep Nodi lymphodei of the lateral head and throat regions. Child, lateral view from the left after the removal of the skin and fascia.

Table 10.17 Lymph nodes of the neck with course and catchment areas.

Lymph nodes	Course	Lymph inward circulation
Nodi lymphoidei cervicales anteriores		
• Nodi lymphoidei cervicales anteriores superficiales – Nodi lymphoidei submentales	Along the V. jugularis anterior	• Skin of the anterior cervical region; drainage goes to the anterior deep lymph nodes • Lower lip, floor of the mouth, teeth, tongue, oral mucosa
• Nodi lymphoidei cervicales anteriores profundi	Along the lower respiratory tract; both collecting and regional lymph nodes	
– Nodi lymphoidei infrahyoidei		• Upper half of the larynx
– Nodi lymphoidei prelaryngei		• Lower half of the larynx
– Nodi lymphoidei thyroidei		• Thyroid gland
– Nodi lymphoidei pretracheales and paratracheales		• Trachea and larynx
– Nodi lymphoidei retropharyngeales		• Hypopharynx, Tuba auditiva, rear sections of the nasal cavity
Nodi lymphoidei cervicales laterales		
• Nodi lymphoidei cervicales laterales superficiales	On the M. sternocleidomastoideus, along the V. jugularis externa	• Regional lymph nodes for: ear lobe, floor of the external acoustic meatus, skin above the mandibular angle and the lower part of the Glandula parotidea • Drainage to the lateral deep lymph nodes

• Nodi lymphoidei cervicales laterales profundi superiores
  – Nodus lymphoideus jugulodigastricus cervicalis
  – Nodus lymphoideus lateralis
  – Nodus lymphoideus anterior
	• Intersection of V. jugularis interna and M. digastricus, Venter posterior	• Regional lymph nodes for:
		  – Tonsilla palatina
		  – Base of the tongue
		  – Tongue
		  – Nodi lymphoidei submentales
		  – Nodi lymphoidei submandibulares
		  – Skin of the anterolateral throat area
		  – Chest wall (mammary gland)
		  – Nape of the neck, shoulder, skin of the lateral throat area
		  – Retroauricular lymph nodes
		  – Occipital lymph nodes

• Nodi lymphoidei cervicales laterales profundi inferiores
  – Nodi lymphoidei juguloomohyoidei
  – Nodus lymphoideus lateralis
  – Nodi lymphoidei anteriores
	• Intersection of the intermediate tendon of the M. omohyoideus with the V. jugularis interna	

• Nodi lymphoidei supraclaviculares	• Along the A. transversa cervicis	
• Nodi lymphoidei accessorii	• Nape of the neck	

regional lymph nodes for the lymph coming from most of the regions of the head. Other lymph node stations, consisting of chain-like rows of Nodi lymphoidei, run vertically in the throat area along the Vv. jugularis and the neck organs; these are the main drainage passages of the head and throat area (➤ Fig. 10.27). As a general rule, they are divided according to their location into frontal **Nodi lymphoidei cervicales anteriores** and lateral cervical lymph nodes (**Nodi lymphoidei cervicales laterales**). In their respective regions, they appear both as superficial (**Nodi lymphoidei superficiales**) and deep nodes (**Nodi lymphoidei profundi**) (➤ Table 10.17).

The deep anterior cervical lymph nodes transfer the lymph they control from the larynx, thyroid gland and trachea to the lateral deep cervical lymph nodes (➤ Fig. 10.28). Analogous to the classification of the American Joint Committee on Cancer (AJCC), on each side of the neck the lymph nodes of the throat area are divided regionally on either side into **6 compartments (I–VI)** (➤ Fig. 10.29).

Clinical remarks

The lymph outflow of the throat area and its organs is complicated, from a clinical perspective; however, the majority of lymph nodes of the neck are easily palpated and suited to the histological diagnosis of tissue (biopsy). In general, an enlargement of multiple cervical lymph nodes (**cervical lymphadenopathy**) can have a variety of causes not necessarily restricted to disease processes of the head and throat area (e.g. lymphoma, viral infections). In case of doubt or where lymphatic metastasis of malignant tumours is present (e.g. in thyroid cancer) the compartmental divisions of the AJCC (➤ Fig. 10.29) are used for the elective surgical removal of the cervical lymph nodes (**neck dissection**).

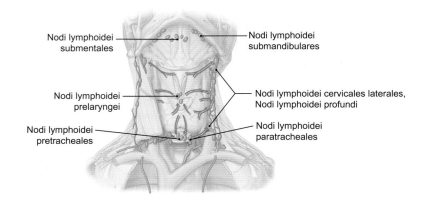

Nodi lymphoidei submentales

Nodi lymphoidei submandibulares

Nodi lymphoidei prelaryngei

Nodi lymphoidei cervicales laterales, Nodi lymphoidei profundi

Nodi lymphoidei pretracheales

Nodi lymphoidei paratracheales

Fig. 10.28 Lymph outflow of the neck organs and the upper airways to the deep lateral cervical lymph nodes (diagram). [E460]

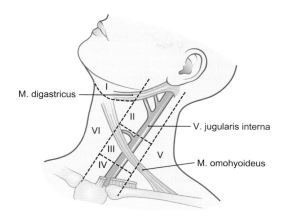

Fig. 10.29 Classification of the head/throat lymphatic drainage areas in 6 compartments (AJCC).

From the lymph vessels coming from the deep cervical lymph nodes (Vasa efferentia) and along the V. jugularis interba, the Trunci jugulares dexter and sinister arise. Via these lymph vessels, the lymph drains to the right via the Ductus lymphaticus dexter into the right venous angle and to the left via the Ductus thoracicus into the left venous angle.

10.5 Thyroid and parathyroid glands
Michael Scholz

─ Skills ─

After working through this chapter, you should be able to:
• explain the embryological development of the thyroid and parathyroid glands
• explain the structure and function of thyroid and parathyroid glands

10.5.1 Location and function

The thyroid gland (Glandula thyroidea) and the parathyroid glands (Glandulae parathyroideae, epithelial bodies) are in the anterior throat area below the larynx (➤ Fig. 10.30).
The **thyroid gland (Glandula thyroidea)** is a large, H-shaped, unpaired gland (weight in adults 20–25 g). It consists of 2 lateral lobes (Lobus dexter and Lobus sinister), which are connected to each other by the unpaired isthmus. This is adjacent to the trachea at approximately the level of the 2nd–3rd tracheal cartilage. The lateral lobes surround the side surfaces of the trachea and are tightly attached to it by the connective tissue of the organ capsule (Capsula fibrosa). Thus the thyroid gland can follow the movements of the larynx and trachea during swallowing. The lateral lobes of the thyroid gland reach the groove between the trachea and oesophagus dorsomedially, where the N. laryngeus recurrens courses. Dorsolaterally the thyroid is adjacent to the carotid sheath (Vagina carotica).

─ Clinical remarks ─

In its course the **N. laryngeus recurrens** is in close proximity to the A. thyroidea inferior. As a result it can be damaged, e.g.

during a thyroid resection. If this occurs (or if it is also simply mechanically irritated), postoperative hoarseness may arise or voice and language formation could be altered. Therefore, nowadays in these operations intraoperative neuromonitoring is used to locate the nerve and identify it with certainty. This is particularly important in cases of enlargement of the thyroid gland (e.g. goitre), because here the normal topography of the N. laryngeus recurrens is elevated (although it maintains its close proximity to the thyroid gland and the A. thyroidea inferior, even though it is no longer as easy to locate). Goitre operations are still the most common causes for paralysis of the laryngeal muscles.

The **parathyroid glands (epithelial bodies, Glandula parathyroidae)** are generally 4 lentil-sized individual organs (2 superior and 2 inferior) located on the rear side (but with exceptionally wide variability) of the thyroid gland. They can also occur within the thyroid gland or the thymus gland (ectopic epithelial bodies). The weight of an epithelial body is approximately 40 mg.
The thyroid and parathyroid glands are part of the endocrine, hormone-forming organs. The **hormones** produced here act on the complete metabolism and intervene to regulate the iodine and calcium balance of the body:
• The thyroid hormones triiodothyronine (T_3) and tetraiodothyronine (thyroxine, T_4) increase the basic metabolic rate and stimulate energy metabolism and growth and differentiation processes.
• The hormone produced by the parafollicular cells (C-cells) of the thyroid, calcitonin is the functional antagonist of the parathormone, which is synthesised in the parathyroid glands. Calcitonin lowers the blood calcium levels, whereas the antagonist parathormone raises it.

10.5.2 Development

Thyroid gland
From around the *24th day* after fertilisation, the site of the thyroid gland is recognisable as a medial thickening of the entoderm at the level of the 2nd pharyngeal arch at the floor of the ectodermal stomodeum (➤ Fig. 10.31a). The epithelial thickening, from which the thyroid bud arises, sprouts caudally lengthwise and stretches as it continues its development passed the hyoid bone in order to reach its final position just below the thyroid cartilage (➤ Fig. 10.31b). The

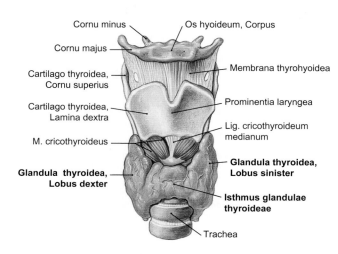

Fig. 10.30 Location of the thyroid gland below the larynx. Ventral view.

ingrown tissue forms an elongated, medially located duct with a narrow lumen (**Ductus thyroglossus**), which is connected to the surface of the tongue. The duct continues to exist up until the *6th week*. At this point in time, the still undivided thyroid bud begins its histological differentiation, even before the formation of the right and left lobes, lateral of the organ system. The median central section (the actual thyroid bud) subsequently remains behind in terms of its growth, later on forming the isthmus of the thyroid gland, while the two side lobes extend somewhat cranially.

In about the *7th week* of embryonic development, the thyroid gland achieves its final shape and its position in the throat area. The isthmus and the lower margins of the two side lobes lie in front of the 2nd and 3rd cartilage rings of the later trachea. At this point, the Ductus thyroglossus has already receded; its proximal opening at the base of the tongue, however, remains as a small medial cavity (**Foramen caecum**) behind the Sulcus terminalis of the tongue (➤ Fig. 10.31b).

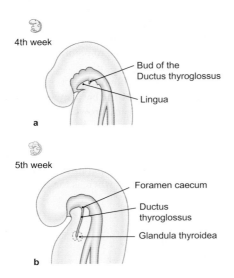

Fig. 10.31 Development of the thyroid gland. a Formation of the thyroid gland bud as an epithelial thickening on the base of the ectodermal Stomodeum in the 4th embryonic week. **b** Descent of the thyroid bud caudally and formation of the Ductus thyroglossus with persisting connection to the base of the tongue. Growth of the two side lobes of the thyroid gland up to the end of the 7th embryonic week. [E838]

NOTE

In almost 50% of people, the distal rudiments of the Ductus thyroglossus do not fully recede, remaining as the **Lobus pyramidalis** running cranially from the isthmus of the thyroid gland. This can even be connected with the hyoid bone via connective tissue fibres and smooth muscles (➤ Fig. 10.32).

Clinical remarks

For the entire length of the Ductus thyroglossus, from the Foramen caecum at the floor of the tongue up to the isthmus or the Lobus pyramidalis, the lumen of the duct may persist and lead to the formation of a **median neck cyst** or (where it connects to the neck surface) a **median neck fistula** (➤ Fig. 10.33a). Both have no clinical significance, as long as they are not inflamed (but can be cosmetically disfiguring). Median neck cysts and fistulas should be differentiated from lateral neck cysts and fistulas. The latter arise when the brachial sulcus or the Sinus cervicalis (a furrow occurring during embryogenesis, which represents the joint opening of the 2nd–4th brachial sulci) are not fully obliterated. **Lateral neck cysts** are noticeable as liquid-filled bulges on the side of the throat area; **lateral neck fistulas** usually open at the anterior border of the M. sterno-cleidomastoideus (➤ Fig. 10.33b).

Parathyroid gland

Unlike the site of the thyroid gland, the parathyroid glands develop as derivatives of the 3rd and 4th pharyngeal pouches. Approximately in the *6th embryonic week* the left and right dorsal buds of the 3rd and 4th pharyngeal pouches are each differentiated into an epithelial body, which are located on the dorsal side of the thyroid gland.

NOTE

Due to the descent of the upper epithelial bodies (3rd pharyngeal pouch) jointly with the thymus, they continue caudally on the posterior of the thyroid gland as the epithelial bodies of the 4th pharyngeal pouch. The epithelial bodies of the 4th pharyngeal pouch are thus found at the upper thyroid pole originating from the 3rd pharyngeal pouch at the lower thyroid pole. This means that their position on the posterior side of the thyroid gland is extremely variable.

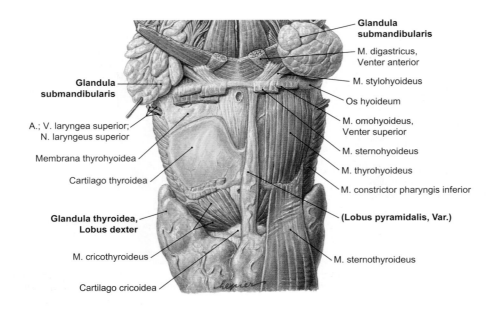

Fig. 10.32 Clearly formed Lobus pyramidalis of the thyroid gland with connection to the hyoid bone (Os hyoideum). Ventral view.

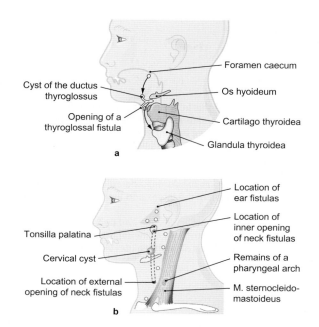

Cyst of the ductus thyroglossus
Opening of a thyroglossal fistula
Foramen caecum
Os hyoideum
Cartilago thyroidea
Glandula thyroidea

a

Tonsilla palatina
Cervical cyst
Location of external opening of neck fistulas
Location of ear fistulas
Location of inner opening of neck fistulas
Remains of a pharyngeal arch
M. sternocleido-mastoideus

b

Fig. 10.33 Cysts and neck fistulae. a Possible location of cysts of the Ductus thyroglossus. The arrows represent the course of the descent of the thyroid gland bud from the Foramen caecum to under the thyroid cartilage of the larynx. **b** Lateral neck fistulas usually perforate through the skin at the leading edge of the M. sternocleidomastoideus. [E581]

10.5.3 Vascular, lymphatic and nervous systems

Arteries

The thyroid gland as an endocrine organ, is very well perfused (➤ Fig. 10.34, ➤ Fig. 10.35). It is supplied on both sides by two arteries coming from different origins:

- The **A. thyroidea superior** runs as the first branch of the A. carotis externa to the upper pole of each thyroid lobe and branches out on the front surface of the thyroid gland.
- The **A. thyroidea inferior** originates from the Truncus thyrocervicalis (➤ Fig. 10.13) and supplies branches to the lower pole and for the supply of the posterior of the thyroid gland (➤ Fig.

10.34). It courses in an arch shape around the neurovascular cord running to the head (A. carotis communis, N. vagus [X], V. jugularis) medially to its supply area.

The 4 parathyroid glands are supplied by branches of the **Aa. thyroideae inferiores**.

Clinical remarks

About 10% of the population have an A. thyroidea ima, mostly arising from the Truncus brachiocephalicus rising in front of the trachea. Individually, their size can vary greatly and can lead to clinical complications within the context of a tracheostomy or thyroidectomy.

Veins

The venous blood from the upper half of the thyroid gland is drained on both sides by the **V. thyroidea superior** into the V. jugularis interna (➤ Fig. 10.36). This contains other venous inflows from the **Vv. thyroideae mediae** which are also paired. The vessels of the **Plexus venosus thyroideus impar** form a venous plexus on the lower poles of the thyroid lobes and the isthmus (➤ Fig. 10.36). They take the blood via the **Vv. thyroideae inferiores** along the front of the trachea into the V. brachiocephalica sinistra. Running caudally, these veins also take with them smaller venous vessels from the trachea and oesophagus.

NOTE

The thyroid hormones leave the thyroid gland and the parathyroid glands via the veins!

Lymph vessels

The lymph from the thyroid and parathyroid glands is drained via the **Nodi lymphoidei thyroidei** along the venous blood vessels to the lateral deep cervical lymph nodes. From the top half of the thyroid gland, lymphatic vessels lead to the **Nodi lymphoidei prelaryngei**. From the lower half, lymphatic vessels run ventrally either via the **Nodi lymphoidei pretracheales** or directly to the caudal **Nodi lymphoidei cervicales laterales profundi** (➤ Table 10.17; ➤ Fig. 10.28).

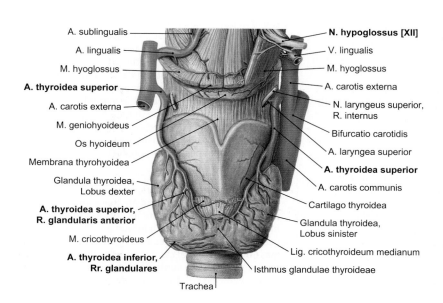

A. sublingualis
A. lingualis
M. hyoglossus
A. thyroidea superior
A. carotis externa
M. geniohyoideus
Os hyoideum
Membrana thyrohyoidea
Glandula thyroidea, Lobus dexter
A. thyroidea superior, R. glandularis anterior
M. cricothyroideus
A. thyroidea inferior, Rr. glandulares
Trachea

N. hypoglossus [XII]
V. lingualis
M. hyoglossus
A. carotis externa
N. laryngeus superior, R. internus
Bifurcatio carotidis
A. laryngea superior
A. thyroidea superior
A. carotis communis
Cartilago thyroidea
Glandula thyroidea, Lobus sinister
Lig. cricothyroideum medianum
Isthmus glandulae thyroideae

Fig. 10.34 Supply areas and course of the arteries of the thyroid gland. Ventral view.

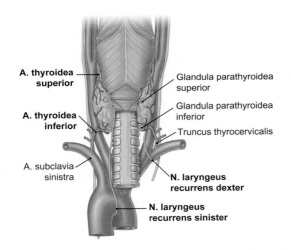

Fig. 10.35 Aa. thyroideae superior and inferior and Nn. laryngei recurrentes sinister and dexter. Dorsal view. [E402]

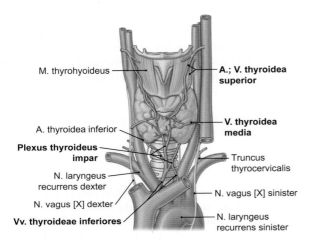

Fig. 10.36 Drainage areas and course of the veins of the thyroid gland. Ventral view. [E402]

Nerves

The thyroid and parathyroid glands are innervated by the **autonomic nervous system**. Postganglionic parasympathetic fibres come from the 3 upper sympathetic trunk ganglia (Ganglia cervicalia superius, medius and inferius or Ganglion cervicothoracicum = Ganglion stellatum → fusion of Ganglion cervicale inferius with the first or the first two thoracic ganglia) and course with the vessels to their target organs. The parasympathetic fibres come from the N. vagus [X] and reach the thyroid and parathyroid glands with the N. laryngeus superior (➤ Fig. 10.34) and the N. laryngeus recurrens (➤ Fig. 10.35).

> N O T E
>
> The thyroid gland has a close spatial relationship with the Nn. laryngei recurrentes (Nn. laryngei inferiores). After its loop around the arterial vessels (left: courses around the aortic arch, to the right: courses around the A. subclavia dexter) the nerves run in the groove between the trachea and the oesophagus cranially to the larynx, where they innervate the inner laryngeal muscles.

10.6 Larynx
Friedrich Paulsen

┌─ **Skills** ─────────────────────────────

After working through this in this chapter, you should be able to:
- describe the essential functions of the larynx, the blood supply, lymph drainage and innervation
- name the skeletal elements and ligaments of the larynx
- present the joints and muscles of the larynx and their function and innervation
- explain terms such as tensioning and adjustment apparatus, the subdivision of the larynx and limits of the entrance to the larynx
- relate the larynx, its blood vessels and nerves to the surrounding structures, and name the important landmarks
- describe the principles of laryngeal development

Clinical case

Carcinoma of the larynx

Case study
A 53-year-old roofer is referred to an ear nose and throat (ENT) specialist by a general practitioner. In patient case history the man says he has been hoarse for some time. He can't say exactly how long it has been. When asked, he admits to smoking at least one pack of cigarettes a day for about 30 years. His alcohol intake is 'normal', without being more specific.

Initial examination
In the laryngoscopy, the ENT specialist sees a large supraglottic tumour in the area of the right vestibular fold, passing continuously into the epiglottis and concealing the anterior commissure and part of the glottis. On the right side of the throat area, he can also clearly palpate a clearly enlarged hard tumour, not painful under pressure, which he classified as enlarged lymph nodes. He then immediately arranges an appointment at the neighbouring university ENT clinic for the patient. He informs the patient that for the purposes of further diagnosis tissue samples need to be taken to rule out a malignant tumour; however, he must consider the possibility of laryngeal cancer.

Further diagnosis
In the university clinic, several tissue biopsies are taken with the patient under local anaesthesia from various superficial sections of the tumour and sent to the pathology department. The histopathological findings in several of the samples confirm the diagnosis of a non-keratinised squamous cell carcinoma. Now a comprehensive tumour staging is undertaken for the patient. This shows a supraglottic malignancy, which has already grown into the fatty material in front of the epiglottis and on the right side has spread to the level of the vocal folds. The anterior commissure and the thyroid cartilage have already been penetrated. The tumour has grown further caudally than the doctors had expected. Ipsilaterally there are already other lymph node metastases, as well as the palpable enlarged lymph nodes. No remote metastases are detectable.

Clinical picture
Malignant laryngeal tumours, at about 40%, are the most common cancers of the head and neck area, with an incidence of 8 out of 100,000 inhabitants per year. They are 5–10 times more common in men than in women. The peak age is 55–65 years old. In 95% of cases they involve squamous cell carcinoma, 60% of laryngeal carcinomas develop in the area of the glottis and 40% are supraglottic tumours. The main causes are exogenic noxious agents, especially tobacco.

Treatment and follow-up
Due to the extensive findings, in this patient the larynx cannot be preserved. This means that he will be informed about the extensive treatment to be carried out and after giving his approval he will be operated on the following day. In the course of the operation, the entire larynx is removed (laryngectomy). The transition to the pharynx is closed and the patient receives a continuous tracheostome in the region of the Fossa jugularis. On the right side, a neck dissection is carried out (removal of the lymph nodes of the throat area) of zones II, III, V and VI according to the classification of the American Academy of Otolaryngology Head and Neck Surgery.
After the operation there is close monitoring, and elaborate speech therapy is planned to learn to speak using the oesophagus (belching speech), as the patient no longer has a larynx. However, 5 days after the operation, the patient is seen once again with a cigarette in his hand in front of the hospital entrance. This time, he is not smoking through the mouth, but through the tracheostome.

10.6.1 Overview

The larynx functionally provides the **reflective protection for the lower respiratory tract** against intrusion by foreign objects and **articulation and voice projection (phonation)**. In addition, it plays a part in abdominal prelum. As part of the airway, the larynx sits between the throat (pharynx) and the windpipe (trachea). Other neck structures such as the thyroid gland, gullet (oesophagus) and neurovascular cord are in close proximity. The larynx is fixed by ligaments and muscles in the throat area in such a way that its location can be changed in the connective tissue spaces of the neck when swallowing and speaking. This is possible due to its close relationship with the hyoid bone (Os hyoideum), with which it is connected by ligaments.

N O T E

The **lower respiratory tract** includes the larynx, trachea and bronchial tree (Arbor bronchialis).

Structure

The larynx consists of a **cartilage skeleton** that partially ossifies over the course of life. The skeletal elements are connected to each other by **true joints** or by connective tissue and are moved by muscles. Some muscles are part of the adjustment apparatus, which expands the glottis, while the other muscles are part of the tensioning apparatus which regulates the length and the tension of the vocal folds in phonation (➤ Chap. 10.6.3).

Functions
Protection

During swallowing, as well as when coughing and sneezing, there is a coordinated interaction of the larynx with all it surrounding structures:

- When **swallowing** the glottis is closed, narrowing the structures lying above, the epiglottis is moved over the entrance to the larynx, and the larynx is pulled forwards and upwards. Thus the airway through the larynx is sealed and protected from the ingress of liquids and food.
- When **coughing** and **sneezing** the vocal ligaments and the higher structures are narrowed for a short time, the larynx is pulled forward and upwards and the glottis is suddenly pulled open by an explosive respiratory breath (cough reflex, ➤ Chap. 10.6.6).

Phonation

For **articulation** many mechanisms, such as the mass, tension and length of the vocal cords, as well as the pressure of blowing, are involved. When doing so, the pitch depends on the frequency of vibration of the vocal folds and the volume of the airflow strength, which in turn is caused by the tension of the diaphragm and the respiratory muscles (blowing pressure).
If one presses the index finger on the Adam's apple and swallows, the upward movement of the larynx can be felt; similarly, one can feel the larynx migrating cranially when a sound is generated and it continues to rise.

Breathing

The width of the lumen of the windpipe can be modified in the larynx by changing the position of the vocal folds.

10.6.2 Development

Prenatal

The development of the larynx is closely linked with the development of the base of the tongue and pharyngeal arches and takes place in the 4th–10th weeks.
Between the 2nd and 4th pharyngeal arches, at the end of the *4th week*, the hypobranchial eminence (Eminentia hypobranchialis) is differentiated from the buccopharyngeal bud. Its lower end overgrows onto the laryngotracheal groove lying medial between the 4th and 5th pharyngeal arches and is differentiated to the **epiglottic eminence**.
Lateral to the laryngotracheal groove, the **arytenoid bulges** develop due to rapid growth from a tracheobronchial bud. They constrict the developing lumen of the trachea from the already separated oesophagus into a T-shape. At this stage *(6th week)* the epiglottis and arytenoid bulges are adjacent to each other and are only separated from each other by a narrow slit (entrance to the larynx) (top bar of the T). There remains between the arytenoid bulges a slit-shaped gap (primitive glottis; lower vertical line of the T). Due to the very rapid growth of the arytenoid bulges, **a short-term closure of the lumen of the larynx** occurs.
In the *10th week* the rest of the laryngeal growth has caught up and the larynx is recanalised again. This creates mucosal pockets on both sides of the larynx (Sinus MORGAGNI), whose upper and lower limits differentiate to the pocket folds and vocal folds.

Clinical remarks

Degenerative disorders of what is usually the short-term closure of the lumen of the larynx can lead to life-threatening partial or complete closure (**congenital stenoses and diaphragms**). Additionally, malformations of the epiglottis are possible (**epiglottic hypoplasia or aplasia, double or split epiglottis**).

The arytenoid cartilage is differentiated from the arytenoid bulges; the epiglottic bulge becomes the epiglottis. Its lateral parts develop into the Plicae aryepiglotticae. Thyroid and ring cartilage originate from the 4th and 5th pharyngeal arches, the inner laryngeal muscles differentiate from the 6th pharyngeal arch. The suspension device develops from the surrounding mesenchyme, the epithelium originates from the entoderm of the foregut.

Postnatal

The infant is able to breathe and drink at the same time, because the larynx is still located relatively high up, and so the epiglottis reaches the nasopharynx. The maternal milk flows through the **Recessus piriformes** (➤ Chap. 10.6.3) of the larynx into the oesophagus, and at the same time, breathing can take place. In the course, due to longitudinal growth, the larynx becomes increasingly caudal (**laryngeal descent**). Now the airway has to be closed when swallowing, in order to prevent aspiration.

During puberty, there is an extensive gender divergent growth spurt of the whole larynx. As a result, the larynx grows significantly within a relatively short time period, in boys much more significantly than in girls, with the laryngeal structures being affected to varying degrees. In boys, the length of the vocal fold increases by an average of 1 cm, in girls by 'only' 3–4 mm. This results in voice changes, which are significantly more pronounced in boys than in girls (**voice break, voice change, mutation**). The cause of the voice break is essentially disruption in the coordination between the different rapidly growing structures involved in phonation.

10.6.3 Laryngeal skeleton

The laryngeal skeleton (➤ Fig. 10.37, ➤ Fig. 10.38) is composed of epiglottic cartilage, thyroid cartilage, ring cartilage, arytenoid cartilage, corniculate cartilage and sphenoid cartilage (➤ Table 10.18).

Cartilage of the laryngeal skeleton
Epiglottis
The foundation of the epiglottis (epiglottis, ➤ Fig. 10.37b) is an apertured plate made of elastic cartilage (**Cartilago epiglottica**). Blood vessels, nerves and excretory ducts of subepithelial glands pass through these holes. The cartilage goes downwards to the front in the stalk of the epiglottis (**Petiolus epiglottidis**).

Table 10.18 Cartilage of the laryngeal skeleton.

Cartilage	Amount	Cartilage histology	Occurrence
Epiglottic cartilage (Cartilago epiglottica)	Unpaired	Elastic	Regular
Thyroid cartilage (Cartilago thyroidea)	Unpaired	Hyaline	Regular
Cricoid cartilage (Cartilago cricoidea)	Unpaired	Hyaline	Regular
Arytenoid cartilage (Cartilago arytenoidea)	Paired	Hyaline (exception: tip of the Proc. vocalis: elastic)	Regular
Corniculate cartilage (Cartilago corniculato, SANTORINI's cartilage)	Paired	Elastic	Variable
Cuneiform cartilage (Cartilago cuneiformis, WRISBERG's cartilage)	Paired	Elastic	Variable

Thyroid cartilage
The thyroid cartilage (Cartilago thyroidea, ➤ Fig. 10.37a) consists of 2 plates, Lamina dextra and Lamina sinistra, sitting like a protective shield in front of the voice-producing part of the larynx. They join together ventrally at a right angle (in men) and at a slightly larger angle (approx. 120° in women). The interface with the **Incisura thyroidea superior** is retracted cranially, and goes up to the furthest point of the ventral side, the **Prominentia laryngea** (Adam's apple). The connection point of the two plates with the Incisura thyroidea inferior is retracted on the lower edge. On the outer side, bulging at the posterior of the thyroid cartilage are a **Tuberculum thyroideum superius** and a **Tuberculum thyroideum inferius**, which are connected via the Linea obliqua. All protruberances serve as zones for tendon insertion. The posterior edges of the side plates each merge cranially into the slightly longer superior horn, the **Cornu superius**, and caudally into the inferior horn, the **Cornu inferius**. On the inside of the Cornu inferius is the articular surface, the **Facies articularis cricoidea**, for articulation with the cricoid cartilage.

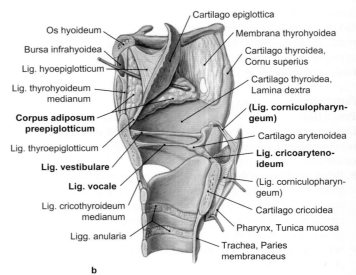

Fig. 10.37 Laryngeal skeleton and ligament arrangement. a Ventral view. **b** Medial view of the sagittal planes of the larynx.

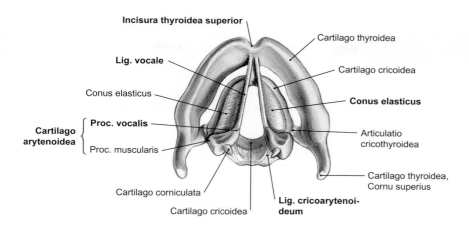

Incisura thyroidea superior
Lig. vocale
Conus elasticus
Cartilago arytenoidea { **Proc. vocalis** / Proc. muscularis }
Cartilago corniculata
Cartilago cricoidea
Lig. cricoarytenoi-deum
Cartilago thyroidea
Cartilago cricoidea
Conus elasticus
Articulatio cricothyroidea
Cartilago thyroidea, Cornu superius

Fig. 10.38 Laryngeal skeleton (without epiglottis) with Conus elasticus. Cranial view.

Cricoid cartilage

Cricoid cartilage (Cartilago cricoidea, ➤ Fig. 10.37) forms the base of the laryngeal skeleton. It is shaped like a signet ring, with the seal being the **Lamina cartalaginis cricoideae** pointing dorsally and carries articular surfaces to the right and left side and on the upper edge: above is the **Facies articularis arytenoidea** to articulate with the respective arytenoid cartilage, and on the side a Facies articularis thyroidea surface to articulate with the thyroid cartilage. At the front, the ring forms a narrow arch, the **Arcus cartilaginis cricoideae.**

N O T E
In adults the cricoid cartilage is at the level of the VI cervical vertebra (C7).

Arytenoid cartilage

The arytenoid cartilage (Arytenoid cartilage, Cartilago arytenoidea, ➤ Fig. 10.37b) are comparable to three-sided pyramids. This means that each cartilage has 4 areas:
- **Facies anterolateralis** (with Colliculus, Crista arcuata, Fovea triangularis and Fovea oblonga)
- **Facies medialis**
- **Facies posterior**
- Base, **Basis cartilaginis arytenoideae** (with Facies articularis for articulation with the cricoid cartilage).

Furthermore, each arytenoid cartilage has 3 processes:
- Anterior **Proc. vocalis**, at its peak consisting of elastic cartilage
- Lateral **Proc. muscularis**
- Above the tip, **Apex cartalaginis arytenoideae**

Corniculate and cuniform cartilage

The corniculate cartilage (Cartilago corniculata, SANTORINI's cartilage) has a hook-shaped structure and can also be absent. It sits on the arytenoid cartilage and protrudes under the mucous membrane as the Tuberculum corniculatum. The cuniform cartilage (Cartilago cuneiformis, WRISBERG's cartilage) also may occur as a variation. It protrudes into the Plica aryepiglottica (see below) as the Tuberculum cuneiforme (➤ Fig. 10.43).

Clinical remarks

From about the age of 20 years, the hyaline laryngeal cartilages (thyroid, cricoid and arytenoid cartilage) start to ossify very slowly and differently according to gender. In men, after the age of 60 years, with very few exceptions the cartilage has almost completely mineralised and ossified; in women only parts of the laryngeal skeleton ossify. Therefore, in men over the age of 50 years the hyaline cartilage should be called bone. Thus, **fractures of the laryngeal skeleton** can occur (e.g. following traffic accidents), accompanied by life-threatening obstruction of the airway, phonation disorders and danger of asphyxiation. Due to the ossification, the operative excision of bone tissue (e.g. in the case of a hemilaryngectomy due to cancer of the larynx) or following a fracture, the fracture ends and/or the remaining parts can be splinted with material used for osteosynthesis.
Rarely, at birth the laryngeal cartilage is too soft **(laryngomalacia)**. This can be associated with respiratory disorders.

Ligaments of the larynx

The laryngeal cartilages (bone) are joined together by joints and a **connective tissue suspension system**. The connective tissue apparatus made up of ligaments and membranes, together with the laryngeal muscles, other muscles and the fascia of the throat area, is essential for the functioning of the mobility of the larynx with breathing, phonation and when swallowing. The ligament apparatus can be divided into **outer and inner laryngeal ligaments** (➤ Table 10.19, ➤ Table 10.20, ➤ Fig. 10.37, ➤ Fig. 10.38).

Ligaments between the larynx and hyoid bone

Top edge of the thyroid cartilage and lower edge of the hyoid bone are connected by the **Membrana thyrohyoidea** which are reinforced in the area of the Incisura thyroidea superior to the **Lig. thyrohyoideum medianum** and in the area of Cornua majora of the hyoid bone at the **Lig. thyrohyoideum laterale** (➤ Fig. 10.37a). In each Lig. thyrohyoideum laterale a triangular cartilage (**Cartilago triticea**) consisting of elastic cartilage can be embedded.

Suspension of the epiglottis

The **Lig. thyroepiglotticum** originates below the Incisura thyroidea superior on the inside of the thyroid cartilage, which attaches the epiglottic stalk (**Petiolus epiglottidis**) to the thyroid cartilage (➤ Fig. 10.37b). The frontal surface of the epiglottis facing the hyoid bone is attached via the **Lig. hyoepiglotticum** to the inner surface of the hyoid bone. Between the Membrana thyrohyoidea and epiglottis, and also at the side of the epiglottis, is the **Corpus adiposum preepiglotticum**, a fatty body which carries out an important role in the distortion of the epiglottis during swallowing by protecting the lower respiratory tract.

Table 10.19 Outer laryngeal ligaments.

Ligament/membrane	Connects	Remarks
Membrana thyrohyoidea	Hyoid and thyroid cartilage	
Lig. thyrohyoideum medianum	Hyoid and thyroid cartilage in the median plane	Reinforcement of the Membrana thyrohyoidea
Lig. thyrohyoideum laterale	Hyoid and thyroid cartilage at the rear edge of the Membrana thyrohyoidea	Reinforcement of the Membrana thyrohyoidea
Lig. cricotracheale	Cricoid cartilage and trachea	Fixes cricoid cartilage to the trachea
Lig. cricopharyngeum	Cricoid cartilage and lower part of the anterior wall of the pharynx	Fixes the cricoid cartilage to the pharynx

Table 10.20 Inner laryngeal ligaments.

Ligament/membrane	Connects	Remarks
Lig. thyroepiglotticum	Thyroid cartilage and stalk of the epiglottis	Fixes the epiglottis to the thyroid cartilage
Lig. cricothyroideum	Thyroid and cricoid cartilage	
Lig. cricothyroideum medianum (Lig. conicum)	Thyroid and cricoid cartilage	Reinforcement of the Lig. cricothyroideum
Lig. ceratocricoideum	Cornu inferior of the thyroid cartilage and outer surface of cricoid cartilage	Reinforces the joint capsule of the Articulatio cricothyroidea
Lig. cricoarytenoideum (posterius)	Posterior of the arytenoid cartilage and lateral posterior of the cricoid cartilage	Contains much elastic material and is used to reset the arytenoid cartilage in the starting position
Membrana fibroelastica	Runs within the wall of the supraglottic and subglottic space and includes the vocal cords and vestibular folds	These include the Conus elasticus, Ligg. vocalia, Membrana quadrangularis and Ligg. vestibularis
Conus elasticus (➤ Fig. 10.38)	Upper edge of the sides of the cricoid ligaments and Lig. vocale	Strong elastic membrane in the wall of the subglottic space; the upper edge of the Conus elasticus thickens towards the Ligg. vocalia, with its width depending on the position of the vocal folds; in phonation, it concentrates and focuses the airstream onto the vocal folds
Lig. vocale	Thyroid cartilage (via vocal ligament and Nodulus elasticus anterior) and Proc. vocalis (via the Nodulus elasticus posterior) of the arytenoid cartilage	Thickened upper edge of the Conus elasticus in the glottis
Membrana quadrangularis	Inside the wall of the supraglottic space, pulls it from the edges of the epiglottis to the vestibular folds	Thinner elastic membrane in the wall of the supraglottal space
Lig. vestibulare	Connects the thyroid cartilage with the respective arytenoid cartilage, cranial of the vocal folds	Thickened lower margin of the Membrana quadrangularis in the vestibular folds

Ligaments of the cricoid cartilage

In the ventral section, the thyroid and cricoid cartilages are connected by the **Lig. cricothyroideum**. This is a syndesmosis, the middle part of which is reinforced by the **Lig. cricothyroideum medianum (Lig. conicum)** (➤ Fig. 10.37). Caudally the cricoid cartilage is attached via the **Lig. cricotracheale** to the first tracheal ring. Dorsally the **Lig. cricopharyngeum** radiates into the pharyngeal wall.

> **NOTE**
>
> Above the Prominentia laryngea (Adam's apple), the Incisura thyroidea superior and the Membrana thyrohyoidea can be palpated. When the person carrying out the test runs their finger from the Prominentia laryngea along the thyroid cartilage in a caudal direction, they reach the clinically significant **Lig. conicum**.

Clinical remarks

If the upper respiratory tract is shifted causing breathlessness, the Lig. cricothroideum medianum (Lig. conicum) serves as a physical landmark. In an emergency measure it can be cut through **(coniotomy)**, together with the underlying Conus elasticus (see below) in order to reach the inner space of the larynx just below the vocal folds.

Laryngeal joints

Thyroid cartilage and cricoid cartilage are linked via the paired **Articulatio cricothyroidea**. Each arytenoid cartilage articulates with the cricoid cartilage via the **Articulatio cricoarytenoidea**. These joints are diarthroses (true joints); however, in a smaller percentage of people, the Articulatio cricothyroidea can also be a synchondrosis.

Articulatio cricothyroidea

The Articulatio cricothyroidea (➤ Fig. 10.37a) is a ball joint. The concave Facies articularis thyroidea of the lateral surface of the cricoid cartilage articulates with the convex Facies articular cricoidea at the lower inner side of the Cornu inferius of the thyroid cartilage. The joint capsule is taut and is reinforced by the **Lig. ceratocricoideum** on the outside. The joint enables shifting movements to take place along the sagittal plane as well as rotational movements around a transverse axis. During rotation, the cricoid cartilage comes close to the thyroid cartilage (➤ Fig. 10.39). The tilting movement leads to tension of the vocal cords (see below; coarse tension of the vocal cords).

Articulatio cricoarytenoidea

In the cricoarytenoid joint the base of the arytenoid cartilage articulates with the posterior side of the upper edge of the cricoid cartilage (➤ Fig. 10.37b). The articular surface of the arytenoid cartilage is more round and concave; the articular surfaces of the cricoid cartilage are convex and oval (cylinder-shaped). Parallel to the cylindrical axis, hinging and sliding movements can be carried out in the cricoarytenoid joint; these serve to open and close the vocal ligaments and maintain the tension of the vocal folds (➤ Fig. 10.37b). When the arytenoid cartilage is guided outwards as part of a hinge movement, this leads to the raising and abduction of the Proc. vocalis, and thus the opening of the glottis. A rotation along the hinge inwards in combination with the lowering and adduction of the Proc. vocalis leads to the closure of the glottis. The hinge movements can be combined with sliding motions. By doing so, the arytenoid cartilage moves in abduction and adduction ventrally

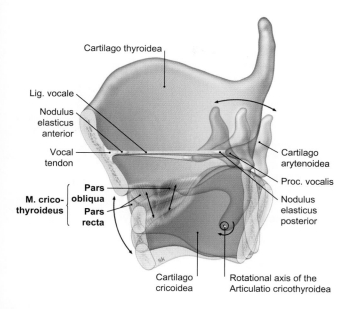

Cartilago thyroidea

Lig. vocale

Nodulus elasticus anterior

Vocal tendon

M. cricothyroideus { **Pars obliqua** **Pars recta**

Cartilago arytenoidea

Proc. vocalis

Nodulus elasticus posterior

Cartilago cricoidea

Rotational axis of the Articulatio cricothyroidea

Fig. 10.39 Outer laryngeal muscles, M. cricothyroideus. Medial view of a lateral sagittal plane of the larynx. Contraction of the M. cricothyroideus tilts the ring cartilage using synchronous movements in the cricothyroid joints. The vocal ligament is extended and is roughly stretched because the arytenoid cartilage sitting on the cricoid cartilage is tilted dorsally.

or dorsally. The joint capsule (Capsula articularis cricoarytenoideae) is broad and taut due to the complex movement options and it has no influence on the joint alignment; however, dorsally the joint capsule is reinforced by the **Lig. cricoarytenoideum (posterius)** made from highly elastic connective tissue (➤ Fig. 10.37b), which functionally aids the alignment of the arytenoid cartilage and counteracts the elastic forces of the Lig. vocalis.

Clinical remarks

The complete paralysis of all the laryngeal muscles leads to the so-called **cadaveric position** of the vocal folds due to the pulling strength of the Ligg. cricoarytenoideae posteriora on the arytenoid cartilages.

Following endotracheal intubation and extubation, laryngoscopy or bronchoscopy, the arytenoid cartilage can be shifted in a dorsolateral or medioventral direction, which is called **arytenoid dislocation**. Because the Lig. vocale on the affected side is unmovable, the patient has a hoarse voice. Causes for this are internal bleeding in the joint cavities or the formation of a reactive effusion after damaging the synovial membranes. Muscle contractures can cause the joint surfaces to subsequently adhere and ankylosis can occur. An arytenoid dislocation should be distinguished from a nerve lesion.

The cricoarytenoid joints are constructed like the large limb joints. That means that here degenerative cartilaginous changes in advanced age are possible **(osteoarthritis)**, affecting the closure of the vocal folds in phonation and thus the quality of the voice, as well as joint infections **(arthritis)** or rheumatoid diseases **(rheumatoid arthritis)**.

Laryngeal muscles

The laryngeal muscles derived from the pharyngeal arches are subdivided according to their origin, location and innervation, into **outer and inner laryngeal muscles**. The striated muscles are extremely densely innervated and very well perfused. Functionally, they serve to open and close the vocal ligaments and maintain the tension of the vocal folds (by lengthening and shortening). Muscles that change the shape of the vocal ligaments belong to the actuator apparatus; muscles that affect their tension are collectively called the tension apparatus.

Outer laryngeal muscles

Apart from the **M. cricothyroideus** sitting directly on the larynx, the **M. constrictor pharyngis inferior** belonging to the muscles of the pharynx (pharyngeal muscles) as well as the **M. thyrohyoideus**

Table 10.21 Outer laryngeal muscles.

Innervation	Origins	Attachment	Function
M. cricothyroideus, Pars interna (➤ Fig. 10.39)			
N. laryngeus superior, R. externus	Anterior inner surface of the cricoid cartilage	Inside of the thyroid cartilage and Conus elasticus	Tenses the vocal folds (coarse tension) by tilting the cricoid cartilage
M. cricothyroideus, Pars externa with a Pars recta and a Pars obliqua (➤ Fig. 10.39)			
N. laryngeus superior, R. externus	Anterior inner surface of the cricoid cartilage	Lower edge of the thyroid cartilage plate (Pars recta), Cornu inferius of the thyroid cartilage (Pars obliqua)	Tenses the vocal folds (coarse tension) by tilting the cricoid cartilage
M. constrictor pharyngis inferior, Pars thyropharyngea			
N. laryngeus superior, R. externus, Plexus pharyngeus	Outer margin of the thyroid cartilage	Pharyngeal wall	Raises the larynx during swallowing, participates in tensing of the vocal folds
M. constrictor pharyngis inferior, Pars cricopharyngea			
N. laryngeus superior, R. externus, Plexus pharyngeus	Outer margin of the cricoid cartilage	Pharyngeal wall	Unclear at the larynx
M. thyrohyoideus			
Radix superior of the Ansa cervicalis (profunda) of the Plexus cervicalis	Lower edge of the thyroid cartilage, outer surface of the thyroid cartilage	Hyoid body, Cornu majus ossis hyoidei	Raises the larynx during swallowing, fixes the larynx during phonation

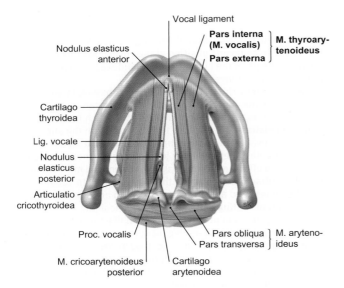

Fig. 10.40 Inner laryngeal muscles, Mm. laryngis. View from above. [L238]

belonging to the infrahyoid muscles are assigned to the outer laryngeal muscles (➤ Fig. 10.39, ➤ Table 10.21).

Inner laryngeal muscles

The central switching points of the inner laryngeal muscles are in the arytenoid cartilage, in which all internal laryngeal muscles attach or originate (➤ Fig. 10.40, ➤ Fig. 10.41, ➤ Fig. 10.42, ➤ Fig. 10.43, ➤ Table 10.22).

Tensioning apparatus

The tensioning apparatus includes the laryngeal joints and the laryngeal muscles, apart from the skeletal elements of the larynx. It influences the volume, shape and length of the vibrating part of the

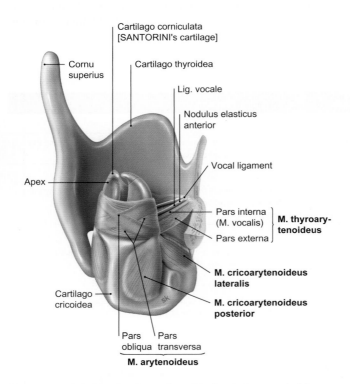

Fig. 10.41 Inner laryngeal muscles, Mm. laryngis. Dorsal oblique view. Thyroid cartilage partially resected. [L238]

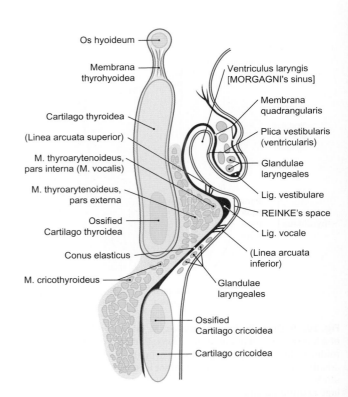

Fig. 10.42 Frontal section through sagittally bisected larynx (diagram). [L126]

vocal folds. The **M. cricothyroideus** regulates the length and tension of the Lig. vocale and Conus elasticus and leads to coarse tension of the vocal folds (➤ Fig. 10.39). The Pars thyropharyngea of the M. constrictor pharyngis inferior contributes to this. The **M. cricoarytenoideus posterior** (posticus) and **Lig. cricoarytenoideum (posterius)** stabilise the arytenoid cartilage, so that it cannot tilt forward. The fine tension is regulated by the **M. vocalis** (Pars interna of the M. thyroarytenoideus ➤ Fig. 10.40, ➤ Fig. 10.42). Its muscle fibres run parallel to the vocal fold and the vocal ligament (Lig. vocale) and are partly attached to the vocal cord. The tension can be strengthened by isotonic muscle contractions and modified even further by isometric contraction, so that the muscle has a decisive impact on tone quality in voice projection. The **Pars cricopharyngea of the M. constrictor pharyngis inferior** (➤ Table 10.23) is able to actively diminish the vocal fold tension.

NOTE

Tension apparatus: structures affecting the volume, shape and length of the vibrating section of the vocal folds: skeletal elements of the larynx, laryngeal joints, laryngeal muscles

Clinical remarks

Voice overloading leads to a loss of tension in the M. vocalis. It is called **laryngeal paralysis**. The glottis can no longer be closed properly, the voice is hoarse. This is also a reduction in mucus production of the laryngeal glands due to voice overload (➤ Chap. 10.6.5).

Actuator apparatus

The **M. cricoarytenoideus posterior** (posticus) is the main muscle of the actuator apparatus (➤ Fig. 10.39, ➤ Fig. 10.40, ➤ Fig. 10.43) since it enables opening of the vocal folds and thus inspiration (➤ Fig. 10.44a) by the abduction and elevation of the Proc.

Table 10.22 Inner laryngeal muscles.

Innervation	Origins	Attachment	Function
M. thyroarytenoideus, Pars interna (M. vocalis) (➤ Fig. 10.40, ➤ Fig. 10.41, ➤ Fig. 10.42)			
N. laryngeus inferior	Lower third of the angle of the thyroid cartilage (radiates over the vocal ligament in thyroid cartilage)	Proc. vocalis, lateral to the Lig. vocale and Nodulus elasticus posterior, Fovea oblonga of arytenoid cartilage	Closes the Pars intermembranacea of the vocal ligaments (shortening or lengthening the vocal folds, isotonic contraction), regulates vocal fold tensioning (vibrating section of the vocal folds, isometric contraction)
M. thyroarytenoideus, Pars externa (➤ Fig. 10.40, ➤ Fig. 10.41, ➤ Fig. 10.42)			
N. laryngeus inferior	Lower third of the angle of the thyroid cartilage, lateral to the vocal ligament	Crista arcuata of the arytenoid cartilage	Closes the Pars intermembranacea of the vocal ligaments by adduction and sinking of the Proc. vocalis
M. arytenoideus transversus (➤ Fig. 10.40, ➤ Fig. 10.41, ➤ Fig. 10.43)			
N. laryngeus inferior	Lateral edge and posterior surface of the arytenoid cartilage	Lateral edge and posterior surface of the contralateral arytenoid cartilage	Closes the Pars intermembranacea of the vocal ligaments by bringing together both arytenoid cartilages
M. arytenoideus obliquus (➤ Fig. 10.41)			
N. laryngeus inferior	Base of the posterior surface of the arytenoid cartilage	Tip of the contralateral arytenoid cartilage	Closes the Pars intercartilaginea by adduction of the arytenoid cartilage; minor lateral rotation of the Proc. vocalis with a slight opening of the Pars intermembranacea
M. arytenoideus obliquus, Pars aryepiglottica (➤ Fig. 10.43)			
N. laryngeus inferior	Arytenoid cartilage tip	Lateral edge of the epiglottis	Slightly lowers the epiglottis
M. cricoarytenoideus lateralis (➤ Fig. 10.40, ➤ Fig. 10.41)			
N. laryngeus inferior	Lateral upper border between Arcus and Lamina of the cricoid cartilage	Proc. muscularis of the arytenoid cartilage	Closes the Pars. intermembranacea of the epiglottis by adduction and elevation of the Proc. vocalis of the artytenoid cartilage, opens the Pars intercartilaginea (whisper triangle)
M. cricoarytenoideus posterior (posticus) (➤ Fig. 10.40, ➤ Fig. 10.41, ➤ Fig. 10.43)			
N. laryngeus inferior	Posterior surface of the lamina of the cricoid cartilage	Proc. muscularis of the arytenoid cartilage	Opens the epiglottis for abduction and elevation of the Proc. vocalis (up to a maximum opening) for inspiration

vocalis of the arytenoid cartilage; however, the **M. cricoarytenoideus lateralis** can also open the glottis to a limited extent: its isolated contraction leads to the formation of the whisper triangle (triangular gap in the posterior region of the glottis). To improve gaseous exchange, in calm expiration the glottis is only opened just enough to allow the exhaled air to escape. It lasts much longer than the short inspiration phase with a wide open glottis. With calm breathing, the width of the glottis is therefore constantly changing. For **phonation** (➤ Fig. 10.44b) the Procc. vocales are brought together and so the glottis is loosely closed. To do this, the **Mm. arytenoidei transversus and obliquus** contract. Furthermore the

Mm. cricoarytenoideus lateralis and thyroarytenoideus and the mucosa on the arytenoid cartilage are also involved. The **fine tension** of the vocal folds that is vital for phonation is undertaken by the Pars interna of the M. thryroarytenoideus (**M. vocalis**), which therefore not only affects the tension but also the actuator apparatus. The Pars externa of the M. thyroarytenoideus has a functional effect on the convergence of the vocal folds. All the muscles can also be contracted so strongly that they ensure the fixed closure of the glottis when there is abdominal pressure (e.g. when defecating) or coughing.

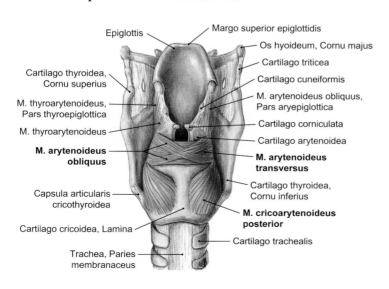

Epiglottis — Margo superior epiglottidis
— Os hyoideum, Cornu majus
Cartilago thyroidea, Cornu superius
— Cartilago triticea
— Cartilago cuneiformis
M. thyroarytenoideus, Pars thyroepiglottica
— M. arytenoideus obliquus, Pars aryepiglottica
M. thyroarytenoideus
— Cartilago corniculata
— Cartilago arytenoidea
M. arytenoideus obliquus
— **M. arytenoideus transversus**
— Cartilago thyroidea, Cornu inferius
Capsula articularis cricothyroidea
— **M. cricoarytenoideus posterior**
Cartilago cricoidea, Lamina
— Cartilago trachealis
Trachea, Paries membranaceus

Fig. 10.43 Inner laryngeal muscles, Mm. laryngis. Dorsal view.

Table 10.23 Pharyngeal constrictors.

Innervation	Origin		Attachment	Function
M. constrictor pharyngis superior				
Rr. pharyngeales of the N. glossopharyngeus [IX] (= Plexus pharyngeus)	• Pars pterygopharyngea:	Lamina medialis of the Proc. pterygoideus and Hamulus pterygoideus	Membrana pharyngobasilaris, Raphe pharyngeus	Together with the M. palatopharyngeus, a bulge arises due to contraction, which blocks the nasopharyngeal space (PASSAVANT's ridge) when swallowing
	• Pars buccopharyngea:	Raphe pterygomandibularis	Membrana pharyngobasilaris, Raphe pharyngeus	Constriction of the throat, transport of food bolus
	• Pars mylopharyngea:	Linea mylohyoidea of the Mandibula		
	• Pars glossopharyngea:	Internal muscles of the tongue		
M. constrictor pharyngis medius				
Rr. pharyngeales of the N. glossopharyngeus [IX] and the N. vagus [X] (= Plexus pharyngeus)	• Pars chondropharyngea:	Cornu minus ossis hyoidei	Raphe pharyngeus	Constriction of the throat, transport of food bolus
	• Pars ceratopharyngea:	Cornu majus ossis hyoidei		
M. constrictor pharyngis inferior				
Rr. pharyngeales of the N. vagus [X] (= Plexus pharyngeus)	• Pars thyropharyngea:	Linea obliqua of the thyroid cartilage	Raphe pharyngeus	Constriction of the throat, transport of food bolus
	• Pars cricopharyngea: – Pars obliqua – Pars transversa	Cartilago cricoidea		

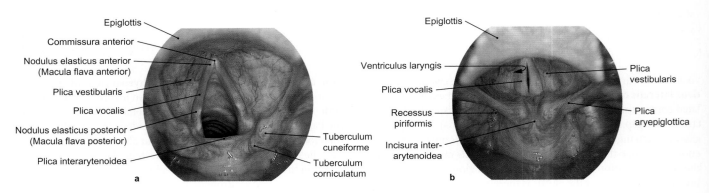

Fig. 10.44 Direct imaging of the larynx (laryngoscopy). a Respiration position. **b** Phonation position. Plica interarytenoidea. [T719]

For phonation air flow is also important; it functions according to the BERNOULLI principle (see textbooks of physiology) on the opening width of the glottis. Since the glottis has a smaller diameter than the trachea, the air coming from the lungs up to the level of the glottis is accelerated and swirled. This results in the mucosa of the vocal folds being set in motion. The vibration can be made visible using stroboscopy (using light flashes creates a virtual slow motion image for the observer's eye). As a rule the vocal folds vibrate in harmony. Through the loose connective tissue of REINKE's space (see below), where there is sufficient basic tension of the vocal folds **edge displacements occur**; these are achieved through the wave-shaped rolling of the mucosa at the free edge of the vocal folds (> Fig. 10.45). Due to the back migration of the mucosal wave towards the subglottis, the mucous membranes on both sides meet each other for a short period and completely stop the air flow. The air flow then forces them away from each other again. This means that there is a permanent alternation between the interruption and liberation of the air flow (vibration), making the vocal folds swing in the air flow.

Clinical remarks

In isolated, **unilateral paralysis of the posticus,** the vocal fold on the affected side is in the paramedian position; **bilateral paralysis** leads to a tightened glottis due to the predominance of the glottis closer and is associated with shortness of breath. **Dysphonia** refers to all disease-related changes in sound formation. This also includes **hoarseness** (hoarseness is a relatively common dysphonia of the voice, recognisable by a rough, broken, husky or silent voice) in unilateral **paralysis of the posticus.** Complete loss of voice is referred to as **aphonia.** It can occur particularly in women due to weakness in the M. arytenoideus transversus **(transversus weakness)** with the whisper triangle and the resulting breathy voice.

NOTE

Actuator apparatus: structures that change the shape of the vocal ligaments.

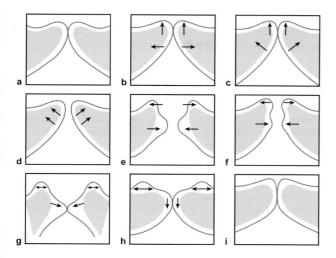

Fig. 10.45 Edge displacements of the vocal fold mucosa during the opening and closing phase. a At the starting position, the vocal folds are closed. **b–d** By increasing the subglottic pressure, a threshold level is reached, pushing the vocal folds apart. This then separates the lower edges. The separation continues further upwards until both vocal folds are completely separated from each other. **e–h** The breath can now pass through the supraglottis and the pharynx as if through a nozzle. The air flow laterally causes a suction effect (BERNOULLI effect), resulting in edge displacement. In doing so, the epithelium and the loose connective tissue in the REINKE's space of the vocal folds are sucked in and pulled together. The lower margins close and the upper edges follow, as soon as the subglottic air flow is cut off. Overall it looks like a rolling of the epithelium on the substrate (Lig. vocale and M. vocalis) from bottom to top. **i** The vocal folds are close together and closed. As a consequence, subglottic pressure begins again, and this starts the phonation cycle again. Repeated cycles lead to regular vibrations. [L126]

Transition between larynx and base of the tongue

The upper edge of the epiglottis (Margo superior epiglottidis) and the base of the tongue are interconnected by the Plica glossoepiglottica mediana and the paired Plicae glossoepiglotticae laterales. The paired Valleculae epiglotticae lie between the folds (this area belongs to the Pars oralis pharyngis, ➤ Fig. 10.47).

Clinical remarks

Swallowed **foreign matter** can get into the Valleculae epiglotticae and, by putting pressure on the epiglottis, can displace the entrance to the larynx and thus the airway. Or it can trigger a **bolus death** via a reflexive cardiac arrest due to vagal stimulation of the sensitive pharyngeal and laryngeal plexus when swallowing large, poorly chewed bits of food (bolus), so that they become jammed in the laryngopharynx, and cannot even be ejected by strong coughing. Fish bones or pieces of chicken bones and other sharp-pointed foreign bodies most often get stuck in the Tonsillae palatinae.

Laryngeal inlet

The laryngeal inlet (**Aditus laryngis**, ➤ Fig. 10.43) is delimited by:
- The upper edge of the epiglottis (Margo superior epiglottidis; ➤ Fig. 10.50): it extends into the oropharynx.
- Aryepiglottic folds (Plicae aryepiglotticae): they range from the lateral edge of the epiglottis up to the arytenoid cartilage tips and each contains a Tuberculum corniculatum and a Tuberculum

cuneiforme, which are raised by the underlying cartilage of the same name.
- The gap between the two arytenoid cartilages (Incisura interarytenoidea, ➤ Fig. 10.44b): its width varies depending on the position of the arytenoid cartilage; the mucosal folds between the arytenoid cartilages are called Plica interarytenoidea, ➤ Fig. 10.44a.

On the right and left of the inlet of the larynx the laryngeal mucosa goes deeper between the aryepiglottal folds on the medial side, as well as between the hyoid bone, Membrana thyrohyoidea and thyroid cartilage on the lateral side to form the **Recessus piriformis**. Within the Recessus the Plica nervi laryngei superioris arising from the N. laryngeus superior can be seen.

Clinical remarks

The structures delimiting the larynx serve as a guide for intubation. **Swallowed foreign matter** can become caught in the Recessus piriformis.

10.6.4 Laryngeal levels

Anatomically, the larynx is divided into
- **Laryngeal vestibule (Vestibulum laryngis);** from the edge of the epiglottis up to the vocal folds
- **Mid-larynx level (glottis);** includes the area between the vocal folds (glottis)
- **Lower larynx level (Cavitas infraglottica);** below the vocal folds to the lower edge of the cricoid cartilage

Clinically the larynx is divided into (➤ Fig. 10.46)
- **Supraglottis (supraglottic space);** from the edge of the epiglottis up to the vestibular folds
- **Transglottic space (glottic space);** of the vestibular folds, including the Ventriculi laryngis up to underneath the vocal folds
- **Subglottis (subglottic space);** from below the vocal folds to the lower edge of the cricoid cartilage

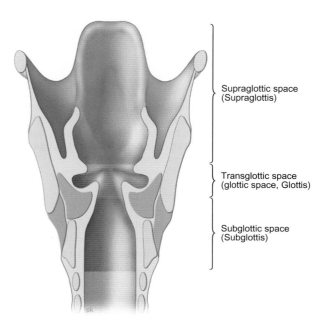

Supraglottic space (Supraglottis)

Transglottic space (glottic space, Glottis)

Subglottic space (Subglottis)

Fig. 10.46 Levels (compartments) of the larynx.

Supraglottis (supraglottic space)

It extends from the inlet of the larynx (Aditus laryngis) up to the level of the vestibular folds (Plicae vestibulares) and includes the epilarynx (laryngeal surface of the epiglottis, Plicae aryepiglotticae and cusps of the arytenoid cartilage).

Clinical remarks

Allergic reactions at the laryngeal inlet can lead to acute oedema with pronounced shortness of breath, as they can expand greatly in the loose connective tissue. Acute bacterial infections of the **epiglottitis,** which particularly occur in children, can very quickly become life-threatening by shifting the airways.

Transglottic space (glottic space)

Included in the transglottic space are

- The paired vestibular folds (Plicae vestibulares or Plicae ventriculares)
- The Tuberculum epiglotticum
- Rima vestibuli (space between the vestibular folds)
- The paired MORGAGNI's ventricules (Ventriculi laryngis); both end in an individually large Sacculus laryngis (Appendix ventriculi laryngis)
- The paired vocal folds (Plicae vocales), which are also referred to as the Labia vocales; they represent the central element of the glottis (glottis, Rima glottidis, voice-forming part of the larynx)

When viewed from above, the vocal folds protrude even further into the lumen of the larynx than the overlying vestibular folds. Due to their covering with squamous epithelium, they appear whitish compared to the red-shimmering vestibular folds.

The **glottis** includes the area of the free edge of the vocal folds. They are contrasted with the transglottic space which includes the space in the area of the glottis, the lower section of the vestibular folds and the laryngeal ventricles. The anterior area of the glottis with the anterior commissure, (Commissura anterior, see below) is referred to as the **Pars intermembranacea** (constitutes around two thirds of the length of the vocal folds); the posterior section of the glottis between the arytenoid cartilages is called the **Pars intercartilaginea.** The vocal folds end at the transition of the Pars intercartilaginea into the Plica interarytenoidea.

Clinical remarks

An extension of the Sacculus laryngis is referred to as a **laryngocele.** If the extension protrudes to such an extent that the Membrana thyrohyoidea is broken, the laryngocele can usually be palpated and visualised from outside **(outer laryngocele).** Complications are infections of the laryngocele and displacement phenomena of the throat area structures.

Subglottis (subglottic space, Cavitas infraglottica)

The subglottis ranges from below the vocal folds to the lower rim of the cricoid cartilage. It is a conically shaped space between the free margin of the vocal folds, the vocal folds, and the lower margin of the cricoid cartilage. The upper boundary is the microscopically locatably Linea arcuata inferior of the Plica vocalis (➤ Fig. 10.42, ➤ Chap. 10.6.5) which can be localised under a microscope. The caudal limit is the lower margin of the cricoid cartilage. Cranial to the side are the Conus elasticus and further caudal of the cricoid cartilage is the boundary. Below, the subglottic space is shaped

like a cylinder and at the top correspondingly tapers to the shape of the Conus elasticus. The anterior boundary is the Lig. cricothyroideum medianum (Lig. conicum); the posterior is the glottis.

Clinical remarks

The lumen of the larynx is for the most part observable by means of various techniques **(examination under laryngoscopy, direct laryngoscopy, indirect endolaryngoscopy)** and therefore, accessible for examination.
The division of the larynx into levels is carried out in clinical imaging for determining the extent (staging) of a tumour-related disease. Although magnetic resonance imaging (MRI) has the highest sensitivity for tumour staging of all imaging techniques, the standard procedure for image-based diagnostics of the larynx is spiral computer tomography (CT) using very thin layers, as with a highly mobile larynx MRI can be associated with significant movement artefacts.

10.6.5 Structure of the Plicae vocales und Plicae vestibulares

Components

In the central area the **Plica vocalis** (➤ Fig. 10.42) is made up of:
- Multilayered non-keratinised squamous epithelium
- Lamina propria made of loose connective tissue
- Lig. vocale (extends cranially into the Membrana quadrangularis and caudally to the Conus elasticus)
- M. vocalis

The **Plica vestibularis** is composed of:
- Multirow respiratory ciliated epithelium
- Lamina propria from loose connective tissue which contains numerous seromucous glands and a lot of lymphatic tissue, which belongs to the mucous-associated lymphoid tissue (LALT = larynx-associated lymphatic tissue)
- Lig. vestibulare (can be viewed as a thickening of the Membrana quadrangularis, in which it is embedded)
- Striated muscle fibre bundles

Epithelium and Lamina propria

Multilayered non-keratinised squamous epithelium is regularly found at the free margin of the vocal cords, on the Plicae aryepiglotticae, on the Plica interarytenoidea, as well as on the top edge of the epiglottis. All other sections of the larynx are covered with **multirow respiratory ciliated epithelium.**

Clinical remarks

In advanced age, increasing amounts of multirow respiratory ciliated epithelium are replaced by squamous epithelium, so that in old people large parts of the mucous membranes are made up of squamous epithelium. Exogenous noxious agents (especially tobacco consumption and alcohol) contribute to **squamous cell carcinoma** originating from here.

The physiological transitions of the squamous epithelium of the Plica vocalis into the ciliated epithelium of the Ventriculus laryngis and the subglottis are referred to as **Linea arcuata superior** and **Linea arcuata inferior** (➤ Fig. 10.42). Below this epithelial transition, the Lamina propria is fixed in place by solid collagen connective tissue at the offshoots of the Lig. vocale, so that the very loose connective tissue below the squamous epithelium of the Plica vocalis forms a closed (virtual) space (REINKE'S space) (➤ Fig. 10.42). Beyond the Linea arcuata superior is the Lamina propria, also made from loose connective tissue and containing many immune cells, lymph follicles and, particularly in the Plica vestibularis, numerous seromucous glands, which secrete their products to the surface of the mucous membranes via fine excretory ducts. Below the Linea arcuata inferior in the loose Lamina propria there are also numerous smaller seromucous glands in the subglottic region.

Attachment structures of the Plica vocalis

Ventrally the vocal folds end in the anterior commissure; dorsally the Pars intercartilaginea goes into the Plica interarytenoidea. The Ligg. vocalia insert in the area of the anterior commissure via 2 structures (➤ Fig. 10.39, ➤ Fig. 10.40, ➤ Fig. 10.41):

- via the **Noduli elastici anteriores** (are visible in examination of the larynx as yellowish thickenings)
- via the **vocal ligament (BROYLES' tendon)** inserted at the thyroid cartilage

The insertion of the Lig. vocale at the Proc. vocalis of the cricoid cartilage is carried out via a **Nodulus elasticus posterior** (also visible when examining the larynx as a yellowish thickening, ➤ Fig. 10.39, ➤ Fig. 10.40). This continuously goes into the elastic cartilage of the **Proc. vocalis** which in turn continues into the hyaline cartilage of the Proc. vocalis. The various structures in the area of the attachment of the vocal ligament serve to attenuate stretching in the vibration of the vocal folds and also enable great mobility within the context of phonation and respiration.

10.6.6 Vascular, lymphatic and nervous systems

Arteries

The main blood vessels of the larynx (➤ Fig. 10.47) are the:
- Aa. laryngeae superiores
- Aa. laryngeae inferiores
- Rr. cricothyroidei

The paired **A. laryngea superior** usually exits close to the upper border of the thyroid cartilage from the A. thyroidea superior

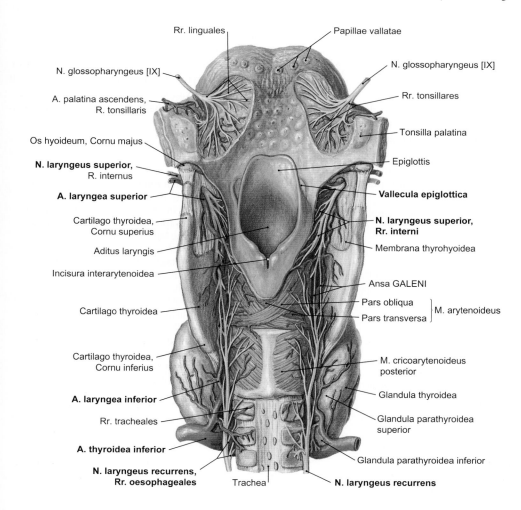

Fig. 10.47 Arteries and nerves of the larynx. Dorsal view.

(branch of the A. carotis externa) (however, it can also directly exit as a stand-alone vessel from the A. carotis interna, the A. lingualis or the A. facialis) and then finally penetrates the membrana thyrohyoidea with the R. internus of the N. laryngeus superior (see below). Rarely it reaches the inner larynx also through a Foramen thyroideum in the thyroid cartilage plate. In the larynx it courses below the mucosa of the Recessus piriformis. Its branches supply the Aditus laryngis and the Vestibulum laryngis.

The blood supply of the glottis is undertaken by the paired **R. cricothyroideus**, a branch of the A. laryngea superior. Together with the branch of the opposite side it forms an arch-shaped arcade before the Lig. cricothyroideum and may, in rare cases, completely replace the A. laryngea superior.

The paired **A. laryngea inferior** is a branch of the A. thyroidea inferior (from the Truncus thyreocervicalis) and, together with the N. laryngeus inferior (see below) rises in the groove between the oesophagus and trachea, These nerves course cranially to the Articulatio cricothyroidea. Here it enters in the space between the thyroid and cricoid cartilages and mainly supplies the dorsally lying muscles (M. cricoarytenoideus posterior and M. arytenoideus). There are many anastomoses between all the laryngeal arteries.

Veins

The veins draining the larynx accompany the arteries. They form an extended mucosla plexus. The blood of the **V. laryngea superior**, together with the blood from the venous R. cricothyroideus, reaches the V. thyroidea superior and from here flows into the V. jugularis. The **V. laryngea inferior** drains into the V. thyroidea inferior, which reaches the Plexus thyroideus impar mostly via the left V. brachiocephalica.

Lymph

The Lamina propria of the laryngeal mucosa is infiltrated by a dense, fine mesh network of lymph capillaries, which join together to major lymph collectors. Lymph vessels above the vocal folds run with the A. laryngea superior and reach the **Nodi lymphoidei infrahyoidei** (Nodi lymphoidei cervicales profundi). Lymph vessels below the Plicae vocales drain into the prelaryngeal (Nodi lymphoidei prelaryngei; DELPHIAN lymph nodes) and to the **Nodi lymphoidei cervicales profundi superiores and inferiores** close to the A. thyroidea inferior (➤ Fig. 10.27). Lymph drainage in the vocal folds is primarily directed dorsally; however there is no separation between the supraglottic and subglottic drainage area and between right and left.

The regional lymph nodes drain via intermediate collection lymph nodes into the Trunci jugularis dexter and sinister.

Innervation

The sensory and motor innervation of the larynx (➤ Fig. 10.47) is taken care of by two branches of the N. vagus [X], the N. laryngeus superior and the N. laryngeus inferior.

NOTE

The **cough reflex** is an involuntarily occurring polysynaptic protective reflex, which is intended to clear the lower respiratory tract of foreign bodies, excess secretions and other potentially harmful stimuli (irritation of the throat). There are many receptors for triggering the reflex in the laryngeal mucosa among other places. The information is passed via viscerosensory nerve fibres of the N. vagus [X] to the cough centre in the Medulla oblongata. The stimulus response is switched to the efferent limb in the Nucleus ambiguus (motor core area of N. vagus [X] and the N. glossopharyngeus [IX]) and is directed to the laryngeal muscles and respiratory muscles, causing a short-term closure of the glottis and explosive exhalation. Ideally the intruding foreign body is thus expelled to the outside.

N. laryngeus superior (➤ Fig. 10.47)

The N. laryngeus superior exits at the level of the Ganglion inferius of the N. vagus [X], runs medially from the A. carotis interna and branches off at the level of the hyoid bone into an outer (R. externus) and an inner (R. internus) branch:

- The **R. externus** of the N. laryngeus superior runs caudal along the side wall of the pharynx to the M. constrictor pharyngis inferior. It penetrates it, innervates it and courses further caudally and ventrally up to the M. cricothyroideus, which it also innervates.
- The **R. internus** of the N. laryngeus superior passes together with the A. laryngea superior through the Membrana thyrohyoidea (➤ Chap. 10.6.3) into the larynx. Here, it runs under the mucosa of the Sinus piriformis (Plica nervi laryngei). It innervates the whole mucosa of the Aditus laryngis, Vestibulum laryngis and the dorsal part of the vocal folds. In most cases it forms an anastomosis (**R. communicans cum nervo laryngeo inferiori; GALEN's anastomosis**).

N. laryngeus inferior (➤ Fig. 10.47)

The N. laryngeus inferior is the terminal branch of the N. laryngeus recurrens. The latter branches off from the **N. vagus [X]** on the left side at the level of the Pars decendens of the aortic arch, runs dorsally beneath the Lig. arteriosum (BOTALLI) and rises in the groove between the trachea and the oesophagus, coursing cranially to the larynx (Fig. 9.40). On the right side, it already leaves the N. vagus [X] at the level of the A. subclavia dextra, crossing beneath it from front to back and so also runs in the groove between the trachea and the oesophagus (Fig. 9.40). At the level of the lower horn of the Cartilago thyroidea and the M. cricoarytenoideus posterior it divides into anterior (R. anterior) and posterior (R. posterior) branches:

- The **R. anterior** innervates the M. thyroarytenoideus and the M. cricoarytenoideus lateralis.
- The **R. posterior** innervates the M. cricoarytenoideus posterior (posticus) and the Mm. arytenoidei transversus and obliquus. It also provides sensory innervation of the front part of the vocal folds, the subglottis and parts of the hypopharynx, the oesophagus and the trachea.

Clinical remarks

Damage to the N. laryngeus superior leads to paralysis of the M. cricothyroideus. As a result, the coarse tension of the vocal fold is insufficient and results in an incomplete closure of the glottis with hoarseness and dysphonia. In addition, sensory disturbances on the inlet of the larynx and in the supraglottis can arise, which can lead to frequent swallowing.

Recurrens paresis refers to **damage to the N. laryngeus recurrens or the N. laryngeus inferior**. There are many causes for this (e.g. malignant tumors, intubation nerve damage due to thyroid surgery). Due to the paralysis of the inner laryngeal muscles, the vocal cords are held on the affected side in a paramedian position **(cadaveric position)**. It results in hoarseness. Bilateral damage may result in a life-threatening shortness of breath.

An A. lusoria, occurring with a frequency of 0.4–2.6% is a vessel variant, with the A. subclavia dextra arising as the last branch from the aortic arch and which in different variants passes behind the oesophagus, between the oesophagus and the trachea or in front of the trachea on the right side of the body. In cases of A. lusoria, the N. laryngeus recurrens is missing on the right side. Instead, the N. laryngeus inferior leaves the N. vagus directly at the level of the larynx and this region is at risk during surgery.

10.7 Pharynx
Wolfgang H. Arnold

The **throat (Pharynx)** is a muscular tube which is attached via the Membrana pharyngobasilaris to the outer surface of the skull base of the Os occipitale. It sits in front of the cervical spine and extends to the level of the VIth cervical vertebra and cricoid cartilage, where it merges into the oesophagus. Its lumen, the **pharyngeal cavity (Cavitas pharyngis)**, is connected to the nasal cavity, the middle ear, the oral cavity, the larynx, and the oesophagus. Within the pharyngeal cavity, respiratory and digestive pathways cross. Functionally, the pharynx is used to transport air, transport food, perceive taste and for immune defence (WALDEYER's tonsillar ring, ➤ Chap. 10.7.7).

10.7.1 Development

The muscles of the throat originate from the 3rd to 5th pharyngeal arches and are in contact with the skeletal elements which previously originated from these pharyngeal arches.

10.7.2 Levels of the pharynx

The pharynx is structured, corresponding to its openings into **3 levels**:

- **Upper level** (Pars nasalis, nasopharynx or epipharynx): it is connected with the nasal cavity through the Choanae and the middle ear via the Tuba auditiva.
- **Middle level** (Pars oralis, oropharynx or mesopharynx): it is the junction between the superior and inferior pharyngeal levels and connects with the oral cavity through the Isthmus faucium.
- **Lower level** (Pars laryngea, laryngopharynx or hypopharynx): it stands at the front, connected with the larynx via the Aditus laryngis and runs caudally into the gullet (Oesophagus).

Epipharynx

The choanae (Choanae nasales) open out from the nose into the epipharynx. Upwards the epipharynx forms the **pharyngeal fornix (Fornix pharyngis)**. Here, the pharyngeal wall consists of taut connective tissue **(Fascia pharyngobasilaris)**, which is fixed to the skull base. It used by the M. constrictor pharyngis as attachment zone. The fascia is attached dorsally at the Tuberculum pharyngeum (➤ Fig. 9.5). From here the connective tissue extends as a median strip of connective tissue, **Raphe pharyngis**, which serves as the attachment zone for the inferior pharyngeal constrictor muscle and reaches caudally to the Pars cricopharyngea. Under the mucosa (respiratory ciliated epithelium) of the rear area, located on the roof of the epipharynx under the skull base, there is lymphatic tissue that bulges forward, particularly in children, known as **Tonsilla pharyngea**. In front of the tonsils, the **pharyngeal hypophysis (Hypophysis pharyngealis)** may be present in the connective tis-

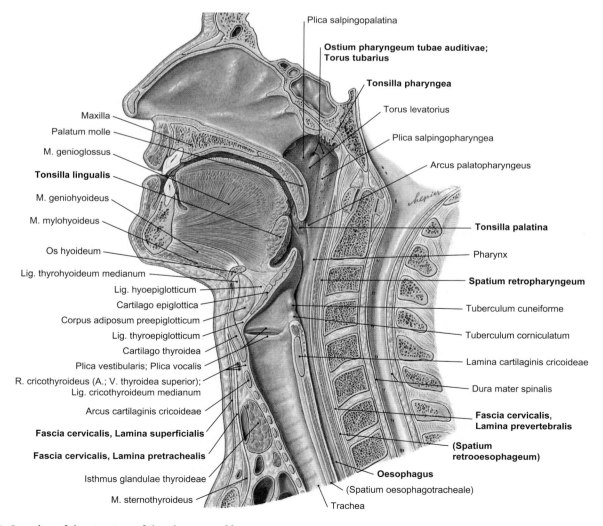

Fig. 10.48 Overview of the structure of the pharynx and larynx.

Plica salpingopalatina
Ostium pharyngeum tubae auditivae; Torus tubarius
Tonsilla pharyngea
Torus levatorius
Plica salpingopharyngea
Arcus palatopharyngeus
Tonsilla palatina
Pharynx
Spatium retropharyngeum
Tuberculum cuneiforme
Tuberculum corniculatum
Lamina cartilaginis cricoideae
Dura mater spinalis
Fascia cervicalis, Lamina prevertebralis
(Spatium retrooesophageum)
Oesophagus
(Spatium oesophagotracheale)
Trachea

Maxilla
Palatum molle
M. genioglossus
Tonsilla lingualis
M. geniohyoideus
M. mylohyoideus
Os hyoideum
Lig. thyrohyoideum medianum
Lig. hyoepiglotticum
Cartilago epiglottica
Corpus adiposum preepiglotticum
Lig. thyroepiglotticum
Cartilago thyroidea
Plica vestibularis; Plica vocalis
R. cricothyroideus (A.; V. thyroidea superior); Lig. cricothyroideum medianum
Arcus cartilaginis cricoideae
Fascia cervicalis, Lamina superficialis
Fascia cervicalis, Lamina pretrachealis
Isthmus glandulae thyroideae
M. sternothyroideus

sue on the under surface of the cuneiform bone as an embryologic relic of the RATHKE's pouch. The Tuba auditiva opens in the lateral wall on both sides, connecting the pharynx to the middle ear. The **Ostium pharyngeum tubae auditivae** is delimited from the back and the top by the **Torus tubarius**. The Torus tubarius is extended downwards and to the rear through the **Plica salpingopharyngea** (➤ Fig. 10.48). It is elevated by the M. salpingopharyngeus. Beneath the orifice of the Tuba auditiva is the **Torus levatorius**, in which the Levator veli palatini courses (➤ Fig. 10.48). Under the epithelium of the tubal opening is lymphatic tissue known collectively as the **Tonsilla tubaria**. The Tonsilla pharyngea and Tonsillae tubariae are part of the lymphatic pharyngeal ring known as (WALDEYER's tonsillar ring, ➤ Chap. 10.7.7).

Clinical remarks

In childhood, a **hyperplasia of the pharyngeal tonsils frequently occurs (adenoids, adenoid vegetation, commonly known as 'polyps')**. This can lead to the pharyngotympanic tube being displaced, reducing the aeration of the middle ear. This results in recurrent middle ear inflammation, which reduces hearing and developmental delays ensue. The treatment of choice in these cases is removal of the tonsils (adenectomy). Sometimes the pharyngeal roof hypophysis (Hypophysis pharyngea) is to be found on the under surface of the cuneiform bone, in the connective tissue in front of the Tonsilla pharyngea. It is left behind during development and in young people can constitute a starting point for a **craniopharyngioma**. Beneath the mucosa between the Tonsilla tubaria and the Tonsilla palatina, there is lymphatic tissue referred to as lateral strands. Especially after removal of the Tonsillae palatinae (tonsillectomy) bacterial infections can occur here as a form of inflammation of the throat area, **pharyngitis**. Commonly, those affected suffer from ear ache and headache, and have difficulty swallowing.

Mesopharynx

The mesopharynx (Pars oralis pharyngis) is connected by the Isthmus faucium with the oral cavity. The base of the tongue, together with the Tonsilla lingualis presses into the mesopharynx (➤ Fig. 10.48). The epiglottis is movably connected with the base of the tongue via the Plica glossoepiglottica mediana and the Plicae glossoepiglotticae laterales. Between the folds are 2 depressions (Valleculae epiglotticae). During swallowing, the Pars oralis is separated from the Pars nasalis by displacement of the soft palate to the posterior pharyngeal wall.

Hypopharynx

The hypopharynx (Pars laryngea pharyngis) is the longest section of the pharynx. At the front it is connected to the **laryngeal inlet (Aditus laryngis)** and ends caudally behind the cricoid cartilage of the larynx, where it joins the oesophagus. This is the location of the first narrowing of the gullet (Constrictio pharyngea oesophagealis). The laryngeal inlet is surrounded by the epiglottis and the Plicae aryepiglotticae. In the lower area, the posterior surfaces of the arytenoid cartilage and subglottis stand out with their muscles. Between the arytenoid cartilages is the Incisura interarytenoidea. The Plica glossoepiglottica lateralis runs from the lateral edge of the epiglottis to the side wall of the larynx. The N. laryngeus superior and the blood vessels of the same name bulge out caudally from the Plicae glossoepiglotticae laterales, towards the Plica nervi laryngei. The **Recessus piriformis** is located between the thyroid cartilage and Plica aryepiglottica, and particularly liquids and liquid nutri-

ents pass through here going from the base of the tongue to the inlet of the oesophagus.

Clinical remarks

Swallowed foreign matter can irritate the delicate neuronal network of the pharynx and larynx and may lead to a vagal reaction with reflex cardiovascular arrest **(bolus death)** when swallowing large, poorly chewed bits of food (bolus), so that they become jammed in the laryngopharynx, and cannot be ejected even by strong coughing and gagging.

10.7.3 Pharyngeal wall

The pharyngeal wall is thin and can be divided into 4 layers:
- **Tunica mucosa** (mucous membrane): in the nasopharynx this is largely made up of respiratory ciliated epithelium, while in the oropharynx and laryngopharynx it is multilayered, non-keratinised squamous epithelium. It contains small salivary glands, Glandulae pharyngeales, and a lot of lymphatic tissue that belongs to the mucosa-associated lymphoid tissue.
- **Tela submucosa** (submucosal connective tissue): it connects with the Tunica adventitia to the Fascia pharyngobasilaris.
- **Tunica muscularis** (musculature): it surrounds the pharyngeal constrictor muscles (Mm. constrictores pharyngis) and the levator pharyngeal muscles (Mm. levatores pharyngis).
- **Tunica adventitia** (adventitia): it creates the connection to the surroundings, dorsally to the Spatium retropharyngeum, a virtual gap attaching the pharynx to the cervical spine, laterally to the Spatium parapharyngeum, virtual spaces creating the connection to the lateral structures of the neck. Virtual means that connective tissue fibres create the connection to neighbouring structures (cervical spine, neck structures), but in the context of pathological processes they can be dissolved, which then creates gaps which can go cranially as far as the skull base and caudally into the mediastinum.

N O T E

Unlike the gastrointestinal tract, the pharyngeal wall has no Lamina muscularis. In the cranial section, a Tunica muscularis is also absent; here, submucosal connective tissue and adventitia merge together with the Fascia pharyngobasilaris.

10.7.4 Pharyngeal musculature

The pharynx is a long outstretched muscle tube consisting of 3 sphincter muscles (pharyngeal constrictors, Mm. constrictores pharyngei) and 3 longitudinal muscles (pharyngeal levators, Mm. levatores pharyngei).

Pharyngeal constrictor muscles
All 3 pharyngeal constrictor muscles (**Mm. constrictores pharyngis**) originate in the anterior region on the structures of the oral cavity wall and the larynx, enclosing in a circular way the lumen of the pharynx, overlapping like roof tiles and coming together dorsally in the centre in the fibrous **Raphe pharyngis** (➤ Fig. 10.49, ➤ Table 10.23). The Raphe pharyngis runs from the Tuberculum pharyngeum of the Os occipitale to the oesophagus. The lowest part (**Pars cricopharyngea**) of the lower pharyngeal constrictor

(M. constrictor pharyngis inferior) consists of 2 muscle units (**Pars obliqua and Pars transversa = Pars fundiformis = KILLIAN's bundle**), which form the weakly muscular KILLIAN's triangle (➤ Fig. 10.49). Below the Pars transversa, another muscle triangle arises (**LAIMER's triangle**) from the obliquely radiating oesophageal muscles. In comparison to KILLIAN's triangle it stands on its head. The Pars transversa forms the basis of both triangles.

Clinical remarks

Within the weak muscle of KILLIAN's triangle a **pulsion diverticulum = hypopharyngeal diverticulum (ZENKER's diverticulum)** frequently occurs in aged men. It involves protrusions of the wall of the pharynx into the retropharyngeal space. If chyme collects in the increasingly expanding diverticulum, it can lead to the regurgitation of undigested food. Problems with swallowing may also occur. A rupture with a life-threatening infection into the peripharyngeal space **(peripharyngeal abscess)** may occur, which can spread to the skull base and into the mediastinum. The same propagation paths also apply to inflammation, which can easily penetrate the thin pharyngeal wall.

Pharyngeal levator muscles

The paired pharyngeal levator muscles (**Mm. levatores pharyngis**) are the **M. stylopharyngeus** (➤ Fig. 10.49), the **M. salpingopharyngeus**, and **M. palatopharyngeus** (➤ Fig. 10.50, ➤ Table 10.24). They pass between the constrictor muscles under the mucosa of the larynx, where they are attached.

10.7.5 Vascular, lymphatic and nervous systems

Arteries and veins

The pharynx is supplied with blood by 4 arteries (➤ Table 10.25):
- The **A. pharyngea ascendens** from the A. carotis externa lies on the lateral pharyngeal wall and runs up to the skull base.
- The **A. palatina ascendens** from the A. facialis supplies the anterior section of the pharynx.
- The **A. sphenopalatina** from the A. maxillaris also supplies the anterior section of the pharynx.
- The **A. thyroidea inferior** supplies the lower part of the pharynx (➤ Fig. 10.49).

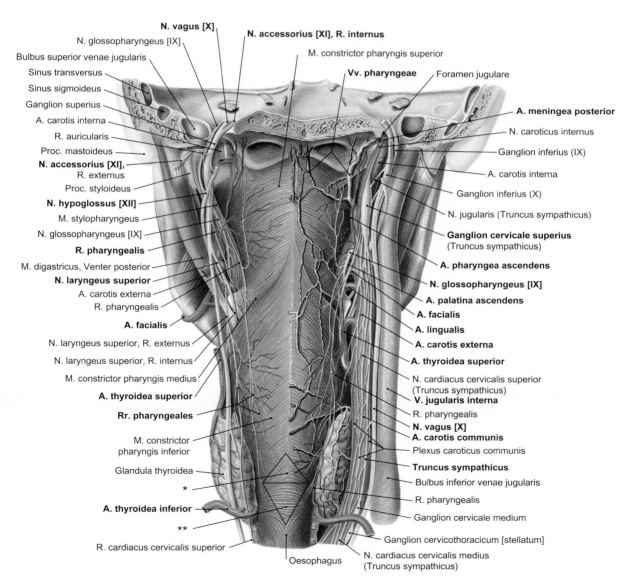

Fig. 10.49 Overview of the constrictors of the pharynx. * KILLIAN'S TRIANGLE, ** LAIMER'S triangle

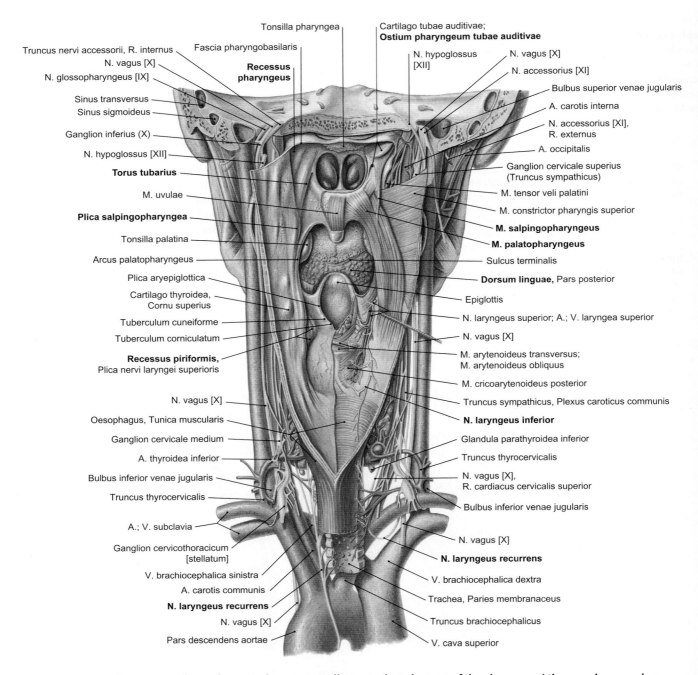

Truncus nervi accessorii, R. internus
N. vagus [X]
N. glossopharyngeus [IX]
Sinus transversus
Sinus sigmoideus
Ganglion inferius (X)
N. hypoglossus [XII]
Torus tubarius
M. uvulae
Plica salpingopharyngea
Tonsilla palatina
Arcus palatopharyngeus
Plica aryepiglottica
Cartilago thyroidea, Cornu superius
Tuberculum cuneiforme
Tuberculum corniculatum
Recessus piriformis, Plica nervi laryngei superioris
N. vagus [X]
Oesophagus, Tunica muscularis
Ganglion cervicale medium
A. thyroidea inferior
Bulbus inferior venae jugularis
Truncus thyrocervicalis
A.; V. subclavia
Ganglion cervicothoracicum [stellatum]
V. brachiocephalica sinistra
A. carotis communis
N. laryngeus recurrens
N. vagus [X]
Pars descendens aortae

Tonsilla pharyngea
Fascia pharyngobasilaris
Recessus pharyngeus

Cartilago tubae auditivae; **Ostium pharyngeum tubae auditivae**
N. hypoglossus [XII]

N. vagus [X]
N. accessorius [XI]
Bulbus superior venae jugularis
A. carotis interna
N. accessorius [XI], R. externus
A. occipitalis
Ganglion cervicale superius (Truncus sympathicus)
M. tensor veli palatini
M. constrictor pharyngis superior
M. salpingopharyngeus
M. palatopharyngeus
Sulcus terminalis
Dorsum linguae, Pars posterior
Epiglottis
N. laryngeus superior; A.; V. laryngea superior
N. vagus [X]
M. arytenoideus transversus; M. arytenoideus obliquus
M. cricoarytenoideus posterior
Truncus sympathicus, Plexus caroticus communis
N. laryngeus inferior
Glandula parathyroidea inferior
Truncus thyrocervicalis
N. vagus [X], R. cardiacus cervicalis superior
Bulbus inferior venae jugularis
N. vagus [X]
N. laryngeus recurrens
V. brachiocephalica dextra
Trachea, Paries membranaceus
Truncus brachiocephalicus
V. cava superior

Fig. 10.50 Pharyngeal levator muscles at the open pharynx, as well as vessels and nerves of the pharynx and the parapharyngeal space, Spatium lateropharyngeum. Dorsal view.

Table 10.24 Pharyngeal levator muscles.

Innervation	Origins	Attachment	Function
M. stylopharyngeus			
Rr. pharyngeales of the N. glossopharyngeus [IX] (= Plexus pharyngeus)	Proc. styloideus	Cartilago thyroidea radiates into the side wall of the pharynx	Raising of the pharynx during swallowing
M. palatopharyngeus			
R. musculi stylopharyngei of the N. glossopharyngeus [IX]	Aponeurosis palatinae, Hamulus pterygoideus	Cartilago thyroidea radiates into the side wall of the pharynx	Raising of the pharynx during swallowing
M. salpingopharyngeus			
Rr. pharyngeales of the N. glossopharyngeus [IX] (= Plexus pharyngeus)	Posterior edge of the Ostium tubae auditivae	Radiates into the side wall of the pharynx	Raising the pharynx during swallowing opens the Tuba auditiva

Table 10.25 Overview of the arterial blood supply to the pharynx.

Arterial trunk	Terminal branch	Supply area
A. carotis externa	A. pharyngea ascendens	Lateral and posterior pharyngeal wall
A. maxillaris	A. sphenopalatina	Superior anterior section of the pharynx
A. facialis	A. palatina ascendens	Medial anterior section of the pharynx
A. subclavia	A. thyroidea inferior	Lower section of the pharynx

Under the mucosa and the pharyngeal muscles is the venous **Plexus pharyngeus**, the blood from which drains into the **Vv. pharyngeae**, which lead to the V. jugularis interna.

Lymph vessels
The entire mucous membrane of the pharynx is interfused with lymph follicles belonging to the mucosa-associated lymphoid tissue. The lymph is discharged from here via the **Nodi lymphoidei retropharyngeales** into the Nodi lymphoidei cervicales profundi.

Innervation
The sensory, motor and secretory innervation of the pharynx is performed by branches of the **N. glossopharyngeus [IX]** and the **N. vagus [X]** (N. laryngeus superior). The branches form the **Plexus pharyngeus**, together with postganglionic sympathetic fibres of the Truncus sympathicus. Fibres from the **N. maxillaris [V/2]** (R. pharyngeus of the Nn. pterygopalatini, ➤ Fig. 10.51) also make a contribution.

N O T E
Afferent and efferent fibres of the Plexus pharyngeus are part of the **swallowing, gag and defensive reflex,** which is also maintained during sleep. The coordination centre for this lies in the Medulla oblongata.

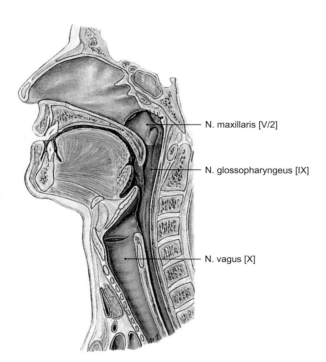

Fig. 10.51 Sensory innervation of the throat.

- N. maxillaris [V/2]
- N. glossopharyngeus [IX]
- N. vagus [X]

10.7.6 Swallowing

In **infants**, the epiglottis reaches from far cranial up to the nasopharynx. Breast milk passes directly into the Sinus piriformis. To do so, the larynx must not be closed, and the soft palate must not to be drawn to the pharynx.
In **children** and **adults**, the airway and gullet cross over each other, which is why when swallowing the airway must be briefly separated from the gullet. To do this, the soft palate is drawn up to the pharyngeal wall and the larynx is briefly closed.

N O T E
Infants can breathe and drink at the same time.

Swallowing takes place in **3 phases**:
- **Oral phase:** this is the voluntary phase of food communition and salivation within the oral cavity. The tongue is pressed against the palate by contraction of the muscles of the floor of the mouth, with the food bolus being transported in the direction of the Isthmus faucium.
- **Pharyngeal phase:** this is the reflex phase, coordinating the safeguarding of the respiratory tract and the transportation of food. Here, initially the M. tensor veli palatini and the M. constrictor pharyngis superior contract to form the PASSAVANT's bar which closes the access to the nasopharynx. The way back to the oral cavity is barred by the sphincter system of the muscles of the Isthmus faucium and the tongue. In addition, the Aditus laryngis and the glottis are closed.
- **Oesophageal phase:** this is characterised by a peristaltic contraction of the pharyngeal muscles from cranial to caudal. At the same time the contraction of the pharyngeal levator raises the larynx, which to a certain extent, draws the pharynx over the bolus. Solid food components are transported by waves of peristaltic contraction; when standing, liquids are passed by jerking contraction of the floor of the mouth and the upper constrictor muscles into the stomach by taking gulps.

10.7.7 Lymphatic pharyngeal ring

The **lymphoid ring (WALDEYER's tonsillar ring)** is understood as a group of lymphatic epithelial tissues, which are located at the transition of the oral and nasal cavities to the pharynx. In its entirety, the tissues form a ring which serves the immune system and belongs to the mucosa-associated lymphoid tissue (MALT). The elements of WALDEYER's tonsillar ring are:
- Lingual tonsil (Tonsilla lingualis, unpaired)
- Palatine tonsil (Tonsilla palatina, paired)
- Lateral cord (paired)
- Tube tonsil (Tonsilla tubaria, paired)
- Nasopharyngeal tonsil (Tonsilla pharyngea, unpaired)

NEURO-ANATOMY

11 General neuroanatomy

11.1 Embryology
Tobias M. Böckers

11.1.1 Overview

Both the central nervous system (CNS) as well as the peripheral nervous system (PNS) are derived from the **ectoderm** of the three-layered germinal disc. This folds into the primitive **neural tube**, which subsequently forms the brain and spinal cord. Here, the cranial section of the neural tube becomes enlarged and thicker, to form the so-called **brain vesicles**, which later form the output structures for the brain parts which differentiate further. The neuroblasts (**neural crest cells**) migrate from the primitive neural tube, forming the PNS, among other structures.

Early development
After fertilisation, the zygote remains for about 30 hours in a quiescent stage before the cells within the surrounding **Zona pellucida** divide in a predominantly synchronous manner (cleavage stages/division without growth phase, ➤ Chap. 2.3.1). The compaction and morula stage follow these cleavage stages (➤ Chap. 2.3.1). The morula reaches the uterus mucosa and the penetrating fluid expands the intercellular spaces. These intercellular spaces coalesce on one side of the embryo where they form so-called **blastocyst cavities**. An outer layer of surrounding **trophoblast cells** are visible (these will form the foetal portion of the placenta), which are differentiated from the inner **embryoblast cells** (the inner cell mass which forms the embryo) (➤ Chap. 2.3.2). Blastocysts finally leave the surrounding Zona pellucida (hatching) and are attached

as 'free blastocysts' between the 5th and 6th day to the mucous membrane of the uterus.

Implantation (syn.: Nidation)
The embryoblast cells 'migrates' first of all to the attachment point, the trophoblast cells dividing very dynamically and merging at the penetration point into large giant cells (**syncytiotrophoblasts,** ➤ Fig. 11.1). Remaining attached to the embryoblast, the single-layered **cytotrophoblast** replenishes through rapid cell division for the further formation of the syncytiotrophoblasts. In this way, **blastocysts** penetrate in the direction of the Zona compacta of the endometrium until finally ending in the epithelial tissue of the endometrium above the implanted embryo. At the site of implantation, surface defects are covered by a final formation of the coagulum (approx. day 7–8). In addition to the invasive growth dynamics of the trophoblasts, the production and secretion of important molecules also begins. Therefore, among other factors, the human chorionic gonadotropin (hCG) is secreted, an analogue of luteinising hormone (LH), which binds to the LH-receptors in the Corpus luteum and induces their conversion into **Corpus luteum graviditatis**. This produces more progesterone, maintaining the pregnancy and preventing the onset of menstrual bleeding. In addition, different signalling molecules are given out that suppress the immune response of the maternal immune system.

Germinal disc development
The *2nd week* of development further differentiates the embryoblast. It creates the **two layers of the germinal disc** (epiblast and hypoblast, ➤ Chap. 2.4.1), and the blastocyst cavity becomes the **primary yolk sac**, lined with hypoblast cells. There is a gap between the trophoblasts and epiblasts that becomes increasingly larger (**primary amniotic cavity**) and which is lined with an epithelium of further differentiated epiblast cells (**definitive amniotic cavity**, ➤ Fig. 11.2b, ➤ Fig. 2.7). Finally, between the germinal system and the rapidly growing trophoblasts, new intercellular spaces are created that become increasingly larger and merge together. This newly created space is referred to as the extra-embryonic coelom, also called the chorionic cavity. The yolk sac splits apart under the growth traction and then closes again to form a secondary yolk sac; an exocoelomic cyst (remnant of the primary yolk sac) often remains behind in the chorionic cavity.

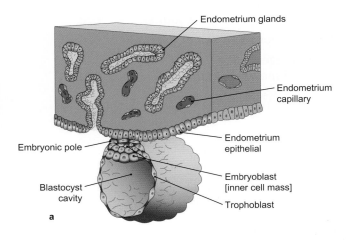

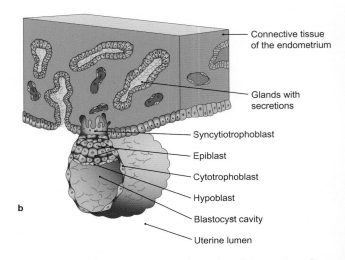

Fig. 11.1 Start of implantation and differentiation of embryoblasts. a Attachment of the blastocyst to the endometrium. **b** Formation of syncytiotrophoblasts and penetrations into the endometrium. [E347-09]

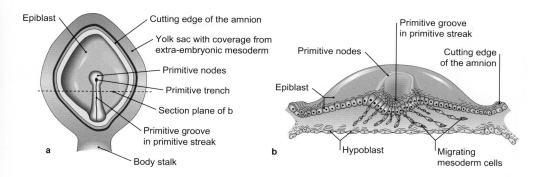

Fig. 11.2 Germinal disc development. a Formation of the primitive streak (view after removal of the amniotic cavity). b Cross-section of the germinal disc, growth movements in the area of the primitive streak, formation of intra-embryonic mesoderms. [E347-09]

At the start of the *3rd week* a strip-shaped thickening, the **primitive streak,** is visible on the epiblasts (➤ Fig. 11.2, ➤ Chap. 2.4.2). It forms from the caudal to the cranial and ends about halfway, where it displays a round enlargement, the **primitive node.** Primitive streaks and primitive nodes form depressions, so that it is possible for the **primitive groove** to be distinguished from the **primitive pit.** These morphological structures suggest dynamic cell migration, directed by in-depth epiblasts (invagination). Epiblast cells detach here from the cell complex and slide between epiblasts and hypoblasts. The resulting germinal layer is thus called the **intra-embryonic mesoderm.** The remaining epiblast cells continue to differentiate from the **ectoderm.** From the primitive node, a cell complex cranially grows as an axial structure and reveals a primitive axis rod, the **Chorda dorsalis** (mesoderm), which is of particular importance for many subsequent development stages. The hypoblast is also replaced by cells of the epiblasts (in particular in the area of the primitive pit); this cell layer is now called the **endoderm.** In 2 positions in the embryo, the ectoderm and endoderm lie directly next to each other as there is no intra-embryonic mesoderm. Cranially, this is the so-called pharyngeal membrane (prechordal plate = later the opening of the mouth) and caudally, the cloaca membrane (= later the anus).

Folding

Dynamic changing in shape in early embryos is described as folding, which ultimately changes the flat embryoblast (germinal disc) into a three-dimensional structure.

- **Lateral folding:** The lateral edges of the germinal disc grow ventrally towards the yolk sac and then merge 'below' the embryo. The lateral and front body wall are thus formed (➤ Fig. 11.3, ➤ Chap. 2.8.2). In addition, this growth movement displaces parts of the definitive yolk sac (entoderm) into the inside of the embryo. These cell layers also merge with each other. This creates a tube structure (**primitive intestinal tube**) on the inside of the embryo, which extends from the pharyngeal membrane to the cloaca membrane.
- **Craniocaudal curvature:** Due to the very rapid growth and further differentiation of the neural tube (➤ Fig. 11.3, ➤ Chap. 2.8.1), the embryo 'bends' into a C-shape and the tail fold can be distinguished from the head fold.
- **Neuronal folding (primary neurulation):** under the influence of messenger substances, which are secreted from the cells of the Chorda dorsalis, a development of a thicker ectodermal cell layer (**neural plate**) in the above-lying ectoderm is induced. Such signal molecules include growth factors such as TGFβ or inhibitors such as chordin or noggin. Via these mediators, specific transcription factors such as neurogenin are activated, which then, for example, induce the differentiation of ectoderm cells in neurons or glial cells. Over the further course of the neurulation, a shallow groove (**neural groove**) forms on the neural plate with lateral raised areas, the **neural cleavage** (➤ Chap. 2.5.2). At this point in time, you can already see a cranio-caudal limit: the section above the 4th somite later becomes the brain, and the sec-

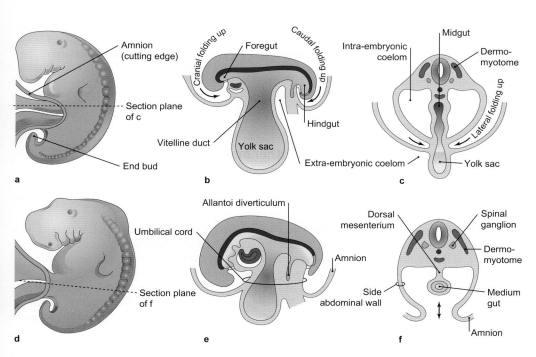

Fig. 11.3 Embryonic folding in the 4th week. The craniocaudal bend (**b, e**) and the lateral folding are visible (**c, f**). [E347-09]

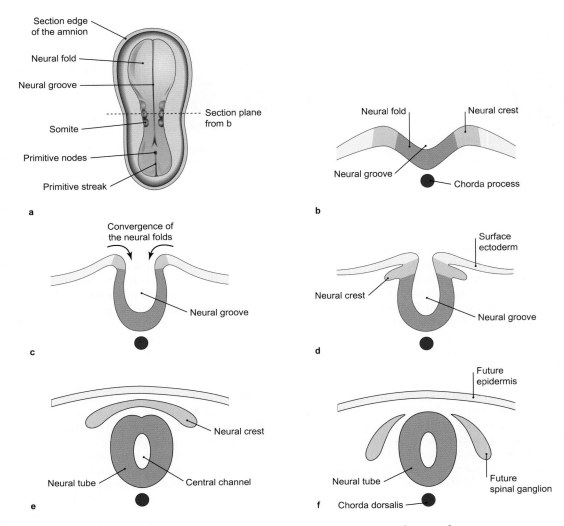

Fig. 11.4 Formation of neural grooves, neural folding, neural tube and neural crests; diagram. [E347-09]
a View from above after removal of the amniotic cavity. **b–f** Illustrated are the cross-sections through embryos in consecutive stages of development. [E347-09]

tion below becomes the spinal cord. The neural folding first begins at the level of the 4th–6th somites to merge with each other and thereby, through the cranial and caudal merger process, form the **neural tube** (➤ Fig. 11.4). At the respective ends, there are still small openings that are called **Neuroporus anterior (rostralis) and posterior (caudalis)**. Through these openings, the lumen of the neural tube is connected with the amniotic cavity, before the Neuroporus anterior closes on the *24th day* and the Neuroporus posterior on the *26th day*. The location of the Neuroporus anterior corresponds to the Lamina terminalis in the adult brain. The Neuroporus posterior is localised in the area of the Filum terminale or at the level of the 31st somite pairs, from which sacral vertebrae I and II are formed. The sections of the spinal cord lying caudally further than S1, are formed by a secondary sprouting of the neural epithelium of the already formed neural tube. This process is also known as **secondary neurulation**. At the edge of the neural plate, in the transition to the surface ectoderm, the **neural crest** system develops, which is formed from cells that migrate laterally from the neural tube and then dorsally into a thin layer of connective tissue between the surface ectoderm and the closed neural tube. The neural crest cells, among other things, form the future PNS.

11.1.2 Further brain development

Further development of parts of the CNS from the neural tube have similarities in all sections, based on an early separation of the neural tube into a dorsal and ventral half:

- The dorsal half consists of the **alar plates**, which are linked with each other through the narrow **roof plate**.
- The ventral half includes the **base plates**, which are linked to each other via the ventrally located **floor plates**.

Alar and base plates are separated from each other by the **Sulcus limitans**. To a large extent this morphological structure also represents a functional structure, insofar as primarily afferent (general somato/visceral afferents or specific somato/visceral afferents)

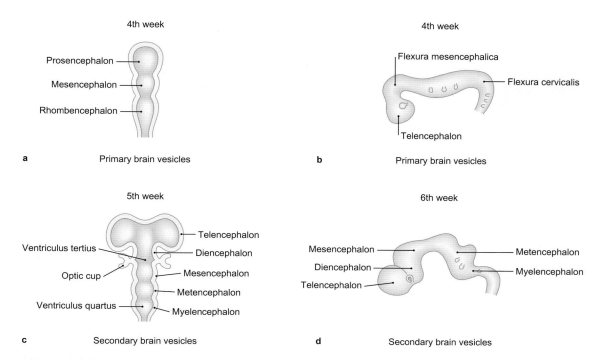

Fig. 11.5 Development of the brain. a Formation of primary brain vesicles; 4th week; horizontal section. **b** The mesencephalic flexure (Flexura mesencephalica) and the cervical flexure (Flexura cervicalis) are visible; 4th week lateral view. **c** Development of secondary brain vesicles; 5th week, horizontal section. **d** secondary brain vesicles; 6th week, the pontal flexure is visible; lateral view. [E838]

nuclei form in the alar plates; in the base plates, efferent (general somato/visceral efferents or specific visceral efferents) nuclei are preferred.

This basic structure is the foundation for further development in all sections of the brain. Histologically speaking, the first homogeneous neuroepithelial part of the neural tube changes to a three-layered structure:

- the outer **marginal zone** (rich in Substantia alba)
- the intermediate **mantle zone** (rich in Substantia grisea)
- the **ventricular zones** lying next to the neural canal (preferentially forming macroglia forms, such as oligodendrocytes, astrocytes and ependymal cells)

At the beginning of the *4th week* the cranial part of the neural tube is certainly already significantly different from the caudal section. Above the 4th somites, after the closure of the Neuroporus anterior, 3 **cerebral vesicles**, the so-called primary brain vesicles, can be detected (from cranial to caudal, ➤ Fig. 11.5a):

- **prosencephalon** vesicles
- **mesencephalon** vesicles
- **rhombencephalic** vesicles

In the *5th week of development,* 5 secondary brain vesicles develop from the 3 primary vesicles. There are 2 extra paired protuberances on the prosencephalon vesicles (**telencephalic** vesicles or endbrain/cerebrum vesicles), the unpaired 'vesicle remnant' later becomes the interbrain (**diencephalon** or diencephalon vesicles). The rhombencephalon vesicles can later be divided into a cranial **metencephalon** and a caudal part, the **myelencephalon** (➤ Fig. 11.5c, d).

With further development, the lumen of the **neural tube** is extended or tapers into the later ventricular system of the CNS. The rapid brain growth and craniocaudal folding of the embryo bend the neural tube so that a **cephalic flexure**, a **ventrally convex pontine flexure** (emerging a little later and located in the area of the rhombencephalon), and a **cervical flexure** (located in the transition between the myelencephalon and the spinal cord), can be dif-

ferentiated in the area of the mesencephalon. The cervical flexure later lies approximately at the level of the Foramen magnum or at the outlet of the 1st spinal nerve (➤ Fig. 11.5b).

Development of the pons and Medulla oblongata

If you change the perspective from the outer structure of the neural tube to the development processes, which can be observed in a cross-section, it can be seen that the development of the pons and Medulla oblongata (parts of the brainstem) is relatively comparable with the myelencephalon vesicles: the **Canalis centralis** extends in this section in which the dorsal alar plate opens out like a book and only the thin roof plate as the cover of the canal or the later IVth ventricle persists (➤ Fig. 11.6b). Thus the alar and base plates end up lying next to each other, separated by the Sulcus limitans. Through these dynamics, the later core areas of the cranial nerves are positioned side by side: nuclei of efferent nerve fibres lie paramedian with a total of 3 groups (general somato/visceral efferent, specific visceral efferent), afferent, the afferent core areas laterally of it (general and specific visceral afferent, general and specific somatoafferent). Neurons of the alar plate migrate in ventrally and form there, for example, the Nuclei olivares, the olive core, or the Formatio reticularis. Also from the alar plates, the so-called **rhombic lips** are formed, from which the cerebellum is developed in a further step (➤ Fig. 11.6, ➤ Chap. 12.4).

Development of the mesencephalon

Mesencephalon vesicles undergo the fewest changes during further development. The lumen of the neural tube narrows due to enhanced growth of the lateral walls and it forms the finely sized Aqueductus mesencephali (SYLVII), which connects the IIIrd and IVth ventricles. The mesencephalon is divided into a roof plate (**tectum**) and a section that covers the ventral two-thirds, the so-called **tegmentum**, to which the anterior portion, the **Pars basilaris mesencephali**, connects. Neuroblasts migrate from the alar plate to the Tectum mesencephali and form the paired **Colliculi superi-**

587

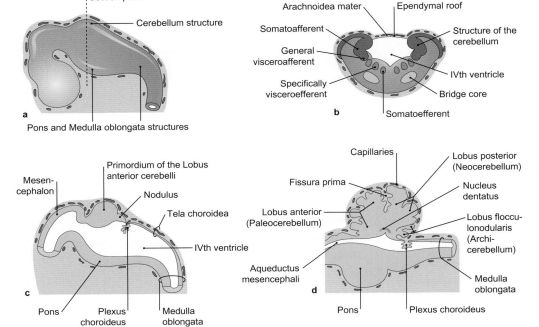

Fig. 11.6 Development of the brain. a Schematic drawing of the brain in the 5th week. **b** Cross-section through the rhombencephalon on which the derivatives of the base plate and alar plate can be seen. **c, d** Sagittal sections of a 6- (c) and 17-(d) week-old rhombencephalon. The ongoing development of the pons and cerebellum is clearly evident. [E347-09]

ores and inferiores (➤ Fig. 11.7b–e). Neuroblasts of the former base plate in turn form motor core groups in the Tegmentum mesencephali (e.g. Nucleus nervi oculomotorii). What is controversial is the origin of the Nucleus ruber and/or the Substantia nigra, which were formed from neuroblasts from either the alar plate or the base plate. Approximately in the *11th week of development* the

structure of the mesencephalon has already reached its final form (➤ Fig. 11.7c–e).

Development of the diencephalon

The **diencephalon vesicles** are the origin of the diencephalon to which the hypothalamus belongs, along with the hypophysis, epi-

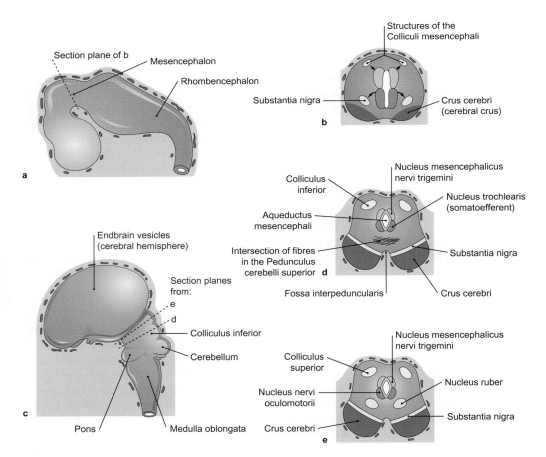

Fig. 11.7 Development of the mesencephalon. a, b 5th week of development. **c–e** 11th week of development. [E347-09]

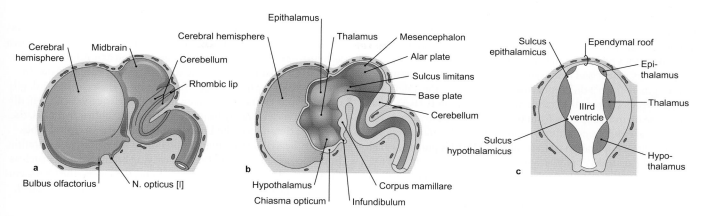

Fig. 11.8 **Development of the brain in the 7th week. a** Surface view of the brain. **b** Corresponding median section with prosencephalon and mesencephalon. **c** Cross-section through the diencephalon, on which the epithalamus can be seen dorsally, the thalamus laterally, and the hypothalamus ventrally. [E347-09]

thalamus, thalamus and the subthalamus (➤ Fig. 11.8b, c). The structure of the eye also grows from the diencephalon. Due to the further growth dynamics of the adult brain – in particular the massive expansion of the telencephalon – diencephalon components are only visible on the basal side of the brain.

The inside of the neural canal will be extended during the early development to the **IIIrd ventricle**. Through massive cell divisions in the lateral wall of the neural tube, the **epithalamus, thalamus** and **hypothalamus are formed**. The **Sulcus epithalamicus** lies between the epithalamus and thalamus; the **Sulcus hypothalamicus** between the thalamus and hypothalamus. The medial cores of the thalamus often bulge in the IIIrd ventricle, so that both touch in the **Adhesio interthalamica** in approximately 70% of people. On the roof plate the **Plexus choroideus** is formed for CSF formation and protrudes into the IIIrd ventricle. On the floor plate, the **Chiasma opticum** lies immediately next to the IIIrd ventricle (➤ Fig. 11.8b).

All neurovascular pathways running to or from the telencephalon have to pass through the diencephalon. Some of these pathways combine to form white matter for the **Capsula interna,** which pushes the subthalamus away laterally. These lateral parts of the di-

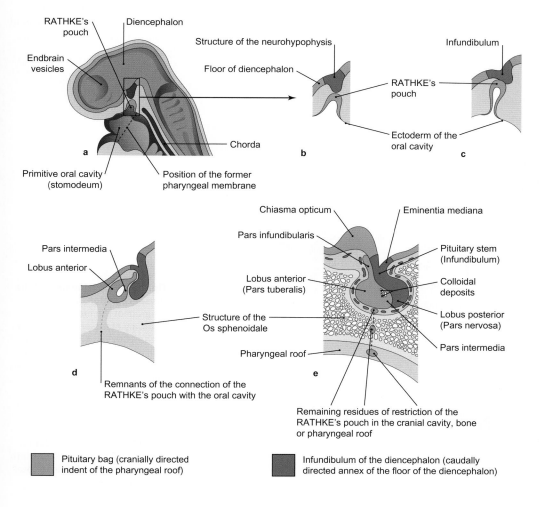

Fig. 11.9 **Development of the pituitary gland. a** Overview in the median section with back of the throat and floor of the diencephalon. **b–d** Folding of the epithelium in the top of the throat (RATHKE's pouch, later adenohypophysis) and fusion with the infundibulum (later neurohypophysis). **e** Position of the pituitary gland. [E347-09]

Pituitary bag (cranially directed indent of the pharyngeal roof)

Infundibulum of the diencephalon (caudally directed annex of the floor of the diencephalon)

encephalon are called **Globus pallidus (pallidum)**. The Globus pallidus thus lies in the telencephalon, but originates from the diencephalic base plates and is integrated into the efferent, precise motor functions or control mechanisms.

The **pituitary gland** is of ectodermal origin, whereby its tissue sections originate from 2 different ectodermal sources: the anterior pituitary develops from the ectoderm of the oral cavity (RATHKE's pouch) the neurohypophysis from the ectoderm of the diencephalon. The oral epithelium folds on approximately the *36th development day* into a duplication (the so-called **RATHKE's pouch**), which grows on the neurohypophysis system, the infundibulum, and finally merges with this to form the pituitary gland (➤ Fig. 11.9).

Development of the telencephalon

The **telencephalic vesicles** consists of a median section and 2 lateral attachments that will evolve into the later cerebral hemispheres. Because the roof plate grows more slowly in comparison to the hemispheres, it sinks into the depths of the Fissura longitudinalis superior and then lies in the area of the later **Corpus callosum**. Developing from the floor and alar plate or the intermediate zone of the neural tube, is the **Substantia grisea**, i.e. the telencephalic cortex, also known as the **pallium**. In the area of the base plate, the parenchyma thickens. Here, at the base of the lateral ventricles, the existing neurons form the **basal ganglia**. **Telencephalon impar** refers to the median-located endbrain section with the Lamina terminalis and the commissural pathways in the area of the former roof and floor plates. In addition, the floor plate of the telencephalon grows significantly more slowly than the walls of the hemispheres, which are divided into a ventral, lateral or dorsal pallium. The medial and dorsal pallium grow outwards and form the neo-(iso-)cortex. As soon as the hemispheres clash medially, further growth is inhibited, causing the flattened shape of the hemispheres in the Fissura longitudinalis cerebri (➤ Fig. 11.10).

The rapid growth of the respective hemispheres is C-shaped, whereby the pallium initially grows ventrally and rostrally and thus forms the **Lobus temporalis**. This growth movement is also known as **hemisphere rotation** whereby the rotation axis is located in the later island (insula) region. The island region is displaced due to the growth of the hemispheres of the surface anatomy in the depth of the fissure, or the Sulcus lateralis. At the telencephalon itself, differentiation can already be made between the **Lobus frontalis**, the **Lobus parietalis** and the **Lobus temporalis**. The **occipital lobes** can only be delineated after completion of the hemisphere rotation. In the described rotation, the deeper lying brain structures such as the ventricular system, the hippocampus, the fornix, the Gyrus cinguli, the Nucleus caudatus and the Corpus callosum are included, which explains their macroscopic C-shaped structure.

Gyrification

At first, the surface structures of the telencephalons are smooth. In later stages of development, the gyri and sulci are formed which significantly increase the surface area of the cortex. **Gyrification** starts around the *26th week,* whereby first the gyri and sulci are formed, which are almost identical in all people (e.g. Sulcus cinguli, Sulcus centralis and lateralis). At the end of the *8th development month* all important primary flutes are created. In the *9th month,* the secondary and tertiary gyri and sulci develop, very often exhibiting quite large inter-individual variations (➤ Fig. 11.11).

Cortex types

According to the phylogenetic development, different cortex types can be identified:

- The **neocortex** is phylogenetically the youngest part of the cerebral cortex. It is found only in mammals. In humans, the neocortex forms the majority of the surface of the cerebrum (around 90%). Opposite it are the phylogenetically older cortical regions, described as the **archicortex** or **'paleocortex'**.

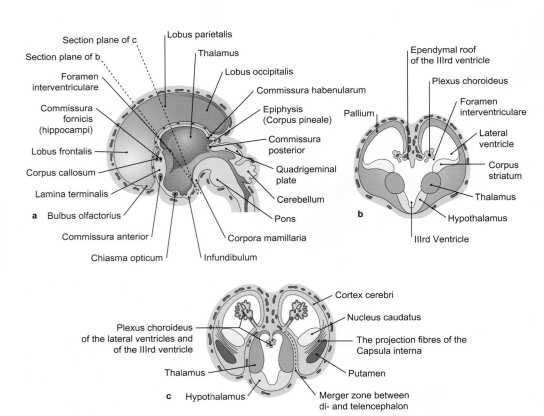

Fig. 11.10 Development of the prosencephalon. a Schematic diagram of the medial surface anatomy of the prosencephalon in the 10th week. **b** Cross-section of the mesencephalon at the height of the Foramina interventriculari that shows the Corpus striatum and the Plexus choroideus of the lateral ventricles. **c** Comparable section in the 11th week. Through the growth of the Capsula interna, the Corpus striatum divides into the putamen and Nucleus caudatus. [E347-09]

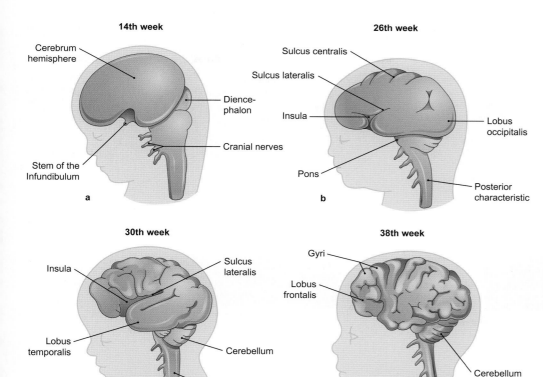

Fig. 11.11 Progression of the development of gyri and sulci (gyrification) in the schematic side view. As part of the growth processes, the island region falls and the Fissura lateralis narrows; the lobi of the cerebrum are increasingly delineated. [E347-09]
a 14th week, **b** 26th week. [E347-09]
c 30th week. **d** 38th week. [E347-09]

- In a division that takes into account the number of differentiable layers, the **isocortex** (classic 6-layer) is differentiated from the **allocortex** (3 layers) and from the **mesocortex** (transition zone).
- The **paleopallium** (Pallium = cortex plus white matter) describes the oldest cerebrum section, in particular the rhinencephalon (olfactory brain). From the **archipallium**, which exhibits a 3-layer archicortex, portions of the limbic system are formed, such as the hippocampus, Indusium griseum or the fornix.

Inner cerebrospinal fluid space

The inner cerebrospinal fluid space (➤ Chap. 11.4.3) originates from the lumen of the neural tube. Above the 4th somites, the lumen expands to the brain vesicles, so that **lateral ventricles** (I and II) in the area of the telencephalon can be differentiated, and which are connected via the Foramina interventricularia with the **IIIrd ventricle** of the diencephalon. The IIIrd ventricle, in turn, tapers towards the **Aqueductus mesencephali**. This passes through the mesencephalon and extends in turn into the area of the metelencephalon and the myelencephalon to the **IVth ventricle**, which is in contact with the outer subarachnoid spaces via median and lateral openings. The ventricles contain the Plexus choroidei responsible for CSF production, also following the rotational movement of the hemispheres. The often closed (obliterated) **Canalis centralis** remains in the section of the Medulla spinalis.

> **NOTE**
>
> The **inner subarachnoid spaces** of the CNS emerge from the lumen of the neural tube. Due to the different growth dynamics of the brain sections, the respective diameter of the subarachnoid spaces is very different. The structure of the Ist and IInd ventricles in the telencephalon is the result of the C-shaped direction of growth of the two cerebral hemispheres. In the spinal cord, the lumen becomes smaller towards the central canal, which is often completely closed.

Postnatal maturation

The brain is one of the few organs which is not yet fully matured after birth. It still has to 'mature' postpartum and later enters a process of further maturation and ageing. The maturation process includes the increasing myelination of axons and a dynamic change in the structure and number of synaptic connections. At 3 years of age, every brain cell has approximately 15,000 contact points (synapses) to other nerve cells, while only 2,500 existed at the time of birth. The maturation process manifests itself, among other things, in that up to the age of 18 years the links between nerve cells – depending on the type of neurons and brain region – are reduced to approximately 10,000 synapses/nerve cells.

11.1.3 Development of the spinal cord

In the embryonic and foetal development of the caudal portion of the neural tube, there is a noticeable thickening of the lateral alar and base plates. Later on, these take on different functions: from the base plate (or the **ventral horn**) the efferent fibres exit and form the **Radix anterior**. Afferent fibres converge towards the alar plate (the **sensory dorsal horn**) and form the subsequent **Radix posterior** (➤ Fig. 11.12). The base and the roof plates clearly lag behind in terms of growth and are eclipsed by other structures or shifted backwards into the depths. In this way, the **Fissura mediana anterior** or the Sulcus medianus posterior are differentiated. In the area of the base and roof plates, fibres cross from one side of the spinal cord to the opposite side. As a result of the depicted proliferation processes, the neural canal visibly narrows and from the *9th/10th development week* becomes a narrow central canal (**Canalis centralis**).

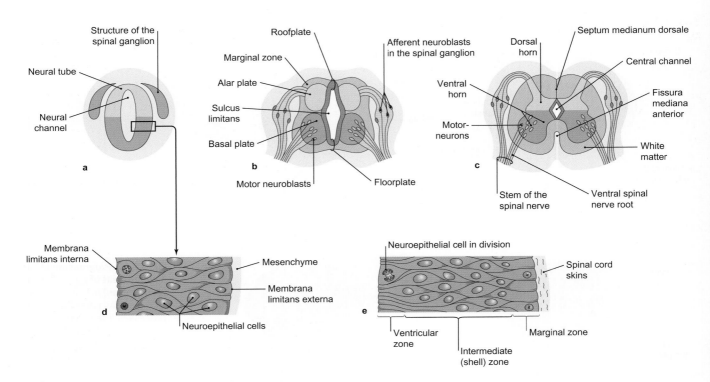

Fig. 11.12 Development of the spinal cord from the caudal portion of the neural tube. **a** 23 days. **b** 6 weeks. **c** 9 weeks. **d, e** The wall of the neural tube becomes thick (d) and can be divided into three zones (e). [E347-09]

Clinical remarks

Particularly impressive are the **(closure) defective malformations** in the area of the Neuroporus anterior or Neuroporus posterior in the lumbar region L5/S1, which can have different longitudinal expansion:

The **dysraphia** exhibit different grades or values and, in addition to the layers of neural tissue, can also affect the tissue layers lying over the top (lack of closure of the vertebral arches, of the vertebral arches and meninges with and without respective involvement of the nerve tissue). Typically, the Proc. spinosus of the vertebral arches is split, from which the clinical description of the disorder **spina bifida** is derived. A distinction is made between:

- **Spina bifida occulta:** 10% of the population, if applicable only proven radiographically or through abnormal hair growth (➤ Fig. 11.13a)
- **Spina bifida cystica:** 0.1%, the most frequent defect in neonates; involvement of the meninges (meningocele) or by meninges and nerve tissue (meningomyelocele, ➤ Fig. 11.13b); the cause is, among other things, folic acid deficiency during pregnancy
- **Spina bifida aperta:** uncovered defect of the myelon (myeloschisis)

Closure defects in the area of the Neuroporus anterior are the most common congenital malformations of the brain. Cranial **meningoencephalocele** and **anencephaly** are included in these. Here, too, the covering tissues, i.e. meninges and the calvaria, are affected:

- In the **Cranium bifidum** these closure defects are in the median plane. Depending on the tissue, one speaks of cranial meningocele, meningoencephalocele or meningohydroencephalocele (with sections of the ventricle in the hernia sac).
- In the case of a particularly early impaired closure of the Neuroporus anterior, the development of the skull bones and the prosencephalon system is disrupted. It leads to **exencephaly**, exposing the brain, which is changed pathologically and ultimately degenerates. The brainstem is, however, often functional, so **'meroanencephaly'** would be the more correct term. The frequency is 1:1,000 with a familial aggregation, so a genetic component is also to be taken into account.

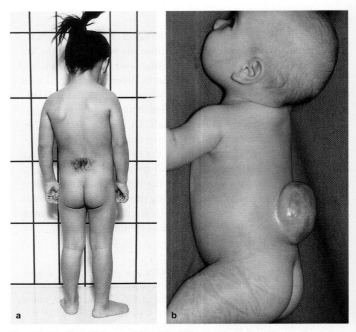

Fig. 11.13 Spinal dysraphia with different degrees of severity. a Spina bifida occulta with hairy skin area. **b** Meningomyelocele in the lumbar region. [E347-09]

11.1.4 Development of the peripheral nervous system

As already described, **neural crest cells** exit during the neurulation of the epithelial complex and finally come to rest on the side of the neural tube below the surface of the ectoderm (formation of neural crest cells). They exhibit a mesenchymal migration behaviour, similar to that of free connective tissue cells. The migration of neural crest cells is closely related to the disappearance of the N-CAM (cell adhesion molecules) formed by the neural tube and the cadherins, as well as to the appearance of membrane-like integrins. The neural crest cells give rise to various cell types that are located in particular in the peripheral nervous system (neurons and glia, formation of the different types of ganglia, adrenal medulla) or as melanocytes in the skin. A loose connective tissue structure, such as the face cartilage or the Pia mater, is also formed.

11.2 Structure of the nervous system

Anja Böckers

Skills

After working through this chapter, you should be able to:
- explain and demonstrate the macroscopic structure of the CNS in its sections on a model of the brain, pointing out the surface structures named here
- explain and demonstrate the core areas and fibre systems named here on a horizontal section of the internal structure of the telencephalon

---

11.2.1 Overview

The nervous system is basically divided into a **peripheral nervous system (PNS)** and a **central nervous system (CNS)**. While the central nervous system is well protected in the vertebral canal and in the bony cranial cavity (➤ Fig. 11.14a), the structures of the PNS exit the protective spine at the Foramina intervertebralia. In addition to this macroscopic border, this subdivision can also be understood microscopically, since the nerve cell fibres are surrounded by different insulating glial cells: in the CNS these are the oligodendrocytes; in the PNS the SCHWANN cells form the myelin sheath. In the same way, the meningeal envelope of the CNS, the Dura mater, transitions into the epineurium of the peripheral nerve in the above-mentioned border area.

In functional terms you can differentiate between an **autonomous** and a **somatic nervous system**, which serve subconscious or conscious control and sensory perception. Both systems either provide the CNS with information (afferents) or relay information from the CNS to the peripheral areas (efferents). This functional organisation of the nervous system (➤ Fig. 11.14b) is not identical in all sections to the morphological structure of the CNS.

Clinical remarks

The **clinical neurological examination** consists of a medical history and physical examination. The medical history will follow the usual procedure, but questions should also be asked in particular about existing neurological disorders, previous

---

traumatic brain trauma, neurological hereditary disorders in the family, risk factors and autonomic body functions. Special examination techniques relating to the functional systems and the cranial nerve functions complement the targeted, symptom-focused history and will be discussed separately in the relevant chapters. In general, for every patient, the overall function of the CNS should be evaluated through a preliminary assessment of consciousness, orientation to time, space and people, as well as with regard to their memory, concentration ability and basic mood. In the clinic, impairments of consciousness, for example, are divided into:
- **Somnolence:** abnormal sleepiness, easily awakened, delayed reaction to verbal communication, prompt response to pain stimuli
- **Stupor:** abnormally heavy sleepiness, difficult to awaken, delayed but targeted defence regarding pain stimuli
- **Coma:** Can no longer be awakened by external stimuli

In addition, the clinical neurological examination assesses the severity of impaired consciousness but also does so quantitatively, by means of the spontaneous behaviour of the patient, reaction to verbal prompts or pain stimuli points **(Glasgow Coma Scale)**. This quantification allows an estimation of the extent to which consciousness is impaired over the course.

Content-related impairment to consciousness can be disorientation, confusion or perception disorders, such as alcohol or drug-related delirium.

11.2.2 Structure of the CNS

Sections

The CNS can be divided into the **Medulla spinalis (spinal cord)** and **encephalon (brain)**. The brain is comprised of 5 sections as per embryological development (➤ Chap. 11.1.1):
- **Medulla oblongata or myelencephalon** ('extended marrow')
- **Pons** (bridge)
- **Mesencephalon** (midbrain)
- **Diencephalon** (interbrain)
- **Telencephalon or cerebrum** (endbrain)

The medulla, pons and mesencephalon together form the brainstem (**Truncus encephali**). The pons attaches dorsally to the **cerebellum**.

Other important designations derived from the development of brain vesicles, are the bringing together of the telencephalon and the diencephalon to form the **prosencephalon** (forebrain) as well as of the pons and the cerebellum to form the **metencephalon**. The metencephalon and myelencephalon in turn form the **rhombencephalon**.

Topographical relationships

The description of relational positions in the CNS (➤ Fig. 11.15) is differentiated from the torso or extremities:
- Structures of the Truncus encephali are described by their position relative to a vertical axis passing through the brainstem, the **MEYNERT's axis**.
- Structures of the telencephalon or diencephalon are described in relation to a longitudinal axis through the earlier forebrain **(FOREL's axis)**.

The Medulla spinalis extends cranially into the adjacent part of the brain, the Medulla oblongata. This passes through the Foramen magnum of the Os occipitale into the interior of the skull. Inside the skull, the front surface of the pons attaches to the clivus, while the cerebellum fits into the posterior fossa and is covered superiorly by the Tentorium cerebelli, a duplication of the Dura mater. The

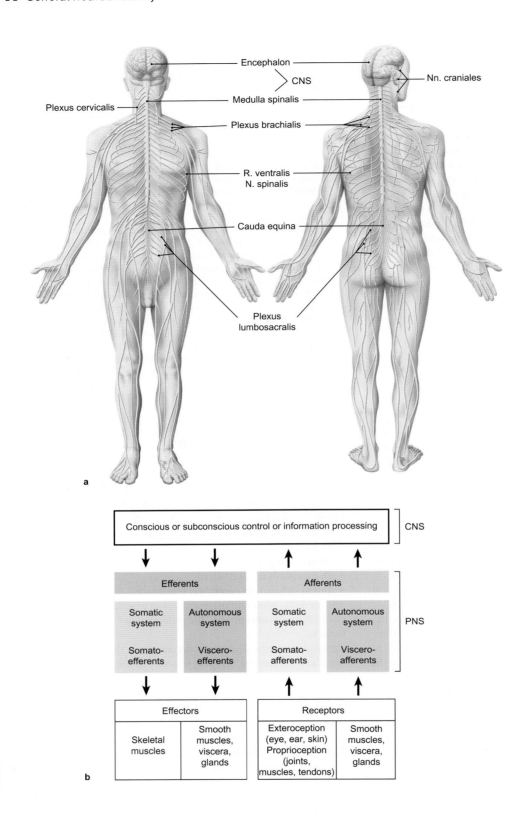

Fig. 11.14 Structure of the nervous system, Systema nervosum; **a** Morphological structure, ventral view and dorsal; **b** Functional organisation. b [L126]

position of the Tentorium cerebelli – and thus the border between the cerebrum and cerebellum – is marked on the outside of the skull by the Protuberantia occipitalis externa. Above this point is the occipital lobe of the telencephalon, while the temporal lobes attach to the middle cranial fossa and the frontal lobes attach to the anterior cranial fossa, and the convex surface of the telencephalons reaches the calotte.

11.2.3 Morphology of the CNS

A description of the outer shape of the CNS is given here. The Medulla spinalis and cerebellum are described in ➤ Chap. 12.6 or in ➤ Chap. 12.4 .

Surface morphology

The external appearance of the brain does not normally lead to conclusions about its general or even individual function. The

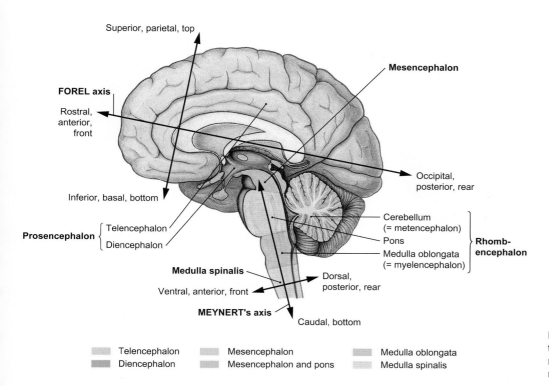

Superior, parietal, top

FOREL axis

Rostral, anterior, front

Mesencephalon

Inferior, basal, bottom

Occipital, posterior, rear

Prosencephalon { Telencephalon / Diencephalon

Cerebellum (= metencephalon)
Pons
Medulla oblongata (= myelencephalon)

Rhomb-encephalon

Medulla spinalis

Dorsal, posterior, rear

Ventral, anterior, front

MEYNERT's axis

Caudal, bottom

Telencephalon
Diencephalon
Mesencephalon
Mesencephalon and pons
Medulla oblongata
Medulla spinalis

Fig. 11.15 Alignment and positional terms of the CNS and spinal cord; structure of the central nervous system.

brain of an adult weighs an average of 1.4 kg with a gender-specific dimorphism that is comparable to differences in height and weight in men and women. The consistency of the brain in a fixed state is often described as 'tofu-like' and its surface colour as greyish. Unfixed, the brain exhibits a lighter, almost rosy colour and has a consistency which is most closely compared to that of unfixed liver tissue. The brain surface presents with regular grooves and shows inter-individual differences.

Telencephalon

The telencephalon is the largest section of the CNS and is the most highly developed part where conscious perception of information takes place. In principle, it is divided into 2 cerebral hemispheres (**Hemispheria cerebri**), which are connected above the **Corpus callosum** and enclose a cerebrospinal fluid-filled cavity system within them. The hemispheres are divided from each other by the **Fissura longitudinalis cerebri**. An outer convex surface, the **Facies superolateralis**, reaches cranially to the **Margo superior (hemispheral rim)** in the **Facies medialis** or caudally to the **Margo inferolateralis** to merge with the **Facies inferior**. These Facies inferior, in turn, border the Facies medialis **of the brain in the frontal section via the Margo inferomedialis**, eventually reaching the Corpus callosum. The ventrally or dorsally reaching endpoints of the convex are described as frontal poles (**Polus frontalis**), temporal poles (**Polus temporalis**) and occipital poles (**Polus occipitalis**) (➤ Fig. 11.16).
The mature brain is characterised by the ridges (**Gyri cerebri**) and grooves (**Sulci cerebri**) on its surface. In doing so, the primary grooves, which are common to all humans and which are already fully established in the 8th embryonic month, can be distinguished from the secondary and tertiary grooves, which exhibit individual variability. The sulci bordering the lobes include:

- the **Sulcus centralis** between the frontal lobe (**Lobus frontalis**) and parietal lobes (**Lobus parietalis**)
- the **Sulcus lateralis (syn.: Fissura lateralis)** between the Lobus frontalis and the temporal lobes (**Lobus temporalis**)

- the **Sulcus parieto-occipitalis**, which according to its name is between the Lobus parietalis and the **Lobus occipitalis**, although it is only clearly definable on the medial hemisphere side (➤ Fig. 11.16d)

The previously mentioned 4 lobes are clearly visible on the Facies superolateralis. In total, the cerebrum has 6 lobes:

- The insular lobes (**Lobus insularis**) lie in the depths of the Sulcus lateralis in the **Fossa lateralis cerebri** and, because it is overgrown during the development of the Lobi frontalis, parietalis and temporalis, it is only visible when you push these to the side (➤ Fig. 11.17).
- The **Lobus limbicus** only becomes visible through a midline section through the Corpus callosum on the Facies medialis of the cerebrum. It includes the **Gyrus cinguli** on the Facies medialis as well as its continuation on the Facies inferior, the **Gyrus parahippocampalis**, through which the **Sulcus collateralis** is separated from the Lobus temporalis (➤ Fig. 11.16c).

> **NOTE**
> The telencephalon is divided into 6 lobes: the Lobus frontalis, Lobus parietalis, Lobus occipitalis, Lobus temporalis, Lobus insularis and the Lobus limbicus.

Lobus frontalis

In the Lobus frontalis, one can distinguish 3 main ridges on the Facies superolateralis: **Gyri frontales superior, medius and inferior** (➤ Fig. 11.18). At its point of contact with the lateral sulcus, the inferior gyrus can be divided from anterior to posterior into the **Partes orbitalis, triangularis and opercularis**. The motor language centre (**BROCA's centre**) is located in the two posterior parts. Just in front of the Sulcus centralis, the only sulcus which cuts into the Margo superior, is the **Gyrus precentralis**, in which the primary motor function centre is located. The Facies inferior of the Lobus frontalis is characterised by irregular Gyri and Sulci orbitales. As a rule, the **Gyrus rectus** is parallel to the Margo infero-

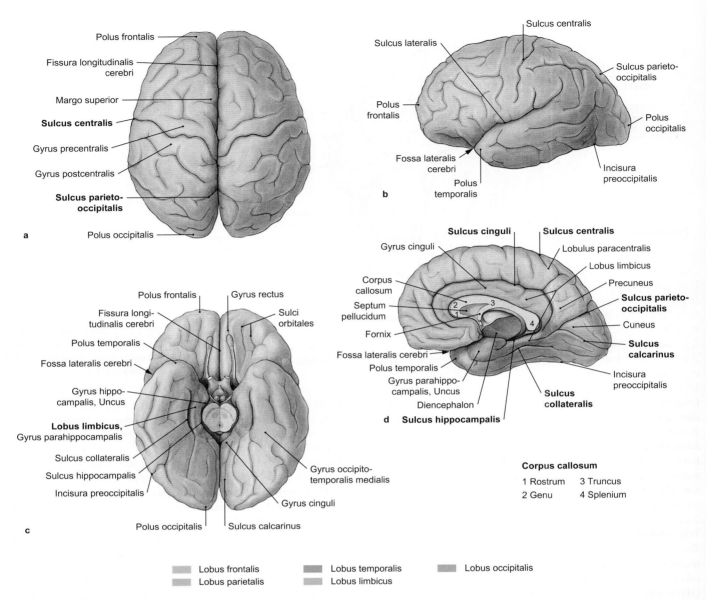

Corpus callosum

1 Rostrum	3 Truncus
2 Genu	4 Splenium

Lobus frontalis Lobus temporalis Lobus occipitalis
Lobus parietalis Lobus limbicus

Fig. 11.16 Lobes of the cerebrum, Lobi cerebri. a View from above. **b** Lateral view with substructure of the cerebrum hemisphere in the Lobus frontalis, Lobus parietalis, Lobus temporalis and Lobus occipitalis. **c** View from below. **d** Medial view.

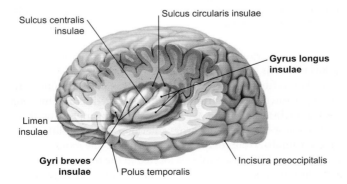

Fig. 11.17 Ridges (gyri) and grooves (sulci) of the cerebral hemispheres. Lateral view of the left-hand Lobus insularis after removal of the opercula of the forehead, parietal and temporal lobes that cover the island region. The Lobus insularis is used for the processing of olfactory, gustatory and visceral information.

medialis. It runs through the **Sulcus olfactorius**, in the Bulbus and Pedunculus olfactorius, bounded laterally (➤ Fig. 11.16c).

Lobus parietalis

In the Lobus parietalis on the Facies superolateralis close to the **Gyrus postcentralis**, in which the primary somatosensory functional centre is located, 2 lobes can be distinguished: **Lobulus parietalis superior and inferior**. At the borderline to the Lobus temporalis, 2 smaller gyri can be described: the **Gyrus supramarginalis**, which lies dome-shaped over the end of the Sulcus lateralis, and the **Gyrus angularis** at the end of the Sulcus temporalis superior. A third lobulus, the **Lobulus paracentralis**, runs in an arch on the Facies medialis around the Sulcus centralis and, because it can be assigned to both the Lobus parietalis and the Lobus frontalis correspondingly, it is divided further into a Pars frontalis and a Pars parietalis. The nearly rectangular cortical area between the Lobulus paracentralis and Sulcus parieto-occipitalis is ultimately called the **precuneus** (➤ Fig. 11.16, ➤ Fig. 11.18).

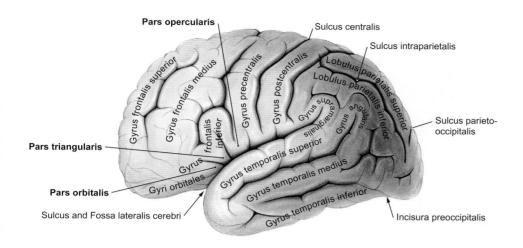

Fig. 11.18 Ridges (gyri) and grooves (sulci) of the cerebral hemispheres. Lateral view of the cerebrum from the left. The Gyrus frontalis inferior is divided into the Pars orbitalis, Pars triangularis and Pars opercularis.

Lobus temporalis

In the Lobus temporalis one can distinguish 3 principal ridges on the Facies superolateralis and frontal lobes: **Gyri temporales superior, medius and inferior**. The Gyrus inferior forms the Margo inferolateralis and continues smoothly to the Facies inferior. Of particular note are the characteristics of the Gyrus temporalis superior: in the Sulcus lateralis are the **Gyri temporales transversi (HESCHL's gyri** or **convolutions)**, which comprise the primary acoustic function centre. In the posterior lateral portion of the Gyrus temporalis superior, in the dominant hemisphere (right side of the left hemisphere), the sensory language centre is located (**WERNICKE's area**). The inferior view of the Lobus temporalis is relatively unspecific in that the Gyri occipitotemporales lateralis and medialis continue from the Gyrus temporalis inferior, separated by the Sulcus occipitotemporales. (➤ Fig. 11.16c, ➤ Fig. 11.18).

Lobus occipitalis

In the Lobus occipitalis the Facies superolateralis exhibits no specific features, so that **Gyri occipitales** are spoken of in only general terms. On the Facies medialis, on the other hand, an area can be seen extending from the Sulcus parieto-occipitalis to the Sulcus calcarinus, which due to its triangular form is known as the **cuneus** ('wedge'). The **Sulcus calcarinus** extends from the Polus occipitalis to the Sulcus parieto-occipitalis in the depths of the lobes. The primary optical functional centre is located in the immediately adjacent cortical areas of the Sulcus calcarinus. The **Gyrus lingualis** joins directly below the Sulcus calcarinus. If the gyri are further traced to the basal side, the Facies inferior of the Lobus occipitalis are thrown up by the Gyri occipitotemporales medialis and lateralis, which exhibit no sharp border with the Lobus temporalis (➤ Fig. 11.16, ➤ Fig. 11.18).

Lobus insularis

The Lobus insularis is characterised by 5–9 fan-shaped ridges, which can be divided into the anterior-lying **Gyri breves** and the rather more posteriorly located **Gyri longi**, each ending at the **Sulcus circularis insulae** (➤ Fig. 11.17).

Lobus limbicus

The Lobus limbicus with its main section, the **Gyrus cinguli**, arches across the Facies medialis via the Corpus callosum and is bordered above by the **Sulcus cinguli** and below by the **Sulcus corporis callosi**. Further on, the Gyrus cinguli narrows and joins with the Gyrus lingualis as the **Gyrus parahippocampalis** and continues to the Facies inferior. At the rostral end, the Gyrus parahippo-

campalis bends slightly medially, so that a small hook, the **Uncus gyri hippocampalis**, forms (➤ Fig. 11.16c).

Diencephalon

> NOTE
>
> The diencephalon extends from the roof of the third ventricle to the exit of the Aqueductus mesencephali (SYLVII). It is divided into a simplified order from cranial to caudal in 4 sections:
> • Epithalamus
> • Thalamus with metathalamus (metathalamus = Corpus geniculatum laterale and mediale)
> • Hypothalamus with hypophysis
> • Subthalamus

The diencephalon is both a hub between the brainstem and cerebral hemispheres and an important point of coordination between the neuronal and endocrine systems. It is hardly visible from the outside, as it is almost completely covered by the extensive growth of the hemispheres during embryonic development of the telencephalon. Visible only in the basal view are small sections (➤ Fig. 11.19): these include the N. opticus [II], of which the intersection of fibres in the **Chiasma opticum** and the **Tractus opticus** evert together with the eye structure from the diencephalon during development. Viewed laterally, the optic tract marks the transition from the diencephalon to the mesencephalon. The tractus becomes thicker along its further posterior pathway to the lateral geniculate body (**Corpus geniculatum laterale**), which together with the medial geniculate body (**Corpus geniculatum mediale**) is to be attributed to the diencephalic thalamus. Both can be seen by pushing the temporal lobes slightly off the brainstem laterally. In front of the Tractus opticus, the **Substantia perforata anterior** can be found on both sides, riddled with a large number of smaller vessels that penetrate here into the depth of the brain. The Tuberculum olfactorium lies underneath it, representing part of the olfactory sensory processing function. Directly behind the Chiasma opticum, in the angle formed by the diverging Tractus optici, the **infundibulum** or the infundibular stalk can be situated in an anterior to posterior arrangement. The hypophysis, the **Tuber cinereum** and the **Corpora mamillaria** are differentiated.

If the Lobus occipitalis and the cerebellum are forced apart, the **pineal gland (Glandula pinealis)** can be recognised occipitally in the depth of the subarachnoid space as part of the diencephalic epithalamus.

The **level structure** of the diencephalon is only visible after a cut in the median plane through the Corpus callosum. With this incision,

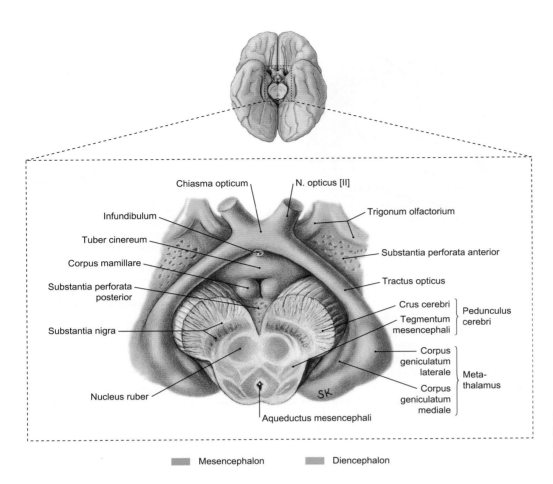

Chiasma opticum
N. opticus [II]
Infundibulum
Trigonum olfactorium
Tuber cinereum
Corpus mamillare
Substantia perforata anterior
Substantia perforata posterior
Tractus opticus
Substantia nigra
Crus cerebri
Tegmentum mesencephali
Pedunculus cerebri
Corpus geniculatum laterale
Meta-thalamus
Nucleus ruber
Corpus geniculatum mediale
Aqueductus mesencephali
SK

Mesencephalon Diencephalon

Fig. 11.19 Diencephalon from below. The brainstem has been separated at the level of the mesencephalon (dotted incision in ➤ Fig. 11.20).

the IIIrd ventricle is opened so that its roof and the outlet of the aqueduct are clearly visible. The lateral wall of the IIIrd ventricle is formed by the diencephalon (➤ Fig. 11.20). The term 'subthalamus' includes several accumulations of nerve cell bodies that originally came from the ventral portion of the thalamus, but which have been forced out of the way in further development of the IIIrd ventricle. The **subthalamus** is therefore not delineated on a median section of the cerebrum.

Truncus encephali

The function of the brainstem comes on the one hand from the cranial nerve cores located in it and on the other hand, functionally, through controlling motor, visual or acoustic reflex activity and the localisation of important life-sustaining centres, such as the respiratory centre. The Truncus encephali is a stalk-shaped structure, with the telencephalon spreading over it like the top of a tree. Dorsally, this 'tree top' has another small 'tree top' in the form of the cerebellum. The surface morphology of the brainstem needs to be studied on the dissection, ventrally and laterally but on the dorsal side the brainstem is largely covered by the cerebellum so that it can only be seen dorsally if the cerebellum is detached from its connecting branches, the **small cerebellar peduncles (Pedunculi cerebellares)** (➤ Fig. 11.21).

NOTE

The Truncus encephali has rostral contact with the diencephalon and extends caudally to the Decussatio pyramidum before continuing into the spinal cord. It is composed in a craniocaudal arrangement of:
• Mesencephalon
• Pons
• Medulla oblongata
Characteristic of the three sections are the exit points of the 12 cranial nerves (see also ➤ Chap. 12.5).

The cerebrum is also connected with the brainstem via strong connecting branches (**Pedunculi cerebri or Crura cerebri**), that run on the ventral side of the mesencephalon (➤ Fig. 11.21c). Between these lies the **Fossa interpeduncularis**. The openings of numerous smaller vessels here give this pit a sieve-like form and its name, **Substantia perforata posterior**. On the dorsal side, the mesencephalon extends caudally from the rostrally located pineal gland (Glandula pinealis) to the upper small cerebellar peduncle (Pedunculi cerebellaris superior). What is striking here is the typical surface relief, characterised by the **quadrigeminal plate (Lamina tecti or quadrigemina)**. In doing so, 2 upper and 2 lower hills (**Colliculi superiores and inferiores**) can be differentiated, each one connected via a **brachium** of the same name with the Corpora geniculata laterale and mediale of the diencephalon (➤ Fig. 11.21a). The triangular area between the lower 'hills' and the Pedunculi cerebellares superiores are also known as **Trigonum lemnisci lateralis**. The swelling at the pons or its transverse running fibres clearly marks the boundary between the mesencephalon and pons. The pons in the **Sulcus bulbopontinus** is just as clearly delineated caudally to the Medulla oblongata. The pons is connected via the middle cerebellar peduncles (Pedunculi cerebellares medii) with the cerebellum. The removal of the cerebellum to expose the dorsal brainstem implicitly implies the removal of the roof of the tent-shaped IVth ventricle. This procedure also means that the floor of the cavity which is filled with cerebrospinal fluid, the **rhomboid fossa (Fossa rhomboidea)**, is visible. The pathway of the **Striae medullares** marks the transverse border area of the pons from caudal to the Medulla oblongata. Finally, the edges of the ventricle roof (Velum medullare inferius) taper down to a point lying in the Sulcus medianus, the **obex**, limiting the rhomboid fossa caudally. The Sulcus medianus continues into the spinal cord and is accompanied by

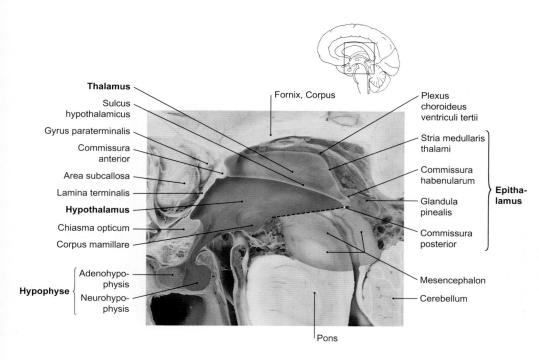

Thalamus
Sulcus hypothalamicus
Gyrus paraterminalis
Commissura anterior
Area subcallosa
Lamina terminalis
Hypothalamus
Chiasma opticum
Corpus mamillare
Hypophyse { Adenohypophysis / Neurohypophysis }

Fornix, Corpus

Plexus choroideus ventriculi tertii
Stria medullaris thalami
Commissura habenularum
Glandula pinealis
Commissura posterior
Mesencephalon
Cerebellum
Pons

Epithalamus

Fig. 11.20 Median section through the IIIrd ventricle (Ventriculus tertius) and level structure of the interbrain (diencephalon) in the epithalamus, thalamus, hypothalamus and subthalamus. Portions of the diencephalon are brown, while those of the mesencephalon are green.

furrows running parallel to it, the Sulcus intermedius posterior and Sulcus posterolateralis. At the level of the obex, there are inconspicuous elevations in the posterior strands, which are described as **Tubercula gracile and cuneatum** (➤ Fig. 11.21a). Ventrally you can see the onion-like bulge of the Medulla oblongata, the **bulbus**, which is also characterised by longitudinal grooves, the Fissura mediana anterior and the Sulcus anterolateralis. Next to the Fissura mediana anterior, the **pyramis** and further laterally, the **olive**, bulges. In the Sulcus anterolateralis, before the olive, and in the Sulcus retro-olivaris, behind the olive, several cranial nerves leave the brainstem. In the **Decussatio pyramidum** there are transverse running pyramidal fibres that ultimately limit the Medulla oblongata caudally.

11.2.4 Distribution of grey matter in the CNS

Telencephalon
A frontal section through the telencephalon makes it clear that along the gyri and sulci of the telencephalon there is an approx. 0.5 cm broad layer of grey matter (Substantia grisea), which is the **Cortex cerebri**. Neuronal perikarya and glial cells are typically arranged in 6 layers so that one speaks of the **isocortex**, in contrast to the **allocortex**, which only consists of 3–4 layers, and in terms of developmental history consists of an older section, the paleocortex (e.g. olfactory outer layer) and archicortex (e.g. hippocampus). The Substantia grisea accumulates in the white matter of the telencephalon, the Substantia alba. In addition to the Cortex cerebri, grey matter is also incorporated in the depths of the white matter of the cerebrum.

The **core areas** of the Nucleus caudatus, the claustrum, the putamen, the Globus pallidus, the amygdala, and the thalamus, which is already attributed to the diencephalon, can here be clearly distinguished macroscopically (➤ Fig. 11.22a).

Truncus encephali
In cross-sections through the Truncus encephali, no superficial cortex layer can be detected. Embedded in the white matter are small accumulations of grey matter in the form of cranial nerve nuclei on the one hand, but also, as macroscopically conspicuous and well-demarcated structures on the other:
- in the Mesencephalon, the Substantia nigra and the Nucleus ruber (➤ Fig. 11.22b)
- in the Pons, the Nuclei pontis (➤ Fig. 11.22c)
- in the Medulla oblongata, the Nucleus olivaris inferior (➤ Fig. 11.22d)

In the Truncus encephali, white and grey matter are more or less arranged in a clearly defined order in 3 longitudinal zones. Starting ventrally, in the first layer are accumulated fibres (e.g. the Crura cerebri), in a middle layer, the cranial nerve cores, and in the dorsal section, the parent reflex centres (tectum, cerebellum). In the mesencephalon, these three layers are also referred to by the terms basis, tegmentum and tectum.

Spinal cord
The mix of grey and white matter is reversed in the spinal cord so that the Medulla spinalis, in contrast to the cerebrum, is characterised by a centrally located Substantia grisea which is surrounded by white matter. In the cross-section, this grey matter of the spinal cord is in a butterfly shape (➤ Fig. 11.22e).

11.2.5 Distribution of white matter in the CNS

While the grey matter includes the nerve cell bodies, the white substance (Substantia alba) is composed of nerve cell fibres, i.e. myelinated or non-myelinated axons of neurons. The axons connect nerve cells of the central nervous system over different distances. Fibres between cortex areas of the same telencephalic hemisphere are **association fibers (Fibrae associationes)**. Adjacent gyri connect these cortex area fibres, thus known as **Fibrae arcuatae cerebri**. So-called fascicles finally connect different lobi of the telencephalon with each other. However, these pathways cannot be delineated on simple horizontal or frontal sections through the cerebrum. Only special preparation techniques, such as the fibrillation of a fixed brain, set these fibres free (➤ Fig. 11.23a).

599

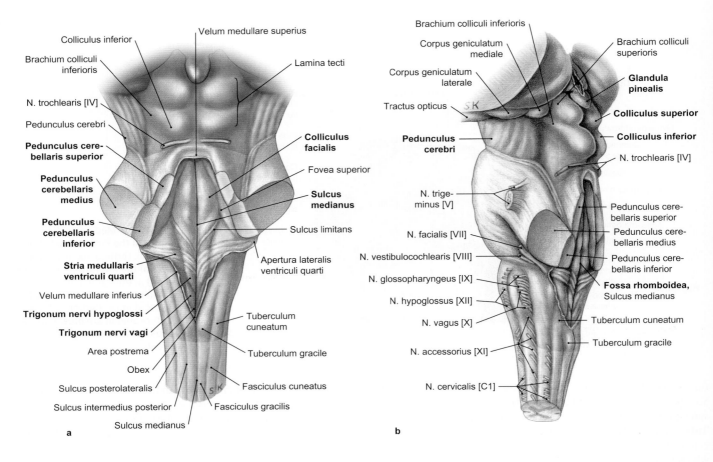

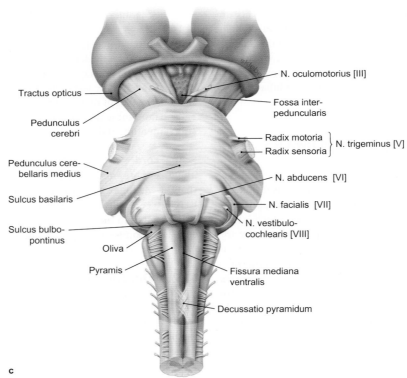

Fig. 11.21 Truncus encephali. a Dorsal view. **b** Lateral view. **c** Ventral view. [L238]

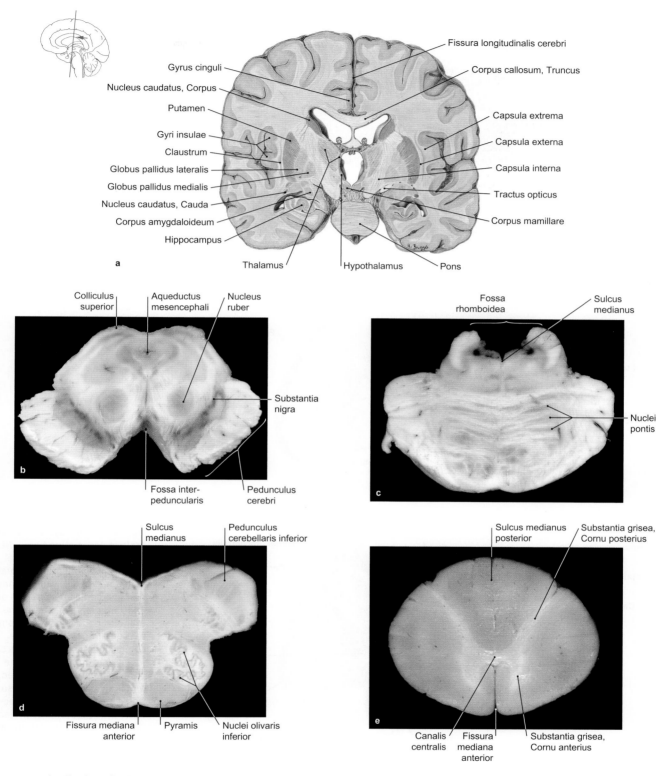

Fig. 11.22 Distribution of Substantiae grisea and alba in the CNS. a In the telencephalon, displayed as a frontal section at the level of the Corpora mamillaria. **b** In the mesencephalon. **c** In the pons. **d** In the Medulla oblongata. **e** In the Medulla spinalis. b–e [R247]

Commissural fibers (Fibrae commissurales) are fibre systems that connect the two hemispheres. Fibres between corresponding brain areas will be referred to as homotopic, whereas those between non-corresponding areas are heterotopic fibres. Commissural pathways can frequently be macroscopically clearly identified on median cuts. These include the strongly formed **Corpus callosum**

and smaller bundles of commissural fibres such as the Commissura anterior, the Commissura posterior or the Commissura fornicis (➤ Fig. 11.23b).

Furthermore, fibre systems are also contained in the white matter connecting brain sections of different altitudes; that is, from the cortex into caudal sections or in the opposite direction from caudal

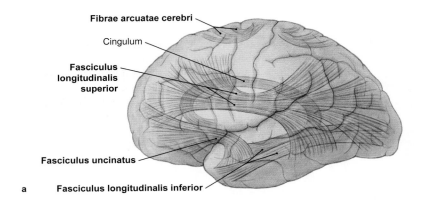

Fibrae arcuatae cerebri
Cingulum
Fasciculus longitudinalis superior
Fasciculus uncinatus
a
Fasciculus longitudinalis inferior

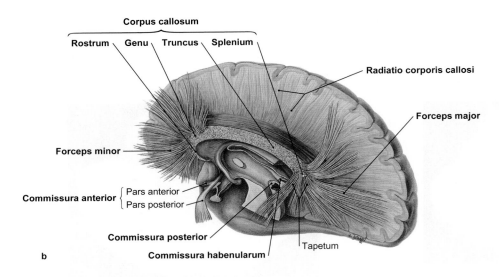

Corpus callosum
Rostrum Genu Truncus Splenium
Radiatio corporis callosi
Forceps major
Forceps minor
Commissura anterior { Pars anterior / Pars posterior
Commissura posterior
Commissura habenularum
Tapetum
b

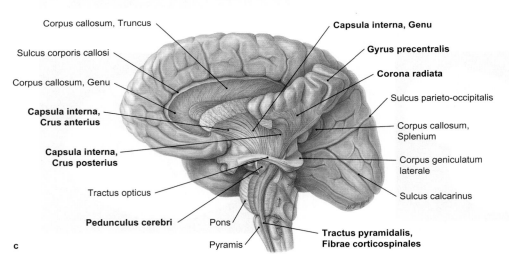

Corpus callosum, Truncus
Sulcus corporis callosi
Corpus callosum, Genu
Capsula interna, Crus anterius
Capsula interna, Crus posterius
Tractus opticus
Pedunculus cerebri
Pyramis
Pons
c

Capsula interna, Genu
Gyrus precentralis
Corona radiata
Sulcus parieto-occipitalis
Corpus callosum, Splenium
Corpus geniculatum laterale
Sulcus calcarinus
Tractus pyramidalis, Fibrae corticospinales

Fig. 11.23 Fibre systems of the brain. a Association fibres (Neurofibrae associationes) and short association fibres (Fibrae arcuatae cerebri), which connect U-shaped adjacent gyri with one another; diagram, view of the brain from the left side. **b** Commissural fibres (Neurofibrae commissurales). The Corpus callosum was, in addition to the median plane, largely divided, and individual Corpus callosum fibres are presented. **c** Projection fibres (Neurofibrae projectiones). The Capsula interna and pyramidal tract have been exposed.

sections, e.g. from the spinal cord to the cortex, in ascending order. Such fibre systems are called **projection fibres**. Macroscopically speaking, the most definable bundling of such projection fibres is the **Capsula interna** in the telencephalon or the Crura cerebri of the mesencephalon (➤ Fig. 11.23c).

NOTE
The most important fibre systems of the CNS are summarised in ➤ Table 11.1.

Clinical remarks

The **absence (agenesis) of the Corpus callosum** is one of the most commonly observed malformations in humans (3–7 cases/1,000 births). Various reasons lead to non-systemic or incomplete formation of the Corpus callosum between the 5th and 16th week of pregnancy, so that the connections between the left and right cerebral hemispheres may be absent or severely underdeveloped. The changes in the brain do not necessarily lead to a change in behaviour. The symptoms depend to a certain extent on the underlying cause of the dysfunction. Frequently exhibited, in addition to neuropsychiatric deficits, are difficulties in solving multimodal tasks such as problem-solving, the understanding of language and grammar, or the description of emotions with words (alexithymia).

Only rarely is a **callosotomy,** the neurosurgical transection of the Corpus callosum, performed today for the treatment of refractory epilepsy. Patients with a separated Corpus callosum, **split-brain patients,** are conspicuous in that information processed in the right hemisphere is not made available to the linguistic centre located in the left (dominant) hemisphere, and subsequently, although the information is for example seen and described, it cannot be named.

Table 11.1 Fibre systems of the Substantia alba.

Fibre system	Connection
Association fibres	
Fasciculus longitudinalis superior	Lobus frontalis with Lobus parietalis and Lobus occipitalis
Fasciculus longitudinalis inferior	Lobus occipitalis with Lobus temporalis
Fasciculus arcuatus	Lobus frontalis with Lobus temporalis (BROCA centre with WERNICKE'S area)
Fasciculus uncinatus	Lobus frontalis with basal Lobus temporalis
Cingulum	Lower sections of the Lobus frontalis with lower sections of the Lobus parietalis and the Lobus parahippocampalis
Commissural fibres	
Corpus callosum	Frontal, parietal and occipital lobes in both hemispheres
Commissura anterior	Tractus olfactorii; front parts of the Lobi temporales (amygdala; Gyrus parahippocampalis) of both hemispheres
Commissura posterior	Nuclei commissurae posteriores of both hemispheres
Commissura fornicis	Hippocampus of both hemispheres
Projection fibres	
Tractus corticospinalis	Cortex (especially Gyrus precentralis) with spinal cord
Tractus corticopontini	Cortex with core areas of the pons
Tractus corticonuclearis	Cortex with core areas of the cranial nerves in the mesencephalon, pons and Medulla oblongata
Fornix	Hippocampus and parts of the limbic system and the diencephalon
Fasciculi thalamocorticales	Thalamus with cortex

11.3 Meninges
Michael J. Schmeißer

11.3.1 Overview

The brain and spinal cord are surrounded by a fibrous envelope system, the **meninges** (brain and spinal membrane), ➤ Fig. 11.24). Here, a distinction is made between hard (**Pachymeninx**) and soft membrane tissue (**Leptomeninx**). The pachymeninx forms the outer membrane and essentially consists of the stiff **Dura mater.** The Leptomeninx is located underneath and consists of the **Arachnoidea mater,** which lies against the dura from the inside, and the **Pia mater,** lying directly on the nervous tissue. There is a physiological gap between the Arachnoidea and the Pia mater, the **subarachnoid space** (Spatium subarachnoideum). It is the outer subarachnoid space and completely surrounds the brain and spinal cord (also ➤ Chap. 11.4.4).

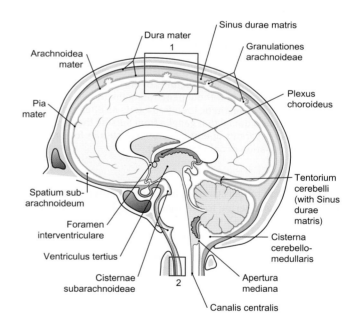

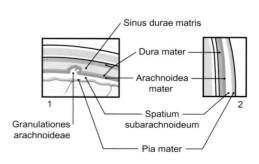

Fig. 11.24 Positions of the meninges within the bony skull as sagittal section. [L126]

11.3.2 Embryology

The membrane of the brain and spinal cord develop from the **Meninx primitiva**. This is mesenchymal connective tissue that originates from the neural crest and the paraxial mesoderm and surrounds the neural tube. With the formation of the dura subchondral plate, the Meninx primitiva is separated into the pachymeninx and leptomeninx.

11.3.3 Pachymeninx – Dura mater

The Dura mater mainly consists of dense, collagenous, fibrous connective tissue and is therefore a kind of 'organ capsule' for the central nervous system. The Dura mater of the brain (**Dura mater cranialis**) fuses directly with the periosteum of the bony skull so that, intracranially, you cannot differentiate a physiological gap between the dura and bony skull. The Dura mater of the spinal cord (**Dura mater spinalis**), on the other hand, forms a tubular sac, which surrounds the spinal cord, and except for its bony attachment points on the Foramen magnum and Os sacrum, is not fused with the bony vertebral canal. Therefore spinally, the majority is present as **epidural space** (Spatium epidurale; syn.: peridural cavity or Spatium peridurale) which surrounds the dural sac and is filled with adipose tissue and a dense venous plexus (Plexus venosus vertebralis internus) (➤ Fig. 11.25).

Clinical remarks

Injecting a local anaesthetic in the epidural or peridural space surrounding the spinal dural sac, is described as **peridural anaesthesia** (PDA for short) (➤ Fig. 11.34). The needle is introduced in the median sagittal alignment between 2 Procc. spinosi through the ligament structures of the vertebral column in the epidural space, without penetrating the Dura mater spinalis. The local anaesthetic therefore exerts its effects on the spinal roots and dorsal root ganglia from outside the dura. The PDA is used in various operations and in obstetrics for perioperative elimination of pain (analgesia).

The Dura mater cranialis consists of 2 superimposed layers: the **Lamina externa** adhering to the bone and the **Lamina interna**,

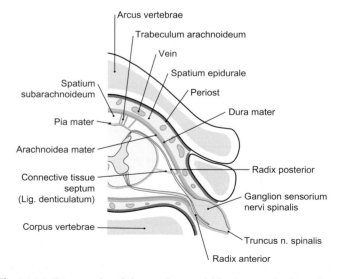

Fig. 11.25 Topography of the meninges within the vertebral canal; at the level of the IVth cervical vertebra in cross-section. [L126]

Labels:
Arcus vertebrae
Trabeculum arachnoideum
Vein
Spatium epidurale
Spatium subarachnoideum
Periost
Dura mater
Pia mater
Arachnoidea mater
Radix posterior
Connective tissue septum (Lig. denticulatum)
Ganglion sensorium nervi spinalis
Corpus vertebrae
Truncus n. spinalis
Radix anterior

which faces the brain. In some places within the bony skull, these two layers split from each other. This thereby creates oblong cavities (**Sinus durae matris**), which are lined with endothelium and in which the venous blood from the brain and meninges is collected and is directed towards the V. jugularis interna (➤ Chap. 11.3.5, ➤ Chap. 11.5.8). In addition, the Lamina interna forms plate-like **duplicatures**, which form the structure of the interior of the skull, separate certain portions of the brain from each other and equally stabilise the position of the brain in the event of mechanical damage to the skull. These include the following structures (➤ Fig. 11.26, ➤ Fig. 11.24, ➤ Fig. 11.27):

- **Falx cerebri** (cerebral falx): This relatively large dural septum is aligned medially sagittally in the Fissura longitudinalis cerebri and separates the two cerebral hemispheres above the Corpus callosum. Its upper margin contains the Sinus sagittalis superior, which fixes it cranially to the calvaria. The falx is positioned rostrocaudally at the Crista galli and the Crista frontalis, occipitally attached to the Protuberantia occipitalis interna. The Sinus sagittalis inferior is situated in its lower free margin, afterwards moving occipitally into the Sinus rectus, which in turn is enclosed by the root of the falx. From here, the Falx cerebri exits on both sides via the Tentorium cerebelli.
- **Tentorium cerebelli** (cerebellar tentorium): This tent-shaped dural septum extends in a horizontal orientation within the Fossa cranii posterior, between the bottom of the Lobi occipitales of the cerebrum and the Facies superior of the cerebellum. Its root is fixed occipitally, together with the Falx cerebri, at the Protuberantia occipitalis interna at the level of the Confluens sinuum; lateral to the margins of the Sinus transversus along the Os occipitale and further forward laterally on the margin of the Sinus petrosus superior at the upper edge of the petrous pyramid. In the medial direction, the root of the Tentorium cerebelli runs up to the Dorsum sellae and is attached to the Procc. clinoidei posteriores and anteriores. Between both sides of the tentorium a slit-shaped gap (tentorium slot, **Incisura tentorii**) remains for the passage of the brainstem (at the level of the mesencephalon), vessels and cranial nerves.
- **Falx cerebelli** (cerebelli falx): The Falx cerebelli is a short, crescent-shaped dural septum, that is attached occipitally to the Crista occipitalis interna and protrudes dorsocaudally into the Incisura cerebelli posterior in a median sagittal alignment.
- **Diaphragma sellae:** This horizontally oriented dural septum is attached to the Procc. clinoidei anteriores and posteriores and spans the Fossa hypophysialis in the Fossa cranii media. It contains a hole in its centre for the passage of the infundibular stalk.

Clinical remarks

With increased intracranial pressure, which can be the result of a cerebral haemorrhage or a brain tumour, sections of the Lobi temporales can be pressed into the Incisura tentorii (**tentorial notch**). This allows the Nn. oculomotorii or the entire mesencephalon to be trapped. It thereby creates a **mid-brain syndrome,** which manifests itself with increasing disorientation, fixed pupils in response to light, and increased and pathological reflexes of the extremities.

11.3.4 Leptomeninx

Arachnoidea mater

The Arachnoidea mater lies flat in the skull and in the vertebral canal of the inner layer of the Dura mater, the so-called neurotheli-

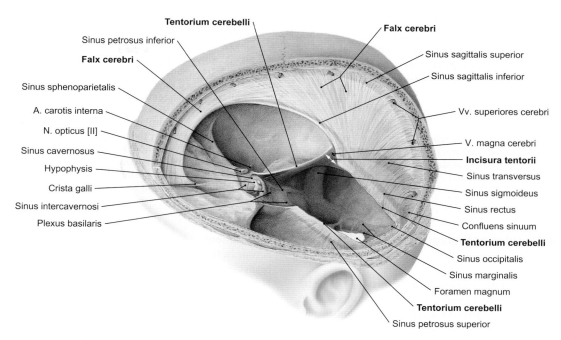

Tentorium cerebelli
Sinus petrosus inferior
Falx cerebri
Sinus sphenoparietalis
A. carotis interna
N. opticus [II]
Sinus cavernosus
Hypophysis
Crista galli
Sinus intercavernosi
Plexus basilaris

Falx cerebri
Sinus sagittalis superior
Sinus sagittalis inferior
Vv. superiores cerebri
V. magna cerebri
Incisura tentorii
Sinus transversus
Sinus sigmoideus
Sinus rectus
Confluens sinuum
Tentorium cerebelli
Sinus occipitalis
Sinus marginalis
Foramen magnum
Tentorium cerebelli
Sinus petrosus superior

Fig. 11.26 Dura mater cranialis and duplicatures. Lateral view.

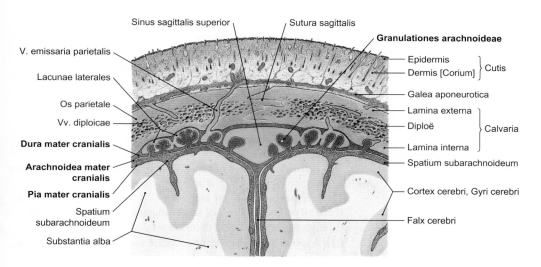

Sinus sagittalis superior
Sutura sagittalis
Granulationes arachnoideae
V. emissaria parietalis
Lacunae laterales
Os parietale
Vv. diploicae
Dura mater cranialis
Arachnoidea mater cranialis
Pia mater cranialis
Spatium subarachnoideum
Substantia alba

Epidermis
Dermis [Corium] } Cutis
Galea aponeurotica
Lamina externa
Diploë } Calvaria
Lamina interna
Spatium subarachnoideum
Cortex cerebri, Gyri cerebri
Falx cerebri

Fig. 11.27 Roof of the skull, meninges and Sinus durae matris. Frontal section.

um. There is therefore no physiological gap between the dura and arachnoid, but there is between the arachnoid and Pia mater. This **Spatium subarachnoideum** (outer subarachnoid space) is filled with cerebrospinal fluid and, in particular in the area of the brain, is threaded through with numerous spidery tissue-like connective tissue trabeculae (**Trabeculae arachnoideae**). In some cases, it is expanded to cisterns, in which, among other things, greater cerebral arteries and some cranial nerve roots run (also ➤ Chap. 11.3.2). Furthermore, in the direction of the dura, you can find villous protuberances of the arachnoid. These mushroom-shaped arachnoidal granulations (**Granulationes arachnoideae**) can penetrate into the lumen of the Sinus durae matris and some even up to the cranial bones and the diploic veins. They are important drainage routes for CSF into the venous system and are particularly numerous and strongly pronounced at the Sinus sagittalis superior (PACCHIONIAN granulations, ➤ Fig. 11.27). In the spinal cord, dorsally in the area of the spinal nerve roots, are arachnoid granulations. These come in contact with the epidural venous plexus and ensure the spinal fluid flow.

Clinical remarks

Meningiomas are slow-growing tumours which are almost always benign, mostly derived from mesothelial cells. They mostly appear in the inter-hemispheric gap, especially in the area of the Sinus sagittalis superior (parasagittal meningioma). Often they remain unnoticed for a long time, because the surrounding tissue adapts and they can thus achieve a significant size before you experience, for example, a sudden seizure. If they can be operated on, meningiomas have a good prognosis if a radically large amount of the tumour tissue can be removed.

Pia mater

The Pia mater cranialis and Pia mater spinalis are directly next to the brain and spinal cord. The **Pia mater cranialis** therefore follows perivascularly – in contrast to the Dura and Arachnoidea mater cranialis – all gyri and sulci down into the deep and large blood vessels and into the brain tissue. These sections are called VIR-

CHOW-ROBIN spaces. A special feature of the **Pia mater spinalis** is the **Lig. denticulatum**. This plate, which is aligned in the frontal plane and consists of tight connective tissue, extends from the Foramen magnum to above the first lumbar nerve on both sides between the spinal cord and Dura mater spinalis and respectively breaks through the arachnoid (➤ Fig. 11.25).

> **NOTE**
>
> Within the bony skull, the Dura and Arachnoidea mater pull together across the surface and thus across the gyri and sulci of the brain. On the other hand, the Pia mater lies directly on the brain tissue and therefore follows the gyri and sulci into the depths without exception (➤ Fig. 11.27).

11.3.5 Neurovascular pathways of the meninges

Arteries and veins

In the vessels of the Dura mater cranialis, a distinction is made between Vasa privata (meningeal vessels, Aa. or Vv. meningeae) and Vasa publica (Sinus durae matris). Vasa privata are responsible for the arterial and venous blood supply of the dura, and Vasa publica carry the venous blood of the brain to the V. jugularis interna. Interestingly, the Arachnoidea mater does not have its own blood supply, but the Pia mater does, the vessels of which in turn are in direct contact with the blood vessels of the brain.

A distinction is made between the following **arteries:**

- **R. meningeus anterior** of the A. ethmoidalis anterior: supplies the Dura mater cranialis of the Fossa cranii anterior
- **A. meningea media** of the A. maxillaris: supplies the largest part of the Dura mater cranialis overall, primarily the Fossa cranii media, and also partly the Fossa cranii anterior
- **A. meningea centralis** of the A. carotis interna: supplies in particular the Tentorium cerebelli
- **A. meningea posterior** of the A. pharyngea ascendens: supplies the largest part of the Dura mater cranialis of the Fossa cranii posterior
- **Rr. meningei** of the A. vertebralis or A. occipitalis: also supply part of the Dura mater cranialis of the Fossa cranii posterior
- **Aa. radiculares** and **Aa. medullares** from the Rr. spinales: supply the Dura mater spinalis

Usually, paired **Vv. meningeae** accompany the above arteries or branches.

> **NOTE**
>
> **Bridging veins** is how the venous sections are defined, connecting the superficial cerebral veins with the Sinus durae matris. They extend from the brain surface through the subarachnoid space, arachnoid and Dura mater cranialis into the respective sinuses.

Clinical remarks

An intracranial **epidural haematoma** describes a collection of blood between the cranial bone and Dura mater cranialis. The cause is often a skull trauma, in which a main vessel supplying the brain, such as the A. meningea media, ruptures. In cerebral computed tomography, an epidural haematoma is hyperdense (denser than the environment) and has a biconvex shape due to the defined attachment sites of the Dura mater to the sutures of the cranial bones. The most important step is early surgery with ligation of the bleeding vessel.

In the event of an intracranial **subdural haematoma**, the blood collects between the Dura mater and the Arachnoidea mater. A subdural haematoma is usually also a result of a traumatic event, but the bridging veins are torn and it may take much longer for the first symptoms to appear. In terms of computer tomography, subdural haematomas are hyperdense and uniconvex. Treatment is by surgery and the insertion of waste drainage.

A **subarachnoid haematoma** usually occurs when an enlargement **(aneurysm)** in an artery in the subarachnoid space ruptures. Such a haemorrhage is also hyperdensed by computed tomography, whereby the accumulation of blood over large parts of the subarachnoid space, depending on how far it extends, can be seen, especially in the cisterns. Again, in terms of prognostics, surgery as early as possible is necessary with closure of the source of bleeding playing an important role.

Innervation

Sensorily, the meninges of the brain are predominantly supplied by branches of the **N. trigeminus [V]**. However, they also involve the **N. glossopharyngeus [IX]** and the **N. vagus [X]** as well as the **cervical spinal nerves** and their sensory innervation.

A topographical distinction is made between:

- N. trigeminus [V]
  - **R. meningeus anterior** of the N. ethmoidalis posterior (branch of the N. nasociliaris; this in turn is the branch of the N. ophthalmicus [V/1]) for the meninges of the Fossa cranii anterior
  - **R. meningeus recurrens (R. tentorius)** of the N. ophthalmicus [V/1] for the Tentorium cerebelli
  - **Rr. meningei** of the N. maxillaris [V/2] or N. mandibularis [V/3] for the meninges of the Fossa cranii media
- N. glossopharyngeus [IX] and N. vagus [X]
  - **Rr. meningei** of the N. vagus [X] and N. glossopharyngeus [IX] for the dura of the Fossa cranii posterior with the exception of the clivus
- cervical spinal nerves
  - **sensory branches of C1–C3** supply the meninges of the clivus after passing through the Foramen magnum

The cerebral meninges are autonomically innervated, **parasympathetically** through **fibres of the head ganglia, sympathetically** through **fibres of the Ganglion cervicale superius**.

In the **spinal cord**, the **Rr. meningei** of each spinal nerve exit segmentally from the sensory and autonomic innervation of the meninges.

Clinical remarks

The meninges are extremely sensitive to pain, in contrast to the brain and spinal cord itself. This sensitivity to pain is particularly evident in inflammatory processes such as **meningitis**. The affected patients have severe headaches and concomitant painful neck stiffness. The latter is caused by an irritation of the membrane that covers the brain and is also known as **meningism**. In a clinical neurological examination, a meningism is determined through the following 2-test procedure:

- **BRUDZINSKI's sign:** In doing this, the patient relaxes lying on their backs with their heads lying passively forward. If the patient's legs act reflexively (to relieve the irritated meninges), the sign is considered positive.
- **KERNIG's sign:** In this case, the stretched leg is raised passively by the patient when lying down. If there is an active flexion in the knee joint due to irritated meninges, the sign is positive.

11.4 Ventricular system and adjacent structures
Anja Böckers

11.4.1 Overview and structure

The brain is surrounded for protection by the cerebrospinal fluid. It is located in the outer (➤ Chap. 11.4.4) and the inner cerebrospinal fluid spaces (➤ Chap. 11.4.3). The **inner cerebrospinal fluid** spaces are in the depths of the cerebral brain and are lined by ependymal cells; they can be referred to as the ventricular system in the narrower sense. They include 4 ventricles and the Canalis centralis (➤ Fig. 11.28):

- **Ventriculi laterales primus** (Ist ventricle, left) and **secundus** (IInd ventricle, right) in the telencephalon
- **Ventriculus tertius** (IIIrd ventricle) in the diencephalon
- **Ventriculus quartus** (IVth ventricle) in the rhombencephalon
- **Aqueductus mesencephali** as a connection between IIIrd and IVth ventricle
- **Canalis centralis** in the spinal cord

The **outer subarachnoid space** is essentially formed by the subarachnoid space surrounding the brain and spinal cord (➤ Chap. 11.4.4). Amongst its extensions are the **cisterns**, including the Cisterna interpeduncularis, Cisterna ambiens and the Cisterna pontocerebellaris.

The cerebrospinal fluid (➤ Chap. 11.4.5) is produced in the Plexus choroidei of the ventricles and is spread over the **Apertura mediana (Foramen MAGENDII)** and the paired **Aperturae laterales (Foraminae LUSCHKAE)** of the IVth ventricle in the outer subarachnoid space, where it is absorbed. Inner and outer cerebrospinal fluid spaces consist of a volume of approx. 140 ml CSF. The cere-

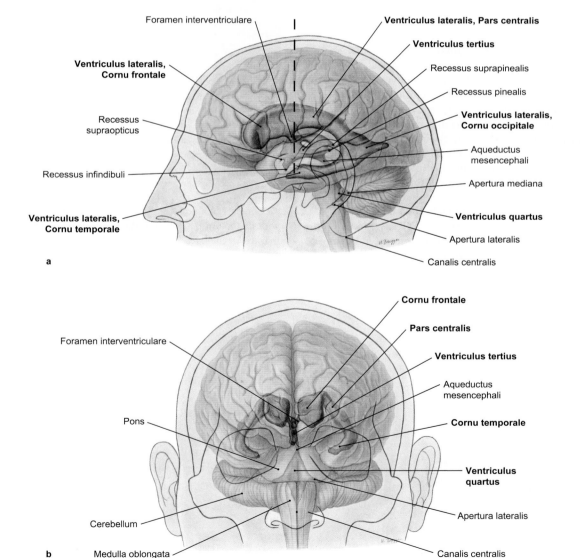

Fig. 11.28 Ventricles of the brain, Ventriculi encephali; a View from the left side. **b** Front view.

brospinal fluid system has a mechanical protection function and transports nutrients and degradation products. It has also been discussed whether the cerebrospinal fluid composition affects circulating substances in the CSF and neurotransmitter hormonal and homeostatic signalling pathways.

11.4.2 Embryology

Ventricular system

With the development of the brain vesicles from the neural tube, there is also simultaneously development of the ventricular system along with the inner cavities of the brain system (➤ Chap. 11.1.1). The two telencephalic vesicles enclose the paired lateral ventricle, and the second of the secondary brain vesicles encloses the IIIrd ventricle of the later diencephalon. After hemispheric rotation, only small-lumen openings remain between the two, the **Foramina interventricularia (Foramina MONROI)**. In the area of the secondary cerebral vesicle located in the mesencephalic part of the brain, the neural tube lumen narrows due to strong growth of the neural tube wall, so that only a narrow passageway between the IIIrd and IVth ventricle, the **Aqueductus mesencephali**, remains. The neural tube lumen of the rhombencephalon becomes the IVth ventricle and the Canalis centralis of the Medulla oblongata or the spinal cord.

Development of the Plexus choroideus

The Plexus choroideus arises from the neuroepithelial of the brain vesicles by blood vessels growing into the ependyme. At these points, the ventricular wall consists of the **epithelial plexus (Lamina epithelialis)** and the connective tissue **Tela choroidea (Lamina propria)**, which differentiates the Pia mater. The vessels grow into the ependymal roof of the IVth ventricle, in the medial wall of the lateral ventricles and in the roof of the IIIrd ventricle. Both of the aforementioned systems develop together in the *7th embryonic week* and are then distributed due to the strong outgrowth of the telencephalon on the lateral ventricles and the IIIrd ventricle. But they remain connected throughout life through the Foramina interventricularia (➤ Fig. 11.29). The choroid plexus is initially created only in the central portion of the lateral ventricles, but expands over the course of hemispheric rotation into the adjacent

Table 11.2 Topography of the lateral ventricles.

Ventricle, section	Wall	Adjacent structures	Plexus choroideus
Ventriculi laterales, Cornu frontale	Roof	Corpus callosum (truncus)	No
	Front wall	Corpus callosum (genu)	
	Medial wall	Septum pellucidum	
	Lateral wall	Caput nuclei caudati	
Ventriculi laterales, Pars centralis	Roof	Corpus callosum	Yes
	Floor	Thalamus	
	Medial wall	Septum pellucidum, fornix	
	Lateral wall	Corpus nuclei caudati	
Ventriculi laterales, Cornu occipitale	Roof	Medulla of the Lobus occipitalis	No
	Floor	Medulla of the Lobus occipitalis	
	Medial wall	Calcar avis	
	Lateral wall	Radiatio optica	
Ventriculi laterales, Cornu temporale	Roof	Cauda nuclei caudati	Yes
	Floor	Hippocampus	
	Medial wall	Fimbria hippocampi	
	Lateral wall	Cauda nuclei caudati	
	Anterior wall	Amygdala	
Ventriculus tertius	Roof	Tela choroidea ventriculi tertii	Yes
	Floor	Hypothalamus	
	Anterior wall	Lamina terminalis ventriculi tertii	
	Lateral wall	Thalamus, epithalamus	
Ventriculus quartus	Roof	Velum medullare superius cerebelli and Velum medullare inferius cerebelli	Yes
	Floor	Fossa rhomboidea	
	Lateral wall	Pedunculi cerebelli	

sections. (➤ Table 11.2). The border between the diencephalon with its thalamic nuclei and the telencephal Nucleus caudatus is marked in the lateral ventricles by the pathway of the V. thalamostriata superior.

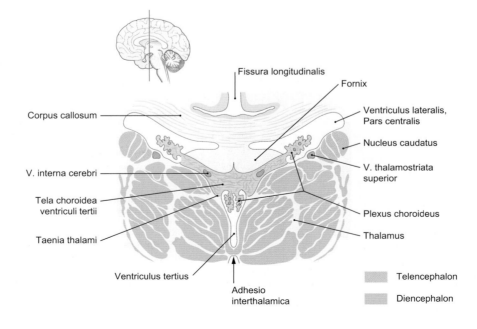

Corpus callosum

Fissura longitudinalis

Fornix

Ventriculus lateralis, Pars centralis

Nucleus caudatus

V. thalamostriata superior

V. interna cerebri

Tela choroidea ventriculi tertii

Taenia thalami

Plexus choroideus

Thalamus

Ventriculus tertius

Adhesio interthalamica

Telencephalon

Diencephalon

Fig. 11.29 Plexus choroideus in the lateral ventricles, Ventriculi laterales, and the IIIrd ventricle, Ventriculus tertius; diagram of frontal section.

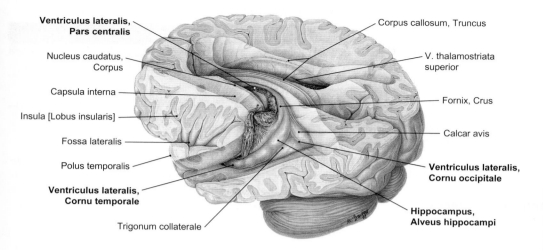

Ventriculus lateralis, Pars centralis

Nucleus caudatus, Corpus

Capsula interna

Insula [Lobus insularis]

Fossa lateralis

Polus temporalis

Ventriculus lateralis, Cornu temporale

Trigonum collaterale

Corpus callosum, Truncus

V. thalamostriata superior

Fornix, Crus

Calcar avis

Ventriculus lateralis, Cornu occipitale

Hippocampus, Alveus hippocampi

Fig. 11.30 Lateral ventricles, Ventriculi laterales. View from the left at the top rear; after removal of the upper parts of the cerebral hemispheres.

11.4.3 Inner cerebrospinal fluid space

Ventriculi laterales primus and secundus

The Ventriculi laterales (➤ Fig. 11.30) each form, viewed laterally, a tube which is bent in a C-shape, whereby the opening of the 'C' points rostrally and has a spur-like bulge posteriorly. The upper arm of the 'C' is the **Cornu frontale [anterius]** in the frontal lobe, continues as the **Pars centralis** in the parietal lobes and with the **Cornu occipitale [posterius]** reaches the occipital lobes of the telencephalon. Via a triangular expansion of the tube, the **Trigonum collaterale,** there is also a wide-lumen connection in the lower leg of the 'C', which in turn penetrates into the temporal lobes (**Cornu temporale [inferius]**).

The lateral ventricles are an important anatomical landmark on sectional images (CT, MRI) through the telencephalon. The core areas of the basal ganglia and clinically important projection fibres which, in their entirety, form the Capsula interna, are located in the immediate vicinity. Knowledge of the ventricle limits is therefore of high clinical relevance. For a basic understanding, it should be remembered that even the Nucleus caudatus of the basal ganglia also reaches its final extent by – like the lateral ventricles – following the hemispherical rotation so that it abuts the lateral wall of the lateral ventricles both in the Crus frontale as well as in the Crus temporale. The thalamus remains as an integral part of the non-rotating diencephalon mediobasal of the lateral ventricle, but lateral to the IIIrd ventricle.

> **N O T E**
> The structures that have accumulated in the walls of the lateral ventricles are listed in ➤ Table 11.2.

Ventriculus tertius

The ventriculi laterales (Ist and IInd ventricle) stand on both sides over the **Foramina interventricularia (MONROI)** with the unpaired IIIrd ventricle. The IIIrd ventricle is located between both parts of the thalami which connect over the **Adhesio interthalamica,** and has characteristic protuberances (➤ Fig. 11.28): in front of the rostrally oriented **Recessus supraopticus**, it binds the Chiasma opticum to the ventricle, including lowering the floor of the IIIrd ventricle in the **Recessus infundibularis** in the infundibular stalk. Closely aligned with the Glandula pinealis (pineal gland) are the **Recessus suprapinealis** and the **Recessus pinealis.**

Aqueductus mesencephali

The IIIrd ventricle communicates through the Aqueductus mesencephali (SYLVII) with the IVth ventricle. The aqueduct begins in the posterior part of the ventricular floor and runs between the Lamina tecti and Tegmentum mesencephali through the mesencephalon to the roof of the IVth ventricle. It is the narrowest point of the inner cerebrospinal fluid spaces. If it narrows or even closes, the Ist–IIIrd ventricles can expand through the CSF congestion (solid) (➤ Fig. 11.31).

Ventriculus quartus

The IVth ventricle has similarities with a tent, with its tip directed to the cerebellum, while the basis points ventrally and is bordered by the rhombus pit (**rhomboid fossa**). The Fossa rhomboidea is bordered by the cerebellar peduncles (Pedunculi cerebelli) from the pons, and – characterised by the horizontally running Stria medullaris ventriculi quarti – by the Medulla oblongata (➤ Fig. 11.21; ➤ Chap. 11.1.2). The IVth ventricle has arm-shaped protuberances on both sides, the **Recessus laterales**. At the ends, the IVth ventricle is connected with the outer subarachnoid spaces via the Aperturae laterales ventriculi quarti (Foraminae **LUSCHKAE**) and via the Apertura mediana ventriculi quarti (Foramen **MAGENDII**), located in the median plane. However, it also continues caudally into the Canalis centralis of the Medulla oblongata or spinalis.

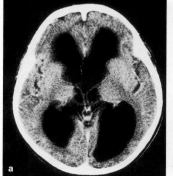
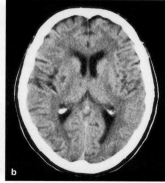

Fig. 11.31 Liquorrhea in the CT. a CT of a patient with liquorrhea through narrowing of the Aqueductus mesencephali. The brain ventricles have been significantly enlarged at the expense of the cerebral parenchyma (hydrocephalus). The patient presented with massive intellectual impairment and significant gait disturbance. **b** CT of a healthy person for comparison. [R317]

Table 11.3 Arterial blood supply of the Plexus choroidei.

Ventricle	Artery
Ventriculi laterales	A. choroidea anterior (from the A. carotis interna) A. choroidea posterior lateralis (from the A. cerebri posterior)
Ventriculus tertius	A. choroidea posterior medialis (from the A. cerebri posterior)
Ventriculus quartus	A. inferior posterior cerebelli (from the A. vertebralis) A. inferior anterior cerebelli (from the A. basilaris)

11.4.4 External subarachnoid fluid spaces – Spatium subarachnoideum

The subarachnoid space is located between the Arachnoidea mater and Pia mater and surrounds the brain and spinal cord. The arachnoidea straddle the irregularities of the brain surface or base so that it results in enhancements of the subarachnoid space. The largest of these cisterns is the **Cisterna cerebellomedullaris**, which spans the cerebellum and Medulla oblongata. It can be penetrated through the Membrana atlantooccipitalis (suboccipital puncture). Above the cerebellum, the **Cisterna quadrigeminalis** expands to the quadrigeminal plate, continuing lateral to the pons in the **Cisterna ambiens**, where it connects rostrally to the **Cisterna interpeduncularis**, located between the Crura cerebri. A multi-chambered system, the **Cisterna basalis**, consists of smaller expansions of the subarachnoid space, especially at the base of the frontal lobe, which also includes the **Cisterna chiasmatica** (➤ Fig. 11.32).

11.4.5 Cerebrospinal fluid

The **Plexus choroideus** and the ependymic cells of the ventricle together form approximately 500 ml CSF a day, i.e., the consistent amount of cerebrospinal fluid (approx. 140 ml) is exchanged approximately three times a day.

Plexus choroideus

The choroid plexus arches out into the ventricular lumen with its numerous vascular fissures, but is in each case attached to the Pia mater via the **Taeniae choroideae.** Like the ependyma, the Plexus epithelium is organised in a one-layered cubic pattern and its surface is covered in microvilli, enlarging it. To protect the brain from possible harmful effects, there is a **blood–CSF barrier** between the

bloodstream and the cerebrospinal fluid: a fenestrated capillary endothelium, the basal membranes of the endothelium or Plexus epithelium, and the choroid plexus epithelial cells connected together via tight junctions. The vessels involved in the formation of the respective vascular bundles of the choroid plexus are shown summarised in ➤ Table 11.3.

The Plexus choroideus of the lateral ventricles and the IIIrd ventricle is 'T'-shaped or '↑'-shaped, with the lateral, almost horizontal limbs of the 'T' or the lateral extensions of the arrowhead extending from the medial side into the Pars centralis and the Cornu temporale of the lateral ventricles, while the long, vertical leg of the 'T' or the arrow shaft is found in the roof of the IIIrd ventricle (➤ Fig. 11.33). The Plexus choroideus of the IVth ventricle partially protrudes from the Aperturae laterales into the subarachnoid space and is clinically described as **BOCHDALEK's flower basket.**

Cerebrospinal fluid formation and absorption

From its place of formation, the Plexus choroidei and the ependymal layer of all the ventricles, the cerebrospinal fluid circulates through the Foramina interventricularia in the IIIrd ventricle through the Aqueductus mesencephali (SYLVII) in the IVth ventricle and finally through the Foraminae laterales and mediana into the subarachnoid space and, thereafter into the outer subarachnoid space (➤ Fig. 11.32). A small portion is directed into the Canalis centralis of the Medulla spinalis, while the main flow passes through the Cisterna basalis and the convexity of the telencephalon hemispheres to the cerebellum and into the spinal canal. The interaction of different transport mechanisms is thereby described: in addition to an oriented cilia impact of the ependymal cells of the ventricular wall, respiratory-dependent pressure fluctuations and a pulsatile flow are also designated by systolic volume changes of the brain. The cerebrospinal fluid circulates to a small extent through the ependyma into the extracellular space of the brain or back into the ventricular system. It is mainly rebsorbed via arachnoid villi, especially via the **PACCHIONIAN's granulations** at the Sinus sagittalis superior, into the venous blood system of the Sinus durae matris. Further drainage paths can

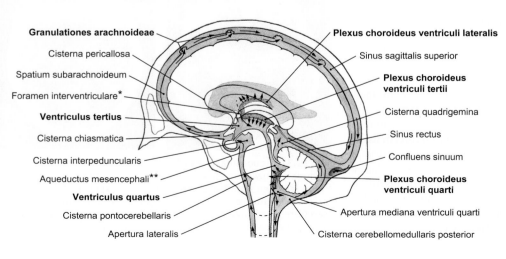

Fig. 11.32 Labels:
Granulationes arachnoideae
Cisterna pericallosa
Spatium subarachnoideum
Foramen interventriculare*
Ventriculus tertius
Cisterna chiasmatica
Cisterna interpeduncularis
Aqueductus mesencephali**
Ventriculus quartus
Cisterna pontocerebellaris
Apertura lateralis

Plexus choroideus ventriculi lateralis
Sinus sagittalis superior
Plexus choroideus ventriculi tertii
Cisterna quadrigemina
Sinus rectus
Confluens sinuum
Plexus choroideus ventriculi quarti
Apertura mediana ventriculi quarti
Cisterna cerebellomedullaris posterior

Fig. 11.32 Diagram of cerebrospinal fluid circulation.
* clinically: Foramen MONROI
** clinically: SYLVIUS canal

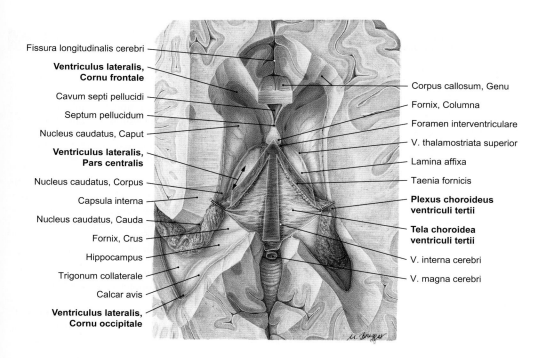

Fissura longitudinalis cerebri

Ventriculus lateralis, Cornu frontale

Cavum septi pellucidi

Septum pellucidum

Nucleus caudatus, Caput

Ventriculus lateralis, Pars centralis

Nucleus caudatus, Corpus

Capsula interna

Nucleus caudatus, Cauda

Fornix, Crus

Hippocampus

Trigonum collaterale

Calcar avis

Ventriculus lateralis, Cornu occipitale

Corpus callosum, Genu

Fornix, Columna

Foramen interventriculare

V. thalamostriata superior

Lamina affixa

Taenia fornicis

Plexus choroideus ventriculi tertii

Tela choroidea ventriculi tertii

V. interna cerebri

V. magna cerebri

Fig. 11.33 Lateral ventricles, Ventriculi laterales. Top view; after removal of the central part of the Corpus callosum and the leg of the fornix.

be found along the blood and lymph canal of the cranial nerves and spinal nerve roots in the spinal canal (➤ Fig. 11.32).

Cerebrospinal fluid composition

The formation of the clear CSF is an active process in which an osmotic gradient is built up via Na^+-K^+-ATPases, in which water can flow through aquaporine canal into the ventricular system. Formation of cerebrospinal fluid can be reduced by inhibition of the enzyme carbonic anhydrase. Usually, CSF contains 99% water with osmolarity comparable to blood, but significantly fewer proteins (0.2%) and only a few cells (less than 4 cells/ml).

Clinical remarks

The composition of the CSF is typically altered in various diseases. In order to be able to explore the cerebrospinal fluid, the subarachnoid space is punctured with a hollow needle **(lumbar puncture)**. In most cases, the puncture site is between the spinous processes of the IIIrd and IVth, or the IVth

and Vth lumbar vertebrae, i.e. much lower than the lower end of the spinal cord (Conus medullaris at the level of the Ist or IInd lumbar vertebra, ➤ Fig. 11.34).

11.4.6 Circumventricular organs

Location

In addition to the ependymal cells, other individual brain cells limit the subarachnoid space. In some locations of the ventricular system, in particular in the IIIrd and IVth ventricles, these types of cells are so numerous and locally concentrated that they are described as the circumventricular organs (CVO) (➤ Fig. 11.35). They are mostly unpaired and are primarily located in the median plane of the brain. Special characteristics of these organs are specialised ependymal cells **(tanycytes)** and fenestrated capillary endothelium that raise the blood–brain barrier at these points. Tanycytes have cilia on their apical cell membrane that can make contact with the cerebrospinal fluid.

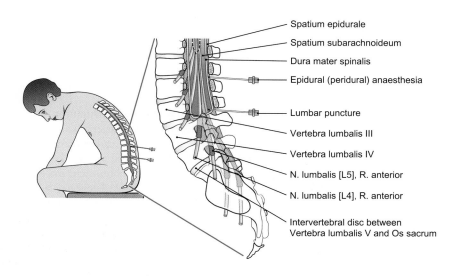

Spatium epidurale

Spatium subarachnoideum

Dura mater spinalis

Epidural (peridural) anaesthesia

Lumbar puncture

Vertebra lumbalis III

Vertebra lumbalis IV

N. lumbalis [L5], R. anterior

N. lumbalis [L4], R. anterior

Intervertebral disc between Vertebra lumbalis V and Os sacrum

Fig. 11.34 Puncture locations for the lumbar puncture and peridural anaesthesia.

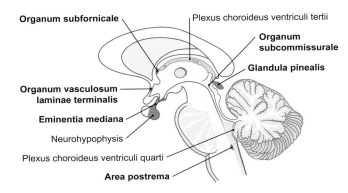

Fig. 11.35 Circumventricular organs. Mid-sagittal section.

The CVOs are divided into:

- **sensory CVOs** in the narrower sense:
  - **Organum subfornicale** in the anterior wall of the IIIrd ventricle
  - **Organum vasculosum laminae terminalis** in the Lamina terminalis immediately dorsal to the Chiasma opticum
  - **Area postrema** at the bottom of the rhombus pit
- **secretory CVOs**
  - **Eminentia mediana** of the pituitary infundibulum
  - **Glandula pinealis**
  - **posterior pituitary**

Organum subcommissurale is formed in humans only in the foetal and newborn phase.

Function

CVOs are a communication interface between the blood flow with its signal substances – such as neuropeptides (including leptin, ghrelin), cytokines, glucose or hormones – and the brain or the cerebrospinal fluid. Through their connections to the brainstem and hypothalamus they are involved in the endocrine and autonomic regulation of food intake, energy and fluid balance, body temperature and sleep. Accordingly, **afferents** are found in the subfornical organ from the hypothalamus and **efferent fibres** which stimulate vasopressin neurons of the Nuclei paraventricularis and supraopticus, thus influencing the regulation of blood volume and blood pressure. The **Organum vasculosum laminae terminalis** is also assigned a special role in the change of body temperature or the development of fever via temperature-sensitive neurons. The **Area postrema** in turn, along with the Nucleus tractus solitarii and the Nucleus dorsalis nervi vagi are also described as a vagal complex. It picks up signals in the blood or cerebrospinal fluid via chemoreceptors and can cause vomiting via this complex.

Clinical remarks

The unique nature of the CVOs opens up a wide variety of pharmacological treatment approaches. Examples are:

- **Salicylic acid**, which acts as a cyclo-oxygenase inhibitor via a reduced fever-reducing prostaglandin formation: with fevers, the sensitivity of temperature-sensitive neurons of the Organum vasculosum laminae terminalis is reduced, e.g. by the body's own prostaglandins. These neurons normally initiate physiological cooling mechanisms, which in the case of fever only functions to a delayed extent or not at all. Acetylsalicylic acid reduces prostaglandin formation, increasing the sensitivity of neurons, readjusts the fever-related set-point adjustment, and clinically reduces fever.
- **Neuroleptics** for treatment of central vomiting (emesis), e.g. due to administration of opioids: neuroleptic drugs bind to dopamine receptors in the Area postrema and thus have an antiemetic effect.

11.5 Cerebral vessels
Thomas Deller

11.5.1 Overview

Clinical significance of the vessel anatomy of the brain

Every doctor will repeatedly come into contact over the course of their professional career with the issues of 'blood supply to the brain', 'stroke' or 'vascular dementia'. It is therefore of great practical importance to know the anatomical pathway of the vessels and their respective supply area: if it should come to the closure of a cerebral artery and thus to a reduced perfusion (ischemia) of the supplied brain area, they can no longer fulfil their function. Accordingly, the patient suffers from neurological symptoms which are typical for this brain area. It is therefore also possible to see, for example, along with a motor weakness in the face and arm area as well as motor speech disturbances, an infarction of the A. cerebri media if one knows that the A. cerebri media supplies the appropriate brain areas.

In addition, however, progress in medicine and especially in the 'neuro-subjects' of neurology, neurosurgery, neuroradiology and psychiatry has led to new imaging techniques (e.g. angio-MRI), invasive treatments (e.g. lysis in the event of a stroke) and innovative neurosurgical techniques that require significantly more knowledge of the vascular anatomy of the brain than a few years ago. The vessel anatomy of the brain is therefore no longer 'specialist knowledge', but is required as basic knowledge for many clinical disciplines.

Overview of the arterial and venous structures

The brain is supplied with blood via 4 arteries with a strong calibre: two **Aa. carotis internae** (from the A. carotis communis) and two **Aa. vertebrales** (from the A. subclavia; ➤ Fig. 11.36). The two Aa. vertebrales join at the level of the brainstem and form the unpaired A. basilaris (A. vertebralis/basilaris system; ➤ Fig. 11.37, ➤ Fig. 11.38, ➤ Fig. 11.39). From the two Aa. carotes internae and the A. basilaris, on the basal side of the brain, the polygonal arterial arches, the Circulus arteriosus cerebri (**WILLISII, circle of WILLIS**) are created; ➤ Fig. 11.37, ➤ Fig. 11.38, ➤ Fig. 11.39. The brain vessels for the two hemispheres exit from these. The supply areas of

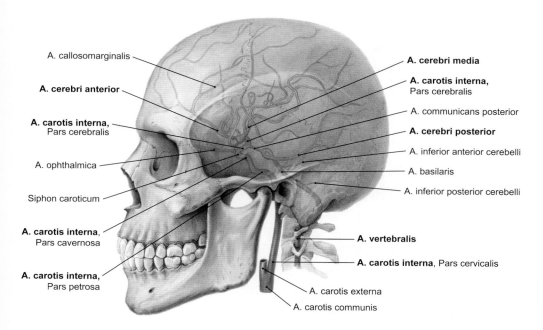

A. callosomarginalis

A. cerebri anterior

A. carotis interna,
Pars cerebralis

A. ophthalmica

Siphon caroticum

A. carotis interna,
Pars cavernosa

A. carotis interna,
Pars petrosa

A. cerebri media

A. carotis interna,
Pars cerebralis

A. communicans posterior

A. cerebri posterior

A. inferior anterior cerebelli

A. basilaris

A. inferior posterior cerebelli

A. vertebralis

A. carotis interna, Pars cervicalis

A. carotis externa

A. carotis communis

Fig. 11.36 Internal arteries of the head. The brain is supplied by 2 Aa. carotes internae and 2 Aa. vertebrales.

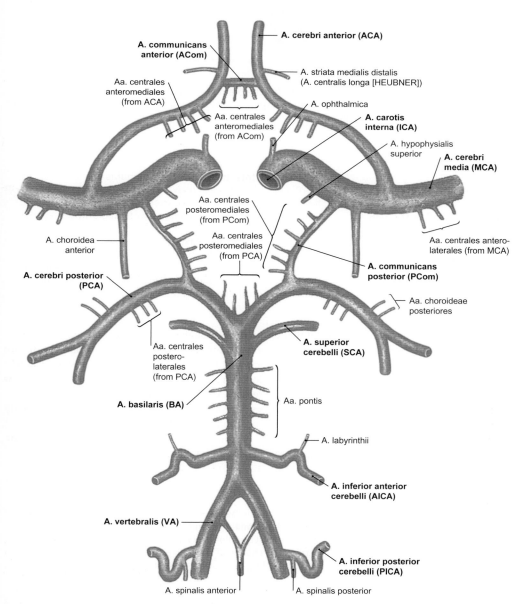

A. communicans anterior (ACom)

A. cerebri anterior (ACA)

Aa. centrales anteromediales (from ACA)

A. striata medialis distalis (A. centralis longa [HEUBNER])

Aa. centrales anteromediales (from ACom)

A. ophthalmica

A. carotis interna (ICA)

A. hypophysialis superior

A. cerebri media (MCA)

Aa. centrales posteromediales (from PCom)

A. choroidea anterior

Aa. centrales posteromediales (from PCA)

Aa. centrales antero-laterales (from MCA)

A. communicans posterior (PCom)

A. cerebri posterior (PCA)

Aa. choroideae posteriores

Aa. centrales postero-laterales (from PCA)

A. superior cerebelli (SCA)

A. basilaris (BA)

Aa. pontis

A. labyrinthii

A. inferior anterior cerebelli (AICA)

A. vertebralis (VA)

A. inferior posterior cerebelli (PICA)

A. spinalis anterior

A. spinalis posterior

Fig. 11.37 Circulus arteriosus cerebri (WILLISII, circle of WILLIS); Diagram.

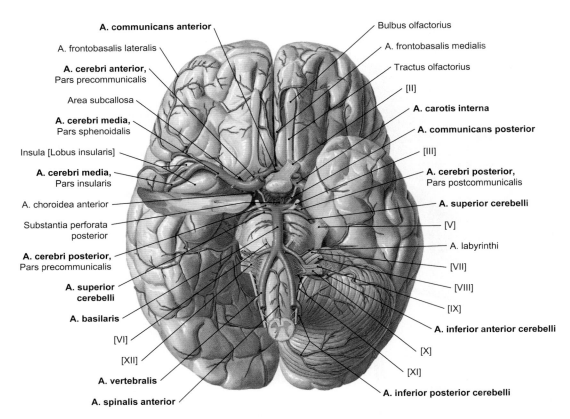

A. communicans anterior

A. frontobasalis lateralis

A. cerebri anterior,
Pars precommunicalis

Area subcallosa

A. cerebri media,
Pars sphenoidalis

Insula [Lobus insularis]

A. cerebri media,
Pars insularis

A. choroidea anterior

Substantia perforata
posterior

A. cerebri posterior,
Pars precommunicalis

**A. superior
cerebelli**

A. basilaris

[VI]

[XII]

A. vertebralis

A. spinalis anterior

Bulbus olfactorius

A. frontobasalis medialis

Tractus olfactorius

[II]

A. carotis interna

A. communicans posterior

[III]

A. cerebri posterior,
Pars postcommunicalis

A. superior cerebelli

[V]

A. labyrinthi

[VII]

[VIII]

[IX]

A. inferior anterior cerebelli

[X]

[XI]

A. inferior posterior cerebelli

Fig. 11.38 Arteries of the brain on the Facies inferior of the brain. The vessels supplying the brain are shown in their typical topographic contexts. For a better illustration of the pathway of the A. cerebri media, a section of the temporal lobe has been separated on the right. For better visibility of the A. cerebri posterior, the right half of the cerebellum was removed.

the cerebral arteries (see below, topography and supply areas of the arteries) are not dependent on the anatomical lobe boundaries. Therefore, for example, the A. cerebri media supplies parts of the Lobus frontalis, Lobus parietalis and the Lobus temporalis.
The supply of the brain depends on the arterial blood flow through the large arteries supplying the brain. In healthy patients with a typical Circulus arteriosus (➤ Fig. 11.37, ➤ Fig. 11.38, ➤ Fig. 11.39), angiographic examinations allow 3 flow sectors to be identified: the **A. carotis interna** therefore supplies the equilateral hemisphere on one side as a rule, with the exception of the Lobus occipitalis and parts of the Lobus temporalis (Carotis-interna flow area). The **A. vertebralis/basilaris system** on the other hand supplies the brainstem, the cerebellum and the remaining hemispherical sections on both sides (vertebralis/basilaris flow area). However, the flow areas of the vessels may differ from this 'normal situation' in individual patients due to congenital vascular variations and/or vascular disease.
The **venous drainage of the blood** from the brain is carried out independently of the arteries via the venous canal of the Dura mater, the **Sinus durae matris** (➤ Fig. 11.40, ➤ Fig. 11.59). These receive the blood via a superficial and a deep venous system: the veins on the brain surface flow directly through **bridging veins**, i.e. through the meninges and on to a sinus, whereas the veins collect blood from the depths of the brain in the unpaired V. magna cerebri (**vein of GALEN**), which is connected to the network of the Sinus durae matris via the Sinus rectus.

Blood flow to the brain
The brain is traversed by approx. 15% of the cardiac output, which gives it a continuous **supply of oxygen and glucose**. Without this blood supply, brain function will fail within minutes as the brain does not have its own oxygen or glucose reserves.

Clinical remarks

The **ischemic tolerance** of the brain amounts to a maximum of 7–10 min. This is of great relevance to the resuscitation of patients in the event of a cardiac arrest.
Even if the blood flow to the brain only temporarily decreases (e.g. when suddenly getting up or standing up straight), there may be a temporary **decreased blood flow to the brain** that could result in a lack of function. The patient drops to the ground (syncope or fainting). Due to the horizontal position of the body, the cerebral blood flow improves rapidly and the patient wakes up after a short time.

The **global blood flow** through the brain is kept constant within certain blood pressure limits (about 80–120 mmHg) by the dilation and contraction of the resistance vessels. This also increases/decreases the blood pressure in the brain. The **regional blood flow** is controlled – regardless of the global blood pressure – by local metabolic factors. These are very closely linked to the local activity of the nerve tissue. Nerve cells are very active, they increase the K^+, the CO_2 and the H^+ concentration (acidosis) in their environment. This leads to localised vessel dilation.

Clinical remarks

The relationship between nerve cell activity and circulation is used in **functional imaging** (functional MRI; fMRT). The BOLD contrast (BOLD = blood oxygenation level-dependent) describes the change of the image signal depending on the oxygen content of erythrocytes: the stronger the nerve cell activity in an area, the more oxygen is consumed there and the more

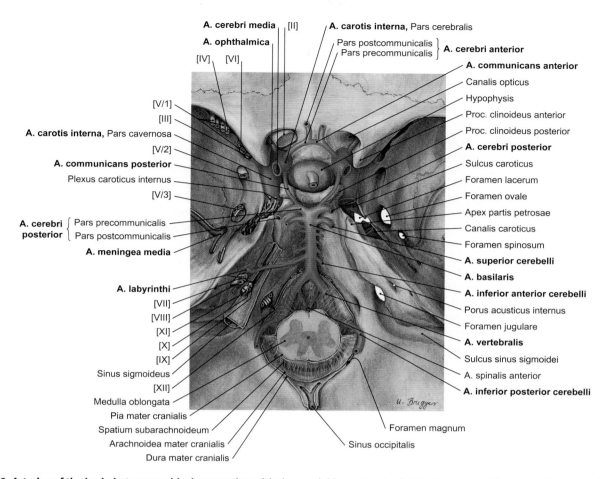

A. cerebri media [II] **A. carotis interna,** Pars cerebralis
A. ophthalmica Pars postcommunicalis
[IV] [VI] Pars precommunicalis } **A. cerebri anterior**
A. communicans anterior
[V/1] Canalis opticus
[III] Hypophysis
A. carotis interna, Pars cavernosa Proc. clinoideus anterior
[V/2] Proc. clinoideus posterior
A. communicans posterior **A. cerebri posterior**
Plexus caroticus internus Sulcus caroticus
[V/3] Foramen lacerum
Foramen ovale
A. cerebri { Pars precommunicalis Apex partis petrosae
posterior { Pars postcommunicalis Canalis caroticus
A. meningea media Foramen spinosum
A. superior cerebelli
A. labyrinthi **A. basilaris**
[VII] **A. inferior anterior cerebelli**
[VIII] Porus acusticus internus
[XI] Foramen jugulare
[X] **A. vertebralis**
[IX] Sulcus sinus sigmoidei
Sinus sigmoideus A. spinalis anterior
[XII] **A. inferior posterior cerebelli**
Medulla oblongata
Pia mater cranialis
Spatium subarachnoideum Foramen magnum
Arachnoidea mater cranialis Sinus occipitalis
Dura mater cranialis

Fig. 11.39 Arteries of the brain in topographical connection with the cranial base. On the right side, a part of the A. carotis interna is removed. In vivo, the underlying Foramen lacerum is closed by a fibrous cartilage plate.

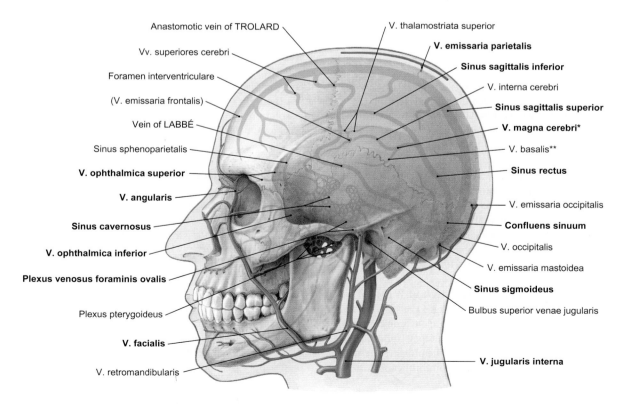

Anastomotic vein of TROLARD V. thalamostriata superior
Vv. superiores cerebri **V. emissaria parietalis**
Foramen interventriculare **Sinus sagittalis inferior**
(V. emissaria frontalis) V. interna cerebri
Vein of LABBÉ **Sinus sagittalis superior**
Sinus sphenoparietalis **V. magna cerebri***
V. ophthalmica superior V. basalis**
V. angularis **Sinus rectus**
Sinus cavernosus V. emissaria occipitalis
V. ophthalmica inferior **Confluens sinuum**
Plexus venosus foraminis ovalis V. occipitalis
V. emissaria mastoidea
Plexus pterygoideus **Sinus sigmoideus**
Bulbus superior venae jugularis
V. facialis
V. retromandibularis **V. jugularis interna**

Fig. 11.40 Inner and outer veins of the brain. The cerebral veins collect the blood in a superficial and deep venous system. From there, it flows into the Sinus durae matris and the V. jugularis interna. * Vein of GALEN, ** Basal vein of ROSENTHAL

the regional blood flow increases (see above), the more oxygenated haemoglobin is supplied to this area. This manifests itself in a measurable increase in signal in the area of activated adjacent brain tissue. With an fMRT, you can thus identify regions of the brain, e.g. it is activated when learning.

Nomenclature

Naming the cerebral arteries is – as is so often the case in anatomy – done according to tradition. The names were usually chosen on the basis of topographical relationships and describe only the approximate area of the CNS that is supplied by the artery. The A. cerebri anterior therefore originates, e.g. in the front (anterior), from the Circulus arteriosus cerebri, but then runs with its main branches dorsally and supplies large areas of the frontal and parietal cortex in the area of the hemispherical rim. Although the A. superior cerebelli runs above the cerebellum, it also supplies functionally important sections of the brainstem with its branches – which is why a combined occlusion of the cerebellum and brainstem occurs when the artery is occluded.

In addition to the international anatomical nomenclature, abbreviations derived from the **English names of the vessels** are often used in clinical practice (e.g. PICAS = posterior inferior cerebellar artery; also ➤ Table 11.6).

Individual differences in the blood supply

The brain shows – as with many other organs – variations in its blood supply. These can either be congenital or acquired. A **congenital variant** is, for example, the duplication of the A. cerebri anterior dextra (the person in question would therefore have 3 Aa. cerebri anteriores). It is also possible that not all the vessels are formed. In the case of **acquired changes** of vessels, the diameter of an existing vessel is normally changed, e.g. if the A. communicans posterior is expanded in the event of an occlusion of the A. carotis interna, and the A. cerebri media is supplied via the vertebral artery/basilaris flow area.

Clinical remarks

The variability of vessels supplying the brain also leads to a variability of the supply areas. Accordingly, it may be the case with **occlusion of an atypical vessel** that clinical stroke symptoms may occur, which cannot be explained initially by 'textbook anatomy'.

Anastomoses and terminal arteries

It is of great practical importance to determine in the case of the under-perfusion of a vessel, how well the blood flow in the capillary bed can be maintained by vascular connections (collaterals) to other vessels. The brain has a whole series of collateral connections, the most important of which are listed below.

Circulus arteriosus cerebri (WILLISII, circle of WILLIS)

The Circulus arteriosus (➤ Fig. 11.37, ➤ Fig. 11.39) is only seen in its ideal form – with all around, end-to-end and communicating vessels – in about half (approx. 45%) of all autopsy studies. In the other cases, variations were observed, with the most frequent changes (about 20–30%) involving the A. communicans posterior and the A. cerebri posterior.

Clinical remarks

A continuous and complete Circulus arteriosus reduces the risk of stroke in patients with an imminent closure of the A. carotis interna.

Connections to the A. carotis externa

The A. ophthalmica is the first major intracranial branch of the A. carotis interna (➤ Fig. 11.36, ➤ Fig. 11.39). Its terminal branch, the A. dorsalis nasi, forms an anastomosis with the A. angularis, a terminal branch of the A. facialis (from the A. carotis externa). Thus, the flow areas of the internal carotid artery and the external carotid artery are connected with each other, with the blood normally flowing from the A. dorsalis nasi into the A. angularis.

Clinical remarks

If the A. carotis interna is closed on one side, the **blood flow in the A. angularis** can reverse direction, i.e., the blood then flows from the A. angularis via the A. dorsalis nasi and the A. ophthalmica into the Circulus arteriosus. This flow reversal can be diagnosed with a doppler ultrasound (➤ Chap. 11.5.9).

Connections of the superficial arteries of the hemispheres

The terminal branches of the superficial arteries supplying the brain form **leptomeningeal anastomoses** in the area of the hemispheres of the cerebellum – even over the Corpus callosum (anastomoses between terminal branches of both Aa. cerebri anteriores, often between the Aa. callosomarginales and Aa. pericallosae of both sides). However, these anastomoses are not sufficient to completely take over the blood supply in the event of acute under-perfusion of a brain-supplying vessel. It leads to ischemic cerebral infarction. These vessels supplying the brain are therefore referred to as 'functional end arteries'. Nevertheless, the leptomeningeal collaterals are not unimportant, because the collateral supply means the area of the infarct is not as large as it would be in the case of a cerebral infarct without this collateral supply. Furthermore, the collaterals supply the surroundings of the infarct (penumbra), so that this tissue, in the event of a re-opening of the closed vessel (e.g. by dissolution of a blood clot, 'thrombolysis'), can survive. However, this has to be done quickly: 'Time is brain'.

NOTE

Functional terminal arteries and end arteries

A vessel without anastomoses with other vessels is regarded as an **end artery** (terminal artery). Its occlusion leads to an infarct of the supplied areas. In the case of an existing but largely insufficient supply by anastomoses with other vessels, one speaks of **functional end arteries**. The brain contains both forms of end arteries.

Central blood supply

After their departure from the main vessel, the central vessels (e.g. Aa. centrales anteromediales) do not form any other significant collateral. They are considered to be terminal arteries in the traditional sense. Their occlusion leads to ischemia and tissue loss in their supply area.

11.5.2 A. carotis interna and its branches

Large parts of the anterior telencephalon and diencephalon are supplied by the A. carotis interna. The anatomy of this vessel is of great clinical importance (duplex ultrasound of the neck vessels; angiography). Anatomically, a distinction is made between 4 sections (➤ Fig. 11.41):

- **Pars cervicalis** – 'throat': from the Bifurcatio carotidis to the skull entry
- **Pars petrosa** – 'rock': in the Bifurcatio carotidis of the temporal bone
- **Pars cavernosa** – 'cavity': in the Sinus cavernosus
- **Pars cerebralis** – 'brain': in the subarachnoid space it is divided into 2 terminal branches, A. cerebri anterior and A. cerebri media

Topography

The **cervical part** begins with the carotid fork, which is usually at the level of the IVth cervical vertebra. The A. carotis interna lies

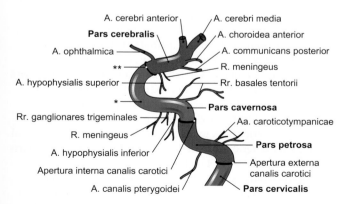

A. cerebri anterior
A. cerebri media
Pars cerebralis
A. choroidea anterior
A. ophthalmica
A. communicans posterior
**
R. meningeus
A. hypophysialis superior
Rr. basales tentorii
*
Pars cavernosa
Rr. ganglionares trigeminales
Aa. caroticotympanicae
R. meningeus
Pars petrosa
A. hypophysialis inferior
Apertura externa canalis carotici
Apertura interna canalis carotici
A. canalis pterygoidei
Pars cervicalis

Fig. 11.41 Sections of the A. carotis interna. No branches exit from the Pars cervicalis, which is why the artery can be safely distinguished from the A. carotis externa during an ultrasound examination of the neck organs. [E402] * Carotid passage, ** through the Dura mater cranialis in the area of the Diaphragma sellae.

dorsolaterally of the A. carotis externa in approx. 50% of the cases. However, because of this variability in the output, it cannot be said with certainty which of the two carotids is 'inside' and which is 'outside' and, in ultrasound examinations, the anatomical fact that the A. carotis interna – in contrast to the A. carotis externa – has no branches in the neck area (➤ Fig. 11.41) is used to identify it.

The **Pars petrosa** starts where it enters the petrous bone. The A. carotis interna runs in the Canalis caroticus and drains over the Foramen lacerum, which is sealed with fibrous cartilage. Along its pathway, there are smaller branches to the tympanic cavity (**Aa. caroticotympanicae;** ➤ Fig. 11.41).

After leaving the petrous bone, the A. carotis interna runs through the venous chamber system of the cavernous sinus (**Pars cavernosa,** ➤ Fig. 11.42). It lies first on the lateral surface of the Corpus ossis sphenoidale and then runs upwards in the Sulcus caroticus. Below the Proc. clinoideus posterior it turns forward and runs horizontally to the Proc. clinoideus anterior. This lies directly underneath the N. opticus. Along its pathway, the A. carotis interna provides smaller **branches to the meninges**, to the **Ganglion trigeminale** and to the pituitary gland (**A. hypophysialis inferior**) (➤ Fig. 11.41).

The **Pars cerebralis** begins where the A. carotis interna leaves the dura and enters an extension (cistern) of the subarachnoid space, which is named after it (Cisterna carotica). It moves back again occipitally and laterally for a short distance and comes to lie under the Substantia perforata anterior. There, it divides into 2 terminal branches. Along its pathway there are 4 vessels (➤ Fig. 11.41):

- **A. ophthalmica** (below the N. opticus; ➤ Fig. 11.39)
- **A. hypophysialis superior**
- **A. choroidea anterior**
- **A. communicans posterior**

The loop-shaped ('S-shaped') pathway of the Pars cavernosa and Pars cerebralis near the Proc. clinoideus anterior resembles a corkscrew or a siphon. Therefore, this section is described as a **carotid siphon**. Approximately at the level of the knee of the siphon or shortly after, the A. ophthalmica exits the A. carotis interna (➤ Fig. 11.41).

NOTE

The **internal carotid artery**
- is formed at the level of the IVth cervical vertebra
- leaves dorsolaterally from the A. carotis communis in 50% of cases
- has no vascular outflow in the throat area
- is divided into 4 anatomically defined sections: Pars cervicalis, Pars petrosa, Pars cavernosa, Pars cerebralis
- forms an S-shaped loop system (carotid syphon)
- has the A. ophthalmica as the first larger vascular branch
- branches into the A. cerebri anterior and the A. cerebri media
- supplies the pituitary gland, the trigeminal ganglion, the eye, and the anterior parts of the telencephalon and the diencephalon

Branches of the A. carotis interna

The branches (direct vessel outflow) of the A. carotis interna are:

- **Aa. hypophysiales:** The A. hypophysialis inferior originates from the Pars cavernosa and essentially supplies the neurohypophysis. The Aa. hypophysiales superiores from the Pars cerebralis (➤ Fig. 11.41) supply the infundibulum. The portal veins of the pituitary gland (Vv. portales hypophysiales) develop from their capillary system, leading to the adenohypophysis (➤ Chap. 11.2.2) and form a second capillary network around their endocrine cells (vascular transport system for hypothalamic control hormones to the adenohypophysis).

617

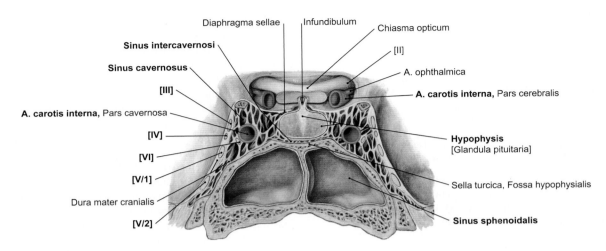

Fig. 11.42 Pars cavernosa of the A. carotis interna. In the chamber system of the Sinus cavernous are the A. carotis interna and N. abducens [VI]. In the wall of the sinus are the N. oculomotorius [III], N. trochlearis [IV], N. ophthalmicus [V/1] and N. maxillaris [V/2]. There are topographical relationships to the pituitary gland and the Sinus sphenoidalis.

- **A. ophthalmica:** The eye and parts of the viscerocranium are supplied via the A. ophthalmica. It is the first major arterial branch of the A. carotis interna. It runs through the Canalis nervi optici together with the N. opticus (➤ Fig. 11.39). One of its terminal branches penetrates into the N. opticus as the A. centralis retinae and reaches the retina of the eye. Another terminal branch (A. dorsalis nasi) forms an anastomosis with the A. facialis.
- **A. communicans posterior** (➤ Fig. 11.37, ➤ Fig. 11.38, ➤ Fig. 11.41): It sends branches into the brain and supplies parts of the thalamus and third ventricle (Aa. centrales posteromediales; A. thalamotuberalis). It extends to the occipital via the Tractus opticus and reaches the A. cerebri posterior anteriorly to the N. oculomotorius [III].
- **A. choroidea anterior** (➤ Fig. 11.37, ➤ Fig. 11.38, ➤ Fig. 11.41): It supplies important parts of the inside of the brain (including the Crus posterius of the Capsula interna) as well as parts of the visual system (Tractus opticus, Corpus geniculatum laterale), the Plexus choroideus, amygdala and hippocampus. There are also branches into the mesencephalon. The A. choroidea anterior runs along the Tractus opticus, winds around the uncus of the temporal lobe and reaches the lateral ventricle.

Bifurcation of the A. carotis interna into its terminal branches

The A. carotis interna crosses the Area perforata anterior and divides into its two main branches at the medial end of the Sulcus lateralis. The midbrain artery, the A. cerebri media, thereby follows the original pathway of the A. carotis interna, while the front brain arteries, A. cerebri anterior, bend almost at a right angle from the A. carotis interna and pull anteromedially towards the Fissura longitudinalis cerebri (➤ Fig. 11.38, ➤ Fig. 11.39).

A. cerebri anterior

The A. cerebri anterior (➤ Fig. 11.38, ➤ Fig. 11.43) provides the front part of the medial hemisphere area and a cortical strip parallel to the hemispheral rim. It sends branches inside the brain to supply the Capsula interna (parts of the Crus anterius) and the basal ganglia. From its distribution site, it runs anteromedially to the Fissura longitudinalis cerebri (➤ Fig. 11.38). It connects there with the A. cerebri anterior of the opposite side via the **A. communicans anterior**. As it continues, it winds around the Corpus callosum and finally splits into two main branches (➤ Fig. 11.43), the **A. pericallosa** (between the Corpus callosum and Gyrus cinguli) and the **A. callosomarginalis** (via the Sulcus cinguli). Branches of the A. cerebri anterior are:

- **Aa. centrales anteromediales:** They branch off early in the initial section of the A. cerebri anterior and pass through the Substantia perforata anterior into the interior of the brain to the hypothalamus, fornix and the Lamina terminalis.
- Backwards-running **A. striata medialis distalis** (recurrent artery of HEUBNER, A. centralis longa): It also originates from the initial section of the A. cerebri anterior (➤ Fig. 11.47) – as a rule, it emerges at the level of the A. communicans anterior or from the immediately adjacent vascular segment of the A. cerebri anterior. It forms a backward loop, runs antiparallel to the A. cerebri anterior back to the Substantia perforata anterior and supplies the anterior horn of the Capsula interna as well as parts of the basal ganglia (➤ Fig. 11.47).
- **A. polaris frontalis:** It flows to the anterior brain sections.

The **A. communicans anterior** (➤ Fig. 11.37, ➤ Fig. 11.38) connects the two Aa. cerebri anteriores with each another. It can be fenestrated dually and is only about 5 mm long. This vessel also supplies the Chiasma opticum with superficial branches and sends central branches into the depths of the brain, e.g., to the Gyrus cinguli, the hypothalamus and the septum region.

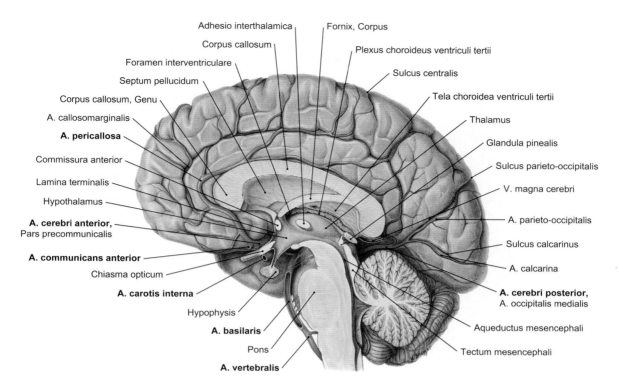

Adhesio interthalamica
Corpus callosum
Foramen interventriculare
Septum pellucidum
Corpus callosum, Genu
A. callosomarginalis
A. pericallosa
Commissura anterior
Lamina terminalis
Hypothalamus
A. cerebri anterior,
Pars precommunicalis
A. communicans anterior
Chiasma opticum
A. carotis interna
Hypophysis
A. basilaris
Pons
A. vertebralis

Fornix, Corpus
Plexus choroideus ventriculi tertii
Sulcus centralis
Tela choroidea ventriculi tertii
Thalamus
Glandula pinealis
Sulcus parieto-occipitalis
V. magna cerebri
A. parieto-occipitalis
Sulcus calcarinus
A. calcarina
A. cerebri posterior,
A. occipitalis medialis
Aqueductus mesencephali
Tectum mesencephali

Fig. 11.43 A. cerebri anterior. The A. cerebri anterior initially provides the A. communicans anterior to the opposite side and then passes dorsally around the Corpus callosum. The Lobus occipitalis is supplied by the A. cerebri posterior.

Clinical remarks

Vascular bulges (aneurysms) are not uncommon in the area of the Circulus arteriosus. The most common are **aneurysms of the A. communicans anterior** (up to 40 %). When performing surgery on an aneurysm in this area, care should be taken that the artery of HEUBNER is not damaged. The central branches of the A. communicans anterior must also be looked after during the operation, as otherwise – fortunately temporary for the most part – a postoperative memory disturbance (A. communicans anterior syndrome) may occur.

A. cerebri media

The A. cerebri media (➤ Fig. 11.44) supplies the largest part of the lateral brain surface, the insula and – with central branches – the Capsula interna (parts of the Crus anterius, genu) and the basal ganglia. At first it continues the pathway of the A. carotis interna

laterally and delivers the **Aa. centrales anterolaterales** in its opening section to supply the inner brain (➤ Fig. 11.37, ➤ Fig. 11.47). Via the medial end of the Sulcus lateralis, it enters the Fossa lateralis and separates into several terminal branches over the island, the insula (➤ Fig. 11.38, ➤ Fig. 11.44, ➤ Fig. 11.45). These vessels are named after their respective supply area (e.g. the A. sulci centralis runs in the Sulcus centralis).

11.5.3 Aa. vertebrales/A. basilaris and their branches

A. vertebralis

The posterior sections of the cortex, the cerebellum and the brainstem are mainly supplied by blood vessels from the vertebrobasilar flow area (➤ Fig. 11.37, ➤ Fig. 11.38, ➤ Fig. 11.39, ➤ Fig. 11.46). Similar to the A. carotis interna, you can differentiate 4 sections in the A. vertebralis:

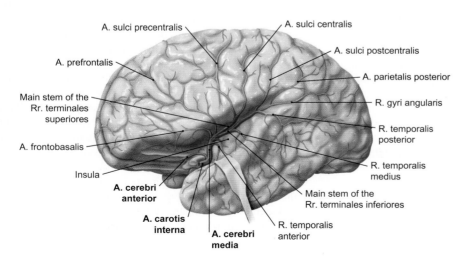

A. sulci precentralis
A. prefrontalis
Main stem of the
Rr. terminales
superiores
A. frontobasalis
Insula
A. cerebri anterior
A. carotis interna
A. cerebri media
A. sulci centralis
A. sulci postcentralis
A. parietalis posterior
R. gyri angularis
R. temporalis posterior
R. temporalis medius
Main stem of the
Rr. terminales inferiores
R. temporalis anterior

Fig. 11.44 A. cerebri media on the Facies lateralis cerebri. The temporal lobes have been pulled down into the Sulcus lateralis with a hook, which gives you a view into the Fossa lateralis with the A. cerebri media and its branches. [L127]

619

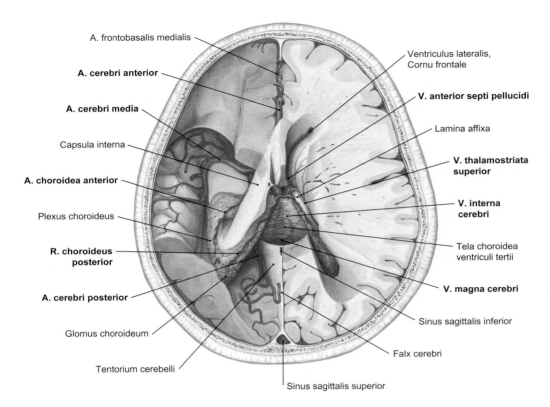

A. frontobasalis medialis

A. cerebri anterior

A. cerebri media

Capsula interna

A. choroidea anterior

Plexus choroideus

R. choroideus posterior

A. cerebri posterior

Glomus choroideum

Tentorium cerebelli

Sinus sagittalis superior

Ventriculus lateralis, Cornu frontale

V. anterior septi pellucidi

Lamina affixa

V. thalamostriata superior

V. interna cerebri

Tela choroidea ventriculi tertii

V. magna cerebri

Sinus sagittalis inferior

Falx cerebri

Fig. 11.45 A. cerebri media, choroidal arteries and internal veins of the brain. By removing large areas of the brain, the Fossa lateralis (left) and the lateral ventricles open up. In the Fossa lateralis, the A. cerebri media branches off. In the lateral ventricles, the A. choroidea anterior (coming from the front below; from the A. cerebri interna) and Aa. choroideae posteriores laterales (coming from dorsal; from the A. cerebri posterior) form a plexus of vessels. The inner venous system is shown on the right side in the vicinity of the Tela choroidea of the third ventricle.

- **Pars prevertebralis:** from the A. subclavia (passing at the level of BWK I) to the Foramen transversarium HWK VI
- **Pars transversaria:** within the Foramina transversaria of HWK VI–II
- **Pars atlantica:** from the transition to the atlas and arch of the atlas to the passage through the Foramen magnum
- **Pars intracranialis:** intracranially up to where it joins the A. basilaris

Topography

The **Partes prevertebralis and transversaria** are described in ➤ Chap. 3.3.2. The **Pars atlantica** starts with the outlet of the vertebral artery from the Foramen transversarium of the IInd cervical vertebra. The artery initially forms an arc ('vertebral siphon', reserve length for movements in the atlantoaxial joint), passes through the Foramen transversarium of the first cervical vertebra, then turns dorsally and finally medially via the Sulcus arteriae vertebralis of the posterior atlas. It breaks through the Membrana atlantooccipitalis posterior and reaches the Foramen magnum (➤ Fig. 11.46). This is the start of the **Pars intracranialis**. The A. vertebralis runs dorsally to anteromedially around the Medulla oblongata and joins approximately at the level of the pontomedullary transition to the unpaired A. basilaris. Along its pathway it provides the **A. spinalis anterior** and the **A. inferior posterior cerebelli** (➤ Fig. 11.38, ➤ Fig. 11.39, ➤ Fig. 11.46).

Clinical remarks

A **doppler examination of the A. vertebralis** is quite possible on the atlas (Pars atlantica). It lies there in the depth of a triangle, spanned by three short neck muscles (M. rectus capitis posterior major; M. obliquus capitis superior; M. obliquus capitis inferior). With the head leaning forward, the direction of blood flow through the A. vertebralis can be easily determined.

NOTE

The **A. vertebralis**
- arises as a branch of the A. subclavia at the level of the first thoracic vertebral body
- is divided into 4 anatomical sections: Pars prevertebralis, Pars vertebralis, Pars atlantica, Pars intracranialis
- merges at the level of the pontomedullary junction with the vertebral artery of the opposite side to the unpaired, central A. basilaris
- supplies the brainstem, the cerebellum and the occipitotemporal sections of the brain
- can be examined by ultrasound in the Trigonum arteriae vertebralis

Branches of the A. vertebralis

Along its pathway, the A. vertebralis provides numerous branches to the neck muscles, to the meninges and to the spinal cord (Rr. spinales; ➤ Fig. 11.37). Critical vessels of the intracranial section are:
- **A. inferior posterior cerebelli** (➤ Fig. 11.38, ➤ Fig. 11.46): This artery is considered to be the most variable cerebral vessel, as the origin and extent of the supply area are very different on an individual basis. They can even be missing. As a rule, it emerges from the A. vertebralis at the level of the olive, travels along the brainstem and forms a radiologically very characteristic loop (caudal loop) in the vicinity of the cerebellar tonsils, before passing through the vallecula of the cerebellum (Vallecula cerebelli) vermis and hemispheres of the lower cerebellum (➤ Fig. 11.46). Along its course it supplies parts of the Medulla oblongata and of the posterior and lower cerebellum (posteroinferior parts). There is often also an **A. spinalis posterior** for the supply of the spinal cord. However, this can also originate directly from the A. vertebralis (about 25%).
- **A. spinalis anterior:** It originates just before the confluence of the Aa. vertebrales (➤ Fig. 11.37, ➤ Fig. 11.48), moves caudally and merges approximately at the level of the Foramen magnum with the A. spinalis anterior of the opposite side. It supplies the ventral parts of the spinal cord (see also, vascular supply of the spinal cord).

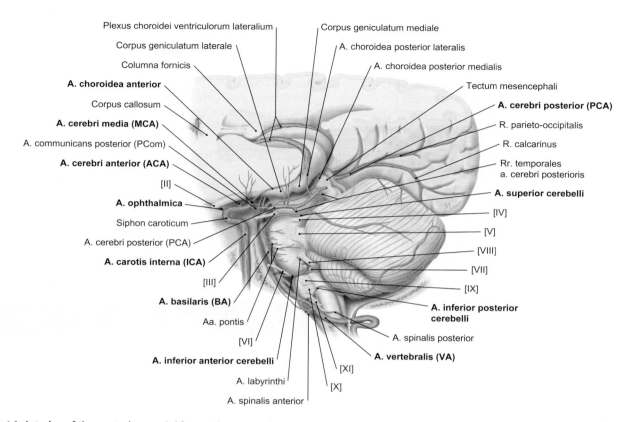

Plexus choroidei ventriculorum lateralium
Corpus geniculatum laterale
Columna fornicis
A. choroidea anterior
Corpus callosum
A. cerebri media (MCA)
A. communicans posterior (PCom)
A. cerebri anterior (ACA)
[II]
A. ophthalmica
Siphon caroticum
A. cerebri posterior (PCA)
A. carotis interna (ICA)
[III]
A. basilaris (BA)
Aa. pontis
[VI]
A. inferior anterior cerebelli
A. labyrinthi
A. spinalis anterior

Corpus geniculatum mediale
A. choroidea posterior lateralis
A. choroidea posterior medialis
Tectum mesencephali
A. cerebri posterior (PCA)
R. parieto-occipitalis
R. calcarinus
Rr. temporales
a. cerebri posterioris
A. superior cerebelli
[IV]
[V]
[VIII]
[VII]
[IX]
A. inferior posterior cerebelli
A. spinalis posterior
A. vertebralis (VA)
[XI]
[X]

Fig. 11.46 Arteries of the posterior cranial fossa. The A. vertebralis, A. basilaris and their branches supply the upper spinal cord, the brainstem and the cerebellum. [L127]

A. basilaris

Topography

The A. basilaris originates from the Aa. vertebrales approximately at the level of the gap between the pons and the Medulla oblongata. It runs along the middle of the pons and its branches supply large parts of the brainstem and the cerebellum. At about the level of the mesencephalon (Cisterna interpeduncularis), it splits back into 2 vessels, the posterior cerebral arteries, **Aa. cerebri posteriores** (➤ Fig. 11.38, ➤ Fig. 11.39).

Branches of the A. basilaris

The branches of the A. basilaris are:

- **A. inferior anterior cerebelli** (➤ Fig. 11.38, ➤ Fig. 11.46): It originates in the lower portion of the A. basilaris and moves posteriorly and externally (posterolateral pathway). In doing so, it usually lies ventrally of the cranial nerves VI, VII and VIII and runs with the N. facialis [VII] and the N. vestibulocochlearis [VIII] to the Meatus acusticus internus. Here it often forms a sling for the outflow of the **A. labyrinthi** (➤ Fig. 11.39). It then moves on to the cerebellum, supplying it underneath and, with branches, the lateral sections of the pons as well. The area of supply of the A. inferior anterior cerebelli depends on the size of the area of supply of the A. inferior posterior cerebelli.
- **Aa. pontis** (➤ Fig. 11.38, ➤ Fig. 11.46): These vessels arise directly from the A. basilaris and supply the ventral portions of the pons as short Rr. mediales or as longer Rr. laterales.
- **A. superior cerebelli** (➤ Fig. 11.38, ➤ Fig. 11.46): This vessel is the least variable small artery. It usually develops shortly before the splitting of the A. basilaris into the Aa. cerebri posteriores. It is first separated from the posterior cerebral artery by the N. oculomotorius [III]. The A. superior cerebelli and the A. cerebri

posterior run parallel laterally and dorsally, while the A. superior cerebelli goes below the tentorium and the A. cerebri posterior above the tentorium. The A. superior cerebelli supplies the upper parts of the cerebellum and, with branches to the brainstem, the dorsal pons.

NOTE

The **A. labyrinthi** runs through the Meatus acusticus internus and supplies the inner ear. As a rule it is a branch of the A. inferior anterior cerebelli, but it can also originate from the other cerebellar arteries or the A. basilaris.

Clinical remarks

Circulatory disorders of the Aa. pontis can cause the motor fibre tracts in the ventral pons to fail and lead to acute paraplegia. Since the dorsal portions of the pons are supplied by branches of the A. superior cerebelli, these sections in which there are important regions for consciousness (e.g. Formatio reticularis) and for eye movements, remain functional.

Locked-in-patients are therefore typically fully aware and not cognitively restricted. They are however completely paralysed and can communicate with their environment only by blinking or eye movements.

The idea of being trapped in one's own body with full mental clarity has led to numerous literary debates on the subject. A famous case is that of the French journalist Jean-Dominique Bauby, who at the age of 43 years suffered a stroke with locked-in syndrome. While in a paralysed state, he wrote the book *Le scaphandre and le papillon* (English: The Butterfly and the Diving Bell) by blinking at letters of the alphabet. He died shortly after the publication of the book.

A. cerebri posterior

The Aa. cerebri posteriores are the terminal branches of the A. basilaris and arise approximately at the level of the Cisterna interpeduncularis (➤ Fig. 11.37, ➤ Fig. 11.38, ➤ Fig. 11.39, ➤ Fig. 11.46). It supplies large parts of the mesencephalon and occipitotemporal parts of the hemispheres with its branches. The Aa. cerebri posteriores run parallel to the Aa. superiores cerebelli laterally and dorsally. They run above the tentorium to the Lobus occipitalis and release several groups of vessels along their pathway. Finally, they branch into their cortical terminal branches, which supply the Lobus occipitalis and parts of the Lobus temporalis and Lobus parietalis (➤ Fig. 11.43, ➤ Fig. 11.46). Branches of the A. cerebri posterior are:

- **Aa. centrales posteromediales** (➤ Fig. 11.37): These vessels emerge from the initial part of the A. cerebri posterior, i.e. before the exit point of the A. communicans posterior. They penetrate – along with the central vascular branches of the A. communicans posterior – through the Substantia perforata posterior and supply large portions of the diencephalon (thalamus, subthalamus, Globus pallidus and the wall of the IIIrd ventricle).
- **Aa. centrales posterolaterales** (➤ Fig. 11.37): These vessels emerge after the exit of the A. communicans posterior from the A. cerebri posterior and supply parts of the diencephalon (epiphysis, thalamus, geniculate body) and mesencephalon.
- **Aa. choroideae posteriores** (➤ Fig. 11.45, ➤ Fig. 11.46): The posterior choroidal arteries are variable in number. They arise after the inflow of the A. communicans posterior and run approximately at the level of the Corpus geniculatum laterale around the diencephalon. Through the Fissura choroidea it reaches the Plexus choroideus of the lateral ventricle, where there are connections to the A. choroidea anterior. Branches of these vessels also supply the Corpus geniculatum laterale, other parts of the thalamus, and the Plexus choroideus of the IIIrd ventricle.

11.5.4 Central blood supply

The inside of the front brain, i.e. the subcortical cores, the medulla with the Capsula interna and the mesencephalon are supplied by central arteries (➤ Fig. 11.37, ➤ Fig. 11.47). Because of their pathway into the depth of the brain, these vessels are known as 'penetrating' vessels. They occur in vascular groups at the base of the brain. If the vessels are removed at this point, numerous small 'holes' remain in the brain tissue, which is why these entry points are referred to as a perforated area (Substantia perforata). A distinction is made between:

- **Substantia perforata anterior:** is located on the Facies inferior of the brain, confined forwards and laterally by the Trigonum olfactorium and to the rear by the Tractus opticus (➤ Fig. 11.19).
- **Substantia perforata posterior:** is located in the depths of the Fossa interpeduncularis of the mesencephalon (➤ Fig. 11.19).

In addition, penetrating vessels also enter the brain tissue in the area of the basal diencephalon. The penetrating vessels are combined in groups to facilitate understanding (➤ Table 11.4):

Table 11.4 Central vessels.

Vessel/vascular group	Entry	Origins	Supply area (including)
Aa. centrales anteromediales	Substantia perforata anterior	• A. cerebri anterior • A. communicans anterior	• Caput nuclei caudati • Globus pallidus • Commissura anterior • Capsula interna
Aa. centrales anterolaterales (Aa. lenticulostriatae)	Substantia perforata anterior	A. cerebri media	• Nucleus caudatus • Putamen • Globus pallidus • Capsula interna (medial vessels)
Aa. centrales posteromediales	Substantia perforata posterior	• A. cerebri posterior • A. communicans posterior	• Thalamus • Hypothalamus • Globus pallidus
Aa. centrales posterolaterales	Substantia perforata posterior	A. cerebri posterior (Pars postcommunicalis)	• Thalamus • Corpus geniculatum mediale • Colliculi • Glandula pinealis

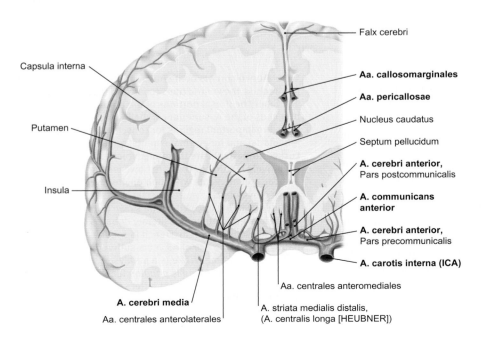

Capsula interna

Putamen

Insula

A. cerebri media

Aa. centrales anterolaterales

A. striata medialis distalis, (A. centralis longa [HEUBNER])

Aa. centrales anteromediales

Falx cerebri

Aa. callosomarginales

Aa. pericallosae

Nucleus caudatus

Septum pellucidum

A. cerebri anterior, Pars postcommunicalis

A. communicans anterior

A. cerebri anterior, Pars precommunicalis

A. carotis interna (ICA)

Fig. 11.47 Central vessels. From the proximal sections of the Aa. cerebrales and the Aa. communicantes, the arteries move into the inner brain. These penetrating vessels are end arteries, which explains why the occlusion of one of these vessels can lead to a cerebral infarction. [L127]

NOTE

The central vessels penetrate basally into the brain and run relatively straight to the dorsal. Accordingly, you can derive the approximate **coverage areas of these central vessels** from the entry point of the vessels and from the location of the core areas to these entry locations:
- anteromedial vessels – anteromedial structures such as the Nucleus caudatus
- anterolateral vessels – anterolateral-lying structures such as the Globus pallidus, Putamen
- posterior vessels – posterior structures such as the Thalamus and Hypothalamus

In addition, portions of the brain's interior are supplied by choroidal vessels. The choroid blood vessels of the lateral ventricles are connected via the Plexus choroideus and form a thin vascular corona or plexus, which connects the tributaries of the A. carotis interna and of the A. vertebralis/basilaris to each other (➤ Fig. 11.45, ➤ Table 11.5).

Clinical remarks

Circulatory disturbances in the area of the A. choroidea anterior lead to a triad of motor, sensory and visual deficits **(Arteria choroidea anterior syndrome):**
- hemiplegia (due to failure of the motor tracts in the Crura cerebri)
- hemisensory disorders (due to failure of the Crus posterius of the Capsula interna)
- hemianopsia (due to failure of the Tractus opticus and parts of the Radiatio optica)

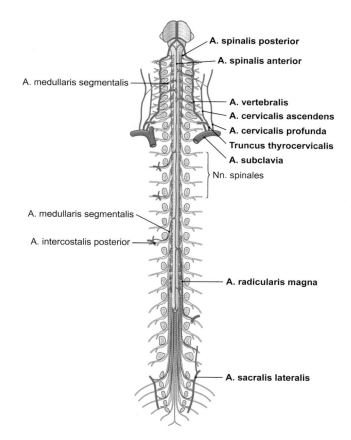

Fig. 11.48 Arteries of the spinal cord. The cervical sections of the spinal cord are supplied by branches of the Aa. vertebrales and in its thoracolumbar sections by branches of the segmental arteries. [E402]

11.5.5 Vascular supply of the spinal cord

The spinal cord is supplied by the following vessels (➤ Fig. 11.48, ➤ Fig. 11.49):
- **A. spinalis anterior** (longitudinal pathway in the Fissura mediana anterior)
- **Aa. spinales posteriores** (paired; longitudinal pathway shortly after the entry point of the Radix posterior)
- **Vasocorona** (transverse connections between spinal arteries on the surface of the spinal cord)

Due to the length of the spinal cord, vessels feed blood at different segment heights into this system (➤ Fig. 11.48).
- **Cervically**, these are the Aa. vertebrales and their branches. The Aa. vertebrales give off a branch ventrally, which becomes the **A. spinalis anterior**. This runs caudally in front of the Fissura spinalis anterior and supplies the anterior horns, the base of the

Table 11.5 Choroidal vessels.

Vessel	Origins	Flow area
A. choroidea anterior	A. carotis interna	• Tractus opticus • Capsula interna (Crus posterius) • Anterior hippocampus • Crura cerebri, Tegmentum mesencephali • Plexus choroideus
Aa. choroideae posteriores	A. cerebri posterior	• Corpus geniculatum laterale • Hippocampus and fornix • Thalamus (posterior sections) • Dorsal mesencephalon • Glandula pinealis

posterior horns and parts of the anterior branch. The Aa. vertebrales can also go into the paired Aa. spinales posteriores (25%). However, these vessels originate far more often from the **A. inferior posterior cerebelli** (normal case). The A. spinalis posterior supplies the posterior threads and posterior horns of the spinal cord. The **vasocorona** mainly forms between these and predominantly supplies the marginal zone on the anterior lateral strands.
- **The thoracolumbar** can, in principle, lead blood to the spinal cord at the level of each spinal nerve (➤ Fig. 11.49). The segmentally created arteries, especially the Aa. intercostales posteriores and the Aa. lumbales, form as branches of their Rr. dorsales, (➤ Chap. 3.3.2) the **Rr. spinales** that enter the spinal canal through the Foramina intervertebralia. There they divide into a R. anterior and a R. posterior, respectively, which lead to the vertebrae and ligaments. A third branch, the **A. medullaris segmentalis**, runs to the structures of the spinal cord. During development and maturation of the spinal cord, approximately 75% of the Aa. medullares segmentales regress and form the thin root arteries, the **Aa. radiculares anteriores and posteriores,** for the supply of the spinal ganglions and the roots. The remaining arteries persist as the Aa. medullares segmentales, providing the Aa. radiculares and reaching the spinal cord with their main branch, which they supply together with the other medullary arteries. The diameter of the Aa. medullares segmentales and their branches can vary. However, at the level of the Intumescentia lumbosacralis, a relatively large root artery is often found, which is often described due to its calibre as the **A. radicularis magna** and usually reaches the spinal cord over the 10th or 11th Foramen interventriculare.

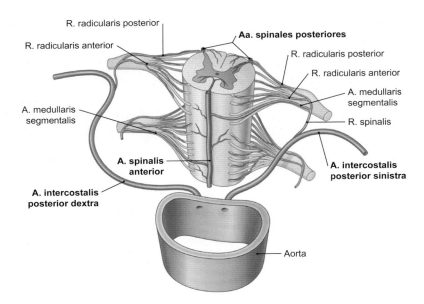

Fig. 11.49 Segmental supply of the spinal cord. The spinal cord is supplied by the A. spinalis anterior (unpaired, middle of the spinal cord), 2 Aa. spinales posteriores (medially of dorsal roots) as well as a vessel circle (vasocorona) between these vessels. At the level of the thoracolumbar, segmental arteries feed blood into this system. [E402]

11.5.6 Topography and supply areas of the arteries

The vasculature supplying the brain is not bound to the lobe boundaries or anatomical structures of the brain. Their names are therefore only an 'approximate' reflection of their situation and their supply areas. In addition, there are significant interindividual differences in the anatomy of the cerebral vessels; in individual cases, the anatomy deviates considerably from the 'standard pathway' of the vessels and their 'standard supply areas' shown here, which explains the variety of neurological deficits in circulatory disorders.

Topography

The anatomical pathway of the individual vessels was described in the previous sections. The most important points are summarised in ➤ Table 11.6. In addition to the descriptions in the Terminologia Anatomica, the arteries are also referred to by the internationally accepted abbreviations based on English-language anatomical terminology, which are used in clinical practice.

Supply areas of the cerebral arteries

The large cerebral vessels supply – with interindividual variations! – characteristic areas of the brain. If there is a reduced blood flow

(ischemia), a combination of neurological symptoms develop that allows conclusions to be drawn about the affected vessel. Knowledge of the supply areas of the arteries is therefore the basis of clinical work. The focus is on the vessels that supply the surface anatomy of the telencephalon, the Capsula interna and the brainstem.

Surface of the telencephalon
The A. cerebri anterior, A. cerebri media and A. cerebri posterior supply the margin of the telencephalon. Their respective supply areas stretch over the Facies superolateralis, Facies medialis and Facies inferior (➤ Fig. 11.50, ➤ Fig. 11.51):
• Direct branches of the **A. carotis interna** supply the pituitary gland, as well as the middle area of the Chiasma opticum. The A. choroidea anterior exiting from it (see below) supplies larger sections within the brain.
• The **A. cerebri anterior** enters the Fissura longitudinalis cerebri anteromedially and runs above the Corpus callosum to approximately the Sulcus parieto-occipitalis. With its branches, it supplies most of the medial surface of the Lobus frontalis and Lobus parietalis, as well as the Corpus callosum (➤ Fig. 11.51). At the Facies superolateralis, it reaches, with its branches, a 2–3 cm wide strip laterally of the hemispheral rim (➤ Fig. 11.50).

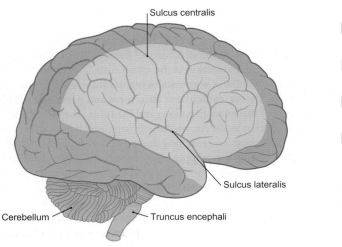

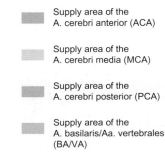

Supply area of the
A. cerebri anterior (ACA)

Supply area of the
A. cerebri media (MCA)

Supply area of the
A. cerebri posterior (PCA)

Supply area of the
A. basilaris/Aa. vertebrales
(BA/VA)

Fig. 11.50 Supply areas of the cerebral arteries (endbrain). Lateral view. [L126]

Table 11.6 Topography of the arteries supplying the brain.

Artery	Topography and special features
A. carotis interna (ICA, 'internal carotid artery')	• Four topographic anatomically defined sections: Pars cervicalis, Pars petrosa, Pars cavernosa, Pars cerebralis • Exit from Sinus cavernosus lateral of the Chiasma opticum
A. ophthalmica	• First major vessel of the A. carotis interna • Emergence below the N. opticus • Passes through the Canalis nervi optici into the eye socket • Anastomosis (A. dorsalis nasi) with A. facialis (A. angularis)
A. choroidea anterior	• Vessel branch of the A. carotis interna • Moves along the Tractus opticus to the inferior horn of the lateral ventricle
A. cerebri anterior (ACA, 'anterior cerebral artery')	• Runs laterally to the Chiasma opticum, to the rostral • Passes to the Fissura longitudinalis cerebri • Runs above the Corpus callosum to the occipital
A. communicans anterior (ACom, 'anterior communicating artery')	• Between the Aa. cerebri anteriores • Location before the Chiasma opticum
A. cerebri media (MCA, 'middle cerebral artery')	• Passes around the Polus temporalis to the Fossa lateralis cerebri • Branching above the insula, leaving the Sulcus lateralis and the pathway of the branches on the lateral surface anatomy of the cerebrum
A. vertebralis (VA, 'vertebral artery')	• Four topographic anatomically defined sections: Pars prevertebralis, Pars transversaria, Pars atlantis, Pars intracranialis • Runs ventrally and forms the A. basilaris (such as the lower rim of the pons)
A. inferior posterior cerebelli (PICA, 'posterior inferior cerebellar artery')	• Exit from A. vertebralis at the level of the olive (but can be missing) • Loop at the level of the cerebellar tonsils (radiological feature) • Entry to the cerebellar valley (Vallecula cerebelli) above the vermis
A. basilaris (BA, 'basilary artery')	• Pathway in the Sulcus basilaris of the pons • Divided into the Aa. cerebri posteriores (approximately at the level of the mesencephalon)
A. inferior anterior cerebelli (AICA, 'anterior inferior cerebellar artery')	• Exit from the lower section of the A. basilaris, ventral of the cranial nerves VI, VII, VIII • Runs to the Meatus acusticus internus with emission of the A. labyrinthi (usually) and from there to the underside of the cerebellum
A. superior cerebelli (SCA, 'superior cerebellar artery')	• Emerges caudally of the N. oculomotorius [III] from the A. basilaris • Runs below the Tentorium cerebelli • Moves posterior to the cerebellum surface
A. cerebri posterior (PCA, 'posterior cerebral artery')	• Emerges cranially of the N. oculomotorius [III] • Runs above the Tentorium cerebelli • Moves posterior to the occipitobasal surface of the cerebrum
A. communicans posterior (PCom, 'posterior communicating artery')	• Connection of the A. carotis interna and A. cerebri posterior • Runs laterally from the hypophysis and Corpora mamillaria

- The **A. cerebri media** enters through the Fossa lateralis and reach the lateral cerebral surface (➤ Fig. 11.50). There it supplies portions of the Lobus frontalis, Lobus parietalis and Lobus temporalis. Their supply area also captures the tip of the Lobus temporalis (Polus temporalis).

- The **A. cerebri posterior** runs to the Lobus occipitalis and supplies on its way large portions of the Facies inferior and Facies medialis of the brain (➤ Fig. 11.51), including the inferior portions of the Lobus temporalis.

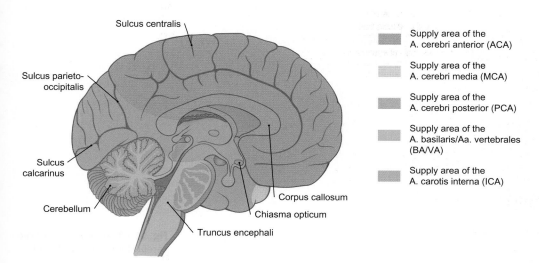

Sulcus centralis

Sulcus parieto-occipitalis

Sulcus calcarinus

Cerebellum

Truncus encephali

Corpus callosum

Chiasma opticum

Supply area of the
A. cerebri anterior (ACA)

Supply area of the
A. cerebri media (MCA)

Supply area of the
A. cerebri posterior (PCA)

Supply area of the
A. basilaris/Aa. vertebrales
(BA/VA)

Supply area of the
A. carotis interna (ICA)

Fig. 11.51 Supply areas of the cerebral arteries (endbrain).
Medial view. [L126]

From the **surface anatomy of the telencephalon** the A. cerebri anterior supplies the anterior two-thirds of the medial surface of the cortex, the A. cerebri media two-thirds of the lateral surface, and the A. cerebri posterior the inferior and occipital surfaces.

Capsula interna and central sections of the telencephalon and diencephalon

The supply of the central telencephalon areas is of particular clinical significance. The fibre tracts from the cortex are bundled and pass between the basal core areas (Nucleus caudatus, thalamus, Globus pallidus, putamen) through the Capsula interna. It is clear that a lack of blood flow in this 'bottleneck' causes severe neurological deficits. Due to the considerable expansion of the Capsula interna in the longitudinal direction of the brain, but also in the dorsobasal direction, several central groups of vessels contribute to their supply. These arise from the A. cerebri anterior, the A. cerebri

Table 11.7 Vascular supply to the Capsula interna.

Capsula interna	Arteries	Origins
Crus anterius	Aa. centrales anteromediales	A. cerebri anterior
	A. striata medialis distalis (A. centralis longa; A. recurrens HEUBNER)	A. cerebri anterior
	Aa. centrales anterolaterales	A. cerebri media
Genu	Aa. centrales anterolaterales	A. cerebri media
Crus posterius	Aa. centrales anterolaterales	A. cerebri media
	A. choroidea anterior	A. carotis interna

media and the A. carotis interna (➤ Table 11.7; ➤ Fig. 11.52, ➤ Fig. 11.53). The anterior limb (Crus anterius) is supplied by branches of the A. cerebri anterior and the A. cerebri media and the knee (genu) and anterior portions of the posterior limb (Crus

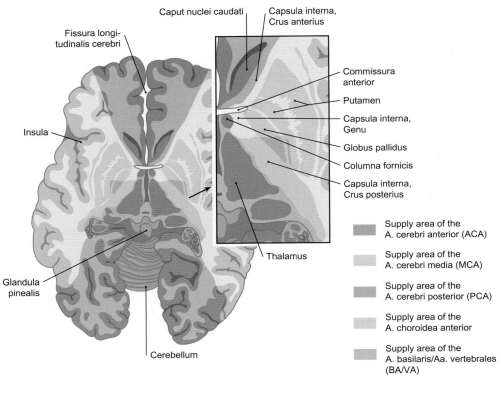

Fig. 11.52 Supply areas of the cerebral arteries (endbrain). Horizontal section. [L126]

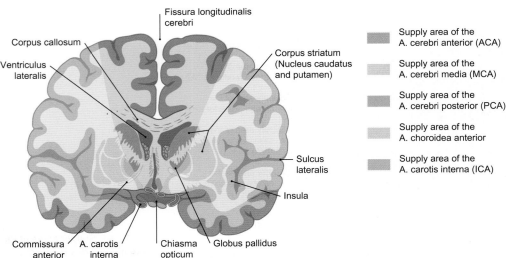

Fig. 11.53 Supply areas of the cerebral arteries (endbrain). Frontal section. [L126]

posterius) by branches of the A. cerebri media. Further occipitally located sections of the hind branch reach the **A. choroidea anterior**, an important central branch of the A. carotis interna. They move into the inner brain and supply central areas of the brain: Crus posterius of the Capsula interna, hippocampus, amygdala and deep cores of the telencephalon and diencephalon (➤ Fig. 11.52, ➤ Fig. 11.53). Their supply area varies greatly.

Clinical remarks

In the case of **a stroke or bleeding in the area of the Capsula interna,** two vessels are very frequently involved:
- A branch of the A. cerebri anterior (part of the Aa. centrales anteromediales): A. striata medialis distalis (syn.: A. centralis longa, A. recurrens, HEUBNER-arteries)
- A branch of the A. cerebri media (part of the Aa. centrales anterolaterales): A. lenticulostriata

---

Brainstem and cerebellum
The brainstem and cerebellum are supplied by branches of the vertebasilar system. It is important to understand that the Aa. cerebellares are not only important for cerebellar care, but also play a crucial role in the supply of the brainstem.

Brainstem
A medial and a lateral supply area can be differentiated on the brainstem. The medial supply area is reached by direct branches of the A. vertebralis, A. basilaris or the A. cerebri posterior, while the lateral supply area is fed by branches of the cerebellar arteries (which, in turn, originate from the vertebrobasilar system). In the Medulla oblongata a posterior supply area can still be delineated; here, the A. spinalis posterior supplies portions of the dorsal medulla. The vessels supplying the brainstem are listed in ➤ Table 11.8 and ➤ Fig. 11.54.

Table 11.8 Arterial supply of the brainstem.

Brainstem section	Medial supply area	Lateral supply area
Mesencephalon	A. cerebri posterior	• A. superior cerebelli • A. cerebri posterior
Pons	A. basilaris (Aa. pontis)	• A. superior cerebelli • A. inferior anterior cerebelli (very variable)
Medulla oblongata	• Aa. vertebrales • A. spinalis anterior • Aa. spinales posteriores	A. inferior posterior cerebelli

Table 11.9 Arterial blood supply of the cerebellum.

Artery	Cortical area	Central area
A. superior cerebelli (SCA; constant)	Upper part of the cerebellum	Nucleus dentatus
A. inferior anterior cerebelli (AICA; variable)	Rear lower part of the cerebellum	
A. inferior posterior cerebelli (PICA; variable)	Front lower part of the cerebellum	The rest of the cores

Table 11.10 Arterial blood supply of the spinal cord.

Artery	Cortical area
A. spinalis anterior	Front horn, base of the dorsal horn, parts of the anterior strand
Aa. spinales posteriores	Rear lower part of the cerebellum
Vasocorona	Border areas of the anterior strand

Cerebellum
The cerebellum is supplied by three arteries. The **A. superior cerebelli** is formed consistently and supplies the upper part of the cerebellum and the Nucleus dentatus. The 2 other small cerebral arteries, the **A. inferior anterior cerebelli** and the **A. inferior posterior cerebelli**, supply the rest of the cerebellum, where they are interdependent in size (i.e., they 'compete' for the rest of the area, hence an increase in, for example, the A. inferior anterior cerebelli leads to a reduction in the A. inferior posterior cerebelli). Unlike the telencephalon, there are anastomoses in the cerebellum between the superficial and central arteries; this reduces the risk of isolated central infarction. The anatomical contexts in the cerebellum (as a rule) are summarised in ➤ Table 11.9 and ➤ Fig. 11.54.

Spinal cord
The supply of the spinal cord can be subdivided into the areas of the A. spinalis anterior, Aa. spinales posteriores and vasocorona. The supply areas are summarised in ➤ Table 11.10 and ➤ Fig. 11.55.

Clinical remarks

An ischemia in the area of the A. spinalis anterior leads to a classic neurological syndrome (**anterior spinal artery syndrome**) with:
- cross-sectional symptoms below the lesion (spinal shock in the early phases/spastic paralysis in later stages; disorders

---

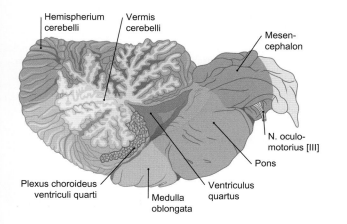

Hemispherium cerebelli — Vermis cerebelli — Mesencephalon — N. oculomotorius [III] — Pons — Ventriculus quartus — Medulla oblongata — Plexus choroideus ventriculi quarti

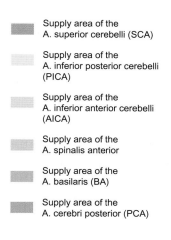

■ Supply area of the A. superior cerebelli (SCA)

■ Supply area of the A. inferior posterior cerebelli (PICA)

■ Supply area of the A. inferior anterior cerebelli (AICA)

■ Supply area of the A. spinalis anterior

■ Supply area of the A. basilaris (BA)

■ Supply area of the A. cerebri posterior (PCA)

Fig. 11.54 Supply areas of the cerebral arteries (brainstem and cerebellum). Sagittal section. [L126]

of the bladder and rectum function) due to the failure of the anterior horns and the anterior lateral strands
- Disorders of pain and temperature perception (lateral strand) in the event of preserved touch and vibration perception (posterior strand); so-called dissociated sensory disturbance. Reason: failure of the anterior lateral strand in the event of an intact posterior strand

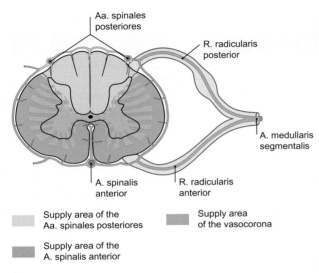

Supply area of the Aa. spinales posteriores

Supply area of the vasocorona

Supply area of the A. spinalis anterior

Fig. 11.55 Supply areas of the spinal cord. Cross-section. [L126]

11.5.7 Clinical description of the vascular sections

In clinical medicine (especially in the Sciences of neurology, psychiatry, neurosurgery and neuroradiology), an alphanumeric nomenclature of the vascular sections of the large cerebral vessels has been adopted in addition to the anatomical designation of the vessels. Due to their clinical relevance, these designations are summarised in ➤ Table 11.11 and juxtaposed with the anatomical terms. For the subdivision of the A. carotis interna, this textbook uses the updated segment name of Bouthillier et al. (1996), which follows the flow of blood of the A. carotis interna and has found its way into the clinical nomenclature of neuroradiology in recent years.

11.5.8 Venous sinuses of the brain

Overview
The venous system of the brain (➤ Fig. 11.40, ➤ Fig. 11.59) takes a back seat in clinical importance compared to the arteries. There are however some important conditions that mainly affect the venous blood vessels of the brain. The pathways of the veins are also important for neurosurgery.
The venous blood vessels can be divided into 2 groups:
- **Sinus durae matris** (➤ Fig. 11.59)
- **Veins**
  - surface of the brain
  - internal areas of the brain
Both have characteristic features compared to the veins of the rest of the body:

Table 11.11 Clinical (radiological) names of the vessel sections of the major blood vessels supplying the brain.

Artery	Segment	Topography/anatomical structures
A. carotis interna, ICA = internal carotid artery	C1 – 'Cervical'	Cervical part
	C2 – 'Petrosal'	Pars petrosa until the end of the Canalis caroticus
	C3 – 'Lacerum'	Up to a ligament between Lingula sphenoidalis and the apex of the Os petrosus ('Lig. petrolingualis')
	C4 – 'Cavernosus'	In the Sinus cavernosus up to the exit point of the dura below the Proc. clinoideus
	C5 – 'Clinoidal'	Between the Proc. clinoideus anterior and the base of the Os sphenoidale
	C6 – 'Ophthalmica'	Up to the outlet of the A. communicans posterior; outlet of the A. ophthalmica
	C7 – 'Communicans'	Up to the bifurcation of the ACI in the Aa. cerebri anterior and media
A. cerebri anterior, ACA = anterior cerebral artery	A1	Pars precommunicalis; from its starting point up to the outlet of the A. communicans anterior
	A2	Pars postcommunicalis; from the A. communicans anterior up to the outlet of the A. callosomarginalis; also: Pars infracallosa
	A3	Pars postcommunicalis; distal from the outlet of the A. callosomarginalis (A. pericallosa); some authors differentiate even more segments (A4 and A5)
A. cerebri media, MCA = middle cerebral artery	M1	Pars sphenoidalis; from its outlet up to where it branches into 2 or 3 main branches
	M2	Pars insularis; in the Fossa lateralis, above the insula
	M3	Pars opercularis; in the Fossa lateralis to lateral routed branches on the cortical surface
	M4	Pars terminalis; after the vessels leave the Sulcus lateralis
A. cerebri posterior (PCA, posterior cerebral artery)	P1	Pars precommunicalis; from its outlet up to the A. communicans posterior; passes through the Cisterna interpeduncularis
	P2	Pars ambiens; from the A. communicans posterior up to the outlet of the Rr. temporales anteriores (upper Cisterna ambiens)
	P3	Pars quadrigeminalis; from the anterior temporal branches up to where it splits into the Aa. occipitales medialis and lateralis (upper Cisterna quadrigeminalis)
	P4	Pars calcarinus; terminal branches: Aa. occipitales medialis and A. occipitalis lateralis
A. vertebralis, VA = vertebral artery	V1	Pars prevertebralis
	V2	Pars transversaria
	V3	Pars atlantis
	V4	Pars intracranialis

- no venous valves
- often run independently of the arteries
- no typical Tunica media (isolated muscle cells), thereby have thin walls (veins)
- rigid walls of the Sinus durae matris, thus protected against a collapse

Drainage of the blood from the brain
Exit points
Venous blood vessels (➤ Fig. 11.40, ➤ Fig. 11.59) are connected to each other and also with extracranial veins. To put it simply, the blood flows from the veins on the surface and inside the brain into the Sinus durae matris. From there, it leaves the inside of the skull in various ways. Important exit points are:
- Sinus sigmoideus to the V. jugularis interna (Foramen jugulare) → the most important!
- Sinus cavernosus via the Foramen ovale to the Plexus pterygoideus
- Vv. emissariae to the V. occipitalis (Foramina emissaria)

In addition, there are smaller intracranial veins that drain into extracranial veins via openings at the base of the skull (including venous outflows via the Foramen magnum, the Foramen ovale, and the Canalis caroticus).

Emissary veins
The Vv. emissariae connect the Sinus durae matris with the diploic veins (= larger venous blood conductors within the diploë of the skull bones) and with the extracranial veins. Because they have no venous valves, they allow for rapid pressure equalisation between internal and external fluctuations in intracranial pressure. Emissary veins can be found in several Sinus durae matris (➤ Fig. 11.40).

Venous anastomosis to the V. facialis
The Sinus cavernosus receives inflows from the Vv. ophthalmicae. These are connected with the V. angularis of the V. facialis via the Fissura orbitalis superior and the Fissura orbitalis inferior. Under certain conditions, the venous blood from the inside of the skull can flow away via these veins to the V. facialis and then to the V. jugularis interna (➤ Fig. 11.40).

Clinical remarks

Because the veins and Sinus durae matris have no venous valves, the blood can also flow into the brain (reverse flow of blood). As a result, infections from the soft tissue of the head are dragged into the Sinus durae matris, e.g. an infection of the upper lip can lead to a bacterial cavernous Sinus thrombosis via the V. angularis.

Veins
Endbrain and diencephalon
A distinction is made between superficial veins, **Vv. superficiales cerebri**, which collect the blood from the surface of the brain, and deep veins, **Vv. profundae cerebri**, via which the blood flows off from the central brain areas:

Superficial veins
Vv. superficiales cerebri drain the blood from the surfaces of the endbrain and diencephalon in the Sinus durae matris (➤ Fig. 11.59, ➤ Fig. 11.60). A distinction is made between three groups that are connected to each other via strong venous anastomoses:

Table 11.12 Venous inflows to the V. magna cerebri.

Vein	Most important inflows	Areas of the brain
V. interna cerebri	V. choroidea superior	Plexus choroideus, Hippocampus
	V. septi pellucidi	Septum pellucidum
	V. thalamostriata	Nucleus caudatus
V. basalis	V. anterior cerebri	Corpus callosum and adjacent gyri
	V. profunda cerebri	Putamen, Globus pallidus

- **Vv. superiores cerebri:** direct inflows to the Sinus sagittalis superior (➤ Fig. 11.59, ➤ Fig. 11.60).
- **V. media cerebri:** collects blood from veins in the vicinity of the Sulcus lateralis; outflow into the Sinus sphenoparietalis and from there into the Sinus cavernosus
- **Vv. inferiores cerebri:** direct inflows to the Sinus transversus

Superficial veins that flow directly into the Sinus durae matris must cross the surface of the brain via the subarachnoid space and pierce the arachnoid and dura to join the Sinus durae matris. They are therefore referred to as **'bridging veins'** (➤ Fig. 11.60). This venous bleeding can lead to a subdural haematoma (➤ Chap. 11.3.5).

Deep veins
Vv. profundae cerebri collect the blood of the central areas and finally lead via the unpaired V. magna cerebri into the Sinus rectus (➤ Fig. 11.61). From each side, the V. magna cerebri receives 2 main inflows each: the **V. interna cerebri** leads blood dorsally from the medullary body and the central cores; the **V. basalis** leads blood basally from the areas at the base of the brain and its central regions:
- **V. interna cerebri:** originates at the level of the Foramen interventriculare due to the confluence of several veins (➤ Table 11.12). In the roof of the IIIrd ventricle it runs to the occipital and joins below the splenium of the Corpus callosum with the V. interna cerebri of the opposite side to the unpaired V. magna cerebri (➤ Fig. 11.61).
- **V. basalis:** originates in the area of the Substantia perforata anterior from several venous tributaries (➤ Table 11.12), including from the basal cortical areas, the insula and dorsally neighbouring central regions. It flows around the Crus cerebri and into the V. magna cerebri or the V. interna cerebri (➤ Fig. 11.61).
- V. magna cerebri (vein of **GALEN**): originates from the confluence of the Vv. internae cerebri and Vv. basales below the splenium of the Corpus callosum (➤ Fig. 11.61). If the veins flow together into one place, this is called the Confluens venosus posterior. The great cerebral vein, V. magna cerebri, is only about 1 cm long and leads blood to the Sinus rectus. At its junction with the sinus, it is attached to the dura.

Clinical remarks

The outflow of blood through the venous system is responsible for the occurrence of **'altitude sickness'**. This occurs in up to 25% of people who go without acclimatisation within a short space of time to a height of 2,500 m. Patients complain especially about headache, dizziness and nausea. Pathophysiologically, it is assumed that the arterial blood flow to the brain is increased to maintain the oxygenation of the brain at a lower partial pressure of oxygen. The larger amount of blood must drain off through the veins, thereby being significantly

---

widened, causing a headache. The more difficult it is for the blood to drain due to the individual anatomy of the venous system, the more the cerebral veins clog up and the more likely headaches are at high altitude.

Brainstem and cerebellum

The venous drainage of the brainstem and cerebellum form numerous anastomoses on the brain surface. As an overview, you can note:

- rostral parts (mesencephalon, upper pons, rostral cerebellum): drain rostrally into the V. basalis, V. magna cerebri, Sinus rectus
- middle parts (pons, lower cerebellum sections): drain laterally into the Sinus durae matris
- caudal parts (Medulla oblongata): drain laterally and caudally to the Sinus durae matris as well as to the spinal venous plexuses

Spinal cord

The veins of the spinal cord form numerous anastomoses at its surface. They connect via the **Vv. radiculares** with the venous plexus of the epidural gap, the **Plexus venosus vertebralis internus**. This venous plexus drains its blood via the Plexus venosus vertebralis externus into the Vv. intervertebrales and from there into the V. cava inferior.

The Vv. radiculares are closely related to the arachnoidea in the root pouches. The cerebrospinal fluid can be reabsorbed via the arachnoid villi, as well as in the Granulationes arachnoideae of the Sinus durae matris. Thus, the spinal cord veins play an important role in CSF circulation.

Table 11.13 Pathway of the Sinus durae matris.

Sinus durae matris	Pathway and characteristics
Sinus sagittalis superior	• Attachment to Falx cerebri up to Protuberantia occipitalis interna • Pathway is anterior–posterior in the Sulcus sinus sagittalis of the skull bones • Bridging veins drain into it or its lateral lacunae • Flows into the Confluens sinuum
Sinus sagittalis inferior	Pathway on bottom edge of the falx to the Sinus rectus
Sinus rectus	Formation at the connection point where the falx and tentorium meet the Sinus sagittalis superior and V. magna cerebri
Confluens sinuum	Confluence of Sinus transversi, Sinus rectus, Sinus sagittalis superior and Sinus occipitalis
Sinus occipitalis	• Lies in the midline of the Os occipitale • Flows toward the Confluens sinuum
Sinus marginalis	• Surrounds the Foramen magnum • Connected to Sinus occipitalis and Plexus venosus vertebralis internus
Sinus transversus	From the Confluens sinuum which emerges from the Os occipitale laterally to the Sinus sigmoideus
Sinus sigmoideus	S-shaped pathway via Pars mastoidea of the Os temporale to the Foramen jugulare and to the V. jugularis
Sinus cavernosus	• Chambered venous space on both sides of the Sella turcica • Connected via the Plexus basilaris on the clivus with the Sinus cavernosus on the opposite side • Topographically very important region (see 'Note' box)
Sinus petrosi superior and inferior	• Pathway at the top or bottom edge of the Pars petrosa ossis temporalis • Connection of the Sinus cavernosus with the Sinus sigmoideus

Sinus durae matris

The venous blood from the cerebral veins flows into the Sinus durae matris (➤ Fig. 11.59, ➤ Table 11.13). These blood vessels lie between the two layers of the Dura mater (➤ Fig. 11.27). They are therefore rigid walls and do not collapse. On the inside, they are lined with endothelium. The Sinus durae matris are directly adjacent to the cranial bones and form shallow pits on their surface. In idealised graphical representations, the Sinus durae matris are often depicted as large, smooth tube systems (➤ Fig. 11.59). They actually arise from intradural venous networks that have joined together. Therefore, there are Corpus callosum structures within the tubes as well as larger lateral lacunae and venous plexuses (➤ Fig. 11.60, ➤ Fig. 11.27). The internal structure of the Sinus durae matris is therefore uneven and there are considerable inter-individual differences.

The venous blood predominantly takes 2 pathways:

- either dorsally to the Confluens sinuum and from there via the Sinus rectus and Sinus sigmoideus to the V. jugularis
- or forward basally to the Sinus cavernosus and via the Sinus petrosi superior and inferior to the V. jugularis (and the Plexus pterygoideus)

N O T E

- running through the **Sinus cavernous**: A. carotis interna, N. abducens [VI]
- running in the lateral wall of the sinus: N. oculomotorius [III], N. trochlearis [IV] and N. ophthalmicus [I]

Clinical remarks

Thrombosis of the Sinus durae matris (Sinus thrombosis) is a rare and serious disease of the brain. This can occur through purulent infections of the face (septic Sinus thrombosis), but also spontaneously when there is an increased tendency for blood to clot (e.g. polycythaemia, but also through the negative impact of contraceptives). The patients suffer from headaches, seizures, paralysis and clouding of consciousness. The diagnosis is made with imaging (MRI, CT).

11.5.9 Presentation of the vasculature

The pathway of the cerebral vessels and the formation of the collateral supply in the area of the Circulus arteriosus are individually different. In the event of an operation it is therefore important to know the individual blood flow situation of a patient before the time, both for the benefit–risk decision and for the surgical planning. Examples are operations on vessels leading to the brain (e.g. operation of a carotid) or intracranial vascular surgery (e.g. aneurysm, angioma).

Angiography, angio-CT and angio-MRI

For the presentation of the vessels, there are various methods. The classic method is the **angiography** (or the digital subtraction angiography). To this end, a catheter is inserted into the A. carotis interna or the A. vertebralis, and an iodine, water-soluble contrast agent is injected as a bolus. Several successive recordings show the blood flow in the arteries, capillaries and veins. A second method is the **angio-CT**, in which an iodine-containing contrast agent is injected into the vein in order to be able to differentiate the vessels more clearly from the tissue. In neuroradiology, this procedure currently plays a rather subordinate role. In contrast, the **an-**

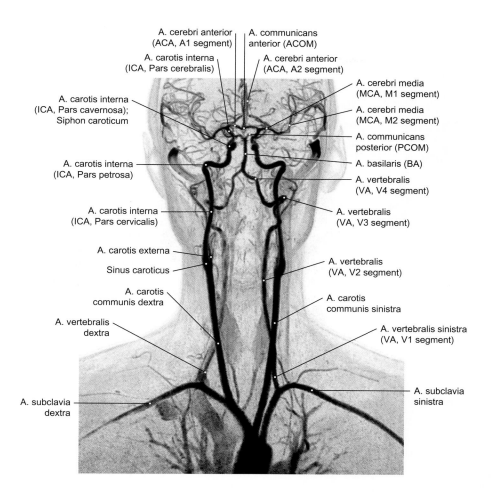

A. cerebri anterior
(ACA, A1 segment)

A. carotis interna
(ICA, Pars cerebralis)

A. communicans
anterior (ACOM)

A. cerebri anterior
(ACA, A2 segment)

A. cerebri media
(MCA, M1 segment)

A. carotis interna
(ICA, Pars cavernosa);
Siphon caroticum

A. cerebri media
(MCA, M2 segment)

A. communicans
posterior (PCOM)

A. carotis interna
(ICA, Pars petrosa)

A. basilaris (BA)

A. vertebralis
(VA, V4 segment)

A. carotis interna
(ICA, Pars cervicalis)

A. vertebralis
(VA, V3 segment)

A. carotis externa

A. vertebralis
(VA, V2 segment)

Sinus caroticus

A. carotis
communis dextra

A. carotis
communis sinistra

A. vertebralis
dextra

A. vertebralis sinistra
(VA, V1 segment)

A. subclavia
sinistra

A. subclavia
dextra

Fig. 11.56 Magnetic resonance angiography of the arteries supplying the brain. Overview. [T786]

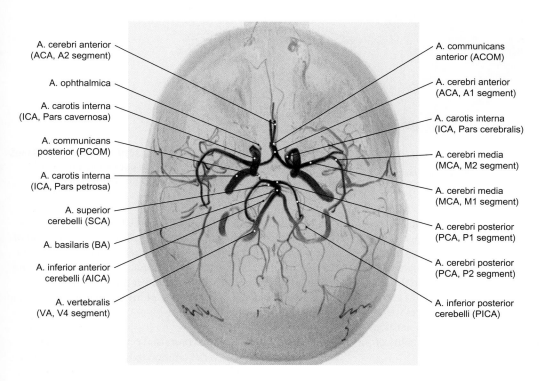

A. cerebri anterior
(ACA, A2 segment)

A. ophthalmica

A. carotis interna
(ICA, Pars cavernosa)

A. communicans
posterior (PCOM)

A. carotis interna
(ICA, Pars petrosa)

A. superior
cerebelli (SCA)

A. basilaris (BA)

A. inferior anterior
cerebelli (AICA)

A. vertebralis
(VA, V4 segment)

A. communicans
anterior (ACOM)

A. cerebri anterior
(ACA, A1 segment)

A. carotis interna
(ICA, Pars cerebralis)

A. cerebri media
(MCA, M2 segment)

A. cerebri media
(MCA, M1 segment)

A. cerebri posterior
(PCA, P1 segment)

A. cerebri posterior
(PCA, P2 segment)

A. inferior posterior
cerebelli (PICA)

Fig. 11.57 Magnetic resonance angiography of the arteries supplying the brain. Caudal view. [T786]

631

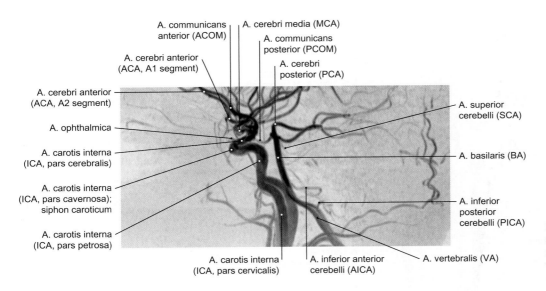

A. communicans anterior (ACOM)
A. cerebri anterior (ACA, A1 segment)
A. cerebri anterior (ACA, A2 segment)
A. ophthalmica
A. carotis interna (ICA, pars cerebralis)
A. carotis interna (ICA, pars cavernosa); siphon caroticum
A. carotis interna (ICA, pars petrosa)
A. carotis interna (ICA, pars cervicalis)
A. cerebri media (MCA)
A. communicans posterior (PCOM)
A. cerebri posterior (PCA)
A. superior cerebelli (SCA)
A. basilaris (BA)
A. inferior posterior cerebelli (PICA)
A. inferior anterior cerebelli (AICA)
A. vertebralis (VA)

Fig. 11.58 Magnetic resonance angiography of the arteries supplying the brain. Lateral view, presentation of the Siphon caroticum. [T786]

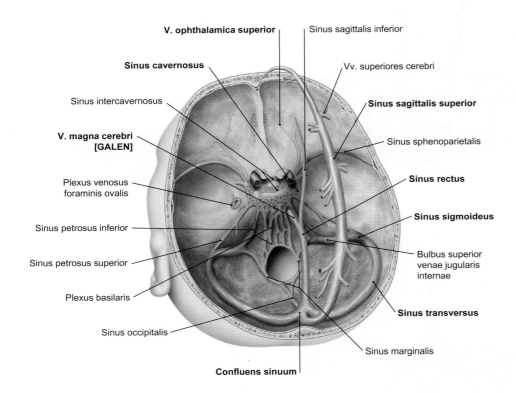

V. ophthalamica superior
Sinus cavernosus
Sinus intercavernosus
V. magna cerebri [GALEN]
Plexus venosus foraminis ovalis
Sinus petrosus inferior
Sinus petrosus superior
Plexus basilaris
Sinus occipitalis
Confluens sinuum
Sinus sagittalis inferior
Vv. superiores cerebri
Sinus sagittalis superior
Sinus sphenoparietalis
Sinus rectus
Sinus sigmoideus
Bulbus superior venae jugularis internae
Sinus transversus
Sinus marginalis

Fig. 11.59 Diagram of the Sinus durae matris in a projection onto the cranial base.

gio-MRI has grown in popularity in the past few years, and is increasingly used. In this procedure, which can be performed with or without MRI contrast agent (iodine-free contrast agent), the cerebral vessels are displayed in three dimensions with high resolution. In this way, the doctor will also gain an insight into the anatomical–topographic relationships (➤ Fig. 11.56, ➤ Fig. 11.57, ➤ Fig. 11.58). It is conceivable that 'stronger' MRI devices (devices with higher magnetic field strengths) and advances in calculation algorithms of MRI data will further improve the quality of the scan.

Ultrasound examination of the vessels supplying the brain

A standard method for the examination of the blood vessels supplying the brain is the Doppler ultrasound. With this technique, the speed of blood flow in vessels can be determined to verify ste-

noses, vascular spasms or of a flow reversal. Combining the Doppler ultrasound with the ultrasound image ('B-scan'; conversion of echo intensity into shades of grey and thereby visualising anatomical structures), is called a 'duplex ultrasound' because 2 ultrasound methods (Doppler and B-scan) are used at the same time. In the duplex ultrasound, the flow direction of the blood is often colour-coded ('Colour Doppler').

Duplex ultrasound of the extracranial cerebral vasculature

The duplex ultrasound is very common in the investigation of the A. carotis and its branches. Stenosis or calcification in the Sinus caroticus or in the proximal A. carotis interna, as well as a decreased blood flow, can thus be detected. The A. carotis interna is distinguished from the A. carotis externa in that it has no vascular branches in the neck area. Using a Doppler ultrasound, a flow re-

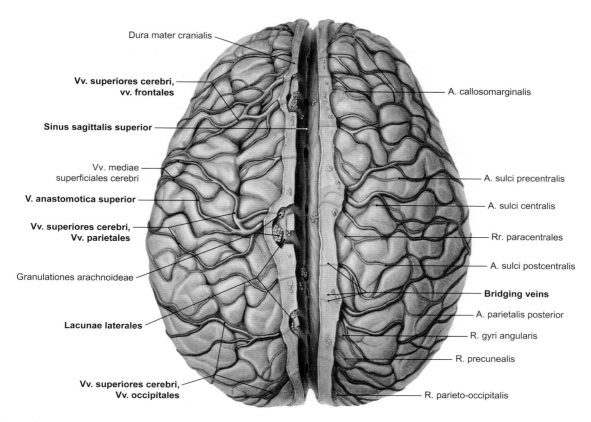

Dura mater cranialis

Vv. superiores cerebri, vv. frontales

Sinus sagittalis superior

Vv. mediae superficiales cerebri

V. anastomotica superior

Vv. superiores cerebri, Vv. parietales

Granulationes arachnoideae

Lacunae laterales

Vv. superiores cerebri, Vv. occipitales

A. callosomarginalis

A. sulci precentralis

A. sulci centralis

Rr. paracentrales

A. sulci postcentralis

Bridging veins

A. parietalis posterior

R. gyri angularis

R. precunealis

R. parieto-occipitalis

Fig. 11.60 Superficial veins of the brain, bridging veins, Granulationes arachnoideae, Sinus sagittalis superior.

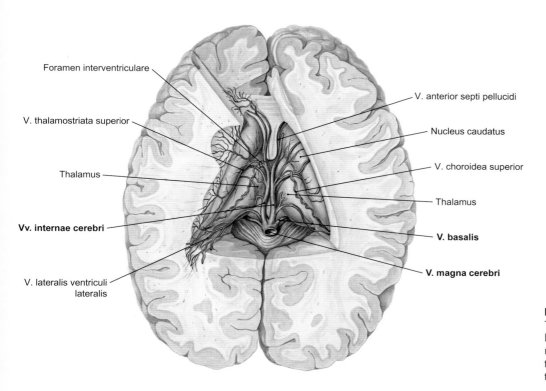

Foramen interventriculare

V. thalamostriata superior

Thalamus

Vv. internae cerebri

V. lateralis ventriculi lateralis

V. anterior septi pellucidi

Nucleus caudatus

V. choroidea superior

Thalamus

V. basalis

V. magna cerebri

Fig. 11.61 Deep cerebral veins.
The blood from the inside of the brain runs through the Vv. internae cerebri and Vv. basales into the V. magna cerebri and from there into the Sinus rectus.

633

versal in the A. vertebralis (Trigonum arteriae vertebralis on the atlas) or in the A. angularis (corner of the eye) can be demonstrated. In the A. angularis, a reverse flow means that the blood that normally flows from the A. angularis into the A. facialis now flows into the A. ophthalmica and from there into the A. carotis interna. The flow reversal in the A. angularis indicates an occlusion of the A. carotis interna.

Doppler ultrasound of intracranial brain vessels
With the ultrasound you can – despite considerable loss of sound – also examine vessels in the skull when the skull bone is thin enough. Important 'sound windows' in this case are:

- the temporal 'sound window' (through the Squama ossis temporalis) for the study of the initial sections of the Aa. cerebri and the intracranial section of the A. carotis interna
- the nuchal 'sound window' (through the Foramen magnum) for the study of the intracranial sections of the Aa. vertebrales and the A. basilaris
- the orbital 'sound window' (through the orbita) for the study of the A. ophthalmica

The transcranial doppler examination also allows the detection of vasospasm of cerebral vessels, for example as a result of a subarachnoid haemorrhage. In acutely ill patients with a subarachnoid haemorrhage, a transcranial examination is therefore carried out on a daily basis as 'vascular monitoring'.

12 Special neuroanatomy

12.1 Telencephalon

Skills

After working through this chapter, you should be able to:
- provide the classification of the telencephalon by its parts, and name the division criteria
- explain the essential fibre connections of the brain and their function
- describe the parts of the neocortex
- explain the position and function of the primary and secondary cortical areas of the individual lobes
- define hemisphere dominance and examples of the clinical impact (in neurological/psychiatric terms)
- identify the macroscopic hippocampus and fimbria-fornix on frontal and horizontal sections and explain their relationship to the ventricular system
- name the areas belonging to the so-called hippocampal formation and describe the signal flow through the hippocampal formation
- indicate the cingulate cortex and its parts in a dissection and talk through your basic knowledge about its function
- indicate the areas of the paleocortex and olfactory cortical areas on the dissection
- explain the connections of the paleocortex with other areas of the brain, especially the limbic system
- explain the position and function of the most important subcortical nuclei and identify them on sections of the brain from a wide range of orientations
- explain, based on the knowledge acquired relating to neuronal configurations within the basal ganglia, the symptoms of PARKINSON's and HUNTINGTON's diseases

12.1.1 Overview
Tobias M. Böckers

The **telencephalon (endbrain, cerebrum)** describes the two **cerebral hemispheres** (Hemispheria cerebri), the **subcortical nuclei** (Nuclei basales) and the **Substantia alba** (pulp of the cerebrum) in the respective cerebrum area. The telencephalon makes up around 80% of the total mass of the human brain, with the grey matter mainly located on the surface anatomy (Cortex cerebri). The grey matter of the cortex, together with the underlying white matter, is referred to as the **pallium**.

Macroscopic examination shows the telencephalon as being by far the greatest part of the brain surface. Even at first glance, the two hemispheres of the brain can be distinguished, separated from each other by the **Fissura longitudinalis cerebri**. Their **hemispheral rim** make the two hemispheres protrude into the Fissura longitudinalis cerebri. The duplication of the Dura mater (Falx cerebri) is embedded within this fissure; on the floor of the fissure, the Corpus callosum is visible. The 6 lobes of the endbrain are distinguished as being separated by other prominent sulci (➤ Chap. 11.2.3, ➤ Fig. 11.16, ➤ Fig. 11.17, ➤ Fig. 11.18):

The endbrain is the youngest portion of the human brain and provides the basis for special human intellectual capacities. It controls language and communication, provides the central control for intentional movements and sensitivity, and it controls or influences the emotions. It is also the part of the brain that is essential for the development of awareness, as well as for memory.

12.1.2 Embryology
Tobias M. Böckers

The telencephalon develops from the **telencephalic vesicles**, which are further differentiated into 2 lateral telencephalic vesicles. These completely grow over the rest of the brain in a ventrocaudal direction in a C-shaped growth curve and remain medially separated by the Fissura longitudinalis. As a result, parts of the lateral cortex are displaced deep into the Sulcus lateralis. This part of the brain is referred to as the insula area; the overlapping brain layers, in particular the frontal lobes, are also called the **opercula**. In later foetal development, the Lobus frontalis can be distinguished from the parietal, temporal and occipital lobes. These cortical areas are initially smooth and then become increasingly gyrified, i.e. the characteristic gyri and sulci of the brain surface are formed; these significantly enlarge the cortex. In the course of development, bundles of fibres grow out of the hemispheres, respectively reaching the corresponding areas of the other hemisphere. These tracts are also known as **commissural tracts** and connect the right and left hemispheres **(Corpus callosum, Commissura anterior, Commissura fornicis)**. In the context of the movement of growth, the lumina of the telencephalic vesicles also expand to reach the winding lateral ventricles of the hemispheres, which are connected via the Foramina interventricularia with the IIIrd ventricle of the diencephalon.

The **subcortical nuclei** are formed from the basal plate in the ventral section of the side wall of both hemispheres. After a massive regional cell division, a swelling (ganglionic hill) arises here, which further develops into the Corpus striatum.

12.1.3 Classification of the telencephalon
Tobias M. Böckers

The telencephalon, due to morphological criteria (the minute structure of the cortex/stratification), can be divided into 3 sections: **neocortex (isocortex)**, **archicortex** and **paleocortex**. The basis for this classification is the comparison of animal brains at various levels of the biological system (i.e. different levels of evolutionary development). This comparative anatomical approach also allows conclusions to be drawn on how the human brain has developed through evolution and which parts of the brain are phylogenetically (Greek: phylon = stem, and genesis = origin) the 'oldest' and the 'youngest'. A phylogenetically older part can thus be demonstrated in the brains of simpler mammals, whereas phylogenetically younger parts of the brain can only be found in the brains of more advanced mammals and, in some cases, only in the human brain (➤ Fig. 12.1).

- Due to histological criteria, the **neocortex** (➤ Chap. 12.1.5) is also referred to as the isocortex. Its volume has greatly increased in the course of human development, so the paleocortex has been shifted to the cranial base and the archicortex likewise to the mediobasal side of the brain. The functions of the neocortex are complex and include motor, sensory and associative tasks. The neurons in these cortex units form predominantly 6 layers.
- The predominantly 3-layered **allocortex** can be further divided into the following sections:
  - The **archicortex** (➤ Chap. 12.1.6) particularly describes parts of the hippocampal formation and histologically shows a 3-layered structure. The archicortex is a younger section of the cortex, tasked with controlling the vegetative functions and learning and memory.
  - The **paleocortex** (➤ Chap. 12.1.8), consists mainly of sections of the olfactory brain, particularly at the base of the brain. This also show a predominantly 3-layered structure.

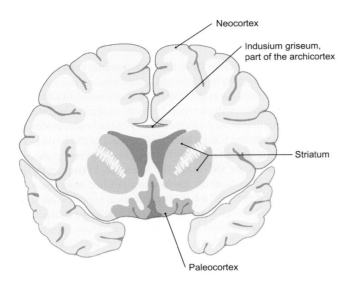

Fig. 12.1 Parts of the telencephalon. [L126]

In addition to these parts of the cortex, developing from the telencephalon there are also the **subcortical nuclei** (Chap. 12.1.9). Amongst them are the striatum (consisting of the Nucleus caudatus and Putamen), of the Nucleus accumbens, the claustrum and parts of the Globus pallidus. Chap. 12.1.9 also describes the amygdala and the Nucleus basalis MEYNERT.

> **N O T E**
> On the basis of histological-morphological and comparative-anatomic criteria, the **cortical sections of the telencephalon** are divided into 3 parts:
> - The **neocortex** is predominantly made up of 6 layers (isocortex) and is by far the largest part of the telencephalon.
> - The **archicortex** includes the largely 3-layered parts (allocortex) of the limbic system.
> - The **paleocortex** is also mostly 3-layered (allocortex) and essentially encompasses the olfactory brain.
> In addition, this includes the subcortical nuclei, embryologically formed from the telencephalon vesicles.

12.1.4 Fibre systems of the telencephalon
Tobias M. Böckers

Cortical and nuclear areas of the telencephalon are in close contact with each other, so that the fibres under the cortex or between the cortex and other parts of the CNS take up a great deal of space (**Substantia alba**, white matter). Because of the source and target structures of the fibre strands, we differentiate between association fibres (Fibrae associationes), commissure fibres (Fibrae commissurales) and projection fibres (Fibrae projectiones) (➤ Fig. 11.23, ➤ Chap. 11.2.5).

Due to their length, **association fibres** can be divided into additional subgroups (➤ Fig. 11.23a):
- short, so-called U-fibres (**Fibrae arcuatae cerebri breves**) connect with adjacent gyri,
- slightly longer fibre strands (**Fibrae arcuatae cerebri longae**) connect gyri which are located further away and
- long association tracts can connect lobes of the same hemisphere.

Examples can also be seen in dissections in the **Fasciculus longitudinalis superior**, connecting the gyri of the Lobus frontalis and the

Lobus parietalis with the Lobus occipitalis. The **Fasciculus longitudinalis inferior** creates the connection between the Lobus temporalis and Lobus occipitalis; the **Fasciculus uncinatus** is found between the Lobus frontalis and the Lobus temporalis; the **Fasciculus arcuatus** connects amongst other things the sensory language area with the motoric BROCA's area (➤ Fig. 11.23a).

The important **commissure tracts** are the Corpus callosum, the Commissura anterior and the Commissura fornicis (➤ Fig. 11.23b):
- The **Corpus callosum** is about 10 cm long and connects the Lobi frontalis, parietalis and occipitalis of the two hemispheres with each other. At the Corpus callosum we can distinguish a front knee (genu) with a tapering Rostrum corporis callosi, a mid trunk and a thickened rear bulge (Splenium). The trunk is connected to the fornix and the Septum pellucidum. The fibre strands turn off sharply in the Corpus collossum, becoming the Forceps frontalis minor (passing in the Lobus frontalis) in the front portion and the Forceps occipitalis major in the rear portion.
- The **Commissura anterior** is in close proximity topographically with the rostrum of the Corpus collossum or the front wall of the IIIrd ventricle and contains, amongst other things, the fibres of the olfactory system.
- The **Commissura fornicis** is the commissural connection of the leg portions of the fornix. Fibre bundles of the hippocampi of both hemispheres pass through this connection.

The **projection fibre systems** form a fibre compartment, also called a **Corona radiata** (fibre strands from or to the cortex). These fibre connections are joined together in the area of the basal nuclei and are canalled through the subcortical nuclear areas at defined points (somatotope classification). The highest density of the projection fibres can be found in the Capsula interna between the Globus pallidus, the thalamus and the Nucleus caudatas. The Capsula interna is divided into a front leg (Crus anterius), a rear leg (Crus posterius) and a knee (genu). The respective fibres pass through the **Capsula interna** to defined points and remain arranged in a somatotopic order. Important descending fibres form the pyramidal tract (➤ Chap. 13.1); large ascending tract systems originate in particular from the thalamus as thalamocortical projections (➤ Chap. 13.2). The **Capsula externa**, a thin plate made of white matter, is situated between the Nucleus lentiformis and the claustrum, and laterally to the claustrum (up to the insular cortex) there is another fine plate of fibre, the **Capsula extrema**.

12.1.5 Neocortex
Tobias M. Böckers

General
The **neocortex (isocortex)** is the uniformly-designed, predominantly 6-layer endbrain cortex, which, in its evolutionary development as a primate has undergone an impressive increase in volume compared to the other parts of the brain. In humans, it accounts for about half of the brain's weight – approximately 90% of all cortex areas of the brain are designed to be isocortex. Overall, the area of the cortex in humans is approximately 2,200 cm².

Functionally, the neocortex is divided into centres, of which the interplay implements the perceptions of all aspects of external stimuli and/or leads to motivated actions. However, the definition of the functional fields serves as a very simplified way of explaining the extremely complex capabilities of the human brain:
- **Primary fields** describe cortex areas, receiving sensory information directly from the thalamus and creating awareness (with the

exception of the olfactory system). They are therefore the primary point at which the corresponding sensory tracts end (e.g., auditory pathway, visual pathway). The Gyrus precentralis is a primary motor field from which direct movement is initiated via the Tractus corticospinalis (pyramidal tract).

- **Secondary fields** are often located directly next to the primary fields. Here, the primary information is processed and brought up to the next level of integration. The information is thus, for example, interpreted and allocated, and the first consequences of what has been experienced are initiated here. In terms of action, movements, for example, are planned and motivated here.
- Polymodal **association fields** are not explicitly allocated to a primary centre, but reciprocally interconnected with several other primary and secondary centres. We can suppose that here, for example, the various experiential components being experienced are reassembled.

Lamination of the isocortex

The cerebral cortex is usually approximately 4 mm thick, but in the primary visual cortex, for example, it is only 2 mm. The laminar **six-layer structure** is best presented in histological dissections that are cut perpendicular to the cortex surface. NISSL-staining is a suitable dyeing method (staining the nuclei and the NISSL-substance), as is myelin-staining (colouration of the myelin), showing such laminations as being either cytoarchitectonic or myeloarchitectonic (➤ Fig. 12.2). The layers are numbered from outside to inside:

- **Molecular layer (Lamina molecularis, lamina I):** In this layer, there are only isolated neurons (no pyramidal cells), with extensions running parallel to the surface anatomy of the cortex and

synaptic contacts. The Pia mater is attached to the Lamina molecularis via a superficial layer (Membrana limitans gliae superficialis). In this layer, small, so-called CAJAL-RETZIUS cells can be identified. These play a special role in the formation and lamination of the cortex (expression of Reelin).

- **Outer nuclear layer (Lamina granularis externa, lamina II):** Characteristically, these are tightly packed, small 'non-pyramidal cells' (mainly GABAergic nuclear cells) with short apical dendrites. In addition, there are a few glutamatergic pyramidal cells.
- **Outer pyramidal layer (Lamina pyramidalis externa, lamina III):** We can distinguish 3 sublaminae with an increasing number of small pyramidal cells (IIIa–c). Apical dendrites can extend up to lamina I, ending as an 'apical cluster'. The laminae IIIa and IIIb are affected in certain neurodegenerative diseases (e.g., particularly in ALZHEIMER's disease).
- **Internal nuclear layer (Lamina granularis interna, lamina IV):** As in the lamina II, here there are small, tightly-packed non-pyramidal cells (nuclear cells) which receive their primary afferents from the thalamocortical neurons.
- **Internal pyramidal layer (Lamina pyramidalis interna, lamina V):** in this layer can be found pyramidal cells of varying sizes, which are very large in some cortex areas and are also called **giant BETZ cells**. The axons of these glutamatergic neurons have strong myelin sheaths, and in the Gyrus precentralis they form the corticospinal and corticonuclear tracts.
- **Multiform layer (Lamina multiformis, lamina VI):** This layer is often divided into the lamina VIa with a high cell density and a lamina VIb which has fewer neurons. Smaller pyramidal cells of varying morphology can be found here.

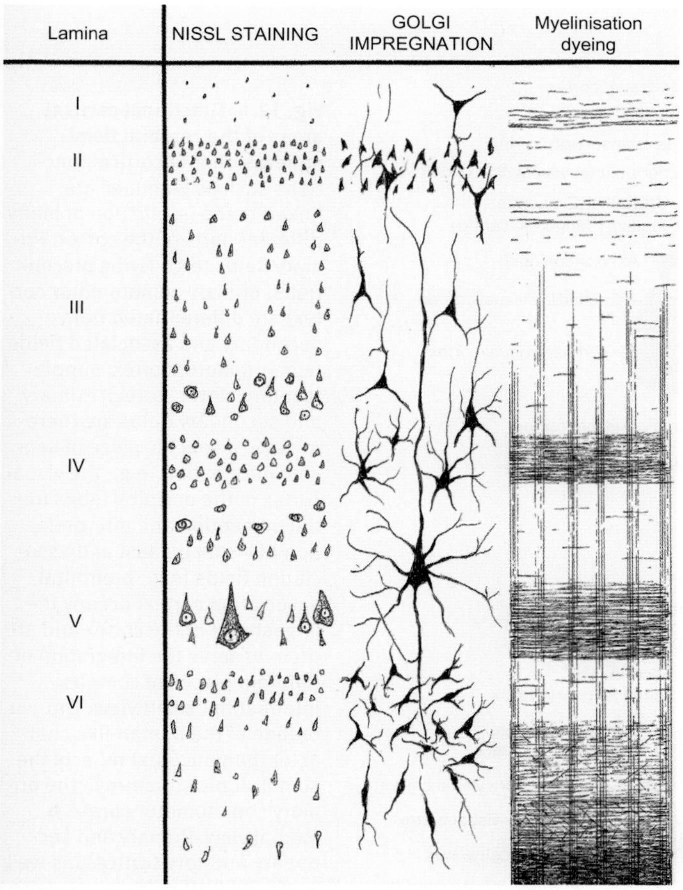

Cortical areas

The essentially uniform layered structure of the isocortex is derived from an initially smooth cortical plate with progenitor cells for neurons and glial cells. The subsequent changes in embryonic development are determined by ingrowing axons and then by the migratory movements of the cortical neurons (proneurons): early developing neurons can be found later in deep layers of the isocortex, with later developing neurons in higher layers (e.g., in the later layer II). This type of layer formation is also known as **'inside-out layering'**.

The six-layered structure of the isocortex may vary significantly: the individual layers can vary in width, and the cells within them can differ in size and density. The layered structure of the human brain has been laboriously analysed, so that areas with equal architectonic layers have been defined, thus creating a mapping of the isocortex, leading to what are known as the **BRODMANN areas** (numbered consecutively) starting at the Gyrus postcentralis, ➤ Fig. 12.3). The individual cortical areas are not only morphologically/histologically similar, but also assume functionally similar tasks. Interestingly, in the cortical fields that serve as projection fields (e.g., the auditory cortex), there are clearly visible granule cell layers, which are almost absent in the motor cortex.

An even smaller unit in the structure of the isocortex is that of fine cell columns, which pass through the layers of the isocortex and are made up of a network of around 100 neurons. These are referred to as **primary modules** and can be grouped into larger organisational units, which thus form larger functional units.

Classification of the neocortex

The neocortex is divided by the well-developed primary grooves (➤ Table 12.1 into 5 externally visible lobi (the 6th Lobus limbicus is only visible through a midline incision through the Corpus cal-

Lamina	NISSL STAINING	GOLGI IMPREGNATION	Myelinisation dyeing

Fig. 12.2 Six-layered structure of the neocortex. [L240/S010-2-16]

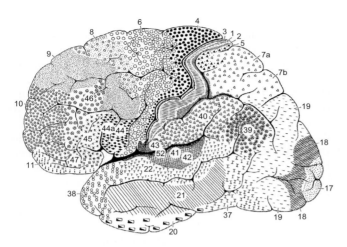

Fig. 12.3 Classification of the brain according to histological criteria (known as the BRODMANN areas). [S010-2-16]

Table 12.1 Primary grooves of the cortex.

Sulcus	Position/course
Sulcus centralis	Runs between the frontal and parietal lobes; thereby separating the (motor) Gyrus precentralis from the (sensory) Gyrus postcentralis
Sulcus lateralis	Separates the frontal, parietal and temporal lobes from each other; the Fossa lateralis and insula lie in the depth
Sulcus parieto-occipitalis	Passes from the Margo superior cerebri on the medial hemisphere area up to the Sulcus calcarinus; separates parietal and occipital lobes
Sulcus calcarinus	Runs like the Sulcus parieto-occipitalis on the medial surface, limiting the cuneus
Sulcus cinguli	Separates the Gyrus cinguli (Lobus limbicus) of the frontal and parietal lobes

losum on the Facies medialis of the cerebrum. It includes the Gyrus cinguli located on the Facies mediales, as well as its continuation on the Facies inferior, the Gyrus parahippocampalis, which is separated by the Sulcus collateralis from the Lobus temporalis):

- Lobus frontalis (frontal lobe)
- Lobus parietalis (parietal lobe)
- Lobus temporalis (temporal lobe)
- Lobus occipitalis (occipital lobe)
- Lobus insularis (insular lobe)

Lobus frontalis

The **frontal lobe (Lobus frontalis)** extends from the frontal pole of the brain to the Sulcus centralis. It can be divided into 3 main areas: the primary motor cortex (BRODMANN area 4), premotor cortex (BRODMANN area 6) and prefrontal areas (including BRODMANN areas 9–12, ➤ Fig. 12.3).

Primary motor cortex

The primary motor cortex corresponds to the Gyrus precentralis, which is directly adjacent to the Sulcus centralis and extends via the Margo superior cerebri to the Fissura longitudinalis cerebri. Within this gyrus, the impulses for the voluntary motor functions are located, which are canalled via the pyramidal tracts (➤ Chap. 13.1) into the periphery of the motor cranial nerve nucleus and the anterior horn cells in the spinal cord. The Gyrus precentralis has a

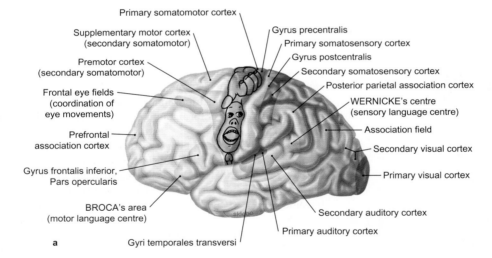

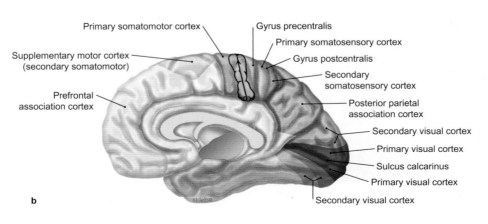

Fig. 12.4 Functional cortical areas of the cerebral hemispheres. Higher cortical functions such as language are linked to the interaction of many different parts of the cortex. Primary fields (e.g., Gyrus precentralis, primary somatomotor cortex) are differentiated from secondary and associated fields (e.g., premotor cortex, supplementary motor cortex). Primary and secondary fields are there to serve a specific piece of sensory information (e.g., the visual cortex in the occipital lobes for the perception and interpretation of visual pulses) and association fields (e.g., prefrontal association cortex) occupy the largest part of the cortex and are there to serve the integration of different pieces of complex information. **a** Left view. The outline of the human-like character (homunculus) reflects the somatotopic structure in the primary somatomotor cortex. **b** Medial view. Primary and secondary auditory cortices, as well as the WERNICKE's area, extend over the top of the temporal lobe, to its inner surface.

clear somatotope structure, which is also referred to as the homunculus and which, for example, illustrates the particularly strong representation of hand and facial muscles (➤ Fig. 12.4). Amongst others, this area receives afferents from the thalamus, the premotor areas, as well as the somatosensory cortical fields.

Premotor cortex

The premotor cortex (area 6) should functionally be a centre for the selection and planning of movement programmes, which are then transmitted to the motor cortex to be implemented. It is additionally assumed that motor programmes are registered in this area, for example, based on the learnt interaction between basal ganglia, the cerebellum and cortex units.

Within the premotor cortex (sometimes also as a separate cortical area), the **frontal eye fields (area 8)** can be delineated, which is crucial for the initiation and planning of conjugated eye movements (eye adjustment movements).

In the Gyrus frontalis inferior of the left (in approximately 95% of people) frontal lobe, the **BROCA's language area** is found in the Pars opercularis and partially in the Pars triangularis. This centre is activated by the concept of sentences and words, terminology, but not the control of speech itself (premotor cortex). Verbal understanding is located in the so-called **WERNICKE's area (area 22)** (located at the transition of the Lobus temporalis [see below] to the Lobus parietalis).

> ### Clinical remarks
>
> With unilateral stimulation, the frontal eye field guides eye movement to the contralateral side. **Lesions of the frontal eye field** (e.g., due to hemorrhage or tumours) which are associated with unilateral failure of area 8, will lead to a deviation of both bulbi to the affected side **(déviation conjugée)**; 'The patient views the lesion.' In failures of the BROCA language area (e.g., within the context of a cerebral infarction) language production is severely limited **(BROCA's aphasia)**. However, the ability to name objects and also to understand speech often remains intact. Syntax in affected patients is often incorrect and there are mistakes with articulation.

Prefrontal area

The prefrontal area (prefrontal cortex) encapsulates the cortex areas rostral of the premotor cortex (up to the Polus frontalis) and is closely associated with the higher intellectual, mental and social performance of the human brain. It seems that here, located in this brain area, are values, ideals and ethical behaviour, as well as the highest parts of cognitive performance such as combinatorial and methodical thinking (and also the development of motivation for actions).

Lobus parietalis

The **parietal lobe (Lobus parietalis)** extends dorsally from the Sulcus centralis to a line defined by the Sulcus parieto-occipitalis. This sulcus is very easily seen on the median side of the brain and it continues on the lateral side. There are several sensory areas in the Lobus parietalis:

- Extending directly behind the Sulcus centralis – parallel to the Gyrus precentralis – the **Gyrus postcentralis** (➤ Fig. 12.4) reaches similarly over the Margo superior cerbri into the Fissura longitudinalis cerebri. This gyrus (S1, BRODMANN areas 3, 1, 2) is the primary somatosensory cortical field of the body. The proprioceptive and somatosensory information from the skin of the opposite side of the body end here, because the associated tract systems cross

over to the opposite side before making contact with various places in the area of the thalamic nuclei (Nucleus ventralis posterior thalami, ➤ Chap. 12.2.3) (➤ Chap. 13.3). As with the Gyrus precentralis, a somatotopy and variable representation of the skin areas are found on the Gyrus postcentralis. The visualisation of these projections is referred to as (somatosensory) homunculus.

- Behind the Gyrus postcentralis, a **secondary sensory cortical field** connects (S2), which is also somatopically divided and is especially significant for the interpretation of the sensitive stimuli.
- In addition, it connects with the Gyrus postcentralis or with the secondary cortical field of the **posterior parietal association cortex** (areas 5 and 7). It receives a wide variety of afferents from other primary and secondary sensory areas and should in particular be meaningful for orientation in a three-dimensional space (non-dominant side).
- The cortical area under the Sulcus intraparietalis and/or around the **Gyrus angularis** (area 39), and the **Gyrus supramarginalis** of the dominant hemisphere is also referred to as the 'mathematical cortex', as here, amongst other things, the ability to deal with numbers is especially represented. The Gyrus angularis seems to be an important connection point between visual and audio information. Accordingly, damage in this area is associated with reading and/or writing problems.
- The **primary vestibular cortex** is delineated close to the Gyrus postcentralis in the hand and mouth area. The afferents from the vestibular nuclear areas of the brainstem terminate here; these can be switched via thalamic nuclear areas (➤ Chap. 13.5).

Lobus temporalis

The **temporal lobe (Lobus temporalis)** is located under the Fissura lateralis of both cerebral hemispheres and merges rostrally without a clear delimitation into the Lobus parietalis.

- An important area in the temporal lobe can be found on the dorsal surface of the Gyri temporales transversi. These are 2 transverse turns, which are also referred to as **HESCHL's gyri** (area 41). This area represents the primary auditory cortex (➤ Fig. 12.4). Terminating here is the auditory system (➤ Chap. 13.4), which, based on relative frequencies, is represented tonotopically on special cortex areas. Lower frequencies are thus located rostrolaterally, with higher frequencies caudomedially along the Fissura lateralis. Its function as the primary cortical field involves perception of auditory stimuli, but these are not interpreted (words are not perceived, for example); moreover, a variable activation could be shown if there are varying sound intensities.
- Lateral to the HESCHL's gyri is the **secondary auditory cortex**, which receives its primary afferents from the primary auditory cortex. In these areas, sound takes on high levels of meaning: tones become melodies, words or phrases. With regard to the two hemispheres, it should be noted that the **WERNICKE's area** is located in the dominant hemisphere; it is also known as the sensory language area. In particular, the interpretation of language is significant. The appreciation for tunes (non-rational auditory impressions) is notably located in the non-dominant hemisphere.

> ### Clinical remarks
>
> When the damage **to the primary auditory cortex** is only on one side, it has a relatively low impact (e.g., impairment of directional hearing, distinguishing between frequency/intensity). **Failure of the WERNICKE's area (WERNICKE's aphasia)** has a significant impact on speech intelligibility. Language production and intonation are retained, but the spoken words often have no meaning and no sentence structure can be identified.

Lobus occipitalis

Occipital lobe (Lobus occipitalis) is the area of the cortex running from the Sulcus parieto-occipitalis up to the rear pole of the brain. In particular, the occipital lobe represents the cortical areas for the visual system (➤ Chap. 13.3).

- On the medial side of the occipital lobe, there is a sulcus (Sulcus calcarinus), the bordering gyri of which contain the **primary visual centre** or the primary visual cortex (area 17). At the occipital pole, these gyri extend slightly into the convexity of the brain (➤ Fig. 12.4). Macroscopically, the cortex stands out relatively finely and contains a white stripe, also known as the lines of **GENNARI** (or the bundle of VICQ D'AZYR). It is produced by association nerve fibres located in the 4th layer of this isocortex area, and the cortical field is also called the **'Area striata'**. The optic radiation ends in the primary vision centre (afferents are conducted primarily from the Corpus geniculatum laterale), i.e., visual stimuli are consciously perceived here. This primary cortical field receives information from the retina in a clear retinotopic structure, so that each retinal area is assigned to an area in the primary visual cortex. The organisational structure of the cortex into what are called columns is particularly obvious in the visual cortex, because the stimulation of the visual cortex affects an entire column per retinal area, running vertically through all the cell layers.
- Around the primary visual cortex are the **secondary visual cortical areas** (areas 18 and 19), arranged in crescent shapes, which receive their afferents mainly from the primary visual centre (area 17). In these areas, the visual impulses are processed (e.g., recognition, memory) and transferred to other cortical areas. Experimentally, it could be demonstrated that certain areas are particularly activated when perceiving colour, while others are used, for example, for identifying faces.

Clinical remarks

Damage to the primary visual cortex of a hemisphere **(cortical blindness)** causes a homonymous hemianopsia. This means that the visual field of the opposite side completely fails. The consequence of damage to the secondary cortical areas is that the patient receives the visual stimuli, but can 'neither identify nor assign' them **(visual agnosia)**.

Lobus insularis

The **insular lobe (Lobus insularis)** is deeply embedded during embryonic development. Located on the floor of the Fissura (Sulcus) lateralis, it is covered with telencephalic structures, which are also known as the **operculum**, consisting of the Operculum frontale, the Operculum parietale and the Operculum temporale. The insular area is triangular in shape and is divided by a Sulcus centralis insulae into an oral and caudal pole (➤ Fig. 11.17). The insular area at the base of the brain passes into the olfactory brain (paleocortex).

In this area of the brain, it is mostly general **viscerosensory information** that is processed, particularly the taste receptors (➤ Chap. 13.6, ➤ Chap. 13.7), as well as the perception of pain, placement and movement. The insular area is closely related to the Corpus amygdaloideum and the hypothalamus, so that visceromotor information also reaches the brainstem from the insula.

NOTE

Important functional centres in the lobi of the neocortex

- **Lobus frontalis (frontal lobe)**
  - Gyrus precentralis (primary motor cortex, BRODMANN area 4)
  - premotor cortex (BRODMANN area 6) with frontal eye fields (area 8, eye adjusting movements) and BROCA language area.
  - prefrontal areas (including BRODMANN areas 9–12, 'higher brain performance')
- **Lobus parietalis (parietal lobe)**
  - Gyrus postcentralis (primary sensory cortex, S1, BRODMANN areas 3, 1, 2)
  - secondary sensory cortical field (early processing of information)
  - posterior parietal association cortex (areas 5 and 7, polymodal association field)
  - Gyrus angularis (area 39) and Gyrus supramarginalis of the dominant hemisphere ('mathematical cortex')
  - primary vestibular cortex (afferents from vestibular nuclear areas of the brainstem)
- **Lobus temporalis (temporal lobe)**
  - Gyrus temporalis transversi (primary auditory cortex, HESCHL's gyri area 41)
  - Secondary auditory cortex (early processing of information)
- **Lobus occipitalis (occipital lobe)**
  - Sulcus calcarinus (and the bordering gyri form the primary visual centre area 17)
  - secondary visual cortex areas (areas 18 and 19, early processing of information)
- **Lobus insularis (insular lobe)**
  - general processing of viscerosensitive information
  - particularly taste receptors, but also pain, position and movement perception

Hemispheric dominance

At first glance, both cerebral hemispheres function in exactly the same way, but on closer inspection, morphological differences can be seen: secondary gyri and sulci in corresponding cerebrum sections are not distributed symmetrically, and their length, depth and shape is different. Furthermore, the left hemisphere has a larger specific weight and in 70% of cases, the SYLVIAN fissure, the Sulcus lateralis, is broader. In addition, functional differences between the two hemispheres have been established. This is referred to as **hemispheric asymmetry**, which is not only observable in humans, but also in other vertebrates. While many somatosensory and somatomotor functions are allocated symmetrically in the two halves of the brain, BROCA had already observed that the hemisphere containing the 'motor centre for speech' is the opposite one to the preferred (dominant) hand – so for a right-handed person it is in the left half of the brain. This is sometimes also referred to as **hemispheric dominance**. It is probably not innate, but may be created and mainly develops in the course of the first years of life alongside language acquisition. This is also reflected in the fact that it is still possible to learn language even after a cerebral hemisphere has been removed (hemispherectomy). After about the age of 15, the non-dominant side is no longer able to learn new linguistic functions. The generalised rule established by BROCA only applies to approximately 95% of right-handed people and 15% of left-handers. In most left-handers, the language area is also sited in the left hemisphere or, in 15% of them, is created bilaterally. Similarly, it was shown that the posterior cortical area behind the primary auditory cortex, known as the **Planum temporale**, where the sensory language area (WERNICKE's area) is located, has been created asymmetrically and is, in the dominant half of the brain (mainly on the left side), significantly more extensive.

The findings on hemispheric asymmetry and the position of important functional centres are shown in the following studies:

- with what is referred to as the WADA method, a transient, pharmacologically-induced hemispherectomy is performed. This procedure has been used before when performing a hemispherectomy to determine the dominant hemisphere by anaesthetising a hemisphere with a one-sided injection of a sedative into the A. carotis interna.
- with 'split-brain' patients, where the Corpus callosum, acting as a unifying element between the two hemispheres, is severed in an operation (e.g., in order to treat an otherwise unmanageable case of epilepsy). Roger SPERRY examined patients such as these and determined that communication between the hemispheres relating to the impulses received and their processing after the operation, was no longer possible following the operation, and for the 'split-brain' patients typically led to malfunctions (see Clinical remarks).

Additional findings also came from the precise examination of patients with brain lesions in only one hemisphere, which led to specific functional failures. Today, functional MRI provides more options for specific research.

Clinical remarks

The functions of the dominant and non-dominant hemispheres are conveyed via a dense neural network to other cortical areas of the same or contralateral hemisphere, the basal ganglia or to the limbic system. Damage to these connections is referred to as disassociative syndrome. An example of this is **'split-brain' patients,** where the hemispheres independently receive and process pulses. These patients are not significantly restricted in their everyday lives, but in experimental situations, certain dissociative symptoms occur: if the image of an object from the left visual field falls on the right retinal halves of both eyes, split-brain patients are not able to name this item. The information will be routed to the primary visual cortex of the right occipital lobe. After separation of the Corpus callossum, this information can no longer reach the language area located in the dominant (left) hemisphere. However, the patients are able to identify an item placed in the dominant (right) hand.

Lesions of the *dominant* half of the brain often lead to problems with speech, and affect both the planning of complex movements (apraxia) as well as analytical thinking. The *non-dominant* hemisphere participates in speech by forming or perceiving affective elements (e.g. speech intonation). In addition, in lesions of the non-dominant hemisphere there are malfunctions of the non-verbal functions, e.g., visual-spatial thinking (parietal association cortex), the emotional comprehension of language and experience, and the appreciation of music. There is evidence that the non-dominant half of the brain is involved in the processing of new, creative situations, while the dominant half of the brain is used instead for known, analytical, and tried and tested situations. While the left half of the brain primarily controls and processes attentiveness to the contralateral environment field (visual field), the non-dominant half of the brain can also do so bilaterally. Since the contralateral environment is predominantly processed in the frontoparietal cortex, lesions – particularly those in the non-dominant hemisphere of the brain – can lead to **hemispatial neglect syndrome**, meaning that the patients do not perceive the contralateral visual field and, to some extent, cannot even see their own contralateral half of the body.

It is generally accepted that hemispheric asymmetry, or the functional lateralisation of the cerebrum, is more pronounced in men than in women. Here also the concentration of sex hormones (the menstrual cycle in women) is thought to have a modulating effect on the level of lateralisation or interhemispheric communication.

12.1.6 Archicortex
Thomas Deller, Andreas Vlachos

General
The term **archicortex** includes a part of the brain phylogenetically located between the paleocortex and the neocortex. It can be identified in reptiles, birds and mammals. In reptiles, the archicortex is the actual control centre of the endbrain. **Histologically**, the archicortex presents a predominantly three-layered structure. It therefore belongs to the allocortex. The archicortex includes, in particular, the **hippocampal formation** and the **cingulate cortex**. The cingulate cortex is cytoarchitecturally a transition zone between the archicortex and the neocortex and is therefore also sometimes referred to as the periallocortex.

Functionally, the archicortex is important for **learning and memory processes**. It is also part of the **limbic system** and is connected intensively via this with brain areas that are important for the control of autonomic and emotional processes. It affects this area and conversely is also influenced by it.

In clinical medicine and research, knowledge of the anatomy of the hippocampal formation has become increasingly important. The hippocampal formation:
- plays a role in neurodegenerative diseases with memory loss (e.g., in ALZHEIMER's disease)
- is involved in the clinical symptoms of major neuropsychiatric disorders (schizophrenia, depression, autism)
- is associated with a common form of epilepsy, temporal lobe epilepsy (see Clinical remarks).
- serves as a landmark in radiological sectional images of the brain
- due to its relatively simple structure it has become a model in research for the study of the cortex. It can be taken from the brains of young rodents and held in cell cultures (organotypical sectional cultures). These brain cultures ('brain in a dish') continue to mature and can be examined in a targeted manner.

Clinical remarks

Temporal lobe epilepsy (TLE) is a common form of epilepsy. It usually starts with an 'aura' (i.e. sensory interferences that prefigure a seizure, e.g., in the form of unpleasant feelings in the stomach), followed by motor symptoms ('focal' seizures, e.g., in the form of smacking and chewing buccal motions, to movements of the whole body) and loss of consciousness. In the hippocampus of TLE patients, there is typically a 'sclerosis', i.e. a nerve cell death and a proliferation of glial cells. The hippocampal CA1 area ('SOMMER sector') is especially common here. To date, it has not been definitively established whether hippocampus sclerosis is the cause or the consequence of seizures.

TLE does not always respond to drugs. Therefore, in some cases that cannot be treated with medication, parts of the hippocampal formation are removed on one side of the brain ('epilepsy surgery'). This significantly reduces the number of seizures, and some patients are seizure-free after the operation.

Hippocampal formation
Overview and terminology
The term 'hippocampal formation' brings together several cortical areas cytoarchitecturally. According to significant neuroscientific authors, the **hippocampal formation includes:**
- Area entorhinalis (also: 'entorhinal cortex')
- Fascia dentata (also: 'Gyrus dentatus')

- Cornu ammonis (also: 'Hippocampus proprius')
- Subiculum
- Pre- and Parasubiculum

These areas of the brain are largely unidirectionally connected to each other and form a functional unit.

The areas of the hippocampal formation are differentiated by their cytoarchitecture, i.e. their microscopic anatomical structure. The superficially identifiable structures of the brain (gyri, sulci) are variable in shape and are only approximate reference points for the position of these cortical areas (➤ Chap. 12.1.5). The cortical areas of the hippocampal formation are located mainly in the macroscopic hippocampus (= bulging structure at the lower horn of the lateral ventricle), the Gyrus dentatus and the Gyrus parahippocampalis (with uncus). Occipitally, the hippocampal formation becomes thinner and finally continues as a thin layer of grey matter, known as Indusium griseum, on the Corpus callossum.

Development and postnatal neurogenesis

The spatial arrangement of the structures of the hippocampal formation is difficult to understand without reviewing the history of its development. Already in the *9th week of pregnancy,* the hippocampal system is found in the developing cerebral hemispheres in the medial area. In the 2nd trimester *(15th–19th weeks of pregnancy)* there is evidence of the characteristic hippocampus subfields that have completely developed up to the Gyrus dentatus at the end of the pregnancy (approximately the *34th week of pregnancy*). In the Gyrus dentatus, the cell count carries on growing until the 6th month of life, i.e., this cortical area develops to a large extent postnatally.

In the Fascia dentata (Gyrus dentatus), forming new nerve cells is a life-long process. This brain area is regarded as a '**neurogenic niche**' of the CNS. However, the ability to form nerve cells decreases with age. It is estimated that in the adult Fascia dentata, up to 700 new nerve cells are formed each day; this means that approximately 1.75 % of the nerve cells of this brain area could be replaced in the course of a year. The newly formed nerve cells play an important role in memory processes.

The hippocampal formation is very characteristically situated in the lower medial temporal lobe. Its shape is created by an **S-shaped fold in the cortex** (➤ Fig. 12.5). In this folding process, the Fascia dentata comes away from the Cornu ammonis and sits on top of it like a cap. Axons of the entorhinal cortex end up at the Dentata fascia by perforating the underlying layer of the subiculum and the hippocampal fissure, and thus reach the surface of the Fascia dentata (➤ Fig. 12.11); these fibres are referred to as the Tractus perforans ('perforating tract'). This unusual projection tract enables a circular flow of information through the hippocampal formation from the entorhinal cortex to the Fascia dentata, and finally via the subiculum back to the entorhinal cortex. (➤ Fig. 12.11).

Attached to the archicortex, the archipallium continues as the cortical structure for the **rotation of the hemispherical vesicle** (➤ Chap. 11.1). In humans, this shifts the main part of the hippocampal formation into the medial temporal lobes. However, sections of the hippocampus are located above and below the Corpus callosum. Thus the hippocampus continues from the temporal lobes onto the Corpus callosum, forming a thin grey layer (Indusium griseum) and white matter (Striae longitudinales medialis and lateralis); it finally reaches the subcallosal area below the Genu corporis callosi. Below the Corpus callosum, the Fimbria hippocampi forms the fornix (➤ Fig. 12.10).

Clinical remarks

There is evidence that **neuropsychiatric disorders** (e.g., schizophrenia, autistic spectrum disorders) go hand in hand with developmental disorders of the hippocampus (as well as other cortical areas).

Macroscopy

The hippocampal formation lies in the medial temporal lobes and migrates in an arch shape above and along the Corpus callosum. Depending on how they relate to the Corpus callosum, a distinction is made between 3 macroscopic **sections:**
- Hippocampus retrocommissuralis: temporal lobe sections
- Hippocampus supracommissuralis: above the Corpus callosum
- Hippocampus precommissuralis: below the Genu corporis callosi

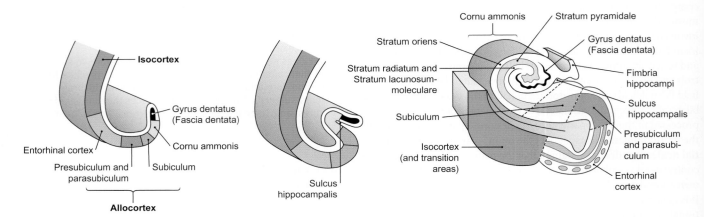

Fig. 12.5 Development of the hippocampal formation. The hippocampal formation is made up of an S-shaped fold of the mediobasal cortex. Fascia dentata = black; Cornu ammonis CA1 = yellow; subiculum complex = green; pre- and parasubiculum = violet; entorhinal cortex = blue; perirhinal cortex = red. [L126]

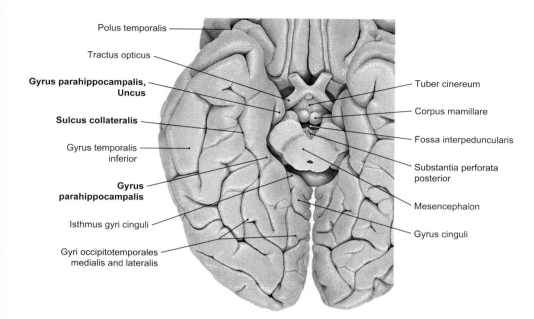

Polus temporalis

Tractus opticus

**Gyrus parahippocampalis,
Uncus**

Sulcus collateralis

Gyrus temporalis
inferior

**Gyrus
parahippocampalis**

Isthmus gyri cinguli

Gyri occipitotemporales
medialis and lateralis

Tuber cinereum

Corpus mamillare

Fossa interpeduncularis

Substantia perforata
posterior

Mesencephalon

Gyrus cinguli

**Fig. 12.6 Ridges (gyri) and
grooves (sulci) of the cerebral
hemispheres.** Ventral view; after
sectioning the mesencephalon.

NOTE
- The hippocampus splits in two around the Corpus callosum: above the Corpus callosum, the grey matter of the hippocampus continues into the Indusium griseum. Below the Corpus callosum, the Fimbria hippocampi continues into the fornix.
- In clinical language (and also in this textbook) we use 'hippocampus' to mean the Hippocampus retrocommissuralis.

Due to their folding (➤ Fig. 12.5), the position of the hippocampal formation can only be partially understood by an analysis of the brain surface ventrally (➤ Fig. 12.6) and medially (➤ Fig. 12.7). Only when opening the lower horn of the lateral ventricle, it becomes possible to view the macroscopically visible hippocampus (➤ Fig. 12.8).

Hippocampal formation from ventral
The **Sulcus collateralis** is located on the ventral side of the temporal lobe, separating the Gyrus occipitotemporalis lateralis from the Gyrus parahippocampalis (➤ Fig. 12.7, ➤ Fig. 12.6). The anterior part of the **Gyrus parahippocampalis** is already a part of the hippocampal formation; the entorhinal cortex is located here. Due to the compact islands of cells in the lamina II of this cortical area, the

brain surface at this point looks bumpy or 'warty' (verrucae) under a magnifying glass.

Hippocampal formation from dorsomedial
In its anterior section, the medial temporal lobe exhibits several smaller gyri and sulci (➤ Fig. 12.7, ➤ Fig. 12.12), making the anatomy of this area relatively complex. These gyri and sulci are frequently observable on the brain surface and are important for neurosurgical procedures in the temporal lobe area.
The Gyrus parahippocampalis is ventromedially delimited by a small hollow, the Sulcus intrarhinalis, from the **Gyrus ambiens**. This, in turn, is separated by the Sulcus semiannularis from the **Gyrus semilunaris**. The Gyrus ambiens and the Gyrus semilunaris contain olfactory cortices and are assigned to the paleocortex (➤ Chap. 12.1.8). Lying caudally of this gyri is the 'hook-shaped' **uncus** of the Gyrus parahippocampalis. The uncus usually raises 3 bulges, referred to from rostral to caudal as the
- Gyrus uncinatus (transition cortex between the hippocampus and the amygdala),
- Limbus GIACOMINI (start of the Gyrus dentatus) and
- Gyrus intralimbicus (CA3 area of the Cornu ammonis)

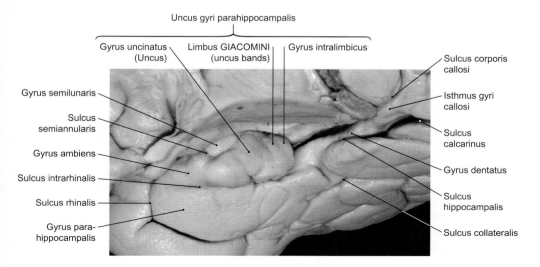

Uncus gyri parahippocampalis

Gyrus uncinatus
(Uncus)

Limbus GIACOMINI
(uncus bands)

Gyrus intralimbicus

Gyrus semilunaris

Sulcus
semiannularis

Gyrus ambiens

Sulcus intrarhinalis

Sulcus rhinalis

Gyrus para-
hippocampalis

Sulcus corporis
callosi

Isthmus gyri
callosi

Sulcus
calcarinus

Gyrus dentatus

Sulcus
hippocampalis

Sulcus collateralis

Fig. 12.7 Temporal lobes. Dorsomedial view. [R247]

645

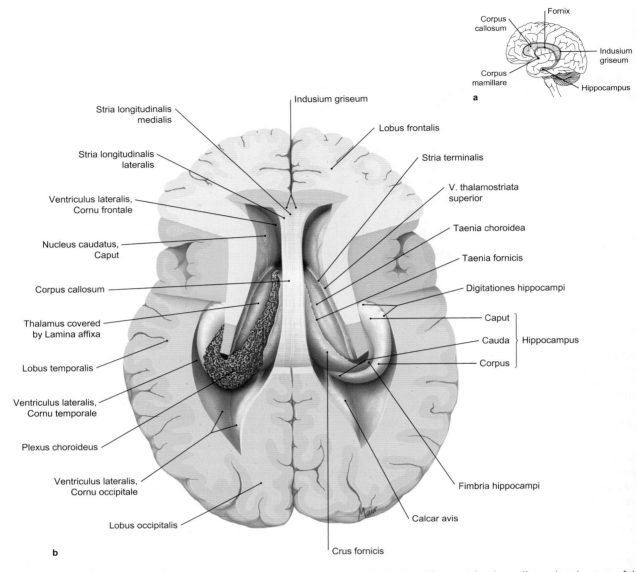

Fig. 12.8 Opened lateral ventricle, hippocampus from dorsal. a Clear presentation of the brain to illustrate the three-dimensional nature of the hippocampus. **b** Top view after opening the lateral ventricles dorsallyl and laterally. The hippocampus lies on the floor of the inferior horn of the lateral ventricle and is covered by the Plexus choroideus on the left. This has been removed on the right side of the illustration. [L127]

Lying deeply caudal of the uncus and medial of the Gyrus parahippocampalis is the Fissura hippocampalis, which is the continuation of the Gyrus dentatus as well as the Fimbria hippocampi. When these structures are followed caudally, we come across 2 horizontally extending bulges, known as the Fasciola cinerea (end of the Gyrus dentatus) and the Gyrus fasciolaris (CA1-area). The latter continues in the Indusium griseum on the Corpus callosum.

Hippocampal formation from dorsal (opened side ventricle)
By opening the side ventricle dorsally and laterally, it is possible to see the cortical bulges that have given the macroscopic hippocampus its name (➤ Fig. 12.8). The hippocampus is thickened at the front (the 'head') and forms the **Pes hippocampi** with multiple elevations, referred to as the **Digitationes hippocampi**. This area is reminiscent of the flipper of the mythological creature, the 'hippocamp.' In its centre, the hippocampus forms a barely structured bulge (the 'body') on the surface anatomy, which extends towards the splenium of the Corpus callosum, becoming thinner (the 'tail'). It passes into the Gyrus fasciolaris and continues into the Indusium griseum. The Fimbria hippocampi is located on the medial side of the hippocampus, aligned with the Fissura hippocampi.

In the macroscopic hippocampus, there are sections of the Fascia dentata, the Cornu ammonis and the subiculum. The characteristic arrangement of these areas can be best understood on frontal sections in the middle of the hippocampus (➤ Fig. 12.9, ➤ Fig. 12.11, see below). Conversely, in the anterior hippocampus, orientation is much more difficult because the hippocampus turns medially here, and therefore some areas on frontal sections have multiple truncations (➤ Fig. 12.9).

Fimbria and fornix (arch)
The axons of the hippocampus form a layer of white matter on its surface anatomy, called the **alveus**. From here they run into the fibre band of the fimbria, located on the hippocampus and the Gyrus dentatus, and which accompanies it caudally (➤ Fig. 12.9, ➤ Fig. 12.10). Below the bar, the fimbria separates from the hippocampus and forms the vaulted columns of fornix, **Columnae fornicis** (➤ Fig. 12.10). Further along, the two Columnae fornices unite, forming the **Commissura fornicis**, in which commissure fibres, as well as other things, interchange between the two hippocampal formations, and more rostrally the **Corpus fornicis**. However, this divides again into 2 columns at the level of the Foramen interven-

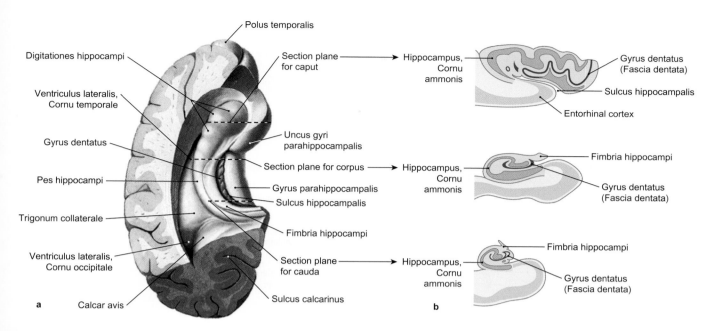

Fig. 12.9 Hippocampus. a Hippocampus in the lower horn of the opened side ventricle. **b** Cross-sections through the hippocampus in the area of the head, body and tail. Differences in the arrangement of the principal cells are notable. In the area at the front, on the frontal sections, the areas of the hippocampus are affected several times, while in the area of the body and tail the 'classic' arrangement of the hippocampus areas is in place. [L127]

triculare (➤ Fig. 12.11a, b), from which 2 separate fibre bundles split off, running in front of and behind the Commissura anterior:

- Fibrae precommissuralis (to septal nuclei, Regio preoptica, hypothalamus)
- Fibrae postcommissuralis (to Corpora mamillaria)

From a superior dorsal point of view, the rear section of the Commissura fornicis with the two Columnae fornicis resembles an ancient harp (David's harp; also: '**Psalterium**', ➤ Fig. 12.10).

Areas and connections of the hippocampal formation
Overview
The hippocampal formation is regarded as an interrelated structure ('formation'), because the cortical areas it includes are very closely related in terms of their anatomy and characteristics. Stimulating nerve cells form a circuit from the entorhinal cortex to the Fascia dentata, to the Cornu ammonis, and via the subiculum back to the entorhinal cortex. Since these connections are located within the hippocampal formation, they are also known as *intrinsic* connections. The commissural axons can be viewed as a special case of these intrinsic connections, as they connect together the areas of the hippocampal formations of both sides.

The connections within or between the hippocampal formations are in contrast to *extrinsic* connections, which on the one hand connect the hippocampal formation with the cortex and on the other with subcortical structures.

Intrinsic connections of the hippocampal formation
Information flow through the hippocampal formation
In the entorhinal cortex, information is collected from cortical areas and the sensory organs. From there they get to the granule cells of the Fascia dentata via the Tractus perforans ➤ Fig. 12.11c). The axons of these cells, known as mossy fibres, project mainly into the CA3 area of the Cornu ammonis, from where the information – still in the Cornu ammonis – gets to the CA1-neurons (via the SCHAFFER collaterals), before they are passed from there to the subiculum and then back to the entorhinal cortex.

The connections of the hippocampal formation (and the flow of information through the hippocampal formation) are most easily understood if one considers them in terms of a histological section made perpendicularly to the longitudinal axis of the hippocampus in the midsection (the 'body') (➤ Fig. 12.8; ➤ Fig. 12.11). In sec-

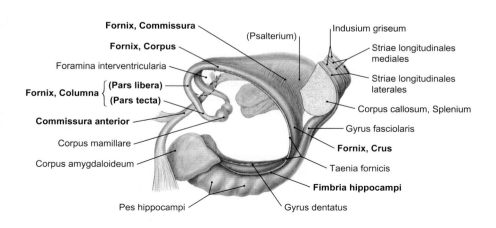

Fig. 12.10 Anterior commissure (Commissura anterior), fornix and hippocampus as well as Indusium griseum. Lateral view.

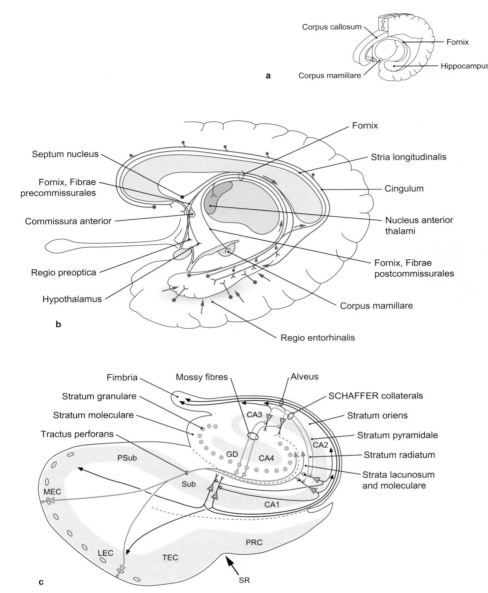

Fig. 12.11 Connections of the hippocampal formation; PAPEZ circuit. a Overview. **b** PAPEZ circuit. **c** Areas of the hippocampal formation and their intrinsic configurations. Frontal section through the middle part ('body') of the hippocampus; CA = Cornu ammonis, GD = Gyrus dentatus, Sub = subiculum, PSub = Pre-subiculum, MEC/LEC = medial/lateral entorhinal cortex, TEC = transentorhinal cortex, PRC = perirhinal cortex, SR = Sulcus rhinalis. a, b [L127], c [L141]

tions such as this, all the areas of the hippocampus and its typical fibre connections are found.

Entorhinal cortex

The entorhinal cortex is the 'gateway to the hippocampus.' On the one hand, it receives direct olfactory inputs (rostral entorhinal cortex) and, on the other hand, inputs from many multimodal sensory association fields (i.e. sensory information that has already been processed). Histologically, it is considered to be allocortex, which means that it is structured differently to the six-layered isocortex. The remarkable point about its structure is its division into a superficial and deep layer which is divided by a cell-free Lamina dissecans. In the superficial layer, there are islands of cells found on the surface anatomy of the Gyrus parahippocampalis, which are visible as small warts (see above). The axons of the superficial nerve cells run as the Tractus perforans to the Fascia dentata and the Cornu ammonis (➤ Fig. 12.11c).

Fascia dentata

The Fascia dentata sits like a cap on top of the Cornu ammonis. Its nerve cells, the granule cells, are located in a densely packed band of cells. The axons of the Tractus perforans reach the dendrites of the granule cells in the molecular layer. The axons of the granule

cells in turn run as mossy fibres into the Cornu ammonis. There they end at the dendrites of the pyramid cells of the CA3 area (➤ Fig. 12.11c).

The area immediately below the granule cells is referred to as the **subgranular zone**. The neurogenic niche is located here, where new nerve cells, even in the adult brain, can be formed.

Cornu ammonis

The Cornu ammonis consists of 1–2 cell layers of pyramidal cells winding around the Fascia dentata (➤ Fig. 12.11c). Due to the cell morphology and cell connections, the Cornu ammonis is divided into 4 sub-areas; of which the CA3 and CA1 areas are of particular importance in understanding the information flow through the hippocampal formation:

- The CA3-pyramidal cells receive information via the mossy fibres of the granule cells. With their axons, they project out of the hippocampal formation (via the alveus in the fimbria), still forming important collaterals, the SCHAFFER collaterals, that move within the hippocampus to the CA1-area.
- The CA1-pyramidal cells behave in a similar manner, also projecting from the hippocampal formation, but also moving with their collaterals to the subiculum complex (➤ Fig. 12.11c).

Subiculum complex

The subiculum, presubiculum and parasubiculum follow on from the CA1 area. The subiculum can be visualised histologically as a wide band of cells. The nerve cells of this area project out of the hippocampal formation and back to the entorhinal cortex (➤ Fig. 12.11c). The function of this area remains unclear.

Commissural connections of the hippocampal formation

Both of the hippocampal formations are closely connected via the Commissura fornicis. In humans, the commissural connections are particularly found in the area of the subiculum complex and the entorhinal cortex. This strong link between the two hippocampal formations is thought to be responsible for ensuring that serious memory impairment only occurs if both hippocampi have failed at the same time.

Clinical remarks

To treat the fits in severe and drug-resistant **temporal lobe epilepsy**, the affected parts of the hippocampal formation can be removed on one side. The removal of *one* hippocampus does not lead to obvious memory impairment. The removal of *both* hippocampi, on the other hand, leads to a serious, mainly anterograde amnesia, i.e. the inability to register new memories and remember them.

Extrinsic connections of the hippocampal formation
Cortical connections

The *afferent* connections of the hippocampal formation with the cortex run via the entorhinal cortex (see above) and the subiculum. The Gyrus dentatus and the Cornu ammonis are 'sealed off' from the neocortex. This ensures that the information is processed sequentially in the areas.

The *efferent* connections of the hippocampal formation with the cortex also run via the entorhinal cortex and subiculum complex. The hippocampal formation projects back to the multimodal areas of the association cortex and reaches the neocortex via these wide areas. In this way, knowledge that has been acquired via the hippocampal formation can be transferred permanently into the long-term memory. In the long term, memory traces are then stored in the neocortex.

Subcortical connections

The hippocampal formation is an 'old' structure of the brain ('archicortex'). In relation to its 'age', it is directly linked with the subcortical nuclear areas of the diencephalon and brainstem which are phylogenetically just as old, frequently with links in both directions. The younger neocortical connections are almost 'mounted' onto this existing system and pass via the entorhinal cortex as its gateway ('interface') into the hippocampal formation.

The close connection with the subcortical structures, which in turn are either part of the 'limbic system', or are in close connection with it, explains why the hippocampus receives information about the autonomic and emotional states of our body and, conversely, can have an influence on them (see below, 'Functions of the hippocampal formation'). Many (but not all) of these subcortical connections reach and leave the hippocampus via the fimbria and the fornix. The main connections are listed below.

- **Septal nuclei:** Fibres from all areas of the Cornu ammonis reach the septum via the Fibrae precommissuralis (see above). Conversely, cholinergic (neurotransmitter: acetylcholin) and GABA-ergic (neurotransmitter: GABA) axons from the septal nucleus

areas to the hippocampus. This connection ('septohippocampal projection') is important for learning and memory.
- **Basal forebrain:** A group of nuclei found basally in the frontal part of the brain, is usually seen as part of the 'basal forebrain'. These include the septal nuclei/diagonal band of BROCA, the **Nucleus basalis (MEYNERT)**, the Substantia innominata as well as the Nucleus accumbens. These nuclei contain many cholinergic fibres, which branch out from the hippocampal formation and many cortex areas, i.e. 'diffusely' innervating with acetylcholine (**'cholinergic system'**). This cholinergic innervation controls the activity level of the nerve cells and is important for neural plasticity and thus for learning and memory.
- **Corpora mamillaria:** A powerful fibre connection runs via the Fibrae postcommissurales from the subiculum to the Corpora mamillaria. Here information from the hippocampus and the amygdala join together and is then transferred to the thalamus (Tractus mamillothalamicus; s. PAPEZ circuit). The exact function of these nuclei and pathways is not understood; they do however play a role in memory formation and the recall of memory content, since the destruction of these nuclei or the Tractus mamillothalamicus is associated with severe **amnesia** (= inability to register the content of new memories or recall them).
- **Amygdala:** Multiple areas of the hippocampal formation, particularly the subiculum and the entorhinal cortex are connected to the amygdala (➤ Chap. 1.10). The amygdala is an important centre for controlling emotional and autonomic reactions and significant for our emotional memory (e.g., fear response).
- **Modulating systems:** The specific processing of information in the hippocampal formation is influenced by pathways from the brainstem. These brainstem afferents end with their axons diffusely distributed via the hippocampal formation and influence the activity status of the overall system. These include, among other things, dopamine (from the Area tegmentalis ventralis), noradrenaline (from the Locus caeruleus), serotonin (from the Raphe nuclei), as well as histamine. The clinical significance of the modulating systems is considerable, as the effect of many psychotropic drugs used in the treatment of neuropsychiatric diseases is based on the interaction of these systems (e.g., selective serotonin re-uptake inhibitors [SSRI] for the treatment of depression).

NOTE

Connections of the hippocampal formation are:
- neocortical connections (via the entorhinal cortex, the 'gateway to the hippocampus'; subiculum complex)
- intrinsic connections (entorhinal cortex – Fascia dentata – CA3 – CA1 – subiculum complex – entorhinal cortex)
- commisural connections (especially entorhinal cortex and subiculum)
- subcortical connections (including septal nuclei, Corpora mamillaria, amygdala, brainstem)

Clinical remarks

A lack of thiamine (vitamin B₁), e.g., due to chronic alcohol abuse, may lead to a bilateral atrophy of the Corpora mamillaria, the thalamus, the cerebellum and the frontal lobe. In the final stage of the resulting **WERNICKE–KORSAKOFF syndrome**, the patients suffer, amongst other things, from severe **amnesia** (= memory disturbance), combined with spontaneous **confabulation** (= the recounting of objectively untrue stories) and **ataxia** (= disturbance in the coordination of movement).

Functions of the hippocampal formation

The hippocampal formation is now one of the most well-researched cortical areas. Comparative neuroscientific research (e.g., examinations of the hippocampus in animals) as well as the functional imaging of the human hippocampus, have contributed to this. As an overview, the following can be differentiated:

- **Learning and memory functions:** The hippocampus is important for a portion of our learning and memory functions. It is needed for our declarative memory. This includes the semantic memory that stores our 'knowledge about the world' (Shakespeare wrote 'Romeo and Juliet'), and the episodic-biographical memory that retains the events of our own life.
- **Spatial representation of the environment** ('satnav in the brain'): parts of the hippocampal formation are responsible for ensuring that we have an 'internal representation' of the room in which we physically find ourselves.
- **Connections to the limbic system:** Our nervous system stores not only events, but also the feelings associated with them. The limbic system takes on the task of coupling hippocampal memory performance with neuroendocrine, autonomic and emotional functions (➤ Chap. 1.10).

Clinical remarks

Neurodegenerative diseases lead to an insidious loss of nerve cells in the brain. The hippocampal formations are affected, and this leads to disturbances of spatial memory and orientation skills. Also the ability to store new experiences and new knowledge is lost.

The best-known neurodegenerative disease which damages the hippocampal formations is **ALZHEIMER's disease**. In the brain of those affected by the disease, there are extracellular protein deposits ('amyloid plaques') and intracellular protein aggregation from hyper-phosphorylated Tau protein ('neurofibrillary changes'). The latter will lead to nerve cell death and atrophy of the cortex. In the early stages of the disease, the hippocampal formation is affected. This results in spatial disorientation (patients 'wander off' and 'get lost') and loss of memory retention. In later stages, the disease takes over the neocortex and also deletes existing memories. At the end, the patient cannot remember himself as a person nor events from his life.

With Alzheimer's disease, the cholinergic system is affected at an early stage. There is therefore a 'lack of acetylcholine' in patients' brains. Since acetylcholine plays a part in learning and memory, the level of acetylcholine is increased at the synapses by treating patients with a course of inhibitors of acetylcholinesterase, the enzyme that degrades acetylcholine. However, this treatment is only effective in the early stages of the disease and generally has only temporary benefits.

Blood supply of the hippocampus

The blood supply to the hippocampal formation is clinically significant for temporal lobe epilepsy surgery. The macroscopic hippocampus is supplied by several vessels, due to its longitudinal extension, which form anastomoses on its surface area. The two critical vessels supplying it are the **A. cerebri posterior** (supply of the occipital two thirds of the hippocampus) and the **A. choroidea anterior** (supply of the rostral third). The relative amount with which these vessels supply the hippocampus varies. This 'variability in detail' is typical of the blood supply to the brain surface (➤ Chap. 11.5).

Clinical remarks

Unilateral circulatory problems of the A. cerebri posterior can result in temporary disturbances to the memory function (amnesia). However, in clinical terms, other symptoms are paramount ('foremost') (e.g., visual disturbances), as unilateral hippocampus damage can be compensated for by the other hippocampus.

Bilateral circulatory disorders of the Aa. cerebri posteriores can lead to equal damage to both hippocampi. The consequences are acute and persistent, mainly involving anterograde memory impairment.

Cingulate cortex

The archicortical areas in the immediate vicinity of the Corpus callosum surround it like a girdle running lengthways (Cingulum, Latin: belt, ➤ Fig. 12.4).

Cytoarchitecturally, multiple areas are differentiated, some of which are aligned to the BRODMANN areas, and to which a variety of functions can be assigned. These include from anterior to posterior:

- Regio subgenualis – sections of the Gyrus cinguli below the genu of the Corpus callosum
- anterior cingulate cortex – rostral section of the Gyrus cinguli
- posterior cingulate cortex – caudal section of the Gyrus cinguli
- Regio retrosplenialis – continuation of the Gyrus cinguli below the splenium of the Corpus callosum

The functions of the cingulate cortex have been studied using functional imaging. In summary, the following has been discovered:

- anterior cingulate cortex: cognitive (identification of errors, reward learning) and autonomous functions (including the linking of emotions and autonomic reactions)
- posterior cingulate cortex: biographical memory, self-confidence, self-reflection

---

Clinical remarks

Disturbances in cingulate cortical areas lead to cognitive change. The **cingulate cortex** is therefore involved in the complex symptoms of neuropsychiatric disorders (depression, schizophrenia, anxiety disorders, impulse control).

12.1.7 Paleocortex
Thomas Deller, Andreas Vlachos

Overview

In phylogenetic terms, the paleocortex is the oldest part of the cortex. In the case of simple mammals, such as the hedgehog, it dominates the brain. It consists mainly of the olfactory cortex and is closely associated with the olfactory system.

The **structures of the paleocortex** are:

- Bulbus olfactorius
- Tractus olfactorius
- Nucleus olfactorius anterior
- Tuberculum olfactorium
- Septal nuclei
- Regio periamygdalaris
- Regio prepiriformis

The Bulbus and Tractus olfactorius derive from the telencephalon and are components of the brain. They are therefore phylogenetic and anatomic-systematic parts of the paleocortex. Histologically, they are clearly differentiated from the six layer isocortex and are allocortex. Details on these paleocortical structures can be found in ➤ Chap. 13.6.

> **N O T E**
>
> Due to the functional importance of the paleocortex for the olfactory sense, the term **rhinencephalon** is often used alongside the term paleocortex. This term usually only covers the olfactory cortex in the narrowest sense, i.e. the paleocortex without the Bulbus and Tractus olfactorius.

Macroscopic structures

Parallel use of nomenclature for macroscopic structures (e.g., gyri) and microscopic areas (e.g. the BRODMANN areas) makes it difficult to get to know the structures in the CNS. The macroscopically identifiable structures are only vaguely identical to the histologically delimited areas. They are however significant practically, since they can become visible using imaging methods and can serve as important landmarks in surgery.

> **N O T E**
>
> The macroscopically visible structures of the cortex (e.g., gyri and sulci) serve as guides in the brain. These structures are variable in shape and are only vaguely identical to the histologically delimitated cortical areas (e.g. the BRODMANN areas).

The basal paleocortex is located on the Facies basalis of the brain (➤ Fig. 12.12). It extends from the basal frontal lobe (Lobus frontalis) to the medial temporal lobes (Lobus temporalis):

Lobus frontalis

Rostrally below the Lobus frontalis is the small, raised, piston-shaped olfactory Bulbus olfactorius. The Tractus olfactorius runs caudally here in the Sulcus olfactorius. It widens and forms the Trigonum olfactorium, from which 2 bundles usually split off as the Stria olfactoria medialis and the Stria olfactoria lateralis. The striae may encompass a small polygonal structure, known as the Tuberculum olfactorium.

Between the Striae olfactoriae lies the Substantia perforata anterior. Here, central blood vessels of the Aa. cerebri anteriores and mediae are found, moving down into the depths and towards the nuclear areas located inside the brain (➤ Chap. 11.5). The Substantia perforata anterior is delimited caudally by the diagonal band of BROCA (nuclear area of the basal forebrain; ➤ Chap. 13.10) and by the Tractus opticus.

Lobus temporalis

Parts of the paleocortex were displaced into the medial temporal lobes during phylogenesis, particularly in the area of the Gyrus parahippocampalis, as well as in 2 smaller gyri medially located to it, known as the Gyrus ambiens and the Gyri semilunaris (➤ Fig. 12.12, ➤ Fig. 12.7). Caudally of these is the uncus in which parts of the hippocampal formation (archicortex) are found (➤ Chap. 12.1.6; ➤ Fig. 12.7).

Olfactory cortical areas

Cortical areas directly connected to the efferent nerve cells (mitral cells) of the olfactory bulb are referred to in their entirety as the ol-

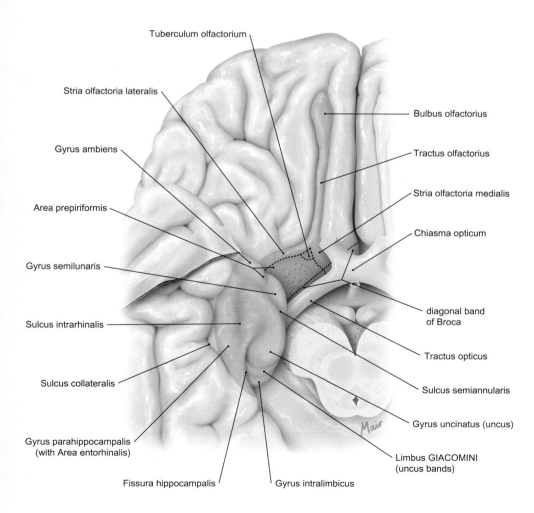

Tuberculum olfactorium
Stria olfactoria lateralis
Gyrus ambiens
Area prepiriformis
Gyrus semilunaris
Sulcus intrarhinalis
Sulcus collateralis
Gyrus parahippocampalis (with Area entorhinalis)
Fissura hippocampalis
Gyrus intralimbicus

Bulbus olfactorius
Tractus olfactorius
Stria olfactoria medialis
Chiasma opticum
diagonal band of Broca
Tractus opticus
Sulcus semiannularis
Gyrus uncinatus (uncus)
Limbus GIACOMINI (uncus bands)

Fig. 12.12 Paleocortical (green) and adjacent archicortical structures (purple) on the Facies basalis of the brain. [L127]

651

factory cortex. These areas include mainly paleocortical as well as other cortical areas. Paleocortical parts are:

- Tuberculum olfactorium
- Septal nuclei and diagonal band of BROCA
- Area prepiriformis
- Area periamygdaloidea

Other areas are:

- Regio entorhinalis (lateral part)
- Nucleus corticalis anterior of the amygdala (part of the cortico-medial nuclear group)

The **Tuberculum olfactorium** corresponds macroscopically with a small bulge, caudal to the Trigonium olfactorium or otherwise sunk down within the Substantia perforata anterior. The **septal nuclei** lie below the Septum pellucidum, which in humans does not contain any nerve cells. The **Area prepiriformis** is found in the Gyrus ambiens and in cortical areas around the Stria olfactoria lateralis; the **Area periamygdaloidea** is located in the Gyrus semilunaris. In addition to these paleocortical areas, axons also run directly from the Bulbus olfactorius to the **Regio entorhinalis** (part of the archicortex), located in the Gyrus parahippocampalis and partly in the Gyrus ambiens, as well as in the **Nucleus corticalis anterior** of the amygdala.

N O T E

Gyrus ambiens and Gyrus semilunaris

In the Gyrus ambiens and the Gyrus semilunaris, there are large parts of the Area prepiriformis and the Area periamygdaloidea. To simplify matters, they are sometimes referred to as the cortical 'olfactory centre' of the human brain.

The term **Area piriformis** is a collective term that includes several cortical areas forming the Lobus piriformis in simpler mammals. Located here is the olfactory cortex, which is particularly well-developed in macrosmatic animals (= animals with a highly-developed sense of smell; e.g., in rodents). The Area prepiriformis, the Area periamygdaloidea and the Area entorhinalis are included as parts of the Area piriformis. In humans (microsmatic beings), these areas also receive a direct input from the Bulbus olfactorius (olfactory cortex).

Connections of the paleocortex

The paleocortex is characterised as a phylogenetically old cortical structure because of 2 special features of its anatomical connections:

- **Direct sensory information from the Bulbus olfactorius:** The olfactory cortical areas at the base of the brain have direct connections to the Bulbus olfactorius. Conversely, the other senses only reach the cortex after interconnecting in the thalamus area. Thus it can be said that 'smells go directly to the brain.'
- **Close ties to different parts of the limbic system** (➤ Chap. 1.10): The brain areas of the limbic system are designed for the central control of autonomic and neuroendocrine bodily functions, basic emotional reactions and specific learning and memory processes. The close connection between the paleocortex and limbic system can be easily understood in phylogenetic terms, since controlling the autonomic processes of the body is a very basic requirement for life as well as being an 'old' brain function. Olfactory cortex areas have an effect on the other areas of the brain via connections to the limbic system, as well as partly via connections to the thalamus and the island area.

Important common **neurodegenerative diseases** (e.g., ALZHEIMER's disease, PARKINSON's disease), are associated early on with olfactory problems.
Examination of the sense of smell by means of standardised olfactory testing is therefore discussed as a diagnostic early marker for neurodegenerative diseases. Additionally, there are hypotheses for the pathogenesis of neurodegenerative diseases that suggest that toxins or infectious particles may penetrate into the central nervous system via the olfactory system. However, these hypotheses remain unproven.

12.1.8 Subcortical nuclei

Michael J. Schmeißer

Overview

Subcortical nuclei refer to the groupings of grey matter created in the white matter of each hemisphere. These include primarily the **basal ganglia**, an important nuclear group of the motor system. In addition, there are other subcortical nuclei such as the **amygdala** (also Corpus amygdaloideum) or the **Nucleus basalis of MEYNERT**. Common to these nuclei is their ability to influence higher brain functions such as learning and memory as well as motivation and the emotions.

Basal ganglia

In a narrower sense, the following nuclear areas can be included in the basal ganglia (➤ Fig. 12.13, ➤ Fig. 12.14):

- **striatum** (also Corpus striatum), consisting of the **caudatus** and **putamen**
- **pallidum** (also called the Globus pallidus)

Ontogenetically, the pallidum does not belong to the telencephalon, but to the diencephalon. In addition, the **Nucleus subthalamicus** of the diencephalon and the **Substantia nigra** of the mesencephalon are functionally associated with the basal ganglia. In academic literature, they are sometimes listed as a direct component of the basal ganglia.

Striatum

The **Nucleus caudatus** is a C-shaped arch that is divided into 3 parts: caput, corpus and cauda (➤ Fig. 12.13b). The rostrally lying caput is somewhat raised, whereas the corpus and cauda gradually become narrower. Topographically, the Nucleus caudatus in its entirety is in the immediate vicinity of the respective side ventricle. In the frontal lobe, the caput forms the base and lateral limit of the Cornu frontale [anterius] (➤ Fig. 12.13c). The corpus is located in the parietal lobe on the floor of the Pars centralis (➤ Fig. 12.13d) and the cauda is in the temporal lobe in the roof of the Cornu temporale [inferius] (➤ Fig. 12.13c, d).

The **putamen** is located somewhat lateral and basal of the Nucleus caudatus and is shaped like an oval disc. In brain sections, it is easy to see that the putamen is located in the medulla of the insular cortex and is flanked laterally by the Capsula externa and medially by the pallidum (➤ Fig. 12.13c, d).

Ontogenetically, the Nucleus caudatus and the putamen arise from the same system and are increasingly separated from each other in the course of their development by the ingrowing fibres of the Capsula interna running from rostral to caudal. The striped rostral connections between the Nucleus caudatus and the putamen are easily recognised in the frontal brain sections, and have been named identically (Corpus striatum = striped body).

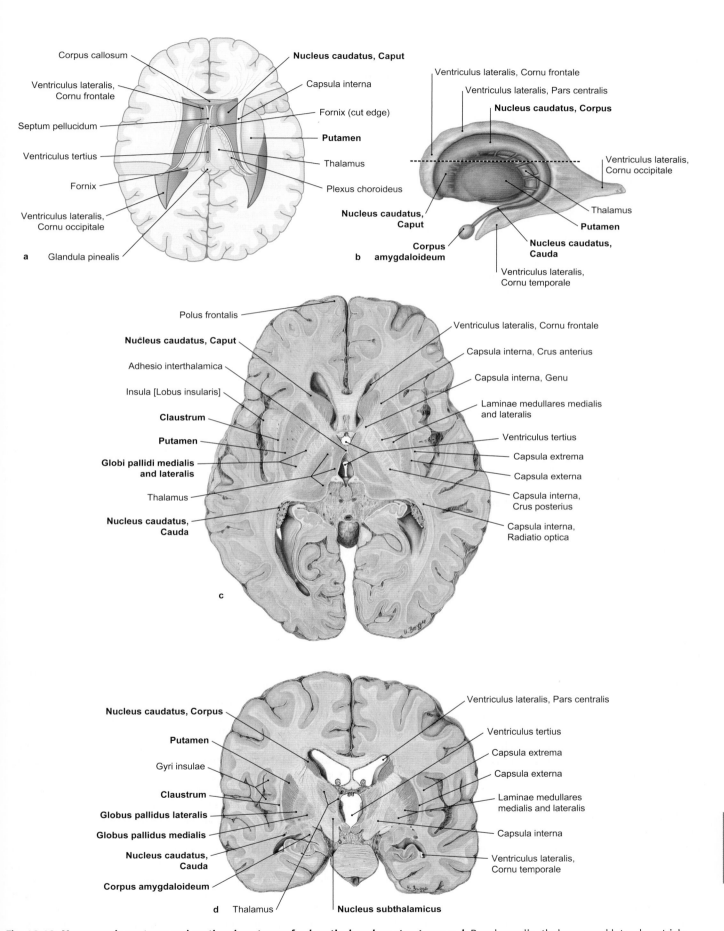

Fig. 12.13 Macroscopic anatomy and sectional anatomy of subcortical nuclear structures. a, b Basal ganglia, thalamus and lateral ventricle.
c Horizontal section through the centre of the IIIrd ventricle. **c** Frontal section at the level of the Corpora mamillaria. a [L126]

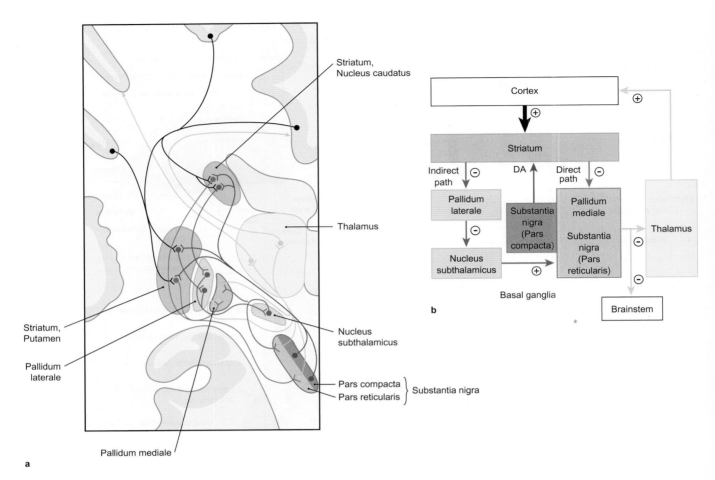

Fig. 12.14 Topography and schematic drawing of the neuronal configurations within the basal ganglia. [L126]

The **striatum** can also be divided into a dorsal and ventral striatum, with the dorsal striatum making up by far the biggest part. The ventral striatum includes only the anteroventral basal sections of the Caput nuclei caudati and of the putamen, which in this area are linked with each other by what is known as the **Nucleus accumbens**. The Nucleus accumbens consists of two visible parts, as is seen in frontal brain sections: a Pars lateralis, the nucleus which resembles the ventral striatum, and a Pars medialis, the 'shell', representing a transition to the neighbouring amygdala.

Pallidum

The pallidum, which appears in brain sections as relatively bright (pale nucleus), is located medially of the putamen and is morphologically delimited from it by a Lamina medullaris lateralis (or externa) (➤ Fig. 12.13). Furthermore, a distinction is made between a lateral and medial section (Pars lateralis or Pars medialis) which is divided by the Lamina medullaris medialis (or interna)(➤ Fig. 12.13c, d).

Nucleus subthalamicus

This is a biconvex nuclear area of the ventral diencephalon, medial to the Capsula interna and situated below the thalamus (➤ Fig. 12.13d).

Substantia nigra

The Substantia nigra is a nuclear area in the mesencephalon and is made up of two parts: the Pars reticularis and the Pars compacta. For more information and details about the position and outer form of the Substantia nigra, consult ➤ Chap. 12.1.8.

Internal structure and fibre connections of the basal ganglia
Dorsal striatum
The striatum, as the main entrance point into the basal ganglia, plays a key role. About 75% of its nerve cells are inhibitory, mid-sized GABAergic neurons, of which the secondary dendrites are filled with many dendritic spines, hence the term '**medium spiny neurons**', **MSNs**. At the end of these spines are:
- primarily the glutamatergic axons of the excitatory projection neurons of the cerebral cortex. These **corticostriatal primary afferents** (➤ Fig. 12.14a, b, black fibres/arrows) originate, depending on where they are located within the dorsal striatum, from the ipsilateral frontal and parietal cortex areas and thus primarily from motor and sensory cortex areas, and they can attract the MSNs.
- also **nigrostriatal primary afferents** (➤ Fig. 12.14a, b, dark grey fibres/arrows). These dopaminergic axons of the projection neurons of the Substantia nigra, Pars compacta, can modulate the activity of the MSNs.

Currently, it is postulated that there are 2 groups and thus **2 projection routes for the MSNs** within the dorsal striatum – direct and indirect routes (➤ Fig. 12.14b). What both routes have in common is the fact that they end in the main output station of the basal ganglia, the **pallidum-medial complex**. This comprises the actual Pallidum medial and the Substantia nigra, Pars reticularis, and contains large inhibitory GABAergic projection neurons, the axons of which go to neurons of the motor thalamic nuclei, and inhibit them (➤ Fig. 12.14a, b, yellow fibres/arrows). Amongst others, the pallidum-medial complex dispatches efferents to the brainstem (➤ Fig. 12.14b, yellow fibres/arrows) and can thus impact the motor centres of the brainstem or the spinal cord. There are important morphological and functional differences between the direct and indirect pathways:

- MSNs of the **direct pathway** (➤ Fig. 12.14a, b, red fibres/arrows) project directly with their axons onto the inhibiting nerve cells of the pallidum-medial complex and can inhibit them. After the corticostriatal activation of the direct pathway MSNs, an 'inhibition of inhibition' occurs– and thus the activation of the motor thalamus nuclei which results in the stimulation of certain cortex areas. In general, this leads to an **increase in motor activity** and 'desirable' movements are encouraged.

- MSNs of the **indirect pathway** (➤ Fig. 12.14a, b, green fibres/arrows) initially project with their inhibitory axons onto inhibitory GABAergic projection neurons of the Pallidum laterale, which are connected with the subthalamic nucleus, and of which the neurons can in turn inhibit. However, the latter are excitatory and project glutamatergically into the pallidum-medial complex. After corticostriatal activation of the indirect pathway MSNs, an 'inhibition of inhibition' occurs – and thus the activation of the Nucleus subthalamicus, which results in the activation of the pallidum-medial complex, an inhibition of thalemic nuclei and finally the inhibition of certain cortex areas. In general, this leads to an **inhibition of motor activity** and 'unwanted' movements are suppressed.

Nigrostriatal dopaminergic fibres (➤ Fig. 12.14a, b, dark grey fibres/arrows) can in this context increase the activity of the direct pathway via corresponding dopamine receptors and inhibit the activity of the indirect pathway.

Clinical remarks

In **PARKINSON's disease,** there is a degeneration of the dopaminergic neurons of the Substantia nigra, Pars compacta, and therefore also a loss of nigrostriatal fibres. As a result, the activity of the indirect pathway is reinforced in the broadest sense, and the activity of the direct pathway is inhibited. This results in the *general inhibition of motor activity,* and impetus or incentive is lost. The resulting symptom is called *akinesia* (physical inactivity), one of the 3 typical symptoms of PARKINSON's disease. In patients affected by the disease, the development is characterised in particular with small, scurrying steps and the absence of arm movement when running. In addition, a one-sided *tremor* develops when the patient is at rest, and generalised muscle stiffness or *rigour.* The underlying reasons for this neurodegenerative disease are not well understood, despite intensive research. For several decades the substance *L-dopa* has been used to treat it, passing through the blood–brain barrier and metabolising in the CNS into dopamine. This is an attempt to compensate for the loss of endogenous dopamine with drugs. Another treatment option is the neurosurgical, stereotactic use of bilateral stimulation electrodes for *deep brain stimulation.* This method is used in the advanced stages of the disease, inhibiting the activity of the subthalamic nucleus which leads to the weakening of the indirect pathway and the strengthening of the direct pathway.

HUNTINGTON's chorea is an autosomal-dominant inherited neurodegenerative disease with changes in the HUNTINGTON gene. The resulting pathophysiological effect on the corresponding nerve cells is still not understood, despite intensive research. Interestingly, in this disease in particular, we find a degeneration of the striatal GABAergic projection neurons, particularly initially affecting the neurons of the indirect pathway. This means that the activity of the direct pathway predominates, expressed clinically by involuntarily exaggerated movements with reduced muscle tone, so-called *choreatic hyperkinesia.*

Where there is a unilateral **malfunction of the Nucleus subthalamicus,** e.g., as a result of ischemia, the activity of the indirect pathway is acutely inhibited. Clinically, this is expressed in proximally accentuated, lightning-fast, darting movements. This *hemiballism* affects the extremities of the contralateral side of the body, because the motor fibres of the Tractus corticospinalis, located downstream of the 'basal ganglia loop' and finally taking control of the muscles of the extremities, cross over in the Medulla oblongata from ipsilateral to contralateral.

Ventrales striatum, Nucleus accumbens

The ventral striatum occupies a special position within the basal ganglia, in which the Nucleus accumbens is most prominent. This part of the striatum also contains MSNs; unlike those primarily found in the dorsal striatum, these MSNs are reached by glutamatergic afferents from the prefrontal cortical and limbic areas such as the hippocampus and amygdala, and by dopaminergic afferents from the Area tegmentalis ventralis of the mesencephalon. MSNs of the ventral striatum project into the ventral pallidum segment, which is connected with thalamic nuclei; these in turn send their efferents into the prefrontal and limbic cortex areas.

NOTE

Due to its involvement with the limbic system, the **ventral striatum** is particularly responsible for the control of emotion- and motivation-related motor behaviour. Here the mesolimbic dopaminergic projection from the Area tegmentalis ventralis plays a special role. The activity of these fibres is always particularly increased when external stimuli are presented, which are predictive of a reward upon completion of a certain motor reaction.

Further subcortical nuclei of the telencephalon
Amygdala

The amygdala or the amygdala complex is located in front of the hippocampus in the medial part of the anterior temporal lobe and laterally borders the Cornu temporale [inferius] of the side ventricle (➤ Fig. 12.13d). Cytoarchitecturally, within the amygdala a distinction is made between morphologically and functionally different nuclei and subnuclei. Particularly 3 nuclear groups are significant here: the superficial, laterobasal and centromedial nuclei:

- The **laterobasal nuclei** are the main entry point for afferents from the limbic system, the thalamus, and from various sensory cortex areas (e.g., auditory, visual, gustatory, visceral).
- The **superficial nuclei** predominantly receive olfactory afferents.
- The **centromedial nuclei** receive afferents from the hypothalamus and the brainstem.

All the above-listed nuclei project efferents back into the same areas from where they receive their afferents; additionally, the laterobasal nuclei project into the dorsal and ventral striatum as well as into the Nucleus basalis of MEYNERT (see below). In addition, there are extensive connections between superficial and laterobasal nuclei, as well as within the centromedial nuclei. Interestingly, in the superficial and laterobasal nuclei, primarily glutamatergic projection neurons are found, and in the centromedial nuclei it is principally GABAergic projection neurons that are found. Functionally, the amygdala is a crucial switching or relay station, especially for emotional reactions, as it can integrate the most diverse afferent impulses and, via its efferent projections, can trigger appropriate and proportionate somatomotoric, endocrine and visceral reactions to a given situation.

Claustrum

The claustrum is a narrow, sagittally positioned area of grey matter located between the Capsula externa and Capsula extrema in the immediate vicinity of the insular cortex (➤ Fig. 12.13c, d). Its actual function has not yet been clarified at the present time. Its established anatomical qualities, however, show that there is a relatively uniform neuron population, as well as extensive reciprocal connections with diverse cortex areas.

Nucleus basalis of MEYNERT

This is a group of cholinergic neurons lying beneath the putamen and pallidum and above the amygdala; this groups sends efferents to the entire cerebral cortex. These projections are very important for selective attention processes in connection with visual stimuli, as well as for the storage of information to learn from long-term memories.

Clinical remarks

In neurodegenerative diseases associated with the development of dementia, e.g., in ALZHEIMER's disease), frontotemporal dementia or LEWY body dementia, **the cholinergic neurons of the Nucleus basalis of MEYNERT degenerate.** We are trying to counteract this loss pharmacologically with the systemic administering of acetylcholinesterase inhibitors, in order to increase the concentration of acetylcholine in the synaptic gap, thus promoting cognitive skills.

12.2 Diencephalon
Tobias M. Böckers

SKILLS

After working through this chapter of the textbook, you should be able to:
• name the components and functional role of the diencephalon
• explain the organisational structure and function of the Thalamus dorsalis
• describe the different parts and functions of the hypothalamus and epithalamus

12.2.1 Overview

Levels of the diencephalon

The **diencephalon (interbrain)** can be divided structurally and functionally into 4 'levels', which in turn contain nuclear areas with specific tasks. A distinction is made between, from dorsal to ventral:

• **Epithalamus** (➤ Chap. 12.2.2): It is on the top level of the diencephalon, lying on the thalamus. Also found here are the pineal gland, the habenulae (Nuclei habenulares, Striae medullares

thalami) and the Commissura posterior. Unlike the other parts of the interbrain, there are virtually no cortical projections leaving the epithalamus.
• **Thalamus dorsalis** (➤ Chap. 12.2.3): It consists of a relatively large, densely-packed nuclear complex, extending bean-shaped on both sides of the IIIrd ventricle from ventral to dorsal. The Corpora geniculata are also called **metathalamus** but they belong – also functionally – to the Thalamus dorsalis.
• **The subthalamus (Thalamus ventralis)** (➤ Chap. 12.2.5): It forms a transitional zone between the diencephalon and the mesencephalon, and is also referred to as the motor zone of the diencephalon. Correspondingly, there are important nuclear areas here for controlling motor skills (Globus pallidus, Nucleus subthalamicus). The nuclear areas of the subthalamus project mainly into the local diencephalic nuclear areas, but they receive afferents from the cortex.
• **Hypothalamus** (➤ Chap. 12.2.4): The lowest level of the diencephalon consists of core areas and fibre tracts, which are found on the floor of the IIIrd ventricle or in the area of the lower side walls of the ventricle. In particular, the neurons of the hypothalamus project within the diencephalon, in the limbic area and up to the brainstem. The hypothalamus also controls the endocrine and autonomous control circuits and modulates emotions and behaviours.

Embryology

The **diencephalon (interbrain)** is formed from the first primitive brain vesicles **(prosencephalon)** during embryonic development, which continues to develop as part of further differentiation in the vesicle of the cerebrum (telencephalon) and of the interbrain (diencephalon) (➤ Chap. 11.1). The actual diencephalon develops out of the interbrain vesicle with its different parts; also in the early stages, the optic vesicle develops from the diencephalon. Embryonic differentiation begins in the area of what will later become the hypothalamus *(5th week)*, then the epithalamus develops *(6th week)* and subsequently the subthalamus (Thalamus ventralis) as well as the Thalamus dorsalis.

Position and external shape

Due to its development, the diencephalon (interbrain), has a close topographical and direct functional relationship with the **telencephalon**, which it borders in particular cranially and rostrally, and into which it merges without any clear margins. Due to the massive growth of the telencephalic vesicles, the diencephalon becomes almost completely covered by the telencephalon. When dissecting the brain, parts of the diencephalon can be found at the base of the brain – after removing the Corpus callosum, the thalamus can be seen deep down and lateral of the IIIrd ventricle. In terms of its developmental history, the Globus pallidus belongs to the diencephalon (subthalamus) and is displaced into the telencephalon in the course of further brain development (➤ Chap. 12.1). Caudally, the diencephalon (interbrain) joins with the **mesencephalon** with no clear boundary.

The diencephalon includes the **IIIrd ventricle** or forms the lateral limit of this inner CSF space. In the interbrain, small, unpaired organs are frequently found in the ventricle walls. These have a specialised ependymium with tanycytes; local vessel plexus are endothelial (known as **circumventricular organs [CVOs]**). In these organs the blood–brain barrier is therefore absent, so that agents from the nervous system can be exchanged directly with the blood (neurohemal area).

The natural expansion of the interbrain and its structured levels is clearly visible in the midsagittal section of the brain

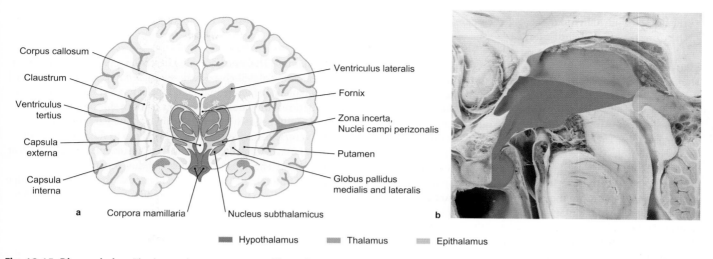

Fig. 12.15 Diencephalon. The layered arrangement and lateral extension of the individual interbrain parts is marked in colour. **a** Extent of the diencephalon in the frontal section (level of the Corpora mamillaria). **b** Diencephalon in midsagittal view. a [L126]

(➤ Fig. 12.15b). The **pituitary gland** or neurohypophysis is connected by the pituitary stem to the hypothalamus, which forms the floor of the IIIrd ventricle. In the transition area, the pituitary stem extends in a funnel-shape to the infundibulum. Ventral to the pituitary stem, the Chiasma opticum can be seen. In addition, the lower sections of the IIIrd ventricle border the hypothalamic nuclear areas laterally up to the **Sulcus hypothalamicus.** This groove marks the edge of the Thalamus dorsalis, the medial nuclear areas of which protrude into the ventricle. On both sides, ventral to these medial nuclei is the **Foramen interventriculare**, which is the connection of the IIIrd ventricle to the lateral ventricle. The pineal gland, Commissura habenularum and the Commissura posterior can be seen over the thalamic nuclei, positioned dorsally ➤ Fig. 12.15. In addition, the choroid membrane of the IIIrd ventricle can be seen, attached to the Taenia thalami.

In a **basal** view of the brain (➤ Fig. 11.19), the outer limit structures of the hypothalamus can be seen: it is located between the Chiasma opticum and the Corpora mamillaria. Between these structures, the funnel of the infundibulum with the suspended pituitary gland can be seen (➤ Fig. 12.16) (during dissection the pituitary gland is often removed, making an open infundibular recess visible).

N O T E

The **interbrain** (diencephalon) has developed embryologically from the first primitive brain vesicle (prosencephalon). Later it is completely overgrown by the telencephalon, so that only very few parts can be recognised immediately at the base of the undissected brain. Due to their specific position and function, the different nuclear areas and fibre tracts of the interbrain play an extraordinarily important role in the modulation and control of the incoming and outgoing nerve impulses to and from the cerebral cortex (particularly the **thalamic nuclear areas**). The diencephalon also acts as the overriding endocrine and autonomic regulation centre for the central control of different hormonal and circadian control circuits for maintaining homeostasis (in particular the **hypothalamus, epithalamus**).

12.2.2 Epithalamus

The epithalamus is located in the dorsocranial diencephalon and also partially forms the roof of the IIIrd ventricle. The epithalamus includes:

- The **Glandula pinealis** (epiphysis or pineal gland)
- the **Commissura posterior**

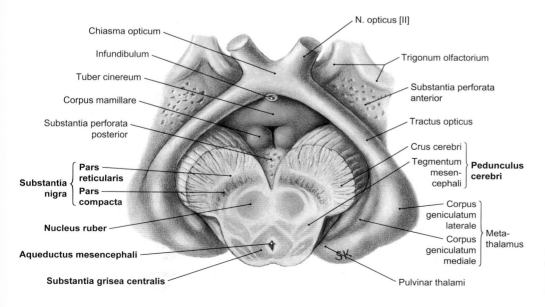

Fig. 12.16 Parts of the hypothalamus viewing the brain from basal (infundibulum, Corpora mamillaria).

- The nuclei of the **habenula** (Nuclei habenulares)
- The **Commissura habenularum**

Glandula pinealis

The Glandula pinealis is a cone-shaped, neuro-endocrine organ where specialised neurons produce the hormone **melatonin**. The pineal gland weighs approximately 100 mg and is located on the dorsal side of the IIIrd ventricle 'over' the quadrigeminal plate (➤ Fig. 12.15b). The production and release of the hormone is organised via a polysynaptic reflex arc (➤ Fig. 12.17). The absence of light/darkness is received through the eye, then the signal is routed primarily via the **Tractus retinohypothalamicus** to the **Nucleus suprachiasmaticus**. From there, the neural reflex arc continues via the **Nucleus paraventricularis** of the hypothalamus, the **Nucleus intermediolateralis** in the spinal cord and the upper cervical ganglion (**Ganglion cervicale superius**) to the Glandula pinealis. Darkness leads to the release of melatonin (darkness hormone), which provides the fine tuning for the day–night rhythm (circadian rhythm) via the Nucleus suprachiasmaticus, induces deep sleep and influences other hormonal reflex arcs (e.g., the reproductive capacity and annual rhythm in the animal world).

Commissura posterior

The Commissura posterior in particular provides a connection between the right and left **Nuclei pretectales** and contains fibres of the dorsal (DARKSCHEWITSCH) nuclei, the Commissura posterior of the dorsal thalamic nuclei and the Colliculi superiores. The particular importance of the Commissura posterior is in the coordination of the bilateral pupillary reflex.

Nuclei habenulares and Commissura habenularum

The **Nuclei habenulares** (medial and lateral) are located under the ependyma of the IIIrd ventricle and receive amongst others afferent fibres from the olfactory brain and the hypothalamus via the **Striae medullares thalami**. There are also connections to the Globus pallidus, the thalamus and the Substantia nigra. The Stria medullaris thalami is formed dorsally on the habenulae, which then emerge as the pineal stalk into the pineal gland. The Nuclei habenulares connects on both sides via the **Commissura habenularum** with the designated afferents.

The function of the habenular complex is predominantly pain processing, endocrine regulation (including reproduction and the sleep–wake rhythm) and reward learning.

12.2.3 Thalamus

Overview

The thalamus (Thalamus dorsalis) describes a part of the diencephalon consisting of densely packed, specialised nuclear areas, separated by fine lamellae of white matter. It is seen as an elongated rectangular structure with parallel alignment on both sides of the IIIrd ventricle. Simultaneously, it forms the floor of the Pars centralis of the lateral ventricle. It spreads out somewhat up to the Foramina interventricularia, delimited laterally by the Capsula interna or by nuclear areas of the telencephalon (Globus pallidus, putamen) (➤ Fig. 12.15). In more than 70% of cases, the medial thalamic nuclei bulge on both sides into the IIIrd ventricle and touch each other (**Adhesio interthalamica**). However, this contact does not represent a neural connection in the sense of a commissural tract.

The thalamus performs key tasks as part of the communication of cortex areas with the periphery, and from the periphery to central brain areas ('gateway to awareness'). All sensory perceptions (up to the olfactory system) are thus switched in the thalamus; specialized nuclear areas are involved in the controlling of motor skills and incorporated into a variety of subcortical reflex arcs (e.g., in the limbic system). In addition, the thalamus participates in autonomic and motor activities (➤ Fig. 12.18).

The thalamus consists of numerous nuclei (Nuclei thalami), which are structurally divided by lamellae (**Lamina medullaris medialis interna**) into 3 core areas or groups (➤ Fig. 12.19):

- ventrolateral group (**Nuclei ventrolaterales**)
- medial group (**Nuclei mediani**)
- anterior group (**Nuclei anteriores**), here the Lamina medullaris medialis interna separates into a Y-shape

Additionally, the **intralaminar nuclei** embedded in the Lamina medullaris medialis interna are distinguished morphologically from the internal medial medullary lamina, the **Nuclei mediani**, the occipitally-positioned **pulvinar** and the **Nuclei reticularis** (separated from the Nuclei ventrolateralis by the Lamina medullaris lateralis). The respective key groups can often be divided into smaller functional units (in total over 100 individual nuclear areas).

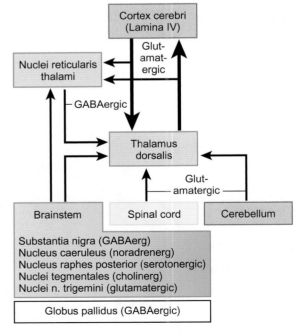

Fig. 12.18 Afferent and efferent compounds of the Thalamus dorsalis. [L126]

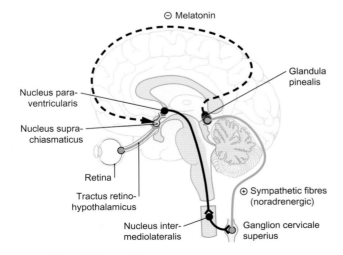

Fig. 12.17 Circuit of the Glandula pinealis.

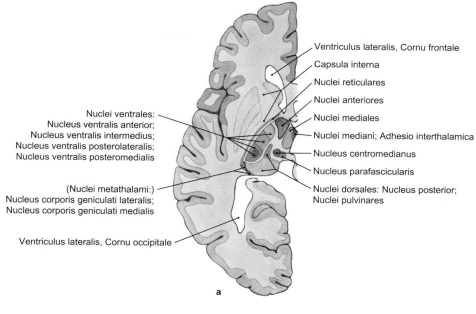

Ventriculus lateralis, Cornu frontale
Capsula interna
Nuclei reticulares
Nuclei anteriores
Nuclei mediales
Nuclei mediani; Adhesio interthalamica
Nucleus centromedianus
Nucleus parafascicularis
Nuclei dorsales: Nucleus posterior;
Nuclei pulvinares

Nuclei ventrales:
Nucleus ventralis anterior;
Nucleus ventralis intermedius;
Nucleus ventralis posterolateralis;
Nucleus ventralis posteromedialis

(Nuclei metathalami:)
Nucleus corporis geniculati lateralis;
Nucleus corporis geniculati medialis

Ventriculus lateralis, Cornu occipitale

a

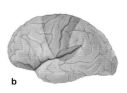
b

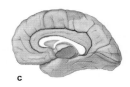
c

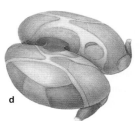
d

Fig. 12.19 Nuclei and cortex projection of the thalamus. The associated nuclei and cortical areas are marked with the same colours in each case. **a** Horizontal section through the left cerebral hemisphere. **b** Left cerebral hemisphere from the left side. **c** Right cerebral hemisphere from medial. **d** View of both thalami – oblique top view.

Here there are specific nuclei (palliothalamus), which control specific cortical areas (primary cortical projection fields and association fields), and unspecific nuclei (Truncothalamus), which project to the brainstem and several diffuse cortical areas (see below).

Important neural connections
Thalamus radiation
The Thalamus dorsalis is central to many connection pathways between the cortex and subcortically-located areas of the brain

(➤ Fig. 12.18). It is assumed that all cortical areas are connected to the thalamus. These fibre trunks, which can be represented macroscopically, are referred to as thalamic radiations (**Radiato thalami**), linking the spinal cord, the brainstem and the cerebellum via the thalamus to the Cortex cerebri. (➤ Fig. 12.20). Within these projection tracts, the **Pedunculus thalami anterior** (to the frontal lobe), the **Pedunculus superior** (to the parietal lobe), the **Pedunculus posterior** (to the occipital lobe) and the **Pedunculus inferior** (to the temporal lobe) can be identified. The corticothalamic and thalamo-

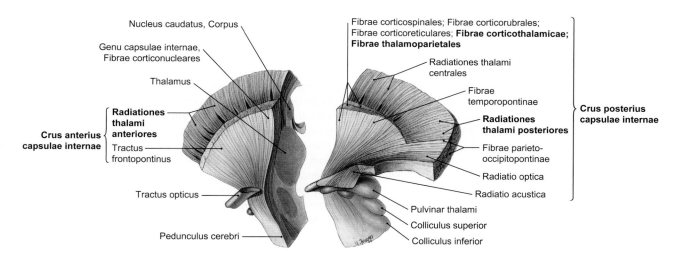

Nucleus caudatus, Corpus
Genu capsulae internae, Fibrae corticonucleares
Thalamus
Radiationes thalami anteriores
Tractus frontopontinus
Crus anterius capsulae internae
Tractus opticus
Pedunculus cerebri

Fibrae corticospinales; Fibrae corticorubrales; Fibrae corticoreticulares; **Fibrae corticothalamicae; Fibrae thalamoparietales**
Radiationes thalami centrales
Fibrae temporopontinae
Radiationes thalami posteriores
Fibrae parieto-occipitopontinae
Radiatio optica
Radiatio acustica
Pulvinar thalami
Colliculus superior
Colliculus inferior
Crus posterius capsulae internae

Fig. 12.20 Thalamus radiation, Radiationes thalami, and internal capsule, Capsula interna. View from the left side; separated into 2 parts by a frontal section. The thalamic nuclei project mainly to the cortex. Their tracts form parts of the Crus anterius and the Crus posterius of the Capsula interna. The tracts include the Radiationes thalami anteriores and posteriores. Other tracts are the Fibrae corticothalamicae and the Fibrae thalamoparietales.

cortical compounds are mainly glutamatergic, flowing into the lamina IV of the cerebral cortex and mainly developing reciprocally; the Thalamus dorsalis particularly receives afferents ➤ Fig. 12.18 from the underlying brain areas (brainstem, spinal cord and cerebellum).

Specific and non-specific nuclei

The functional classification of the thalamus has not been consistently described and according to current research results, it undergoes constant change. A basic distinction is made between the palliothalamus and the truncothalamus:

- The **palliothalamus** describes the thalamus nuclei which are specifically and systematically in contact with specialized cortex areas (**specific nuclei**).
- The **truncothalamus**, on the other hand, includes nuclear areas which receive afferents from the brainstem and the basal ganglia (e.g., Nucleus centromedianus and intralaminar nuclei) and send their efferents to individual cortical areas or to the hippocampal formation, as well as to other nuclear areas of the limbic system (**non-specific nuclei**). Amongst others, they play a role in learning and memory processes.

Important specific nuclei are:

Nuclei anteriores

They are the hub between the Gyrus cinguli (limbic system) and the Tractus mamillothalamicus. Macroscopically, they are located between the short arms of the Y-shaped split of the Lamina medullaris medialis interna. The nuclei can be further differentiated into the Nuclei anterodorsalis, anteromedialis and anteroventralis. The Tractus mamillothalamicus ends in these nuclear areas ipsilaterally and contralaterally. Other afferents originate from the cortex (fornix), the brainstem and the Globus pallidus. Important efferents pass into the Gyrus cinguli and the Gyrus parahippocampalis. It is significant in the modulation of emotional behaviour and attention.

Nuclei mediodorsales and Nuclei mediani

These thalamic nuclei project into the prefrontal cortex. They are divided into a large cell and small cell nuclear segments. Both parts receive important afferents from the olfactory brain and the amygdala. In particular, the efferents reach the frontal cortex areas and the Gyrus cinguli. Its function should principally be the modulating of emotions, but its importance in learning and memory processes has also been shown.

Pulvinar

The pulvinar is the hub between the visual system and associative visual cortex areas. It is a relatively large nuclear area taking up approximately one third of the Thalamus dorsalis. Important primary afferents come from other diencephalon neurons (integration nucleus) and there are important reciprocal links with the parietal and temporal lobes. The pulvinar is considered to be particularly important for symbolic thinking and speech comprehension in the context of integrating optical and acoustic impulses.

Nucleus ventralis lateralis, Nucleus ventralis anterior and Nuclei ventrobasales

These nuclear areas carry out the specific projection onto the primary motor cortex with information from the basal ganglia, Substantia nigra and the cerebellum (also referred to as the motor thalamus), and thus are the most important relay stations of the motor system in the brain. The ventral nuclei contain large and small cell neurons, each receiving afferents from the Substantia nigra, pallidum or from the Nuclei cerebelli. The nucleus-specific efferents reach the motor, pre-motor or supplementary motor cortex.

Nucleus ventralis posterolateralis and Nucleus ventralis posteromedialis

These nuclear areas have a specific projection onto the primary somatosensory cortex (via the upper thalamus stem). Both nuclei get afferents from the Lemniscus medialis (sensory information) or from the Lemniscus spinalis (temperature, pain). The efferents reach the primary (Gyrus postcentralis) and the secondary, somatosensory cortex. The somatotopy is retained in this circuitry chain and can be seen at each level of routing. These nuclei are therefore essential for the cortical routing of the information and the modulation of sensations (e.g., the pain experience).

Blood supply

The arterial blood supply of the thalamus is carried out via multiple arteries supplying the brain. The **A. thalamoperforans anterior** originates from the A. communicans posterior, mainly supplying the rostral thalamus. The **A. thalamoperforans posterior** supplies a range of nuclear areas of the thalamus; a lesion results in severe cognitive disorders. The **A. thalamogeniculata** originates from the A. cerebri posterior; here a blockage leads to sensory disturbances and restlessness.

Clinical remarks

Bleeding in the thalamic nuclear areas due to lesions in the specific nuclear areas can lead to personality changes, motor failures, as well as to cramping pain and discomfort (dysesthesias). The painful attacks are also known as **thalamic pain syndrome**. If non-specific nuclear areas are affected, this often leads to a reduction in consciousness.

12.2.4 Hypothalamus

Overview and classification

The **hypothalamus** is located on both sides of the IIIrd ventricle below the thalamus nuclei groups, as described in ➤ Chap. 12.2.3, ventrally of the subthalamus, and extends over the infundibulum to the posterior pituitary. This also forms the floor of the IIIrd ventricle. The hypothalamus includes specific **hypothalamic nuclear areas** and the **pituitary gland** (more precisely: the posterior pituitary). Topographically, the hypothalamus is in close contact with the Nn. optici and/or the Chiasma opticum. At the base of the brain, the expansion of the hypothalamus defines the Chiasma opticum, the respective Tractus optici and the Corpora mamillaria (➤ Fig. 12.15, ➤ Fig. 12.16). The hypothalamus is only about 0.3 % of the human brain; but, as a central control, regulates significant basal functions of the human body, such as temperature, fluid and electrolyte balance, food intake, the sleep–wake rhythm and hormone levels (homeostasis). To a large extent, it also influences social behaviour (including emotions and sexual behaviour) and also the autonomic nervous system with the sympathicus and the parasympathicus. It controls and coordinates almost all neural and humoral communication systems. The special feature of the hypothalamus is, amongst others, that neurons of the hypothalamic nuclear area adopt a neurosecretory function and thus can transform stimuli into humoral signals.

Areas and zones

The grey matter of the hypothalamus is very densely packed in some areas (**nuclei** of the hypothalamus), as well as less dense in others (**areas** of the hypothalamus). Areas consisting mainly of grey matter are also referred to as being non-myelinated, whereas areas which are predominantly white matter (tractus) are referred to accordingly as myelinated.

A regulatory structure in the hypothalamus is created, initially by organising the grey matter into areas from rostral to caudal in the sagittal section. As a result, the pre-optical or chiasmatic area is above the Chiasma opticum, followed by the intermediary (tuberale) area, then the posterior zone (➤ Fig. 12.21, ➤ Table 12.2):

- The **chiasmatic nuclei group** includes the Nucleus suprachiasmaticus (central pace setter for the circadian rhythm, sleep–wake cycle, body temperature, blood pressure), the Nuclei paraventricularis and supraopticus (production of anti-diuretic hormone [ADH] and oxytocin and axonal transport [Tractus hypothalamo-hypophysialis]) in the neurohypophysis) and the Nuclei preoptici (participation in the regulation of blood pressure, body temperature, sexual behaviour, menstrual cycle, gonadotropin).

- The **intermediate nuclei group** comprises the Nuclei tuberales, dorsomedialis, ventromedialis and arcuatus [infundibularis = semilunaris] (production and secretion of releasing and release-inhibiting hormones, participation in the regulation of water and food intake).

- The **posterior nuclear group** includes the Nuclei corporis mamillaris in the Corpora mamillaria, which are integrated by afferents from the fornix and efferents from the thalamus (Fasciculus mamillothalamicus) into the limbic system. They modulate sexual functions and play an important role in activities related to memory and emotions. They are connected via the Fasciculus mamillotegmentalis with the Tegmentum mesencephali.

In the frontal section, the lateral expansion of these zones is also divided into periventricular, medial and lateral zones.

Functional division

The functional division of the nuclear areas of the hypothalamus is the result of their specific functions in key hormonal reflex arcs. In this case, a distinction is made between magnocellular and a parvocellular neuroendocrine system.

Magnocellular neuroendocrine system

In this system, nuclear areas of neurosecretory neurons are encapsulated, synthesising the pituitary hormones from the pituitary posterior lobe (Pars neuronalis), and transporting them along their axons. These include the **Nucleus paraventricularis** and the **Nucleus supraopticus** (above the N. opticus) which produce the peptide hormones vasopressin (anti-diuretic hormone, ADH or Adiuretin) and oxytocin and bring them into the posterior pituitary gland via the Tractus hypothalamohypophysialis. These hormones are modified translationally in the axon endings, then stored and finally released on receiving specific signals. During histological dissection, the stored shape of these hormones stands out in the form of a **HERRING body**. **Vasopressin** particularly regulates diuresis in the kidneys and is therefore significantly involved in the regulation of water and electrolyte balance, and **oxytocin** stimulates smooth muscle cell contraction (including milk production in the mammary gland, and the postpartum contraction of the uterus).

Table 12.2 Structure of the hypothalamus into areas, zones, important areas and nuclei.

Periventricular zone	Medial zone	Lateral zone
Pre-optical/chiasmatic area		
• Nucleus preopticus medianus • Nuclei periventriculares preopticus and anterior • Nucleus suprachiasmaticus	• Area preoptica medialis (Nucleus preopticus medialis) • Area hypothalamica anterior (Nucleus anterior hypothalami) • Nucleus paraventricularis • Nucleus supraopticus • Nuclei interstitiales hypothalami anteriores	• Area preoptica lateralis • Area hypothalamica lateralis • Nuclei interstitiales hypothalami anteriores
Intermediary (tuberal) area		
• Nucleus arcuatus	• Nucleus ventromedialis • Nucleus dorsomedialis	• Area hypothalamica lateralis • Nuclei tuberales laterales • Nucleus tuberomamillaris
Posterior (mamillary) area		
• Nucleus periventricularis posterior • Area hypothalamica posterior (Nucleus posterior hypothalami)	• Nuclei mamillares medialis and lateralis	• Area hypothalamica lateralis • Nucleus tuberomamillaris

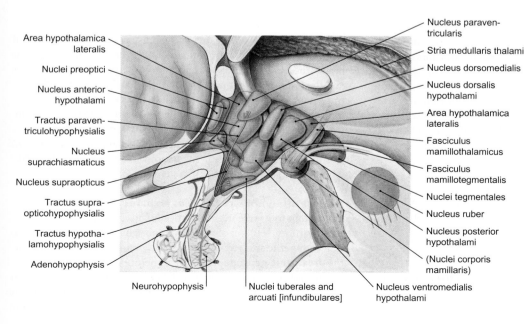

Area hypothalamica lateralis

Nuclei preoptici

Nucleus anterior hypothalami

Tractus paraventriculohypophysialis

Nucleus suprachiasmaticus

Nucleus supraopticus

Tractus supraopticohypophysialis

Tractus hypothalamohypophysialis

Adenohypophysis

Neurohypophysis

Nuclei tuberales and arcuati [infundibulares]

Nucleus ventromedialis hypothalami

Nucleus paraventricularis

Stria medullaris thalami

Nucleus dorsomedialis

Nucleus dorsalis hypothalami

Area hypothalamica lateralis

Fasciculus mamillothalamicus

Fasciculus mamillotegmentalis

Nuclei tegmentales

Nucleus ruber

Nucleus posterior hypothalami

(Nuclei corporis mamillaris)

Fig. 12.21 Hypothalamus with nuclei (drawn transparently). Medial view. The nuclear areas of the hypothalamus are divided into chiasmatic, intermediate and posterior nuclear groups.

Changes in hypothalamic hormone concentrations can have serious effects on the body's homoeostasis. For example, **central diabetes insipidus** can arise when the pituitary gland stem (Tractus hypothalamohypophysialis) is torn by a skull fracture. This disrupts the production or release of vasopressin (antidiuretic hormone, ADH) from the pituitary posterior lobe. ADH is a peptide hormone (9 amino acids), which reduces diuresis in the urine by promoting the incorporation of aquaporins in the collecting ducts of the kidneys. Central diabetes must be differentiated from **renal diabetes insipidus,** which is expressed for example by a congenital or acquired resistance of the kidney to ADH.

Parvocellular neuroendocrine system

This system includes nuclear areas which control the secretion activity of the anterior and mid-pituitary lobe **(anterior pituitary)** via the releasing or inhibiting hormones (liberins and statins, e.g., thyrotropin-releasing hormone [TRH] or corticotropin-releasing hormone [CRH]). In terms of its historical development, the anterior pituitary gland does not originate from the diencephalon; instead it accumulates as an adherence of epithelium from the back of the throat of the posterior pituitary. Thus the anterior pituitary cells are regulated by a fine mesh of venous vessels **(portal vascular system)**, located at the bottom of the **infundibulum** and the **median eminence**. Here the axons of parvocellular neurosecretory neurons end, so the peptide hormones which are produced reach the fine blood flow of the portal vessels (from the A. hypophysialis superior) (no blood–brain barrier!). The subsequent second drainage area of the portal vein is found in the anterior pituitary; thus its hormone-producing cells are reached by the respective liberins and statins. The production and secretion of the hormone cells of the anterior pituitary are under close hypothalamic control. In terms of hormonal 'feedback mechanisms', the system is autonomously regulated according to the circulating hormone concentrations.

The parvocellular system includes the **Nucleus infundibularis** (or Nucleus arcuatus), of which the cricoid shape surrounds the funnel entrance to the pituitary gland. The neurons of the Nucleus infundibularis form a protrusion on the basal side of the hypothalamus (Tuber cinereum). With its thin, myelin-free axons, these nerve cells represent the main contingent of the small cell hypothalamohypophyseal system **(Tractus tuberoinfundibularis)**. Hypothalamic hormones are brought to the portal vascular system at the Eminentia mediana via this tract. In addition, the **Nucleus ventromedialis**, which borders the Nucleus infundibularis dorsally and laterally, can be attributed to the system. It predominantly receives afferents from the limbic system and plays a role in the regulation of hunger and satiety. Finally, the **Nucleus periventricularis**, the **Nucleus paraventricularis** (small cell content), the **Nucleus suprachiasmaticus** and the **Nucleus dorsomedialis** are included in the parvocellular system.

NOTE

The **portal vein circulation** of the pituitary gland is supplied by the A. hypophysialis superior. The first venous drainage area is located on the Eminentia mediana of the hypothalamus, the terminal zone of the neurosecretory axons of the parvocellular neurons). They release their statins and liberins here (the releasing and inhibiting hormones) into the blood of the portal vascular system. The second drainage area is found in the anterior pituitary. Here, the secretion-active hormone cells are achieved in their entirety, and fine adjustment takes place.

Important hypothalamic nuclei and neural connections
Nucleus suprachiasmaticus

The Nucleus suprachiasmaticus found directly above the Chiasma opticum (periventricular zone), is central to the regulation of the **circadian rhythm** in the organism. Neurons of the Nucleus suprachiasmaticus can synthesise different peptide hormones (e.g., ADH, TRH). They both express what are known as clock genes and melatonin receptors. On the basis of melatonin levels in the blood, they integrate day–night information, but are also directly neurally connected with retinal neurons. Neurons of the Nucleus suprachiasmaticus can generate an endogenous, genetically fixed rhythm of spontaneous activity (the internal clock), which can be transmitted via hormonal and neural pathways to other brain structures (synchronisation). **Afferents** are received by the nucleus from the Tractus retinohypothalamicus as well as from the limbic cortex and the Raphe nuclei. The **efferents** remain largely local and innervate the neurons of other hypothalamic nuclei.

Nuclei tuberomamillares

The Nuclei tuberomamillares can be found in the posterior or mamillary part of the hypothalamus. Here there are histamine and adenosine-producing neurons, which are particularly involved in the reflex arcs of sleeping, waking, alertness and the circadian rhythm. **Afferents** reach the Nuclei tuberomamillares from the Medulla oblongata, the hypothalamus and the forebrain. Their **projections** reach other hypothalamic nuclei, the cerebellum and cortex areas, which are thereby activated. Specific hypothalamic neuropeptides associated with sleep (e.g., orexin), may influence the activity of the neurons of the Nuclei tuberomamillares.

Narcolepsy is a condition mainly characterised by excessive daytime sleepiness, cataplexy (sudden loss of muscle tone), sleep paralysis and hypnagogic hallucinations. The reason is very likely due to the selective loss of hypocretin/orexin cells in the hypothalamus. In the brain of the affected patient, only very low levels of orexins (orexin 1 and 2) can be measured. Interestingly, narcolepsy is also known in dogs, accompanied by a mutation of the hypocretin-(orexin-)2 receptor.

Nuclei mamillares

The Nuclei mamillares (lateralis and medialis) are neuron groups in the posterior part of the hypothalamus, which raise the external structure of the Corpora mamillaria bodies on the basal side of the brain. These nuclear areas receive **afferents** from the hippocampus and the brainstem via the fornix and the Pedunculus mamillaris. Important **efferents** leave these nuclear areas via the Fasciculi mamillothalamicus and mamillotegmentalis, moving to the Nuclei anteriores thalami and the Nuclei tegmentali anterior and posterior. Via these afferents and efferents, these nuclei are part of the PAPEZ circuit or the limbic system. The neurons are involved in the regulation of the subcortical motor system.

Nucleus infundibularis/Nucleus arcuatus

In addition to its role in the parvocellular regulation system (see above), the nuclear area also has an important function in the regulation of appetite and growth. In this way, neurons which synthesise the **orexigenic neuropeptides** NPY (neuropeptide Y) and AgRP (agouti-related protein) can be identified. It is believed that, due to the expression of leptin receptors, these neurons are involved in the regulation of hunger and/or satiety. They are directly distributed in proportion to the levels of ghrelin and leptin in the blood. **Primary afferents** receive neurons from other hypothalamic nuclear areas and from the limbic system.

Food intake (feelings of hunger) is regulated by a complex interplay of peripheral and centrally-produced and secreted signal molecules. One of these signal molecules is **leptin**, which is produced in fatty tissue. A lack of leptin is received centrally in the hypothalamus via specific binding sites and triggers sensations of hunger. There is an interplay between various nuclear areas in the hypothalamus in an **orexic network**. Also included in this are the Nucleus paraventricularis and the Nucleus arcuatus. Other peptides involved in the regulation of food intake are the peptide **galanin**, which reinforces fat intake, and opioid peptides which increases protein intake. **Neuropeptide Y (NPY)** is arguably the most well-known stimulator for food intake. The corticotropine-releasing hormone (CRH) is one of the known antagonists of NPY in regulating hunger.
Orexigen's (appetite-stimulating) effect: neuropeptide Y (NPY), agouti-related peptide (AgRP), galanin, orexin A and B, opioids, melanin-concentrating hormone (MCH), noradrenaline (α_2 receptor), gamma-amino-butyric acid (GABA), ghrelin, β-Endorphin.
Anorexigen's (appetite-limiting) effect: melanocyte-stimulating hormone (α-MSH), corticotropin-releasing factor (CRF), glucagon-like peptide 1 (GLP-1), glucagon, cocaine- and amphetamine-regulated transcript (CART), thyrotropin-releasing hormone (TRH), interleukin β (IL-β).

Anterior hypothalamic area

This area includes the **Nuclei anteriores hypothalami** and the **Area preoptica medialis**. The nuclear areas are included in the chiasmatic part of the hypothalamus, and, among their other roles, are involved in heat regulation and sexual behaviour. Interestingly, it was shown that these nuclear areas are not of the same size in men and women, so it is thought that they contribute to gender identity.

Areae hypothalamicae lateralis and posterior

They are found in the posterolateral hypothalamus. The **Area hypothalamica lateralis** is the name given to the border between the hypothalamus and the telencephalon. Here, there are afferents and efferents on the brainstem, cerebellum and spinal cord. The **Area hypothalamica posterior** (AHP) is located in the posterior part of the hypothalamus and has fibre connections to the mesencephalon. These nuclear areas are also involved in the regulation of food intake and respond, for example, to changes in the glucose concentration in the blood.

The core areas of the **hypothalamus** are connected via many afferent/efferent (mostly reciprocal) connections with other areas of the brain (in particular parts of the limbic system). The main configurations are shown in ➤ Table 12.3.

Pituitary gland

The pituitary gland is located in the Fossa hypophysialis of the Sella turcica and is separated by a Dura mater (**Diaphragma sellae**) from the actual central nervous system. The pituitary stem acts as a connecting structure for the hypothalamus (made up of axons of magnocellular neurons) which runs through a fine recess of the Diaphragma sellae.

The pituitary gland develops from various parts of the brain (also ➤ Chap. 11.1.2):
- The pituitary posterior lobe (**Pars nervosa**) grows from the diencephalon and forms the neurosecretory release area for oxytocin and vasopressin (anti-diuretic hormone, ADH) of the axons from the Nuclei supraoptici and paraventriculares.
- The anterior pituitary lobe (**adenohypophysis**) accumulates as an enfolding of the posterior pituitary by epithelial cells from the back of the throat. In its mid-section, cystic structures are frequently found; these are residues of the lumen of RATHKE's pouch.

Table 12.3 Afferents and efferents of the hypothalamus.

Important afferents of the hypothalamus	Important efferents of the hypothalamus
<ul><li>Limbic system</li><li>Hippocampus<ul><li>Corpus amygdaloideum</li><li>Septum area</li><li>Olfactory cortex</li></ul></li><li>Formatio reticularis, horn of the spinal cord, sensitive cranial nerve nuclei</li><li>Retina</li><li>Within the hypothalamus</li><li>Insular cortex</li></ul>	<ul><li>Cerebral cortex, thalamic core areas</li><li>Cranial nerve nuclei, Formatio reticularis</li><li>Spinal cord</li><li>Within the hypothalamus</li><li>In the framework of the magnocellular system for the posterior pituitary</li></ul>

Table 12.4 The anterior pituitary (adenohypophysis) hormones.

Hormone	Staining characteristics	Function	Hypothalamic regulation via
Pars distalis			
Prolactin (PRL)	Acidophilic	Milk synthesis	Prolactostatin (dopamine)
Growth hormone (GH, STH)	Acidophilic	Growth	GHRH (somatoliberin)
Corticotropin (ACTH)	Basophilic	Stimulation of the adrenal gland	CRH (corticoliberin)
Melanotropin (α-MSH)	Basophilic	Skin pigmentation	CRH (corticoliberin)
β-endorphine	Basophilic	Opioid receptor	CRH (corticoliberin)
Follicle-stimulating hormone (FSH)	Basophilic	Maturation of ovum/sperm	GnRH
Luteinising hormone (LH)	Basophilic	Ovulation, formation of Corpus luteum	GnRH
Thyroid-stimulating hormone (TSH)	Basophilic	Stimulation of thyroid cells	TRH (thyroliberin)
Pars intermedia			
Corticotropin (ACTH)	Basophilic	Stimulation of the adrenal gland	CRH (corticoliberin)
Melanotropin (MSH)	Basophilic	Skin pigmentation	CRH (corticoliberin)
β-endorphin	Basophilic	Binds to opioid receptors	CRH (corticoliberin)
Pars tuberalis			
Pars tuberalis specific cells	Chromophobic	Circadian/circannual rhythm	? (melatonin)

The **anterior pituitary gland** is also a central endocrine organ and can be divided into 3 parts (Pars distalis, Pars intermedia, Pars tuberalis). Hormone production (➤ Table 12.4) and secretion is controlled by the neurons of the hypothalamus (liberins, statins) which reach the anterior pituitary via the portal circulatory system:

- **Pars distalis:** It makes up the largest part of the anterior pituitary. Within it there are cells capable of the production and secretion of hormones (➤ Table 12.4). ACTH, α-MSH and β-endorphin are produced in a cell type of the anterior pituitary from a common precursor molecule (pro-opiomelanocortin, POMC, which is split into the respective active peptides).
- **Pars intermedia:** The Pars intermedia consists of an irregular cell band, and in humans is often only rudimentary.
- **Pars tuberalis:** The Pars tuberalis wraps itself around the pituitary stem (Tuber cinereum) and attaches itself to the hypothalamus. The chromophobic specific cells express melatonin receptors and produce subunits of thyreotropin.

Clinical remarks

There are various kinds of benign or malignant **tumours of the anterior pituitary gland**, which can be functionally or histologically/anatomically classified. The most common secretory tumours secrete prolactin, followed by growth hormone (GH) and corticotropin (CRH). There are also hormonally inactive tumours:

- Prolactinomas (**prolactin**-producing adenomas) lead to infertility in women with signs of masculinisation (change of hair distribution, hirsutism), cessation of periods (amenorrhoea) and milk production in the mammary gland (galactorrhoea).
- The hypersecretion of **growth hormone** (GH or STH) in the early growth stages of the body can lead to extreme body growth (gigantism). In adults, this is shown by acromegaly with enlarged nose, tongue, jaw, hands and feet (➤ Fig. 12.22).
- The rare **ACTH**-producing tumours stimulate the adrenal cortexes with signs of excessive steroid hormone production (including cortisol). The clinical pattern is referred to as central Cushing's syndrome and is accompanied by hypertension, striae, abdominal obesity and redness of the cheeks.

Large tumours can compress the Sinus cavernosus or the Chiasma opticum as they are topographically very closely-related areas:

- A compression of the **Sinus cavernosus** can be observed, for example, in cranial nerves III or IV
- When there is compression of the **Chiasma opticum**, the crossing fibres of the optic nerve are selectively interrupted and this creates a bitemporal hemianopsia (tunnel vision).

Surgery can be undertaken for the tumours described, initially using nasal access, then using keyhole surgery to reach and remove the tumour.

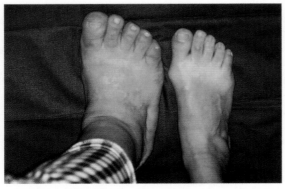

Fig. 12.22 Acromegaly. The foot of a patient with acromegaly (left) compared to the foot of a healthy patient of the same height. [R236]

12.2.5 Subthalamus

The subthalamus can be found beneath the thalamus, behind the hypothalamus and caudally of the epithalamus (➤ Fig. 12.15a). Caudally, however, it borders the mesencephalon. The neurons of the subthalamus are in close contact with the Thalamus dorsalis. The **Nucleus subthalamicus** is important for the coordination of movement and is closely connected by fibres to the **pallidum** (in terms of its developmental history it is also part of the diencephalon, ➤ Chap. 12.1.8).

12.3 Brainstem
Michael J. Schmeißer, Stephan Schwarzacher

SKILLS

After working through this chapter, you should be able to:
- name the 3 parts of the brainstem and describe their respective embryological, topographical and morphological features
- explain the functional systems of the brainstem, including the most important brainstem reflexes and neurotransmitter systems
- explain the importance of the two clinical terms 'midbrain syndrome' and 'WALLENBERG's syndrome', using basic anatomical terms

The brainstem (**Truncus encephali**) consists of the midbrain (**mesencephalon**), the **pons** and extended marrow (**Medulla oblongata**). This macroscopic division is located opposite the division derived from the brain's development. Ontogenetically, the mesencephalon (➤ Chap. 12.3.1) therefore arises from the middle vesicle of the brain's 3 primary vesicles; conversely the pons and the Medulla oblongata (➤ Chap. 12.3.2) (and the cerebellum, ➤ Chap. 12.4) arise from the lower vesicle.

The inside of the brainstem consists of nuclei (grey matter) and tracts (white matter). In the nuclei, there are essentially the primary sensory and motor **cranial nerve nuclei** (III–XII). In addition there are relay nuclei, processing information to and from the cranial nerve nuclei (e.g., the nuclei for eye movement coordination, the auditory system, the vestibular system), but also important **autonomic centres** such as the respiratory and circulatory centres and the so-called **Formatio reticularis**. In addition, there are relay nuclei for cerebellum afferents and nuclei that are **monoaminergic neurotransmitter systems** (serotonin, noradrenaline, dopamine).

12.3.1 Mesencephalon

Overview

The **midbrain (mesencephalon)** borders the diencephalon to cranial and caudal as the top section of the brainstem and continues to the pons. It is divided into three sections, which are clearly differentiated when seen in cross-section:

- **Basis mesencephali:** It is in an anterior position and contains the **Crura cerebri**, where large descending tracts, such as the pyramidal tracts, run.
- **Tegmentum mesencephali:** The covering of the mesencephalon borders the base of the midbrain and contains, amongst others, the **Substantia nigra** with dopaminergic neurons and the **Nucleus ruber**, both important nuclei of the extrapyramidal motor system, and the **nuclei of cranial nerves III and IV**, the **mesencephalic Raphe nuclei**, the **Substantia grisea centralis** and the **Aqueductus mesencephali,** the connection between the IIIrd and IVth ventricles.

- Quadrigeminal plate of the **Tectum mesencephali:** It is positioned at the posterior, and contains important relay stations for the visual and auditory systems in its **colliculi**.

Embryology

The mesencephalon develops from the middle vesicle of the 3 primary brain vesicles, the **mesencephalon vesicle**. Measured against the other sections of the brain, the mesencephalon grows less quickly in the course of the brain's development, and thus remains close to the isthmus (**Isthmus cerebri**). The delimiting of the mesencephalic vesicle and the caudal rhombencephalic vesicle is the first early embryological structuring of the rostral neural tube and is regulated by morphogenes of the embryonic **isthmic organiser**.

It is fundamentally important for the structure of the brain and the positioning of the brain in the skull.

NOTE

Morphogenic or transcription factors such as the pax genes are also involved in the further differentiation of the CNS and the formation of various nuclear areas. In research, the expression pattern of these genes is taken into account for determining detailed nuclear groups.

Seen in the horizontal plane looking inwards, the wall of the tube thickens due to the migration of cells from the base and alar plate, and the formation of nuclear areas. The neural canal later becomes

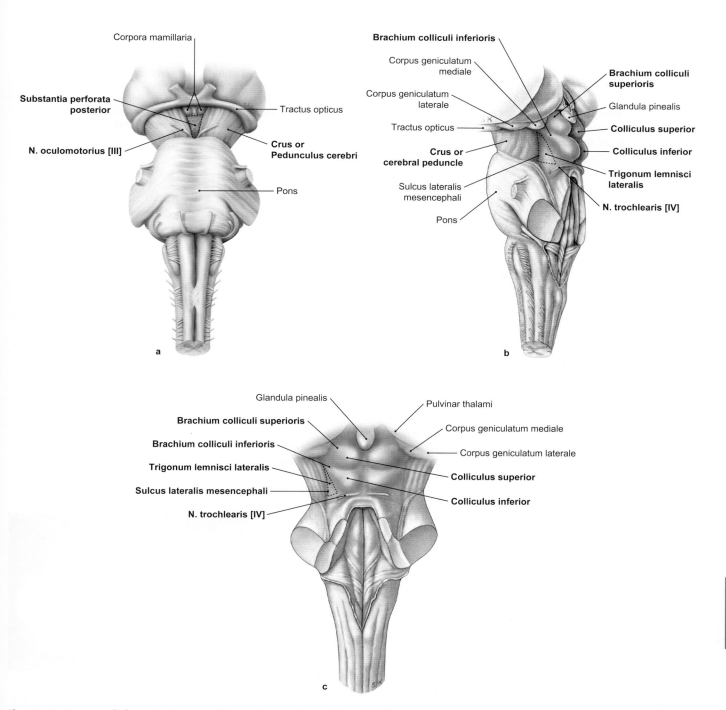

Fig. 12.23 Mesencephalon. a Ventral view. **b** Lateral view. **c** Dorsal view. [L238]

the Aqueductus mesencephali. Neuroblasts from the alar plate form the colliculi in the Tectum mesencephali, while neuroblasts from the base plate form the nuclear motor groups in the Tegmentum mesencephali (e g., Nucleus ruber, Substantia nigra, oculomotor cranial nerve nuclei [III and IV]). The corticopontine, corticonuclear and corticospinal fibres running within the Basis mesencephali arise from the cerebral cortex and thus ontogenetically from the telencephalon. Thus they follow the general principle that axons always sprout from the somata of nerve cells, and that the fibres (axons) of all tracts arise ontogenetically from their associated somata. It follows that tracts (with white matter) generally arise later as nuclear areas (with grey matter). Accordingly, after they arise, nuclear areas are often crossed through by fibres (e.g., taking the ascending fibres of the **Lemniscus medialis** from the rhombencephalon through the Tegmentum mesencephali).

Location and external appearance

Observed ventrally or basally, (➤ Fig. 12.23a) we can see the two caudally converging crura or **Pedunculi cerebri** at the mesencephalon, with the **Fossa interpeduncularis** lying between them. The oculomotor nerve [III] exits and the Aa. centrales posteriores enters in the Fossa interpeduncularis. If the meninges are removed during the dissection of the brainstem, these entry points create an area with small holes, referred to as the **Substantia perforata posterior**. Rostral from here are the medially-positioned Corpora mamillaria, as well as the Tractus optici of the diencephalon running a little further laterally; caudal of the Crura cerebri is the transversally running fibre bundle of the pons.

Viewed laterally (➤ Fig. 12.23b), each Crus cerebri is detached by the Sulcus lateralis mesencephali, forming the externally-visible demarcation of the Tegmentum mesencephali. On the dorsal side is the **Trigonum lemnisci lateralis**, under the surface of which are parts of the auditory system (**Lemniscus lateralis**).

Viewed dorsally, (➤ Fig. 12.23c) the Tectum mesencephali can be recognised by its signature surface relief, known as the quadrigeminal plate (**Lamina quadrigemina** or **Lamina tecti**). Here, a distinction is made between the two larger 'upper hills' (**Colliculi superiores**) and the two smaller 'lower hills' (**Colliculi inferiores**). On each side, the Colliculus superior is connected via the **Brachium colliculus superioris** with the **Corpus geniculatum laterale** (optic tract), and the Colliculus inferior via the **Brachium colliculi inferioris** with the **Corpus geniculatum mediale** (auditory system) of the thalamus. Directly caudal to the Colliculi inferiores, the N. trochlearis [IV] exits as the only cranial, dorsal nerve emerging on both sides from the brainstem, running around the lateral surface of the mesencephalon in the Cisterna ambiens to the front.

Rostrally, the mesencephalon borders the diencephalic Pulvinar thalami as well as the habenulae with the Glandula pinealis; caudally the upper cerebellar peduncles, together with the upper cerebellar sail, form the demarcation with the pons.

Clinical remarks

The mesencephalon pushing through the Incisura tentorii is surrounded in this area by the free edge of the Tentorium cerebelli and by fluid from the Cisterna ambiens. Due to the topography, medial parts of the temporal lobes can be compressed into the respective gaps between the mesencephalon and the Tentorium cerebelli and become trapped (**'upper entrapment'**) where there are supratentorial processes demanding space (e.g., bleeding, tumor). This may result in numerous neurological symptoms, such as:

- failure of the ipsilateral N. oculomotorius [III] with widening of the pupils
- compression of the pyramidal tract in the Crura cerebri with accompanying motor paralysis, spasms of the extremities and exaggerated proprioceptive reflexes
- a compression of the internal pathways and autonomous centres of the Substantia grisea centralis of the mesencephalon, which may lead to circulatory dysregulation, autonomic lapse or loss of consciousness, known as **midbrain syndrome**.

Internal structure

In cross-sectional images (➤ Fig. 12.24), the three sections of the mesencephalon are clearly delimited from ventral to dorsal:

- Basis mesencephali with the Crura cerebri
- Tegmentum mesencephali
- Tectum mesencephali

Basis mesencephali with the Crura cerebri

The Crura cerebri consist of projection fibres. These can be assigned to specific tracts. In each crus, the following can be basically distinguished:

- Projection fibres of the cerebrum to the **Fibrae corticopontinae**
- Projection fibres of the pyramidal tract, which pass from the cerebrum to the cranial nerve nuclei or to the spinal cord (**Fibrae corticonucleares and corticospinales**)

Within a Crus cerebri, these fibres are arranged by somatopes. Fibrae corticopontinae run quite medially from the frontal cortex; they are then joined laterally by Fibrae corticonucleares, then by Fibrae corticospinales, and running completely laterally are Fibrae corticopontinae from the parietal and occipital cortex. In this way,

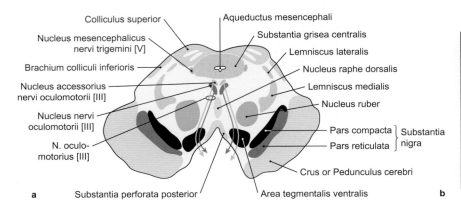
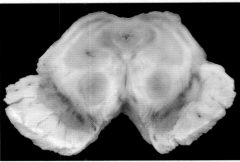

Fig. 12.24 Cross-section through the rostral mesencephalon at the level of the exit of the N. oculomotorius. **a** Diagram [L126]. **b** Anatomical dissection [R247].

the projection fibres of the pyramidal tract are flanked within the Crura cerebri by the respective corticopontine fibre system.

Tegmentum mesencephali
Substantia nigra
Directly dorsal of the Crura cerebri is the Substantia nigra, an important nuclear area, especially for the dopaminergic system. Macroscopically it appears to be black due to the high melanin content in the perikarya of the local dopaminergic neurons and can therefore be easily recognised in mesencephalic segment dissections. Microscopically, 2 parts are distinguished:

- The **Pars compacta** is the larger part of the Substantia nigra, lying further dorsally. Here the dopaminergic neurons are found, tightly packed together.
- The **Pars reticulata** is the smaller part of the Substantia nigra, located further ventrally. The GABAerg neurons are located here and are not as tightly packed as in the Pars compacta.

The Substantia nigra receives afferents from both the motor and the premotor areas of the cerebral cortex as well as from the striatum. Efferent is projected by the dopaminergic neurons of the Pars compacta into the striatum (**Fibrae nigrostriatales**), and by the GABAergic neurons of the Pars reticulata, primarily into the thalamus.

Clinical remarks

In **PARKINSON's disease,** neuropathological dissection reveals a definite blanching of the Substantia nigra (Pars compacta). This is caused by the morphological loss of the local dopaminergic neuron population.

Area tegmentalis ventralis
Medial to the Substantia nigra there is another primarily dopaminergic neuronal population, the so-called Area tegmentalis ventralis. From here, primarily efferent projection fibres go into the cortical and limbic areas, such as the prefrontal cortex, the hippocampus, amygdala and the Nucleus accumbens, and form the mesocorticolimbic dopaminergic system.

Nucleus ruber
Directly dorsal of the Area tegmentalis ventralis is a nuclear area that appears reddish in a freshly sectioned dissection, due to the high iron content of the neurons found there, called the Nucleus ruber, stretching rostrocaudally from the approximate border of the diencephalon up to the caudal margin of the Colliculi superiores. Microscopically, 2 parts are distinguished:

- The **Pars parvocellularis** is located further rostrally and contains small neurons, which are primarily reached via the Capsula interna by afferents from the ipsilateral cerebral cortex (**Tractus corticorubralis**), and also to a small extent via the upper cerebellar stem by afferents from the contralateral Nucleus dentatus of the cerebellum. The neurons project efferents via the **Tractus tegmentalis centralis** ipsilaterally to the lower olive, thereby belonging to the extrapyramidal-motor cortico-rubro-olivo-cerebellar system.
- The **Pars magnocellularis** lies caudally and in humans tends to be poorly formed. It is reached via the upper cerebellar stem, particularly by afferents from the contralateral Nuclei globosus and emboliformis of the cerebellum. To a lesser extent, afferents from the ipsilateral cerebral cortex end here. The neurons of the Pars magnocellularis project via the **Tractus rubrospinalis** (which in humans tends to be poorly formed) into the contralateral spinal cord in particular.

Aqueductus mesencephali and Substantia grisea centralis
Exactly in the middle of the dorsal tegmentum is the **Aqueductus mesencephali**. This canal like structure links the IIIrd ventricle within the diencephalon to the IVth ventricle within the rhombencephalon.

The Aqueductus mesencephali is surrounded by a collection of grey matter, the periaqueductal grey (**Substantia grisea centralis**). This is a complex integration centre for primarily autonomic functions. Morphologically, it mostly maintains numerous reciprocal connections with the hypothalamus and structures of the limbic system, with the autonomic nerve centres of the pons and Medulla oblongata and various cranial nerve nuclei. Functionally, the Substantia grisea centralis is involved, amongst others, in the central autonomous control and coordinates anxiety and, fight or flight, reflexes, as well as various cranial nerve nuclei for voice projection. It has another central role in endogenous pain inhibition because its corresponding neurons project via Raphe nuclei into the spinal cord, in order to inhibit pain impulses by activating inhibitory interneurons (also ➤ Chap. 13.8).

Clinical remarks

Pharmacologically, the neuroanatomical circumstances of the Substantia grisea centralis are used in central pain treatment, as the endorphinogenic afferents of the endogenous pain-relieving system end at the local nerve cells. Endorphins are effective via opiate receptors. In the context of **central pain treatment**, opiates such as morphine or derivatives of morphine can target these receptors and, by stimulating neurons in the Substantia grisea centralis, activate the endogenous pain inhibition system.

Nucleus raphe dorsalis
Ventral of the Substantia grisea centralis, the serotonergic mesencephalic Raphe nuclei, also referred to as the Nucleus raphe dorsalis, lie in the midline (➤ Chap. 12.3.3). They project locally into the mesencephalon, mainly ascending into the diencephalon and telencephalon.

Cranial nerve nuclei and pathways
In the rostral mesencephalon, the **Nucleus nervi oculomotorii [III]** are located ventrally of the Aqueductus mesencephali next to the midline and directly dorsal of the **Nucleus accessorius nervi oculomotorii EDINGER-WESTPHAL**. The **Nucleus nervi trochlearis [IV]** is located in the caudal mesencephalon, lateral to the mesencephalic Raphe nuclei. Directly lateral to the Substantia grisea centralis is the **Nucleus mesencephalicus nervi trigemini [V]** with its characteristically large somata seen in a histological dissection. This is the perikarya of the proprioceptive pseudo-unipolar neurons from the chewing muscles. The following **systems or ducts** also pass through the Tegmentum mesencephali: Formatio reticularis, Lemniscus medialis, Lemniscus lateralis, Tractus spinothalamicus, Tractus tegmentalis centralis, Tractus tectospinalis, Fasciculi longitudinales medialis and posterior, Decussationes pedunculorum cerebellarium superiorum.

Tectum mesencephali
The Tectum mesencephali consists of the Lamina quadrigemina. This, in turn, is constructed from the two Colliculi superiores and the two Colliculi inferiores.

Colliculi superiores

The Colliculi superiorus each consist of 7 layers and are an important optic reflex centre. Respectively, they primarily receive afferents from the visual system via the Brachium collicullis superior, including retinotectally directly from the N. opticus and/or the Tractus opticus, from the occipitally located visual cortex and from the frontal field of vision, as well as from the spinal cord and the Colliculi inferiores. The Colliculi superiores are connected efferently with the motor nuclei of the brainstem via the **Tractus tectobulbaris**, and via the **Tractus tectospinalis** with the motor neurons of the spinal cord.

Due to these links, in the case of acute visual stimuli such as a flash of light, the Colliculi superiores can cause the eyelids to close and/or the head to turn away. On the other hand, they also play a decisive role in turning the head and eyes towards an acoustic stimulus. In addition, they are very important for the coordination of rapid eye movement, known as saccades. The integration function of the Colliculi superiores means that a look can be directed as quickly as possible to corresponding targets and that the eye is assisted in following moving objects.

Colliculi inferiores

The Colliculi inferiores are an important relay station in the auditory system and consist respectively of one large and 2 smaller nuclei: Nucleus centralis, Nucleus pericentralis and Nucleus externus. The Lemniscus lateralis of the auditory system ends afferently at the tonotopically-structured Nucleus centralis; its efferents pass via the Brachium colliculi inferioris to the Corpus geniculatum mediale of the thalamus, where they are switched onto the neurons of the auditory system that reach the auditory cortex.

12.3.2 Pons and Medulla oblongata

Overview

The **pons** and the extended medulla (**Medulla oblongata**) is assigned along with the **cerebellum** to the **rhombencephalon**. The rhombencephalon received its name from the **Fossa rhomboidea**, the rhomboid-shaped confined dorsal surface of the pons and Medulla oblongata, forming the 'floor' or the front wall of the IVth ventricle. Rostrally, the rhombencephalon is marked-off topographically from the mesencephalon by the Tentorium cerebelli. Caudally, it merges at the Foramen magnum with the spinal cord. The pons and Medulla oblongata are reached and infused by the rising and descending ducts connecting the rostral brain sections with the cerebellum and the spinal cord. They contain the nuclei of the subtentorial cranial nerves (V–XII), vital autonomous centres for respiration, circulation and digestion, the caudal sections of the hearing and balance system as well as the nuclei of the afferent cerebellar pathways.

> ### Clinical remarks
>
> Clinically, **injury to the pons and Medulla oblongata** is frequently dramatic, as they may often lead to life-threatening disturbances of breathing and circulation, as well as the interruption of descending motor control or the ascending sensory pathways.

Embryology

Ontogenetically, the rhombencephalon originates from the most caudal of the 3 primary brain vesicles, the **rhombencephalic vesicle**. Its delimitation from the mesencephalon occurs very early on.

It is the first rostrocaudal segmentation of the neural tube in the brain structure. Initially, the rhombencephalon is arranged in 8 rostrocaudally arranged **rhombomeres**. But this structure is largely lost during development, in contrast to the somite-induced segmental structure of the spinal cord. The cerebellum only forms relatively late on dorsally. Parallel to it, the Nuclei pontis develops in the ventral rostral area. Later on, these form the characteristic ventral swelling at the Pars basilaris pontis. Laterally, they continue into the middle cerebellar peduncles (**Pedunculi cerebellares medii**) which span the original rhombencephalon (the dorsal part of the pons) like a bridge, to pass dorsally into the cerebellum. Corresponding with its later shape, the pons and cerebellum are referred to as the hindbrain (**metencephalon**) and is delimited from the afterbrain (**myelencephalon** and/or Medulla oblongata).

Pons

Position and external appearance

The pons is above the clivus and is cranially adjacent to the Crura cerebri and caudally adjacent to the bulbus of the Medulla oblongata, from which it is separated by the transverse Fissura pontomedullaris. At the ventral surface (➤ Fig. 12.25a), transverse fibre bundles dominate, and these each merge laterally into the middle cerebellar peduncle (**Pedunculus cerebellaris medius**). Medially, there is a longitudinal furrow, the Sulcus basilaris, in which the A. basilaris runs. Right and left of this sulcus, there are 2 horizontal bulges generated by the longitudinally-running pyramidal fibres. Laterally, on each side at the transition from the pons to the middle cerebellar peduncle, the N. trigeminus exits with its Radix motoria and Radix sensoria; exiting ventrally at the lower edge of the pons in the medial area of the Fissura pontomedullaris are the N. abducens and, at the lateral margin of the pons, the N. facialis and N. vestibulocochlearis in the so-called cerebellopontine angle (➤ Fig. 12.25b). This is positioned between the lower margin of the pons, the lower edge of the middle and lower cerebellar peduncle (**Pedunculus cerebellaris inferior**), as well as rostral and dorsal of the lower olive of the Medulla oblongata.

The dorsal surface of the pons (➤ Fig. 12.25c) is the rostral half of the rhomboid fossa and is only visible after removal of the cerebellum. Among other things, the **Colliculus facialis**, is notable here as a protrusion caused by the bend in the facial nerve (Genu nervi facialis).

Internal structure

The pons and the Medulla oblongata emerged ontogenetically as a single unit; accordingly, the internal structures show continuity and the Fissura pontomedullaris is not a clear internal boundary. The pons is divided into a front section, the **Pars basilaris pontis**, and a rear section, the **Pars dorsalis pontis**. This can be particularly clearly visualised in cross-section (➤ Fig. 12.26). The Pars basilaris, which determines the mighty ventral swelling at the pons, takes up around two-thirds of the ventral surface. Dorsally, the original pontine part of the rhombencephalon joins with the Pars dorsalis, forming the rostral continuation of the Medulla oblongata.

Pars basilaris pontis

In the white matter of this pons section there are fibres running in both a longitudinal and transversal direction (**Fibrae pontis longitudinales and transversae**), and in the grey matter embedded in between them, there are numerous **Nuclei pontis**. The Fibrae pontis longitudinales continue the fibre tracts of the Crura cerebri and therefore contain the pyramidal tracts routed through the pons and corticopontine projections that end at the neurons of the Nuclei pontis. In turn, their axons run as Fibrae pontis transversae to the opposite sides and reach the cerebellar cortex via the Pedunculus

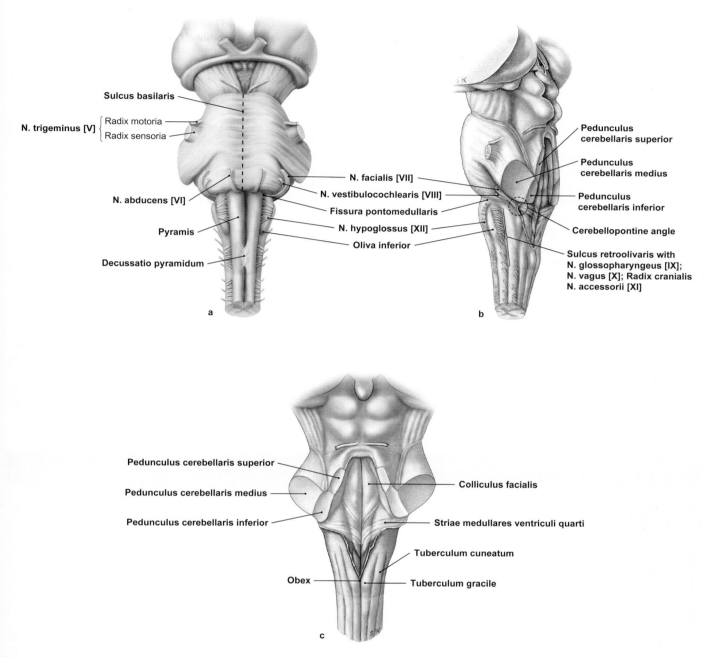

Sulcus basilaris

N. trigeminus [V] { Radix motoria / Radix sensoria

N. abducens [VI]

Pyramis

Decussatio pyramidum

N. facialis [VII]

N. vestibulocochlearis [VIII]

Fissura pontomedullaris

N. hypoglossus [XII]

Oliva inferior

Pedunculus cerebellaris superior

Pedunculus cerebellaris medius

Pedunculus cerebellaris inferior

Cerebellopontine angle

Sulcus retroolivaris with N. glossopharyngeus [IX]; N. vagus [X]; Radix cranialis N. accessorii [XI]

Pedunculus cerebellaris superior

Pedunculus cerebellaris medius

Pedunculus cerebellaris inferior

Obex

Colliculus facialis

Striae medullares ventriculi quarti

Tuberculum cuneatum

Tuberculum gracile

Fig. 12.25 Pons and Medulla oblongata. a Ventral view. **b** Lateral view. **c** Dorsal view. [L238]

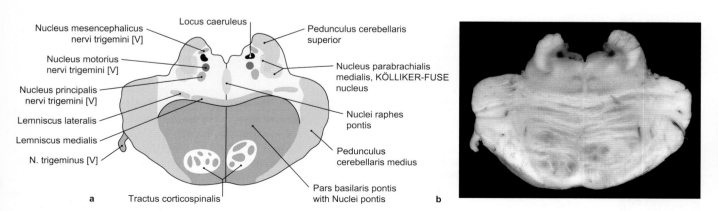

Nucleus mesencephalicus nervi trigemini [V]

Locus caeruleus

Nucleus motorius nervi trigemini [V]

Nucleus principalis nervi trigemini [V]

Lemniscus lateralis

Lemniscus medialis

N. trigeminus [V]

Tractus corticospinalis

Pedunculus cerebellaris superior

Nucleus parabrachialis medialis, KÖLLIKER-FUSE nucleus

Nuclei raphes pontis

Pedunculus cerebellaris medius

Pars basilaris pontis with Nuclei pontis

Fig. 12.26 Cross-section through the rostral pons at the level of the exit of the N. trigeminus. **a** Diagram [L126]. **b** Anatomical dissection. [R247]

cerebellaris medius. At its entry point at the Pars basilaris pontis, the pyramidal tract separates into numerous fascicles, which push through the grey matter, and after passing through the pons reunite into a common structure, the pyramid.

Pars dorsalis pontis
The dorsal part of the pons, like the caudally-joining Medulla oblongata, is divided into a medial raphe and lateral parts, containing numerous nuclear areas of the brainstem system, the Formatio reticularis and the pontine cranial nerve nuclei (V–VIII). Laterally, it includes the area of the cerebellar peduncle. In contrast to the Pars basilaris, which has a similar cross-section structure at all levels, significant differences can be found in the Pars dorsalis pontis, depending on the level of the relevant cross-section:

- In the **rostral half**, trigeminal nuclear complexes are found. These include the dorsolaterally located Nucleus motorius nervi trigemini, and further laterally, the Nucleus principalis nervi trigemini. Dorsal from here are the Tractus mesencephalicus nervi trigemini and the caudal sections of the Nucleus mesencephalicus nervi trigemini. In the area of the midline are the **Nuclei raphes pontis** as well as caudally and ventrally of the upper cerebellar peduncle (**Pedunculus cerebellaris superior**), the pigmented **Locus caeruleus**, an essential part of the central catecholaminergic system. In addition, directly lateral and also ventral of the upper cerebellar peduncle are the **Nuclei parabrachiales medialis and lateralis** and the **KÖLLIKER-FUSE nucleus**. These nuclear areas form the pontine respiratory group for the central regulation of breathing.

- In the **caudal half**, directly dorsal of the Nuclei pontis of the Pars basilaris, is the **Corpus trapezoideum** and lateral from here lies the upper olive (**Nucleus olivaris superior**), both being nuclear areas of the auditory system (➤ Table 12.5, also ➤ Chap. 13.4). Positioned ventrally along the midline is the **Raphe pontis** with the pontine serotonergic Raphe nuclei positioned caudally. Located ventrolaterally is the **Nucleus nervi facialis [VII]**. The axons of the motor neurons localised within the pons run initially dorsally and then entwine the **Nucleus nervi abducentis [VI]**, which sits on the dorsal surface, caudally and medially, subsequently running laterally to the ventral surface of the pons, and exiting from the brainstem together with the N. vestibulocochlearis in the cerebellopontine angle. The **vestibular nuclei** lie dorsally on the floor of the rhomboid fossa in the pontomedullary transition area. We can differentiate between 4 subnuclei – the Nuclei vestibularis medialis, lateralis, superior and inferior, all of which receive nerve fibres from the vestibular part of the N. vestibulocochlearis and send axons to the cerebellum (➤ Table 12.5, also ➤ Chap. 13.5). Ventral of the Nuclei vestibulares are the Nuclei cochleares dorsalis and ventralis (also ➤ Chap. 13.4).

The following **systems or ducts** pass through the Pars dorsalis: Lemniscus medialis, Lemniscus lateralis, Tractus tegmentalis centralis, Fasciculi longitudinales medialis and posterior, Tractus mesencephalicus and spinalis nervi trigemini. The fibres of the **Lemniscus medialis**, which cross in the Decussatio lemniscorum of the Medulla oblongata, initially pass dorsally along the Corpus trapezoideum in the caudal pons right next to the midline. Along their rostral pathway, they move increasingly laterally, reaching the dorsolateral surface in

Table 12.5 Overview of the functional anatomy of the brainstem.

Centre/system	Function/reflex		Nuclear area or brain area	Participating afferent cranial nerves	Participating efferent cranial nerve nuclei or spinal cord
Eyes/Vision	Pupillary reflex		Area pretectalis	N. opticus [II]	Nucleus accessorius nervi oculomotorii
	Ocular motor function		Pre-occular motor centres, Colliculi superiores	N. opticus [II]	Nucleus nervi oculomotorii [III], Nucleus nervi trochlearis [IV], Nucleus nervi abducentis [VI]
	Corneal reflex, eyelid movement			Nucleus principalis nervi trigemini [V]	Nucleus nervi facialis [VII]
Ears/hearing	Directional hearing, movement of the head towards the source of the sound		Nucleus olivaris superior, Corpus trapezoideum, Colliculi inferiores	Nuclei cochleares [VIII]	Spinal cord (cervical anterior horn)
Balance	Posture, spatial orientation		Nucleus olivaris inferior, cerebellum	Nuclei vestibulares [VIII]	Spinal cord
Nose	Sneezing reflex		Respiratory centre, ventrolateral Medulla oblongata	Nucleus principalis nervi trigemini [V/2]	Nucleus ambiguus (IX, X), spinal cord (anterior horn)
Gastrointestinal tract	Taste, saliva			Rostral part of the Nucleus tractus solitarii (VII, IX, X)	Nucleus salivatorius superior [VII] and inferior [IX]
	Swallowing		Swallowing centre, ventrolateral Medulla oblongata	Nucleus principalis nervi trigemini (V/2, V/3), medial Nucleus tractus solitarii (IX, X)	Nucleus motorius nervi trigemini [V/3], Nucleus nervi facialis [VII], Nucleus ambiguus (IX, X), Nucleus Nervi hypoglossi [XII]
	Vomiting		Area postrema	Medial Nucleus tractus solitarii [X]	Nucleus dorsalis nervi vagi [X]
	Digestion (including secretion of gastric juices, bile, pancreatic juices and peristalsis)			Medial Nucleus tractus solitarii [X]	Nucleus dorsalis nervi vagi [X]
Breathing	Respiratory reflexes (including lung expansion reflex, cough reflex)		Respiratory centre, ventrolateral Medulla oblongata	Lateral Nucleus tractus solitarii [X]	Nucleus ambiguus (IX, X), Nucleus nervi hypoglossi [XII], spinal cord (ventral horn)
Heart/circulation	Circulatory reflexes (including baroreceptor and chemoreceptor reflexes)		Circulation centre, rostral ventrolateral Medulla oblongata (RVLM)	Dorsolateral Nucleus tractus solitarii (IX, X)	Nucleus ambiguus, external formation [X], sympathicus, spinal cord: lateral horn

the caudal mesencephalon. In the rostral pons, they incorporate the fibres of the Nucleus principalis nervi trigemini. The Lemniscus lateralis joins laterally. Ventrally the **Fasciculus longitudinalis medialis** runs near the midline on the floor of the rhomboid fossa.

Medulla oblongata
Position and external appearance
The Medulla oblongata is the caudal part of the rhombencephalon. Ventrally it sits on the clivus and extends caudally to the Foramen magnum. The ventral surface (➤ Fig. 12.25a) of the bulbus is characterised medially by the longitudinal tracts of the pyramid, **Pyramis**. Both the pyramids taper caudally, and the majority of descending fibres of the Tractus corticospinalis cross over in the **Decussatio pyramidum**, which marks the boundary with the spinal cord. Directly to the side of the pyramid, the **lower olive (Oliva inferior)** joins; it is well-defined on the outer surface as an ovoid nuclear area. It serves as a good ventral landmark: its expansion corresponds exactly with the 'open' rostral Medulla oblongata, i.e. it starts at the Fissura pontomedullaris and extends caudally to the obex. Between the pyramid and lower olive, the roots of the N. hypoglossus [XII] exit; dorsally of the lower olive in the **Sulcus retroolivaris**, the roots of the N. glossopharyngeus [IX] and the N. vagus [X], as well as the Radix cranialis of the N. accessorius [XI] (➤ Fig. 12.25a, b) exit. Dorsally, the Medulla oblongata lies on the cerebellum, with which it is connected via the two lower cerebellar peduncles (Pedunculi cerebellares inferiores). In the area of the Medulla oblongata, the IVth ventricle narrows caudally to the central canal – in this way a rostral section (open part of the Medulla oblongata = caudal half of the Fossa rhomboidea) can be distinguished from the caudal section (closed part of the Medulla oblongata) (➤ Fig. 12.25c). The entrance point to the central canal is known as the **obex**. It serves as an important landmark to determine the rostrocaudal level of cross-sections through the rhombencephalon. Laterally and caudally, the Fossa rhomboidea is bordered by protrusions of the Nuclei gracilis and cuneatus (**Tubercula gracile and cuneatum**), which pass to the spinal cord in the corresponding longitudinal bulges of the Funiculi gracilis and cuneatus of the posterior column tracts.

Internal structure of the Medulla oblongata
The Medulla oblongata (➤ Fig. 12.27), is structured like the pons as a median raphe (**Nuclei raphes medullae**) with lateral parts, containing numerous nuclear areas of the brainstem systems and the Formatio reticularis, as well as the medullar cranial nerve nuclei (IX–XII). Laterally, the area of the cerebellar peduncle is included.

Rostral half
In the rostral half (open part of the Medulla oblongata = caudal half of the Fossa rhomboidea), the pyramid and the lower olive are notable ventrally. Positioned dorsally are the nuclei of the posterior column tract, the Nuclei gracilis and cuneatus, and laterally, the Pedunculi cerebellares inferiores pass to the cerebellum.

On the cross-section, the **lower olive** is highly visible macroscopically as the largest nuclear area of the Medulla oblongata. The winding, snake-like tracts are characteristic, formed from numerous small and densely-packed somata, wherein a number of sub-nuclei can be distinguished. Overall, the lower olive is a relay nucleus in front of the cerebellum, primarily processing spinal and vestibular information.

Directly around the central canal or at the bottom of the IVth ventricle is the **Nucleus nervi hypoglossi [XII]**. It consists of ventral and dorsal subnuclei representing different tongue muscles. Dorsally of the Nucleus nervi hypoglossi is the **Nucleus dorsalis nervi vagi [X]** and dorsally thereof is the **Nucleus tractus solitarii (IX, X)**, which also contains taste buds in the rostral section.

Located directly on the obex, medially dorsal of the central canal, is the small **Area postrema** with right and left lateral offshoots which are in direct contact with the Nucleus tractus solitarii. The Area postrema contains vagal visceroafferents and is the central vomiting centre. In the Area postrema, the blood–brain barrier is suspended.

Located dorsolaterally are the sensory **Nuclei principalis and spinalis nervi trigemini [V]**. Dorsal of the Nucleus spinalis nervi trigemini, in the rostral Medulla oblongata, are the caudal parts of the **Nuclei vestibulares**, as well as the **Nucleus salivatorius inferior [IX]**. In the ventrolateral medulla is the **Nucleus ambiguus**, which comprises the motor neurons of the branchiogenic muscles of the 3rd–6th pharyngeal arch (IX, X, medullary section of XI), i.e. the muscles of the larynx and the pharynx. It forms a longitudinal rostrocaudal Pars compacta, which passes through the entire Medulla oblongata as the actual Nucleus ambiguus, as well as individual para-ambigualis nucleus groups ventral of this Pars compacta, including the external formation which includes parasympathetic neurons for the innervation of the heart (➤ Table 12.5, also ➤ Chap. 13.9). In the immediate vicinity and ventrally of the Nucleus ambiguus are the groups of medullary breathing regulation with the **pre-BÖTZINGER complex** as the medullary respiratory centre. Medial to the respiratory centre the nuclei of the medullary cardiovascular entre is positioned in the rostral ventrolateral Medulla oblongata, which, amongst others, sends adrenergic neurons to the sympathetic neurons of the spinal cord.

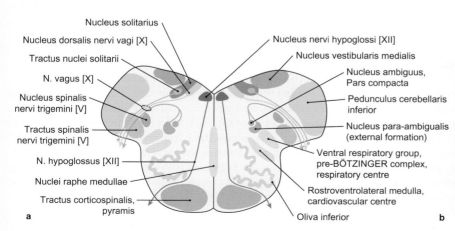
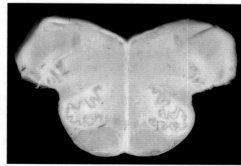

Nucleus solitarius
Nucleus dorsalis nervi vagi [X]
Tractus nuclei solitarii
N. vagus [X]
Nucleus spinalis nervi trigemini [V]
Tractus spinalis nervi trigemini [V]
N. hypoglossus [XII]
Nuclei raphe medullae
Tractus corticospinalis, pyramis

Nucleus nervi hypoglossi [XII]
Nucleus vestibularis medialis
Nucleus ambiguus, Pars compacta
Pedunculus cerebellaris inferior
Nucleus para-ambigualis (external formation)
Ventral respiratory group, pre-BÖTZINGER complex, respiratory centre
Rostroventrolateral medulla, cardiovascular centre
Oliva inferior

a   b

Fig. 12.27 Cross-section through the rostral Medulla oblongata at the level of the exit point of the N. vagus. **a** Diagram [L126]. **b** Anatomical dissection [R247].

Caudal half

In the caudal half (closed part of the Medulla oblongata = transition to the spinal cord) the lower olive is no longer visible and the cross-section is significantly reduced. The tapered caudal offshoots of the **nuclear areas** of the rostral Medulla oblongata are truncated (Nucleus ambiguus, Nucleus dorsalis nervi vagi, Nucleus tractus solitarii, Nucleus nervi hypoglossi), which partially extend to the spinal cord or continue in tracts to/from the spinal cord. The transition from the caudal Medulla oblongata to the spinal cord is fluid and is called a transitional zone. However, the anterior and dorsal horn of the spinal cord are clearly delimited by the rostrally entering and/or exiting spinal roots of the C1.

The following **tract systems** go to or pass through the Medulla oblongata: Lemniscus medialis, Tractus tegmentalis centralis, Fasciculi longitudinales medialis and posterior, Tractus spinalis nervi trigemini, Tractus corticonuclearis and corticospinalis, Tractus spinothalamicus, Tractus spinocerebellaris. Axons from the posterior column nuclei pass ventrally and medially and cross in the midline, ventrally of the Nucleus nervi hypoglossi, in the Decussatio lemniscorum, and finally ascend.

Clinical remarks

Bilateral **damage to the motor cranial nerve nuclei** in the Medulla oblongata causes **bulbar paralysis**. The tongue and throat muscles are paralysed by atrophy, so that those affected clinically display slurred speech and difficulty swallowing. A possible cause is a neurodegenerative motor neuron disease, such as Amyotrophic Lateral Sclerosis (ALS).

NOTE

In order to inspect the **Fossa rhomboidea**, the cerebellum is detached at the 3 cerebellar peduncles and the rear side of the pons and Medulla oblongata (➤ Fig. 12.25c) can be seen. You can see the diamond-shaped, identically named 'floor' or the front panel of the IVth ventricle. The rostral arms of the Fossa rhomboidea are bordered by the cerebellar peduncles; the caudal arms are bordered by the adhesion site of the Tela choroidea of the IVth ventricle at the Medulla oblongata. In between, where the IVth ventricle has its largest lateral expansion, the Recessus laterales are on the left and right with the Aperturae laterales. This lateral expansion marks the dorsal border between the pons and the Medulla oblongata. Additionally, this limit is indicated by the Striae medullares ventriculi quarti which crosses the floor of the Fossa rhomboidea and belongs to the auditory system. Rostrally, the surface of the Fossa rhomboidea provides reference points for the position of the pontine cranial nerve nuclei (V–VIII), and caudally for the position of the medullary cranial nerve nuclei (IX, X, XII).

12.3.3 Functional systems of the brainstem

The anatomical configuration of the functional system of the brainstem is as complex as the range of functions it performs. The brainstem contains relay nuclei which process information to and from the nuclei of cranial nerves III–XII (e.g., the nuclei for eye movement coordination, the auditory system, the vestibular system, but also important autonomic centres such as the respiratory and circulatory centres, which amongst others relay autonomous afferents and efferents of the N. vagus). In addition, there are relay nuclei for cerebellar afferents and nuclei of the monoaminergic neurotransmitter systems (serotonin, noradrenaline, dopamine). The functional relationships are presented in the respective chapters (sensory systems, cranial nerves, cerebellum, autonomic nervous system).

Brainstem reflexes

Learning about brainstem function, and particularly about basic configurations, helps with the orientation of brainstem reflexes and their afferent and efferent reflex limbs into the corresponding cranial nerves (➤ Table 12.5). Additionally, the testing of brainstem reflexes or cranial nerve reflexes is of central, vital importance when taking any medical history (e.g., first aid for unconscious people). Also applying to the brainstem as for the entire CNS is the distinction between

- a somatosensory nervous system, the response to environmental stimuli via the afferent senses and efferent skeletal muscle movements
- an autonomic nervous system, the control and maintenance of body functions by autonomic primary afferents and efferents

For both systems, there are essential rules for their organisation: the principle of rostrocaudal hierarchy or the overall impact of higher centres is opposed by the principle of local control or the shortest possible oligosynaptic interconnection between primary afferents and efferents, i.e. of the rapid reflex arches. This results in the model of the 'rope ladder' nervous system, with ascending and descending systems side by side, which are configured with each other on all rostrocaudal levels (from the spinal cord to the cerebral cortex) while at the same time being subject to rostrocaudal hierarchical control. It also derives from the principle that the first central nervous configuration always takes place at the entry point level of the afferents, such as controlling the respiratory movements at the level of the Medulla oblongata (breathing reflex).

An overview of the brainstem functions or brainstem reflexes and their configuration is shown in ➤ Table 12.5.

Formatio reticularis

The parts of the brainstem referred to as the Formatio reticularis are those which histologically do not have clearly defined fibre tracts or nuclear areas. The area of the Formatio reticularis lies in the inner part of the brainstem (Tegmentum mesencephali, Pars dorsalis pontis, Medulla oblongata) between the median raphe and the outer adjacent nuclear areas and tracts. Characteristically, there are varying numbers of loosely-bundled groups of nerve cells of different sizes, as well as fibre bundles, which pass through the area of the Formatio reticularis in all directions. From this it has been concluded that the Formatio reticularis is a diffuse network of multiple relay neurons, which passes through the entire brainstem, and according to some authors, also through the diencephalon and the cervical spinal cord. To this quasi-intrinsic network of the brainstem, certain functions have also been assigned, such as the ascending reticular activating system (**ARAS**). Under the influence of serotonergic Raphe nuclei, this causes an activation of the motor system ascending from the spinal cord, as well as the central autonomous nuclear areas up to the hypothalamus and limbic system. As a result, the body is in a state of increased alertness and awareness.

With such a diffuse definition, the Formatio reticularis by its very nature resists this kind of clear distinction. The more that is known about individual nuclear groups and their functions (for example, due to evidence from specific transmitters and receptors), the more this perception is replaced by a detailed description of individual areas and systems. However, the apparently disorganised diversity of the systems in the brainstem is an expression of the phylogenetically old, 'matured' and complex regulation of vital autonomous bodily functions.

Raphe and Raphe nuclei, serotonin system

In all sections of the brainstem, numerous **commissure fibres** cross the midline, which do not only belong to the long ascending and

Table 12.6 Monoaminergic neurotransmitter systems of the brainstem.

Name of the nuclear area	Position in the brainstem	Neuro-transmitters used	Projection goals
Substantia nigra, Pars compacta	Borders between Basis and Tegmentum mesencephali	Dopamine	Striatum
Area tegmentalis ventralis (VTA)	Tegmentum mesencephali	Dopamine	Cerebral cortex, limbic system, Nucleus accumbens
Nucleus or Locus caeruleus	Part of the Formatio reticularis in the Tegmentum pontis	Noradrenaline	Cerebral cortex, limbic system, thalamus, hypothalamus, cerebellum
Raphe nuclei	Nuclear groups in the area of the Mesencephalon up to the Medulla oblongata	Serotonin	Total CNS

descending tracts, but are also mostly axons of local nuclear groups that are coordinated bilaterally. All of the fibres crossing in all directions over the midline are referred to as **raphes**. Depending on the segment of the brainstem, a distinction is made between the mesencephalic, pontine and medullar raphes. In all raphe segments, there are serotonergic neurons embedded in different groups of nuclei, referred to as mesencephalic, pontine and medullar **raphe nuclei**. Typical of the **serotonergic system** (but also of other monoaminergic systems, such as the dopamine, histaminergic or noradrenergic systems, ➤ Table 12.6) is the concentration of serotonergic somata on a few, relatively small nuclear areas in the brainstem, from where large parts of the brain and spinal cord are reached by deep axonal fibres. In the case of the serotonergic system, all areas of the CNS without exception and microscopically almost all neurons are reached directly by a dense network of axonal terminals. These terminals are often enlarged presynaptic boutons and are therefore referred to as varicose terminals. They release serotonin into the extracellular spaces, from where it can act on postsynaptic serotonin receptors of the target neurons. This brings to mind a scattergun approach, i.e. the seemingly random distribution of serotonin to all nerve cells of the central nervous system. However, the effect is completely different:

- Postsynaptic stimulation is also achieved very specifically at individual target cells by numerous, highly-varied and partly counteracting serotonin receptors.
- Raphe nuclei neurons have different target areas: the dorsal and medial mesencephalic Raphe nuclei send axons in 2 concurrent systems to the mesencephalon, diencephalon and telencephalon; the pontine and medullary Raphe nuclei supply the rhombencephalon and spinal cord.
- Even more striking is a particularly strong innervation of the primary somatic afferent nuclei in the brainstem and the spinal cord, especially the pain pathway, as well as the primary somatoefferent nuclei, i.e. the motor neurons. This increases awareness of incoming (afferent) environmental stimuli and reinforces the somatic response, i.e. the activation of the skeletal muscle.

Clinical remarks

According to current understanding, both the noradrenergic projections of the Nucleus caeruleus and the serotonergic projections of the Raphe nuclei are clinically highly significant in the pathogenesis of **mood disorders**, such as depression. In our society, this is a very common psychiatric illness, and is assumed to be due to a lack of noradrenaline and/or serotonin in the synaptic gap. This deficiency can be antagonised by the continuous use of selective noradrenaline re-uptake inhibitors and/or selective serotonin re-uptake inhibitors, leading to a significant improvement in many patients' symptoms.

12.3.4 Blood supply to the brainstem

All parts of the brainstem get their arterial blood from the posterior **vertebrobasilar basin**. The individual arterial vessels originate either directly from the Aa. vertebrales or the A. basilaris (e.g., Rr. ad pontem) or from their respective branches, e.g., the cerebellar arteries (➤ Chap. 12.4.6). Although the arterial vascular network of the brainstem may be superficially highly variable, in the horizontal section we can distinguish 3 relatively consistent, pronounced supply areas: a posterior, a lateral and an anterior vascular territory. The following parts of the brainstem are supplied by the respective vascular territory:

- anterior: paramedially located tract systems such as the pyramidal tract and the medial part of the Lemniscus medialis, cranial nerve nuclei III, IV, VI, XII
- lateral: laterally-located tract systems and cranial nerve nuclei V, VII, IX, X, XI
- posterior: posterior column nuclei, Nuclei vestibulares, Pedunculi cerebellares, Tectum mesencephali

---
Clinical remarks

Disorders of the arterial supply of the brainstem, due to the close proximity of the most varied vital nuclear areas and tracts, often lead to wide-ranging symptoms of deficit and are frequently life-threatening. One example is the **WALLENBERG's syndrome.** This is a unilateral infarction of the dorsolateral Medulla oblongata due to a circulatory disorder in the A. inferior posterior cerebelli (PICA = 'posterior inferior cerebellar artery'). The symptoms are wide-ranging and highly variable: vertigo and postural instability to the damaged side (Nuclei vestibulares, lower olive), ipsilateral hemiataxia (Pedunculus cerebellaris inferior, cerebellum), contralateral dissociated sensory disturbances (Nuclei gracilis and cuneatus, Tractus spinothalamicus), dysphagia and hoarse voice (Nucleus ambiguus), HORNER'S syndrome and rapid pulse (central sympathicus and cardiovascular centre of the rostroventrolateral Medulla oblongata), as well as respiratory disorders (respiratory centre of the ventrolateral Medulla oblongata with pre-BÖTZINGER complex).

12.4 Cerebellum
Michael J. Schmeißer

SKILLS

After working through this chapter, you should be able to:
- use a macroscopic dissection or an anatomical model to describe the surface anatomy of the cerebellum and explain its functional organization
- name the corresponding anatomic sections through the cerebellum, cerebellar nuclei and cerebellar peduncles, and explain their respective involvement in relay circuits or fibre systems
- explain which clinical neurological tests can be used to test parts of the cerebellum which have a functional-anatomical meaning

12.4.1 Overview

The cerebellum, in a similar way to the pons, is part of the rhombencephalon, forming with it the hindbrain (**metencephalon**). It is located in the posterior cranial fossa (**Fossa cranii posterior**), is positioned dorsally on the brainstem and is connected with it on each side by 3 stems (**Pedunculi cerebellares**). The pedunculi contain afferent and efferent tracts by which the cerebellum is connected directly or indirectly with other areas of the brain. Macroscopically the strikingly furrowed cerebellum is divided into **3 sections:**
- the cerebellar vermis (**Vermis cerebelli**) in the middle,
- which is flanked by a cerebellar hemisphere (**Hemispherium cerebelli**) to the right and left.

Grey matter is predominantly found in the triple-layered cerebellar cortex (**Cortex cerebelli**) as well as in the cerebellar nuclei (**Nuclei cerebelli**); **white matter** fills the **Pedunculi cerebellares**, surrounds the cerebellar nuclei (**Corpus medullare cerebelli**) and penetrates into the winding coils of the cortex.

Functionally, the cerebellum is primarily responsible for the subconscious fine-tuning and coordination of movement, and the maintenance of muscle tone and balance.

A midsagittal section through the vermis (➤ Fig. 12.28) shows the image of the **Arbor vitae**. This nomenclature is based on the characteristic arrangement of grey and white matter, which is visible in this section. Starting from the 'trunk-shaped' Corpus medullare, increasingly fine lamellae of marrow 'branch off' from it, with distinct 'leaf-shaped' coils in the cerebellar cortex (**Folia cerebelli**).

12.4.2 Embryology

The development of the cerebellum starts in the 2nd half of the embryonic period between the *5th and 6th weeks*. It consists mainly of the metencephalic section of the **rhombencephalon** and also partly of caudal parts of the mesencephalon. In this context, the dorsolateral parts of both alar plates are critical; from these the so-called **rhombic lips** are formed. These superior sections provide the majority of the original neuroepithelial tissue of the two cerebellum systems (**Primordia cerebellares**), which merge with each other in the course of their growth in the median plane and finally form a transversal dorsally-curved bulge, the **cerebellum plate**. Its lateral parts show the strongest growth and develop later into the Hemispheria cerebelli; the mid-section becomes the Vermis cerebelli. Due to the formation of the first horizontal furrow of the cerebellum, the **Fissura posterolateralis**, the caudal portions of the cerebellum plate can be distinguished in the *12th week* as the **Lobus**

flocculonodularis (phylogenetically: **archicerebellum**). In the *14th week*, due to the formation of another horizontal furrow in the cranial part, the **Fissura prima, Lobus anterior** arises (phylogenetically: **paleocerebellum;** in which the Vermis cerebelli is included) and the **Lobus posterior** (phylogenetically: **neocerebellum**). After the *16th week*, as a result of the development of further horizontally-aligned fissures, there is segmentation into lobes, lobuli, and leaf-shaped coils or folia.

12.4.3 Position and external appearance

Topographical relationships

The cerebellum lies in the Fossa cranii posterior and borders the pons, Medulla oblongata and the IVth ventricle ventrally. Cranially, it borders the Lobus occipitalis and the posterior part of the Lobus temporalis of the cerebrum – separated by the cerebellar tentorium (**Tentorium cerebelli**) consisting of Dura mater; dorsocaudally, the Os occipitale or the Cisterna cerebellomedullaris. It also encompasses the Medulla oblongata dorsally and laterally, and ranges from laterally thereof up to the pons, so that it completely covers the IVth ventricle.

> **Clinical remarks**
>
> An anatomical knowledge of the positional relationships of the cerebellum plays a crucial role in the surgical treatment of tumours of the posterior cranial fossa. **Surgical access** to **infratentorial tumours** (e.g., to a schwannoma of the N. vestibularis = 'acoustic neuroma' in the cerebellopontine angle) is usually undertaken by opening the Fossa cranii posterior after the temporary removal of parts of the Os occipitale. Depending on the entity and position of the tumour (cerebellar vs. extra-cerebellar), non-affected parts of the cerebellum are moved aside using a spatula, as are any parts in the way of the surgical field, and thus are spared.

Surface area anatomy

The slender, leaf-shaped coils of the cerebellum (**Folia cerebelli**) are separated from each other by a variety of deeply indented, virtually parallel furrows (**Fissurae cerebelli**). The **Fissura posterolateralis** divides the cerebellum into two main parts: the **Lobus flocculonodularis** and the **Corpus cerebelli**. The latter is further divided by the Fissura prima into the **Lobus anterior** and the **Lobus posterior**. Additional furrows subdivide these lobes into lobules (**lobuli**). On the cerebellum surface, a distinction is made between 3 sections.

Superior surface anatomy

This area (➤ Fig. 12.29) is directed towards the Tentorium cerebelli or the cerebrum. The boundaries between the vermis and cerebellar hemispheres are difficult to recognise on the surface. However, the **Fissura prima** and the **Fissura horizontalis** are clearly visible. The latter furrow is not a functional border; instead it forms a dividing line between the superior and inferior surface areas.

Inferior surface anatomy

The inferior surface anatomy (➤ Fig. 12.30) is directed towards the Os occipitale or Cisterna cerebellomedullaris. On it can be seen in particular the two cerebellar tonsils (**Tonsillae cerebelli**), adjacent to the clearly defined vermis and the two cerebellar hemispheres. As the most caudal components of the hemispheres, they include

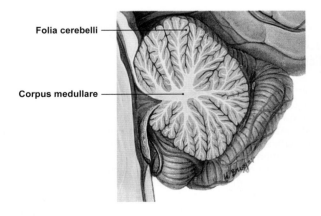

Folia cerebelli

Corpus medullare

Fig. 12.28 Midsagittal section through the cerebellum.

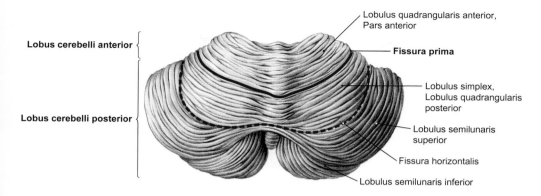

Lobus cerebelli anterior

Lobulus quadrangularis anterior, Pars anterior

Fissura prima

Lobus cerebelli posterior

Lobulus simplex, Lobulus quadrangularis posterior

Lobulus semilunaris superior

Fissura horizontalis

Lobulus semilunaris inferior

Fig. 12.29 Superior surface anatomy of the cerebellum.

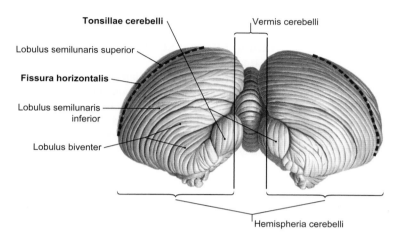

Tonsillae cerebelli

Vermis cerebelli

Lobulus semilunaris superior

Fissura horizontalis

Lobulus semilunaris inferior

Lobulus biventer

Hemispheria cerebelli

Fig. 12.30 Inferior surface anatomy of the cerebellum.

the dorsolateral section of the Medulla oblongata and are thus located directly on the edge of the Foramen magnum.

Clinical remarks

In the case of increased intracranial pressure (e.g., due to oedema, hemorrhages or tumours) the cerebellum can be moved caudally. Its caudal structures, such as the cerebellar tonsils, are then pressed into the greater Foramen magnum and trapped between the Medulla oblongata and the bony structures **(tonsillar entrapment)**. A possible consequence is the compression of the Medulla oblongata with **bulbar paralysis** (failure of the brainstem reflexes, ➤ Chap. 12.3.3). If brain pressure is not relieved, this may result in damage to the respiratory and circulatory centre in the brainstem, and in death.

Anterior surface anatomy

The anterior surface of the cerebellum (➤ Fig. 12.31) is directed to the IVth ventricles and to the brainstem. On this surface area, it is primarily the cerebellar peduncles **(Pedunculi cerebellares superior, medius and inferior)** which serve to identify where the cerebellum is separated from the brainstem. The Pedunculi cerebellares superiores border the unpaired superior medullary velum **(Velum medullare superius)** medially on both sides, a thin fibre plate made of white matter, representing the connection between the cerebellum and quadrigeminal plate and forming the upper roof of the IVth ventricle. A second pair of lamellae, the lower medullary velum **(Velum medullare inferius)**, connects the cerebellum with the Medulla oblongata, making it the lower roof of the IVth ventricle. Additionally, we can see the **flocculus** ('little flake', positioned below the medial cerebellar peduncle) and the **nodulus** ('little nodule', section of the vermis below the Velum medullare superius), which, together as the Lobus flocculonodularis, are separated from the rest of the cerebellum by the Fissura posterolateralis. The floc-

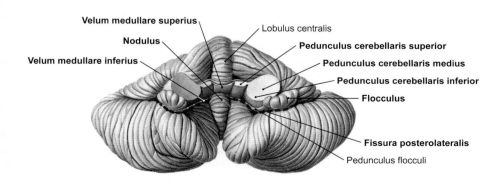

Velum medullare superius

Nodulus

Lobulus centralis

Velum medullare inferius

Pedunculus cerebellaris superior

Pedunculus cerebellaris medius

Pedunculus cerebellaris inferior

Flocculus

Fissura posterolateralis

Pedunculus flocculi

Fig. 12.31 Inferior surface of the cerebellum.

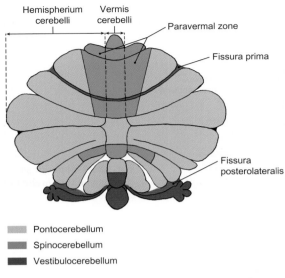

Pontocerebellum
Spinocerebellum
Vestibulocerebellum

Fig. 12.32 Functional-anatomical classification of extended small cortex. [R247]

culus and nodulus are connected via nerve fibres in the **Pedunculi flocculi.**

Functional classification

Functionally, we divide the cerebellum into 3 sections (➤ Fig. 12.32).

Vestibulocerebellum

This part consists of the Lobus flocculonodularis, and it is both afferently and efferently closely connected with the vestibular apparatus of the inner ear. In addition, there are efferent connections to the oculomotor centres of the Formatio reticularis and the eye muscle nuclei. The vestibulocerebellum serves primarily for the **controlling of supporting motor skills** (stabilisation of standing and walking), **fine-tuning of eye movement** as well as the coordination of both functions with the vestibular system (**maintenance of balance**).

Spinocerebellum

This part consists of the vermis (without the nodulus), the paravermal zone of both hemispheres (Partes intermediae) as well as the largest part of the Lobus cerebelli anterior. The spinocerebellum receives direct afferents from the spinal cord and is indirectly efferently connected via the Nucleus ruber and Formatio reticularis with the spinal cord. It is largely responsible for the **regulation of muscle tone** and, together with the vestibulocerebellum, controls **supporting motor functions.**

Pontocerebellum

This part contains the largest area of the cerebellum, the parts of the cerebellar hemispheres which lie lateral to the paravermal zone. It is mainly afferently connected with the pons (and thus indirectly with the cerebrum) and partly efferently connected with the olive and with the Nucleus ruber and thalamus. The primary role of the pontocerebellum is the **coordination of fine motor activities and the speech muscles.**

12.4.4 Internal structure

The fundamental micro-cellular structure of the cerebellar cortex is crucial to understanding the configurations and tracts of the cerebellum. The grey matter, i.e. the accumulation of nerve cell bodies, is predominantly found within the cerebellum in the cerebellar cortex (Cortex cerebelli) and in the cerebellum nuclei (Nuclei cerebellares).

Cerebellar cortex

The Cortex cerebelli, in contrast to the Cortex cerebri, reveals a three-layered structure. From the outside in, these are:

- The molecular layer (**Stratum moleculare**, outermost layer): low density of neurons, high levels of nerve cell appendages (especially PURKINJE cell dendrites and axons of granular cells) and synapses
- The PURKINJE cell layer (**Stratum purkinjense** or ganglionic middle layer): predominantly nerve cell bodies of the PURKINJE cells and BERGMANN glial cells (specialised astrocytes)
- The granular cell layer (**Stratum granulosum**, innermost layer): predominantly nerve cell bodies of the granular cells

NOTE

The cerebellum contains more than 50% of the **neurons in the brain** and hence more neurons than the cerebrum. In percentage terms, the granular cells in the granular layer of the cerebellar cortex form the majority (approximately 99% of all the neurons in the cerebellar cortex).

The cerebellum receives **afferent inputs,** either via the so-called **mossy fibers** (axonal appendages of neurons from the Pons nuclei, the spinal cord, the Formatio reticularis or the vestibular nuclei) or via **climbing fibres** (axonal appendages from the lower olive nucleus complex of the Medulla oblongata). This input in both cases is **excitatory/glutamatergic:**

- Mossy fibre axons end in the Stratum granulosum and stimulate mainly granular cells. These granular cells, in turn, send their axonal appendages, known as parallel fibres, into the Stratum moleculare and form, amongst others, excitatory/glutamatergic synapses at the distal dendritic tree of the PURKINJE cells.
- Climbing fibre axons pass directly into the Stratum moleculare and form, as in the case of the parallel fibres, excitatory/glutamatergic synapses on PURKINJE cell dendrites.

The function of the **PURKINJE cells is significant.** They are the only neurons of the cerebral cortex which send an axon which then leaves the Cortex cerebelli again. Thus, PURKINJE cells are a **central inte-**

gration element of all the neuronal circuits; this includes the cerebellum cortex as a 'relay station'. Interestingly, PURKINJE cells are **inhibitory** and end with their axons at the neurons of the cerebellar nuclei, where they form inhibiting, **GABAergic synapses**.

> **Clinical remarks**
>
> Contrary to previous assumptions, malfunctions of the cerebellum and its circuits also appear to be accompanied by a decline in higher brain activities, such as social interaction and communication. In this context, the integrity of the PURKINJE cells play a highly crucial role. So for example we often find a lower number of PURKINJE cells in certain cortical sections of the cerebellum in cross-sections of patients with **autism**.

Cerebellar nuclei

Embedded in the Corpus medullare cerebelli of the pontocerebellum, there is a total of 4 cerebellar nuclei (**Nuclei cerebelli**) on each side, which can be particularly recognised in oblique or flat sections through the upper cerebellar peduncles on the basis of their macroscopically characteristic shapes. Listed below from lateral to medial, they are (➤ Fig. 12.33):
- **Nucleus dentatus** (dentate nucleus): positioned furthest laterally, looks like a U-shaped, serrated, pleated tape; its anteromedial aperture is referred to as the Hilum nuclei dentati
- **Nucleus emboliformis** (emboliform nucleus): elongated, lying medial of the Hilum nuclei dentati
- **Nucleus globosus** (globose nucleus): round, lying medial of the Nucleus emboliformis; often divided in two
- **Nucleus fastigii** (fastigial nucleus): egg-shaped, lying furthest medial

The cerebellar nuclei mainly receive afferent input from the PURKINJE cells of the cerebellar cortex. Due to the fact that each cerebellar nucleus receives afferents from a topographically different area of the cerebellar cortex, functional attributions can be made:
- Nucleus dentatus – pontocerebellum
- Nucleus emboliformis – spinocerebellum
- Nucleus globosus – spinocerebellum
- Nucleus fastigii – vestibulocerebellum, spinocerebellum

> **NOTE**
>
> The Nucleus emboliformis and Nucleus globosus of the cerebellum are functionally very similar, because both receive their primary afferents from the spinocerebellum. They can therefore be combined with a nucleus, the so-called **Nucleus interpositus cerebelli**.

In the cerebellar nuclei, multipolar nerve cells are particularly found, projecting efferently into other areas of the brain. These projection fibres form primarily excitatory/antiglutamatergic synapses in their target area.

Cerebellar peduncles

The cerebellum is connected with the brainstem on each side by 3 cerebellar peduncles (**Pedunculi cerebellares**); this is where all the afferent and efferent tracts of the cerebellum pass. The volumes of the individual cerebellar peduncles and thereby also their fibre contents, are visible from the front, especially after dissection when viewing the Facies anterior (➤ Fig. 12.31).
- **Pedunculus cerebellaris superior:** The superior cerebellar peduncle contains mainly efferent fibres from all 4 cerebellar nuclei, which primarily pass to the Nucleus posterior ventrolateralis of the thalamus (Tractus cerebellothalamicus) and to the Nucleus ruber into the mesencephalon (Tractus cerebellorubralis). In addition, afferent fibres from the spinal cord (Tractus spinocerebellaris anterior, superior, cervicospinocerebellaris) run into it.
- **Pedunculus cerebellaris medius:** The middle cerebellar peduncle is the most pronounced and lies furthest laterally, containing only afferent fibres (Fibrae pontocerebellares), which arise from the Nuclei pontis.
- **Pedunculus cerebellaris inferior:** the lower cerebellar peduncle lies medial of the middle peduncle and is divided into 2 sections: an external fibre tract, the so-called **Corpus restiforme**, containing only afferent fibres (Tractus spinocerebellaris posterior, Fibrae cuneocerebellares, Tractus trigeminocerebellaris, Tractus olivocerebellaris, Tractus reticulocerebellaris), and a medially connecting section referred to as the **Corpus juxtarestiforme**, with efferent (Tractus cerebellovestibularis) and afferent fibres (Tractus vestibulocerebellaris).

> **NOTE**
>
> Within the cerebellar peduncles, the ratio between afferent and efferent fibres is approx. 40 : 1. This underlines the central role played by the cerebellum within the complex integration of afferent signals.

12.4.5 Neurovascular pathways

Afferent neurovascular pathways

With the afferent neurovascular pathways of the cerebellum (➤ Fig. 12.34), a distinction is made between the climbing fibre system and the mossy fibre system.

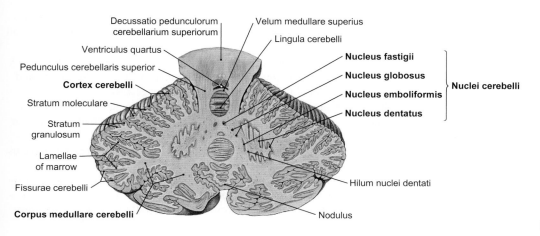

Decussatio pedunculorum cerebellarium superiorum
Velum medullare superius
Ventriculus quartus
Lingula cerebelli
Pedunculus cerebellaris superior
Nucleus fastigii
Cortex cerebelli
Nucleus globosus
Stratum moleculare
Nucleus emboliformis
Nuclei cerebelli
Stratum granulosum
Nucleus dentatus
Lamellae of marrow
Fissurae cerebelli
Hilum nuclei dentati
Corpus medullare cerebelli
Nodulus

Fig. 12.33 Cerebellar nuclei.

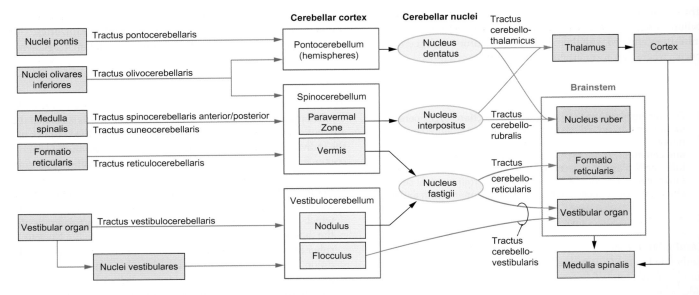

Fig. 12.34 Afferent and efferent compounds of the cerebellum. [L141]

Climbing fibres are derived from the lower olive nuclear complex (**Complexus olivaris inferior**), run as the **Tractus olivocerebellaris** through the inferior cerebellar peduncle and cross to the opposite side, partly to the cerebellar nuclei, but above all to the PURKINJE cell populations of the cerebral cortex in their entirety. **Mossy fibres** originate from several different areas. Common to all mossy fibres is the characteristic that they end at the granular cells of the cerebellar cortex:

- **Spinocerebellar mossy fibres** derive from the spinal cord and all end ipsilaterally in the spinocerebellum. The first one is the **Tractus spinocerebellaris anterior**, running through the superior cerebellar peduncle. The **Tractus spinocerebellaris posterior** and the **Tractus cuneocerebellaris** run conversely in the lower cerebellar peduncle.
- Trigeminocerebellar mossy fibres arise from the 3 somatoafferent nuclei of the N. trigeminus [V] and, like the spinocerebellar mossy fibres, run via the inferior cerebellar area into the ipsilateral areas of the spinocerebellum.
- **Pontocerebellar mossy fibres** arise from the **Nuclei pontis**, then cross to the opposite side as the **Tractus pontocerebellaris** at the middle cerebellar peduncle, thus ending in the contralateral pontocerebellum.
- **Reticulocerebellar mossy fibres** arise from the Formatio reticularis, run as the **Tractus reticulocerebellaris** through the lower cerebellar peduncle and end in the spinocerebellum bilaterally.
- **Vestibulocerebellar mossy fibres** run partially directly out of the Nuclei vestibulares, partially as the **Tractus vestibulocerebellaris** via the Corpus juxtarestiforme of the lower cerebellar peduncle and bilaterally into the vestibulocerebellum.

Efferent pathways

With the exception of a few fibres of the homeostatic system, all other efferent fibres of the cerebellar cortex (> Fig. 12.34) **are relayed in the cerebellum nuclei**. Here, the following principles are important:

- Efferents from the **pontocerebellum** or the **cerebellum hemispheres** project in particular onto the Nucleus dentatus, and efferents from the **paravermal zone** project onto the **spinocerebellum** on the Nucleus interpositus. They are there relayed onto projection neurons, primarily reaching the contralateral thalamus via the **Tractus cerebellothalamicus** or reaching the contralateral Nucleus ruber via the **Tractus cerebellorubralis**.
- Efferents from the **spinocerebellum** or the **vermis** as well as from the **vestibulocerebellum** or the **nodulus** project onto the Nucleus fastigii, where principally a relay to the vestibular nuclei and to the Formatio reticularis takes place on both sides. These fibre connections are known as the **Tractus cerebellovestibularis** and the **Tractus cerebelloreticularis**.
- Most efferents from the **vestibulocerebellum** or the **Lobus flocculonodularis**, however, go directly to the Nuclei vestibulares without being relayed into the cerebellum nuclei.
- Nucleo-olivary fibres take all cerebellar nuclei to the lower olive nuclear complex.

12.4.6 Blood supply

The cerebellum receives 3 arteries, all of which originate from the rear, vertebrobasilar basin:

- **A. superior cerebelli** from the A. basilaris: supplies the upper parts of the hemispheres and the Vermis cerebelli, as well as the Nucleus dentatus
- **A. inferior anterior cerebelli** from the A. basilaris: supplies the flocculus and peripheral areas of the lower surface of the hemispheres
- **A. inferior posterior cerebelli** from the Pars intracranialis of the A. vertebralis: supplies the lower parts of the hemisphere and the Vermis cerebelli, as well as the Nuclei emboliformis, globosus and fastigii

The veins of the cerebellum run independently of the arteries and can be assigned to the following drainage areas:

- Blood from the anteromedial and superomedial surface-drainage area V. magna cerebri: **V. precentralis cerebelli, V. superior vermis, Vv. superiores cerebelli mediales**
- Blood from the superolateral surface-drainage area, Sinus rectus: **Vv. superiores cerebelli laterales**
- Blood from the inferolateral surface-drainage area Sinus petrosus superior: **V. petrosa**
- Blood from the inferomedial surface-drainage area Sinus transversus: **V. inferior vermis, Vv. inferiores cerebelli**

The expansion of supply and/or drainage pathways depends on the calibre of their respective vessels and shows strong inter-individual differences. In addition, there are numerous anastomoses, both between arteries and between veins.

12.5 Cranial nerves
Anja Böckers, Michael J. Schmeißer

Note: the cranial nerves are also presented in ➤ Chap. 9.3.

12.5.1 Overview

Cranial nerves (**Nn. craniales**) are 12 nerves arranged in pairs, which exit the central nervous system at the base of the brain or at the brainstem. To make it easier to understand, they can primarily be seen in the same way as the spinal nerves, which exit the spinal cord in pairs towards the periphery. However, the N. olfactorius [I] and the N. opticus [II] do not fit into a scheme like this due to their ontogenous origins as separate parts of the brain. There are also other differences between the spinal and cranial nerves (➤ Table 12.7): while the spinal nerves primarily spread out segmentally, the cranial nerves do not run segmentally and, in part, run in such a complex manner between the meninges or through certain cranial cavities and apertures to their target organs in the head/neck area, that a significantly wider topographical understanding is required in order to understand their pathway. While almost all cranial nerves have their target organs in the head/neck area, part of the fibres of the N. vagus [X] pass into the abdominal cavity to the CANNON's point on the Flexura coli sinistra.

Spinal nerves carry 4 different fibre qualities, whereas in the cranial nerves a total of 7 fibre qualities can be distinguished, but not all cranial nerves carry 7 fibre qualities. Altogether we can distinguish, in the same way as for the spinal nerves:

• **general somatoefferent** fibres for the innervation of the skeletal muscles
• **general somatoafferent** fibres, which take impulses from the skin (exteroception), the GOLGI tendon organs or the muscle spindle (proprioception)
• **general visceroefferent** fibres for the parasympathetic innervation of smooth muscle fibres and glands
• **general visceroafferent** fibres which take impulses from the mucous membranes, viscera and the blood vessels to the CNS

In addition, the cranial nerves are distinguished as having further fibre qualities, or 'special' fibres, according to their embryological development from the pharynx. Thus, the following can also be found in the cranial nerves:

• **special visceroefferent** fibres for the innervation of the striated muscles, pharyngeal arch muscles, e.g., mastication muscles
• **special visceroafferent** fibres, which take impulses from the sensory epithelial cells of the smell and taste receptors

The fibres of the sensory epithelia of the eye and the ear are exceptions, and are therefore not referred to as being specially visceroafferent, but as being **specially somatoafferent**. However, in academic literature, the fibre qualities are often inconsistently assigned. Correspondingly, the fibres of the N. olfactorius are also in part referred to as specially visceroafferent.

The autonomic nerve fibres exiting the Medulla spinalis leave the spinal cord through the ventral root and are relayed onto a second postganglionic neuron in the sympathetic system as they continue into the paravertebral or prevertebral ganglia. This relay onto the second neuron occurs in the parasympathetic system, mostly in the intramural ganglia, e.g., in the intestinal wall. The same principle of configuration applies to the **autonomic fibres** of the cranial nerves.

Table 12.7 Characteristics of the cranial nerves in comparison with the spinal nerves.

Spinal nerve	Cranial nerve
Segmental arrangement	Non-segmental arrangement
(Mostly) 31 paired spinal nerves	12 paired cranial nerves
Exit from the Medulla spinalis	Exit from the Truncus encephali
Passes through segmentally arranged Foramina intervertebralia	Passes through non-segmentally arranged openings of the internal surface of the cranial base
4 functional fibre qualities	7 functional fibre qualities
Primary target organs below the upper thoracic aperture	Primary target organs above the upper thoracic aperture

From a topographical point of view, the relay to the sympathetic ganglia occurs remotely from organs, so that the postganglionic fibres show a divergent course and travel as fine nerve plexus with the arterial vessels to their target organs in the head and throat area.

N O T E

In the cranial nerves, 7 different fibre qualities (➤ Table 12.8) can be distinguished; however, not every cranial nerve carries fibre qualities.

A total of 12 pairs of **Nn. craniales** can be distinguished, the structure of which is laid out in the following chapter (➤ Fig. 12.35). The cranial nerves are numbered from rostral to caudal using Roman numerals. This means that the first 4 cranial nerves (I–IV) have their exit point in the mesencephalon or further rostral from there, the medial 4 cranial nerves (V–VIII) exit in the pons and the caudal 4 cranial nerves (IX–XII) exit in the Medulla oblongata (**4th rule**).

The **exit points of the cranial nerves** are arranged on the ventral side in a medial and in a lateral row in the brainstem:

- The medial range extends the exit points of the ventral roots of the spinal nerves cranially. Following this line, the N. oculomo-

Table 12.8 Fibre qualities, distinguished by efferents and afferents.

Fibre quality	Innervation
Efferents	
General somatoefferent	Motor: skeletal muscles
General visceroefferent	Parasympathic: glands, smooth muscles
Special visceroefferent	Branchiomotoric: pharyngeal arch muscles
Afferents	
General somatoafferent	Proprioceptive (joints, muscles) and exteroceptive (sensitivity – skin)
General visceroafferent	Enteroceptive (sensitivity – mucosal, blood vessels)
Special visceroafferent	Odour and taste organ
Special somatoafferent	Sensory: vision, hearing and balance organ

torius [III], the N. abducens [VI] and the N. hypoglossus [XII] all leave the CNS.
- The lateral series forms the extension of the Sulcus posterolateralis, the recess through which the Radix posterior leaves the spinal cord. Thus, in the Medulla oblongata, the lateral exit points of the N. glossopharyngeus [IX], the N. vagus [X] and the N. accessorius [XI] are located in the Sulcus retroolivaris. Further

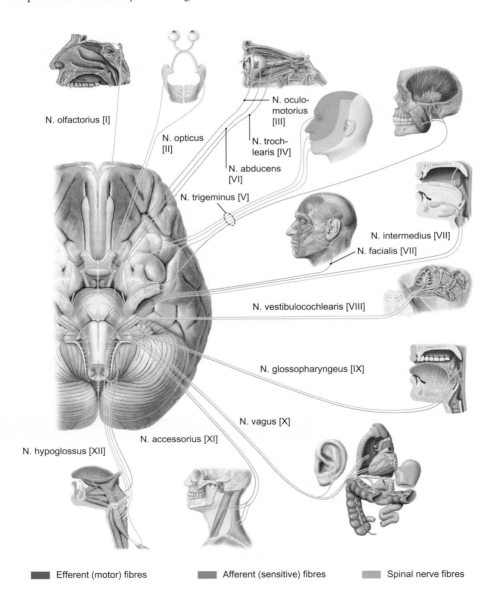

N. olfactorius [I]

N. opticus [II]

N. oculo-motorius [III]

N. troch-learis [IV]

N. abducens [VI]

N. trigeminus [V]

N. intermedius [VII]

N. facialis [VII]

N. vestibulocochlearis [VIII]

N. glossopharyngeus [IX]

N. vagus [X]

N. accessorius [XI]

N. hypoglossus [XII]

■ Efferent (motor) fibres   ■ Afferent (sensitive) fibres   ■ Spinal nerve fibres

Fig. 12.35 Cerebrum, brainstem and cerebellum with the exit points of the 12 pairs of cranial nerves, which are numbered in the order of their exit from rostral to caudal, using Roman numerals (I–XII). View from basal. The Ist cranial nerve is a part of the cerebrum which was displaced during development, corresponding to the N. opticus [II], which is a prolapsed protrusion of the diencephalon.

cranially the exit points of the N. trigeminus [V] and the N. facialis [VII] join.

The N. trochlearis [IV] is an exception in this regard, as it is the only cranial nerve on the dorsal side of the mesencephalon which leaves the CNS and has the longest intratradural course (➤ Fig. 12.36).

The **names of the 12 cranial nerves** can easily be remembered or repeated in the correct order based on a mnemonic such as 'On old Olympus's towering top a Finn and German viewed some hops,' meaning that their exit points are localised on the brainstem according to the 4th rule described above. Furthermore, the 4th rule also includes the following:

- *4 cranial nerves generally carry visceroefferent fibres (III, VII, IX and X)
- *4 cranial nerves, of which the numbers are factors of 12, possess somatoefferent nuclear areas within the brainstem (III, IV, VI and XII)

The 12 cranial nerves are uniformly covered, from ➤ Chap. 12.5.4 to Chap. 12.5.16:

- The 1st section describes the respective cranial nerve exit point from the basal side of the brain or brainstem.
- The 2nd section largely consists of a summarised graphic presentation of the cranial nerves with its target organs (➤ Fig. 12.37) – the corresponding peripheral nerve pathway is described in ➤ Chap. 9.3.
- In the 3rd section, the respective cranial nerve nuclei, their positions, qualities and features are described as well as their afferent and efferent links to other central brain sections or systems.
- Finally, for each of the 12 cranial nerves, we will describe how their function can be checked in the context of a clinical neurological examination.

12.5.2 Embryology

For a topographical situational awareness of the cranial nerve nuclei in the brainstem, it is essential to be able to report their longitudinal arrangement. It must be borne in mind that cranial nerve nuclei should not be thought of as being round or spherical accumulations of neurons, but – in the same way as the spinal cord – they are arranged in intermittent columns of nuclei that can also expand over a distance, e.g., from the pons to the Medulla oblongata. For a three-dimensional understanding of their position, this image must then be expanded to include the mediolateral arrangement of the individual cranial nerve nuclei. This mediolateral arrangement is derived from the embryological development of the rhombencephalon.

From early on in development, we can already distinguish in the neural tube a base plate pointing ventromedially to the Chorda dorsalis and a **roof plate** for the neural tube pointing dorso-medially. Between these two plates, in the dorsal half of the neural tube, are the **alar plates**, which are separated by the **Sulcus limitans** from the ventral half of the neural tube, known as the **base plates** (➤ Fig. 12.38a). The ongoing differentiation of the neurons in the alar and base plates is controlled by the chordal process which suppresses dorsalising genes with specific substances. Subsequently, motor neurons form from the neuroblasts near the chord of the neural tube (in the base plates), while with an increasing concentration gradient of these substances, from ventral to dorsal, visceroefferent, visceroafferent and somatoafferent neurons are differentiated. Finally, the development of the pontine flexure brings about the expansion of the central canal to the IVth ventricle, so that the roof plate for the ependymal ventricle roof thins out and the alar and base plates open like the pages of a book, with the spine of the book being formed by the former base plate (➤ Fig. 12.38b). Dorsal parts of the neural tube wall thus go to lateral and

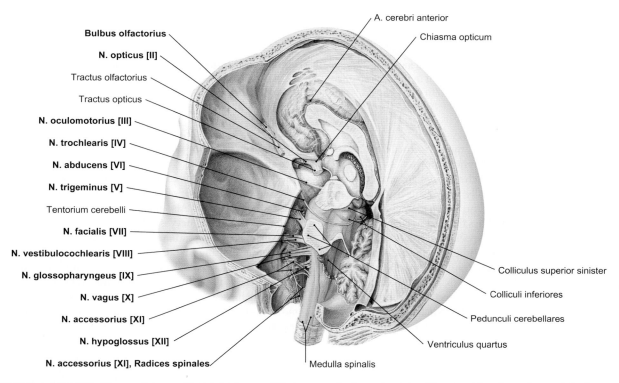

Fig. 12.36 Exit points of the Nn. craniales on the brainstem and their course in the subarachnoid space. View from the top left after removal of the left halves of the cerebrum and cerebellum as well as of the Tentorium cerebelli. The N. abducens has the longest intracranial extradural pathway up to the point where it passes through the cranial base.

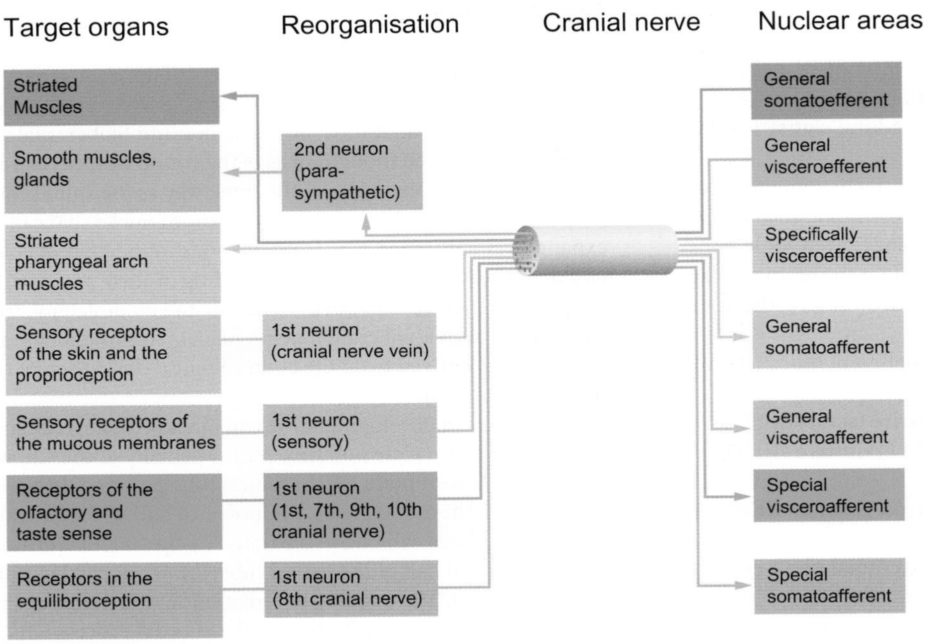

Target organs   Reorganisation   Cranial nerve   Nuclear areas

Fig. 12.37 Fibre qualities of the cranial nerves (nuclei) with possible configurations or reorganisation points and the respective effectors. [L127]

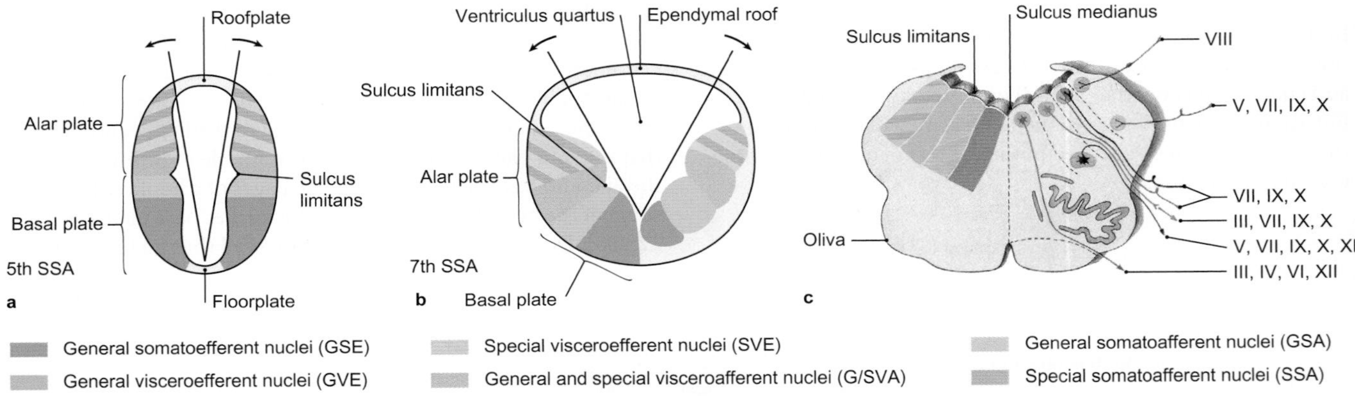

Fig. 12.38 Development of the rhombencephalon and of the mediolateral arrangement of the cranial nerve nuclei, according to their function. **a** Originally there is a dorsoventral arrangement in the neural tube (5th week of development. **b** This arrangement is changed by the expansion of the Canalis centralis to the IVth ventricle (7th week of development) into a mediolateral arrangement. **c** The individual fibre qualities are attributable to the respective cranial nerve nuclei. a,b [L126]

to ventral followed by visceroafferent, then visceroefferent and, finally, furthest medial by somatoefferent neurons.

The respective column nuclei are in the immediate proximity of the floor of the IVth ventricle. Specifically, this means that the special somatoafferent columnar nuclei of the VIIIth cranial nerves (**Nuclei vestibulares and cochleares**) lies furthest to lateral, followed medioventrally by the general and special visceroafferent nuclei (**Nucleus tractus solitarii**) of the VIIth, IXth and Xth cranial nerve (➤ Fig. 12.38c). Medial to the Sulcus limitans, the general visceroefferent columnar nuclei of the IIIrd, VIIth, IXth and Xth cranial nerve joins with the **Nuclei accessorii nervi oculomotorii, Nuclei salivatorii superior and inferior** and the **Nucleus dorsalis nervi vagi**, (see above, 4th rule). However, the general visceroefferent nucleus of the IIIrd cranial nerve has no direct contact with the IVth ventricle; it has a rather more cranial position in the mesencephalon. Finally located between this nucleus column and the Sulcus medianus is the general somatoefferent nucleus column formed by the nuclei of the IIIrd, IVth, VIth and XIIth cranial nerve, the **Nucleus nervi oculomotorii, Nucleus nervi trochlea-**

ris, **Nucleus nervi abducentis** and the **Nucleus nervi hypoglossi** (see above, 4th rule).

The general somatoafferent nucleus column also lies lateral, but does not reach the floor of the IVth ventricle, but instead runs inside of the brainstem. Also included are neurons of the Vth, VIIth, IXth and Xth cranial nerves, which are arranged longitudinally in the **Nuclei mesencephalicus, pontinus and spinalis nervi trigemini** longitudinal alignment. The same applies to the specially visceroefferent nucleus columns of the Vth, VIIth, IXth, Xth and XIth cranial nerves, the neurons of which innervate branchiogenic muscles of the head and throat area and include those of the **Nucleus motorius nervi trigemini, Nucleus nervi facialis, Nucleus ambiguus** and the **Nucleus nervi accessorii** (➤ Fig. 12.39).

The last nuclear group (V, VII, IX, X and XI) is closely developmentally linked with the development of the oropharyngeal arches. This means that the entire musculature of a pharyngeal arch is innervated by one of these cranial nerves, the 'pharyngeal arch nerve'. Accordingly, each of the above-mentioned cranial nerves can be assigned to a pharyngeal arch (➤ Table 12.9). With its N. accessorius

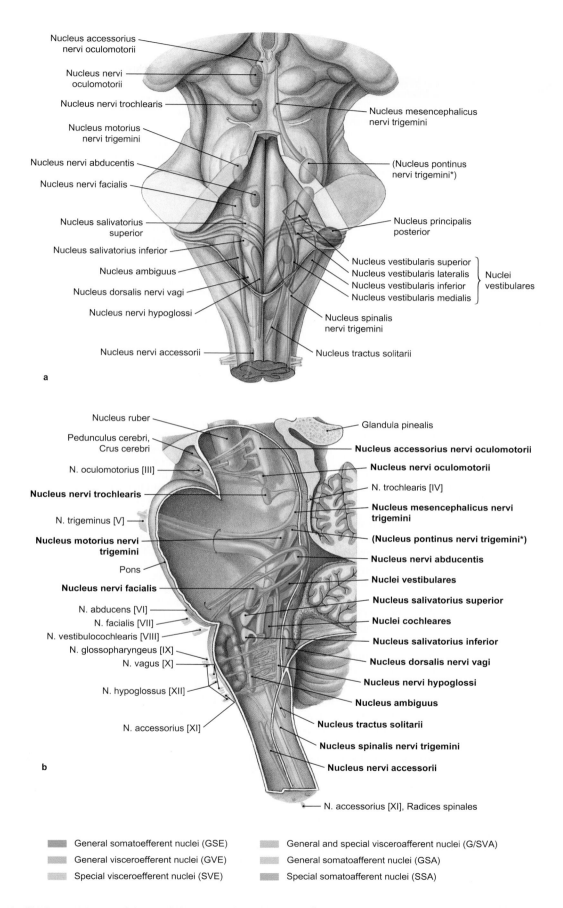

Nucleus accessorius nervi oculomotorii

Nucleus nervi oculomotorii

Nucleus nervi trochlearis

Nucleus mesencephalicus nervi trigemini

Nucleus motorius nervi trigemini

Nucleus nervi abducentis

Nucleus nervi facialis

(Nucleus pontinus nervi trigemini*)

Nucleus salivatorius superior

Nucleus principalis posterior

Nucleus salivatorius inferior

Nucleus ambiguus

Nucleus dorsalis nervi vagi

Nucleus nervi hypoglossi

Nucleus vestibularis superior
Nucleus vestibularis lateralis
Nucleus vestibularis inferior
Nucleus vestibularis medialis
} Nuclei vestibulares

Nucleus spinalis nervi trigemini

Nucleus nervi accessorii

Nucleus tractus solitarii

a

Nucleus ruber

Glandula pinealis

Pedunculus cerebri, Crus cerebri

Nucleus accessorius nervi oculomotorii

N. oculomotorius [III]

Nucleus nervi oculomotorii

Nucleus nervi trochlearis

N. trochlearis [IV]

Nucleus mesencephalicus nervi trigemini

N. trigeminus [V]

Nucleus motorius nervi trigemini

(Nucleus pontinus nervi trigemini*)

Pons

Nucleus nervi abducentis

Nucleus nervi facialis

Nuclei vestibulares

N. abducens [VI]

Nucleus salivatorius superior

N. facialis [VII]

Nuclei cochleares

N. vestibulocochlearis [VIII]

Nucleus salivatorius inferior

N. glossopharyngeus [IX]

Nucleus dorsalis nervi vagi

N. vagus [X]

Nucleus nervi hypoglossi

N. hypoglossus [XII]

Nucleus ambiguus

Nucleus tractus solitarii

N. accessorius [XI]

Nucleus spinalis nervi trigemini

Nucleus nervi accessorii

b

N. accessorius [XI], Radices spinales

General somatoefferent nuclei (GSE)

General and special visceroafferent nuclei (G/SVA)

General visceroefferent nuclei (GVE)

General somatoafferent nuclei (GSA)

Special visceroefferent nuclei (SVE)

Special somatoafferent nuclei (SSA)

Fig. 12.39 Longitudinal arrangement of the cranial nerve nuclear areas III–XII). a Nuclear areas of the cranial nerves III–XII with a dorsal view of the brainstem or the rhombus pit. The right side of the image shows the Nuclei terminationes (end nuclei) of the afferent tracts, the left side of the image half the Nuclei originis (nuclei of origin) of the efferent tracts. **b** Spatial overview of efferent and afferent nuclear areas of cranial nerves III–XII and their pathway in the brainstem viewed from the median plane; * clinically: Nucleus sensorius principalis nervi trigemini.

Table 12.9 Assignment of the most important cranial nerves for the respective pharyngeal arches and the corresponding branchiogenic muscles.

Pharyngeal arch	Pharyngeal arch nerve	Muscles
1st pharyngeal arch (mandibular arch)	N. trigeminus [V]; N. mandibularis [V/3]	• Chewing muscles • M. mylohyoideus • Venter anterior musculi digastrici • M. tensor tympani • M. tensor veli palatini
2nd pharyngeal arch (hyoid arch)	N. facialis [VII]	• Mimic muscles • M. stylohyoideus • Venter posterior musculi digastrici • M. stapedius
3rd pharyngeal arch	N. glossopharyngeus [IX]	• Pharyngeal muscles • M. stylopharyngeus • M. levator veli palatini
4th pharyngeal arch (laryngeal arch)	N. vagus [X] with N. laryngeus superior	• Laryngeal muscles • Pharyngeal muscles: M. cricothyroideus
5th pharyngeal arch	– Regresses –	– Regresses –
6th pharyngeal arch	N. vagus [X] with N. laryngeus inferior (N. recurrens)	• Inner laryngeal muscles • Upper oesophageal muscles

having a cranially-oriented course, the Radix spinalis is referred to partially inconsistently as being specially visceroefferent or as somatoefferent.

12.5.3 Arterial blood supply

A disruption in arterial perfusion can result in brainstem infarctions, leading to resulting tissue death in the perfusion area of localised neuronal structures and thus leading to a corresponding loss of function. The symptoms observed enable conclusions to be drawn about the localisation of the affected brainstem area and the affected vessel.

To simplify, the **brainstem** belongs to the cranial nerve nuclei contained within it to the supply area of the Aa. vertebrales, which come together at the level of the transition from the Medulla oblongata to the pons to the A. basilaris. Accordingly, nuclear areas of the **Medulla oblongata** are supplied to some extent by the A. vertebralis or its branches, such as the **pons** to some extent from the A. basilaris and its branches. It is not possible to allocate one single vessel so clearly to the **mesencephalon**, but here again there is a constant arterial blood supply of the cross-section of the brainstem by an anterior, posterior and lateral inflow area:

- With its branches, the anterior supply area takes blood paramedially into the brainstem and thus reaches the general somatoefferent nuclear areas of the IIIrd, IVth, VIth and XIIth cranial nerve (➤ Chap. 12.5.1, 4th rule). Depending on the position of the level, the inflow takes place from the A. spinalis anterior or the Rr. paramediani of the A. vertebralis, the Rr. mediales of the Aa. pontes of the A. basilaris and from the A. superior cerebelli and from the Rr. interpedunculares of the A. cerebri posterior in the area of the mesencephalon.
- The lateral supply area reaches the nuclei of the Vth, VIIth, IXth, Xth and XIth cranial nerves via branches of the A. inferior anterior cerebelli from the A. basilaris and Rr. laterales (differentiated as Rr. circumferentes breves and longi) of the Aa. pontes from the A. basilaris.

- The posterior supply area is ultimately fed by the A. spinalis posterior of the A. vertebralis or by branches of the A. inferior posterior cerebelli and reaches, among others, the Nuclei vestibulares.

The close topographical proximity of the cranial nerves with the basal brain arteries along their intracranial pathway up to the point when it breaks through the bone is often the cause of clinical symptoms or malfunctions of the cranial nerves. For example, a vessel may compress a directly neighbouring cranial nerve due to an aneurysmal enlargement.

NOTE
- The N. oculomotorius [III] passes through the Fossa interpeduncularis and here lies in the immediate proximity to the A. cerebri posterior or, further along its pathway, to the A. communicans posterior.
- At the Meatus acusticus internus, the A. inferior anterior cerebelli leaves the A. labyrinthi and at the cerebellopontine angle is found in the immediate vicinity of the N. facialis [VII] and N. vestibulocochlearis [VIII].
- The strongest branch of the A. vertebralis, the A. inferior posterior cerebelli, runs initially near the olive in the immediate vicinity of the N. hypoglossus or to the cranial nerve roots along the Foramen jugulare.

Clinical remarks

In the case of the **functional failure of a cranial nerve**, it is initially important for the purposes of ongoing diagnosis to distinguish whether it is a central (supranuclear) lesion or a lesion of the cranial nerve nucleus, or whether the cranial nerve is damaged in its peripheral pathway. To do so, it is crucial to know the exact position of the cranial nerve nuclei, its exit point and its adjacent structures, in order to be able to localise the lesion precisely. Clinically, due to the close topographical relationships of the cranial nerves with each other, diseases involving combined cranial nerve lesions are frequently found – for example, if caudal cranial nerves run very closely together as they pass through the openings in the base of the internal surface of the cranial base (e.g., through the Foramen jugulare). Isolated cranial nerve lesions – especially of the IIIrd to VIIIth cranial nerves – are frequently causally affected due to hemorrhage or lesions of the brainstem arteries.

12.5.4 N. olfactorius (1st cranial nerve, N. I)
Michael J. Schmeißer

SKILLS
After working through this chapter, you should be able to:
- describe the special position of the N. olfactorius in comparison to cranial nerves III–XII and explain the difference between a primary and a secondary sensory cell
- clinically distinguish a lesion of the N. olfactorius from a lesion of the N. trigeminus

N. olfactorius [I] is the term given to approximately 20 fine nerve fibres, surrounded by meninges (**Fila olfactoria**). These contain unmyelinated axons of the bipolar olfactory neurons and from the olfactory mucosa in the upper nasal cavity, they pass through the Lamina cribosa of the Os ethmoidale up into the anterior cranial fossa and the **Bulbus olfactorius** (➤ Fig. 9.32). Thus the N. olfactorius [I] is not a classic cranial nerve fibre with a peripheral fibre pathway and a central nuclear area; instead it corresponds to the first part of the olfactory system of the CNS (➤ Chap. 13.6.2) and so it is assigned to the telencephalon. As before, we are still not in agreement about the quality of its fibres: basically, the fibres taking impulses from the sensory epithelial cells of the olfactory receptors are referred to as specially visceroafferent fibres. However, in academic literature, the fibres of the N. olfactorius are also partially stated as being specially somatoafferent (➤ Chap. 12.5.1). Olfactory neurons are **primary sensory cells**, which receive impressions of the sense of smell via its dendrites and transfer them via their axons to the central nervous system. Secondary sensory cells also receive impulses; these cannot however be transferred directly to the central nervous system.

Clinical remarks

Examination

When taking a detailed patient medical history, we ask firstly about **disturbances in smell and taste**. An olfactory sensory disorder is hard to diagnose in a patient's history because it often presents as a disruption of the sense of taste. To objectively carry out a **functional test** for the sense of smell, the patient closes their eyes and, isolated under each nostril, various aromatic substances are proffered to test their smell. In this context it is very important for the subsequent 'odour samples' to be carried out using irritants such as ammonia, because it is not perceived by the N. olfactorius [I], but via the branches of the N. trigeminus [V] supplying the nasal mucosa. If the affected person fails to perceive either the aromatic or the irritating substances, the nasal mucosa may be affected. If the affected person reacts to the irritating substance but not to the aromatic substances, a neurogenic disorder, e.g., a disorder of the N. olfactorius [I], is very likely.

Damage to the nerve

In the case of a fracture of the base of the skull, the N. olfactorius can be torn off from the nasal cavity in the bony area where it penetrates into the anterior cranial fossa. This may result in olfactory impairment **(hyposmia)** or a complete failure of the ability to smell **(anosmia)**.

12.5.5 N. opticus (2nd cranial nerve, N. II)
Michael J. Schmeißer

SKILLS

After working through this chapter you should be able to:
- describe the special position of the optic nerve in comparison with cranial nerves III–XII
- explain what a Stasis papilla is and consider the possible causes for it

In a similar way to the N. olfactorius, the **N. opticus [II]** is also not a classic cranial nerve; instead it is a CNS structure of the optic tract, assigned to the diencephalon, and is enveloped by meninges and oligodendrocytes. Its exclusively special somatoafferent fibres are the bundled axons of the multi-polar ganglion cells of the retina; initially these axons are unmyelinated and subsequently become myelinated (➤ Chap. 9.3.2). These transfer visual information and predominantly end in the Corpus geniculatum laterale (CGL) of the thalamus. The optic nerve papilla **(Discus nervi optici)** is seen in the ocular fundus reflection as a yellowish disc, and it marks the beginning of the N. opticus at the dorsal pole of the Bulbus oculi. As it continues its slightly S-shaped course, the N. opti-

cus is initially embedded in the retrobulbar fat body of the orbita, then passes through the anulus of ZINN (Anulus tendineus communis) and is then fed as the only nerve via the Canalis opticus into the middle cranial fossa, where it joins with the N. opticus of the opposite side in the Chiasma opticum above the pituitary gland (for Optic Tract see ➤ Chap. 13.3.1). The A. and V. centralis retinae run directly behind the Bulbus oculi, inside the N. opticus [II], on their way to the retina.

Clinical remarks

Examination

The patient is initially questioned about his general **vision**, as detrimental effects on the N. opticus may only be accompanied by a partial loss of vision ('blurred vision', 'dark spots'), but may sometimes lead to blindness. You should therefore direct the examination – separately for each eye – towards acuity (using an eye chart) and the field of vision (using finger perimetry). In addition, it is essential to examine the **pupillary reflex** because the afferent reflex largely runs via the N. opticus. In case of damage it is not possible to trigger a light reaction (contraction of the pupil = miosis) either ipsilaterally or contralaterally when shining a light in the affected eye, whereas the reflex response is normal in both eyes when a light is shone in the healthy eye.

Damage to the nerve

An acute inflammation of the optic nerve (**Neuritis nervi optici** or retrobulbar neuritis) is primarily identified by a potentially reversible one-sided loss of vision. Affected patients report seeing a 'veil', but imaging of the ocular fundus, including an evaluation of the optic nerve papilla, often reveals no abnormalities ('the patient cannot see anything and the doctor cannot see anything either'). In about one third of the cases, optical nerve neuritis in young people is the first symptom of multiple sclerosis (MS), a relatively frequent autoimmune disease of the central nervous system.
Due to increased intracranial pressure (e.g., due to a brain tumour or a cerebral haemorrhage) the optic nerve can be compressed on both sides. This is accompanied by a venous backflow, entailing an ophthalmoscopically-visible oedema of the optic papilla, which has now protruded into the bulbi. This is called **papilloedema**.

12.5.6 N. oculomotorius (3rd cranial nerve, N. III)
Michael J. Schmeißer

SKILLS

After working through this chapter, you should be able to:
- name the target organs of the N. oculomotorius
- enumerate the cranial nerve nuclei of the N. oculomotorius, explain their topographical position and clarify their respective functions correctly
- describe the clinical findings in a case of oculomotoric paralysis and identify possible causes

The **N. oculomotorius [III]** is a classic cranial nerve and, as well as the N. trochlearis [IV] and the N. abducens [VI], is one of the 3 cranial nerves that control the movements of the eyeball ('eye muscle nerve'). Due to its general somatoefferent innervation of almost all the striated extra-ocular eye muscles, it is able to move the Bulbus oculi medially downwards, medially upwards and laterally upwards. In addition, its general somatoefferent fibres are mainly responsible for lifting the eyelids. It innervates generally visceroefferently the smooth intra-ocular muscles. It ensures the contraction of the pupil (miosis) and intensifies the curvature of the lens (➤ Fig. 12.41).

Course and branches

The N. oculomotorius exits from the brainstem medially on the Crus cerebri in the Fossa interpeduncularis of the mesencephalon (➤ Fig. 12.40). It initially runs between the A. superior cerebelli and the A. cerebri posterior, and laterally of the A. communicans posterior and the Proc. clinoideus posterior it breaks through the Dura mater. After that, it enters the Sinus cavernosus and passes through its side wall as the uppermost nerve (➤ Fig. 12.46). From here it passes through the mediocaudal part of the Fissura orbitalis superior into the orbita, entering through the Anulus tendineus communis (annulus of ZINN), where it divides into further branches:

- **R. superior:** This smaller branch supplies the M. rectus superior (elevation of the Bulbus oculi, combined with mild adduction and internal rotation) and the M. levator palpebrae superioris (lifting of the upper lids) general somatoefferent.
- **R. inferior:** This larger branch supplies the M. rectus medialis (adduction of the Bulbus oculi), the M. rectus inferior (depression of the Bulbus oculi, combined with mild adduction and external rotation) and the M. obliquus inferior (elevation of the Bulbus oculi, combined with mild abduction), generally somatoefferent.
- **R. ad ganglion ciliare:** This general visceroefferent branch passes to the Ganglion ciliare (➤ Chap. 9.3.3). Its parasympathetic fibres are relayed from pre- to postganglion and continue to the M. sphinchter pupillae (contraction of the pupil = miosis) and the M. ciliaris (relaxation of the zonular fibres and resulting strengthening of the lens curvature in short-distance visual accommodation).

Cranial nerve nuclei and central links

Corresponding to its 2 fibre qualities, the N. oculomotorius has 2 specific cranial nerve nuclei: the general somatoefferent **Nucleus nervi oculomotorii** and the general visceroefferent **Nucleus accessorius nervi oculomotorii** (Nucleus EDINGER-WESTPHAL).

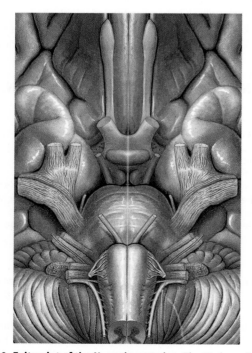

Fig. 12.40 Exit point of the N. oculomotorius. The IIIrd cranial nerve exits directly above the pons; Ventral view.

Both nuclei are adjacent to each another in the mesencephalon at the level of the Colliculi superiores (➤ Fig. 12.41). The Nucleus nervi oculomotorii is located ventrally of the aquaduct and posterior to the Nucleus ruber close to the midline. It consists of several sections; particularly noteworthy here is the unpaired Nucleus caudalis centralis, which contains the somata of the motoneurons for the M. levator palpebrae superioris from both sides. The Nucleus accessorius nervi oculomotorii is located mediodorsally of the Nucleus nervi oculomotorii, even closer to the midline.

The **configurations of the 'eye muscle nuclei'** with each other and their associations with supranuclear, pre-oculomotor centres are extremely complex (➤ Chap. 13.3.3). Amongst others, the **inter-nuclear neurons** are important here. These are found in addition to the classic general somatoefferent motoric projection neurons in the 'eye muscle nuclei'. The individual 'eye muscle nuclei' in the brainstem are relayed via them. The most studied internuclear projection runs in the **Fasciculus longitudinalis medialis (FLM)** and connect internuclear neurons of the Nucleus nervi abducentis with inter-nuclear neurons of a contralateral subnucleus of the Nucleus nervi oculomotorii. In addition, the Nucleus accessorius nervi oculomotorii plays a crucial role in the pupillary and accommodation reflex as well as in the convergence reaction (➤ Chap. 13.3.2).

Clinical remarks

Examination

In a **general inspection**, the position of the eyelids is noted first, then on closer inspection the position of the bulbi and the pupil – always comparing both sides. Additionally, the patient should be asked about double vision. In the event of failure of the N. oculomotorius, this would lessen on the damaged side looking downwards and outwards, but it would never quite disappear. For a general and combined **examination of the oculomotor system**, including the 'eye muscle nerve', N. oculomotorius [III], N. trochlearis [IV] and the N. abducens [VI], the patient is asked to focus his eyes on an index finger held approximately 20–30 cm away at eye level and to follow its course. The eye movement is then tracked while moving the index finger to all lines of sight (cranial-caudal, medial-lateral and combinations of these). If there is damage to the N. oculomotorius, the Bulbus oculi on the affected side deviates downwards and outwards from the start of the examination and is usually unable to follow the index finger. The **convergence reaction** is checked by moving the index finger towards the patient's nose at eye level. Here, it is important to check whether both eyeballs move towards the centre, and that reflexive miosis occurs simultaneously in both eyes. Lastly, the **pupillary reflex** is checked. In the event of a failure of the N. oculomotorius, the efferent reflex fails, so that there is neither a direct or indirect light reaction in the affected eye.

Damage to the nerve

The complete picture of **oculomotoric paralysis** is characterised by the following 3 key symptoms:
- Ptosis (drooping eyelid) due to the paralysis of the M. levator palpebrae superioris
- Incorrect outwards positioning of the bottom of the Bulbus oculi due to the loss of the Mm. rectus superior, rectus medialis, rectus inferior and obliquus inferior
- Mydriasis (widening of the pupil) due to the failure of the M. sphincter pupillae

On closer examination, it also emerges that near-point accommodation (due to the failure of the M. ciliaris) and the convergence reaction (due to the failure of one of the two Mm. recti mediales) are no longer possible. Affected patients also report double vision. The following should be taken into account in cases of oculomotor paralysis or excluded by imaging techniques:

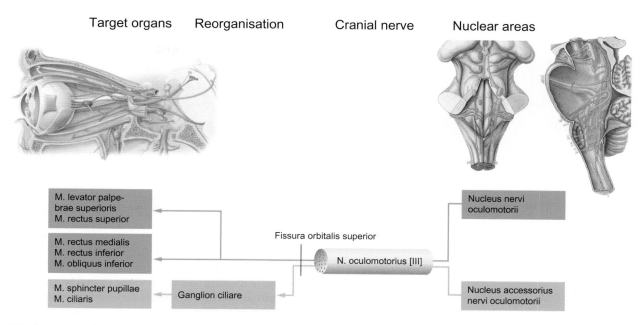

Target organs   Reorganisation   Cranial nerve   Nuclear areas

M. levator palpe-
brae superioris
M. rectus superior

M. rectus medialis
M. rectus inferior
M. obliquus inferior

Fissura orbitalis superior

N. oculomotorius [III]

M. sphincter pupillae
M. ciliaris

Ganglion ciliare

Nucleus nervi
oculomotorii

Nucleus accessorius
nervi oculomotorii

Fig. 12.41 Pathway, branches and fibre qualities of the N. oculomotorius, left. Lateral view. [L127]

- bulges or aneurysms of the intracranial vessels that run close to the nerve, such as the Aa. cerebri posterior or communicans posterior
- a thrombosis of the Sinus cavernosus
- Tumours of the internal surface of the cranial base and/or the orbita
- Skull fractures
- Inflammation of the meninges that cover the brain in the area of the cranial base

Furthermore, intracranial pressure and the subsequent displacement of the brain mass into the tentorium slot ('upper entrapment') can lead to what is called **clival syndrome**. Here, the N. oculomotorius is compressed against the bony edge of the clivus due to the brain mass displacement, gets into a state of irritation (small pupils ipsilaterally initially) and finally fails (open, non-responsive pupils ipsilaterally).

12.5.7 N. trochlearis (4th cranial nerve, N. IV)
Michael J. Schmeißer

SKILLS

After working through this chapter, you should be able to:
- name the target organ and cranial nerve nuclei of the N. trochlearis
- precisely explain the topographical pathway of the N. trochlearis
- describe the clinical findings of a trochlear paralysis and give the possible causes

The **N. trochlearis [IV]** is a purely general somatoefferent cranial nerve. It is the thinnest of all the cranial nerves and is responsible for the motor innervation of the M. obliquus superior (➤ Fig. 12.43). In its primary position (looking straight ahead), this muscle can roll the Bulbus oculi inwards and move it laterally downwards. However, when the eye is positioned in the adduction position, the M. obliquus superior is mainly responsible for the lowering of the eyeball laterally downwards.

Pathway
The N. trochlearis exits dorsally as a single cranial nerve from the brainstem directly below the Colliculi inferiores (➤ Fig. 12.42). It runs within the Cisterna ambiens between the A. superior cerebelli and the A. cerebri posterior around the cerebral crus and basally forwards and finally penetrates the Dura mater in order to enter into the side wall of the Sinus cavernosus. Here, it runs directly below the N. oculomotorius (➤ Fig. 12.46). Finally, it runs through the laterocranial part of the Fissura orbitalis superior furthest laterally and arrives outside of the Anulus tendineus communis (annulus of ZINN) under the roof of the orbit to the M. obliquus superior.

Cranial nerve nuclei and central links
Since the N. trochlearis only has one fibre quality, there is also only one nuclear area, the general somatoefferent **Nucleus nervi trochlearis**. This is located in the mesencephalon at the level of the Colliculi inferiores ventrally of the aquaduct (➤ Fig. 12.43). Its efferent fibres cross over to the opposite side before exiting the brainstem dorsally. In the same way as has already been mentioned for the N. oculomotorius, the **configurations of the 'eye muscle nuclei'** with each other, and their connection with supranuclear, pre-oculomotor centres, are extremely complex (➤ Chap. 13.3). A tract that is solely or principally assigned to the N. trochlearis has not been described here.

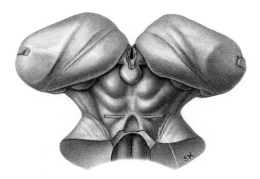

Fig. 12.42 Exit point of the N. trochlearis. The IVth cranial nerve exits below the Colliculi inferiores; dorsal view.

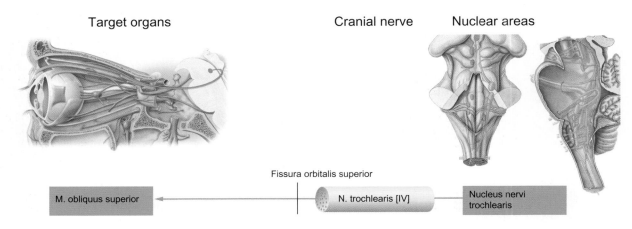

Target organs   Cranial nerve   Nuclear areas

Fissura orbitalis superior

M. obliquus superior ← N. trochlearis [IV] ← Nucleus nervi trochlearis

Fig. 12.43 Pathway, branches and fibre qualities of the N. trochlearis, left. Lateral view. [L127]

Clinical remarks

Examination

When examined, the patient may already present with a tilted head position. Similarly to the examination of the other two 'eye muscle nerves', the position of the bulbi is noted, the clinical examination for eye-tracking movements, as already described for the N. oculomotorius, is carried out and the patient is asked about double vision. Where there is isolated damage to the N. trochlearis, the eye can still be moved in all the main directions. Therefore, the clinical diagnosis of an isolated lesion of the N. trochlearis where there is no tilted head position is singularly difficult to make.

Damage to the nerve

In case of a **trochlear paralysis**, the affected bulb is turned medially upwards and slightly outwards. The resulting obliquely distorted double images lie over each other and are primarily perceived when looking medially downwards. Occasionally the affected patient develops a posture where the head is permanently tipped to the healthy side. This position is adopted to compensate for the fact that the Bulbus oculi can no longer turn inwards. The causes of trochlear paralysis is the same as for oculomotoric paralysis, because both nerves run adjacent to each another. Therefore, whatever the cause, nerve damage to both nerves is identified.

12.5.8 N. trigeminus (5th cranial nerve, N. V)
Anja Böckers

SKILLS

After working through this chapter, you should be able to:
• name the target organs of the three trigeminal branches
• correctly describe the neuronal stations of the trigeminoafferent system
• clinically differentiate between peripheral and central trigeminal lesions

The name of the **N. trigeminus [V]** results from its splitting into 3 main branches to innervate the head: the **N. ophthalmicus [V/1]**, the **N. maxillaris [V/2]** and the **N. mandibularis [V/3]**. The N. trigeminus is a mixed cranial nerve made from general somatoafferent and specially visceroefferent fibres, since it is supplied by the muscles developing from the first pharyngeal arch. These include the masticatory muscles, parts of the muscle of the floor of the mouth (M. mylohoideus, Venter anterior musculi digastrici) and smaller

muscles of the Tuba auditiva or in the Cavitas tympani (M. tensor veli palatini, M. tensor tympani). General somatoafferent fibres carry, in particular, the sensitivity as well as the temperature and pain sensations of the facial skin. However, the mimic muscles radiating into the facial skin are innervated by the N. facialis [VII].

Pathway and branches
The division of the N. trigeminus into both of its fibre qualities can already be macroscopically visualised when it exits the brainstem in the area of the lateral pons (➤ Fig. 12.44). This can be distinguished as a larger **Radix sensoria nervi trigemini (syn.: Portio major)** and a **Radix motoria nervi trigemini (syn.: Portio minor)**. Both cranial nerve parts pass via the Margo superior of the temporal bone, to form the **Ganglion trigeminale (GASSER's ganglion)**, in a pouch-shaped dural duplicature called the **Cavum trigeminale**. The Ganglion trigeminale is located at the Facies anterior at the tip of the Pars petrosa ossis temporale in the Impressio trigeminalis. This ganglion contains most of the perikarya of pseudo-unipolar sensory neurons, which are somatotopically ar-

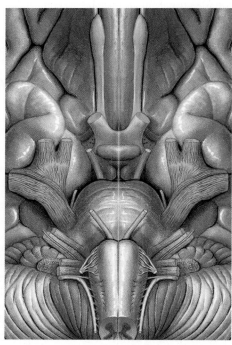

Fig. 12.44 Exit point of the N. trigeminus. The cranial nerve vein exits at the lateral side of the pons; Ventral view.

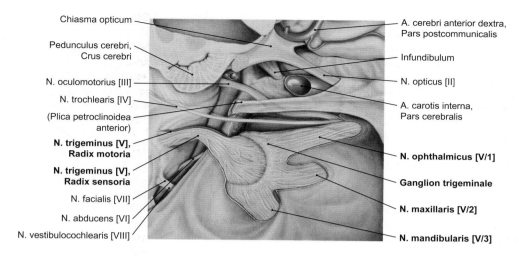

Chiasma opticum
Pedunculus cerebri, Crus cerebri
N. oculomotorius [III]
N. trochlearis [IV]
(Plica petroclinoidea anterior)
N. trigeminus [V], Radix motoria
N. trigeminus [V], Radix sensoria
N. facialis [VII]
N. abducens [VI]
N. vestibulocochlearis [VIII]

A. cerebri anterior dextra, Pars postcommunicalis
Infundibulum
N. opticus [II]
A. carotis interna, Pars cerebralis
N. ophthalmicus [V/1]
Ganglion trigeminale
N. maxillaris [V/2]
N. mandibularis [V/3]

Fig. 12.45 Inside view of the right Fossa cranii media. The Cavum trigeminale (MECKEL's cavity) is opened after removing the Dura mater and the arachnoidea. You can see the Ganglion trigeminale with its crescent shape and its split into the three branches of the trigeminal nerve: the N. ophthalmicus with its passage through the Fissura orbitalis superior into the orbit, the N. maxillaris nerve and its passage through the Foramen rotundum into the Fossa pterygopalatina, as well as the N. mandibularis with its passage through the Foramen ovale in the Fossa infratemporalis.

ranged according to their supply areas in a dorsoventral direction. Immediately after the ganglion, the N. trigeminus divides into its three main branches which exit the mid cranial fossa via various openings in the internal surface of the cranial base (➤ Fig. 12.45).

NOTE

For a simplified functional understanding, you should note the following rough division of the innervation areas of the head for the three trigeminal branches:
- **N. ophthalmicus [V/1]:** Area above the lower eyelid, which is the forehead up to the lambdoid suture, including the skin area as well as the head cavities, i.e. the orbita and the eye
- **N. maxillaris [V/2]:** Area between lower eyelid and upper lip, which is the skin area including the body openings, i.e. nasal cavity and adjacent upper jaw area
- **N. mandibularis [V/3]:** Area between the bottom lip and chin line, which is the skin area including the adjacent body opening, i.e. oral cavity and adjacent lower jaw area; the N. mandibularis is the only trigeminal branch which carries special visceroefferent fibres to the muscles of the 1st pharyngeal arch.

A ganglion adheres to each of the three branches of the trigeminal nerve. Here, however, the sensory fibres are *not* switched, but the general visceroefferent fibres of the other cranial nerves are. They include:
- **N. ophthalmicus [V/1]:** the Ganglion ciliare adheres in the orbita with the switching over of the general visceroefferent fibres of the N. oculomotorius [III].
- **N. maxillaris [V/2]:** the Ganglion pterygopalatinum adheres in the Fossa pterygopalatina with the switching over of the general visceroefferent fibres of the N. facialis [VII]
- **N. mandibularis [V/3]:** the Ganglion oticum adheres at the Foramen ovale with the switching over of the general visceroefferent fibres of the N. glossopharyngeus [IX]

Each of the three branches of the trigeminal nerve supplies one section of the Dura mater in sensory terms. To simplify matters, the innervation of the Dura mater can be described as follows:
- **N. ophthalmicus [V/1]:** Dura mater of the anterior cranial cavity
- **N. maxillaris [V/2]** and **N. mandibularis [V/3]:** Dura mater of the middle cranial cavity; the Dura mater of the posterior cranial cavity is not innervated by the N. trigeminus [V], but by the Rr. meningei of the N. vagus [X] and the N. glossopharyngeus [IX].

The special visceroefferent fibres arise from the Nucleus motorius nervi trigemini located in the pons, and the general somatoafferent fibres end in an elongated nuclear pillar which begins in the mesencephalon as the Nucleus mesencephalicus nervi trigemini and reaches up to the Nucleus principalis (syn.: Nucleus pontinus) in the pons, continuing via the entire Medulla oblongata into the Nucleus spinalis nervi trigemini.

Clinical remarks

Sharp, shooting, stabbing pain is mostly limited to the face, and is referred to as **trigeminal neuralgia**. These fits typically only last for a few seconds, rarely for more than 2 minutes. Between the bouts, the patient is usually pain-free, although the overall trend is progressive. The cause is frequently pathological neurovascular contact between the A. superior cerebelli and the N. trigeminus (where it leaves the brainstem). Trigeminal neuralgia is initially treated with drugs, but if this is unsuccessful, invasive procedures can be considered. These include percutaneous puncture through the cheek and/or through the Foramen ovale to perform a thermocoagulation of the Ganglion trigeminale. This procedure is destructive and therefore also reduces touch sensations in the area of one or more branches of the trigeminal nerve (hypoaesthesia). Another therapeutic method is microvascular decompression. Here, the above-mentioned pathological neurovascular contact is resolved by the use of an interponate, such as a small Teflon sponge.

N. ophthalmicus

The N. ophthalmicus [V/1] is a purely afferent nerve, carrying impulses from the area of the orbita, the Bulbus oculi, including the cornea, the skin of the face up to the lambdoid suture and the back of the nose (➤ Fig. 12.49, but also of the mucosa of the ethmoidal sinuses, the sphenoidal sinus, of the nasal septum and the dura of the anterior cranial cavity. It forms the basis of the corneal reflex.

Clinical remarks

The **corneal reflex** is a reflexive protective mechanism of the eye, with stimulation of the cornea leading to closure of the opening between the eyelids (palpebral fissure). The corneal reflex is a polysynaptic reflex, which should be particularly noted when checking the neurological status of an unconscious patient (see below). It can be absent in peripheral nerve lesions, as well as in cases of severe brainstem lesions. The reflex is usually triggered by touching the cornea with a cotton swab, but it is also possible to trigger the reflex here using glaring lights or acoustic stimuli. The stimulatory impulses are routed through fibres of the N. ophthalmicus. After central configuration in the trigeminal nucleus complex, the reflex arch runs polysynaptically via the Colliculi superiores, the Formatio reticularis, and finally to the nuclear complex of the N. facialis. From here, the efferent pulses travel via the N. facialis to the facial muscles (M. orbicularis oculi), which generate eyelid movement.

After the Ganglion trigeminale, the N. ophthalmicus [V/1] continues on its way to the Fissura orbitalis superior through the **Sinus cavernosus** or in its lateral limit, through the Dura mater. The Sinus cavernosus nestles laterally on both sides of the Corpus ossis sphenoidalis with the Sinus sphenoidalis located within it (➤ Fig. 12.46). Still in the Sinus cavernosus, the N. ophthalmicus emits an **R. meningeus recurrens** (syn.: **R. tentorius**) for the dura of the anterior cranial cavity and the Tentorium cerebelli. Before its passage through the Fissura orbitalis superior, the N. ophthalmicus splits into its three main branches (➤ Fig. 12.47, light green-coloured nerve branches):

- **N. nasociliaris** (1st main branch): It passes through the Anulus tendineus to the medial orbital wall. Here it divides into both the **Nn. ethmoidales anterior and posterior**:
  The **N. ethmoidalis anterior** reaches the anterior cranial cavity with its **R. meningeus** via the identically named foramen of the orbita, then passes through the Lamina cribrosa in order to enter the nasal cavity. Its **Rr. nasales anteriores laterales and septi** innervate the anterior part of the nasal cavity and of the nasal septum and the anterior ethmoidal sinuses. Its terminal branches leave the nasal cavity again as **Rr. nasales externi** for the area of the dorsum of the nose to the tip of the nose.
  The **N. ethmoidalis posterior** also passes through the identically named foramen of the orbita, reaching the posterior ethmoidal sinuses.
  The pathway of the N. nasociliaris is eventually continued by the **N. infratrochlearis,** with its branches innervating the medial eye angle. Sensory branches of the Ganglion ciliare run along with the **Nn. ciliares breves and longi** to the Bulbus oculi and supply the cornea and the conjunctiva.
- **N. frontalis** (2nd main branch): It runs around the roof of the orbit in order to innervate the **N. supraorbitalis** and the **N. supratrochlearis,** of the forehead, sinus and upper eyelid via its two end branches.
- **N. lacrimalis** (3rd main branch): It runs along the lateral orbita above the M. rectus lateralis to the lacrimal gland. Postganglionic general visceroefferent fibres of the N. facialis [VII] from the Ganglion pterygopalatinum accumulate here via the **R. communicans cum nervo zygomatico.** Sensory fibres also accumulate at the lateral eye angle, upper eyelid and conjunctiva.

N. maxillaris
The N. maxillaris [V/2] is a purely afferent nerve, carrying impulses from the area of the lower eyelid, the cheek skin and the upper lip. Its cutaneous innervation area also includes the skin above the zygomatic bone and the temporal area (➤ Fig. 12.49). In addition, it also carries afferents from the mucous membranes of the rear and lower nasal cavity, the maxillary sinus, the palate and the maxilla, including the associated upper teeth and the meninges of the middle cranial fossa. After passing through the Ganglion trigeminale, it runs together with the N. ophthalmicus through the Sinus cavernosus, but further basolaterally it is located in the lateral boundaries of the sinus (➤ Fig. 12.46) before it goes through the Foramen rotundum into the Fossa pterygopalatina. The ramifications of the N. maxillaris [V/2] are presented in ➤ Fig. 12.47 in orange:

- An **R. meningeus** leaves the N. maxillaris intracranially for the dura of the middle cranial fossa. In the Fossa pterygopalatina, the following branch off from the N. maxillaris:

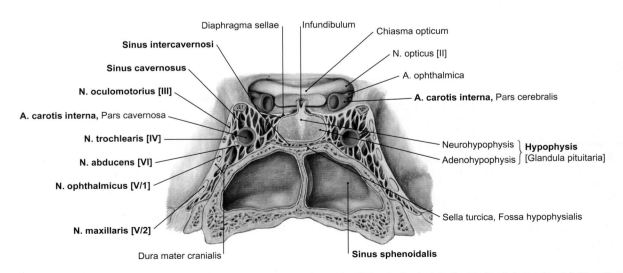

Fig. 12.46 Frontal section through the Sinus cavernosus at the level of the Glandula pituitaria (pituitary gland, hypophysis). View from posterior. The Sinus cavernosi surrounds both sides of the Corpus ossis sphenoidalis with the Sella turcica and the Fossa hypophysialis. The N. oculomotorius [III], the N. trochlearis [IV], the N. ophthalmicus [V/1] and the N. maxillaris [V/2] run within the lateral wall of the Sinus cavernosus. The N. abducens [VI] and the A. carotis interna are centrally located in the Sinus cavernosus.

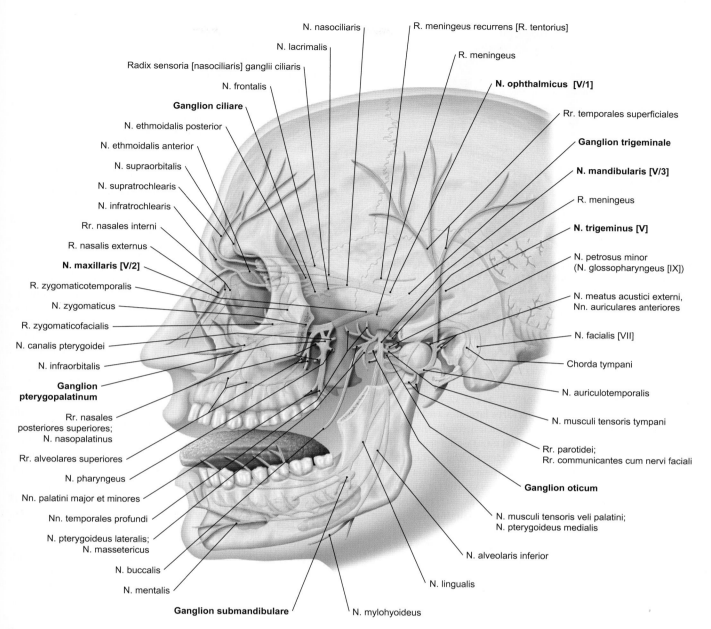

N. nasociliaris
N. lacrimalis
Radix sensoria [nasociliaris] ganglii ciliaris
N. frontalis
Ganglion ciliare
N. ethmoidalis posterior
N. ethmoidalis anterior
N. supraorbitalis
N. supratrochlearis
N. infratrochlearis
Rr. nasales interni
R. nasalis externus
N. maxillaris [V/2]
R. zygomaticotemporalis
N. zygomaticus
R. zygomaticofacialis
N. canalis pterygoidei
N. infraorbitalis
Ganglion pterygopalatinum
Rr. nasales posteriores superiores; N. nasopalatinus
Rr. alveolares superiores
N. pharyngeus
Nn. palatini major et minores
Nn. temporales profundi
N. pterygoideus lateralis; N. massetericus
N. buccalis
N. mentalis
Ganglion submandibulare

R. meningeus recurrens [R. tentorius]
R. meningeus
N. ophthalmicus [V/1]
Rr. temporales superficiales
Ganglion trigeminale
N. mandibularis [V/3]
R. meningeus
N. trigeminus [V]
N. petrosus minor (N. glossopharyngeus [IX])
N. meatus acustici externi, Nn. auriculares anteriores
N. facialis [VII]
Chorda tympani
N. auriculotemporalis
N. musculi tensoris tympani
Rr. parotidei; Rr. communicantes cum nervi faciali
Ganglion oticum
N. musculi tensoris veli palatini; N. pterygoideus medialis
N. alveolaris inferior
N. lingualis
N. mylohyoideus

Fig. 12.47 N. trigeminus left with a split into the main branches N. ophthalmicus [V/1] (bright green), N. maxillaris [V/2] (orange) and N. mandibularis [V/3] (turquoise). Lateral view.

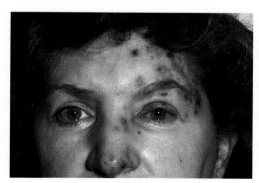

Fig. 12.48 Zoster ophthalmicus. The skin is affected in the innervation area of the 1st trigeminal branch, as well as the epithelium of the surface of the eye such as the cornea and the conjunctivae. The conjunctiva becomes clearly reddened and the eyelids narrowed. [E943]

- The **N. zygomaticus** incorporates postganglionic general viscerofferent fibres of the N. facialis [VII], passes through the Fissura orbitalis inferior in the orbita and releases these fibres here via the **R. communicans cum nervo zygomatico** in the direction of the Glandula lacrimalis. The trigeminal general somatoafferent fibres run along the lateral orbital wall and, with the **Rr. zygomaticotemporalis and zygomaticofacialis**, pass through canals of the same name via the cheekbone to the surface of the face, in order to innervate the skin of the temple above the cheekbone and of the lateral eye angle.
- **Rr. alveolares superiores posteriores** supply the molars of the upper jaw with adjacent areas of the Sinus maxillaris and the gingiva. The **Rr. alveolares superiores medii and anteriores** from the N. infraorbitalis (see below) accordingly innervate the premolars, canines and incisors. The Rr. alveolares superiores are collectively referred to as the **Plexus dentalis superior**.
- The **N. infraorbitalis** is the terminal branch of the N. maxillaris [V/2]. Unlike the previous branches, it initially runs via the Fissura orbitalis inferior into the orbita, but leaves again immediately via

691

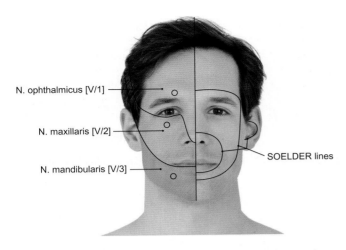

N. ophthalmicus [V/1]

N. maxillaris [V/2]

N. mandibularis [V/3]

SOELDER lines

Fig. 12.49 Innervation areas of the facial skin by the N. trigeminus, exit points and protopathic sensitivity. On the left side of the face (right side on the illustration) the somatotopic structure of the protopathic sensibility is shown, on the right side of the face are the innervation areas and nerve exit points for the 3 peripheral trigeminal branches. [K340]

the Canalis infraorbitalis, in order to move forward in the roof of the Sinus maxillaris and to exit below the eye at the Foramen infraorbitale (trigeminal pressure point V/2, ➤ Fig. 12.49, left side).

- The **Rr. nasales posteriores superiores laterales and mediales** pass through the sphenopalatine foramen medially into the nasal cavity, to the mucosa of the lateral nasal wall, the nasopharynx and the Tuba auditiva. A branch descending to the septum, the **N. nasopalatinus**, finally reaches the oral cavity via the Canalis incisivus or the mucous membranes via the Os incisivum of the hard palate and a small section of the nasal septum. These branches are collectively referred to as **Rr. ganglionares ad ganglion pterygopalatinum**.
- The **N. palatinus major** and the **Nn. palatini minores** leave caudally in identically named canal in the Fossa pterygopalatina and reach the corresponding Foramina palatina major and minores to the mucosa of the hard and soft palates.

N. mandibularis

The N. mandibularis [V/3], in contrast to the other two branches of the N. trigeminus, is a mixed nerve. It forms the strongest outgoing part of the Ganglion trigeminale, which joins the Radix motoria before they pass through the Foramen ovale of the middle cranial fossa in the Fossa infratemporalis. In summary, the N. mandibularis is responsible for the general somatoafferent innervation of the entire mandibular area. It supplies sensory innervation to the chin and anterior ear area (➤ Fig. 12.49), the adjacent lower jaw area with the bottom teeth, as well as the mucosa of the cheek and of the dorsum of the tongue (anterior two-thirds) as well as the meninges of the middle cranial fossa. The special visceroefferent fibres innervate the muscles leading from the 1st pharyngeal arch myotome. These include the masticatory muscles, but also parts of the mouth floor muscles and the 'tensors' at the Tuba auditiva and the tympanic membrane (M. tensor veli palatini and M. tensor tympani). Only after leaving the cranial cavity, the N. mandibularis [V/3] releases a

- descending **R. meningeus** which, together with the A. meningea media, gets to the interior of the skull of the dura via the Foramen spinosum. Directly below the Foramen ovale, the Ganglion oticum accumulates medially on the N. mandibularis (➤ Fig. 12.47, turquoise nerve fibres), before it divides into anterior and posterior parts.

- The anterior nerve trunk is also known as the **N. masticatorius (chewing nerve)**, as mostly special visceroefferent fibres for mastication muscles originate from it:
  - The **Nn. pterygoidei lateralis and medialis** are fine branches that run directly to the masticatory muscles. The N. pterygoideus medialis usually releases the special visceroefferent fibres for the M. tensor veli palatini and M. tensor tympani.
  - The **Nn. temporales profundi** for the M. temporalis and the **N. massetericus** for the M. masseter, the special visceroefferent supply of the maxillary-closing muscle.
  - The only afferent nerve of the N. masticatorius is the **N. buccalis**: it penetrates the M. buccinator and innervates the buccal mucosa with adjoining buccal sections of the gingiva.
- The posterior main trunk of the N. mandibularis contains mixed fibre qualities:
  - **N. auriculotemporalis:** On its lateral pathway, it forms a loop around the A. meningea media. Its general somatoafferent fibres ultimately go to the skin of the ear and, with a small branch, the **N. meatus acustici externi**, to the external ear canal and the eardrum. Together with branches of the A. temporalis superficialis, its branches reach the temple cranially. In addition, postganglionic general visceroefferent fibres of the N. glossopharyngeus [IX] accumulate onto the N. auriculotemporalis from the Ganglion oticum for the innervation of the Glandula parotidea.
  - **N. alveolaris inferior:** It runs between both the Mm. pterygoidei to caudal. At the Foramen mandibulae it enters the bony Canalis alveolaris inferior of the mandibula and with the fine branches of the **Plexus dentalis inferior,** it supplies the teeth of the lower jaw with the adjacent gingiva. At the Foramen mentale, the N. alveolaris inferior passes as the **N. mentalis** to the surface anatomy (trigeminal pressure point V/3, ➤ Fig. 12.49, left-hand half of the image) and here supplies the skin of the chin and the lower lip. Shortly before entering the Foramen mandibulae, the **N. mylohyoideus** branches off for special visceroefferent innervation of the identically named muscle and of the Venter anterior musculi digastrici.
  - **N. lingualis:** It runs medially of the N. alveolaris inferior and almost parallel to it caudally, although it does not enter the Foramen mandibulae, but instead reaches the root of the tongue. With generally somatoafferent fibres, it innervates the anterior two-thirds of the tongue mucosa and the Glandula sublingualis. Already in its cranial section, the N. lingualis accumulates preganglionic general visceroefferent fibres and special visceroafferent taste fibres from the Chorda tympani of the N. facialis [VII]. Further along the Ganglion submandibulare pathway, the general visceroefferent fibres are relayed and control the hypersecretion of the Glandulae sublingualis and submandibular. The taste fibres of the Chorda tympani come from taste buds at the back and tip of the tongue, accumulating on the lingual nerve and ultimately pass via the Fissura petrosquamosa to the N. facialis [VII].

Cranial nerve nuclei of the N. trigeminus

The N. trigeminus itself only carries 2 fibre qualities, with general visceroefferent fibres accumulating on it only peripherally. This makes it possible to differentiate special visceroefferent fibres with a corresponding cranial nerve nucleus and general somatoafferent fibres with an associated nucleus complex. The latter forms the rostral processing of neurons of the spinal dorsal horn, resulting in similarities between the spinoafferent system and the trigeminoafferent system. In both systems, depending on the sensory modality, there are different neural pathways for relays: here, the epicritical, proprioceptive and protopathic (management of mechanoreceptors, thermal receptors and nociceptors) stimuli management of the skin and mucous membranes can be separately observed. Unlike the usual cranial nerve nuclei, this trigeminal complex can therefore be differentiated into 3 subnuclei, according to the description of their sensory modality (➤ Fig. 12.50).

Nucleus of the special visceroefferent fibres
The **Nucleus motorius nervi trigemini** lies in the Pars dorsalis pontis and reaches the lateral area of the periaqueductal zone, as well as the lateral angle of the IVth ventricle. It contains the perikarya of special visceroefferent fibres, which go to the muscles of mastication as the Radix motoria with the N. mandibularis.

Nuclei of the general somatoafferent fibres
Nucleus mesencephalicus nervi trigemini
The proprioceptive afferent fibres from the muscle spindles of the masticatory muscles accumulate onto this Radix motoria. In the brainstem, these form the **Tractus mesencephalicus nervi trigemini** and pass to the **Nucleus mesencephalicus nervi trigemini** within the mesencephalon. The perikarya of these proprioceptive primary afferents do not lie within the Ganglion trigeminale, but directly within the Nucleus mesencephalicus. Thus the Nucleus mesencephalicus nervi trigemini is also referred to as a single **central ganglion**.

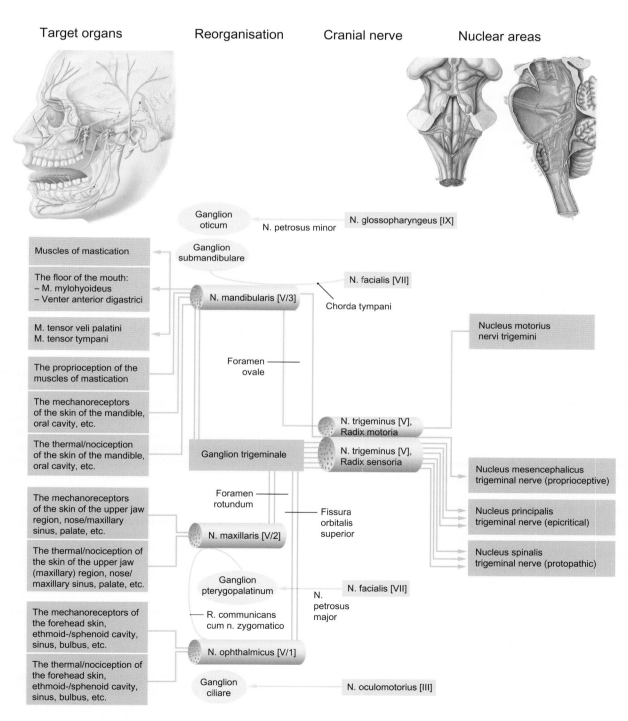

Fig. 12.50 N. trigeminus with fibre qualities, cranial nerves nuclei and target organs (diagram). [L127]

Nucleus principalis [pontinus] nervi trigemini

The perikarya of the other primary afferents lie within the Ganglion trigeminale. Impulses of the fine discrimination of mechanoreceptors are carried via the central axon from here to the 2nd neuron in the **Nucleus principalis [pontinus] nervi trigemini** in the cranial pons, approximately at the level of the exit point of the N. trigeminus.

Nucleus spinalis nervi trigemini

Poorly discriminating mechanoreceptors are also projected via the Ganglion trigeminale, as well as again to a 2nd neuron in the **Nucleus spinalis nervi trigemini**. The fibres of the trigeminal thermoreceptors and nociceptors end in the Pars caudalis of the Nucleus spinalis nervi trigemini. The entire Medulla oblongata penetrates relatively far laterally of the elongated Nucleus spinalis nervi trigemini and continues caudally to the horn of the spinal cord (C6). Thus it is somotopically divided in a ventrodorsal direction, with the afferent fibres or neurons of the N. mandibularis [V/3] furthest dorsally, the afferent fibres or neurons of the N. ophthalmicus [V/1] furthest ventrally, with an intervening section for the N. maxillaris [V/2]. The somatotopy of this cranial nerve nucleus in a rostrocaudal direction is clinically even more important: afferents from the perioral zone are furthermost rostrally within the nucleus while the afferents end further caudally in the nucleus, increasingly far from the cleft lip. This somatotopy of the trigeminal fibres corresponds to concentric boundary lines, **SÖLDER's lines**, the central sensory innervation areas of the facial skin (➤ Fig. 12.49, right half of the illustration).

Clinical remarks

In the case of a nuclear **central lesion of the N. trigeminus,** we therefore note a somatosensory disorder similar to an onion skin, whereas typically in a peripheral lesion of the trigeminal nerve, the supply areas of the N. ophthalmicus [V/1], of the N. maxillaris [V/2] and N. mandibularis nerve [V/3] are affected in an isolated or combined manner.

Central links of the N. trigeminus

The central neuronal configurations of the cranial nerve nuclei of the trigeminal nerve include, on the one hand, the regulation of masticatory function, e.g., chewing pressure, the control of reflexes, as well as voluntary perception of sensations of skin and mucous membranes in the head area.

Nucleus mesencephalicus nervi trigemini

For these control mechanisms, the neurons of the Nucleus mesencephalicus form direct synapses with the neurons of the Nucleus motorius nervi trigemini. Proprioceptive impulses from the muscles of mastication are projected through these directly onto motoneurons. This kind of monosynaptic configuration in the motoric system is ultimately comparable to a proprioceptive muscle reflex (➤ Chap. 12.6.7) such as the patellar tendon reflex. Accordingly, this is referred to as a **masseter muscle reflex.**

Nucleus motorius nervi trigemini

The Nucleus motorius nervi trigemini also receives afferent impulses from the face and oral cavity, which arrive secondarily via neurons of the sensory trigeminal nuclei and interneurons of the Formatio reticularis. Via the Formatio reticularis, the limbic system has an influence on the activity of the Nucleus motorius. But the nucleus receives the most important afferents for arbitrary motor control via the Fibrae corticonucleares, which reach the nucleus complex bilaterally, going from the motoric cortex via the Capsula interna. One-sided lesions of these fibres, such as in the context of a stroke, often remain asymptomatic due to the bilateral innervation of the nucleus, whereas direct damage to the nucleus complex leads to ipsilateral muscle atrophy.

Nucleus principalis [pontinus] nervi trigemini

The body is consciously aware of impulses of fine point discrimination, vibration and the perception of the chewing pressure on the periodontium, by being transferred from the 2nd neuron in the Nucleus principalis nervi trigemini into the somatosensory cortex via the thalamus. These efferent axons of the main nucleus mostly cross onto the opposite side and form the **Tractus trigeminothalamicus anterior**, which joins the Lemniscus medialis and, in the thalamus, reaches the 3rd neuron in the **Nucleus ventralis posteromedialis** (conversely spinoafferent fibres reach the Nucleus ventralis posterolateralis in the thalamus). Via the **Tractus trigeminothalamicus posterior**, uncrossed fibres reach the ipsilateral thalamus, before being transferred to the cortex. Additionally, this posterior tract conducts touch and pressure sensations from the oral cavity, including the teeth.

Nucleus spinalis nervi trigemini

The configuration of impulses of pain and temperature sensations in the head area (protopathic sensibility) is organised in the same way as in the spinothalamic system of the spinal cord. Rather than being in the spinal ganglion, here the perikaryon of the 1st neuron is found within the **Ganglion trigeminale** and carries the impulses of the 2nd neuron in the **Nucleus spinalis nervi trigemini**. The central efferents of this nucleus cross over to the opposite side and then run together with the efferents of the Nucleus principalis nervi trigemini in the **Tractus trigeminothalamicus anterior** to the **Nucleus ventralis posteromedialis** of the thalamus (3rd neuron), but also to the intralaminar thalamic nuclei. The impulses of this sensory modality are also stimulated via thalamocortical projections. Other neuronal links of the Nucleus spinalis nervi trigemini can be found at the **Formatio reticularis**. Functionally, a general increase in activity in the central nervous system results from this configuration. This is well-illustrated, for example through the irritation of the nasal trigeminal fibres with smelling salts (ammonia), which in the 18th century was used as a standard treatment for dizziness and fainting. Strong trigeminal ganglion stimulation by odours in the nasal cavity [V/2], 'sharp' flavouring agents in the oral cavity [V/3] or eyes [V/1], e.g., when slicing onions, often leads to a reflex-related increase in saliva production or lacrimation, so we assume that there are neuronal links to the general visceroefferent nuclear areas (Nucleus salivatorii superior and inferior).

NOTE

In the case of **lesions of the brainstem,** e.g., in a brainstem stroke, there are frequently combined lesions of the nucleus and Tractus spinalis nervi trigemini and the Tractus spinothalamicus, as both are located in close proximity to each other in the lateral brainstem. Usually temperature and pain perceptions of the ipsilateral side of the face cease and at the same time, the temperature and pain sensations are disrupted on the contralateral side of the body, as these spinal fibres already cross at the segmental level.

Clinical remarks

An examination of the N. trigeminus is always **carried out comparing both sides,** and should provide clues that make it possible to distinguish between a peripheral nerve lesion and a nuclear central lesion. To do this, the following are checked:

- pain perceptions at the exit points of the 3 peripheral branches of the trigeminal nerve using bilateral pressure of the thumb (pressure sensitivity at what are normally non-painful exit points is a sign of nerve irritation)
- sensitivity in the innervation area of the 3 branches of the trigeminal nerve and according to the nuclear boundary lines with a cotton swab
- the functional capability of the mastication muscles by palpation and assessment of the M. masseter and the M. temporalis in a closed jaw position (with a lesion of the Mm. pterygoidei, the lower jaw typically deviates to the affected side when opening)
- the corneal reflex by delicately touching the cornea with a cotton bud
- the masseter reflex by hitting the M. masseter with a reflex hammer

12.5.9 N. abducens (6th cranial nerve, N. VI)
Michael J. Schmeißer

SKILLS

After working through this chapter, you should be able to:
- name the target organ and cranial nerve nuclei of the N. abducens
- precisely explain the topographical pathway of the N. abducens
- describe the clinical findings of abducens paralysis and identify possible causes

The **N. abducens [VI]** carries general somatoefferent fibres and is responsible for the motor innervation of the M. rectus lateralis, which can abduce the Bulbus oculi (➤ Fig. 12.52).

Pathway and branches
The N. abducens passes directly below the pons near the midline from the brainstem (➤ Fig. 12.51). It then runs forwards through the Cisterna pontis, arrives at the clivus under the dura, crosses over the tip of the temporal bone on its further extradural course, and enters the Sinus cavernosus, where it does not run around its edge as the only cranial nerve, but instead passes through it. (➤ Fig. 12.46). In the orbita, it travels mediocaudally through the Fissura orbitalis superior between the superior branch of the N. oculomotorius and the N. nasociliaris of the N. ophthalmicus. Finally, it passes through the Anulus tendineus communis to the M. rectus lateralis (➤ Fig. 12.52).
Two aspects should be emphasised in the topographical anatomy of the N. abducens:

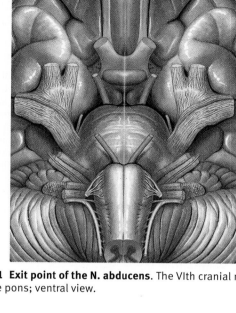

Fig. 12.51 Exit point of the N. abducens. The VIth cranial nerve exits below the pons; ventral view.

- Of all the cranial nerves, it has the longest intracranial, extradural course.
- As the only cranial nerve, it passes right through the Sinus cavernosus.

Cranial nerve nuclei and central links
Due to its fibre composition, the N. abducens has a general somatoefferent cranial nerve nucleus, the **Nucleus nervi abducentis**. This is located in the Pars dorsalis pontis under the floor of the rhomboid cavity. Fibres of the N. facialis [VII] curving dorsally round the Nucleus nervi abducentis, easily seen in horizontal cross-sectional images, is topographically important. This is called the '**inner genu of the facial nerve**' (see below).
The **configurations of the 'eye muscle nuclei'** with each other, and their connection with supranuclear, pre-ocular motor centres, are extremely complex (➤ Chap. 13.3). Particularly significant for conjugated horizontal eye movements is the **Fasciculus longitudinus medialis (FLM)** which connects the Nucleus nervi abducentis nerve with a contralateral subnucleus of the Nucleus nervi oculomotorii (➤ Chap. 12.5.6).

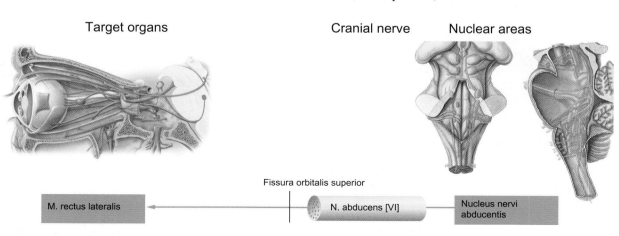

Target organs

Cranial nerve   Nuclear areas

Fissura orbitalis superior

| M. rectus lateralis | ← | N. abducens [VI] | ← | Nucleus nervi abducentis |

Fig. 12.52 Pathway, branches and fibre qualities of the N. abducens, left. Lateral view. [L127]

Clinical remarks

Examination

As with the examination of the other 'eye muscle nerves', we firstly observe the position of the bulbi when examining the N. abducens, then carry out a clinical examination of the eye tracking movements as described for the N. oculomotorius and ask about double vision.

Abducens nerve palsy

In the case of an abducens nerve palsy, the eye on the affected side can no longer be abducted due to the failure of the M. rectus lateralis and is directed medially inwards. This results in double vision, which increases especially when looking sideways. The N. abducens is particularly at risk from fractures of the skull on its long intracranial, extradural pathway along the clivus. In addition, a thrombosis of the Sinus cavernosus can lead to abducens nerve palsy (usually combined with other eye muscle paralysis).

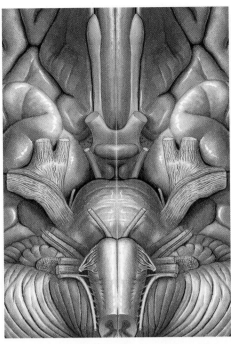

Fig. 12.53 Exit point of the N. facialis. The VIIth cranial nerve exits in the cerebellopontine angle. Ventral view.

12.5.10 N. facialis (7th cranial nerve, N. VII)

Michael J. Schmeißer

SKILLS

After working through this chapter, you should be able to:
- name the target organs of the N. facialis
- describe the cranial nerve nuclei of the N. facialis, explain their topographical position and correctly explain their respective functions
- describe the clinical findings of facial paralysis, distinguish between peripheral and central facial paralysis and explain possible causes

One of the main jobs of the **N. facialis [VII]** is the motor innervation of the mimic muscles. It also explains the name 'facial nerve'. Both the facial nerve and the mimic muscles arise from the 2nd pharyngeal arch, so the corresponding motor nerve fibres are specially visceroefferent. As well as this, the fibres of the N. facialis contain other qualities that can be summarised as the so-called **nervus-intermedius part** of the N. facialis:

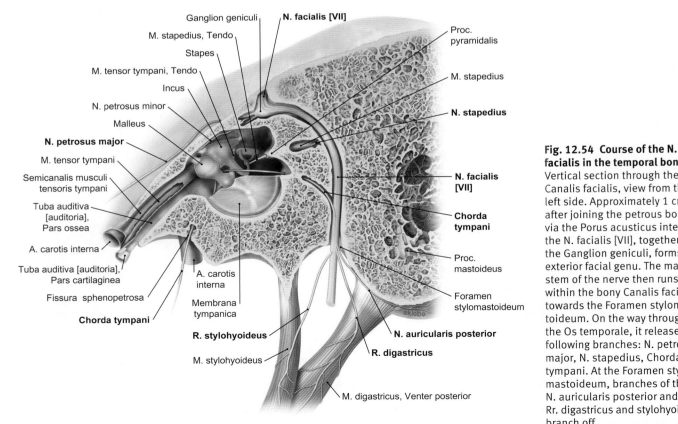

Ganglion geniculi
M. stapedius, Tendo
Stapes
M. tensor tympani, Tendo
Incus
N. petrosus minor
Malleus
N. petrosus major
M. tensor tympani
Semicanalis musculi tensoris tympani
Tuba auditiva [auditoria], Pars ossea
A. carotis interna
Tuba auditiva [auditoria], Pars cartilaginea
Fissura sphenopetrosa
Chorda tympani
M. stylohyoideus
R. stylohyoideus
M. digastricus, Venter posterior
A. carotis interna
Membrana tympanica
R. digastricus
N. facialis [VII]
Proc. pyramidalis
M. stapedius
N. stapedius
N. facialis [VII]
Chorda tympani
Proc. mastoideus
Foramen stylomastoideum
N. auricularis posterior

Fig. 12.54 Course of the N. facialis in the temporal bone. Vertical section through the Canalis facialis, view from the left side. Approximately 1 cm after joining the petrous bone via the Porus acusticus internus, the N. facialis [VII], together with the Ganglion geniculi, forms the exterior facial genu. The main stem of the nerve then runs within the bony Canalis facialis towards the Foramen stylomastoideum. On the way through the Os temporale, it releases the following branches: N. petrous major, N. stapedius, Chorda tympani. At the Foramen stylomastoideum, branches of the N. auricularis posterior and the Rr. digastricus and stylohyoideus branch off.

- general visceroefferent fibres for the parasympathetic innervation of the lacrimal gland and salivary glands (up to the Glandula parotidea)
- special visceroafferent taste fibres of the anterior two-thirds of the tongue
- general somatoafferent fibres from the outer ear (➤ Fig. 12.56).

Pathway and branches

Intermedius and actual facial parts of the N. facialis leave the brainstem rostral of the olive in what is called the cerebellopontine angle (➤ Fig. 12.53). They pass via the Porus or Meatus acusticus internus with the N. vestibulocochlearis [VIII] into the petrous pyramid and then run as a common nerve root inside a bony canal, the so-called **Canalis nervi facialis**. About 1 cm after entering this canal, the nerve root in the geniculate ganglion (**Ganglion geniculi**) turns towards dorsolateral and runs arch-shaped in the rear wall of the tympanic cavity caudally to the **Foramen stylomastoideum**, through which it leaves the cranial base. Finally, it divides into its terminal branches within the Glandula parotidea which is however neither efferently nor afferently innervated by it. As it runs through the Canalis nervi facialis, the N. facialis provides the following branches from proximal to distal (➤ Fig. 12.54):

- **N. petrosus major:** This general visceroefferent branch leaves the trunk of the N. facialis at the Ganglion geniculi, passes

through the Hiatus canalis nervi petrosi majoris to the front surface of the temporal bone and arrives in its own groove, covered by Dura mater, through the Foramen lacerum into the Canalis pterygoideus of the Os sphenoidale. Here it combines with the sympathetic N. petrosus profundus. Both nerves pass together into the Fossa pterygopalatina as the **N. canalis pterygoidei**. In the Ganglion pterygopalatinum, the general visceroefferent fibres of the N. petrosus major are relayed from preganglionic to postganglionic. The postganglionic, secretory fibres partially accumulate in the continued course of the N. zygomaticus of the N. maxillaris [V/2] and pass with it into the orbita and via the N. lacrimalis of the N. ophthalmicus [V/1] to the Glandula lacrimalis, or they run as Nn. palatini and Nn. nasales posteriores to the upper palate or rear nasal glands.

- **N. stapedius:** This is a special visceroefferent branch, which provides the motor innervation for the M. stapedius of the middle ear.
- **Chorda tympani** or tympanic string: This facial branch predominantly contains general visceroefferent and special visceroafferent taste-related fibres. The Chorda tympani passes retroactively back from the Canalis nervi facialis through its own bony canal to the middle ear. Here it runs medially of the tympanic membrane between the hammer and the anvil. Finally it runs via the Fissura sphenopetrosa or the Fissura petrotympanica (various information in the literature) in the Fossa infratemporalis and

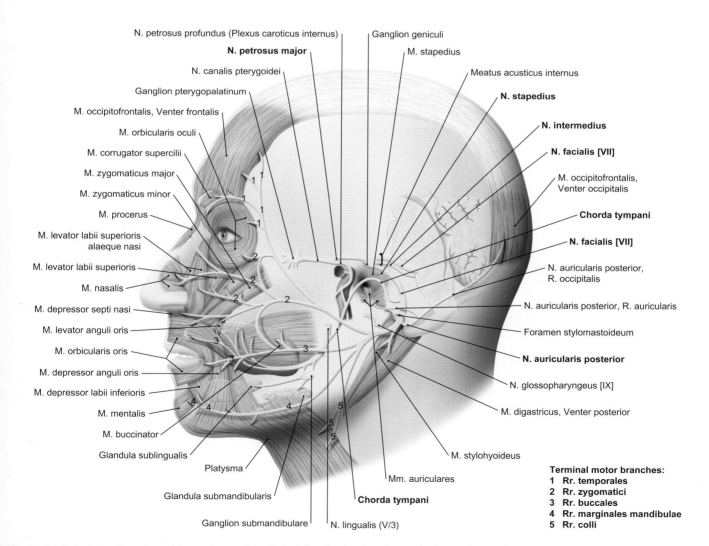

N. petrosus profundus (Plexus caroticus internus)
N. petrosus major
N. canalis pterygoidei
Ganglion pterygopalatinum
M. occipitofrontalis, Venter frontalis
M. orbicularis oculi
M. corrugator supercilii
M. zygomaticus major
M. zygomaticus minor
M. procerus
M. levator labii superioris alaeque nasi
M. levator labii superioris
M. nasalis
M. depressor septi nasi
M. levator anguli oris
M. orbicularis oris
M. depressor anguli oris
M. depressor labii inferioris
M. mentalis
M. buccinator
Glandula sublingualis
Platysma
Glandula submandibularis
Ganglion submandibulare
N. lingualis (V/3)

Ganglion geniculi
M. stapedius
Meatus acusticus internus
N. stapedius
N. intermedius
N. facialis [VII]
M. occipitofrontalis, Venter occipitalis
Chorda tympani
N. facialis [VII]
N. auricularis posterior, R. occipitalis
N. auricularis posterior, R. auricularis
Foramen stylomastoideum
N. auricularis posterior
N. glossopharyngeus [IX]
M. digastricus, Venter posterior
M. stylohyoideus
Mm. auriculares
Chorda tympani

Terminal motor branches:
1 **Rr. temporales**
2 **Rr. zygomatici**
3 **Rr. buccales**
4 **Rr. marginales mandibulae**
5 **Rr. colli**

Fig. 12.55 N. facialis. Overview of the pathway of the N. facialis after leaving the cerebellopontine angle up to where it branches off into the Glandula parotidea (diagram).

accumulates dorsally on the N. lingualis [V/3] so that its fibres pass to the Ganglion submandibulare or to the anterior two-thirds of the tongue. In the Ganglion submandibulare, the general visceroefferent fibres are relayed from preganglionic to postganglionic. The latter ensures the secretory supply of the Glandulae sublingualis and submandibularis.

At the Foramen stylomastoideum, the **N. auricularis posterior**, the **R. digastricus** and the **R. stylohyoideus** branch off from the N. facialis. Via its special visceroefferent fibres, the N. auricularis posterior supplies the M. occipitofrontalis (R. occipitalis), and via its general somatoafferent fibres (R. auricularis) supplies the skin above the outer ear. The Rr. digastricus and stylohyoideus innervate the Venter posterior of the M. digastricus and stylohyoideus by special visceroefferent means (➤ Fig. 12.55).

After the N. facialis [VII] leaves the Canalis nervi facialis through the Foramen stylomastoideum, it forms a network of special visceroefferent fibres, the **(Plexus intraparotideus)** within the Glandula parotidea in the Fossa retromandibularis. From this, 2 main nerve trunks are formed, of which the one lying furthest cranially (R. temporofacialis, clinically: 'frontal branch') innervates the muscles of the forehead and the eyelids together with the **Rr. temporales**, and the one lying further caudally (R. cervicofacialis) innervates the muscles of the cheeks, lips and chin with the **Rr. zygomatici and buccales**, via the **R. marginalis mandibulae** and the **R. colli** (➤ Fig. 12.55). These branches all arise in a fan shape from the front edge of the parotid gland and pass subcutaneously to the mimic (facial) muscles.

Cranial nerve nuclei and central links

Corresponding with its 4 fibre qualities, the N. facialis has 4 cranial nerve nuclei (➤ Fig. 12.56):

- The special visceroefferent fibres supplying the facial muscles and the Mm. stapedius, digastricus and stylohyoideus originate in the **Nucleus nervi facialis**. This nuclear motor complex, which has an upper and a lower cell group, is located in the caudal part of the Pars dorsalis pontis. Its efferent fibres run initially dorsally and, from caudal, loop dorsally around the abducens nucleus ventrolaterally, thereby forming the so-called **inner facial genu** (Genu nervi facialis). The facial genu forms a swelling, the Colliculus nervi facialis, which can be observed in a dorsal view of the brainstem or the rhomboid fossa.
- The original neurons of the general visceroefferent fibres are located in the parasympathetic **Nucleus salivatorius superior**, which lies in the immediate vicinity of the Nucleus nervi facialis in the pons.
- The special visceroafferent taste fibres of the N. facialis end in the upper section of the Solitarius nucleus complex, also referred to as the **Nucleus ovalis** of the **Nuclei tractus solitarii**, and which is located in the Medulla oblongata.
- In the **Nucleus spinalis nervi trigemini**, a few general somatoafferent fibres from the skin of the outer ear terminate.

The special visceroefferent Nucleus nervi facialis receives direct and indirect afferents from key areas of the **motor system**, including from the motor cortex, from the motor brainstem centres and from the spinal cord. **Voluntary facial expression** is controlled, for example, by direct projections that originate from the motor cortex and run via the Tractus corticonuclearis into the Nucleus nervi facialis. **Emotional facial expression**, on the other hand, appears to be controlled by indirect projections into the Nucleus nervi facialis from the limbic system. The lateral zone of the Formatio reticularis in the brainstem acts as an intermediate switching station.

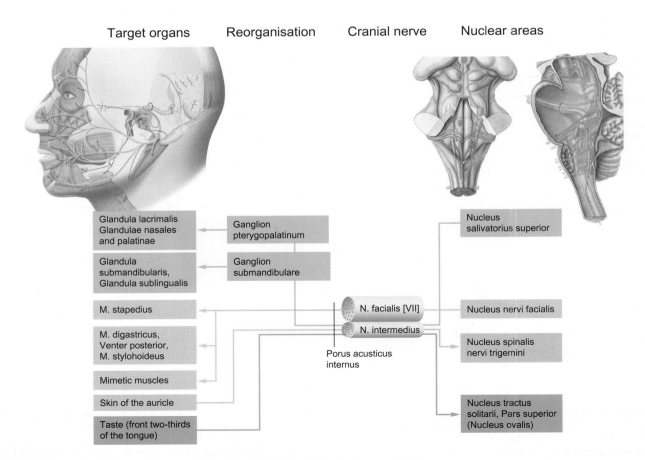

| Target organs | Reorganisation | Cranial nerve | Nuclear areas |

Glandula lacrimalis, Glandulae nasales and palatinae ← Ganglion pterygopalatinum

Glandula submandibularis, Glandula sublingualis ← Ganglion submandibulare

M. stapedius

M. digastricus, Venter posterior, M. stylohoideus

Mimetic muscles

Skin of the auricle

Taste (front two-thirds of the tongue)

N. facialis [VII]
N. intermedius

Porus acusticus internus

Nucleus salivatorius superior

Nucleus nervi facialis

Nucleus spinalis nervi trigemini

Nucleus tractus solitarii, Pars superior (Nucleus ovalis)

Fig. 12.56 Pathway, branches and fibre qualities of the N. facialis, left. Lateral view. [L127]

In addition, the Nucleus nervi facialis includes afferent input from **acoustic relay nuclei**, e.g., from the upper olivary nucleus complex. Where there is a lot of noise, this acts to contract the M. stapedius which is innervated by the N. stapedius and stabilises the movement of the stapes, thus attenuating the transmission of sound to the inner ear.

There is another important link between the Nucleus ovalis of the Solitarius nucleus complex, the Formatio reticularis and the Nuclei nervi facialis, motorius nervi trigemini and salivatorii. This is highly important in the making of food choices (**gustatory signal transduction** via the Chorda tympani of the N. facialis) and food intake (e.g., the induction of saliva secretion via the Chorda tympani of the N. facialis).

Clinical remarks

Examination

By examining and comparing the two sides of the face, facial symmetry can be checked, as well as the function of the special visceroefferent branches of the mimic muscles. A drooping corner of the mouth gives the first indication about which side is affected. Now the patient is asked to close their eyes and furrow their forehead (checking the function of the cranially located R. temporofacialis of the Plexus intraparotideus with the Rr. temporales – clinically known as the 'frontal branch'), inflate the cheeks, purse the lips to whistle, and show their teeth (checking the function of the caudally located R. cervicofacialis of the Plexus intraparotideus with Rr. zygomatici, buccales, marginalis mandibulae and colli). Special care must be taken here to observe whether the patient can still furrow their forehead on both sides and if both eyes are able to close or not:

- If there is **central facial paralysis**, the frown often remains intact on both sides, in contrast to the rest of the facial muscles on the affected side.
- On the other hand, if there is **peripheral facial paralysis**, all of the mimic muscles on the affected side are paralysed. When trying to furrow the forehead, it remains smooth, and when trying to close the eyes, the physiological upwards rotation of the Bulbus is visible (BELL's palsy) due to the incomplete closure of the lids (lagophthalmus).

Where a central facial palsy is clinically excluded, characteristic associated symptoms can suggest the location of the damage in the peripheral pathway of the N. facialis. These include:

- dry eyes due to a reduction of lacrimation (damage before the exit of the N. petrosus major)
- increased sensitivity to acoustic stimuli (damage before the exit of the N. stapedius)
- taste and saliva secretion disorders (damage before the exit of the Chorda tympani).

Facial paralysis/palsy

A basic distinction is made between peripheral and central facial palsy. The main clinical symptom in both forms is the drooping paralysis of the facial muscles, whereby the contralateral side is affected by a central, supranuclear paralysis and the eye and forehead muscles are spared (see above). This is due to the fact that the upper nuclear group of the respective Nucleus nervi facialis, which control the eye and forehead muscles via the 'frontal branch', are innervated by corticonuclear fibres on both sides of the brain. Therefore, in the event of damage to the contralateral side, central innervation is ensured by the fibres of the ipsilateral side (➤ Fig. 12.57).

It is extremely important clinically to be able to differentiate between central and peripheral facial paralysis, because in contrast to peripheral paresis, central paralysis is almost always due to a stroke (ischemia or bleeding in the area of the Capsula interna) affecting the supranuclear fibres. Diagnostic and therapeutic measures must be rapidly initiated to limit the extent of brain damage. Conversely, peripheral facial palsy occurs for example due to traumatic brain trauma with fractures of the petrous bone or infections in the middle and inner ear and the temporal bone. Often, however, no clear cause can be determined. In this case it is referred to as idiopathic nerve paralysis.

12.5.11 N. vestibulocochlearis (8th cranial nerve, N. VIII)
Michael J. Schmeißer

SKILLS

After working through this chapter, you should be able to:
- give an accurate outline of the fibre qualities of the N. vestibulocochlearis
- describe the clinical symptoms which can arise in acoustic neuroma

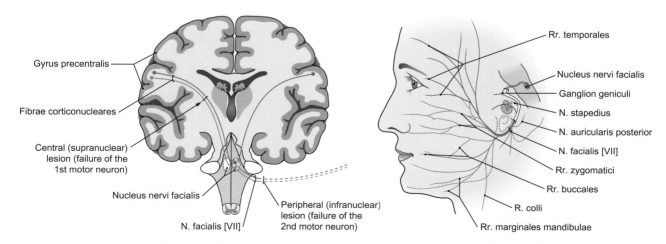

Fig. 12.57 Corticonuclear compounds and peripheral course of the N. facialis. On the left, the central connections to the Nucleus nervi facialis are presented in simplified form. The corticonuclear tracts to the upper part of the nucleus derive from both hemispheres (green). The lower part is only reached by the contralateral hemisphere (red). On the right, the fibres leaving from the top and bottom nuclear section are presented correspondingly up to the peripheral. On the left is an example of possible locations for damage in the context of central (supranuclear) and peripheral (infranuclear) facial palsy.

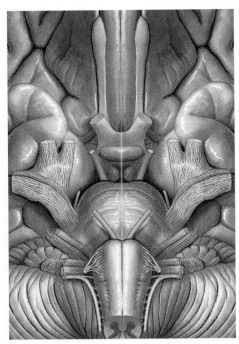

Fig. 12.58 Exit point of the N. vestibulocochlearis. The VIIIth cranial nerve exits in the cerebellopontine angle. Ventral view.

The **N. vestibulocochlearis [VIII]** (syn.: N. statoacusticus) consists of both the N. vestibularis (vestibular or 'balance' nerve) and the N. cochlearis (cochlear or 'auditory' nerve) and includes both special somatoafferent and efferent fibres. The special somatoafferent fibres:

- of the **N. vestibularis** are central afferent projections of the 1st neuron of the balance system (bipolar, perikaryon in the Ganglion vestibulare in the Meatus acusticus internus, ➤ Chap. 13.5)
- of the **N. cochlearis** are central afferent projections of the 1st neuron of the auditory system (bipolar, perikaryon in the Ganglion spirale in the cochlea, ➤ Chap. 13.4).

A characteristic is the efferent fibers of the N. vestibulocochlearis. These efferent axonal projections of neurons from the upper olivary complex are responsible for the efferent innervation of the hair cells of the inner ear. They are known as the **olivocochlear bundle**. Initially, the fibres run in the N. vestibularis and then,

within the Meatus acusticus internus, they pass over to the N. cochlearis, with which they reach the hair cells (➤ Fig. 12.59).

Pathway and branches

The N. vestibulocochlearis arises somewhat caudolaterally of the N. facialis nerve [VII] from the brainstem rostral of the olive in the so-called cerebellopontine angle (➤ Fig. 12.58) and runs together with the N. facialis after branching off into the N. vestibularis and N. cochlearis through the Porus and Meatus acusticus internus of the temporal bone (➤ Fig. 12.59).

Cranial nerve nuclei and central links

Six nuclei are assigned to the N. vestibulocochlearis:

- Two **cochlear nuclei** lie within the pons (Nuclei cochleares posterior and anterior, ➤ Chap. 13.4). Their most important central efferents run in the **Lemniscus lateralis** – the part of the auditory system that connects the cochlear nuclei with the Colliculi inferiores of the mesencephalon.
- Four **vestibular nuclei** lie in the pons and in the Medulla oblongata (Nuclei vestibularis superior [BECHTEREW], vestibularis inferior [ROLLER], vestibularis lateralis [DEITER's nucleus] and vestibularis medialis [SCHWALBE], ➤ Chap. 13.5). Centrally, they have a much more complex configuration than the cochlear nuclei. They receive primary afferents from the vestibular organ, the spinal cord and the cerebellum and project efferent via the thalamus to the cortex, to the pre-oculomotoric centres and the eye muscle nuclei, and back to the cerebellum and into the spinal cord. Ultimately, these numerous fibre connections are used to keep the body balanced and able to follow objects with the eyes, even when the body position changes.

Clinical remarks

Examination

Hearing can be checked by a one-sided or two-sided simultaneous snap at ear level. In order to make the findings more objective, it is possible to differentiate between a conductive and a sensorineural hearing disorder with a tuning fork. Where there is damage to the cochlear part, it is probably a sensorineural hearing disorder.

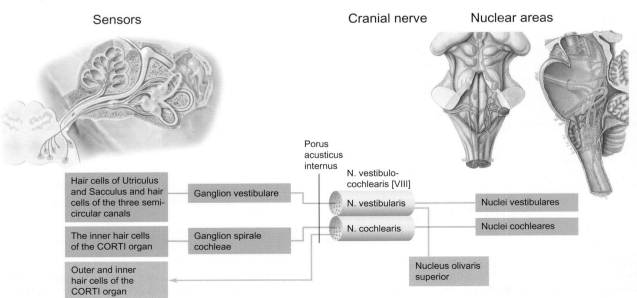

Fig. 12.59 Pathway, branches and fibre qualities of the N. vestibulocochlearis. [L127]

The vestibular part is tested using a balance test (e g. ROM-BERG's test, ➤ Chap. 12.4.6) and detailed analysis of eye-tracking movements. Where there is a lesion or failure of the vestibular part, falling and nystagmus can occur.

Acoustic neuroma

An acoustic neuroma is a benign tumour which grows out of the SCHWANN cells of the nerve sheath of the N. vestibulo cochlearis and grows slowly but progressively. Due to the resulting compression of the nerve, gradual hearing loss, dizziness, nausea, a tendency to fall to the affected side and pathological nystagmus occur. Often the compression not only affects the N. vestibulocochlearis, but also the N. facialis running in the immediate topographical vicinity, so that in addition, a peripheral facial palsy may occur.

12.5.12 N. glossopharyngeus (9th cranial nerve, N. IX)
Anja Böckers

SKILLS

After working through this chapter, you should be able to:
- name the target organs of the N. glossopharyngeus
- list the cranial nerve nuclei of the N. glossopharyngeus and correctly explain their function
- recognise a one-sided paralysis of the N. glossopharyngeus with a simultaneous examination of the mouth and phonation

The name of the IXth cranial nerve already identifies its target organs: the **N. glossopharyngeus [IX]** is a branchiogenic cranial nerve of the 3rd pharyngeal arch, particularly responsible for the innervation of the rear third of the tongue ('glosso') and the contiguous area of the pharynx ('pharyngeus'), including the soft palate. It undertakes critical functions in the coordination of the swallowing process, especially in the prerequisite separation of the windpipe and the digestive tract at the soft palate, in language formation, in the perception of bitter tastes on the dorsal third of the tongue, and in the regulation of breathing and circulation.

Pathway and branches

The nerve leaves the brainstem together with the N. vagus [X] and the N. accessorius [XI] in the Sulcus retroolivaris between the olive and the lower cerebellar stem (➤ Fig. 12.60). Together with these nerves, it leaves the cranial cavity in the Foramen jugulare. The N. glossopharyngeus is a mixed cranial nerve with 5 different fibre qualities. Disregarding the subdivision of the Nucleus tractus solitarii [Nucleus solitarius] into a Pars superior and a Pars inferior, 4 cranial nerve nuclei can be distinguished (➤ Fig. 12.61). As with the N. vagus, the N. glossopharyngeus forms 2 ganglia at the Foramen jugulare:

- The **Ganglion superius** is the smaller of the two and contains the Perikarya pseudounipolarer, general somatoafferent nerve cells.
- The **Ganglion inferius** is slightly larger and contains perikarya of general and special visceroafferent pseudo-unipolar nerve cells.

The main trunk of the nerve passes in an arc-shape between the M. stylopharyngeus, its 'guiding' muscle, and the medially-positioned M. styloglossus to caudal, reaching the root of the tongue (➤ Fig. 12.62). On its route, it releases branches to the middle ear, to the parotis and to the Glomus and Sinus caroticus:

- **N. tympanicus:** The N. tympanicus leaves the N. glossopharyngeus at the Ganglion inferius with general visceroefferent and

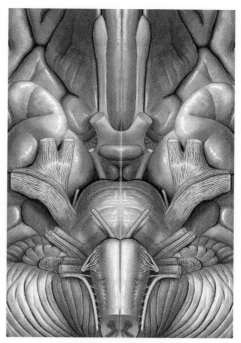

Fig. 12.60 Exit point of the N. glossopharyngeus. The IXth cranial nerve exits in the Sulcus retroolivaris between the olive and the lower cerebellar stem in the Medulla oblongata.

general visceroafferent fibres. It passes into the middle ear via the **Canalis tympanicus** to form the **Plexus tympanicus** on the promontorium, together with the sympathetic fibres, the Nn. caroticotympanici:

- From here, the **R. tubarius** reaches the Tuba auditiva to provide its sensory innervation.
- The **N. petrosus minor** leaves the Cavitas tympani again by penetrating the Tegmen tympani through the **Hiatus** or **Canalis nervi petrosi minoris** and returning to the internal surface of the cranial base. It proceeds on the front side of the Pars petrosa, the petrous bone of the Os temporale, to the **Foramen lacerum**, in order to get into the Fossa infratemporalis by this route. The relay onto postganglionic general visceroefferent fibres takes place in the **Ganglion oticum**, lying directly on the Foramen ovale, medial of the N. mandibularis [V/3]. This connection between the N. tympanicus and the Ganglion oticum is also known as the JACOBSON's anastomosis. Ultimately, the postganglionic fibres accumulate on the N. auriculotemporalis from the N. mandibularis [V/3] passing via this and the N. facialis [VII] to the parotid gland. Smaller branches reach the small salivary glands in the mouth of the cheek and lips, the Glandulae buccales and labiales.
- **R. sinus carotici:** It runs to the chemoreceptors and baroreceptors in the Glomus caroticum and the Sinus caroticus.
- **R. musculi stylopharyngei:** It innervates the guiding muscle of the N. glossopharyngeus, the M. stylopharyngeus.
- **Rr. pharyngei:** Together with the nerve branches of the N. vagus [X], they form the **Plexus pharyngeus** for the motor and sensory innervation of the pharynx. Additional motor fibres reach the Mm. palatoglossus and palatopharyngeus, the M. salpingopharyngeus as well as the muscles and mucosa of the soft palate.
- **Rr. tonsillares:** They are responsible for the sensory innervation of the tonsils, the tonsillar fossa and the Isthmus faucium.
- **Rr. linguales:** With sensory fibres, they reach the rear third of the tongue with the Papillae vallatae at the Sulcus terminalis.

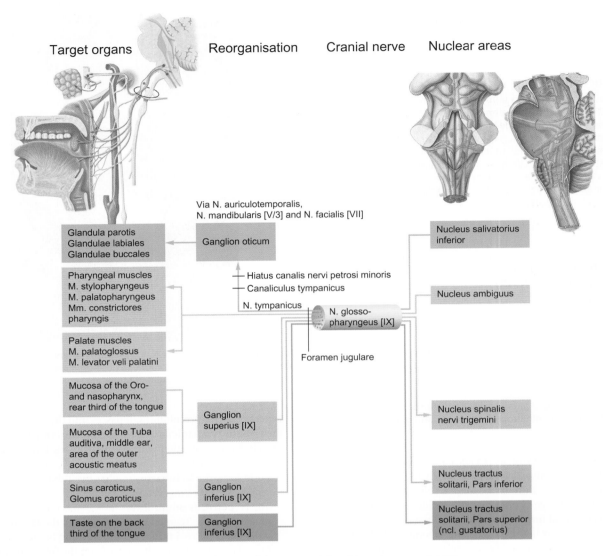

Target organs   Reorganisation   Cranial nerve   Nuclear areas

Fig. 12.61 N. glossopharyngeus with its fibre qualities, cranial nerve nuclei and target organs. [L127]

Clinical remarks

The N. glossopharyngeus runs from its exit point on the brainstem in topographical proximity to the A. inferior anterior cerebelli. The **aberrant pathway of the A. inferior anterior cerebelli**, e.g., between the exit points of the N. glossopharyngeus and the N. vagus, can lead to pathological impulse control. This can cause incipient, stabbing, one-sided pain in the tongue, the soft palate or throat with drinking and swallowing problems **(Glossopharyngeus neuralgia)**. The pathological stimulation can also be transferred via the Nucleus tractus solitarius to the N. dorsalis nervi vagi and can in rare cases lead to reflex bradycardia or reflex asystole (cardiac arrest). The treatment is to separate vessels and nerves from each other microsurgically.

Cranial nerve nuclei and central links

There are 4 different cranial nerve nuclei:
- The motor neurons of the special visceroefferent fibres of the N. glossopharyngeus are located (together with those of the N. vagus [X] and the N. accessorius [XI]) in the **N. ambiguus**. This nuclear area lies in the ventrolateral Formatio reticularis of the Medulla oblongata.

- The nuclear area of the general visceroefferent fibres, the **Nucleus salivatorius inferior**, is responsible for the innervation of the salivary glands and is positioned furthest caudal in the brainstem. This nuclear area is located on the border between the pons and the Medulla oblongata.
- The taste fibres of the N. glossopharyngeus as well as those of the N. facialis [VII] and the N. vagus [X] end in the **Nucleus tractus solitarii**. The Tractus solitarius extends caudally from the facial nucleus to the pyramidal intersection. It shows somatotopic and functional organisation. The target neurons of the Chorda tympani and the N. petrosus major from the N. facialis [VII] are located in the rostral section, while the target neurons of the N. glossopharyngeus are arranged caudally from here, followed by those of the N. vagus [X]. The upper part, die **Pars superior** or the **Nucleus gustatorius** for the taste fibers, can thus be differentiated from the **Pars inferior** of the Nucleus tractus solitarii, which is responsible for the general visceroafferent fibres, including the baroreceptors and chemoreceptors of the Sinus and Glomus caroticus.
- The perikarya of general somatoafferent fibres are located in the Ganglion superius of the N. glossopharyngeus and end in the **Nucleus spinalis nervi trigemini**. This nuclear area extends rostrally from the border area between the pons and the medulla and the Nucleus principalis nervi trigemini far caudally, merging by

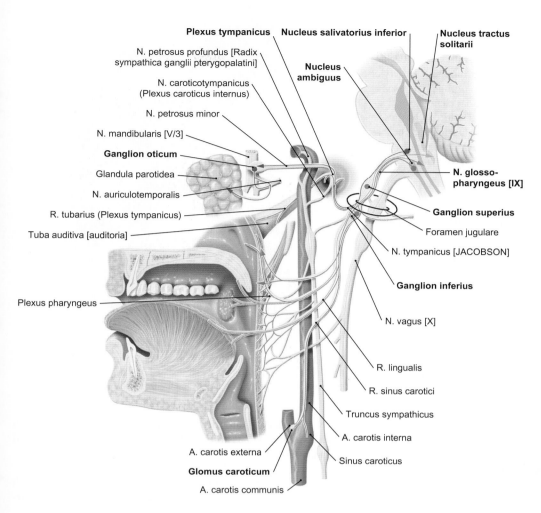

Plexus tympanicus
Nucleus salivatorius inferior
Nucleus tractus solitarii

N. petrosus profundus [Radix sympathica ganglii pterygopalatini]

Nucleus ambiguus

N. caroticotympanicus (Plexus caroticus internus)

N. petrosus minor

N. mandibularis [V/3]

Ganglion oticum

Glandula parotidea

N. auriculotemporalis

R. tubarius (Plexus tympanicus)

Tuba auditiva [auditoria]

Plexus pharyngeus

N. glosso-pharyngeus [IX]

Ganglion superius

Foramen jugulare

N. tympanicus [JACOBSON]

Ganglion inferius

N. vagus [X]

R. lingualis

R. sinus carotici

Truncus sympathicus

A. carotis interna

Sinus caroticus

A. carotis externa

Glomus caroticum

A. carotis communis

Fig. 12.62 Pathway of the N. glossopharyngeus. Schematic representation in the median section.

flowing into the laminae I–V of the spinal cord. The general somatoafferent fibres also end here, originating from the N. facialis [VII] and the N. vagus [X], but taken primarily via the N. trigeminus as a 'service provider'.

The cranial nerve nuclei of the N. glossopharyngeus receive primary afferents from the cortex, as well as from the Formatio reticularis. Efferent impulses, particularly the taste management, are redirected, starting from the Nucleus tractus solitarii to reach the Nucleus ambiguus and, ultimately, the ipsilateral Nucleus basalis ventralis medialis thalami via the tegmental tract. After another relay in this nuclear area, the taste fibres reach the parietal operculum or the insular cortex.

Due to its neuronal connections, the Nucleus tractus solitarii is also a crucial hub in the regulation of the circulation as well as the basis of the **baroreflex**: increased blood pressure activates the baroreceptors in the Sinus caroticus. Via the hub of the Nucleus tractus solitarii, afferent fibres project onto cardio-inhibiting neurons in the ventral part of the Nucleus ambiguus. From there, the descending tracts reach the N. intermediolateralis in the thoracic spine and the ascending tracts reach the hypothalamus, which results in the inhibition of the sympathetic nervous system. As a result, the heart rate and peripheral vascular resistance decreases and the blood pressure is lowered.

What is referred to as the **respiratory centre** is closely associated with the nuclear areas which regulate the circulation, and it is located in the ventrolateral section of the Nucleus tractus solitarii or of the ventrolateral medulla; it is the rhythm generator for inspiration and expiration. These rhythmogenic respiratory neurons are re-

ferred to as the pre-BÖTZINGER complex and transfer impulses to the N. phrenicus and the Nn. intercostales. The respiratory drive and therewith the impulses of the supplying afferents to these neurons come from central and peripheral chemoreceptors for the measurement of the pH of fluids and blood or they arise non-chemically as a result of the stimulation of expansion receptors in the lungs. Respiration is also regulated by the Nuclei parabranchiales in the pons, which on the basis of impulses from the limbic system, e.g., with anxiety-inducing situations, signal an increase in the respiratory rate to the respiratory centre.

Clinical remarks

Damage to the respiratory centre, e.g., when there is increased intracranial pressure, can lead to a centrally modified breathing pattern. For example, a breathing pattern where adequate, even and deep breathing is always interrupted by pauses in breathing, is referred to as **BIOT's respiration**.

The N. glossopharyngeus is also an important component of the **swallowing reflex** (see below). The act of swallowing itself requires coordinated interaction between the tongue (N. XII), mucosal sensitivity in the mouth and throat (N. trigeminus [V] and the N. glossopharyngeus [IX]), the pharynx (N. glossopharyngeus [IX]), the larynx (N. vagus [X]) and the oesophagus. The neurons involved are activated and inhibited in a coordinated manner by close links between the involved cranial nerve nuclei via the lateral and intermediate Formatio reticulares in the Medulla oblongata.

Furthermore, an important role is played by the N. glossopharyngeus and/or the Nucleus tractus solitarii in the process of the **vomiting reflex**. The vomiting reflex is a protective reflex, the aim of which is to protect the body from harmful substances. A variety of stimuli can trigger it: the mechanical irritation of the pharynx via the N. glossopharyngeus, intoxication, hormonal changes, or triggered by optical, vestibular or olfactory stimuli. Ultimately, these afferent pulses stimulate the Nucleus tractus solitarius and the Area postrema ('vomiting or emetic centre'), to activate the required target organs for vomiting via the Formatio reticularis.

Clinical remarks

The function of the N. glossopharyngeus can be tested by the gag reflex. The gag reflex is a foreign reflex, of which the afferent impulses trigger a reflex response via the N. vagus, after touching the oropharynx. By doing so, the absence or weakening of the gag reflex can be evaluated by comparing both sides. Since the N. glossopharyngeus, as well as the N. vagus is involved in the innervation of the soft palate muscles, care should be taken to examine both cranial nerves on the soft palate contour and the position of the uvula (➤ Chap. 12.5.13). When saying 'aaah', an asymmetrical contraction of the soft palate can be observed with a displacement to the healthy side. This symptom is known as **uvular deviation**. The taste function of the nerve can be checked using bitter substances (such as quinine) and thereby the sense of taste in the rear third of the tongue can be determined.

12.5.13 N. vagus (10th cranial nerve, N. X)
Anja Böckers

SKILLS

After working through this chapter, you should be able to:
- name the target organs of the N. vagus
- list the cranial nerve nuclei of the N. vagus nerve and correctly explain their function
- indicate the pathway of the N. vagus on a dissection or on ➤ Fig. 12.65 and explain it in your own words

The **N. vagus [X]** (Lat. vagari = wander around, spread out) spreads out from all the cranial nerves furthermost caudally and thus reaches the thoracic and abdominal cavities. It is the largest parasympathetic nerve in the body and includes the upper portion of the parasympathetic autonomic nervous system. It is also a branchiogenic cranial nerve, formed from the merger of the 4th, (5th) and 6th pharyngeal arch nerves. The N. vagus shares its cranial nerve nuclei for the most part with the N. glossopharyngeus [IX], resulting here in neuroanatomical and functional similarities or overlaps.

The N. vagus ensures the special visceroefferent innervation of the larynx, as well as partially that of the pharynx (M. constrictor pharyngis inferior) and that of the soft palate (M. levator veli palatini). Without it, stable breathing and speech functions are impossible. Its general visceroefferent fibres supply the smooth muscles and glands from the throat area down to the Flexura coli sinistra, the CANNON's point by which it controls hypersecretion and peristalsis in the gastrointestinal tract. In addition, it ensures important functions in the regulation of respiration – as does the N. glossopharyngeus [IX] – via the impulse management of extension receptors in the lungs or in the regulation of circulation, via receptors in the right atrium and in the aortic wall. Together with

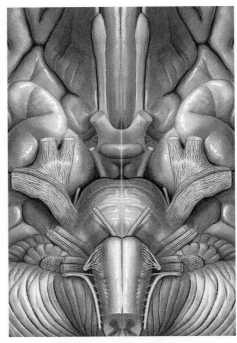

Fig. 12.63 Exit point of the N. vagus. The Xth cranial nerve exits in the Sulcus retroolivaris between the exit points of the N. glossopharyngeus [IX] (cranial) and the N. accessorius [XI] (caudal).

the N. facialis [VII] and the N. glossopharyngeus [IX], it also leads special visceroafferent fibres, taste fibres, from receptors of the caudal pharynx and of the epiglottis. To summarise, the N. vagus is a mixed cranial nerve with 5 different fibre qualities, which in the brainstem, disregarding the subdivision of the Nucleus tractus solitarii into a Pars superior and a Pars inferior, are expressed as 4 different cranial nerve nuclei (➤ Fig. 12.64).

Course and branches
Similar to the N. glossopharyngeus [IX], the N. vagus [X] leaves the Medulla oblongata in the Sulcus retroolivaris (➤ Fig. 12.63), passes through the subarachnoid space and leaves the internal surface of the cranial base together with the N. glossopharyngeus and the N. accessorius [XI] through the Foramen jugulare. Here, the N. vagus thickens into a **Ganglion superius** (syn.: **Ganglion jugulare**) and a **Ganglion inferius** (syn.: **Ganglion nodosum**). In the same way as for the N. glossopharyngeus [IX], there are perikarya of the general somatoafferent neurons in the upper ganglion, and perikarya of the general and specific visceroafferent pseudo-unipolar neurons in the lower ganglion. The N. vagus runs caudally together with the internal jugular vein, and its continuing course divides correspondingly into a **Pars cervicalis**, a **Pars thoracica** and a **Pars abdominalis**.

Directly at the level of the Foramen jugulara at the Ganglion superius, the N. vagus starts 2 general somatoafferent branches (➤ Fig. 12.65):
- **R. meningeus:** It innervates the Dura mater in the posterior cranial fossa.
- **R. auricularis:** It passes through the Canaliculus mastoideus and the Fissura tympanomastoidea to the Canalis acusticus externalis, to which it provides sensory innervation.

A little further caudally at the Ganglion inferius, the cervical part of the N. vagus nerve releases the two following branches:
- **R. pharyngeus:** This is essentially formed from fibres of the Radix cranialis of the N. accessorius nerve [XI], initially adhering to the N. vagus, but radiating later into the **Plexus pharyngeus**.

Target organs   Reorganisation   Cranial nerve   Nuclear areas

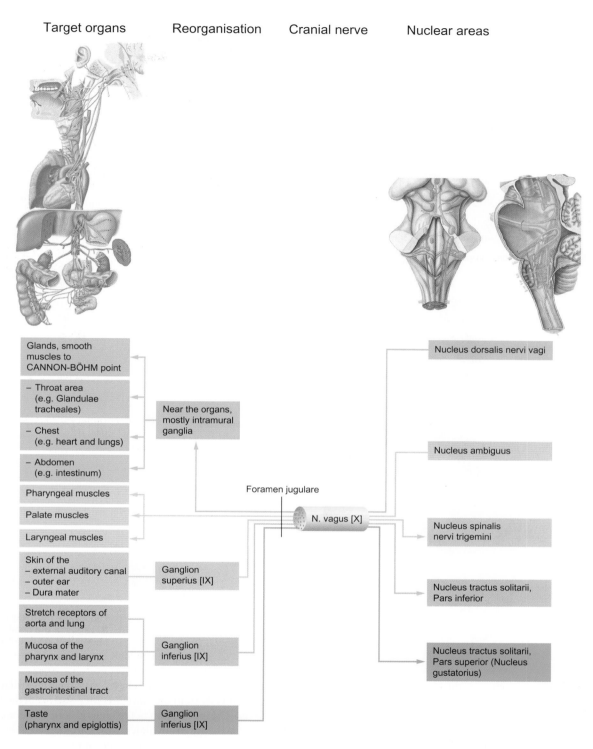

Fig. 12.64   The N. vagus with its fibre qualities, cranial nerve nuclei and target organs. [L127]

Together with the N. glossopharyngeus [IX], the general vis-ceroefferent fibres of this nerve branch reach the pharyngeal glands, the special visceroefferent fibres reach the pharyngeal muscles, and the general visceroafferent fibres of this branch reach the pharyngeal mucosa.

- **N. laryngeus superior:** This divides into an R. externus and an R. internus. The **R. externus** innervates the single outer larynx muscle, the M. cricothyroid. The **R. internus** passes through the Membrana thyrohyoidea and supplies the sensory innervation of the mucosa above the Rima glottis.

On its continued caudal route between the V. jugularis interna and the A. carotis interna, the N. vagus branches off into:

- **Rr. cardiaci cervicales superiores and inferiores:** They run to the **Plexus cardiacus**, accumulating on the aortic arch from the rear. Cardioinhibitory impulses reach the atrial muscles via these fibres. Thus the fibres of the right N. vagus nerve have a prefer-ential effect on the sinus nodes, and fibres of the left N. vagus have a preferential effect on the AV nodes of the impulse con-duction system. The N. vagus has an overall negative chrono-tropic effect and a negative inotropic effect on the heart. Afferent

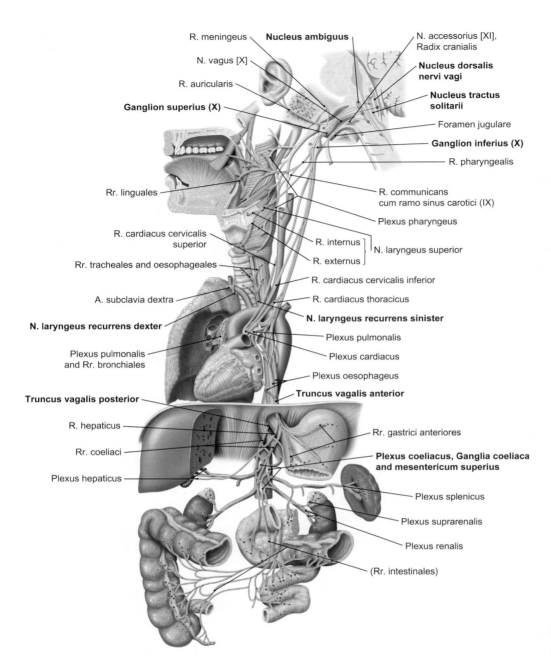

R. meningeus

Nucleus ambiguus

N. accessorius [XI],
Radix cranialis

N. vagus [X]

**Nucleus dorsalis
nervi vagi**

R. auricularis

**Nucleus tractus
solitarii**

Ganglion superius (X)

Foramen jugulare

Ganglion inferius (X)

R. pharyngealis

Rr. linguales

R. communicans
cum ramo sinus carotici (IX)

Plexus pharyngeus

R. cardiacus cervicalis
superior

R. internus
R. externus

N. laryngeus superior

Rr. tracheales and oesophageales

R. cardiacus cervicalis inferior

A. subclavia dextra

R. cardiacus thoracicus

N. laryngeus recurrens dexter

N. laryngeus recurrens sinister

Plexus pulmonalis

Plexus cardiacus

Plexus pulmonalis
and Rr. bronchiales

Plexus oesophageus

Truncus vagalis posterior

Truncus vagalis anterior

R. hepaticus

Rr. gastrici anteriores

Rr. coeliaci

**Plexus coeliacus, Ganglia coeliaca
and mesentericum superius**

Plexus hepaticus

Plexus splenicus

Plexus suprarenalis

Plexus renalis

(Rr. intestinales)

**Fig. 12.65 Pathway of the
N. vagus in the head, chest and
abdominal area.**

fibers of these nerve branches conduct impulses from the pressure receptors of the aortal vessel wall or of the right atrium, thus forming the afferent femoral anti-hypertensive reflexes of the N. vagus.

- **N. laryngeus recurrens:** In terms of its historical development, it is seen as the nerve of the 6th pharyngeal arch. It leaves the N. vagus in the area of the upper thoracic aperture. The N. laryngeus recurrens sinister loops from ventral to dorsal around the aortic arch, and in the same way, the N. laryngeus recurrens dexter loops around the A. subclavia dextra. Both nerve branches then emerge again between the trachea and oesophagus to cranial and release the identically named branches to the adjacent organs of the throat area. Finally, the N. laryngeus recurrens reaches the interior of the larynx as the N. laryngeus inferior, by passing between the Cartilago cricoidea and the Cartilago thyroidea of the larynx skeleton, and there supplies the sensory innervation of the mucosa below the Rima glottis and all the remaining laryngeal muscles.

As they continue through the chest cavity, the **Rr. cardiaci thoracici** depart directly from the N. vagus. They also reach the **Plexus cardiacus.** The innervation of the lungs is done bilaterally by both Nn. vagi via the **Rr. bronchiales**, which accumulate dorsally on the main bronchi, forming the **Plexus pulmonalis**.

Around the oesophagus, the N. vagus forms another neuronal network, the **Plexus oesophageus,** which converges caudally with the Trunci vagales. In accordance with the embryological rotation of the stomach by 90° to the right, the left N. vagus thus forms the **Truncus vagalis anterior**, running on the ventral side of the oesophagus and accordingly the N. vagus dexter forms the **Truncus vagalis posterior** on the dorsal side. Both leave the chest cavity through the Hiatus oesophageus and reach the anterior and posterior sides of the stomach. The anterior truncus only supplies the stomach (up to the pylorus) and the liver, whereas the Truncus vagalis posterior also reaches the Ganglion coeliacum and, together with the sympathetic nerve fibres, reach the abdominal organs up to the CANNON's point (transition is in the middle to the lower third of the transverse colon). Unlike the N. glossopharyngeus or the N. facialis in the head area, the preganglionic parasympathetic fibres are usually only relayed onto postganglionic fibres close to organs in intramural ganglia. Aboral from the CANNON's point, the parasympathetic innervation of sacral neurons takes place in the lateral horn of the spinal cord.

Cranial nerve nuclei and central links

In the same way as the N. glossopharyngeus [IX], the N. vagus [X] is a mixed nerve of which the fibre qualities are also assigned 4 cranial nerve nuclei (➤ Fig. 12.64):

- Neurons in the **Nucleus ambiguus** are responsible for the special visceroefferent innervation of the pharyngeal arch muscles of the pharynx, larynx and soft palate. This nucleus lies in the Medulla oblongata and can be divided into a dorsal and ventral nucleus column:
  - The **dorsal nucleus column** encompasses the visceroefferent neurons in that, the N. vagus is shared with the N. glossopharyngeus [IX] and the N. accessorius [XI], thereby presenting a roughly somatotopic structure.
  - The **ventral nuclear column** does not contain any branchiomotor neurons, but instead is functionally assigned to the Nucleus dorsalis nervi vagi due to its cardioinhibitory neurons.
- The general visceroefferent fibres of the N. vagus derive from the **Nucleus dorsalis nervi vagi.** This cranial nerve nucleus reaches from the rostral medulla to caudal, to the pyramidal tract intersection. This nuclear area forms the **Trigonum nervi vagi** near the obex and laterally to the Trigonum nervi hypoglosi on the floor of the rhomboid fossa.
- The perikarya of the special visceroafferent neurons are located in the Ganglion inferius of the N. vagus and send their centrally targeted axon to the **Nucleus tractus solitarii** [Nucleus solitarius]. In the same way as the N. facialis [VII] and the N. glossopharyngeus [IX], these taste fibres end in the rostral section of the nuclear complex, the **Nucleus gustatorius.** In the caudal part of this cranial nerve nucleus, the centrally-directed axons of the general visceroafferent neurons, of which the perikarya are located in the Ganglion inferius nervi vagi, are relayed synaptically. Here, impulses from the viscera (e.g., intestinal pain due to the activation of pain receptors, 'bloating' due to the activation of stretch

receptors), the pharynx and the larynx are passed on. Likewise, subconscious information is also conveyed which is essential for respiratory regulation (HERING-BREUER reflex) or for circulatory regulation (baroreceptors in the right atrium, in the wall of the aorta or in the Sinus caroticus). Up to 80% of the N. vagus is made up of afferent nerve fibres, illustrating the high value of this afferent information from inside the body.

- To a lesser extent, the N. vagus also carries general somatoafferent impulses of the sensations of touch, pain and temperature from small areas of skin of the external ear, the rear wall of the external acoustic meatus and the hard meninges in the posterior cranial fossa. The central axons of the 1st neurons form synapses in the **Nucleus spinalis nervi trigemini** with the corresponding 2nd neuron. In a somatopic arrangement, the N. trigeminus [V], the N. facialis [VII], the N. glossopharyngeus [IX] and the N. vagus [X] share this section of the vein of the Vth cranial nerve nucleus. This nucleus forms the rostral progression of the laminae I–V of the dorsal horn of the spinal cord and ends rostrally at the Nucleus principalis nervi trigemini (➤ Chap. 12.5.8).

The **Nucleus ambiguus** – in the same way as the N. glossopharyngeus [IX] – is closely associated in neuronal terms with the **Nucleus tractus solitarii**. In addition, it receives afferent impulses from the Formatio reticularis and via corticonuclear tracts from the cortex. The Nucleus tractus solitarii is a central hub for both the glossopharyngeal nerve and the N. vagus for controlling respiratory and circulatory functions. In addition, the Nucleus ambiguus also sends fibres to the **Nucleus dorsalis nervi vagi**. The latter, in turn, receives afferents from the Nuclei salivatorii and is controlled by hypothalamic centres (Nucleus paraventricularis thalami) and by the limbic system (Nucleus centralis amygdalae). These neuronal connections are the basis for the regulation of food intake and digestion: even before food intake occurs, in what is called the cephalic phase, impulses from the Formatio reticularis act to stimulate the Nucleus dorsalis nervi vagi. During actual food intake, chemo- and mechanoreceptors in the stomach and small intestine are stimulated and take impulses via vagal afferents to the Nucleus tractus solitarii. Neurotransmitters (glutamate), as well as enteroendocrine hormones, such as cholecystokinin, thus act on the Nucleus tractus solitarii. This projects in an inhibitory way into the Nucleus dorsalis nervi vagi, the axons of which reach the intramural ganglia in turn. Together these neuronal configurations are referred to as **vagovagal reflexes**.

The **Nucleus spinalis nervi trigemini** is part of the somatosensory system or more correctly, the trigeminoafferent system. From here, amongst others, impulses of pain and temperature sensation cross and are projected into the thalamus to the Nucleus ventralis posteromedialis (3rd neuron) (trigeminothalamic fibres), passing from here to the somatosensory cortex.

12.5.14 N. accessorius (11th cranial nerve, N. XI)
Anja Böckers

The **N. accessorius [XI]** is a branchiogenic cranial nerve which supplies special visceroefferent innervation to the M. trapezius and the M. sternocleidomastoideus. It is however controversial as to whether it is a real cranial nerve, because its spinal nuclear area, the **Nucleus nervi accessorii**, lies in the cervical anterior horn cells of the spinal cord, whereas its cranial nuclear area is assigned to the basal section of the **Nucleus ambiguus** and and thereby to the N. vagus. Accordingly, the fibres derived from C1–7 are encapsulated in a **Radix spinalis nervi accessorii** and the fibres from the Nucleus ambiguus in a **Radix cranialis nervi accessorii**.

Pathway and branches
The Radix spinalis nervi accessorii rises to cranial behind the olive between the anterior and posterior root of the spinal cord and passes through the Foramen magnum to the internal surface of the cranial base. After merging with the Radix cranialis in the Pars nervosa of the Foramen jugularis, the N. accessorius exits outwards again via the cranial base (➤ Fig. 12.66).
Immediately after exiting – usually between the Ganglia superius and inferius nervi vagi – the fibres of the Radix cranialis leave the N. accessorius again as the **R. internus** and adhere to the N. vagus, in order to innervate with this pharyngeal and laryngeal muscle (➤ Fig. 12.67, ➤ Fig. 12.68). The main trunk of the **R. externus** eventually reaches the Regio cervicalis lateralis and there releases the visceroefferent branches of the M. sternocleidomastoideus. It continues along the M. levator scapulae further dorsally to the M. trapezius. However, both muscles also receive direct fibres from the cervical segments (C1–C4); via these, proprioceptive impulses of these muscles are transferred to the Nucleus nervi accessorii.

Cranial nerve nuclei and central links
In addition to the primary afferents from the actual muscles, the Nucleus nervi accessorius receives reticospinal fibres of the extrapyramidal motor system, as well as pyramidal afferents via corticospinal or nuclear fibres from the pre-central area of the cortex. The central connections of the Nucleus ambiguus have already been given for the N. glossopharyngeus [IX] (➤ Chap. 12.5.12) and the N. vagus [X] (➤ Chap. 12.5.13).

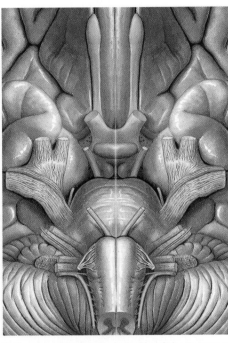

Fig. 12.66 Exit point of the Radix spinalis of the N. accessorius. The XIth cranial nerve exits at the ventral side of the brainstem, dorsal of the olive.

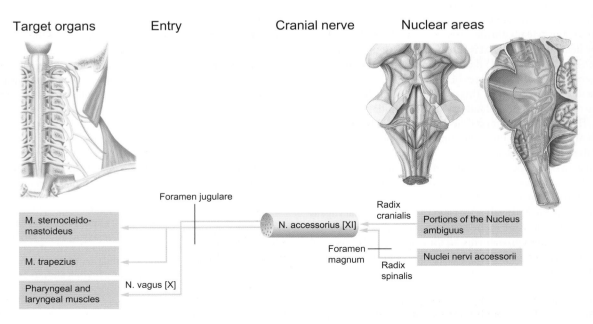

Fig. 12.67 N. accessorius with its fibre qualities, cranial nerve nuclei and target organs. [L127]

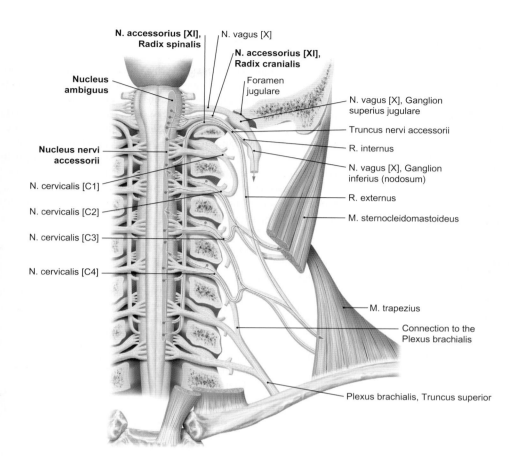

N. accessorius [XI], Radix spinalis

N. vagus [X]

N. accessorius [XI], Radix cranialis

Nucleus ambiguus

Foramen jugulare

N. vagus [X], Ganglion superius jugulare

Truncus nervi accessorii

R. internus

Nucleus nervi accessorii

N. vagus [X], Ganglion inferius (nodosum)

N. cervicalis [C1]

R. externus

N. cervicalis [C2]

M. sternocleidomastoideus

N. cervicalis [C3]

N. cervicalis [C4]

M. trapezius

Connection to the Plexus brachialis

Plexus brachialis, Truncus superior

Fig. 12.68 N. accessorius. Frontal view, vertebral canal and skull are opened.

Clinical remarks

Examination

One-sided contraction of the M. sternocleidomastoideus leads to a turning of the head to the opposite side and a tilting of the head to the same side. The functional capability of the M. sternocleidomastoideus is checked by the examining doctor by turning the head against the pressure of his/her own hand. Consequently, the functionality of the Pars descendens of the M. trapezius can be measured by raising the shoulder girdle (by shrugging) and pushing against the hand carrying out the examination or by abduction of the arm over an angle of 90°. Following a longer standing lesion of the N. accessorius, consideration should be given to muscular atrophy, which in extreme cases can lead to a twisted neck or to a Scapula alata.

12.5.15 N. hypoglossus (12th cranial nerve, N. XII)
Anja Böckers

SKILLS

After working through this chapter, you should be able to:
- name the organs of the N. hypoglossus
- indicate the position of the Trigonum nervi hypoglossi on a model or a dissection of the Fossa rhomboidea
- extrapolate a one-sided lesion of the N. hypoglossus, using an illustration or a description of the findings of a clinical investigation

The 12th cranial nerve, the **N. hypoglossus [XII]**, is a cranialised spinal nerve, which arises from the anterior branches of the upper cervical segment.

Pathway and branches
It leaves the brainstem on the ventral side of the Medulla oblongata between the pyramid and the olive as a single cranial nerve in the Sulcus anterolateralis (➤ Fig. 12.69). It runs in the **Canalis nervi hypoglossi** through the base of the skull to innervate both the internal and the external tongue muscles as a general somatoefferent nerve, with the exception of the M. palatoglossus (➤ Chap. 9.7.5). After leaving the bony skull, the N. hypoglossus passes dorsolaterally in an arc-shaped course into the **Spatium lateropharyngeum** and loops around the N. vagus and the A. carotis externa. It then crosses below the Venter posterior of the M. digastricus and ends up in the cranial section of the Trigonum caroticum, before finally reaching the tongue between the Mm. hyoglossus and mylohyoideus. For 3–4 cm on its peripheral pathway, it accumulates onto fibres of the ventral branches of the upper 2 cervical nerves (C1–2), then exits these again as the so-called **Radix superior** of the **Ansa cervicalis nervi hypoglossi**. Some of these fibres will however also continue in the N. hypoglossus to innervate the M. thyrohyoideus and the M. geniohyoideus. Together with fibres from segments C2–3, of the **Radix inferior**, the Radix superior forms the **Ansa cervicalis nervi hypoglossi** at the level of the transition from the Venter superior to the Venter inferior of the M. omohyoideus. This is important for the innervation of the infrahyoid muscles. There is however a wide range of deviations from this simplified course, such as in approximately 15% of the cases, where there is an additional root arising from the N. vagus (➤ Fig. 12.70).

Cranial nerve nuclei and central links
The nuclear area of the N. hypoglossus, the **Nucleus nervi hypoglossi**, lies in the Medulla oblongata, paramedially of the Sulcus medianus near the floor of the Fossa rhomboidea. Subjacent to the

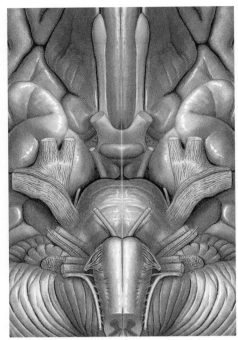

Fig. 12.69 Exit point of the N. hypoglossus. The XIIth cranial nerve exits at the ventral side of the brainstem in the Sulcus anterolateralis between the olive and the pyramid.

nucleus area on the floor of the Fossa rhomboidea is the **Trigonum nervi hypoglossi**. The Nucleus nervi hypoglossi is surrounded by small groups of neurons, known collectively as perihypoglossary nucleus groups. In the main nuclear itself, several subgroups can be distinguished which can be assigned to the respective branches and target muscles of the N. hypoglossus, according to their arrangement.

Unlike the spinal nerves, the Nucleus nervi hypoglossi does not receive direct somatoafferents from its target muscles. Hence there are also no monosynaptic reflex arches, although there are disynaptic or polysynaptic reflex arches which are important for coordinating the chewing process. Their afferents are taken to the Nucleus nervi hypoglossi via the trigeminal nucleus complex or conducted via the Nucleus tractus solitarii. Other afferents originate from the Formatio reticularis and the motor cortex, of which the impulses reach the cranial nerve nuclear primarily by crossing over via corticonuclear fibres running in the Capsula interna. Therefore lesions of these central afferents result in contralateral tongue weakness, whereas lesions of the Nucleus nervi hypoglossi nerve itself lead to ipsilateral tongue weakness.

Clinical remarks

Examination

To evaluate the functional capability of the N. hypoglossus, the patient is asked to stick out the tongue (saying 'aaah' simultaneously is part of the clinical examination for the N. vagus). This helps you to evaluate whether there is atrophy or fasciculations (muscle twitching/shaking) of the tongue muscles or whether the tongue can be stuck straight out or deviates to one side. In addition, language formation ('slurred speech'), drinking and swallowing should be assessed.

Damage to the nerve

In case of damage to the *peripheral* nerve section or the *cranial nerve nucleus,* the tip of the tongue deviates to the paralysed side due to the predominant pull of the N. genioglossus to the healthy side. In case of a supranuclear lesion, the contra lateral tongue muscles are damaged, so that the *central defect* is in the half of the brain controlling the tip of the tongue. A bilater-

---

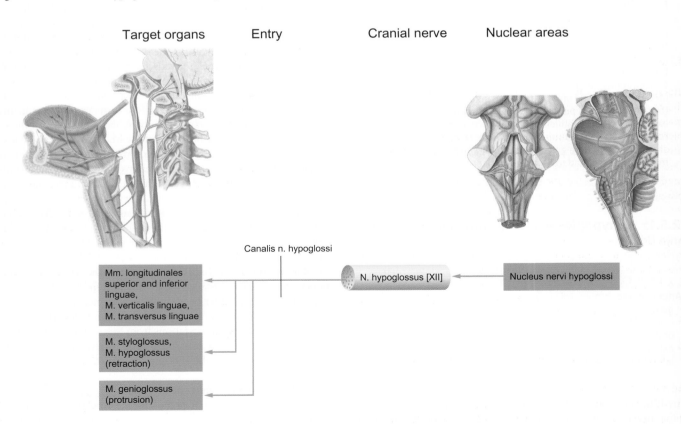

Fig. 12.70 N. hypoglossus with its fibre qualities, cranial nerve nuclei and target organs. [L127]

al lesion of the Nuclei nervi hypoglossi is common due to the close paramedial position.

In addition to an isolated lesion of the N. hypoglossus, such as following surgery on the A. carotis externa, systemic diseases of inflammatory, vascular or neoplastic origin can also be causing the symptoms. Because the N. accessorius, together with the N. vagus [X], the N. glossopharyngeus [IX] and the V. jugularis exits the cranial base through the Foramen jugulare, all 3 nerves can frequently be affected simultaneously by lesions at the Foramen jugulare. This results in a combination of symptoms, indicated by difficulty with swallowing or paralysis of the M. trapezius, as well as in clinical examination by a positive uvular deviation (➤ Chap. 12.5.12) or by failure of the gag reflex. Because the meningeal branch of the A. pharyngea ascendens goes through the Foramen jugulare into the interior of the skull, patients' symptoms may be accompanied by headaches which may be due to reduced circulation in the meninges. Overall, it is referred to as **Foramen jugular syndrome.** If the N. hypoglossus is also affected, this combined damage to the caudal cranial nerves is also referred to as **COLLET-SICARD syndrome.**

12.6 Spinal cord
Anja Böckers

12.6.1 Overview

The spinal cord, the **Medulla spinalis**, is located in and protected by the vertebral canal, wrapped in meninges. In adults, it is approximately 40–45 cm long and as thick as a pencil, but cervically and sacrally there is a thickening, the **Intumescentiae cervicalis and lumbosacralis.** Cranially it borders the Medulla oblongata in the Decussatio pyramidum area and with its caudal end, the **Conus medullaris**, it goes up to the Ist or IInd lumbar interbody. As with all brain sections of the CNS, the inside of the spinal cord is hollow but it only consists of a narrow, occluded tube called the **Canalis centralis.** Characteristic for the spinal cord, it is divided into Substantia grisea and Substantia alba, into a somatic and autonomous nervous system, as well as into efferent and afferent fibre systems. Efferent fibres refer to the superior, controlling descending tracts which, for example, control motor functions. Afferent fibres are, correspondingly, ascending tracts to the brain which, for example, transfer impulses from the interior of the body or the body surface.

12.6.2 Segmental structure of the Medulla spinalis

Spinal cord segments
Already by the 4th week of pregnancy, the spinal cord starts to develop from the neural tube (➤ Chap. 12.5.2). Under the influence of the mesoderm, which accumulates on the neural tube and ex-

hibits a metameric segmentation in somites, a segmental structure of the spinal cord is also induced. This segmental structure of the spinal cord is not visible from the outside, but can be understood by referring to the branches of the exiting spinal roots. The spinal roots are assigned to the mesodermal structures of their original segment, called dermatomyotomes. In terms of development, on the one hand, afferents are derived from receptors of the segmentally assigned skin areas, the dermatomes, and, on the other hand, their association with segment-specific muscles, known as indicator muscles (➤ Fig. 12.71, ➤ Table 12.10).

A total of 31–33 spinal cord segments can be distinguished, divided into
• 8 cervical (**Pars cervicalis**)
• 12 thoracic (**Pars thoracica**)
• 5 lumbar (**Pars lumbalis**) and
• 5 sacral (**Pars sacralis**)
spinal cord segments and an irregular number of coccygeal segments (**Pars coccygea**).

Fila radicularia
Each segment releases strands of multiple root threads, the **Fila radicularia**, which come together as the front and rear root, **Radices anterior and posterior**, forming a spinal nerve. The cervical Radices posterior and anterior demonstrate a virtually horizontal course to their exit point from the vertebral canal, the Foramen intervertebrale. Here the first spinal nerve (C1) leaves the spinal cord canal between the occiput and the atlas. The roots of the spinal cord segments, which are located further caudally, run increasingly vertically, because after the relative ascent of the spinal cord they have a long journey inside the vertebral canal, in order to reach the Foramen intervertebrale associated with their segment. Thus the lumbar spinal cord segments are generally at the level of the thoracic vertebrae X–XI. It should be noted that in the living, the vertebral body itself cannot be palpated, only its Proc. spinosus, the tip of which is mostly at the vertebral level of 1.5 further caudally. The spinal cord segments Co1–3 lying furthest caudally correspond to the level of the Conus medullaris (vertebral body height LI/LII). However, the associated spinal nerve roots run up to the end of the dura sac (vertebral body height SI/SII), here leaving the vertebral canal or the Hiatus sacralis. Collectively, these lumbar and sacral Fila radicularia form the **Cauda equina.** Their fila float in the fluid-filled Cisterna terminalis and – unlike the spinal cord itself – are not at risk of injury by lumbar puncture. The Conus medullaris is

Table 12.10 The most common clinically-examined spinal cord segments, Segmenta medullae spinalis, and their associated indicator muscles.

Spinal cord segment	Indicator muscle	Dermatome
C5	M. deltoideus	Lateral upper arm; shoulder area
C6	M. biceps brachii; M. brachioradialis	Thumb; thenar area
C7	M. triceps brachii	Middle finger
C8	Mm. interossei of the hand	Digitus minimus; hypothenar area
L3	Quadriceps femoris; M. iliopsoas	Inner knee
L4	M. tibialis anterior	Medial lower leg side
L5	M. extensor hallucis longus	Big toe area
S1	M. triceps surae	Lateral foot and leg area

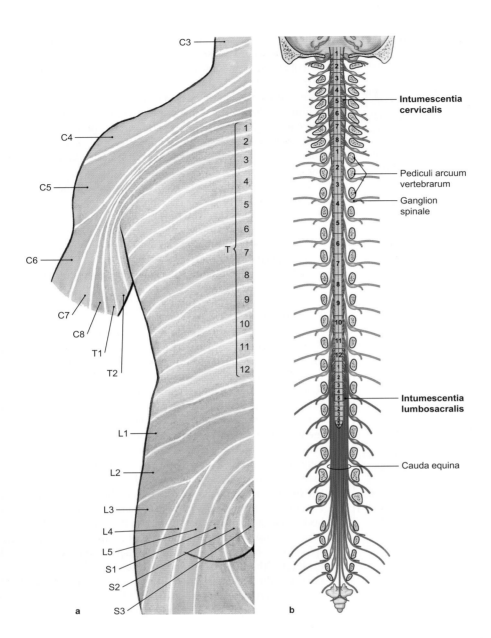

Fig. 12.71 Spinal cord segments, Segmenta medullae spinalis, and their associated dermatomes. b [E402]

Labels on figure: Intumescentia cervicalis; Pediculi arcuum vertebrarum; Ganglion spinale; Intumescentia lumbosacralis; Cauda equina

attached by a delicate strand of fibrous connective tissue containing glial cells, called the **Filum terminale**, attached to the dura sac (vertebral body height SI/SII) or via its Pars duralis at the vertebral canal (vertebral body height CoI/CoII) (➤ Fig. 12.72a).

12.6.3 Surface and cross-sectional anatomy

Surface anatomy
The surface anatomy of the Medulla spinalis is characterised by longitudinally-running furrows. The deepest furrow, the **Fissura mediana anterior**, is found in the median plane of the anterior surface of the medulla. On the dorsal side, it superficially forms the longitudinal furrow, so is referred to as a **Sulcus medianus posterior**. Even flatter and marked by the exit of the respective Fila radicularia, the **Sulcus anterolateralis** is positioned on the lateral side of the Fissura mediana anterior with the exiting Radix anterior or motoria, and the **Sulcus posterolateralis** is correspondingly positioned laterally of the Sulcus medianus posterior with the exiting Radix posterior or Radix sensoria. In the cervical section a **Sulcus intermedius** is the distinct separation between the Sulci mediani

posterior and posterolateralis, dividing the **Fasciculi gracilis and cuneatus** from each other (➤ Fig. 12.72b).

Cross-sectional anatomy
Cross-sections through the Medulla spinalis clarify the typical distribution of grey and white matter (➤ Fig. 12.72b): unlike in the encephalon, the Substantia grisea here is shaped like a butterfly on the inside of the spinal cord and is enveloped by white matter.

Substantia grisea
In the grey matter, particularly in the thoracic-lumbar section, we differentiate a **posterior horn (Cornu posterius)**, a **lateral horn (Cornu laterale)** and an **anterior horn (Cornu anterius)**. In the same way, if one wishes to describe this area in three-dimensional terms one also talks of the **Columna posterior** (posterior column), **Columna intermedia** (side column) and **Columna anterior** (anterior column), (➤ Fig. 12.74). The Cornu posterius is divided from ventral to dorsal into the **basis, cervix, caput** and **apex** and finally reaches the Sulcus posterolateralis dorsally via the so-called **Substantia gelatinosa**. Both Cornua lateralia are connected to each other by a bridge of grey matter positioned in front of and behind

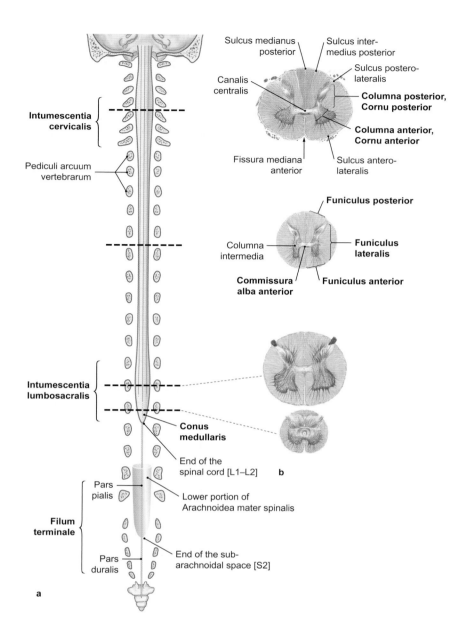

Intumescentia cervicalis

Sulcus medianus posterior

Sulcus inter-medius posterior

Sulcus postero-lateralis

Canalis centralis

Columna posterior, Cornu posterior

Columna anterior, Cornu anterior

Fissura mediana anterior

Sulcus antero-lateralis

Pediculi arcuum vertebrarum

Funiculus posterior

Columna intermedia

Funiculus lateralis

Commissura alba anterior

Funiculus anterior

Intumescentia lumbosacralis

Conus medullaris

End of the spinal cord [L1–L2]

b

Pars pialis

Lower portion of Arachnoidea mater spinalis

Filum terminale

Pars duralis

End of the sub-arachnoidal space [S2]

a

Fig. 12.72 Spinal cord, Medulla spinalis and cross-sections.
a Ventral view. **b** Cross-sections at the level of the dotted lines in the Pars cervicalis, Pars thoracica, Pars lumbalis and Pars sacralis. a[E402]

the Canalis centralis, the **Commissurae griseae anterior and posterior**.

Substantia alba
The Substantia alba is divided into:
- an **anterior funiculus (Funiculus anterior)** between the Fissura mediana anterior and the Sulcus anterolateralis
- a **lateral funiculus (Funiculus lateralis)** between the Sulcus anterolateralis and the Sulcus posterolateralis
- A **posterior funiculus (Funiculus posterior)** between the Sulcus posterolateralis and the Sulcus medianus posterior

The two anterior funiculi – like the structure in the grey matter – are connected with each other by fibres which overlap the midline, known as the **Commissura alba anterior**.

By comparing the cross-sections of the spinal cord at different heights, as well as seeing the varying diameters of the spinal cord, it is also possible to recognise that the amount of Substantia alba decreases from cranial to caudal. It is formed primarily in the cervical spine, which explains on the one hand why there is an increase in the number of sensory pathways accumulating at the spinal cord from caudal to cranial, and that on the other hand, the number of

motor pathways leaving the spinal cord decreases. At the Intumescentiae cervicalis and lumbosacralis, the Cornu anterioris is particularly large and broad due to a large number of α-motor neurons for the innervation of the muscles of the extremities. In a thoracic cross-section, the Cornu laterale is particularly recognisable with the sympathetic nerve cells found there (➤ Fig. 12.72b).

Spinal roots, spinal nerves and plexus
In the **Radix anterior** there are axons of nerve cells of the anterior and lateral horn which leave the spinal cord at the Sulcus anterolateralis and are therefore described as being efferent. Since these axons arise, amongst others, from motor neurons lying in the Cornu anterius, the Radix anterior is also known as the **Radix motoria**.
The **Radix posterior** conversely contains axons of pseudounipolar nerve cells of the spinal ganglion (**Ganglion sensorium nervi spinalis**), which is located in the Foramen intervertebrale at the transition point from the CNS into the PNS (➤ Fig. 12.73a). These axons forward impulses to the spinal cord, so are therefore afferent; this is called a **Radix sensoria**.
Immediately after the spinal ganglion, the fibres of the Radices motoria and sensoria join together to form the root of the spinal

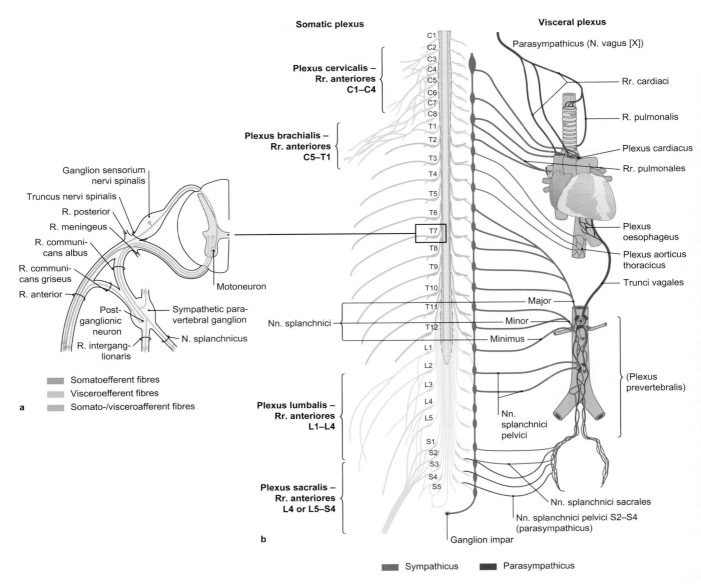

Somatic plexus

C1
C2
C3
C4
C5
C6
C7
C8

**Plexus cervicalis –
Rr. anteriores
C1–C4**

T1
T2
T3
T4
T5
T6
T7
T8
T9
T10
T11
T12

**Plexus brachialis –
Rr. anteriores
C5–T1**

Ganglion sensorium
nervi spinalis
Truncus nervi spinalis
R. posterior
R. meningeus
R. communi-
cans albus
R. communi-
cans griseus
R. anterior
Post-
ganglionic
neuron
R. intergang-
lionaris

Motoneuron

Sympathetic para-
vertebral ganglion
N. splanchnicus

Nn. splanchnici

Somatoefferent fibres
Visceroefferent fibres
Somato-/visceroafferent fibres

a

L1
L2
L3
L4
L5
S1
S2
S3
S4
S5

**Plexus lumbalis –
Rr. anteriores
L1–L4**

**Plexus sacralis –
Rr. anteriores
L4 or L5–S4**

b

Visceral plexus

Parasympathicus (N. vagus [X])
Rr. cardiaci
R. pulmonalis
Plexus cardiacus
Rr. pulmonales
Plexus
oesophageus
Plexus aorticus
thoracicus
Trunci vagales
Major
Minor
Minimus
(Plexus
prevertebralis)
Nn.
splanchnici
pelvici
Nn. splanchnici sacrales
Nn. splanchnici pelvici S2–S4
(parasympathicus)
Ganglion impar

Sympathicus   Parasympathicus

Fig. 12.73 Spinal nerve and plexus. a Composition and branching of a thoracic spinal nerve [L126]. **b** Somatic (left half of image) and autonomous (right half of image) nerve plexus. [E402]

nerve, which thus contains mixed fibre qualities (somatic motor, somatosensory and autonomous). This spinal nerve root quickly divides into its terminal branches: **R. meningeus, R. posterior, R. anterior** and in the thoracic-lumbar area as a **R. communicans albus**, which carries preganglionic fibres to the sympathetic chains (**Truncus sympathicus**). Conversely, sympathetic impulses are conducted back to the spinal nerve via a less stongly myelinised **R. communicans griseus** (➤ Fig. 12.73a).

The R. posterior of the spinal nerve is responsible for the motor innervation of the autochtonous back muscles and the sensory innervation of the overlying skin area, whereas the R. anterior innervates the ventral abdominal wall or forms nerve plexus in the cervical and lumbosacral section to innervate the extremities; these are called **somatic nerve plexus**. Here the following plexus can be distinguished (➤ Fig. 12.73b, left half):

• Plexus cervicalis (C1–4)
• Plexus brachialis (C5–T1)
• Plexus lumbalis (L1–L4)
• Plexus sacralis (L4–S4)

The original unisegmental association of a spinal cord segment with a dermatomyotome disappears in these areas, since the nerve

fibres from various segments become mixed. As a result, a spinal cord segment may innervate several muscles or dermatomes and vice versa, a muscle or dermatome can be associated with several spinal cord segments (plurisegmental).

Clinical remarks

Irritation or damage to the nerve roots is referred to as a pinched spinal nerve or **radiculopathy**. One of the most common causes for this is disc problems, where most of the Nucleus pulposus of a Discus intervertebralis presses on the nerve roots running in the immediate vicinity. The most frequently affected intervertebral discs are in the lower cervical spine (C4–C7) and the lumbosacral transition (e.g., L4/5 and L5/S1). Typical symptoms are loss of sensitivity, muscle weakness or paralysis and the loss of muscle reflexes. In clinical practice, from a differential diagnostic viewpoint, it is critical to make a distinction between a radicular localisation and a peripheral position of a nerve lesion. Radicular symptoms follow the segmental structure of the spinal cord, i.e., a lesion of the nerve root L4 displays loss of sensitivity in dermatome L4 or a weakness of the reference muscle for the segment L4, the M. tibialis anterior. If peripheral nerves lying distally of the plexus formation become damaged, along with fibres from several segments, the symptoms no longer follow segmental classification; instead they follow the innervation pattern of the peripheral nerve.

In addition to the formation of somatic plexus, **autonomic nerve plexus** are also formed (➤ Fig. 12.73b, right half). The nerve cell bodies of the sympathetic fibres are located in the Cornu laterale of the spinal cord (C8–L3), leaving the Medulla spinalis via the Radix anterior and reaching the Truncus sympathicus via the Rr. communicantes albi (➤ Fig. 12.73b). This is composed of 21–25 paravertebrally-arranged ganglia connected together with **Rr. interganglionares**. Via these compounds and the returning Rr. communicantes grisei, the sympathetic impulses are also distributed via segments C8–L3 further cranially and caudally (divergence circuit). Ultimately, the spinal nerves in all segments are fed by sympathetic fibres, thereby also autonomically supplying the glands and blood vessels of the extremities, e.g., for perspiration or vasoconstriction. Further non-configured efferent fibre pathways of sympathetic trunk ganglia are the **Nn. splanchnici**, which form visceral prevertebral plexus, particularly in the chest and abdomen. In addition to sympathetic fibres, these nerve plexus also contain parasympathetic fibres, which either come from the upper part of the parasympathetic nervous system, the N. vagus [X], or from nerve cell bodies of the Cornu laterale of the sacral spinal cord segments S2–4.

12.6.4 Structure of the Substantia grisea

The Substantia grisea of the spinal cord consists of nerve cell bodies, but also from interconnections of glia cell processes, dendritic cells and myelinised and non-myelinised axons. Collectively this network is referred to as **neuropile**.

Classification by target structures
The various nerve cells can be differentiated into 3 groups, according to the respective target structure of its axons: root cells, intermediate cells and tract cells:

- The **root cells** are within the Columna anterior or intermedia; their fibres are somatoefferent or visceroefferent and form the Radix anterior.
- The nerve cell processes of **intermediate cells** do not leave the Substantia grisea. Intermediate cells frequently act as glycinergic inhibitory interneurons of the spinal cord.
- The nerve fibres of the **tract cells** combine together into fibre pathways or tracts which then remain within the spinal cord, i.e. forming a part of the **proprioceptive apparatus** of the spinal cord, or producing an ascending connection to higher-level structures of the CNS and thus forming a part of the **association fibres**. This third type of nerve cell in grey matter, the tract cells, are located mainly in the Columna posterior.

The functional differentiation of neurons in tract or root cells or the division into a front and rear horn is induced during embryological development by the Chorda dorsalis or by the signal molecules released by it.

Classification by cyto-architecture
The Substantia grisea of the spinal cord is also classified according to REXED on the basis of the specific cyto-architecture. According

to REXED, a total of 10 layers, **laminae**, are distinguished, numbered from dorsal to ventral. To simplify, the Columna posterior is assigned to laminae I–VI, the intermediate column is assigned to lamina VII and the area around the Canalis centralis is assigned to lamina X while the Columna anterior includes laminae VIII and IX (➤ Fig. 12.74).

The significant laminae are presented below in terms of their anatomical or clinical relevance. The Columna posterior receives somato- and visceroafferents. The nerve cell bodies of the pseudounipolar neurons which convey these sensory qualities (e.g., pain and temperature sensations), are in the spinal ganglion. This 1st neuron takes exteroceptive impulses, e.g., from pain receptors in the skin, interoceptive impulses from the intestines or proprioceptive impulses from the skeletal muscles or from joint and tendon receptors (see ➤ Fig. 12.76). The centrally-oriented axon of the spinal ganglion cells reaches the laminae I–III via the posterior root in the Cornu posterior. Here there are tract cells, such as the **Nucleus marginalis** (in the **lamina I, Substantia spongiosa,** or in laminae II–III, **Substantia gelatinosa**). These tract cells are therefore the 2nd neuron for pain sensation (nociception) and send their centrally-oriented axons to cranial spinal cord segments or to nuclear areas of the brain (e.g., the thalamus). In laminae I and II, not only does pain management occur, but also the processing of pain sensation, e.g., meaning the inhibition of pain transfer to the 2nd neuron (➤ Chap. 13.8).

Proprioceptive impulses of depth sensitivity also pass via the posterior root of the Cornu posterior. The tract cells or the 2nd neuron are located in the **Nucleus proprius** in laminae III and IV, and also in the thoracic lumbar spine in the nuclear pillar of the **Nucleus thoracicus posterior (Nucleus dorsalis,** Nucleus STILLING-CLARKE) of the laminae V–VI, an area of origin for spinocerebellar pathways. Lamina VII includes the majority of the Columna intermedia. Here there are two important key groups: on the one hand, in the thoracic spine, the perikarya of the 1st sympathetic neuron is found in the **Nucleus intermediolateralis**, and on the other hand, in the 2nd or 3rd sacral spine, the 1st parasympathetic neuron is found in the **Nuclei parasympathici sacrales**.

In laminae VIII and IX of the Cornu anterior, as well as intermediate cells and interneurons, there are root cells, the α and γ-motoneurons. The cell groups or pillars located in these laminae show a somatotopic arrangement, which is of vital importance for localisation diagnosis in case of damage to the spinal cord. The motor neurons of the axial muscles, i.e. those near the torso, are located furthest medially near the Fissura mediana anterior, whereas motor neurons of the distal body parts, such as the hand and foot, are located furthest laterally. The neurons of the extremity muscles are

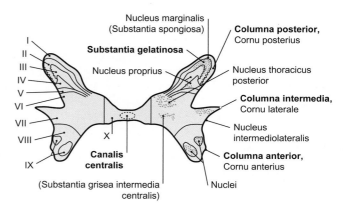

Fig. 12.74 Laminar structure of the Substantia grisea. Cross-section through a thoracic spinal cord segment (T10).

also somatotopically arranged in the sagittal direction, so that neurons of the extensor muscles are more likely to be found in the ventral portion of the Cornu anterior and the neurons of the flexor muscles accumulate here dorsally.

12.6.5 Structure of the Substantia alba

The fibres running in the Substantia alba can be sub-divided into those that remain in the spinal cord (**proprioceptive fibres**), and those that connect to the other sections of the CNS (**association fibres**). The latter makes up the main mass of the Substantia alba, while the fibres of the proprioceptors envelop the Substantia grisea with a thin layer of **Fasciculi proprii**, and manufacture intersegmental connections (➤ Fig. 12.75).

Proprioceptors

The proprioceptors control the internal work done by the spinal cord, which takes place involuntarily and independently of supraspinal centres. However, supraspinal centres can have an influence on the internal working of the spinal cord, modulating via descending pathways, in the sense of strengthening or inhibiting. Included in the work done by the spinal cord in the narrower sense are spinal reflexes, such as muscle proprioceptive reflexes, flexor reflexes and visceral reflexes. Morphologically, in addition to the Fasciculi proprii which are divided according to their position into anterior, lateral and posterior groups, the **Tractus posterolateralis** is demarcated at the tip of the Cornu posterior by intersegmental fibres. Also assigned to the proprioceptors are the descending collaterals of the Funiculus posterior which push into the cervical marrow as the **Fasciculus interfascicularis (comma tract of SCHULTZE)** between the Fasciculus cuneatus and gracilis or into the thoracic marrow as the **Fasciculus septomarginalis (FLECHSIG field)**, in the median plane of the Funiculus posterior.

Association fibres

The association fibres include the fibre pathways, which from a functional viewpoint either rise from the spinal cord to the brain (afferents) or vice versa descend from the brain to the spinal cord (efferents). Both pathway systems are allocated to the Funiculi medullae spinalis as described above. Both ascending and descending pathway systems display a somatotopic structure, which was clearly evident in the cervical medulla.

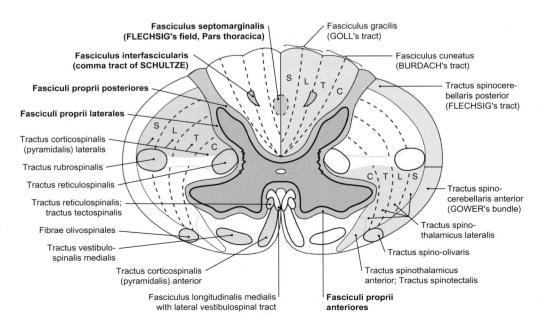

Fasciculus septomarginalis (FLECHSIG's field, Pars thoracica)
Fasciculus interfascicularis (comma tract of SCHULTZE)
Fasciculi proprii posteriores
Fasciculi proprii laterales
Tractus corticospinalis (pyramidalis) lateralis
Tractus rubrospinalis
Tractus reticulospinalis
Tractus reticulospinalis; tractus tectospinalis
Fibrae olivospinales
Tractus vestibulo-spinalis medialis
Tractus corticospinalis (pyramidalis) anterior
Fasciculus longitudinalis medialis with lateral vestibulospinal tract
Fasciculi proprii anteriores
Fasciculus gracilis (GOLL's tract)
Fasciculus cuneatus (BURDACH's tract)
Tractus spinocerebellaris posterior (FLECHSIG's tract)
Tractus spinocerebellaris anterior (GOWER's bundle)
Tractus spinothalamicus lateralis
Tractus spino-olivaris
Tractus spinothalamicus anterior; Tractus spinotectalis

Fig. 12.75 Structure of the Substantia alba. Cross-section through a cervical spinal cord segment.
Blue = ascending tracts, pink = descending tracts, purple = proprioceptive fibres.

Table 12.11 Efferent and afferent tract systems of the association fibres of the Substantia alba of the spinal cord.

Type	Tracts/ systems	Tractus/Fasciculi
Descending (efferent) tract systems		
Autonomic fibres	➤ Chap. 13.9	
Motor nerve fibres	Pyramidal tracts	• Tractus corticospinalis lateralis • Tractus corticospinalis anterior

	Extrapyra-midal tracts	• Lateral tract: Tractus rubrospinalis
		• Medial tract:
		  – Tractus tectospinalis
		  – Tractus reticulospinalis
		  – Tractus vestibulospinales medialis and lateralis

Ascending (afferent) tract systems		
Propriocep-tive fibres	Posterior funiculus system	• Fasciculus gracilis • Fasciculus cuneatus
Pain con-ductive fibres	Spinotha-lamic sys-tem	• Tractus spinothalamicus lateralis • Tractus spinothalamicus anterior • Tractus spinoreticularis • Tractus spinotectalis
	Spinocere-bellar sys-tem	• Tractus spinocerebellaris posterior • Tractus spinocerebellaris anterior • Tractus spinocerebellaris superior • Tractus spinoolivaris

In this context, the Funiculus posterior is an exception, with the fibres being arranged from medial (sacral fibres) to lateral (cervical fibres). The following description of the association fibres follows the functional structure in descending or ascending fibre tracts.

Descending tracts

Principally motor and autonomous descending tract systems can be distinguished (➤ Table 12.11). The functioning of the peripheral autonomic nervous system is controlled by numerous nuclear areas in the brainstem and hypothalamus, where influence is exerted on the preganglionic nerve cells in the Cornu lateralis of the spinal cord via the descending tract systems (➤ Chap. 13.9). The motor fibres, in turn, can be divided into **pyramidal** and **extrapyramidal fibres** (➤ Chap. 13.1). Both directly or usually indirectly have an influence via the interneurons on the root cells, the α and γ-motor neurons. The main mass of these motor tracts lies in the Funiculi anterior and lateral, which are also combined with the **Funiculus anterolateralis** (➤ Fig. 12.75).

Pyramidal tract

The extrapyramidal fibres, the **Tractus pyramidalis**, on the one hand, contain **Fibrae corticonucleares**, i.e., fibres that end at the motor cranial nerve nuclei of the brainstem and, on the other hand, contain **Fibrae corticospinales** up to the spinal cord. The pyramidal tract originates in the somatotopically-structured primary motor cortex (Gyrus precentralis), as well as in the secondary premotor cortex areas of the frontal lobe and a lower proportion (20%) in the sensory cortex of the parietal lobe. Fibres from the primary sensory cortex have no motor function; instead they end in the Cornu posterior of the spinal cord and modulate sensory perceptions. The axon fibres of the pyramidal tract are derived from the motor cortex, and are consistently arranged somatotopically on their pathway through the Capsula interna of the telencephalon and the Crura cerebri of the mesencephalon. Once the Fibrae corticonucleare in the brainstem have left the pyramidal tract, the re-

maining fibres reach the pyramis in the Medulla oblongata, where 70–90 % of their fibres cross over to the opposite side in the **Decussatio pyramidum**, which lies slightly caudal, and continue in the spinal cord as the **Tractus corticospinalis lateralis** (➤ Fig. 12.75). The uncrossed fibres reach the spinal cord segments as the **Tractus corticospinalis anterior** (➤ Fig. 12.75) in the Funiculus anterior next to the Fissura longitudinalis anterior, in order to initially cross over to the opposite side via the Commissura anterior of the Substantia alba (➤ Chap. 13.1). The Tractus corticospinallis anterior ends in the cervical spinal cord, whereas the fibres of the lateral tract go as far as the sacral spine (S4). Functionally, the pyramidal tract controls, in particular, the fine motor skills of the distal extremity muscles. In addition, the Tractus corticospinalis has a control function over the proprioceptors and so can attenuate proprioceptive reflexes, or it can suppress primitive reflexes, such as the BABINSKI reflex which, due to the immature myelination of the pyramidal tract in newborn babies, can still be triggered.

Extrapyramidal system

The term **extrapyramidal system (EPS)** covers all motor projection fibres not running in the pyramidal tract. However, both systems are closely interlinked and should not be considered independently of each other.

> **NOTE**
>
> In contrast to the monosynaptic pyramidal fibres, the EPS is polysynaptic, has different areas of origin, does not consistently cross over to the other side of the body, and most importantly ends at the γ-motor neurons.

The origin areas of the EPS are located in subcortical nuclear areas, although they have tight connections with the cortex and the cerebellum. The areas of origin in the Nuclei vestibulares medialis and lateralis, the Nucleus ruber, the Nucleus olivaris inferior, the Lamina tecti of the midbrain and the Formatio reticularis are correspondingly differentiated from the Tractus vestibulospinales medialis and lateralis, the Tractus rubrospinalis, the Tractus olivospinalis and the Tractus tectospinalis and reticulospinalis (➤ Fig. 12.75). Based on their main features, they can also be grouped into medial and lateral groups (➤ Table 12.11).

As a **lateral tract**, the **Tractus rubrospinalis** originates from the Nucleus ruber in the mesencephalon. It is divided somatotopically. Its fibres cross in the tegmental decussation (**Decussatio tegmentalis anterior**) to the opposite side before passing caudally in the Funiculus lateralis anterior, directly anterior to the Tractus corticospinalis lateralis in the spinal cord. In a comparable way to the pyramidal fibres, impulses of the Tractus rubrospinalis activate a contraction of the flexors and inhibit a contraction of the extensors. In the same way, it influences the muscle tone of the distal extremity muscles and controls the skeletal muscles of the distal extremity sections – particularly the arms, which is significant after a malfunction of the pyramidal tract.

The **medial tracts** preferentially allow control over muscle tone and major movements of the trunk and the proximal extremity muscles. The main function of these tracts is to stabilise the body position and balance. To enable this, these tracts influence basic muscle tension, the holding and supporting of motor skills required in the relevant body position, and the coordination of movement processes. A change in head or body posture and the perception of acoustic or visual signals usually require the body to make a rapid motor adaptation. The posture and supporting motor system is controlled by an increased contraction of the extensors and the corresponding inhibiting of the inversely acting flexors.

The receptive impulses of the vestibular organs (vestibular system) in the inner ear take control of the support motor skills via the relay or interconnection in the vestibular nuclei. The **Tractus vestibulospinales medialis and lateralis** respectively originate in the Nuclei vestibulares medialis and lateralis and pass caudally into the mid-thoracic spine, with the medial tract being significantly less developed and located near the Commissura alba anterior. The Tractus vestibulospinalis lateralis in the Funiculus anterior of the spinal cord runs purely ipsilaterally and is divided somatotopically (➤ Chap. 13.5).

The **Tractus reticulospinalis** comes from both the upper (pontine) and the lower (bulbar) nuclei of the Formatio reticularis. Its fibres run both ipsilaterally and contralaterally in the Funiculus anterior and end at α and γ-motor neurons, in particular in those of the axial trunk muscles and proximal limb muscles.

The fibres of the **Tractus tectospinalis** originate in the Lamina tecti of the mesencephalon. The Lamina tecti receives optical impulses via the Colliculi superiores, and receives acoustic impulses via the Colliculi inferior, which acts as a protection mechanism, e.g., when there is a loud bang, resulting in head and neck reflex movements. The fibres of the Tractus tectospinalis cross in the **posterior tegmental decussation (Decussatio tegmentalis posterior)**, run in the Funiculus anterior of the spinal cord and indirectly reach the motor neurons of the neck muscle there.

Ascending tracts

The ascending tract systems take afferent impulses from the periphery or the interior of the body to the brain. The perikaryon of the 1st neuron of this functional system is located in the spinal ganglia, the fibre tract systems themselves – therefore the axons of this 1st neuron or, with synaptic relays in the Cornu posterior, of the 2nd neuron – run in the Funiculus anterolateralis or the Funiculus posterior centrally. In general, we differentiate here a **posterior funiculus system**, a **spinothalamic (anterolateral) system** and a **spinocerebellar system** (➤ Fig. 12.75).

Posterior funiculus system

The posterior funiculus system is located, as its name indicates, in the Funiculus posterior. The sensory property transferred here includes:
- sensory perceptions, such as pressure and vibrations
- fine touch sensations of the skin
- depth perception from the interior of the body with information about body positions (from muscle, tendons and joint receptors)

The posterior funiculus system consists of 2 fasciculi:
- The **Fasciculus gracilis (GOLL)** is positioned medially. It begins in the sacral spine and ensures pulse management for the lower extremity.
- The **Fasciculus cuneatus (BURDACH)** joins laterally and continues in a wedge shape up to the Cornu posterior. It starts in the thoracic spine (T3) and carries the sensory qualities mentioned above for the upper limbs.

The tracts of the Funiculus posterior do not cross in the spinal cord, they do so only after their ipsilateral switching in the **Nuclei gracilis and cuneatus** of the Medulla oblongata (➤ Chap. 13.2.3). The tracts of the Funiculus posterior are arranged somatotopically on their pathway.

Clinical remarks

One of the most common vitamin deficiency disorders in Western Europe is Vitamin B$_{12}$ deficiency. Women are particularly affected during pregnancy as they have a higher vitamin consumption; as are patients who abuse laughing gas, or chronic alcoholics, of whom the parietal cells in the stomach can no longer form sufficient 'intrinsic factor' for the uptake of Vitamin B$_{12}$ in the ileum due to chronic inflammation. As a result, a systemic disease with anaemia occurs and, above all, a spinal manifestation causing the demyelisation of the myelin sheath, primarily affecting the tract of the Funiculus posterior and the pyramidal tract in the cervical and thoracic spine. In 90% of patients, proprioception disorders dominate at the onset of the disease: symmetrical paresthesia, unsteady gait and later, along with the sensory symptoms, motor symptoms such as paralysis or increased proprioceptive muscle reflexes. Upon being administered replacement vitamin B$_{12}$, 50% of patients demonstrate a complete regression of their symptoms.

Spinothalamic system

The spinothalamic system is a part of the **anterolateral system**, to which the smaller tract systems such as the **Tractus spinoreticularis and spinotectalis** are additionally assigned. In a narrow sense, the spinothalamic system is made up of the **Tractus spinothalamici lateralis and anterior**. Major pressure and tactile sensations (mechanical sensory system), as well as pain perception (nociception) and temperature perception are carried via this system of tracts (➤ Chap. 13.2.3, ➤ Chap. 13.8):
- The **Tractus spinothalamicus lateralis** is structured somatopically so that the cervical fibres are located centrally near the Cornu anterius.
- The **Tractus spinothalamicus anterior** accumulates medial to the lateral tract, with its fibres mixing with those of the Tractus spinotectalis.

Spinocerebellar system

This system carries proprioceptive information from muscle spindles and GOLGI tendon organs to the ipsilateral cerebellum. In this way, the cerebellum receives information about the position of joints and limbs. The **Tractus spinocerebellaris posterior (FLECHSIG)** and the **Tractus spinocerebellaris anterior (GOWER)** are significant parts of the system (➤ Fig. 12.76, ➤ Chap. 13.2.3). Both tracts do not occur in the cervical spine, and information of the sensory quality mentioned above for the upper half of the body is conducted via smaller fibre tracts, the **Fibrae cuneocerebellares** and the **Tractus spinocerebellaris superior**, to the cerebellum (➤ Chap. 13.2.3). Indirect fibre connections between the spinal cord and the cerebellum arrive as the **Tractus spinoolivaris** in the contralateral funiculus, anterior to the olive, and cross back as the **Tractus olivocerebellaris** to the ipsilateral hemisphere of the cerebellum. Other relays for these fibres within the cerebellum are described in ➤ Chap. 12.4.

N O T E
- The long, ascending tract systems access the spinal cord via the Radix posterior. The perikarya of the 1st neuron are located in the spinal ganglia.
- The 2nd neuron is normally located in the Cornu posterius – with the exception of the posterior funiculus system, in which the relay to the 2nd neuron only occurs in the Medulla oblongata.

Clinical remarks

The neurologist BROWN-SÉQUARD was the first to describe the symptom complex of unilateral complete damage of the spinal cord **(BROWN-SÉQUARD syndrome)** in 1851. Unlike what is found in a complete cross-sectional lesion, the picture

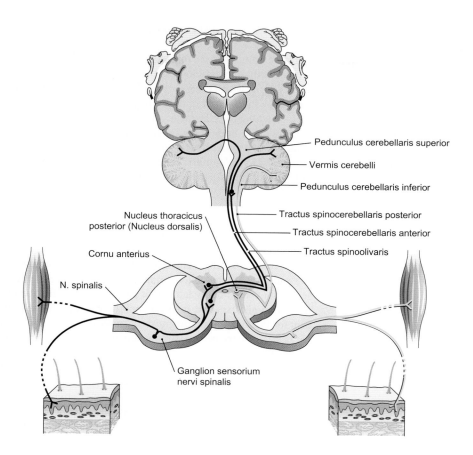

Pedunculus cerebellaris superior

Vermis cerebelli

Pedunculus cerebellaris inferior

Tractus spinocerebellaris posterior

Tractus spinocerebellaris anterior

Tractus spinoolivaris

Nucleus thoracicus posterior (Nucleus dorsalis)

Cornu anterius

N. spinalis

Ganglion sensorium nervi spinalis

Fig. 12.76 Management of the subconscious depth sensitivity (afferent neurovascular pathways); spinocerebellar system.

is inconsistent in one-sided damage of the spinal cord. This can be explained by the differing locations of the fibre tract intersections. On the damaged side, the pyramidal tract is severed, leading to equilateral, homolateral, firstly slack, then spastic paralysis at the location and caudally from there. Similarly, the Funiculus posterior tracts and most of the spinocerebellar tracts leave the spinal cord uncrossed, so that a homolateral set of symptoms with loss of fine tactile sensation and depth sensitivity can also be observed. Conversely, the Tractus spinothalamicus – and therefore the perceptions of temperature and pain – already crosses at the segment height of the spinal cord, so that on the contralateral side and downwards from there, there is a corresponding sensory disturbance. Autonomous descending tracts to the sympathetic and parasympathetic reflex centres run bilaterally, so that the bladder and rectum functions generally survive a one-sided lesion.

12.6.6 Blood supply

Arterial blood supply
Spinal cord arteries
The spinal cord is supplied arterially by a fine network of vessels fed by 3 longitudinally running vessels. A distinction is made between the frontal A. spinalis anterior running in the Fissura mediana anterior, and the paired but less-developed Aa. spinales posterior, located medially of the Radix posterior.

- The **A. spinalis anterior** is formed at the level of the spinal cord segment C1–2 from branches of both the Aa. vertebrales. Via the **Rr. medullares mediales (Aa. sulci)**, which run in the depth of the Fissura mediana anterior, it supplies the anterior two-thirds of the spinal cord with the Cornu anterior, the Commissura alba,

the Commissura grisea anterior, the Funiculus anterolateralis as well as the base of the Cornu posterior with the Nucleus dorsalis.
- The **Aa. spinales posteriores** mostly arise from the bilateral A. inferior posterior cerebelli, which originates from the A. vertebralis. They supply the remaining dorsal third.

All 3 arteries are connected via the vasocorona, transversely running fine vessels on the surface of the spinal cord. The vessel branches entering the spinal cord are regarded as functional terminal arteries.

Segmental inflows
The spinal arteries receive segmental inflows from the supply areas of the A. subclavia (A. vertebralis, A. cervicalis ascendens, A. cervicalis profunda), the Aorta thoracica (Aa. intercostales posteriores) and the Aorta abdominalis (Aa. lumbales). For the Conus medullaris and the Cauda equina, the A. sacralis lateralis as well as the A. ileolumbalis from the A. iliaca interna are also specified (➤ Fig. 11.48, ➤ Fig. 11.49 in ➤ Chap. 11.5). Between the above-mentioned supply areas, the blood vessels are often very thin and only receive restricted segmental inflows. Circulatory disorders therefore particularly arise in spinal cord segments T4 and L1. Conversely, at the level of the intumescences, the arterial blood supply is fairly well-ensured by many segmental inflows. Clinically significant and therefore worth mentioning is the arterial blood supply to the Intumescentia lumbosacralis via the **A. radicularis magna (ADAMKIEWICZ)**, mostly at the level of T9–L5, originating from the left A. intercostalis posterior. Its diameter measures between 0.7 and 1.3 mm, so that compared to the spinal artery which is only 0.3–0.5 mm wide, it can actually be described as 'magna'.
The segmental arterial blood supply of the spinal cord is undertaken by the **R. spinalis**, receiving blood via the R. dorsal branch of the A. intercostalis posterior. The spinal branch passes through the Foramen intervertebrale and divides at the level of the Radix poste-

rior into short **Aa. radiculares anterior and posterior**, both of which provide the blood supply to the spinal ganglion and Radix posterior, while the **A. medullaris segmentalis** ensures the actual supply of the spinal cord matter and takes blood to the Aa. spinales anterior and posterior (➤ Fig. 11.49, ➤ Chap. 11.5).

Venous drainage

In the same way as for arterial blood supply, the venous blood of the radially-oriented internal veins of the spinal cord flows into the **V. spinalis anterior** or the larger **V. spinalis posterior**, found in the Sulcus medianus posterior (➤ Fig. 12.77). Drainage continues through the **Vv. radiculares** along the Radix posterior to the venous plexus of the epidural space, the **Plexus venosus vertebralis internus**. The **Vv. intervertebrales** leave the vertebral canal via the Foramina intervertebralia. They carry blood from the spinal cord, the dura and the Plexus venosus vertebralis internus and provide a connection to the **Plexus venosus vertebralis externus** on the front and back sides of the spine. They are however also connected to the Vv. intercostales, the Vv. lumbales and the veins which are assigned to the previously mentioned arteries. Intervertebral veins form anastomosis tissue without valves between the inner and outer Plexus venosus of the spine. Considered together, this venous system is an important intercaval anastomosis.

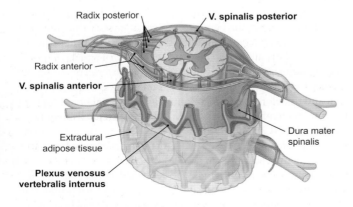

Fig. 12.77 Veins of the vertebral canal. [E402]

12.6.7 Motor functions of the spinal cord

Intrinsic and extrinsic reflexes

A reflex is the subconscious unchanging response from specific effector organs where there is receptor activation. A **reflex arc** is then formed by the afferent fibres leading to the CNS and the efferent fibres reaching the effector organ.

Reflexes occur both in the somatic and the autonomic nervous systems with the **visceral reflexes** of the autonomic nervous system, in contrast to the **somatic reflexes**, which are usually polysynaptically relayed and are therefore assigned to extrinsic reflexes (see below).

Intrinsic reflexes

An intrinsic reflex is characterised by a stimulus-receiving receptor with the stimulus response found in the same organ, hence there is only a single relay from afferent onto efferent tracts (monosynaptic) and the reflex arrangement takes place via a single spinal cord segment (➤ Fig. 12.78, left half of page). The examination of somatic, segment-specific intrinsic muscle reflexes is highly significant for the localisation diagnosis of spinal cord lesions (➤ Table 12.12). The triggering stimulus for an intrinsic muscle reflex is the stretching of muscle spindles, e.g., by hitting the muscle tendon with a reflex hammer. Ia-afferents of the muscle spindles reach the α-motoneurons (monosynaptically) directly and trigger a muscle contraction. At the same time, collaterals of Ia-afferents arrive along with inhibiting interneurons, which ensure a reciprocal inhibition of the antagonistic muscle (polysynaptically). Although such a reflex takes place completely as a motor function of the spinal cord, the reflex arcs are however also subject to supraspinal control and thus, for example, can be facilitated. This becomes clear when via a muscular tensing of the arms, the leg reflexes are triggered more easily. This facilitation takes place via the convergence of multiple subliminal stimuli, which then together ensure a depolarisation of motor neurons. This phenomenon of facilitation in the form of the **JENDRASSIK manoeuvre,** named after a Hungarian neurologist, is useful in a clinical neurological examination.

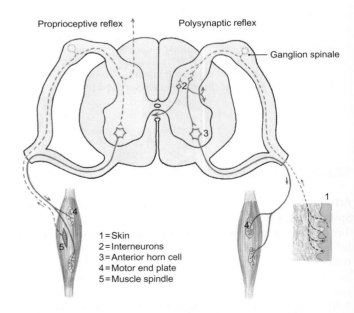

1 = Skin
2 = Interneurons
3 = Anterior horn cell
4 = Motor end plate
5 = Muscle spindle

Fig. 12.78 Reflexes of the Medulla spinalis. Monosynaptic proprioceptive reflex (on the left side of the image) and polysynaptic extrinsic reflex (on the right half of the image).

Table 12.12 Somatic intrinsic and extrinsic reflexes with appropriate allocation of the spinal cord segments for clinical neurological diagnosis.

Reflex	Triggering stimulation	Reflex response	Spinal cord segments
Intrinsic reflexes			
Biceps tendon reflex	Impact on the biceps tendon	Contraction of the M. biceps brachii (flexion in the elbow joint, supination)	C6 (C5–C6)
Triceps tendon reflex	Impact on the triceps tendon	Contraction of the M. triceps brachii (extension in the elbow joint)	C7 (C6–C8)
Patellar tendon reflex	Impact on the patellar ligament	Contraction of the M. quadriceps femoris (extension in the knee joint)	L3 (L2–L4)
Achilles tendon reflex	Impact on the Achilles tendon	Contraction of the M. triceps surae (plantar flexion of the foot)	S1 (L5–S2)
Extrinsic reflexes			
Cremasteric reflex	Stroking of the skin on the inner thigh	Contraction of the M. cremaster (retraction of the testis into the torso)	L1–L2
Abdominal skin reflex	Stroking of the lateral abdominal skin	Contraction of the ipsilateral abdominal wall musculature (e.g., M. obliquus externus abdominis)	T6–T12
Anal reflex	Stroking of the anal skin	Contraction of the M. sphincter ani externus	S3–S5

Extrinsic reflexes

An extrinsic reflex is characterised by the fact that the stimulus and its response are not located in the same organ, so there are always several relays of afferent onto efferent tracts (polysynaptic) and the reflex arrangement takes place in several spinal cord segments (➤ Fig. 12.78, right half of image, ➤ Table 12.12). We can distinguish between purely somatic, purely visceral and mixed reflexes:

- **Somatic reflexes** usually involve sensory motor stimuli, i.e., an activation of receptors of the skin (e.g. temperature, pain) leading to a motor response. **Fight or flight reflexes** fall into this category such as the **flexor reflex:** a pain stimulus, for example in the foot leads to a reflexive activation of the ipsilateral flexors and thus to a retraction of the foot. At the same time, the body posture is also strengthened by the activation of contralateral extensors on the standing leg.
- In the same way as for purely somatic reflexes, there are also purely **visceral reflexes** of the autonomic nervous system. These are called **viscerovisceral reflexes (gut reflexes)**, when afferent and efferent tracts are located in the autonomic nervous system. These unconsciously occurring reflexes are relayed at the spinal cord level, as well as at the brainstem level since the parasympathetic visceral innervation takes place up to the CANNON's point via the N. vagus located in the brainstem. Here, amongst others, the impulses of the stretch receptors in the wall of hollow organs have an influence on the function of the organ muscles. For example, the expansion of the stomach wall after food intake leads to increased gastric peristalsis.

Mixed reflexes can be either **viscerosomatic** or **somatovisceral**. A clinically significant example of a segmentally organised viscerosomatic reflex is the development of the **muscular defence** reflex, a 'rock hard' tensing of the ventral abdominal wall musculature when the bowels, for example, are irritated due to inflammation. Conversely, the **application of heat,** a skin stimulation by a somatovisceral (cutivisceral) reflex via visceroefferent tracts leads to a relaxation of the abdominal muscles.

Spinal function centres

In the spinal cord there are several important **spinovisceral reflex centres** of the autonomic nervous system, controlled via the viscerovisceral reflexes. Examples of this are:

- in the cervical spine, the **Centrum ciliospinale (C8–T1)**, which activates the dilation of the pupils via its sympathetic efferents to the M. dilatator pupillae
- in the thoracic lumbar spinal cord segments (T11–L1) is a **sympathetic reflex centre,** which innervates male and female pelvic organs with its efferents and is vital for functions such as the ejaculation process and the long-term function of maintaining continence for the anal and bladder sphincters
- in the Cornu lateralis of the sacral spine, the **parasympathetic centre for the pelvic organs (S2–S4),** controls the bodily functions of erection as well as stool and urination controls – as an antagonist of the sympathetic centre for the pelvic organs mentioned above.

In physiological terms, the spinal reflex level for controlling micturition and defecation is superior to that of the supraspinal control centre.

Clinical remarks

In the case of **paraplegia** due to damage to these connection pathways, the micturition reflex initially goes and is eventually replaced by spinal reflexes. Depending on the level of the lesion in the spinal cord and the associated damage to the autonomous reflex centres, there is a spinal *reflex bladder* (in the case of damage above the sacral reflex centre) or a spinal *overflow bladder* (in the case of damage to the sacral reflex centre).

The **cauda equina syndrome** denotes a lesion below the IInd lumbar vertebra in the area of the Cauda equina with damage to one or more nerve roots. The most common causes are tumours, disc problems or trauma. Typically, patients complain about flaccid paralysis of the legs, with the hip muscles usually unaffected. As well as bladder or rectal disorders with an overflow bladder (since the efferent fibres of the parasympathetic reflex centre can be affected), there is what is known as *saddle anaesthesia,* i.e. a sensory disturbance of the inner thigh and the anal area. In treatment terms, immediate neurosurgical decompression is required by removal of the mass-forming process.

13 Functional systems

Stroke

Medical history

A 63-year-old man comes to the emergency department in the early morning, as he first noticed while shaving that the right corner of his mouth was drooping. While drinking coffee, it ran out of his mouth again without him noticing, and in the meantime he is finding it difficult to lift his right arm. He could no longer walk independently from the taxi to the door of the hospital. His wife reports that she has noticed the drooping mouth previously, but that it always passed within a few hours and so she did not call in a doctor. History of medication shows that the patient has been treated for many years with antihypertensives, diuretics and low-dose acetylsalicylic acid. Up to about 10 years ago, the patient used to smoke around 40 cigarettes per day.

Initial examination

The night-duty doctor notices that the man's speech sounds 'frozen'. During a further physical examination it becomes clear, amongst other things, that it is not possible for the man to close his mouth completely; he does however manage to wrinkle both sides of his forehead ('frown'). The arm muscles (right) are flaccidly paralysed and the maximum power development in the right leg is only around 10% of the left leg. With forceful stroking of the lateral right sole, the big toe is particularly abducted (positive 'BABINSKI sign').

Probable diagnosis

The patient shows many symptoms of a stroke (apoplex). From the pre-history it is known that there were already common episodes of slight functional failures, all of which cleared up. Such episodes are referred to as transient ischaemic attacks (TIA).

Clinical picture

Possible causes of stroke are either arterial supply restriction (ischaemia) or haemorrhages, which often occur in the area of the Capsula interna. They are often traced back to pathological changes of the vascular wall of cerebral arteries, which frequently accompany risk factors such as long-term hypertension and/or heavy smoking. If – as in this case – corticonuclear tracts and the N. facialis are affected, this shows in a weakness of the mimetic muscles on the contralateral side ('drooping mouth'). Because of the double motor innervation of the central motor nuclei for supplying the forehead muscles, the mimetic muscles above the eye are not affected. The additional flaccid paralysis of the right arm and right leg indicates that the left Tractus corticospinalis is also affected (a few weeks or months later this paralysis turns into spastic paralysis). The triggering of pathological reflexes (here the BABINSKI reflex) also indicates central damage.

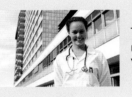

The above-mentioned case is decribed to you during the patient presentation whilst you are on rotation in neurology. Your objectives are 'risk factors and classification of cerebral ischaemia'. You decide to create an index card on this.

<u>Cerebral ischemia</u>
First risk factors   (THE classic vascular expansion – here as well!)
Arterial hypertension, smoking, obesity, diabetes mellitus, heavy alcohol consumption, physical inactivity, hyper cholesterol-emia, possible family history of stroke, age, male Gender
In addition: atrial fibrillation, stenosis of the A. carotis int.
2nd classification of cerebral circulatory disorders
▫ **Asymptomatic stenosis:** stenosis, but Ø symptoms
▫ **TIA** (Transient Ischemic Attack): symptoms < 24 h
▫ **Progressive stroke:** symptoms increase over the course of the stroke, only partially reversible
▫ **Complete stroke:** irreversible damage of brain tissue

13.1 Somatic nervous system
Tobias M. Böckers

Skills

After working through this chapter, you should be able to:
- define the pyramidal and extrapyramidal systems and specifically describe the corresponding tractus in its pathway and function
- name structures involved in the execution of voluntary movements
- explain the symptoms of a stroke

13.1.1 Overview

The somatic nervous system (also known as the voluntary nervous system) generates and forwards signals for controlling movements or movement processes and body positions via the innervation of striated skeletal muscles. Belonging to this system are specific cortical areas for the planning, coordination and execution of movement: relaying, descending tracts in the brain and spinal cord (e.g., the pyramidal tract) as well as the neuronal switching stations in the brainstem or spinal cord (motorneurons) with the consecutive cranial nerves or spinal nerves (peripheral nerves). This configuration cascade is grouped together as the **pyramidal system**.

It must be taken into account however that further areas of the brain and/or nuclei are essential for targeted movements. The ax-

ons from these areas also end in the spinal cord and form defined tracts. These regulate the signals and movement planning of the pyramidal system, but can also initiate or change movements itself. Particular examples are the cerebellum, the basal ganglia, the Nucleus ruber, the Substantia nigra, and the Formatio reticularis. These areas of the brain and their tract systems are grouped together as the **extrapyramidal system**. Due to the close functional interweaving of the pyramidal and extrapyramidal systems (both systems are important, e.g., for balance as well as physiological body posture and movement processes), but also due to the innervation of parts of the extrapyramidal system by the pyramidal tract, there does not yet appear to be a clear separation between these systems. However, this chapter presents the anatomy of the parts of the somatomotor system in its classic division – also due to its application in clinical medicine.

13.1.2 Central section

Pyramidal system
The motor system is divided into a pyramidal and an extrapyramidal system, whereby both work together functionally and are activated together, so that a clear separation of their functions is not possible.

A slightly closer look at the pyramidal system shows that further cortical areas are involved. In addition to the **primary motor cortex,** the **premotor area** and the **parietal association cortex,** which feed descending fibres into the pyramidal tract, the other areas are the **frontal eye field** (BRODMANN area 8), the **BROCA's area** (BRODMANN areas 44 and 45), as well as the **supplementary**

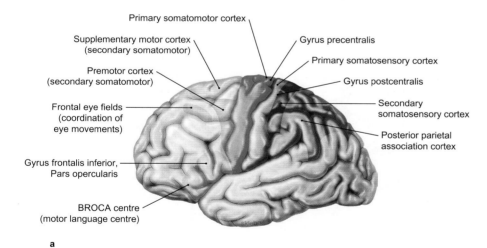

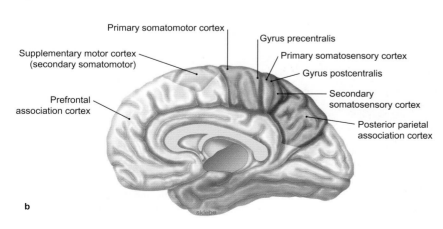

Fig. 13.1 Cortex areas that are involved in the coordination of motor skills. a Lateral view. **b** Medial view.

Table 13.1 Pyramidal system

Neuron chain	Groups of neurons
1st neuron	Neurons of the primary motor cortex, M1 (Gyrus precentralis, BRODMANN area 4), but in some cases also neurons from the premotor area (BRODMANN area 6 on the convexity) or from the parietal association cortex (BRODMANN area 5; ➤ Fig. 13.1, ➤ Fig. 13.2).
2nd and 3rd neuron respectively	Spinal α-motorneurons (but also γ-motorneurons); in most cases these are however reached via the innervation of spinal interneurons in the spinal cord segment (the spinal α-motorneurons then innervate the peripheral skeletal muscles)

motor cortex (BRODMANN area 6, medial cortex; ➤ Table 13.1, ➤ Fig. 13.1). In addition, as part of a 'feedback loop', sensory areas (primary and secondary cortical areas) influence the execution of movements. These cortical areas, which are also integrated into the pyramidal system, are important, amongst other things, for the mediation of conjugate eye movements (**Tractus corticomesencephalicus**), important for speech and fine-tuning of complex movement processes.

Pyramidal tract

The pyramidal tract (Tractus pyramidalis) consists of the **Tractus corticospinalis** (running to the respective motorneurons in the spinal cord) and the **Tractus corticonuclearis** (running to the cranial nerve nuclei). The efferents mainly originate from the Gyrus precentrali of the right and left halves of the brain, which then converge on both sides to medial in the direction of the basal ganglia (➤ Fig. 13.2, ➤ Fig. 13.3).

The tract systems exhibit a clear **somatotopic arrangement,** which can be tracked in a corresponding arrangement into the spinal cord (➤ Chap. 12.6.5). Located on the Gyrus precentralis in the lateral view is the large representation of hand, face and tongue muscles. Attaching cranially at the junction with the Fissura longitudinalis cerebri is the torso with the legs 'hanging' over the mantle edge into the Fissura longitudinalis cerebri (➤ Fig. 13.1). The selected depiction reflects not only the somatotopic representation, but also the size of each respective cortical field for the individual skeletal muscle or for the respective muscle groups. Hereby the areas with particularly pronounced innervation density become clear, and it shows the importance of the hand and facial muscles in the evolutionary development of humans. The representation shown in this way on the Gyrus precentralis is referred to as the '**homunculus**' (➤ Fig. 13.3).

The two parts of the pyramidal tract then run caudally between the basal ganglia via the Capsula interna (Tractus corticospinalis: Crus posterior; Tractus corticonuclearis: genu; ➤ Fig. 13.4, ➤ Table 13.2) and run inside the midbrain into the Crura cerebri in the direction of the pons. On this pathway, the **Tractus corticonuclearis** then ends partially uncrossed, also after crossing into the contralateral nuclei of the cranial nerves (V, VII, IX–XII).

The **Nucleus nervi facialis [VII]** has a special feature in that the mimetic forehead muscles are innervated on both sides by fibres from both the right and left Tractus corticonuclearis; the rest of the mimetic muscles are only innervated by crossed fibres. In the case of a one-sided failure of the corticonuclear tracts, the forehead muscles are thus still innervated ('**central facial paresis**', ➤ Chap. 12.5.10).

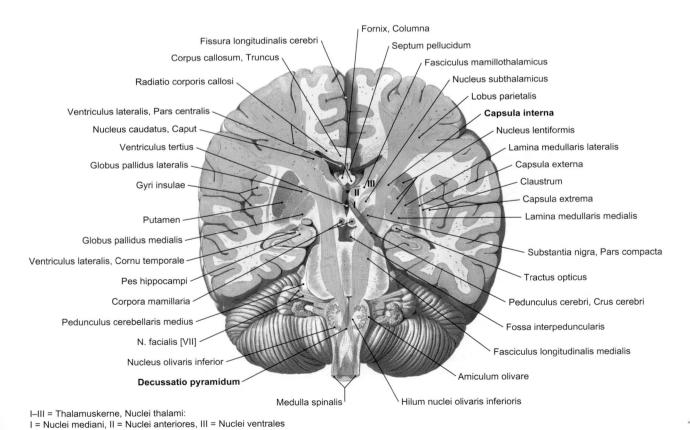

I–III = Thalamuskerne, Nuclei thalami:
I = Nuclei mediani, II = Nuclei anteriores, III = Nuclei ventrales

Fig. 13.2 Pyramidal tract, Tractus pyramidalis, and basal ganglia, Nuclei basales. Oblique layered section through the posterior limb of the internal capsule, the cerebral peduncles, and the Medulla oblongata. Anterior view; pyramidal tract highlighted in colours, right: pink, left: green.

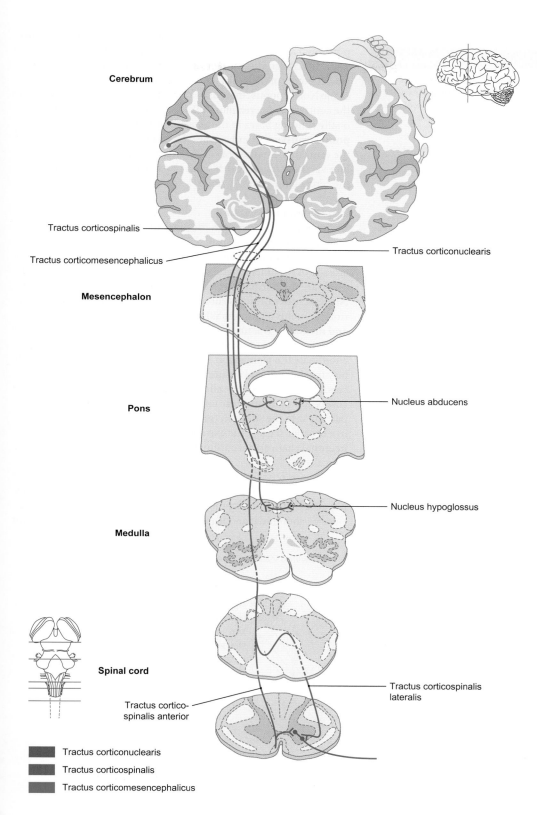

Cerebrum

Tractus corticospinalis

Tractus corticomesencephalicus

Tractus corticonuclearis

Mesencephalon

Pons

Nucleus abducens

Nucleus hypoglossus

Medulla

Spinal cord

Tractus corticospinalis lateralis

Tractus cortico-spinalis anterior

Tractus corticonuclearis

Tractus corticospinalis

Tractus corticomesencephalicus

Fig. 13.3 Parts and pathway of the pyramidal tract. The Tractus corticospinalis (red) passes through the Capsula interna and forms the Tractus corticospinales anterior and lateralis at the height of the pyramids. The Tractus corticonuclearis ends crossed and uncrossed at the cranial nerve nuclei. Belonging to the Tractus corticomesencephalicus (green) are the fibres from the central eye field, which end at the nuclei of the cranial nerves III, IV and VI (example here: Nucleus abducens). [L127]

A special part of the Tractus cortinuclearis is the **Tractus corticomesenephalicus,** the fibres of which originate from area 8 (the central optical field) of the cortex. These fibres run mainly crossed to the nuclei of the oculomotor nerves (cranial nerves III, IV, VI), which perform there synergistically after stimulation (conjugate eye movement).

In the pons, the **Fibrae corticospinales** are less densely packed, but then integrate in turn below the pons to the ventral side of the Medulla oblongata into a fibre bundle that is visible from the outside as a triangular **pyramid.** Roughly at the level of the junction from the Medulla oblongata to the spinal cord, the tractus divides and, after crossing around 80% of the fibres, forms the **Tractus corticospinalis lateralis** on the contralateral side. The uncrossed fibres run as the **Tractus corticospinalis anterior** through the spinal cord and eventually cross at the level of the respective spinal cord segments. Finally, the respective α-motorneurons are innervated via them (mostly via interneurons) in the anterior horn of the spinal cord (also ➤ Chap. 12.6.5).

Table 13.2 Tracts and arterial blood supply to the Capsula interna.

Localisation	Tracts	Blood supply
Front limb (Crus anterius)	• Tractus frontopontinus • Radiatio anterior thalami	Aa. centrales anteromediales (from the A. cerebri anterior)
Genu	• Tractus corticonucleares	Aa. centrales anterolaterales (from the A. cerebri media) = Aa. lenticulostriatae
Posterior limb (Crus posterius)	• Tractus corticospinalis • Tractus corticorubralis and Tractus corticoreticularis • Radiatio centralis thalami (from rostral thalamus muscles to the motor cortex • Radiatio posterior thalami (from the Corpus geniculatum laterale and from further thalamus muscles to the parietal and occipital lobes) • Tractus parietotemporopontinus and Tractus occipitopontinus • Radiatio optica (optic radiation; from the Corpus geniculatum laterale to the occipital lobes) • Radiatio acustica (acoustic radiation; from the Corpus geniculatum mediale to the temporal lobes)	Rr. capsulae internae (from the A. choroidea anterior)

Tractus corticopontini

The Tractus corticopontini cannot be assigned to either the classic pyramidal nor the extrapyramidal system, but belong to the motor system due to their function. They originate from defined cortical areas and end mainly in the pons. These are fibres which originate from the Lobi parietalis and temporalis (**Tractus parietotemporo-** **pontinus**) as well as from the Lobus occipitalis (**Tractus occipito-** **pontinus**) and the Lobus frontalis (**Tractus frontopontinus).** These fibres also run through the Capsula interna and end in the Nuclei pontis of the pons. After synaptic conversion onto neurons of the Nuclei pontis, their axons run via the middle cerebellum into the contralateral cerebellum (Tractus pontocerebellaris). The diagonally running fibres in the area of the pons are named **Fibrae pontis transversae** and can also be identified macroscopically on the ventral side of the pons. Efferents are directed to the cerebellum via these tracts, which reach in particular the corneal cells of the cerebellum as mossy fibres.

Extrapyramidal system

Phylogenetically older than the pyramidal tract system, the extrapyramidal system consists of descending fibre systems which originate in different nuclei of the brainstem and run crossed or uncrossed in the anterolateral chain of the spinal cord (➤ Fig. 13.5). These are the **Formatio reticularis** (Tractus reticulospinalis), the **Nucleus ruber** (Tractus rubrospinalis), the **tectum** (Colliculi superiores, Tractus tectospinalis) and the **Nuclei vestibulares lateralis and medialis** (Tractus vestibulospinalis). These nuclei are, for their part, directly or indirectly influenced by the cortical fibres. They coordinate the planning of movement, control most of the involuntary movements and ensure muscle tone and balance. In the process, they in turn receive afferents from the cerebellum and the cortex and there are close connections to the basal ganglia, here in particular to the striatum (grouped as the extrapyramidal system in a broader sense). The extrapyramidal system is organised as a neuronal chain and accordingly integrates several nuclei multi-synaptically.

The Tractus reticulospinalis, vestibulospinalis and tectospinalis form an anatomically functional **medial system,** which innervates in particular the medial motorneurons, located in the Cornu anterius, for abdominal and leg muscles, (including the standing motor

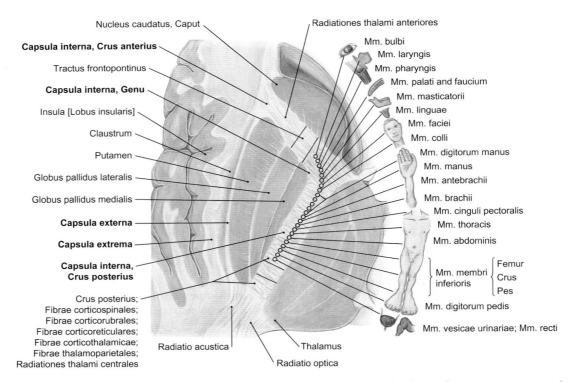

Fig. 13.4 Capsula interna, internal capsule; functional structure. Within the Capsula interna, the descending tracts are structured somatotopically. The corticonuclear fibres run in the genu of the capsule; the corticospinal fibres for the upper extremity, torso and lower extremity are arranged somatotopically from anterior to posterior in the posterior limb.

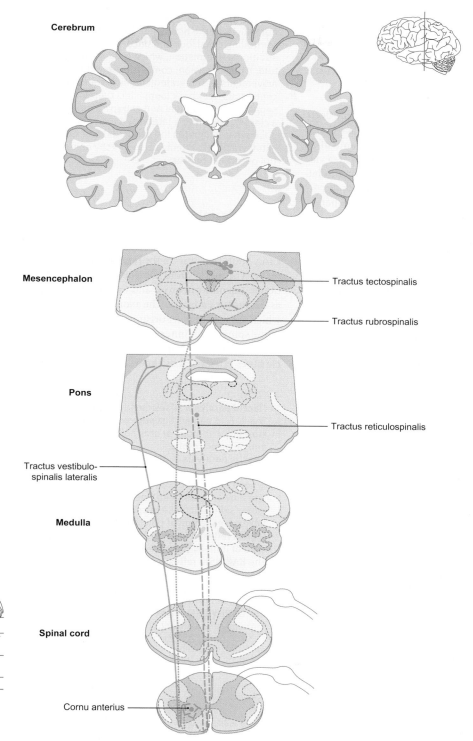

Cerebrum

Mesencephalon — Tractus tectospinalis

Tractus rubrospinalis

Pons — Tractus reticulospinalis

Tractus vestibulo-spinalis lateralis

Medulla

Spinal cord

Cornu anterius

Fig. 13.5 Extrapyramidal system. [L127]

function). Like the corticospinal tracts, the rubrospinal tract belongs to the **lateral system** and, located laterally in the Cornu anterius via the motorneurons, predominantly innervates the distal muscles, particularly those of the upper extremity, and supports movement patterns of the arms and hands.

Cortex

The areas of the motor cortex influence the extrapyramidal system directly or indirectly via the innervation of the basal ganglia (**Tractus corticostriatalis**, striatum and pallidum), which then regulate the neuronal activity of the Formatio reticularis, the tectum (Col-

liculi superiores) or the Nucleus ruber via the cerebellum or the Substantia nigra. The Tractus corticospinalis also has collaterals, which directly innervate the Substantia nigra and the respective extrapyramidal nuclei in the brainstem.

Tractus reticulospinalis, Fibrae reticulospinales
The Tractus reticulospinalis has its starting point in the Formatio reticularis of the pons and Medulla oblongata respectively. Therefore, a distinction is made between the **Tractus pontoreticulospinalis** (origin in the pons) and the **Tractus bulboreticulospinalis** (origin in the Formatio reticularis of the Medulla oblongata). The

former runs uncrossed in the anterior column of the spinal cord, the latter is found crossed and uncrossed in the lateral column. These fibre systems innervate α- and γ-motorneurons in the anterior horn of the spinal cord directly or indirectly and coordinate posture and movement through the integration of cortical and sensory signals.

Tractus tectospinalis

The fibres of the Tractus tectospinalis have their origin in the deep layers of the **Colliculus superior** of the quadrigeminal plate (Lamina tecti), run on the contralateral side in the anterior column of the spinal cord and innervate the motorneurons in the throat area via interneurons. In this way, they convey stimulation of the contralateral neck muscles and inhibition of the ipsilateral neck muscles – and control the movement reflexes of head and neck (e.g., when turning the head to look at something).

Tractus vestibulospinalis

The Tractus vestibulospinalis can be further divided into a Tractus vestibulospinalis lateralis and a Tractus vestibulospinalis medialis:

- The **Tractus vestibulospinalis lateralis** originates from neurons of the Nucleus vestibularis lateralis. Its fibres run uncrossed up into the lumbosacral spinal cord. The stimuli which are forwarded here are for the conveying of position and balance information of particular importance. There is a very close connection to the cerebellum via cerebellar afferents, which reach the Nucleus vestibularis lateralis. Unlike in the case of the pyramidal tract or the Tractus rubrospinalis, α- and γ-motorneurons are stimulated or inhibited in such a way that the extensors are tensed and the flexors relaxed.
- The fibres of the **Tractus vestibularis medialis** originate from the Nucleus vestibularis medialis and run ipsilaterally and contralaterally up into the thoracic spinal cord.

Tractus rubrospinalis

Emerging from the Nucleus ruber in the mesencephalon, the Tractus rubrospinalis runs somatotopically divided into the spinal cord. It crosses onto the opposite side (**Decussatio tegmentalis ventralis**, ventral tegmental decussation), is connected via further dispersed tract systems associated with other areas of the brain (e.g., cerebellum, cranial nerve nuclei) and then runs in the spinal cord in the Funiculus lateralis. The tracts also end directly or indirectly at α- and γ-motorneurons. They have a stimulatory effect on flexors and inhibit extensors.

13.1.3 Peripheral section

The above-mentioned descending motor systems innervate the α- and γ-motorneurons in the brainstem and spinal cord mainly indirectly (via interneurons), but also directly. This synaptic connection to the motorneurons and their efferents are grouped together as the **motor endplate**. The axons of the respective motorneurons, which are functionally organised in columns in the Cornu anterius of the spinal cord, innervate the striated skeletal muscles (➤ Fig. 13.6). The anterior horn cell, the corresponding axon and the muscle fibres innervated by them form the **motor unit**.

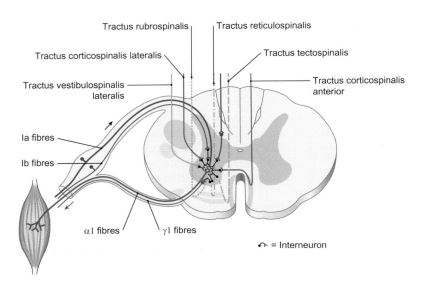

Tractus rubrospinalis
Tractus reticulospinalis
Tractus corticospinalis lateralis
Tractus tectospinalis
Tractus vestibulospinalis lateralis
Tractus corticospinalis anterior
Ia fibres
Ib fibres
α1 fibres
γ1 fibres
↷ = Interneuron

Fig. 13.6 Motor endplate and motor unit. α- and γ-motorneurons in the spinal cord are innervated – usually via interneurons – by fibre tracts of the pyramidal and extrapyramidal systems. Individual motorneurons, their axons and the muscle fibres innervated by them are referred to as a motor unit. Via afferent fibres, motorneurons also receive information from the relevant muscle fibres (e.g., about stretch receptors). [L127]

Examination

In the framework of a neurological examination, the functionality of the motor system is examined in particular by looking at muscle tone, muscle strength and reflex status. In addition, loss of muscle mass is noted as well as involuntary muscle contractions (fasciculations, possibly tics) or muscle contractions (myoclonus).

- **Muscle tone** in a relaxed patient is explored via passive movement of the extremities. In the process, possible pathological changes can arise such as, e.g., *spasticity* (cramp-like increased muscle tone), *rigor* (increase of muscle tone with abrupt, staccato movements, cogwheel phenomenon) or, in the case of complete or incomplete *paresis* (paralysis), *hypotonia* or *atonia* (reduced or absent muscle tone).
- **Muscle strength** is determined by the resistance of a muscle or a whole muscle group against tension provided by the examiner and can be evaluated on a scale of 1 to 5. Latent paralysis in the extremities can also be determined by holding up the arms or legs for approximately 20 seconds, because the affected limb will then drop.
- **Monosynaptic or polysynaptic reflexes,** which cause uncontrollable muscle contractions upon stimulus, give additional information on possible impairment of motor control circuits. For example, in case of damage to the tracts before the motor neuron of the spinal cord (e.g., pyramidal tract system), monosynaptic reflexes are increased by activity of the extrapyramidal system; in contrast, polysynaptic reflexes, which are relayed via several segments, often decrease or are lost.

Important diseases of the somatomotor system

As far as they affect motorneurons, neurodegenerative diseases are differentiated in the English language into **'upper motor neuron disease'** and **'lower motor neuron disease':**

- If the 1st motor neuron in the motor cortex or the axon of this neuron is affected, it gives a predominant clinical picture of a flaccid paralysis (e.g., stroke, multiple sclerosis, traumatic brain injury). It should be noted that in the case of isolated lesions of the 1st motor neuron (e.g., due to local cortical infarction in the Lobus precentralis), flaccid paralysis ensues.
- If the 2nd motor neuron is affected, flaccid paralysis results (e.g., in the case of **polio, GUILLAIN–BARRÉ syndrome** or damage to a plexus or a peripheral nerve.)

However, there are also motor neuron diseases in which both motorneurons are affected (e.g., **amyotrophic lateral sclerosis,** which can present as a combination of spastic and flaccid paralysis). In addition, diseases in areas of the brain that are involved in motor function can lead to motor neuron diseases. These include in particular the cerebellum (➤ Chap. 12.4) and the basal ganglia (➤ Chap. 12.1.8), which are centrally involved in the symptoms of **PARKINSON's disease, HUNTINGTON's disease** and **hemiballism.**

13.1.4 Execution of voluntary movements

The anatomical structures depicted work closely together during the execution of voluntary movements. In the process, movement execution is theoretically mapped in a series of processes that are localised in different areas of the brain. The **stimulus** for movement originates in the limbic system; the **planning** then takes place in the prefrontal cortex and in the association cortex. This stimulus is subsequently passed on to the premotor cortex and supplementary motor cortex. Here, the first planned movements will now be **programmed.** Finally, the stimulus reaches the primary motor cortex, which **executes** movement. Parallel to these stations, the cerebellar hemispheres and basal ganglia in particular are integrated within a 'feedback loop' into the processes in order to consistently control the movement, e.g., in intensity and orientation. With each activation of the pyramidal tracts, the extrapyramidal system is also involved and thus, with simultaneous activation of various fibres, executes a movement via motorneurons in the spinal cord. The movement to be executed is, due to constant somatosensory information (e.g., muscle tone, joint position) being fed to the various functional brain centres, and is further controlled, refined and corrected during its sequence (➤ Fig. 13.7).

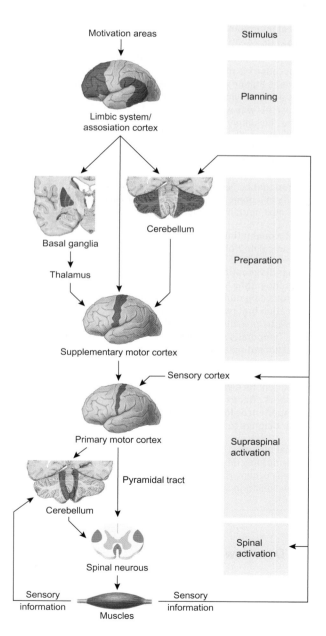

Fig. 13.7 Planning and execution of voluntary movements. [L127]

13.2 Somatosensory system
Anja Böckers

Clinical case

Cortical infarction

Medical history
A 45-year-old man (right-handed) presents at a medical practice because his right arm 'had gone missing'. When asked, he describes that he woke up in the morning and thought that his wife's arm was lying across his chest. This was actually unlikely because his wife was lying with her face away from him. Nonetheless, he simply moved the arm away and was able to get back to sleep. About one hour later he woke up again and found his way in semi-darkness to the bathroom. He was however not able to find the door handle to the bathroom by feeling for it. He noticed that his arm felt as if it didn't belong to him and that he no longer had a sense of touch. He then called his wife in a panic and found that his speech was slurred. Within the next hour, however, the symptoms all disappeared.

Initial examination
The clinical neurological examination is completely normal.

Further diagnostics
Ultrasonography and an MRI show a dissection of the left A. carotis communis artery with a thrombotic occlusion of the bifurcation that reaches into the left A. carotis interna. In the follow-up, an acute myocardial infarction in the cortical area of the Temporalis superior (dorsal section) is detected. ECG and echocardiography are normal.

Treatment and follow-up
The patient receives thrombolytic medication (heparin). Several months after experiencing the acute symptoms, he still often experiences for brief moments the feeling that his arm no longer belongs to him.

Clinical picture
The symptoms described are referred to as **asomatognosia**. It typically occurs in the event of malfunctions in the somatosensory association areas, especially in the parietal lobes.

13.2.1 Overview

The somatosensory system serves the purpose of receiving, forwarding and processing sensations from the body's surface area (skin) and from the interior of the body (deep sensitivity). Exteroceptors of the skin detect mechanical, thermal and pain stimuli (nociception). In addition, there are special receptors and tract systems for **proprioception** (Latin 'proprius' = own), self-awareness of the body. Here, a distinction is made between **exteroceptive** per-

ception of the body's surface area and **interoceptive** perception from the interior of the body. Depending on the type of sensory quality, reference is made to the:
- **spinothalamic system** for perception of pain and temperature (formerly also **the protopathic** system)
- **posterior funiculus system** (formerly **epicritic system**) for the mechanical perception of touch, pressure and vibration sensations, but also for a small part of proprioception
- **spinocerebellar system** for a main part of proprioceptive impulse conduction

These sensory perceptions are conducted to the cortex either via the **spinal afferent system** (➤ Chap. 12.6.5) or from the head area via the **trigeminal afferent system**.

13.2.2 Peripheral section

A somatosensory irritation of the skin leads to the stimulus of various **cutaneous mechanoreceptors,** where a distinction is made between free and corpuscular nerve endings according to their morphology:
- Via **free nerve endings** of Aδ- or C-fibres, different sensory qualities such as pressure, pain, temperature or itchiness are conveyed. *Temperature sensation* takes place via 2 types of thermal sensors, which are distributed in various densities in the skin and usually exhibit a maximum activity at cold (25°C) or warm (34–45°C) temperatures. *Nociception* is served by other free nerve endings that react to mechanical stimuli, but also to polymodal stimuli (mechanically, chemically, thermally). *Itchiness* is again perceived via its own group of 'itchiness' receptors in the skin.
- **Corpuscular nerve endings** conduct sensations of touch in the narrower sense (epicritical sensitivity) via fast Aβ fibres. On the one hand, these mechanoreceptors are located in the superficial layers of hairless skin (MERKEL nerve endings and MEISSNER's corpuscles) or in deeper layers of the dermis (VATER–PACINI corpuscles and RUFFINI nerve endings) and form mainly an action potential. Depending on the type of mechanosensor and the location of the cutaneous area, these sensors vary in their density distribution, resulting in differently sized receptive fields. These have, e.g., an average size of 1–2 mm on the finger pad, but 40 mm on the thigh.

Also included amongst the sensors of proprioception are the muscle spindles, GOLGI tendon organs and afferents from the joints, which convey the impulses of deep sensitivity and sense of location.

13.2.3 Central section

Overview
From each respective sensation-specific receptor, the fibres run via a pseudounipolar 1st neuron, the perikaryon of which is located in the spinal ganglion or in the Ganglion trigeminale, centripetally (➤ Table 13.3). Via different funiculi of the spinal cord, the central redirection reaches the thalamus and finally the primary somatosensory cortex in the Lobus parietalis (➤ Table 13.3). Here, sensations are consciously perceived. Assigned to the primary function cortex are BRODMANN areas 1, 2, as well as 3a and b. Typically, the primary somatosenory cortex is structured somatopically so that the image of an inverted sensory homunculus emerges, based on the size of the receptive fields. (➤ Fig. 13.8). Since efferents radiate into other cortical areas in turn from the primary somatosensory cortex, these areas should not be understood as nerve endings of the somatosensory system areas, but as a switching point in a neu-

Table 13.3 Somatosensory system.

Neuronal chain	Localisation
1st neuron	Perikarya of pseudounipolar ganglion cells in the Ganglion spinale or Ganglion trigeminale
2nd neuron	In the Cornu posterius
	In the Nucleus cuneatus or Nucleus gracilis of the Medulla oblongata
	In the Nucleus dorsalis
	Or in the Nucleus spinalis nervi trigemini
3rd neuron	Perikarya in the contralateral Nucleus ventralis posterolateralis of the thalamus
4th neuron	Primary somatosensory cortex: Gyrus postcentralis and Lobulus paracentralis
5th neuron	Secondary somatosensory cortex: Operculum parietale

ronal circuit, which, e.g., has influence on motor function via projections in the pyramidal tract. In addition, some of the efferents project respectively into the secondary somatosensory cortex in the area of the Operculum parietale or into the somatosensory association cortex (BRODMANN areas 5 and 7) for an interpretive allocation of the perceived sensations. Here, amongst others, vestibular impulses also converge, which determine sensory information.

Spinal afferent system
Assigned to the spinal afferent system are the **posterior funiculus system**, the **spinothalamic (anterolateral) system** and the **spinocerebellar system** (➤ Fig. 13.8, ➤ Fig. 13.9) which respectively conduct sensations from the upper and lower extremity or from the torso. Sensations from the head area are not conveyed via spinal nerves or the spinal afferent system, but via cranial nerves, especially via the trigeminal afferent system (see below).

Posterior funiculus system
The posterior funiculus system (formerly: epicritic system) is located in the **Funiculus posterior** of the spinal cord. The sensory qualities transferred here firstly include sensations like pressure and vibrations from the skin and the skin's sensitivity to touch. A failure of the posterior funiculus tracts, however, causes surprisingly few deficiencies for patients, probably because some mechanosensitivity is also conveyed via the anterolateral system. Typically, patients have difficulties in tactile recognition of numbers or letters that are drawn on the skin.

--- Clinical remarks ---

In the context of a **neurological examination,** functionality of the posterior funiculus system can be tested by comparing the touch sensitivity of a cutaneous area with the corresponding unaffected half of the body. Another possibility is a comparison of touch sensitivity between proximal and distal extremities. Orientation is roughly possible through touching with a cotton ball with closed eyes. A second, more precise method, which also enables a comparison with set values, is **two point discrimination.** In this case, one calculates the minimum distance between 2 stimulus points, in which the patient still perceives 2 separate sensation stimuli (normal value at the fingertip 3–5 mm).

In the same way, **vibration perception (pallaesthesia)** can be checked by setting off a tuning fork (128 Hz), and then setting the base of the tuning fork onto bone protuberances (e.g., Proc. styloideus or Malleolus medialis) and the patient states when s/he can no longer feel any vibrations. At this moment, the current value on the tuning fork is taken on a scale from 0 to 8.

To check the **sense of location (proprioception),** the toes or ankles of the patient are held from the side and flexed or extended lightly, with the patient stating the direction of movement of the toe or ankle with closed eyes.

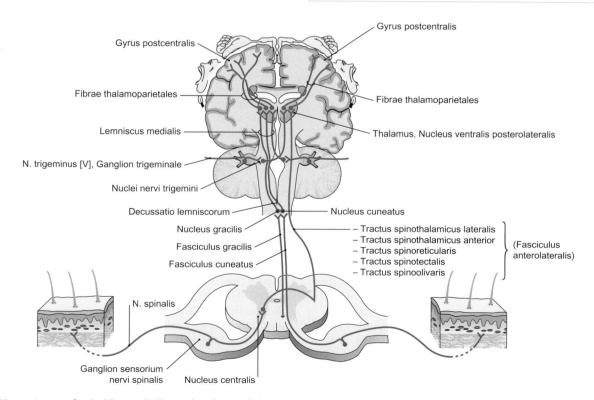

Fig. 13.8 Management of epicritic sensibility and pathway of the posterior funiculus system (blue), the spinal afferent system and the trigeminal afferent system. Management of pain/temperature and pathway of the neospinal thalamic system (green) as well as of the spinal and trigeminal afferent systems.

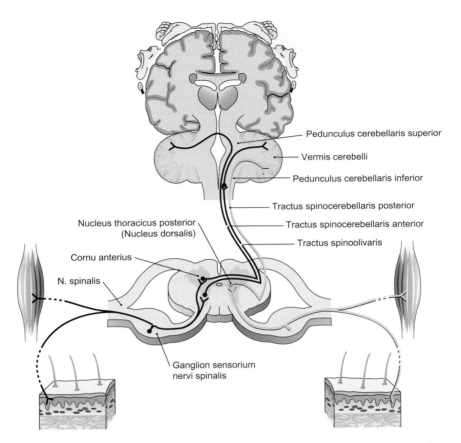

Pedunculus cerebellaris superior

Vermis cerebelli

Pedunculus cerebellaris inferior

Tractus spinocerebellaris posterior

Tractus spinocerebellaris anterior

Tractus spinoolivaris

Nucleus thoracicus posterior (Nucleus dorsalis)

Cornu anterius

N. spinalis

Ganglion sensorium nervi spinalis

Fig. 13.9 Management of subconscious proprioception (afferent vascular, lymphatic and nervous systems). Anterior spinocerebellar tract (Tractus spinocerebellaris anterior, black) and posterior cerebellar tract (Tractus spinocerebellaris posterior, yellow).

Proprioception from inside the body – from muscle, tendon and joint receptors – is also transmitted in the posterior funiculus in order to provide information on the body's position in the sense of proprioception. Impulses of mechanoreceptors are routed to the spinal cord via the fast conducting Aβ fibres. Mono- and polysynaptic reflexes are connected via intersegmental collaterals in the propriospinal system (➤ Chap. 12.6.7); the majority of the fibres, however, run without being switched in the ipsilateral posterior funiculus (➤ Chap. 12.6.5). Both tracts do not cross in the spinal cord, but only after their ipsilateral switching in the **Nuclei gracilis and cuneatus** of the Medulla oblongata as the **Fibrae arcuatae internae** (➤ Fig. 13.10). At this intersection point (**Decussatio lemnisci medialis),** as well as within the **Lemniscus medialis (medial lemniscus)** itself, somatotopy always remains in the thalamic nuclei and in the primary somatosensory cortical area (Gyrus postcentralis of the parietal lobe). In the Decussatio, fibre bundles of the lower extremity are located ventrally to those of the upper extremity. In the pons, the fibres of the Lemniscus medialis rotate by 90°, so that the fibres of the lower extremity come to lie laterally and those of the upper extremity to lie medially. The axons of the 2nd neuron, as the **Tractus bulbothalamicus,** reach the 3rd neuron behind the posterior funiculus tract, the **Nucleus ventralis posterolateralis** in the thalamus. The axons of this neuron run as thalamocortical fibres (Fibrae thalamoparietales) through the Crus posterior of the Capsula interna and make the connection to the cortex. While the primary somatosensory cortex only receives impulses from the contralateral half of the body, the secondary somatosensory cortex (BRODMANN areas 5 and 7) also receive bilateral impulses.

Spinothalamic system

The spinothalamic system (formerly: protopathic system, ➤ Chap. 12.6.5) can be divided into a paleospinothalamic and a **neospinothalamic system**. Both systems are essential for pain perception. At this point, only the neospinothalamic system will be considered, while all the fibres relevant for pain perception and processing as a whole are illustrated in ➤ Chap. 13.8.

Rough pressure and touch sensations (mechanosensory functions) are conducted to this tract system via weakly myelinated Aδ and C fibres, as are pain perception (nociception) and temperature. The perikaryon of the **1st neuron** of this tract system is located, as in the posterior funiculus system, in the spinal ganglion (➤ Fig. 13.8) or in the Ganglion trigeminale. The centrally-directed axon reaches the spinal cord also via the Radix posterior, where in the Cornu posterius – particularly in laminae I and II – it is converted directly or conducted via interneurons to funiculus cells (**2nd neuron**). Already at this first conversion point, pain perception can be increased or inhibited (➤ Chap. 13.8). In the **LISSAUER's tract (Tractus posterolateralis)** these axons give off collaterals to the respective cranially and caudally located segments. The axonal fibres of the 2nd neuron finally cross to the opposite side at the same segment height in the **Commissura alba anterior,** so that in the Funiculus lateralis they reach as the Tractus spinothalamicus without further switching and after adhering to the **Lemniscus medialis,** the **3rd neuron** in the thalamus (**Nucleus ventralis posterolateralis**) (➤ Fig. 13.8, ➤ Chap. 13.8).

The **Tractus spinothalamicus** consists of a lateral and an anterior tract (➤ Chap. 12.6.5). They differ not only in their location and size, but also in their general function:

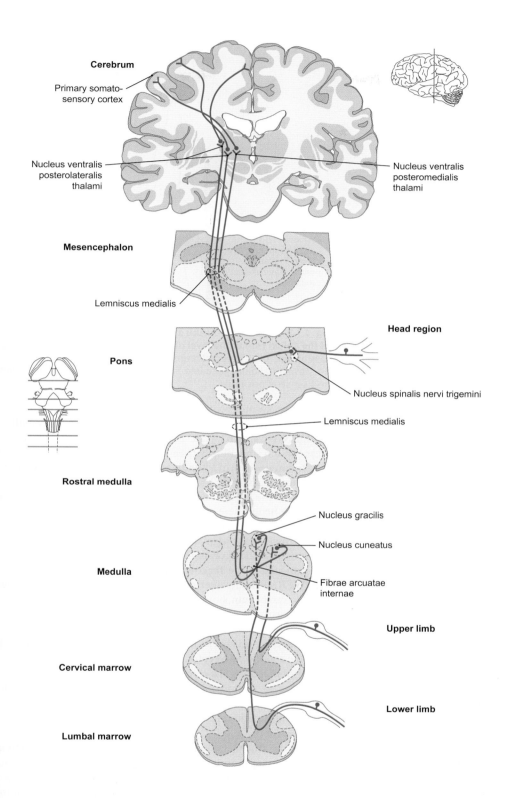

Cerebrum

Primary somato-
sensory cortex

Nucleus ventralis
posterolateralis
thalami

Nucleus ventralis
posteromedialis
thalami

Mesencephalon

Lemniscus medialis

Head region

Pons

Nucleus spinalis nervi trigemini

Lemniscus medialis

Rostral medulla

Nucleus gracilis

Nucleus cuneatus

Medulla

Fibrae arcuatae
internae

Upper limb

Cervical marrow

Lower limb

Lumbal marrow

**Fig. 13.10 Epicritic sensitivity
of the spinal afferent posterior
funiculus system and/or for the
head area of the trigeminal
afferent system.** [L127]

- The **lateral tract** contains primarily axons of the projection neurons of lamina I and conducts the impulses for pain perceived as quick and sharp and for the perception of temperature.
- The **anterior tract**, in contrast, preferentially leads the axons of the projection neurons from lamina V and, correspondingly, the impulses for pain perceived as slow and dull as well as crude mechanosensory functions. Its fibres can run crossed as well as uncrossed. Due to these polymodal receptor impulses in the Tractus spinothalamicus anterior, it also conducts impulses of minimally discriminating mechanosensory functions (which are

usually conducted via the posterior funiculi) so that a failure of the posterior funiculi can be well compensated clinically.

After switching over in the thalamus, a majority of the fibres of the spinothalamic system reach the **primary somatosensory cortex** via the Capsula interna. Many fibres, however, also end at **subcortical nuclei,** which undertake a significant function in pain processing (➤ Chap. 13.8). This is particularly true for fibres of the anterior tract and of the smaller tract systems, the Tractus spinoreticularis and spinotectalis, which end at the Formatio reticularis or the Tectum mesencephali of the brainstem. At this point, these are usually axons from the projection neurons of the laminae VII and VIII, which run uncrossed and end at the medial and intralaminar thalamic nuclei.

Spinocerebellar system

Proprioception (deep sensitivity) comprises the sense of position, movement and power of the body. While consciously perceived proprioception is conducted via the posterior funiculus tracts (see above), essential unconscious proprioception for movement processes run via the spinocerebellar systems, which constitute decisive afferent fibre tracts to the cerebellum. The impulses of proprioceptors of the lower extremity are conducted via the anterior and posterior spinocerebellar tracts (**Tractus spinocerebellares anterior [GOWER] and posterior [FLECHSIG]**), while those of the upper extremity reach the spinocerebellum via the **Fibrae cuneocerebellares** and the superior spinocerebellar tract (**Tractus spinocerebellaris superior**).

Even in this ascending tract system, pseudounipolar perikarya of the **1st neuron** in the spinal ganglia can be found. Their centrally-directed axons run via the Radix posterior into the posterior horn and axonal collaterals reach the adjoining spinal cord segments in the posterior funiculus. However, the main mass of the

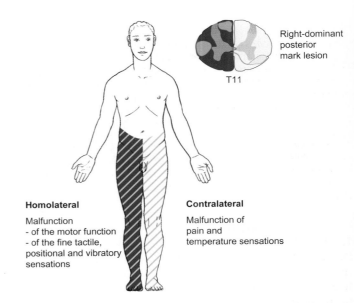

Right-dominant posterior mark lesion

T11

Homolateral

Malfunction
- of the motor function
- of the fine tactile, positional and vibratory sensations

Contralateral

Malfunction of pain and temperature sensations

Fig. 13.11 BROWN-SÉQUARD syndrome in the case of hemisection of the spinal cord at the level of Th11 with consecutive hemiplegia, loss of sensitivity to temperature and pain on the contralateral side and ipsilateral damage to fine haptic sensitivity, vibration sensation and sense of position.

fibres form synapses with tract cells in lamina VII (according to REXED), which as a whole form the columnar **Nucleus dorsalis STILLING–CLARKE** (syn.: Nucleus thoracicus posterior), a nuclear column stretching between segments T1 and L2. The axons of this **2nd neuron** form a bundle at the **Tractus spinocerebellaris posterior (FLECHSIG)**, which runs ipsilaterally in the lateral funiculus via the Pedunculus cerebellaris inferior into the equilateral cerebellar hemisphere.

Another part of the fibres is switched in laminae V–VII, but already crosses at the segmental level to the opposite side via the Commissura alba in order to run cranially in the contralateral lateral funiculus as the **Tractus spinocerebellaris anterior (GOWER)**. Prior to entering via the superior cerebellar peduncle into the cerebellum, however, these fibres cross a second time ('double crosser'), so that they ultimately end as mossy fibres in the ipsilateral cerebellar hemisphere as well.

Both tracts are divided somatotopically, but they differ in the quality of the conducted receptor impulses and their function: via the posterior funiculus, the cerebellum receives impulses for the control of the interaction of individual muscle groups of a limb, while the anterior tract (with larger receptive fields and therefore more general information) has more influence on the motor activity of a complete limb.

As with the Tractus spinocerebellaris anterior for the lower extremity, a **Tractus spinocerebellaris anterior** can be delineated for the upper extremity, of which the 2nd neurons lie in the inferior 4 neck segments and whose axons run via both cerebellar peduncles into the cerebellum. The equivalent to the posterior cerebellar lateral tract for the upper extremity are the **Fibrae cuneocerebellares.** Their afferents also run ipsilaterally in the posterior funiculus and in the Medulla oblongata, reaching the **Nucleus cuneatus accessorius (MONAKOW)**, where they, after conversion into the 2nd neuron as the **Fibrae arcuatae externae posteriores**, reach the ipsilateral vermal and paravermal cerebellar areas via the superior cerebellar peduncle.

In addition to these direct spinal projection fibres into the cerebellum, there are also **indirect proprioceptive tract systems,** which run, e.g., via the inferior olivary bodies into the cerebellum (➤ Fig. 13.10).

Trigeminal afferent system

Sensory information from the head area is not conducted via the spinal cord, but rather via afferent fibres of 4 cranial nerves. Exteroceptive somatosensitivity of the skin is primarily conveyed via the N. trigeminus [V], while the N. facialis [VII], the N. glossopharyngeus [IX] and the N. vagus [X] preferentially convey visceral sensitivity.

Sense of touch

The perikarya of the 1st neuron do not lie correspondingly in the spinal ganglion, but in the **Ganglion trigeminale (GASSERI)** (➤ Fig. 13.10). The centripetally directed axon reaches the Pons nucleus of the N. trigeminus, the **Nucleus principalis nervi trigemini.** The axons of the 2nd neuron then run either crossed in the **Tractus trigeminothalamicus anterior** or uncrossed in the **Tractus trigeminothalamicus posterior** to the thalamus. Both together form the **Lemniscus trigeminalis,** which adheres to the Lemniscus medialis and finally reaches the **Nucleus ventralis posteromedialis.** There, a conversion onto the 3rd neuron takes place, the fibres of which also reach the Gyrus postcentralis via the Capsula interna.

Proprioception

The conduction of proprioceptive afferents from the mastication muscles is an exception: the perikarya of these pseudounipolar neurons are *not* typically located in the Ganglion trigeminale. Rather, these fibres directly reach the **Nucleus mesencephalicus nervi trigemini** via the Radix motoria in the CNS so that we can also refer to a single, centrally-located ganglion of the body. Via the efferents, which run from the Nucleus mesencephalicus to the Nucleus motorius nervi trigemini, the muscles of mastication are managed reflexively, which is necessary, e.g., for an appropriate level of power when biting down.

Pain and temperature sensation

The afferent fibres also reach the Ganglion trigeminale (1st neuron), to then reach the Pars caudalis of the **Nucleus spinalis nervi trigemini** (2nd neuron), which, in principle, corresponds to the posterior horn structure of the spinal cord. This nucleus stretches as an elongated nuclear column from the superior cervical medulla up into the caudal sections of the pons and is divided somatotopically. After switching, the fibres run crossed as an attachment to the Tractus spinothalamicus and analogically reach the epicritic sensitivity of the 3rd neuron in the **Nucleus ventralis posteromedialis** of the thalamus, in order to finally end in the Gyrus postcentralis. Trigeminal cerebellar fibres can also be specified, originating from all 3 somatoafferent trigeminal nuclei and, as mossy fibres, reach the ipsilateral spinocerebellum via the superior and inferior cerebellar peduncles.

Somatosensory cortex

In the periphery, various sensory modalities are perceived by different receptors and are forwarded in the CNS via separated tract systems. Functionally, the cortex undertakes the integration of these sensations in order to develop a coherent perception. The **primary somatosensory cortex** comprises BRODMANN areas 1, 2 and 3a and b in the Gyrus postcentralis of the parietal lobe. Here, too, a separation of the modality specific projections from the ventrobasal thalamus can be detected, whereby mechanoafferents of the sense of touch primarily project into lamina IV of BRODMANN areas 1 and 3b; in contrast, proprioceptive afferents project into BRODMANN areas 2 and 3a instead, as well as temperature and pain perception into BRODMANN area 3. Especially in BRODMANN area 2, various sensation modalities converge onto a nerve cell column. Corresponding to the size of the peripheral receptive fields, the image of a sensory homunculus is formed in the primary somatosensory cortex, whereby the cortical receptive fields are larger than those of the peripheral receptor due to divergence and convergence configurations. In addition, the cortical receptive fields can also expand or reorganise themselves through learning procedures and frequently repeated movement processes. In extreme cases proprioception can be affected in the process, and motor function can fail in the affected area of the body. For exam-

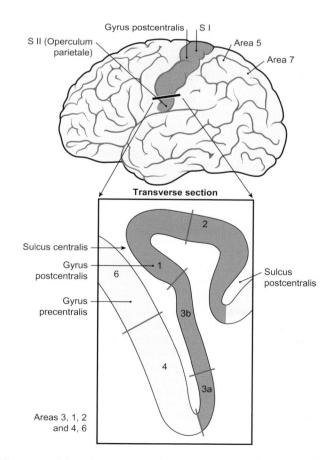

Fig. 13.12 Primary somatosensory cortical field (SI: BRODMANN areas 3, 1, 2), secondary somatosensory cortical area in the Operculum parietale (SII) and somatosensory association cortex (BRODMANN areas 5 and 7) of the Lobus parietalis. [L126]

ple, in 14–16% of professional musicians, focal dystonia (movement disorder) of the fingers occurs, in which involuntary, sustained contractions lead to a malfunction.

Via mechanisms that have not yet been definitively researched, a subjective sensory perception also occurs in the primary somatosensory cortex in addition to the primary perception of sensations. However, the main interpretation of somatosensory information first follows in the **secondary somatosensory cortex,** a small area at the Sulcus lateralis (Fissura SYLVII), the Operculum parietale (➤ Fig. 13.12). Here – connected via the Corpus callosum – stimulus impulses from both halves of the body also converge. A lesion of this area can lead to the loss of the ability to recognise objects by feeling them (tactile agnosia).

Efferent projections run from the secondary somatosensory cortex, on the one hand, into the **somatosensory association fields** (postparietal cortex, BRODMANN areas 5 and 7), and on the other hand, also to the island area and to the limbic system. In the association fields, visual stimuli are linked with the somatosensory stimuli or they exert influence over motor control via efferent fibres of the precentral area.

An intact sense of touch and proprioception is essential in early childhood development for the correct development of motor skills such as walking or grasping. It has moreover also been shown that tactile stimuli are decisive for healthy development of communication and social skills.

13.3 Visual system
Michael J. Schmeißer

Skills

After working through this chapter of the textbook, you should be able to:
- list the anatomical structures of the visual tract, including neuronal configuration in the correct order and, according to the localisation of a visual tract injury, describe their clinical consequences
- list the anatomical structures of the pupil and accommodation reflexes, each with their neuronal configuration in the correct order, and describe the clinical consequences for each after a localised injury
- name the supranuclear centres for the control of oculomotor function as well as explaining possible causes and clinical consequences of horizontal and vertical ocular pareses

---

Clinical case

Neuritis nervi optici
Medical history
A 25-year-old female student presents at a walk-in centre of the university eye clinic. She is currently studying for an exam and for a couple of days when reading her textbooks has had the impression that vision in her left, but not right, eye has been blurry. Similar symptoms had already emerged a year ago – even if somewhat less pronounced – and went away of their own accord. When asked, she denies having headaches or double vision.

Initial examination
The doctor's ocular examination is normal apart from slight pain when moving the left eyeball.

Further diagnostics
After an EEG of visual evoked potentials (VEP) for determining that the sensory stimuli conduction falls within the optic tract, a significant delay in nerve conduction velocity is detected after stimulation of the left eye.

Diagnosis
Due to the left-sided blurred vision and the pathological VEP findings with delay of nerve conduction velocity within the optic tract, a diagnosis of Neuritis nervi optici is made, which has probably occurred repeatedly.

Treatment and further steps
Over 3 days, the patient receives 1 g of methylprednisolone per day given intravenously. Since Neuritis nervi optici – especially occurring repeatedly and in young patients – can be an indication of multiple sclerosis, an MRI examination of the entire CNS and a lumbar puncture are carried out on the patient in order to rule out typical MS findings.

13.3.1 Optic tract

The optic tract is an afferent system of the CNS, which serves the purpose of conveying optical impressions to the consciousness. The tract has no peripheral section, but starts in the **retina** and ends in the **visual cortex** in the occipital lobes of the cerebrum.

NOTE
Depending on whether the first neuron is a cone or a rod, the neuronal chain of the optic tract consists of 4 (cone) or 5 (rod) cells. The first 3 or 4 neurons are thereby located within the retina; the respective 4th or 5th neuron lies in the Corpus geniculatum laterale (CGL) of the diencephalon.

Retina
On the retina (Tunica interna bulbi, ➤ Chap. 9.4.4) an image is formed of the part of the environment which is perceived with the stationary eye, the visual field. The largest part of the visual field is identical in both eyes; only a small, outer part of the visual field can be perceived by each respective eye. The imaging of the visual field on the retina is mirror inverted and upside-down.

The retina contains the first 3 or 4 neurons of the optic tract (➤ Fig. 13.13):
- 1st neuron: **photoreceptor cell** (cone or rod)
- 2nd neuron: **bipolar cell** (follows both cones and rods)
- 3rd neuron of the cone bipolars: **ganglion cell**
- 3rd/4th neuron of the rod bipolars: **amacrine cell/ganglion cell**

In the ganglion cells, a distinction is made between **magnocellular** and **parvocellular** neurons according to their size, forming the **M-** or the **P-system** respectively. The M-system is responsible for recognition of movements; the P-system for recognition of colours and shapes.

Pathway of the optic tract
N. opticus
The 3rd and 4th neuron of the optic tract have a relatively long process, which runs initially in the N. opticus [II]. This cranial nerve is formed from the merging of all the axons of the retinal ganglion cells, runs through the orbita and after entry into the middle cranial fossa, and merges with the N. opticus of the opposite side to the Chiasma opticum (➤ Chap. 9.3.2, ➤ Chap. 12.5.5).

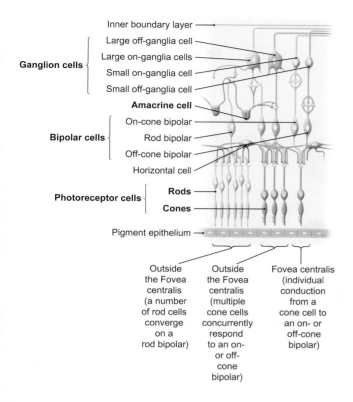

Ganglion cells
- Inner boundary layer
- Large off-ganglia cell
- Large on-ganglia cells
- Small on-ganglia cell
- Small off-ganglia cell

Amacrine cell

Bipolar cells
- On-cone bipolar
- Rod bipolar
- Off-cone bipolar
- Horizontal cell

Photoreceptor cells
- **Rods**
- **Cones**

Pigment epithelium

| Outside the Fovea centralis (a number of rod cells converge on a rod bipolar) | Outside the Fovea centralis (multiple cone cells concurrently respond to an on- or off-cone bipolar) | Fovea centralis (individual conduction from a cone cell to an on- or off-cone bipolar) |

Fig. 13.13 Neuronal configuration of the retina.

Chiasma opticum

In the Chiasma opticum, approximately half of all fibres running in the optic nerve cross to the opposite side. In this case, these are fibres from the nasal halves of the retina (which map the temporal visual fields) – the fibres from the temporal half of the retina do not cross. Clinically important are the narrow topographic relationships of the Chiasma opticum to the pituitary gland, which is located below the chiasma, as well as to the A. carotis interna, which is respectively located laterally of the chiasma.

Tractus opticus

Running in the Tractus opticus, which passes the Crura cerebri of the mesencephalon anterolaterally, are the fibres of the temporal half of the retina that originate from the ipsilateral eye, as well as the fibres of the nasal half of the retina that originate from the contralateral eye. Each Tractus opticus therefore receives the fibres of the corresponding halves of the retina – the right tractus receives the fibres of the right halves of the retinas of both eyes and thus information from the left visual field; the left tractus receives fibres of the left halves of the retinas of both eyes and thus information from the right visual field. The majority of the fibres end respectively as the Radix lateralis in the CGL of the thalamus; the minority, **extrageniculate projections,** however, branch off beforehand. These include, e.g., the retinohypothalamic projection, which extends to the Nucleus suprachiasmaticus of the thalamus and is thus involved in the regulation of day-night rhythm; or the Radix medialis, which runs via the Brachium colliculi superioris to the Colliculus superior and to the Area pretectalis of the mesencephalon and is thus integrated into visual reflexes and into ocular motor function.

Corpus geniculatum laterale

The extension of the 3rd/4th neuron ends in the Corpus geniculatum laterale (CGL) as does the switch-over to the 4th/5th neuron of the optic tract, and it is called a **geniculocortical projection neuron.** The CGL is structured in 6 layers whereby the neurons of the first two layers are particularly large and belong to the M-system. The neurons of layers 3–6 are rather small and belong functionally to the P-system. Due to the pathway of the fibres of the retinal axons in the Tractus opticus, the CGL receives visual information from each respective contralateral visual field.

Radiatio optica

The axon of the 4th/5th neuron of the optical tract runs in the Radiatio optica or GRATIOLET's optic radiation, which runs initially in the temporal lobes and subsequently via the rear part of the Crus posterius (Pars retrolenticularis) of the Capsula interna up into the occipital lobes.

Visual Cortex

The geniculocortical fibres finally end in the primary visual cortex (BRODMANN area 17). This is located at the occipital pole on both sides of the **Sulcus calcarinus.** Similarly to the CGL, the visual cortex of each side receives visual information of the respective contralateral visual field. In the process, the superior part of the visual field is cortically below the Sulcus calcarinus, which represents the inferior part of the visual field above the Sulcus calcarinus. BRODMANN area 17 is enveloped shell-like by areas 18 and 19, which belong to the secondary visual cortex and process the visual stimuli further.

NOTE

The entire optic tract is **retinotopically** divided. This means that neighbouring fields of the retina are mapped onto neighbouring neurons within the optic tract. In addition, parts of the retina that are important for visual impression are represented by particularly large areas within the optic tract: in this way, the projection, which originates from the Fovea centralis retinae – the area with the sharpest vision – takes up the largest area both within the CGL as well as within the visual cortex directly at the occipital pole.

Clinical remarks

If the optic tract is damaged at defined points, failures in the field of vision occur (**scotoma;** ➤ Fig. 13.14). A vascular occlusion of the A. centralis retinae or a severe traumatic brain injury with orbit involvement can, e.g., cause total damage of the retina or of the optic nerve before reaching the Chiasma opticum, and thus results in the affected eye going blind (**amaurosis**). In the case of further lesions of the optic tract, the type of scotoma can be determined clinically by the location of the damage. If the patient only retains, e.g., the respective nasal portions of the visual fields of both eyes (tunnel vision), then there is a median damage of the nasal fibres that cross in the Chiasma opticum, which represent the temporal visual field units (**bitemporal hemianopsia**). Otherwise, if only one visual field is perceived, there is damage either to the Chiasma opticum from lateral, to the contralateral Tractus opticus or to the entire contralateral Radiatio optica or the contralateral visual cortex (**homonym hemianopsia**).

In practice, there are also partial failures, e.g., quadrantanopia or very rare findings, such as, e.g., binasal hemianopsia caused by bilateral damage to the Chiasma opticum from lateral. The extent of a scotoma can be determined by an ophthalmologist by systematically measuring the visual field (**perimetry**). The causes can be manifold, e.g., the Chiasma opticum can be damaged by a pituitary tumour or by an aneurysm of the A. carotis interna. The Tractus opticus, the Radiatio optica or the visual cortex can be functionally affected because of circulatory disorders, inflammatory changes (e.g., in multiple sclerosis) or by primary brain tumours. Therefore, for diagnostic evaluation of a scotoma, cerebral imaging (CT or MRI) is usually essential.

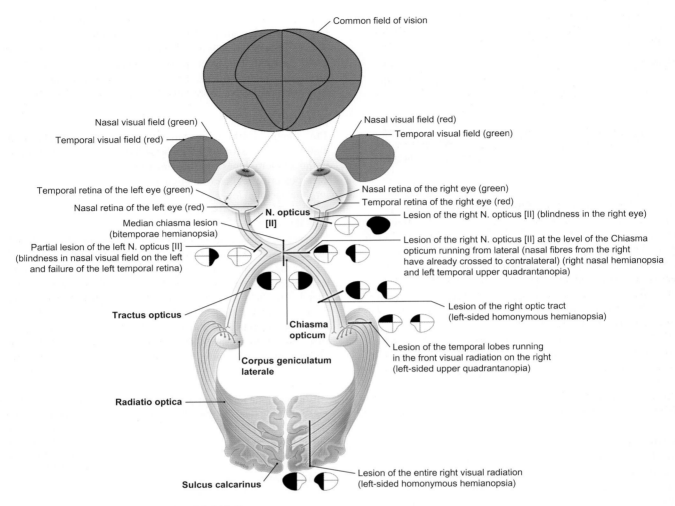

Common field of vision

Nasal visual field (green)

Temporal visual field (red)

Nasal visual field (red)

Temporal visual field (green)

Temporal retina of the left eye (green)

Nasal retina of the left eye (red)

Nasal retina of the right eye (green)

Temporal retina of the right eye (red)

N. opticus [II]

Lesion of the right N. opticus [II] (blindness in the right eye)

Median chiasma lesion (bitemporae hemianopsia)

Partial lesion of the left N. opticus [II] (blindness in nasal visual field on the left and failure of the left temporal retina)

Lesion of the right N. opticus [II] at the level of the Chiasma opticum running from lateral (nasal fibres from the right have already crossed to contralateral) (right nasal hemianopsia and left temporal upper quadrantanopia)

Tractus opticus

Chiasma opticum

Lesion of the right optic tract (left-sided homonymous hemianopsia)

Corpus geniculatum laterale

Lesion of the temporal lobes running in the front visual radiation on the right (left-sided upper quadrantanopia)

Radiatio optica

Sulcus calcarinus

Lesion of the entire right visual radiation (left-sided homonymous hemianopsia)

Fig. 13.14 Optic tract and possible visual field failures.

13.3.2 Visual reflexes

In addition to conveying visual impressions to the consciousness, the light reflex, the near-far response, and the line of sight are of great importance for an intact visual process. These functions are regulated by the **pupillary reflex** as well as by the **accommodation-convergence reflex**.

Pupillary reflex

The pupillary or light reflex leads to a narrowing of the pupils (**miosis**) in both eyes when light falls into one eye (➤ Fig. 13.15):

- The afferent reflex limb consists of axons of retinal ganglion cells, which branch off before reaching the CGL from the Tractus opticus, and run via its Radix medialis into the Area pretectalis of the mesencephalon. There, they are converted into prevertebral neurons, which run to both the ipsilateral as well as – via the Commissura posterior – the contralateral, generally visceroefferent Nucleus accessorius nervi oculomotorii (hence the narrowing of the pupils of both eyes when light falls into just one eye: **consensual light reaction**).
- The preganglionic neurons there send their axons, which run in the actual N. oculomotorius [III], via the efferent, parasympathetic reflex limb to the Ganglion ciliare within the orbita, where the final switching takes place. The postganglionic fibres finally run into the Nn. ciliares breves to the M. sphincter pupillae.

Pupils dilate in the dark (**mydriasis**). In contrast to miosis, this is conveyed sympathetically:

- Here, too, the afferent reflex limb consists of retinal pretectal axons. However, a further configuration of the corresponding neurons runs from the Area pretectalis outwards via the Substantia grisea centralis up to the Centrum ciliospinale in the Nucleus intermediolateralis of the Zona intermedia in the lateral horn of the spinal cord at the level of C8–T3.
- This is where the efferent sympathetic reflex limb begins. Preganglionic fibres run from the Centrum ciliospinale via the Rr. communicantes to the Ganglion cervicale superius. After being converted, the postganglionic fibres then run along the arterial neurovascular pathways and finally via the Plexus caroticus internus all the way to intracranial. The majority of the fibres initially run together with the N. ophthalmicus via the Fissura orbitalis superior into the orbita, then pass without switching through the Ganglion ciliare and finally reach the M. dilatator pupillae via the Nn. ciliares breves.

Clinical remarks

In the case of a lesion of the retina or of the N. opticus, the afferent limb of the pupillary reflex is interrupted. Therefore, not only does blindness occur, but it can also lead to **amaurotic pupil rigidity.** This means that the direct light reaction of the affected eye is destroyed. However, when shining a light into the healthy eye, the indirect, consensual light reaction in the affected eye is triggered because the efferent reflex limb is intact.

In the case of a lesion of the efferent reflex limb, e.g., within the framework of damage to the N. oculomotorius [III], both direct as well as indirect light reaction is destroyed in the affected eye. This is called **absolute pupil rigidity.**

In the case of damage to the mesencephalon, a loss of any light reaction in both eyes can occur due to bilateral interruption of connections between the Area pretectalis and the Nucleus nervi oculomotorii. This is called **reflexive pupil rigidity.**

Accommodation reflex and convergence reaction

In order to fix the eyes on a nearby object, the refractive power of the lens must be increased by means of the **accommodation reflex**. By means of the **convergence reaction,** the lines of vision are directed towards the centre, and through narrowing of the apertures by means of **miosis**, depth acuteness is increased (➤ Fig. 13.15):

- The afferent reflex limb of each side corresponds to the entire optic tract right up to the visual cortex and therefore contains the information of both eyes.
- Neurons of the visual cortex project in the efferent reflex limb via the Brachium colliculi superioris into the Area pretectalis and are configured in the same way as during a light reflex (crossed or uncrossed). An increase in the refractive power of the lens is carried out by a contraction of the M. ciliaris, which is innervated by the general efferent fibres of the N. oculomotorius

[III]; miosis is achieved by contraction of the M. sphincter pupillae, which is innervated by the same fibres.

The convergence reaction is also conveyed via the N. oculomotorius [III], but also via the general somatoefferent fibres to the eye muscles. For this, neurons of the Nucleus nervi oculomotorii must be stimulated from the Area pretectalis, the axons of which reach the M. rectus medialis via the N. oculomotorius nerve in order to move the respective Bulbus oculi towards the middle. At the same time, atony of the M. rectus lateralis is achieved from the Area pretectalis via the Fasciculus longitudinalis medialis and its connections to the Nucleus nervi abducentis.

13.3.3 Management of ocular motor function

For the correct execution of quick eye movements (saccades) and slower eye-tracking movements, as well as fixing onto objects while the head and body move, coordinated attunement of the individual eye muscle nuclei in the brainstem is essential. Corresponding impulses from various nervous and muscular structures such as from the retina, the proprioceptors of the external ocular muscles, the vestibular apparatus, the cerebral cortex and from the cerebellum run firstly to the **supranuclear centres,** in which a pre-integration of these impulses takes place. At the connection point, these centres send out targeted signals to the corresponding eye muscle nuclei. The supranuclear centres include:

- **Colliculi superiores:** This is an optical reflex centre in the mesencephalon, which helps the eye to discover and track moving

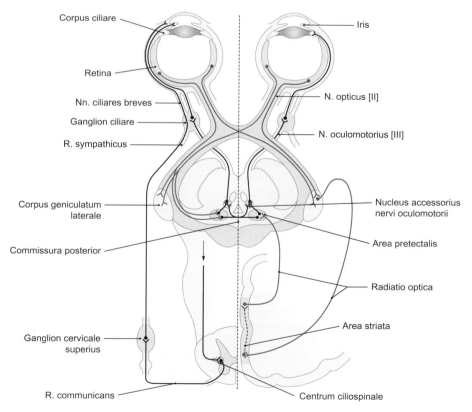

Fig. 13.15 Pupil reflex (left) and accommodation reflex (right). [L126]

objects. It has a superficial sensory area that is reached by fibres from the retina, the visual cortex and frontal eye fields. In addition, it has a deep area which receives extremely varied afferent impulses from numerous areas of the brain (somatoafferent, auditory, motor) and therefore serves as a multi-modal integration centre. Neurons of the superficial area project efferently to the Corpus geniculatum laterale and, via the Pulvinar thalami, to the secondary visual cortex. Neurons of the deep area project efferently to the brainstem and into the spinal cord.

- **Area pretectalis:** Functionally, the Area pretectalis is important for the pupillary reflex, the accommodation reflex and for vergence eye movements (convergence reaction) (➤ Chap. 13.3.2). This area of the mesencephalon lies rostrally of the Colliculi superiores and receives afferents from the retina, CGL and Colliculi superiores. Efferent projections run either reciprocally to the primary afferents or reach other supranuclear centres as well as eye muscle nuclei, such as, e.g., the Nucleus accessorius nervi oculomotorii.
- **Nucleus interstitialis CAJAL:** This mesencephalic nucleus lies laterally of the rostral pole of the Nucleus nervi oculomotorii and is particularly involved in the triggering of vertical eye and head movements. It is connected afferently to the Area pretectalis, but also to other supranuclear centres. Its efferents run via the Commissura posterior mainly into the contralateral Nucleus nervi oculomotorii as well as into the Nucleus nervi trochlearis.
- **Nucleus interstitialis rostralis of the Fasciculus longitudinalis medialis (riMLF):** This nucleus also lies in the mesencephalon and coordinates vertical eye movements, especially downwards. It is located rostrally of the Nucleus interstitialis CAJAL and dorsomedially of the Nucleus ruber. It receives afferents from the PPRF (see below) and from the Colliculi superiores. Efferent projections are dispatched to the ipsilateral Nuclei nervi oculomotorii and trochlearis.
- **Paramedian pontine reticular formation (PPRF):** This part of the Formatio reticularis belongs to the cell groups of the medial zone in the pons, receives cortical afferents from contralateral, and projects efferently onto the ipsilateral Abducens nucleus. Functionally, therefore, the PPRF is important for horizontal eye movements.
- **Vestibular nuclear complex** and **Fasciculus longitudinalis medialis (FLM):** The combination of these structures enables the vestibulo-ocular reflex (➤ Chap. 13.5). Efferent projections of the vestibular nuclei to the eye muscle core nuclei via the FLM are decisive here.
- **Nucleus prepositus hypoglossi:** This nucleus lies in the Medulla oblongata rostrally of the Nucleus nervi hypoglossi and is of great importance for the planning and execution of eye movements. It is also assumed that it integrates movement signals to maintain eye position. The Nucleus prepositus receives afferents from the frontal visual centres of both sides, out of the ipsilateral Nucleus interstitialis CAJAL, the riMLF and the Area pretectalis. Efferent projections run to all eye muscle nuclei, ipsilaterally and contralaterally.

Clinical remarks

Clinically, a distinction is made between horizontal and vertical gaze palsy. Both types are usually determined by damage to the corresponding central ocular motor coordination and integration centres.
Horizontal gaze palsy arises in the case of a supranuclear or nuclear lesion of the PPRF. A supranuclear lesion can affect cortical areas such as the frontal eye field or subcortical structures, such as the Capsula interna. Since the relevant decreasing tracts cross on their way to the pons, the contralateral PPRF is less activated by a supranuclear lesion and the ipsilateral PPRF more so. This results in conjugate eye deviation with a bias to the right. In contrast, in a unilateral injury of the PPRF at the level of the pons, activity of the contralateral PPRF predominates and results in a gaze palsy to the left.
Vertical gaze palsy arises in the case of a lesion of the Tegmentum mesencephali, and specifically either of the Nucleus interstitialis CAJAL, of the Commissura posterior or of the Nucleus interstitialis rostralis of the FLM (riFLM). In the case of a lesion of the two former structures, a vertical gaze palsy upwards on the contralateral side occurs since the fibres to the corresponding eye muscle nuclei cross. A lesion of the riFLM, in contrast, leads to an ipsilateral gaze palsy downwards because the fibres to the corresponding eye muscle nuclei do not cross.

The 'eye muscle nuclei' in the brainstem must also be densely interconnected with each other, so that movements of the individual eye muscles can be coordinated with each other. Serving this purpose are the internuclear neurons already mentioned in ➤ Chap. 12.6, which can be found piled up within certain 'eye muscle nuclei', e.g., in the Nucleus nervi oculomotorii and Nucleus nervi abducentis. These two nuclei are connected to each other via a reciprocal fibre connection, which runs in the **Fasciculus longitudinalis medialis** (FLM). This internuclear tract coordinates the M. rectus lateralis (innervated by the N. abducens) and the M. rectus medialis (innervated by the N. oculomotorius) in conjugated horizontal eye movements (contraction of the ipsilateral M. rectus lateralis of the contralateral M. rectus medialis when looking ipsilaterally). In implementation of the convergence reaction, this connection in the FLM is, however, inhibited, so that both bulbi can be directed inwards by a simultaneous contraction of both Mm. recti mediales.

Clinical remarks

In the case of multiple sclerosis, an inflammatory centre in the brainstem may cause, depending on the degree, mono- or bilateral damage to the Fasciculus longitudinalis medialis. This results in **internuclear ophthalmoplegia** (INO).
At this point, the eye of the damaged side cannot be adducted when looking to the contralateral side of the damage and double vision results. Clinically, it is important that the convergence reaction remains extant and there are no eyeball disorders when looking straight ahead. Peripheral innervation of the M. rectus medialis is namely completely intact through the N. oculomotorius [III]; only coordination of the simultaneous contraction of this muscle fails in the case of contraction of the contralateral M. rectus lateralis.

13.4 Auditory system
Anja Böckers

Skills

After working through this chapter of the textbook, you should be able to:
- describe the auditory function system (direct/indirect auditory system) on the basis of the neuronal chain given in ➤ Fig. 13.17

- name at least 3 key functions of the auditory system (e.g., conscious perception of acoustic stimuli, directional hearing, acoustic reflex configuration)
- explain the functions of the secondary auditory cortex for formation and understanding of language in the case of specific lesions

---

Clinical case

Lesion of the Corpus trapezoideum

Medical history
A 45-year-old female patient reports to her ENT specialist that she is having trouble following conversation in rooms with a lot of people, and she has also noticed that she often cannot distinguish which telephone in the office is actually ringing. Similarly, she is having problems making out which direction the sound of a moving object is coming from. She can therefore not say without looking, when standing on a platform, from which direction a train is pulling into a station. When asked, she reports that she has suffered for 10 years from right-sided headaches and right-sided tinnitus.

Initial examination
The neurological examination is normal.

Further diagnostics
The symptoms described by the patient are identified with a special test, in which the difference in signal transit time from both ears is measured. This also shows a slight asymmetric hearing loss in the low-frequency range (500 Hz). Finally, diagnostic imaging (MRT) shows a pontine lesion between the tegmentum and the ventral pons, which is most likely explained by a capillary vascular malformation and anatomically matches the area of the Corpus trapezoideum.

Clinical picture
The damage to the Corpus trapezoideum affects the afferents to the superior olivary complex of the opposite side and thus the binaural impulse exchange that is important for directional hearing.

13.4.1 Overview

The auditory system is divided into a sound-receiving, a conducting and a processing section. The sound is initially received through the air by the auricle, then conducted to the eardrum, reinforced by the auditory ossicle chain, and finally broadcast to the inner ear. The central section of the auditory system begins at the stimuli receptive sensory cells of the **Organum spirale (organ of CORTI)** in the inner ear, and via a chain of at least five neurons it reaches the primary auditory cortex in the Lobus temporalis of the telencephalon. Further processing and interpretation of the tones perceived here as language or melody takes place in the adjacent secondary cortical areas.

The perception of acoustic stimuli from one's surroundings is an important sensory function that secures survival in the sense of a protective function. Moreover, the auditory system is important for the conveying of information and emotions. The close link between hearing and speech is particularly evident in early childhood development, when language development can be delayed or even made impossible by damage to the auditory system. Serving as acoustic stimuli are sound waves, which are characterised by their frequency (measured in hertz [Hz]) and their amplitude (measured in decibels [dB]). The healthy ear can perceive frequencies between 18 Hz and 18 kHz, with the main speech range lying between 250 and 4,000 Hz at an intensity of 40–80 dB. 'Sound intensities' above 140 dB can cause permanent hearing damage and even deafness.

13.4.2 Peripheral section

Located in the organ of CORTI are the cochlear sensory cells which are arranged in one row of inner hair cells and 3 rows of outer hair cells. These hair cells are specialised epithelial cells and not nerve cells; they are also referred to, therefore, as secondary sensory cells. On the apical cell membrane, the hair cells carry approximately 50–120 stereocilia arranged according to size, which are connected to each other by protein filaments ('tip links') and thus always react together. Adequate stimulus for a depolarisation and transmitter dispersal of the sensory cells is the kinking of the stereocilia in the direction of the longest stereocilium by contact with the tectorial membrane which lies above the organ of CORTI. 10–20 of the inner hair cells then conduct their impulses together onto a bipolar ganglion cell in the **Ganglion spirale**, which lies in the modiolus of the bony spiralis and at the base of which the N. cochlearis or the **Pars cochlearis of the N. vestibulocochlearis [VIII]** are respectively formed (➤ Fig. 13.16).

The outer hair cells are, on the one hand, innervated afferently via pseudounipolar type II ganglion cells. These however as a whole only account for 5% of all ganglion cells of the Ganglion spirale, and their centrally-directed axons, for the most part, do not enter into the N. cochlearis, but take on intrinsic cochlear coordination functions (➤ Fig. 13.16).

It is important to realise, in contrast to the general basic understanding of a stimulus-receiving organ, that the Pars cochlearis not

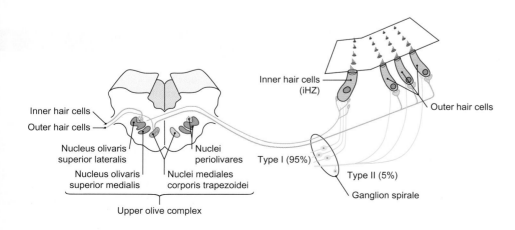

Fig. 13.16 Origins and termination areas of bipolar type I and pseudounipolar type II ganglion cells as well as olivocochlear efferent fibres. [L126]

Inner hair cells
Outer hair cells
Nucleus olivaris superior lateralis
Nucleus olivaris superior medialis
Nuclei periolivares
Nuclei mediales corporis trapezoidei
Upper olive complex
Inner hair cells (iHZ)
Outer hair cells
Type I (95%)
Type II (5%)
Ganglion spirale

only contains afferent fibres, but also efferent fibres which build synapses with the afferent fibres of the inner hair cells and with the cell bases of the outer hair cells (see ➤ Chap. 12.5.11, N. vestibulocochlearis [VIII]). These efferents originate from the superior olivary complex and are referred to as the **olivocochlear bundle**. After leaving the brainstem these fibres run initially in the N. vestibularis, then switch in the inner ear canal to the N. cochlearis (**OORT anastomosis**). In the process, the fibres ending at the inner hair cells come out of the ipsilateral part of the lateral superior olivary complex; the fibres of the outer hair cells have their origins instead in the contralaterally located medial superior olivary complex. Each tone produces a sound pressure, which firstly sets the perilymphatic fluid into a wave motion and finally also starts the sensory cell-bearing organ of CORTI oscillating on the basilar membrane. Typically, the basilar membrane at the base of the cochlea is smaller, (0.1 mm), more solid and more elastic than the membrane at the apex of the cochlea (0.5 mm), so that, depending on the sound frequency, different sections of the basilar membrane start oscillating: sections near the base at high frequencies (16,000 Hz), but sections at the apex at low frequencies (20 Hz). This results in a tonotopic impulse release, which is also represented over the ganglion cells as a tonotopic stimulus transmission in the whole auditory system as well as in the primary auditory cortex. However, at lower volumes, the oscillations of the basilar membrane are not sufficient to induce a depolarisation so that they must first be micromechanically reinforced by a cochlear mechanism of the outer hair cells in order to stimulate the inner hair cells.

Clinical remarks

In an ENT medical practice, a distinction is made between different types of hearing loss. In the case of a **conductive hearing loss,** conduction of sound in the outer ear or in the middle ear is adversely affected. Here, the air conduction of the sound is affected, while the bone conduction remains intact. The air or bone conduction is checked diagnostically by the tuning fork test described by RINNE and WEBER.
If, however, there is damage to the inner ear itself, then it is a case of **sensorineural hearing loss.** Strictly speaking, this hearing loss can have a sensory cause (inner ear in the narrower sense) or a neuronal cause, i.e. retrocochlear. For function testing of the inner ear and of central impulse processing, **'auditory brainstem response (ABR) audiometry'** can be carried out in toddlers even before the development of speech. For this, an **auditory evoked potential** (AEP) response is deduced according to a standardised acoustic stimulation of the inner ear using surface electrodes placed on the scalp and their latency and amplitude, amongst other things, are evaluated.

13.4.3 Central section

The perikarya of the first neuron of the central auditory system are located in the **Ganglion spirale** in the modiolus of the cochlea (➤ Fig. 13.17, ➤ Table 13.4). The centrally-directed axon runs in the **N. vestibulocochlearis** through the inner ear canal and in the cerebellopontine angle it reaches the brainstem together with the N. facialis [VII]. Located here in the Recessus lateralis of the IVth ventricle are special somatoafferent cochlear nuclei, which are divided into an anterior and a posterior group and form the 2nd neuron of the auditory system. Each cochlear nucleus exhibits tonotopy with an ascending frequency arrangement from low to high in an anterior–posterior orientation.

NOTE
The **auditory system** is structured tonotopically throughout:
• In the stimulus receiving organ, the cochlea, the area near the base, is stimulated by high frequencies, the area near the apex by low frequencies.
• In the primary cortical area, the Gyri temporales transversi (HESCHL), high frequencies are represented more laterally and low frequencies more medially.

The **Nucleus cochlearis anterior** transmits the impulses received by it, almost unchanged, towards the ipsilateral and contralateral superior olivary complex. The crossing fibres thereby form a strong fibre bundle, the **trapezoid body (Corpus trapezoideum)**, so that in individual nuclei, the **Nuclei corporis trapezoidei**, a further conversion, can be carried out. The axons of the **Nucleus cochlearis posterior**, in contrast, cross completely to the opposite side and directly reach the **Colliculi inferiores** in the Tectum mesencephali via the **Lemniscus laterales**, without being converted (**direct auditory system**). Already at the level of the brainstem or in the **superior olivary complex**, information from both inner ears converges respectively, which forms the anatomical basis for directional hearing. The superior olivary complex is the crucial hub of the **indirect auditory system** and is composed of the **Nuclei olivares superiores** and the **Nuclei periolivares**. The nuclear complex is anterior to the Nucleus nervi abducentis [VI] in the internal facial genu and consists of a lateral and a medial part. The lateral part sends out the following efferents:
• to the Colliculi inferiores
• for acoustic reflexes also to the middle ear muscles, to the M. stapedius and to the M. tensor tympani
• the olivocochlear bundle (described above) back to the hair cells of the cochlea

Among other things, directional hearing is based on the determination of the binaural interaural time difference in the medial and/or the binaural level difference in the lateral part of the complex. The crossed fibres ascend in the brainstem in the **Lemniscus lateralis**, which, via the **Decussatio lemniscorum lateralium (PROBST)**, facilitates a further fibre exchange between the halves of the body, and they then reach the **Nucleus centralis**, the 3rd neuron (direct auditory system) or the 4th/5th neuron respectively (indirect auditory system) of the inferior colliculus.

The **Colliculi inferiores** are divided tonotopically from lateral to medial according to the ascending frequency arrangement. They are connected via the Commissura colliculi inferiores, so that a binaurally perceived impulse stimulus can be exchanged. The Colliculi inferiores are also referred to as the auditory reflex centre, in which responses from the body, which are triggered by noises, e.g., flinching in the case of a bang, are configured. Via the **Brachium colliculi inferiores** the efferents of this 3rd neuron continue to the

Table 13.4 Auditory system

Neuronal chain	Groups of neurons
1st neuron	Type I ganglion cells in the Ganglion spirale
2nd neuron	Nuclei cochleares anterior and posterior in the passageway between the pons and the Medulla oblongata in the Recessus lateralis of the 4th ventricle
(Indirect auditory tract)	(Nuclei olivares superiores, if necessary via the Nuclei corporis trapezoidei)
3rd neuron	Nucleus centralis colliculi inferioris in the Tectum mesencephali
4th neuron	Corpus geniculatum mediale of the metathalamus
5th neuron	Gyri temporales transversi (HESCHL), BRODMANN area 41 in the Lobus temporalis

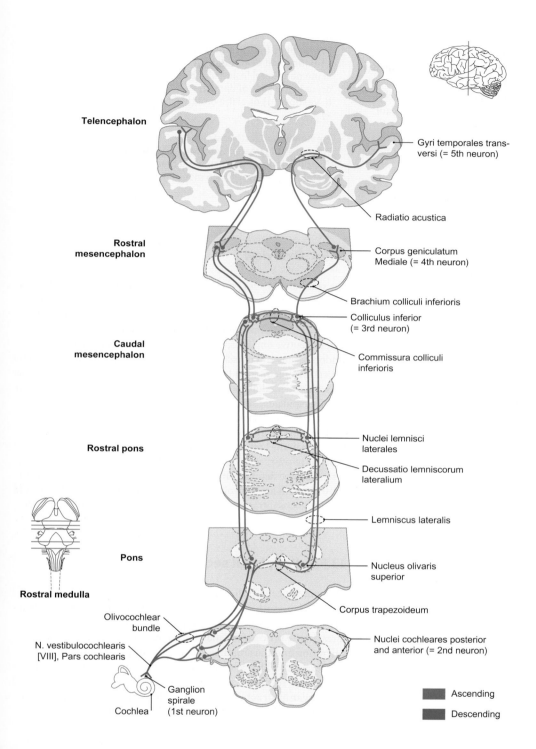

Telencephalon

Gyri temporales trans-
versi (= 5th neuron)

Radiatio acustica

Rostral
mesencephalon

Corpus geniculatum
Mediale (= 4th neuron)

Brachium colliculi inferioris

Colliculus inferior
(= 3rd neuron)

Caudal
mesencephalon

Commissura colliculi
inferioris

Nuclei lemnisci
laterales

Rostral pons

Decussatio lemniscorum
lateralium

Lemniscus lateralis

Nucleus olivaris
superior

Pons

Rostral medulla

Corpus trapezoideum

Olivocochlear
bundle

Nuclei cochleares posterior
and anterior (= 2nd neuron)

N. vestibulocochlearis
[VIII], Pars cochlearis

Ganglion
spirale
(1st neuron)

Cochlea

Ascending

Descending

**Fig. 13.17 Most important neu-
ronal stations and intersections
of the central auditory pathway**
(diagram). [L127]

Commissura colliculi inferiores (CGM) of the metathalamus in
the interbrain (➤ Fig. 13.17).
The 4th (5th/6th) neuron is located in the **Nucleus dorsalis** of the
CGM and again manifests tonotopy with ascending frequencies
from lateral to medial in the same way as the Colliculus inferior.
The axons of this nuclear group eventually, via **acoustic radiation
(Radiatio acustica)** in the posterior section of the Capsula interna,
reach the primary auditory cortex, the **Gyri temporales transversi
(HESCHL)** (➤ Fig. 13.17). This cortical area (BRODMANN area
41) includes the 5th (6th/7th) neuron of the auditory system in the
cortical layers III and IV and it takes up the preceding tonotopic
structure from lateral to medial again. It is here that awareness of
tones, sounds and simple acoustic patterns takes place. Words, language or melodies are only processed in the adjacent secondary au-

ditory cortex. Belonging to the secondary auditory cortex are
BRODMANN areas 42 and 22 and the **sensory language centre
(WERNICKE)**. This is located in the dominant hemisphere, while
the analogue area in the nondominant hemisphere tends to serve
nonrational processing and interpretation of speech. Hearing and
speaking are thereby closely linked: efferents from WERNICKE's
area run to the **motor language centre (BROCA)** via the **Fibrae
arcuatae** (syn.: Fasciculus arcuatus). Further close links to the telencephalic function centres, e.g., to the visual cortex, run via the
Gyrus angularis – at the parietal end point of the Sulcus temporalis – and form the neural basis of reading.
In addition to the auditory system, described in the narrower
sense, it should also be pointed out that **descending cortical tracts**
connect all stations of the auditory system to each other. There are

therefore fibres which run preferentially from lamina V of the primary auditory cortex to the ipsilateral Colliculus inferior. It is thought that these corticofugal fibres – triggered by acoustic learning processes – induce a restructuring of subcortical structures, contributing to the selective processing of acoustic stimuli which is important for behaviour. They can filter out or 'dampen' irrelevant noises and enhance important noises.

Clinical remarks

A failure in WERNICKE's area of the dominant hemisphere is referred to as **sensory aphasia** and is associated with damage to speech comprehension, which causes incomprehensible language. In the process, speech production is fluid and pronunciation normal. Words and phrases, however, are often altered pointlessly (paraphasia) or even invented (neologisms), while the sentence melody and emphasis remain extant. Patients can often hardly make themselves understood, but are often not aware of their speech disorder and therefore leave a false impression of general confusion.

In **motor aphasia**, due to a failure of BROCA's area, formation of speech and articulation is adversely affected in received understanding of speech.

A failure of the Gyrus angularis of the dominant hemisphere means that the affected person cannot name optically perceived structures with words. This applies to objects, but of course also in abstract form to the written word, which is seen, but can no longer be read correctly. The latter describes a reading disorder **(alexia)** and, consequently, also a writing disorder **(agrafia)**.

13.5 Vestibular system
Anja Böckers

Skills

After working through this chapter of the textbook, you should be able to:
- describe in your own words which afferent and efferent fibre connections are shown by the Nuclei vestibulares
- explain how the central configuration of the vestibular system fulfils functions of balance control and gaze stabilisation

---

Clinical case

Peripheral lesion of the vestibular system

A 45-year old patient presented in a clinic with vertigo and vertical double vision. He states he is no longer able to hear anything on the left side. When asked, he denies pre-existing conditions of eyes, ears or brain.

Initial examination
During the examination, in addition to a spontaneous onset of horizontal nystagmus (typically a two-phase, involuntary eye movement) to the right, a downwards-oriented squinting of the left eye as well as a left inclination of the head are also noted. These symptoms are grouped clinically as an 'ocular tilt reaction'.

Further diagnostics
A caloric testing of the left vestibular system shows no response. No central lesion can be identified in the MRT.

Diagnosis
The findings (nystagmus of the healthy side as well as the squinting and head-tilting to the side of the lesion) suggest an acute peripheral lesion of the vestibular system, such as can occur in the case of damage in the peripheral course of the N. vestibularis or of the otolithic dysfunction of the vestibular system.

Treatment and further steps
The patient is treated with intravenous steroid administration. The symptoms of the 'ocular tilt reaction' are almost completely reversible within 6 months by central compensation mechanisms.

13.5.1 Overview

The vestibular system particularly serves the purpose of maintaining the body's balance with changes in body position or with body movements. It perceives changes in location and movement in the inner ear; functionally, the transmitted impulses become closely linked to proprioceptive impulses, which are forwarded from the GOLGI tendon organs and muscle spindles via the spinal cord, and also to the optical system, in order to guarantee gaze stabilization. The vestibular nuclei in the Medulla oblongata form a key integration centre, which enables rapid adaptation in the case of a modified body position or movement. This adaptation is carried out unconsciously and also without direct cortical configuration. A further configuration via the thalamus to the cortex is necessary for awareness of visual impressions, as in other sensory systems too. However, no primary cortical system can be definitely named for the vestibular system. Instead, up to 10 different areas involved in impulse handling are debated, including the Sulcus intraparietalis, the parieto-insular cortex, the somatosensory cortex or the hippocampus.

13.5.2 Peripheral section

The sensory cells of the vestibular system are located in the membranous labyrinth of the inner ear in the **Macula sacculi,** the **Macula utriculi** and the **Cristae ampullares** of the Canales semicirculares. In the process, the macular sensory cells perceive linear acceleration and the ampullary sensory cells perceive rotational acceleration, which are registered via the flow of endolymphatic fluid in the vestibular system. The sensory cells are hair cells, which are similar in structure to the hair cells of the organ of CORTI in the cochlea. They correspond to modified epithelial cells and are referred to as **secondary sensory cells**. A deflection of apical stereocilia through the fluid movement of the endolymph in the direction of the edge of the marginal kinocilium of the sensory cells leads to hyperpolarisation, deflecting away from the kinocilium to a depolarisation. The vestibular hair cells are innervated by bipolar ganglion cells of the **Ganglion vestibulare**, of which the centrally-directed axon runs in the **N. vestibularis** of the N. vestibulocochlearis [VIII] to the cerebellopontine angle of the CNS.

13.5.3 Central section

Overview
The N. vestibularis conveys its afferent fibres to the Nuclei vestibulares (➤ Fig. 13.18, ➤ Table 13.5). Via the inferior cerebellar peduncle (Corpus juxtarestiforme), however, a small part of the fibres

Table 13.5 Vestibular system

Neuronal chain	Groups of neurons
1st neuron	Ganglion cells in the Ganglion vestibulare
2nd neuron	Nuclei vestibulares superior, lateralis, inferior and medialis in the passageway between the pons and Medulla oblongata
3rd neuron	Thalamus (Nucleus posterior ventrolateralis)
4th neuron	Cortex: Sulcus intraparietalis, parieto-insular area, Gyrus postcentralis, BRODMANN area 7 and hippocampus

from the vestibular system also directly reach the vestibular cerebellum or the Lobus flocculonodularis (direct sensory cerebellar tract) respectively. In its initial part, the N. vestibularis also conducts efferent fibres of the auditory system (olivocochlear bundle). But these fibres do not have – as far as is known – any functional importance for the vestibular system. Finally, the Nuclei vestibulares are important integration nuclei for proprioceptive, optical and vestibular impulses.

A distinction is made between 4 main vestibular nuclei, the **Nuclei vestibulares superior (BECHTEREW), lateralis (DEITERS), inferior (ROLLER)** and **medialis (SCHWALBE).** They project from their location into the Medulla oblongata or into the caudal section of the pons ventral to the Pedunculus cerebellaris inferior and superior respectively. All 4 nuclei receive primary afferents from the vestibular apparatus. In the vestibular nuclei, however, other afferents also converge, particularly from the Nuclei fastigii from the vestibulocerebellum, bilateral projections from the spinal cord (which, amongst others, run in the tracts of the posterior funiculus), and afferents from the Nucleus spinalis nervi trigemini. Likewise, from a great variety of parts of the central nervous system, optical impulses are for example transmitted indirectly via the Formatio reticularis to the vestibular nuclei. Incoming information is processed in the vestibular nuclei in order to ultimately influence holding and supporting motor function. This manifests itself morphologically in the efferent tract systems to the spinal cord:

- **Tractus vestibulospinalis lateralis:** This tract is also attributed to the extrapyramidal motor system (EPMS) and originates preferentially in the Nucleus vestibularis lateralis. Uncrossed and somatotopically structured, it runs right up into the sacral spinal cord and ends directly or indirectly at the α- or γ-motorneurons in the anterior horn. Its fibres serve the purpose of securing balance by increasing the tone of extensors and simultaneously inhibiting the antagonistic flexors.

- **Tractus vestibulospinalis medialis:** This tract begins in the Nucleus vestibularis medialis, runs initially in the Fasciculus longitudinalis medialis and finally both ipsilaterally as well as contralaterally reaches the motorneurons in the cervical and thoracic spine. This tract system is also assigned to the extrapyramidal system and makes it possible to react to the positional changes of the body with counterbalancing head movements.

In addition to direct vestibulocerebellar fibres, there are also fibres that run via the Nuclei vestibulares as an indirect sensory cerebellar tract (mossy fibres) via the inferior cerebellar peduncle to the vestibulocerebellum. A decisive factor for the coordination of eye movements or for gaze stabilisation is the fast configuration of impulses from the vestibular nuclei onto eye muscle nuclei that lie in the brainstem (cranial nerve cores III, IV, VI) and onto the **Nucleus interstitialis** (CAJAL; see below). These efferents originate from all 4 vestibular nuclei and run ventrally in the medial longitudinal fascicle, running ventrally in the aquaduct (**Fasciculus longitudinalis medialis**) to cranial. Also important for gaze stabilization, particularly for the control of horizontal eye movements, are the reciprocal connections of the vestibular nuclei with the paramedian pontine Formatio reticularis.

Via the ventral portion of the medial loop tract (Lemniscus medialis), efferent fibres of the medial and upper vestibular nuclei finally reach both sides of the posterolateral and posteromedial thalamus (**Nucleus posterior ventrolateralis**) as the **Tractus vestibulothalamicus,** and are conducted from there, e.g. onto the **parietoinsular vestibular cortex,** for a voluntary perception of body position, sense of space and own body awareness. Projections into the hypothalamus are seen as responsible for, amongst other things, the occurrence of nausea and vomiting associated with dizziness or, e.g., being sea sick.

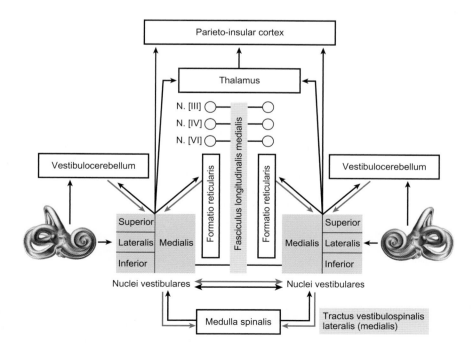

Fig. 13.18 Important afferents and efferents of the Nuclei vestibulares functioning as integration nuclei (diagram). [L126]

Vestibulo-ocular reflex

An essential function of the vestibular organ is to adapt eye positioning during head movements in such a way that the resulting picture in both eyes is mapped at the same time at the point of sharpest vision (Fovea centralis). This adjustment process occurs reflexively using the aforementioned fibre connections and nuclei, particularly via the **Fasciculus longitudinalis medialis**. Stimulation of the sensory cells in the Cristae ampullares of the lateral archway when turning the head (to the left) results in an increased impulse frequency in the left N. vestibularis (➤ Fig. 13.19). Via the Nuclei vestibulares, motoneurons in the contralateral Nucleus nervi abducentis and thereby the right M. rectus lateralis, are activated. Interneurons to the ipsilateral oculomotor core, in turn, activate the left M. rectus medialis. Likewise, the antagonistic eye muscles are inhibited via the correlating semicircular canal system and the Nucleus vestibularis medialis. Movements of the head result in eye movement in the opposite direction. Via the Formatio reticularis, there is also an indirect way to coordinate the eye movements.

The **Nucleus interstitialis (CAJAL)** lies at the cranial end of and lateral to the Fasciculus longitudinalis medialis in the immediate vicinity of the Nucleus nervi oculomotorii. As well as afferents from the Nucleus vestibularis, it also receives afferents from the retina, which, amongst other things, are important for the configuration of the light reflex of the pupil (➤ Chap. 13.3.2). It is an important connection point between the optical and vestibular system, including for coordination of vertical eye and head movements.

13.6 Olfactory system
Michael J. Schmeißer

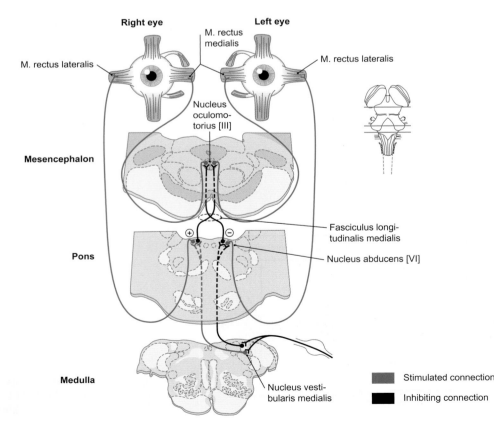

Fig. 13.19 Configuration of the vestibulo-ocular reflex with stimulation of the left lateral archway, e.g., when the head is turned to the left. [L127]

Diagnosis

In the cranial CT that had been carried out after the accident, amongst other things, a distinct fracture of the Lamina cribrosa was described. Running through this bony structure are the Fila olfactoria of the olfactory tract. Therefore, an interruption of the olfactory tract due to tearing of the Fila olfactoria is suspected. A smell test with odour samples is carried out, whereby the samples are tested separately on each side by closing the right or the left nostril, respectively. This test reinforces the suspected diagnosis and with the greatly reduced sense of smell, post traumatic hyposmia is diagnosed.

Follow-up

The prognosis is relatively poor. On the basis of clinical observations, only around 10% of affected patients recover in the long-term.

The **olfactory tract** is an afferent neuronal system that conveys the sense of smell to the brain. It starts in the nasal mucosa (**Regio olfactoria**) and ends in the primary **olfactory cortex**, which is located fronto- or temporobasally in the cerebrum. Interestingly, the olfactory tract is the only sensory tract which is not switched in the thalamus on its way to the cortex, and for the most part runs uncrossed.

NOTE

The neuronal chain of the olfactory tract consists of 2 cells. The 1st neuron is located within the olfactory mucosa of the nasal cavity, the 2nd neuron in the Bulbus olfactorius.

The individual stations of the olfactory tract and the corresponding **neuronal chain** are described below. ➤ Fig. 13.20 is used for illustration purposes.

13.6.1 Regio olfactoria

The **olfactory mucosa** in humans stretches across a part of the nasal mucosa that is only a few square centimetres. It is located above the upper nasal concha at the lateral nasal wall and on the section lying opposite to the Septum nasi. The **olfactory epithelium** of the olfactory mucosa, which is turned towards the nasal cavity, comprises the **olfactory sensory cells** or **olfactory neurons**. This is the first neuron of the olfactory tract. Olfactory neurons are bipolar **primary sensory cells.** With their dendrites, they receive the stimulus – an odorous substance – via chemoreceptors and transmit this excitation pattern directly to the CNS themselves.

13.6.2 Pathway of the olfactory tract

Fila olfactoria

The bundled axons of the olfactory neurons, which run in the form of approx. 20 fine unmyelinated nerve fibres through the Lamina cribrosa of the Os ethmoidale, are referred to as the Fila olfactoria or the N. olfactorius [I] (➤ Chap. 9.3.1, ➤ Chap. 12.5.4), and end on each side in the olfactory bulb (**Bulbus olfactorius**) that lies directly opposite.

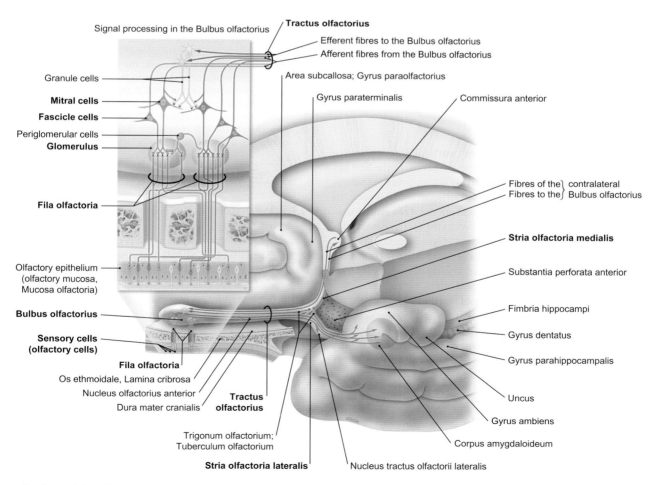

Fig. 13.20 Stations of the olfactory tract.

Bulbus olfactorius

The Bulbus olfactorius is structured in six layers. The axons of the olfactory neurons end in specialized structures, the **glomeruli.** There, they primarily form **excitatory glutamatergic synapses** with primary dendrites of **tufted** and **mitral cells,** the 2nd neurons of the olfactory tract. Their axons leave the bulbus as afferent fibres via the Tractus olfactorius.

In addition to tufted and mitral cells, **GABAergic interneurons** can also be found in the Bulbus olfactorius, such as, e.g., **periglomerular neurons** and **granule cells.** These interneurons have inhibiting synaptic contacts with the tufted or mitral cells and can influence signal transmission in the olfactory tract. In turn, they are reached by efferent fibres, which run from nuclei in the telencephalon and in the brainstem to the Bulbus olfactorius. In this way the activity of the bulbar interneurons can be influenced.

Tractus olfactorius

The Tractus olfactorius is located in the **Pedunculus olfactorius** and contains, amongst other things, the axons of the tufted and mitral cells of the Bulbus olfactorius. In the Trigonum olfactorium, the Tractus olfactorius is divided into the Striae olfactoriae medialis and lateralis:

- The **Stria olfactoria lateralis** runs laterally off to the **Substantia perforata anterior** and reaches the olfactory cortex.
- The **Stria olfactoria medialis**, in contrast, ends in the Tuberculum olfactorium and in the septum area.

Located within the Tractus olfactorius proximally of the Trigonum olfactorium is a further nucleus, the **Nucleus olfactorius anterior.** The precise function of this structure for signal processing within the olfactory tract is not yet sufficiently understood. It is however strongly associated with ipsilateral and contralateral structures of the olfactory system. In this way, the axons here are configured from the ipsilateral Bulbus olfactorius into neurons, of which the projections run via the Commissura anterior to the contralateral Bulbus olfactorius and sometimes also to the contralateral cortex.

13.6.3 Olfactory cortex

Included amongst the **primary olfactory cortical areas** are several frontobasal or temporobasal areas of the cerebrum. In the first instance this includes the **Cortex piriformis** (also Cortex prepiriformis), which is located basally in the transition area between the frontal and temporal lobes; also included are the **Area entorhinalis,** which attaches dorsally and is located in the Gyrus parahippocampalis, the **Cortex periamygdaloideus** (Gyrus semilunaris and Gyrus ambiens), as well as the anterior areas of the **insular cortex.** The Cortex periamygdaloideus is a particularly important interface to the limbic system, as well as to the autonomic system, via amygdalohypothalamic connections. Sense of smell impressions are perceived in **secondary olfactory cortical areas** and are further processed (analysis, recognition, interpretation, evaluation), including in the limbic cortex (e.g., the hippocampus) and the **posterior orbital frontal cortex.** In particular, the latter has a crucial role in the perception and differentiation of odours.

NOTE

Central structures of the olfactory tract such as the bulbus and the Tuberculum olfactorium, septum, Area entorhinalis and Cortex piriformis, are assigned to the **paleocortex,** the phylogenetically oldest part of the cerebrum. In contrast, secondary olfactory cortical areas belong to the neocortex (posterior orbitofrontal cortex) or the archicortex (hippocampus).

13.7 Gustatory system
Anja Böckers

Skills

After working through this chapter of the textbook, you should be able to:
- give an impromptu description of the gustatory function system with the neuron chain depicted in ➤ Fig. 13.21.

Clinical case

Taste disorder in vertebrobasilar embolism

Medical history

A 32-year-old man without any significant pre-existing conditions is brought into the emergency department with sudden left-sided hemiparesis and vertical double vision. With the suspicion of a stroke, the patient is treated immediately according to the guidelines. With thrombolytic treatment (dissolving of blood coagulation), the neurological symptoms significantly improve, but the patient spontaneously reports that he can no longer perceive whether food or drink is sweet or sour.

Diagnostics

The CT findings show an infarct area in the right (non-dominant hemisphere) thalamus and midbrain. This infarct also affects the ipsilateral Tractus tegmentalis centralis and thus the 2nd neuron of the gustatory tract and the 3rd neuron in the Nucleus ventralis posteromedialis of the thalamus.

Diagnosis

The findings illustrate a unilateral taste disorder, but it is also made clear that in humans some fibres may possibly cross to the opposite side. In this case, the cause can be diagnosed as an embolic vascular occlusion in the vertebrobasilar basin. In a transesophageal echocardiogram, a 4 mm large, previously undiagnosed Foramen ovale is identified so that an embolism from the venous circulation was able to run via the right atrium directly into the left atrium and thereby end up in the arterial outflow to the A. vertebralis.

13.7.1 Peripheral section

Serving sensory perception in the peripheral area are approximately 2,000 **taste buds (Caliculi gustatorii),** which are located on the tongue in particular, but also on the soft palate and the epiglottis. The taste buds are located in the papillae, where a distinction is made between 3 forms of papillae: **Papillae vallatae, Papillae fungiformes** and **Papillae foliatae.** Each taste bud is made up of various cell types. Functioning as the actual receptor cells are epithelial sensory cells, which perceive the 5 primary taste categories – sweet, sour, salty, bitter and 'umami' (glutamate). Sensations like piquancy or the cold feeling from menthol, in contrast, originate from a stimulation of thermal receptors on the tongue that transmit their impulses via the N. trigeminalis [V]. With their unmyelinated fibres, the actual taste bud sensory cells form synapses with the axonal plexuses that lie on the basal side of the taste buds. These are also referred to as **secondary sensory cells,** because the sensory cells do not generate an action potential; this potential first originates at the synapse with the first afferent neuron.

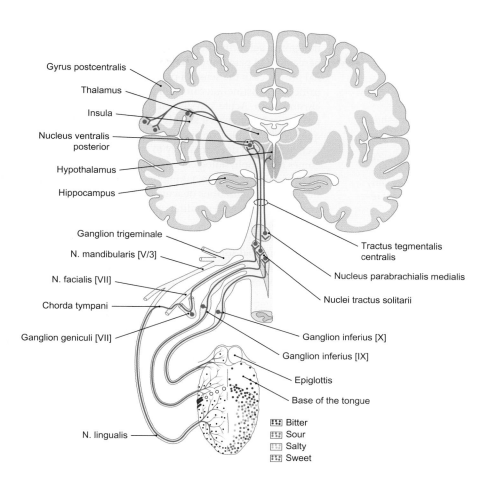

Gyrus postcentralis

Thalamus

Insula

Nucleus ventralis posterior

Hypothalamus

Hippocampus

Ganglion trigeminale

N. mandibularis [V/3]

N. facialis [VII]

Chorda tympani

Ganglion geniculi [VII]

N. lingualis

Tractus tegmentalis centralis

Nucleus parabrachialis medialis

Nuclei tractus solitarii

Ganglion inferius [X]

Ganglion inferius [IX]

Epiglottis

Base of the tongue

Bitter
Sour
Salty
Sweet

Fig. 13.21 Human tongue with epiglottis and taste buds. [L127]

The mucosa of the oral-pharyngeal space is innervated by 3 different cranial nerves, which conduct the resulting action potential to the **Nucleus tractus solitarii** that lies centrally in the Medulla oblongata:

- Taste buds of the anterior two-thirds of the tongue conduct nerve impulses via the facial nerve, Pars intermedius [VII] (➤ Chap. 9.3.7, ➤ Chap. 12.5.10).
- Taste buds of the rear third of the tongue conduct nerve impulses via the N. glossopharyngeus [IX] (➤ Chap. 9.3.9, ➤ Chap. 12.5.12).
- Taste buds of the epiglottis conduct nerve impulses via the N. vagus [X] (➤ Chap. 9.3.10, ➤ Chap. 12.5.13).

The perikarya of the 1st neuron are located as pseudounipolar ganglion cells in the **Ganglion geniculi** [VII], in the **Ganglion inferius** [IX] (syn.: Ganglion petrosum) of the N. glossopharyngeus or in the **Ganglion inferius** (synonym: Ganglion nodosum) of the N. vagus [X] (➤ Fig. 13.21).

13.7.2 Central section

The respectively centrally-directed axon of the ganglion cells runs via the Meatus acusticus internus (for the N. facialis [VII]) or via the Foramen jugulare (for the N. glossopharyngeus [IX] and vagus [X]) into the interior of the skull and finally reaches the Nucleus tractus solitarii – especially its cranial section, the **Pars gustatoria (Nucleus gustatorius)**, where conversion into the 2nd neuron takes place. The Pars gustatoria is structured somatotopically, so that the afferents of the Pars intermedius of the N. facialis can end

rostrally, those of the N. glossopharyngeus below them and those of the N. vagus caudally. Interneurons within the nucleus establish connections to subdiaphragmatic branches of the N. vagus which, amongst other things, also controls the gastric motility.

The fibres of the 2nd neuron run ipsilaterally in the **Tractus tegmentalis centralis** or attached to the **Lemniscus medialis** of the 3rd neuron in the **thalamus (Nucleus ventralis posteromedialis)**. The conscious perception of taste results from thalamocortical projections into the – corresponding to the location of the homunculus – inferior section of the Gyrus postcentralis, but also into the **anterior insular cortical area** of the temporal lobe and the operculum of the frontal lobe. Also these primary gustatory cortex areas are divided somatotopically. A minority of the fibres runs directly from the thalamus or indirectly from the Nucleus tractus solitarii via the **Nucleus parabrachialis medialis** to the hypothalamus and the amygdala as well, and there influences autonomic body functions such as appetite, feeling sated or linking the taste perception with emotions (➤ Fig. 13.21).

Clinical remarks

Taste perception is age-dependent, because the excitation threshold for the development of an action potential in taste receptors increases with age. A complete loss of taste perception is known as **ageusia** and the reduction in the way things taste is known as **hypogeusia.** The taste and olfactory system interact closely, which is also represented by a joint secondary cortical field in the orbitofrontal cortex.

13.8 Nociceptive system
Anja Böckers

┌─ Clinical case ──────────────────────────────────┐

CIPA syndrome

Medical history
During a clinical traineeship in Iran during walk-in hours, a
12-month-old toddler is presented with recurring episodes of
fever, diarrhoea and dry skin. The girl is the second child of
parents who are blood relatives. Pregnancy and birth were
normal, and the physical and mental development were normal. The parents have however noticed for some months that
the child seldom cries and does not adequately respond to
painful stimuli.

Initial examination
The little girl shows deep ulcers on the fingertips, lips and
tongue. The clinical neurological examination shows slightly
weakened muscle reflexes and a rather unremarkable tactile
sensitivity with temperature perception, but clearly shows no
response to pain stimuli.

Diagnosis
The main symptoms of insensitivity to superficial and deep pain
stimuli and of autonomic dysfunction with anhidrosis (an absence of sweat secretion), diarrhoea and dry skin can be explained by a very rare inherited disease which is referred to as
CIPA syndrome (congenital insensitivity to pain with anhidrosis).

Clinical picture
The cause is an autosomal recessive mutation of the neurotrophic tyrosine kinase receptor type I gene with a connected
malfunction of the formation of NGF (nerve growth factor) in
the embryonic phase. Pain insensitivity often leads to
self-harming behaviour, which begins with initial dentition
through bite injuries to the lips, cheek, tongue and fingers.
Patients often suffer life-long trauma with bone fractures and
complicating osteomyelitis (bone marrow inflammation). Therapeutically, in addition to family counselling, symptomatic
treatment is required, aimed at avoidance of self-harming behaviour and the resulting, often mutilating, complications.
However, anaesthetic is still necessary during operations because tactile sensation remains intact.

└──┘

13.8.1 Overview

Pain is defined as '*an unpleasant sensory or emotional experience
that is associated with actual or potential tissue damage or described
in such a way by the person concerned as if such damage were the*

cause' (International Association for the Study of Pain). Pain is
therefore a subjective perception that is determined not only by the
perception of pain impulses, but also results from complex neuronal processes in the sense of pain processing or modulation. In
principle, a distinction can be made between **acute pain** and
chronic pain. Acute 'physiological' pain undertakes an important
protective function as it signals to the body to remove itself as
quickly as possible from a dangerous situation. However, this protective function does not apply to chronic pain and it therefore becomes a pathophysiological symptom instead.

In the following section, taking into account pain processing, the
neuronal configurations of acute physiological pain will be considered in particular. Depending on the site of origin, various forms of
pain can be defined:
* peripherally-triggered pain
  - **superficial somatic pain,** caused by nociceptors in the skin
    and muscles
  - **deep somatic pain,** conducting impulses from joints and ten-
    dons
  - **visceral pain,** triggered by chemical stimuli, by distension of
    the visceral hollow organs or by spasms of the smooth visceral
    muscle
* centrally-conveyed pain such as **thalamic pain, psychosomatic
  pain** or **referred pain** on the spinal level

13.8.2 Pain conduction

Pain is an indispensable signal for survival and maintenance of the
body's integrity. Pain perception and impulse conduction are
therefore created early on in phylogenetic development. Three different ascending pain pathways can be differentiated.

Archispinothalamic tract
This tract forms the oldest tract system and runs mainly in the pro-
priosinal system. The perikarya of the 1st neuron are located in the
spinal ganglion (pseudounipolar neurons; ➤ Table 13.6). Pain impulses then run in the posterior horn into lamina II (Substantia gelatinosa), so that after configuration into the local 2nd neuron they
reach several of the adjoining segments in a multisynaptic ascending and descending manner. The fibres of this rather diffusely applied tract system run to cranial, both crossed as well as uncrossed,
right up into the **periaqueductal grey** (PAG) of the brainstem
(**Substantia grisea periaqueductalis,** syn. **Substantia grisea centralis**) and to the intralaminar nuclei of the thalamus (Nucleus

Table 13.6 Stations of the nociceptive system.

Neuronal chain	Groups of neurons
1st neuron	Perikarya of pseudounipolar ganglion cells in the Ganglion spinale or Ganglion trigeminale
2nd neuron	In the Cornu posterius (laminae II, IV–VIII) or Nucleus spinalis nervi trigemini
3rd neuron	Perikarya of the thalamus: • Ipsilateral Nucleus ventralis posterolateralis (for the Tractus spinothalamicus) • Contralateral Nucleus ventralis posteromedialis (for the Tractus trigeminothalamicus) • Perikarya of intralaminar nuclei
4th neuron	• Primary somatosensory cortex: Gyrus postcentralis • Hypothalamus, limbic system • Brainstem (Substantia grisea centralis, tectum, Formatio reticularis)

centromedianus and Nucleus parafascicularis). Via projections to the hypothalamus and to the limbic system, collateral fibre tracts of this system convey visceral, emotional and autonomic pain reactions.

Paleospinothalamic tract

Together with the archispinothalamic tract, these fibres preferentially convey dully perceived slow somatic and deep pain, which is often associated with autonomic reactions. In addition, this tract forms a neural network or a matrix structure, which is decisively involved at various levels – particularly subcortical – in pain processing. This matrix structure makes clear, in particular, the affective and motivational component of nociception (➤ Fig. 13.22). The axons also reach the 1st neuron of the posterior horn of the spinal cord here; they are likewise multimodal and also conduct

mechanosensory and thermosensory impulses. The fibres of the 2nd neuron predominantly cross to the opposite side and eventually form the **Tractus spinothalamicus anterior,** which reaches various subcortical areas in ascending order; amongst them are mainly the intralaminar and medial nuclei of the thalamus, but also the periaqueductal grey **(Tractus spinomesencephalicus).** Further subcortical destination areas are the mesencephalic Formatio reticularis **(Tractus spinoreticularis),** the tectum **(Tractus spinotectalis)** and the Nuclei parabrachiales in the pons. The latter project directly into the hypothalamus and the amygdala and thus are connected to autonomic and affective pain processing.

The above-mentioned tracts, together with the Tractus spinothalamicus lateralis (see below), are referred to as the **anterolateral system.** After conversion in the thalamus they reach various cortical areas, including BRODMANN area 3 and the frontal cortex. In

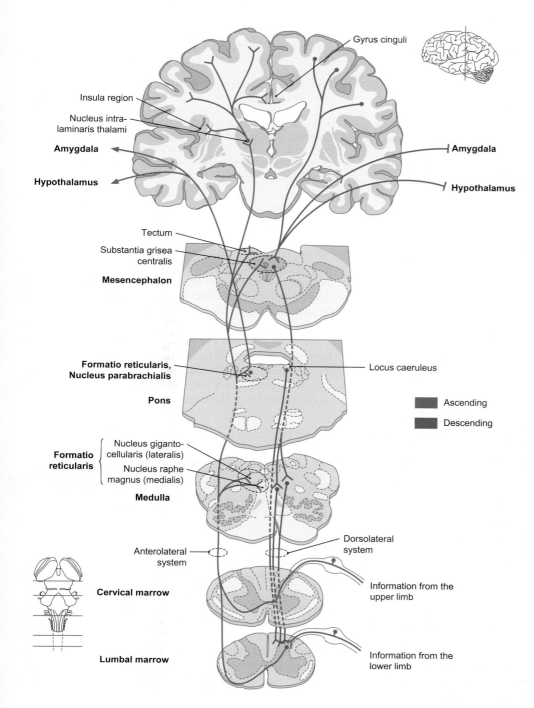

Gyrus cinguli

Insula region

Nucleus intra-laminaris thalami

Amygdala

Hypothalamus

Amygdala

Hypothalamus

Tectum

Substantia grisea centralis

Mesencephalon

Formatio reticularis, Nucleus parabrachialis

Locus caeruleus

Pons

Ascending

Descending

Formatio reticularis ⎰ Nucleus giganto-cellularis (lateralis)
⎱ Nucleus raphe magnus (medialis)

Medulla

Dorsolateral system

Anterolateral system

Cervical marrow

Information from the upper limb

Lumbar marrow

Information from the lower limb

Fig. 13.22 Ascending tracts of the paleospinothalamic tract for pain management (left half of image) and descending pain modulating fibre tracts (right half of image) in a simplified diagram. [L127]

doing so, the tracts ascending from the spinal cord run both crossed as well as uncrossed, and thus reach the thalamic nuclei of both hemispheres.

In addition to this 'main tract' there are however also 'accessory tracts', which run predominantly from the Formatio reticularis via the intralaminar thalamic nuclei to reach the Gyrus cinguli (part of the limbic system) and the insular cortex. In turn, projections of the limbic system into the hypothalamus are made responsible for autonomic reactions to a pain stimulus (sweat secretion, nausea). Regressive projections from the frontal cortex into the limbic system are connected functionally to emotional reaction to a pain stimulus.

Neospinothalamic tract

This tract conducts 'classic' – perceived as sharp and fast – somatic pain from the skin and muscles of the upper and lower extremity. It makes it possible to differentiate pain according to localisation, intensity and quality. The central axons of the 1st neuron end in the Cornu posterius (Lamina I) and are conducted after conversion and the crossing of fibres in the Commissura anterior in the anterolateral bundle as the **Tractus spinothalamicus lateralis** to the thalamus, in particular to the **Nucleus ventralis posterolateralis** and the **Nucleus ventralis posterior inferior.** A pain stimulus is localised precisely and consciously via cortical projections into the somatotopically structured primary sensory cortex (Gyrus postcentralis). Pain conduction from the head and throat area run via the 1st neuron, of which the perikaryon is located in the **Ganglion trigeminale.** The centrally-directed axons reach the Nucleus spinalis nervi trigemini in the Medulla oblongata; there they are converted into the 2nd neuron and reach the **Nucleus ventralis posteromedialis** of the thalamus via the contralateral **Tractus trigeminothalamicus** in the Lemniscus medialis. Ending here first and foremost are quick Aδ fibres, while slower C fibres are configured synaptically with the intralaminar nuclei of the thalamus.

Conduction of visceral pain

Visceral pain, e.g., of the abdominal organs, also reaches the CNS via nerve fibres of pseudounipolar neurons in the spinal ganglia and run after conversion in the **anterolateral system** to the supraspinal centres. To a certain extent, these afferents also form synaptic contacts with neurons that are located at the base of the Cornu posterior near the Canalis centralis. The axons of these neurons do not run in the anterolateral system, but in the medial parts of the posterior funiculus. Configuration into the 3rd neuron then takes place in the **Nuclei gracilis and cuneatus** in the Medulla oblongata. From there, the axons project via the Lemniscus medialis into the ventroposterior nuclei of the thalamus.

Clinical remarks

These projections in the posterior funiculus are seen as the main way in which visceral pain is conveyed. Their separation **(midline myelotomy)** can therefore be used alongside other neurosurgical methods for treating treatment-resistent pain, e.g., in cancers of the abdominal and pelvic spaces.

13.8.3 Pain processing

Knowledge of pain processing and the structures involved open therapeutic approaches for the treatment of pain. Pain can be triggered peripherally as a nociceptor which can be irritated directly or indirectly. An example of an indirect irritation is an inflammatory tissue reaction to an injury: substances in the injured tissue such as protons, arachidonic acid, histamines or prostaglandins lead to an increased sensitivity to pain. Pain-relieving (analgesic) treatment is applied either at the site of the pain's origin (peripherally) or at further pain conduction (centrally).

Clinical remarks

Peripherally, prostaglandins lead to increased pain sensitivity by binding to G-protein coupled receptors and increasing the intracellular cAMP levels in the nociceptors. Via a further point of application at the sodium channels, they simultaneously lower the depolarisation threshold of the nociceptors. **Non-steroidal anti-inflammatory drugs** (NSAIDs) such as acetylsalicylic acid or ibuprofen inhibit cyclooxygenase – the key enzyme in the biosynthesis of prostaglandins – and thereby develop their peripherally acting analgesic (and anti-inflammatory) power. For central analgesic treatment, highly effective **opioids** are used (derivatives of opium, which is obtained from the dried latex of the opium poppy). They act predominantly centrally by binding to 3 different classes of opiate receptors (μ-receptor, λ-receptor and κ- receptor). A particularly high density of these receptors are found, amongst others, in the spinal cord (lamina I), in the Substantia grisea centralis, in the hypothalamus, in the Nuclei raphes and caudatus and in the hippocampus. However, opioids also influence other important central functions such as respiratory drive, cardiovascular functions, appetite, intestinal peristalsis and mood, and they have a high potential for addiction.

In the following section, the focus will be on central pain processing and the general options for analgesic treatment.

Spinal modulation of incoming pain impulses

As early as the 1960s, MELZACK and WALL proposed a designated mechanism of spinal pain processing as a **gate control theory**: inhibitively acting interneurons thereby regulate the incoming pain impulses at a segmental level. They are activated by collateral sensory fibres from the skin and project onto the 2nd neuron of pain conduction in the lamina I of the Cornu posterior or the Nucleus spinalis nervi trigemini. Typically, they use glycine, GABA or opioids as inhibiting transmitters and thus effect a presynaptic inhibition of pain fibres. A non-painful perception on the skin suppresses the conduction of pain stimuli ('closes the gate').

Clinical remarks

The gate theory is the physiological basis for the method of pain treatment called **transcutaneous electrical nerve stimulation (TENS)** or for acupuncture. Since the lamina I is rich in opioid receptors, local or systemic **application of opiates** also has an analgesic effect in this case.

Central modulation via descending tracts

Descending tracts also have an influence via interneurons at a spinal level on pain processing. Primarily, pain is suppressed in the process (see above), but can also be increased in some situations. These supraspinal projections of the brainstem originate from the Formatio reticularis (Nucleus raphes magnus) and the **periaqueductal grey** (PAG) in the mesencephalon. They run in the **dorsolateral funiculus** to caudal and end excitatorily at inhibiting interneurons or at spinal neurons, which reach the thalamus monosynaptically (➤ Fig. 13.22).

The PAG receives afferent fibres and dispatches efferent fibres to the **Nucleus raphes magnus.** This nucleus, as well as the **Nucleus gigantocellularis,** subsequently create via serotonergic projection connections to the Cornu posterius of the spinal cord and there inhibit pain transmission. Likewise, both centres communicate with the Locus caeruleus, which dispatches noradrenergic fibres into the posterior horn. The central switching points of pain processing set out here are typically rich in opiate receptors. These opiate receptors are the actual target structure for neurotransmitters, endogenous opiates (β-endorphins, enkephalins or dynorphine), that are distributed in situations of acute stress, or for exogenously conducted opiates – e.g., by systemic or intrathecal routes (in the space between the Pia mater and the arachnoidea) – in order to effect pain relief.

The described descending tract system or the PAG is activated, amongst others, by fibres ascending from the spinal cord, which reach the PAG via the Nucleus gigantocellularis and in this way complete a pain modulating neuronal circuit.

Central modulation via superordinated centres

The descending tract system of the PAG is also activated via cortical fibres. These originate from the hypothalamus, the prefrontal cortex and the amygdala, which, in this context, is regarded as indispensable for emotional and motivational processing of pain, in that they make a significant contribution to emotional integration of pain and trigger reactions such as fear and anxiety upon pain stimuli. The influence of central processing mechanisms also becomes clear from the example of the placebo effect: the effect, that a placebo medication leads to subjective pain relief, is detectable in approximately one-third of all people and can be connected to an increase in μ-opioid receptor activity in the Gyrus cinguli, amongst others.

13.9 Autonomic nervous system
Thomas Deller

Skills

After working through this chapter of the textbook you should be able to:
- divide the nervous system into various parts (somatic, autonomic, central, peripheral)
- schematically map the configuration of the visceromotor function
- name the neurotransmitters of the sympathetic and parasympathetic nervous system
- describe the structure of the sympathetic nervous system (thoracolumbar system) and thereby differentiate between configurations into paravertebral and prevertebral ganglia
- map a schematic diagram of sympathetic fibres from the spinal cord via the spinal nerve up to the target organ
- identify sympathetic ganglia on a specimen
- describe the structure of the parasympathetic nervous system (craniosacral system)
- name the course of parasympathetic fibres in the head area, the cranial ganglia in which they are configured and their target organs, and identify them on a specimen
- explain the autonomy of the enteric nervous system
- explain visceral motor function and its importance for autonomic reflex arches and autonomic control systems
- name central portions of the autonomic nervous system and roughly localise the position of important 'centres' (e.g. respiratory centre, cardiovascular centre) on a specimen
- identify the hypothalamus in the brain and classify its role as the highest control centre of the autonomic nervous system

13.9.1 Overview

Homeostasis

Human life is reliant on the maintenance of a constant internal milieu of the body. The body has a physiological 'set value' for a stable body equilibrium (homeostasis). 'Sensors' (e.g., chemoreceptors) measure the current value of a body's parameter ('actual value') and transmit this information to a 'controller' (e.g., the respiratory centre in the brainstem). This 'controller' compares the set and actual values with each other and via appropriate 'adjustable values' (e.g., respiratory drive) counteracts a deviation of balance (➤ Fig. 13.23).

Control systems of the body

A disruption of homoeostasis can occur due to stimuli from the environment (e.g., outside temperature), from the interior of the body (e.g., increase of pCO_2), or from the CNS (e.g., emotional reactions). The autonomic nervous system is involved in many of the control circuits, which bring the system back into a state of equilibrium. It responds quickly (within seconds) to changes of the set value and adjusts the body's functions to the new requirements. In addition, it is closely connected via the hypothalamus with the endocrine system and the immune system, which play central roles in the long-term maintenance of homoeostasis and a possibly longer-term required adjustment of the 'set value'. Activity of the autonomic nervous system is generally not consciously controlled. The system controls the internal milieu of the body independently, which is why it is referred to as 'autonomic'.

Anatomy

Parts of the autonomic nervous system are located in the CNS (e.g., hypothalamus, brainstem and spinal cord (neurons) and in the PNS (e.g., autonomic ganglia). It has an afferent part, which conducts information from the interior of the body to the CNS ('viscerosensory afferents'), and efferent parts, which control the function of corporeal cells ('visceromotor efferents'). The target cells of the visceromotor axons are – corresponding to the diverse functions – markedly varied (smooth muscle cells, glandular cells, adipose cells, immune cells and more). In comparison, the somatomotor axons of the somatic nervous system 'only' control the skeletal muscles.

> **NOTE**
> With its visceromotor axons, the autonomic nervous system reaches a wide range of body cells (smooth muscle cells, glandular cells, fat cells, immune cells and more). In contrast, the skeletal muscles are innervated by somatomotor axons.

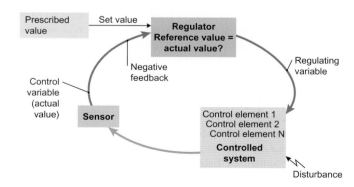

Fig. 13.23 Homeostatic control circuit. The actual value of a variable is measured via a sensor or 'feeler'. The controller compares the measured value with the physiological set value and adjusts variables in the case of a deviation, counteracting any deviation from the set value. This form of regulation is called negative feedback. [L127]

Autonomic reflex arches

Maintenance of homeostasis requires simple control circuits (e.g., negative feedback loops), which proceed predominantly at the levels of the ganglia, of the spinal cord and of the brainstem (➤ Fig. 13.23, ➤ Fig. 13.25). For this purpose, as is also the case in the somatic nervous system – visceroafferent information is processed and converted into visceromotorneurons: **visceroafferent axons** are generally formed by pseudounipolar ganglion cells, which are located in the spinal and cranial sensory ganglia. These send their peripheral process to the organs and their central process into the spinal cord or into the brainstem. Via further central configurations, information from the interior of the body finally reaches the **visceroefferent neurons,** which in turn can adapt organ function (polysynaptic autonomic reflex arc).

Central control

The autonomic control circuits that descend largely autonomically at the levels of the spinal cord and of the brainstem are influenced by decreasing tracts from the brain (➤ Fig. 13.29). To put it simply, 2 central hierarchy levels can be distinguished:

- **Autonomic control centres in the brainstem:** these include, e.g., the cardiovascular centre and the respiratory centre in the Medulla oblongata. Neurons in these areas receive visceroafferent information from the periphery and control the cardiovascular system and breathing in a complex way.
- **Autonomic control centres in the hindbrain and interbrain:** these include, e.g., the hypothalamus and amygdala, which process information from the interior of the body and can trigger behavioural changes, e.g., drink or food intake. In addition, these areas of the brain have interfaces to other control systems such as the endocrine system. Via a chain of autonomic nerve cells in various nuclei of the brainstem (➤ Fig. 13.29), the higher autonomic control centres finally have an effect on the function of the visceroefferent neurons in the brainstem and spinal cord.

13.9.2 Visceromotor function

Overview

The **visceromotor part** of the autonomic nervous system is divided at the levels of the brainstem and the spinal cord as well as the PNS into 2 functionally and structurally different parts (➤ Fig. 13.24). This is referred to as the **'sympathetic nervous system'** and the **'parasympathetic nervous system'.** For several years, the enteric (more commonly known as the 'enteric') nervous system, the nervous system of the gastrointestinal tract, has been delineated from these two. The sympathetic and parasympathetic nervous systems act opposingly to each other in many situations. They can be understood as 2 controls of a single system that can direct the system in either one or the other direction. While the enteric nervous system is affected by these two systems, it controls the intestinal functions largely independently. Thus, based on their main functions, a distinction is made between 3 systems.

- **Sympathetic nervous system:** is activated in order to improve performance capability (e.g., during physical exertion or in emergency situations; 'fight/flight'). It is therefore known as an ergotropic (energy releasing) system. It controls, amongst other things, temperature regulation (sweat glands of the skin), vascular tone and the expansion of the pupil; it stimulates heart activity, expands the bronchi and increases the activity of numerous sphincters of internal organs (➤ Fig. 13.26). The sympathetic nervous system reaches all the areas of the body, including those of the abdominal wall and the extremities (e.g., for vessel and skin innervation). When the sympathetic nervous system is activated, the integral system can adjust or prepare for a 'fight/flight' state. The body is placed temporarily into a particularly powerful 'state of alarm'. At the same time and 'concordantly', heart activity, blood pressure and sweat production increase, the pupils widen and the bronchi expand. The body can therefore react to external dangers as quickly as possible.
- **Parasympathetic nervous system:** is activated in order to replenish the energy storage areas of the body (e.g., in a resting phase). It is therefore called a trophotropic (focused on nutrition, energy-building) system. It controls the glands of the head, pupil constriction and lens accommodation in the eye, stimulates intestinal glandular activity, slows the heart, narrows the bronchi and regulates micturition and genital erection. In contrast to the sympathetic nervous system, the parasympathetic nervous system supplies neither the extremities nor the abdominal wall (➤ Fig. 13.26). Rather, it conveys organ-specific reflexes and does not adjust the 'whole system'.
- **Enteric nervous system:** controls motility (peristalsis) and digestive activity (e.g., glandular function) of the intestine. It functions predominantly autonomously (intramural autonomic plexus, Plexus submucosus and myentericus), but is influenced by the sympathetic and parasympathetic nervous systems. The parasympathetic nervous system performs a constructive effect on intestinal motility and intestinal gland secretion, while the sympathetic nervous system increases the tone of the sphincters (e.g., the pylorus).

Clinical remarks

Negative stress (distress) and the autonomic nervous system

As a result of negative stress, mental or physical stimuli (stressors) can develop that are perceived as negative, threatening or annoying. The body reacts to such stimuli, amongst other things, with an increase in tension, i.e. an enhanced activation of the sympathetic nervous system. If the negative stress situation persists, the sympathetic nerve system can be activated and strengthened permanently, accompanied by an increased release of so-called stress hormones (e.g., glucocorticoids, catecholamines). This, in turn, induces functional autonomic symptoms (e.g., increase in heart rate, cardiac arrhythmia, increase in blood pressure, nervousness), which are perceived and felt by a person as additional strain ('Circulus vitiosus'). A very long-lasting activation of the sympathetic nervous system and a long-lasting increased secretion of stress hormones can lead to physical and mental exhaustion.

NOTE

The **sympathetic and parasympathetic nervous system** form the visceromotor limb of the autonomic nervous system. They work in many situations as opposing 'controls' to counteract the body's reaction in the direction of 'fight/flight' or 'rest/digestion'. The two systems can be easily distinguished at the spinal cord level and in the peripheral nervous system. However, they are only a part of the entire autonomic system to which the enteric nervous system, the visceroafferent leg as well as the higher autonomic centres also belong.

Configuration principles and neurotransmitters
General principle

If one compares somatomotor innervation of the skeletal muscles with the visceromotor innervation of the various autonomic target

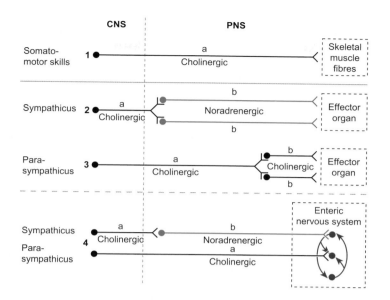

Fig. 13.24 Circuit diagram of the peripheral motor innervation in the somatic and autonomic nervous systems. [L141] 1 = somatomotor neuron, 2 = visceromotor neuron of the sympathetic nervous system, 3 = visceromotor neuron of the parasympathetic nervous system, 4 = visceromotorneurons and their impact on the enteric nervous system; a = 1st neuron, b = 2nd neuron. [L141]

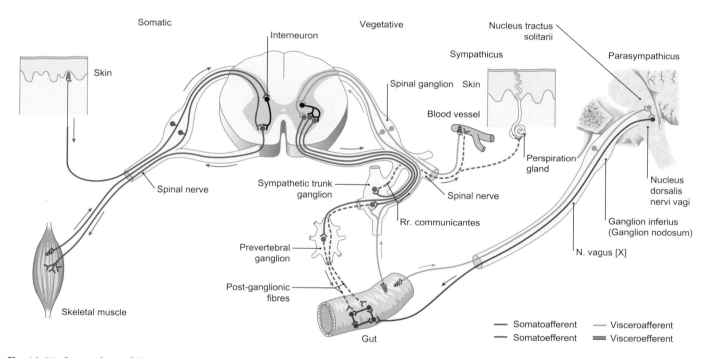

Fig. 13.25 Comparison of the organisation of the somatic with the autonomic nervous systems (spinal cord and PNS). In the somatic nervous system (left), afferent information reaches the α-motorneurons of the anterior horn via the processes of the spinal ganglion cells either directly (monosynaptic reflex arc) or indirectly. In the case of the sympathetic nervous system, visceroafferent information initially reaches the interneurons of the spinal cord via spinal ganglion cells. Via one or more switching stations they finally reach the visceroefferent neurons of the lateral horn. From there, the preganglionic visceroefferent axons (green, solid line) run either to the paravertebral ganglia of the sympathetic trunk or to the prevertebral ganglia in the area of the aorta. After they have been converted in the ganglia, the postganglionic axons (green, dotted line) run to their target organs. In the case of the parasympathetic nervous system (here: the N. vagus), visceroafferent information about the Ganglion inferius of the N. vagus initially reaches the Nucleus tractus solitarii in the brainstem. There, they are converted into the Nucleus dorsalis nervi vagi. Via the N. vagus, visceromotor fibres pass back into the body's periphery (vasovagal reflex arc). [L127]

cells, a major difference in the peripheral configuration of the two systems becomes clear (➤ Fig. 13.24): while somatomotor innervation of skeletal muscle fibres runs directly, i.e. without further configuration, via the axons of α-motorneurons of the spinal cord, the visceromotor axons are converted at least once in an autonomic ganglion (exception: adrenal medulla). In both the sympathetic and the parasympathetic nervous system, the 1st neuron is located in the CNS (spinal cord or brainstem) and is referred to as a **preganglionic neuron**. Its axon (preganglionic axon) reaches an auto-

nomic ganglion, where it is converted into a 2nd neuron (**postganglionic neuron**). Finally, its axon (postganglionic axon) reaches the target organ.

NOTE

In autonomic ganglia, preganglionic axons are converted into postganglionic neurons (multipolar ganglion cells). In contrast, no conversion takes place (pseudounipolar ganglion cells) in sensory ganglia (craniospinal ganglia).

Sympathetic and parasympathetic nervous system

The sympathetic and parasympathetic nervous systems can be differentiated into the spinal cord and the brainstem as well as the PNS, based on the location of the 1st and 2nd neurons (➤ Fig. 13.26):

- In the sympathetic nervous system, the 1st neuron is located in the lateral horn of the spinal cord at the level of segments C8–L3, which is why the sympathetic nervous system is also referred to as the 'thoracolumbar system' (➤ Fig. 13.25, ➤ Fig. 13.26, ➤ Fig. 13.27).
- In the parasympathetic nervous system, the 1st neuron is located in the brainstem as well as in the sacral area of the spinal cord in segments S2–5, which is why the parasympathetic nervous system is also called the 'craniosacral system' (➤ Fig. 13.26, ➤ Fig. 13.28).

The location of the 2nd neurons of the two systems also differs:

- In the sympathetic nervous system they are not close to the organs (sympathetic trunk or prevertebral ganglia).

- In the parasympathetic nervous system they are located in individual ganglia (head) or in the vicinity of a target organ (rest of the body); in many cases they are even located within the organ. These are therefore also referred to as 'intramural' ganglia ('within the walls' of an organ; ➤ Fig. 13.24).

Enteric nervous system

The enteric nervous system lies in the intestinal wall. Located there are autonomic ganglion cells in the Plexus myentericus and in the Plexus submucosus. These form a largely autonomous circuit, which, nevertheless, can be influenced by the parasympathetic and sympathetic nervous systems. The sympathetic and parasympathetic nerve connections to the intestine, in turn, follow the above illustrated switching principle (➤ Fig. 13.24).

Neurotransmitters

The sympathetic and parasympathetic nervous systems sometimes differ partly in terms of their chemical transmitters. Both systems

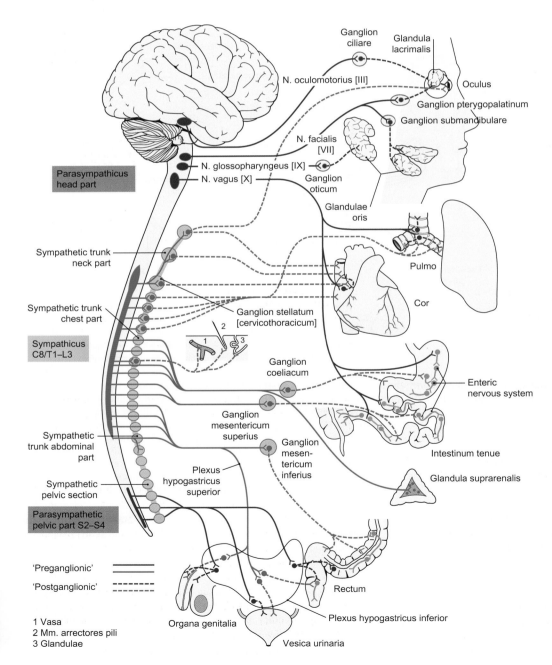

Fig. 13.26 Sympathetic and parasympathetic nervous systems. Depicted here are the two visceromotor parts of the autonomic nervous system from the spinal cord to their peripheral effector organs. Neurons of the sympathetic nervous system are found in the spinal cord at the level of segments C8/T1–L3 (thoracolumbar system) and reach the paravertebral (sympathetic trunk) or prevertebral sympathetic ganglia with their axons. After conversion, the sympathetic axons run either with nerves or vessels to their target organs. Neurons of the parasympathetic nervous system are found in the brainstem and in the sacral spinal cord (craniosacral system). Their axons run to parasympathetic ganglia in the area of the head or to ganglia in the body near to the organs. After switching onto a 2nd neuron, they also innervate their target organs. [L106]

Labels in figure:
Ganglion ciliare
Glandula lacrimalis
N. oculomotorius [III]
Oculus
Ganglion pterygopalatinum
Ganglion submandibulare
N. facialis [VII]
N. glossopharyngeus [IX]
N. vagus [X]
Ganglion oticum
Glandulae oris
Parasympathicus head part
Sympathetic trunk neck part
Pulmo
Sympathetic trunk chest part
Cor
Ganglion stellatum [cervicothoracicum]
Sympathicus C8/T1–L3
Ganglion coeliacum
Enteric nervous system
Ganglion mesentericum superius
Ganglion mesentericum inferius
Sympathetic trunk abdominal part
Intestinum tenue
Plexus hypogastricus superior
Glandula suprarenalis
Sympathetic pelvic section
Parasympathetic pelvic part S2–S4
Rectum
'Preganglionic'
'Postganglionic'
Plexus hypogastricus inferior
1 Vasa
2 Mm. arrectores pili
3 Glandulae
Organa genitalia
Vesica urinaria

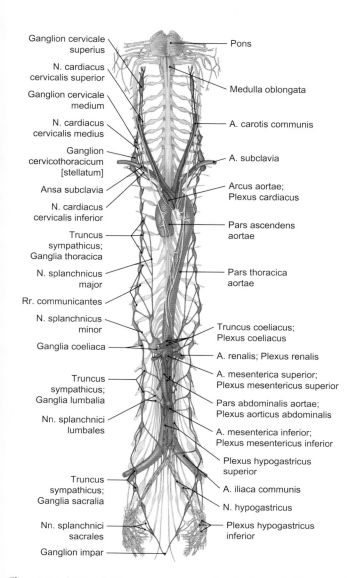

Fig. 13.27 Sympathetic nervous system. Semi-schematic diagram of the sympathetic nervous system in a topographic-anatomical context. Sympathetic axons emerge with the Nn. spinales from the spinal cord, reach the ganglia in the sympathetic trunk or emerge prevertebrally and finally run with vessels or nerves to the target organs.

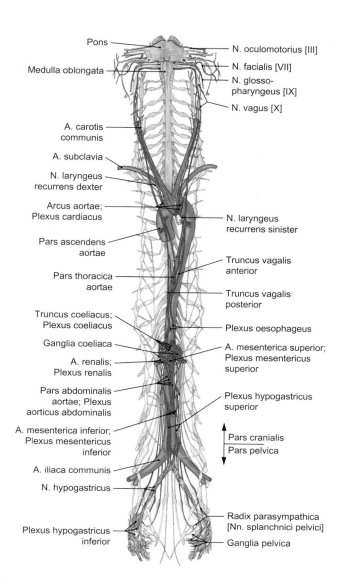

Fig. 13.28 Parasympathetic nervous system. Semi-schematic diagram of the parasympathetic nervous system in a topographic-anatomical context. Parasympathetic axons in the head area run with cranial nerves to parasympathetic ganglia and from there to their target organs. The thoracic and abdominal organs are mainly innervated by the N. vagus [X]. The last section of the intestine and the pelvic organs receive their parasympathetic innervation from the sacral medulla.

use acetylcholine between the 1st and 2nd neurons. However, at the synapse between the postganglionic axon and the target cell, the axons of the sympathetic nervous system largely use noradrenaline, while the parasympathetic nervous system, in contrast, uses acetylcholine. An exception to this rule are the sympathetically innervated sweat glands and a few specialised blood vessels; here the sympathetic nervous system also resorts to acetylcholine.

> **NOTE**
>
> The sweat glands of the skin are innervated by the sympathetic nervous system. The neurotransmitter of these postganglionic sympathetic axons is acetylcholine (exception!).

Receptors

The target cells of the visceromotor axons are filled with different receptors and receptor subtypes for the respective neurotransmitters. Through these differences in the receptors contained in the target cells, a neurotransmitter can have different effects on differ-

ent target cells. This is of particular importance for medical treatment, as drugs have been developed which can selectively influence the function of particular internal organs (e.g., 'cardioselective' drugs that work particularly on the heart) via different receptors.

Adrenal medulla

Playing a special role in the circuitry of the autonomic nervous system is the adrenal medulla. It contains cells that correspond to modified sympathetic neurons and in 'fight/flight' situations can release catecholamines into the blood ('adrenaline rush'). It derives evolutionarily from the neural crest and the paraganglia. It is therefore also regarded as the 'largest paraganglion of the body'.
In the logical context of the circuitry of the sympathetic nervous system (➤ Fig. 13.24), the adrenal medulla corresponds to a sympathetic ganglion, of which the ganglion cells do not form axons, but rather issue their neurotransmitters directly into the blood. Accordingly, the adrenal medulla is also directly innervated by preganglionic axons of the sympathetic nervous system.

Sympathetic nervous system
Preganglionic neuron

The **1st neuron** is located in the lateral horn of the grey matter of the spinal cord in the spinal cord segments C8–L3. Here, the preganglionic neurons which run to the extremities and the abdominal wall are located further laterally, and the neurons which run to the internal organs further medially.

The **myelinated axon** runs with the ventral root fibres of the segment and with these finally forms the spinal nerve (➤ Fig. 13.25). As the **R. communicans albus,** it then leaves the spinal nerve again and runs into the sympathetic trunk (Truncus sympathicus).

Postganglionic neuron

The **2nd neuron** can be found at various places (➤ Fig. 13.25, ➤ Fig. 13.26, ➤ Fig. 13.27):
* in the sympathetic trunk ganglia
* in the prevertebral ganglia outside of the sympathetic trunk
* in the pelvic ganglia (special case)

In addition, smaller sympathetic ganglia can also be detected in some autonomic plexuses or nerves, which will not be dealt with here.

The **postganglionic axons** leave the sympathetic ganglia and run as unmyelinated axons to the target organs. The exact pathways will be discussed below. In principle, the following applies:
* A group of axons from the sympathetic trunk ganglia runs via the **Rami communicantes grisei** to all the spinal nerves and via these to the wall of the body and the extremities.
* A second group of axons from the sympathetic trunk ganglia run via the vascular plexus to the target organs in the area of the head and via autonomic nerves (e.g., Nn. cardiaci) to the thoracic viscera.
* Axons from the prevertebral ganglia run to the abdominal and pelvic viscera.
* Axons from the pelvic ganglia run to the genitalia.

Anatomical position of the ganglia
Sympathetic trunk ganglia

The ganglia of the sympathetic trunk (Truncus sympathicus) lie on both sides adjacent to the spinal column (➤ Fig. 13.26, ➤ Fig. 13.27). Due to their location they are also called 'paravertebral ganglia'. They are connected to each other lengthways along the spinal cord via the **Rr. interganglionares.** Via these connection bridges, preganglionic autonomic nerve fibres reach the ganglia above or below their respective entry segment.
* **Thoracic and lumbar area (C8–L3):** here there is a ganglion in front of each Caput costae. Via the Rr. communicantes albi, the ganglia receive preganglionic fibres from the spinal cord (➤ Fig. 13.25).
* **Cervical sympathetic trunk:** Above C8, the sympathetic trunk receives no direct access from the spinal nerves (i.e. no Rr. communicantes albi). It continues, however, via the Rr. interganglionares in the 3 respective cervical ganglia (➤ Fig. 13.26, ➤ Fig. 13.27). These cervical ganglia receive their preganglionic fibres from C8 and the upper chest segments, which occur at this level in the sympathetic trunk and ascend via the Rr. interganglionares up into the throat area.
* **Pelvic sympathetic trunk:** Below L3, the sympathetic trunks no longer receive any direct forms of access from the spinal nerves (i.e. no Rr. communicantes albi) either. The sympathetic trunks continue with their own lumbar and sacral ganglia up into the pelvis and finally merge at their caudal end in the **Ganglion impar** (➤ Fig. 13.26, ➤ Fig. 13.27). The pelvic sympathetic trunks receive their preganglionic fibres from neurons of the upper

lumbar spine, which run at the level of their respective spinal nerves into the sympathetic trunk and from there descend into the pelvis via the Rr. interganglionares.

> **NOTE**
> Often the Ganglion cervicale inferius merges with the Ganglion thoracicum I and is then referred to as the Ganglion cervicothoracicum **(Ganglion stellatum).** It is located in front of the first Caput costae.

Prevertebral ganglia

These ganglia are located approximately in the midline of the body in front of the aorta and their outlets to the abdominal organs and kidneys. Due to their location in front of the spine they are also referred to as the 'prevertebral ganglia'. They are located in the middle of a dense autonomic nerve plexus on the ventral surface anatomy of the abdominal aorta (sometimes this plexus is also referred to as the solar plexus or the Plexus solaris). The location, size and exact number of individual ganglia is variable. They are often named as groups located around an aortic vessel outlet:
* Ganglia coeliaca
* Ganglion mesentericum superius
* Ganglia aorticorenalia
* Ganglion mesentericum inferius

The ganglia receive preganglionic fibres from the spinal cord. These run with the Rr. communicans albi to the sympathetic trunk, but instead of being converted there, proceed as the **Nn. splanchnici** to the prevertebral ganglia (➤ Fig. 13.26). According to their location (segment height), a distinction is made between:
* Nn. splanchnici thoracici (thorax)
* Nn. splanchnici major and minor (abdomen and upper retroperitoneum)
* Nn. splanchnici lumbales (lower retroperitoneum and pelvis)

Pelvic ganglia

The Ganglia pelvica are mixed ganglia which contain parasympathetic and sympathetic nerve cells. They are, therefore, a special case. They are located in autonomic nerve plexuses on both sides of the pelvic organs and primarily supply the genitalia. The ganglion next to the Cervix uteri is called the Ganglion paracervicale uteri (FRANKENHÄUSER's ganglion). Even if nerve cells of the parasympathetic and sympathetic nervous systems lie next to each other in these ganglia, they can easily be separated by modern detection methods (e.g., immunohistochemistry).

Arteries – conductors for the sympathetic nervous system

The ganglia of the sympathetic nervous system are not located directly at the organ. For bridging the distance between the ganglia and the target organs, the postganglionic sympathetic fibres use the neighbouring arteries. On the one hand, these vessels are innervated by sympathetic fibres (nerve plexuses around the vessels), but, on the other hand, they are also used as conductors in order to reach the actual target organs. The close relationship of the sympathetic nervous system to the vessels is particularly noticeable at some points of the body where nerve loops (ansae) are formed around vessels (e.g., Ansa subclavia). There, nerves and vessels exchange autonomic fibres. The sympathetic nerve plexuses around the vessels are named systematically with the name of the vessel, e.g., Plexus vertebralis or Plexus hepaticus.

Parasympathetic nervous system

The structure of the parasympathetic nervous system corresponds in principle to that of the sympathetic nervous system. Also in this system, there are 2 neurons that are configured sequentially. In practice, it is useful to divide the parasympathetic nervous system into 3 parts:

- cranial parasympathetic nervous system – cranial nerves III, VII, IX: supplying the head glands
- cranial parasympathetic nervous system – cranial nerve X: supplying cervical, thoracic and abdominal viscera (up to the CANNON's point)
- sacral parasympathetic nervous system: supplying the abdomen (from the CANNON's point) and the pelvic viscera

Although individual ganglia of the parasympathetic nervous system can be detected in the head and pelvis, the parasympathetic ganglion cells in the rest of the body are located mostly near to organs or intramurally.

Cranial parasympathetic nervous system – cranial nerves III, VII, IX

The preganglionic neuron (1st neuron) of the cranial parasympathetic nervous system lies in the nucleus of the brainstem (➤ Table 13.7). The preganglionic fibres attach to the respective cranial nerves and reach the parasympathetic ganglia. From there, they run via postganglionic fibres to their target organs.

Cranial parasympathetic nervous system – N. vagus [X]

The N. vagus differs from the other cranial nerves with parasympathetic nerve fibres because it does not develop its properties in the head, but in the throat, chest and abdomen areas. It runs as a 'vagabond' nerve through the body (➤ Chap. 12.5.13) and reaches the transverse colon (CANNON ventralis posteromedialis point) via the foregut. Preganglionic neurons are located in two nuclei:

- The neurons that originate from the **Nucleus dorsalis nervi vagi** reach the abdominal viscera (➤ Table 13.8).
- The neurons that originate from an anatomically delineated part of the **Nucleus ambiguus** (also referred to as 'external formation' or 'ventral column') reach the organs in the throat and chest area and control the attenuation of cardiac activity as well as the narrowing of the bronchi.

In its target organs, the preganglionic fibres are finally switched over. Together with fibres of the sympathetic nervous system, the postganglionic fibres form the autonomic plexuses within the organs (autonomic terminal path, see below).

Table 13.7 Cranial parasympathetic nervous system (cranial nerves III, VII, IX).

Cranial nerve	1st neuron	2nd neuron	Target organs
N. oculomotorius [III]	Nucleus accessorius nervi oculomotorii (EDINGER–WESTPHAL)	Ganglion ciliare	• M. ciliaris • M. sphincter pupillae
N. facialis [VII]	Nucleus salivatorius superior	Ganglion pterygopalatinum	• Glandula lacrimalis • mucous membranes
		Ganglion submandibulare	• Glandula submandibularis • Glandula sublingualis • mucous membranes
N. glossopharyngeus [IX]	Nucleus salivatorius inferior	Ganglion oticum	• Glandula parotidea • mucous membranes

Table 13.8 Cranial parasympathetic nervous system (N. vagus [X]).

Cranial nerve	1st neuron	2nd neuron	Target organs
N. vagus [X]	Nucleus ambiguus (external formation)	Intramural ganglia	Neck structures, heart and lungs
	Nucleus dorsalis nervi vagi	Intramural ganglia	Abdominal glands
		Ganglia of the enteric nervous system	Intestine

Sacral parasympathetic nervous system

The preganglionic neurons are located in segments S2–4. They run with the Nn. splanchnici pelvici (old name: Nn. erigentes) to the pelvic ganglia (containing both sympathetic as well as parasympathetic ganglion cells) or to intramural ganglia in the area of the organs (e.g., urinary bladder, rectum). They control the intestinal, genital and bladder function (➤ Table 13.9).

Terminal end pathway
Autonomic organ plexus

The sympathetic and parasympathetic nervous systems reach their target organs via the autonomic plexuses of the arteries (sympathetic) or via nerves or nerve plexuses (sympathetic and parasympathetic nervous system). In the organs, the postganglionic autonomic nerve fibres of both systems mix together and jointly form autonomic nerve plexus. In these autonomic nerve plexus the sympathetic and parasympathetic nervous system are no longer macroscopically separable from each other. However, this can be done with appropriate detection methods on a microscopic level (e.g., histochemical techniques, immunostaining).

Autonomic synapses

The postganglionic fibres form at or in the vicinity of their target cells (e.g., smooth muscle cells or glandular cells) small distensions (varicosities). These can end directly at the target cell or at some distance. In the latter case, it is called an **'en passant synapse'**, which can reach a larger number of cells in a volume of tissue via a transmission 'en distance' (see below).

Neurotransmitters, neuromodulators, receptors

The specific effects of autonomic synapses at their target cells can be explained by the different neurochemical conditions at the autonomic synapses. There are differences with regard to:

- Neurotransmitters (e.g., acetylcholine vs. noradrenaline)
- Composition of neurotransmitter-receptors (e.g., muscarinic and nicotinic acetylcholine receptors, α- and β-adrenoreceptors)
- Neuromodulators

Neuromodulators are substances that are distributed by a synapse; they are usually diffused through the tissue and can thereby reach several synapses. Particularly 'en passant synapses' of the autonomic nervous system use this form of information transfer. In contrast to the neurotransmitters, which convey quick answers, neuromod-

Table 13.9 Sacral parasympathetic nervous system

Part	1st neuron	2nd neuron	Target organs
Sacral parasympathetic nervous system	S2–4	Ganglia pelvica	Genitalia
		Intramural ganglia	• Distal colon • Rectum, urinary bladder • Parts of the ureter

ulators work more slowly and modulate the excitability of the target cells over a longer period of time. Important neuromodulators of the autonomic nervous system are:

- Sympathetic nervous system: neuropeptide Y (NPY), ATP
- Parasympathetic nervous system: vasoactive intestinal peptide (VIP), Substance P

Enteric nervous system

The enteric nervous system forms a largely autonomous neuronal circuit in the wall ('intramurally') of the digestive tract. It controls peristalsis (propelling the contents of the intestine and the aboral transport of chyme), glandular activity (e.g., stomach acid secretion) and resorption. Here there are 2 groups of ganglion cells:

- Plexus myentericus (AUERBACH) in the Tunica muscularis for controlling the Tunica muscularis and intestinal motor function
- Plexus submucosus (MEISSNER) in the Tela submucosa for controlling mucous membrane functions (Laminae muscularis mucosae; glandular secretion; circulation of the mucosa)

The enteric nervous system works independently, but receives modulating influences from postganglionic neurons of the sympathetic and parasympathetic nervous systems (➤ Fig. 13.24).

Local control of intestinal peristalsis

To control intestinal peristalsis, only a simple, local control circuit is required, which is located entirely within the intestinal wall. In this way, a sensory neuron perceives stretching of a wall section by means of chyme. In order to transport it further aborally, it reaches stimulating motorneurons intestinally upwards (towards oral) via interneurons and inhibiting motorneurons intestinally downwards (towards aboral). In this way, on the oral side there arises a contraction of the intestine and on the aboral side an atony of the muscles. In this way the chyme is guided to carry on flowing. Interestingly, the intestinal nervous system in this functional respect is 'directed'. If one took, e.g., an intestinal segment, rotated it and deployed it again in the 'wrong direction', it would function as a delaying element. This can be usefully applied in certain diseases of the gastrointestinal tract.

Reflex arcs via sympathetic ganglia

The above described mechanism for controlling intestinal peristalsis is a local mechanism. Expanding processes in an intestinal section can however also affect intestinal peristalsis of sections of the intestine located further away. For this purpose, the intestinal nervous system uses autonomic reflexes which are configured via sympathetic ganglia. In this case (exception!), visceroafferent fibres come from ganglion cells of the intestinal wall and run to the prevertebral sympathetic ganglion cells. With visceral motor fibres, these in turn inhibit peristalsis in intestinal sections located in an oral direction and they prevent overfilling of the already distended distal intestinal segments.

> **NOTE**
> Visceroafferent ganglion cells can be found in spinal ganglia, brain nerve ganglia and the intestinal wall.

Central influences of the sympathetic and parasympathetic nervous system

Intestinal peristalsis is adapted by central visceroafferents to the needs of the whole organism. In addition, psychological influences on intestinal function are conveyed in this way. The central visceral motor systems thus have a somewhat different function from the local regulatory active element of the enteric nervous system. The

sympathetic nervous system inhibits intestinal activity and increases the tone of the sphincters, while the parasympathetic nervous system stimulates intestinal activity and causes the sphincters to relax.

The parasympathetic nervous system is characteristic in its configuration: while the sympathetic nervous system reaches prevertebral ganglia via the Nn. splanchnici and postganglionic fibres of the sympathetic nervous system innervate intestinal ganglia (typically), in the parasympathetic nervous system, preganglionic fibres directly innervate intestinal ganglion cells.

13.9.3 Viscerosensory function

Overview

Viscerosensory function is just as important as visceromotor function for the functionality of the autonomic nervous system. Viscerosensory function perceives stimuli from the periphery, which are processed at either an organ, ganglia, spinal cord or brain level, and constitutes the afferent limb of the predominantly reflexive control of the viscera. Similar to the somatic nervous system, sensory function forms a unit with motor function and they can be referred to as **viscerosensory motor function** (analogue to sensory motor function in the somatic nervous system).

> **NOTE**
> Unlike the visceral motor part of the autonomic nervous system, the viscerosensory part *cannot* be compartmentalised into the sympathetic and parasympathetic nervous system.

Viscerosensory nerve cells

Viscerosensory neurons are located:

- in the spinal ganglia
- in the cranial ganglia (especially IX, X)
- partially intramurally in the organs (especially intestine, heart)

Viscerosensory neurons in the spinal ganglia

Located in the spinal sensory ganglia are pseudounipolar ganglion cells that are assigned to the autonomic nervous system. With their peripheral process they run to the viscera and with their central process they reach the posterior horn of the spinal cord (➤ Fig. 13.25). The functions and configurations of the peripheral processes of the viscerosensory neurons are more complex than those of the somatosensory neurons. In essence, somatosensory neurons conduct sensory information to the CNS, whereas the peripheral processes of the viscerosensory neurons release messaging material (local regulation) at the site of stimulation and/or can form collaterals with the autonomic ganglion cells of the sympathetic and parasympathetic nervous system. Via these direct connections to the ganglia, short reflex arcs originate initially underneath the spinal cord level, via which the viscera functions are regulated.

Viscerosensory neurons in cranial ganglia

Viscerosensory information from the interior of the body reaches the higher control centres of the brainstem via visceroafferent fibres of the N. glossopharyngeus [IX] and the N. vagus [X]. In comparison, ascending tracts from the spinal cord play a much smaller role (an important difference compared to the somatosensory system). Viscerosensory neurons of these two cranial nerves are located in their own viscerosensory ganglia (➤ Table 13.10).

- **N. glossopharyngeus [IX]:** It conducts afferents from the Sinus caroticus and the Glomus caroticus as well as from other glom-

Table 13.10 Viscerosensory afferents of the brainstem.

Nerve	Ganglion	Central nucleus	Organs of origin
N. glossopha-ryngeus [IX]	Ganglion inferius	Nucleus tractus solitarii	• Glomus caroticum • Sinus caroticus
N. vagus [X]	Ganglion inferius (Ganglion nodo-sum)	Nucleus tractus solitarii	• Glomera in the throat and thoracic area • Thoracic viscera • Gastro-intestinal tract

era in the area of the head. Located in the Sinus caroticus are baroreceptors, which are important for the control of blood pressure (baroreceptor reflex). Located in the Glomus caroticus are chemoreceptors that measure oxygen and carbon dioxide in the blood.

- **N. vagus [X]:** In addition to afferents from smaller glomera in the throat and chest area (chemoreceptors), the N. vagus receives the majority of viscerosensory afferents of the internal organs. In this way, it conducts information from the thoracic viscera (heart, lungs) and the gastrointestinal tract to the brain.

In the Medulla oblongata, the central processes of both cranial nerves reach the **Nucleus tractus solitarii.** This is a type of 'gate' for the visceroafferents of the internal organs to the brain (see below).

NOTE

The N. vagus [X] is the most important visceroafferent nerve in the body for central organ regulation.

Viscerosensory ganglia in the organs

Unlike the somatic nervous system, viscerosensory nerve cells can also be found in a number of organs in the autonomic nervous system. Particularly in the intestine, there are numerous viscerosensory nerve cells, which run with their central processes to prevertebral ganglia and control through them motility of the intestine through large sections. Viscerosensory neurons are also described in the heart.

13.9.4 Autonomic reflex arcs and control circuits

Visceral function is regulated at different levels. Common to all levels is the fact that stimuli are perceived and then follow a set response (➤ Fig. 13.23). The levels are:
- organ level (local reactions of peripheral fibres and local reflexes within the organ)
- reflexes at the level of the autonomic ganglia
- reflexes at the level of the spinal cord
- control circuits including higher centres

Local reactions and reflexes at an organ level are facilitated by:
- visceroafferent axons, which can directly issue transmission material according to a stimulus and thus give the most straightforward and immediate stimulus response
- visceroafferent neurons (especially in the enteric nervous system), which are configured with nearby visceromotorneurons and regulate peristalsis

Reflexes at a ganglion level are referred to when afferent fibres establish contact directly with the ganglia and, bypassing the spinal cord, control visceral functions. These reflexes occur both in the sympathetic nervous system as well as in the parasympathetic nervous system, e.g., in the above-mentioned control of intestinal peristalsis via visceroafferent axons from intestinal ganglion cells.

With their extensions, these reach the prevertebral ganglia and control the motility of the intestine over larger sections.

Reflexes at the level of the spinal cord are common. Visceroafferent neurons in the spinal ganglia run with their axons into the posterior horn of the spinal cord. There, they are configured via interneurons into visceroafferent neurons, which can be located in various segments (heights) of the spinal cord. These autonomic reflex arcs of the spinal cord are similar in their configuration (via interneurons; polysynaptically; several spinal cord segments are connected to each other) to the polysynaptic reflex arcs of the somatic nervous system. The spinal cord has a special position for reflexes of the pelvic organs. Since, in addition to the sympathetic neurons in the lumbar spinal cord, parasympathetic neurons in the sacral spinal cord are involved, this leads to extensive autonomy of the lumbar sacral spinal cord, roughly regulating the emptying of the urinary bladder or defecation.

> **Clinical remarks**
>
> Control of emptying the urinary bladder, which is predominantly controlled at the level of the spinal cord, is partially retained in the case of paraplegia above the lumbar sacral spinal cord. Although voluntarily controlled emptying of the bladder is not possible in this case, reflexive emptying of the bladder due to external stimuli (e.g., by percussion of the abdomen) can be trained. Reference is then made to a **'reflex bladder'.**

Control circuits including higher centres often emanate from the internal organs. Their visceroafferent information runs primarily with the N. vagus to the Nucleus tractus solitarii and reaches – proceeding from this visceroafferent nucleus – other autonomic nuclei and centres in the brain (see below). In these, information is processed, i.e. is compared with the set value and reconciled with information from higher control centres. Finally, via the sympathetic and parasympathetic nervous systems, they once again influence visceral functions. Via the hypothalamus they also manage to connect to the endocrine system, whereby long-term set value adjustments become possible (see below).

Vagovagal reflexes are a simple example of reflexes at the level of the brainstem. Among other things, they are important for the control of the gastrointestinal functions (glandular secretion, gut motility). Via the N. vagus, afferents run initially to the Nucleus tractus solitarii. From there, they are switched over to the visceral motor nuclei of the N. vagus (Nucleus dorsalis nervi vagi or Nucleus ambiguus). Via these, the vagal efferents run back again to the target organs.

> **Clinical remarks**
>
> In the case of 'fainting' **(vasovagal syncope)**, there is a sudden drop in heart rate and thus cardiac output. At the same time, vascular tone is reduced and blood pressure is lowered. The brain is no longer sufficiently supplied and the patient loses consciousness. This phenomenon, that can be triggered by various physical and psychological factors (e.g., too little to drink, gastrointestinal infection, pain, stress), is conveyed via the N. vagus. Afferents of the N. vagus reach the brainstem. From there, they reach the visceral motor vagal nuclei and the depressor areas of the cardiovascular centre (➤ Chap. 13.9.5). On the one hand, vagally conveyed bradycardia ensues and, on the other hand, vasodilation conveyed by a reduction in sympathetic tone. Both together finally lead to syncope.

13.9.5 Central regulation of the autonomic nervous system

Central control of the autonomic nervous system takes place at various levels of the CNS, each of which are closely configured to each other (➤ Fig. 13.29):

- **Spinal cord:** Located here are the neurons of sympathetic and parasympathetic nervous systems in the thoracolumbar or in the sacral anterior horn.
- **Inferior brainstem** (nuclei and areas in the Medulla oblongata and pons): Located here are the higher control centres for reflexive control of the cardiovascular system, breathing, gastrointestinal function and bladder control.
- **Superior brainstem** (especially the mesencephalon): Here, pain perception and autonomic control are coordinated.
- **Prosencephalon** (nuclear areas and areas in the diencephalon and telencephalon): Via these nuclei, autonomic control and the endocrine system are coordinated. Autonomic requirements lead to behavioural changes (hypothalamus). Conversely, psychological and emotional processes are connected via the limbic system to the central autonomic nervous system (➤ Chap. 1.10).

Spinal cord level and brainstem

In addition to autonomic nuclei of the spinal cord and the parasympathetic nuclei of the brainstem (➤ Chap. 12.2.4), there are other areas at the level of the brainstem which are seen as control centres for certain organ systems.

Nucleus tractus solitarii

This nucleus is the most important assembly point for visceroafferents of the brainstem areas and of the higher centres. Here, the viscerosensory afferents from cranial nerves IX (information from barometers and chemoreceptors) and X (information from the throat, chest and stomach viscera) are amalgamated. The nucleus is structured viscerotopically and is divided into 3 sections:

- cranial section (gustatory afferents)
- intermediate section (afferents from the gastrointestinal tract)
- caudal section (afferents from the vessels and from the heart, lungs and chemoreceptors)

The Nucleus tractus solitarii transmits its autonomic information to the neighbouring cardiovascular and respiratory control centres as well as other centrally located nuclei. Gastrointestinal afferents are processed in it or in its immediate vicinity, for which reason it can also be seen as a medullary centre of gastrointestinal control.

Emetic centre

The emetic centre is located directly adjacent to the Nucleus tractus solitarii in the area of the obex. It is innervated directly by vagal afferents. In addition, the blood–brain barrier in this area is functionally suspended. Direct stimulation of the N. vagus ('peripheral vomiting'), toxins ('central vomiting'), but also an increase in intracranial pressure, vestibular irritations or disgust can trigger a strong antiperistaltic contraction of the gastrointestinal tract via this area of the brainstem.

Respiratory centre

The respiratory centre lies in the **Formatio reticularis** of the ventrolateral Medulla oblongata as well as in parts of the pons. It controls the breathing largely independently. Suprapontine centres exert a modulating effect, e.g., when singing and speaking.

Location of neurons

The respiratory nerve cells form a longitudinally arranged chain of nerve cells in the Formatio reticularis, which stretches from the ventrolateral Medulla oblongata right up to the pons. The respiratory nerve cells within the Formatio reticularis can only be identified with special dyes and on the basis of their functional characteristics (in animals). Within this nerve cell chain, in turn, several functional groups can be differentiated, all with different breathing functions.

Functional anatomy

The muscles involved in breathing are controlled directly by inspiratory and expiratory neurons. These effector neurons are, in turn, controlled by nerve cells that generate the actual breathing rhythm (rhythm generators). This rhythm, a regular sequence of inspiration and expiration, already originates intrauterine before birth, and from birth until death ensuring oxygen supply. The most important rhythm generator is the **pre-Bötzinger nucleus**, a group of neurons in the Medulla oblongata section of the Formatio reticularis.

Respiratory reflexes

These reflexes are of central importance for lung function. Their structural basis is the anatomical configuration of respiratory cells in the brainstem. Put simply, they originate from an afferent limb, central processing and an efferent limb. Autonomic afferents reach the **Nucleus tractus solitarii** of the brainstem ('gateway for autonomic afferents') via the N. vagus [X] and the N. glossopharyngeus [IX]. The **N. vagus** transmits, amongst others, information for lung expansion, which is the basis of the HERING–BREUER reflex. The **N. glossopharyngeus** conducts, amongst others, information from the chemoreceptors that is important for respiratory drive. Via the nerve cells of the Nucleus tractus solitarii, this information is distributed to various respiratory groups. They process the information and converge with their axons, in turn, onto inspiratory and expiratory effector neurons that ultimately control respiratory muscle contraction and thereby respiratory rate and respiratory depth.

Cardiovascular centre

The cardiovascular centre lies mainly in the Formatio reticularis of the rostral ventral Medulla oblongata. It controls blood pressure and cardiac functions and coordinates all nerve influences on the cardiovascular system. These come from the periphery of the body, but also from autonomic centres in the hypothalamus, in the mesencephalon (Substantia grisea centralis) and in the pons (Nucleus parabrachialis). The neurons of the cardiovascular centre have pacemaker properties and receive valid basic innervation from the vessels ('medullary blood pressure').

Anatomical location

The nerve cells of the cardiovascular centre are located somewhat medially of the more ventrolaterally located respiratory areas. As with the respiratory centre, special dyes are needed to identify the related nerve cell groups in the brainstem. Put simply, it can be noted that neurons which increase blood pressure (pressor neurons) are located predominantly rostrally and laterally, while the neurons which lower blood pressure (depressor neurons) are predominantly found caudally and medially.

Functional anatomy and reflexes

Via the cardiovascular centre, important cardiovascular reflexes are conveyed (e.g., baroreflex, cardiac reflexes, cardiopulmonary reflexes, chemical reflexes). As in the respiratory centre, an afferent limb, the central processing and an efferent limb are differentiated in the cardiovascular centre. The afferents reach the cardiovascular centre via the **Nucleus tractus solitarii** ('gateway for autonomic afferents'). The **N. vagus** conducts information from the heart, baroreceptors and chemoreceptors from the aortic arch and its branches; the **N. glossopharyngeus** conducts information from chemoreceptors in the Glomus carotid. From the Nucleus tractus solitarii, autonomic information is distributed from the periphery

- to the hypothalamus,
- into the mesencephalon (Substantia grisea centralis),
- to the dorsolateral pons (Locus caeruleus, Nucleus parabrachialis) and
- to the ventral Medulla oblongata.

These areas of the brain process the information and act on the cardiovascular centre, which, in turn, controls the parasympathetic and the sympathetic nervous system. The effects of the **parasympathetic nervous system** are conveyed via connections to the N. vagus; those of the **sympathetic nervous system** (vascular tone and cardiac function) are conveyed via connections to the preganglionic sympathetic nerve cells in the lateral horn of the spinal cord.

To summarise, this means that cardiovascular functions are measured via peripheral sensors, reconciled with the set values in the cardiovascular centre of the inferior brainstem and adjusted via the sympathetic and parasympathetic nervous systems. This principal control circuit is influenced by higher centres in the brain (e.g., tachycardia in emotional excitement).

Pontine micturition centre

The bladder function is controlled spinally and via a nucleus in the rostral pons ('BARRINGTON's nucleus'):

- At a **spinal** level, sphincter contraction increases reflexively when the bladder fills (**continence reflex**).
- If the filling of the bladder exceeds a certain volume, the cells of the **pontine micturition centre** are activated via ascending spinal tracts and the '**spinobulbospinal micturition reflex**' is triggered, whereby 3 groups of spinal cells are influenced:
  - Preganglionic sympathetic cells in the lumbar spinal cord are inhibited, decreasing the tone of the M. sphincter urethrae internus.
  - Preganglionic parasympathetic cells in the sacral spinal cord are activated, which causes contraction of the M. detrusor vesicae.
  - Nerve cells that innervate the striated (arbitrary) M. sphincter urethrae externus are inhibited, and thus urine flow is released. These nerve cells are located in the sacral spinal column and are referred to as ONUF's nucleus. They run with their axons into the N. pudendus.

The pontine micturition centre is controlled by higher centres that can manage and prevent the sequence of the micturition reflex. In this way, a person can determine the timing of the micturition him/herself.

Nucleus parabrachialis

The Nucleus parabrachialis lies in the rostral pons in the vicinity of the Pedunculus cerebellaris superior (formerly: Brachium conjunctivum; hence the name of the nucleus). On the one hand, it receives afferents from the autonomic part of the Nucleus tractus solitarii and transmits these in a central direction ('relay station' or 'interface'); on the other hand, central afferents from the amygdala are transmitted to it. Via efferents to the Medulla oblongata and to the spinal cord, it conveys autonomic reactions that are connected to strong emotional states (e.g., anxiety). To put it simply, it can be said that it prepares the 'fight/flight' reactions of the body.

Mesencephalon – Substantia grisea centralis

In the Substantia grisea centralis there is an assembly of nerve cells which are located in the immediate vicinity of the Aqueductus mesencephali (hence also: 'periaqueductal grey'). It is a switching point between the autonomic brainstem centres and the hypothalamus. Their main function is the integration of autonomic and somatic reactions to pain and stress – it is decisively involved in the perception and modulation of pain at the spinal cord level. In addition, its stimulation triggers a defence behaviour and associated autonomic and somatic reactions (e.g., increase in blood pressure, tachycardia, increase in muscle tone). In this way, the Substantia grisea centralis prepares the body for a dangerous situation with its autonomic and somatic organ functions.

Clinical remarks

After stimulation of the **Substantia grisea centralis**, strong **analgesia** occurs at the level of the spinal column. A chain of neurons is responsible for this, beginning in the periaqueductal grey, running via the serotonergic Raphe nuclei of the brainstem, and ending in the Substantia gelatinosa of the spinal cord. There, afferent pain fibres are inhibited via presynaptic receptors, whereby pain transmission to the 2nd sensory neuron is suppressed. This phenomenon, in which non-painful afferents close the 'doors' for the painful afferents, is also called the '**gate control theory of pain**'.

In central analgesia with opiates, the neurons of the periaqueductal grey (but also other neurons), which contain numerous opioid receptors, are activated. In this way, the body's own 'anti-pain system' can be stimulated with medication and induce analgesia.

Prosencephalon

Located in the prosencephalon are nuclei and cortical areas which, on the one hand, have a substantial impact on the function of the autonomic nervous system, but, on the other hand, also perform functions that cannot be directly attributed to the autonomic nervous system (e.g., amygdala – emotional memory). These nuclei are generally integrated into several central circuits (e.g., within the limbic system) and also fulfil several functions. This makes it clear that the separation of the nervous system into an 'autonomic' and a 'somatic' nervous system, introduced for didactic and systematic reasons, is no longer useful starting from a particular level of complexity in the areas of the brain.

The purpose of the close interlinking of nuclei, which have an influence on the autonomic nervous system, with other parts of the nervous system is because complex behavioural changes are also required to maintain homeostasis. For example, the organism begins to search for water when experiencing strong thirst, and suspends all other activities until water has been found and the thirst is quenched.

Being aware of the problem of functional categorisation of 'central autonomic brain structures', the hypothalamus can be interpreted very pragmatically as the 'foremost control centre' of the autonomic nervous system. In addition to its role as the foremost autonomic regulator, it is simultaneously the foremost regulator of the endocrine system and thus can harmonise both systems, which serve the purpose of maintaining homeostasis. Its connections to higher cognitive levels (e.g., emotional and psychological experience) allow it to also trigger more complex behaviours of the whole organism, which also serve the purpose of homeostasis (see below).

Hypothalamus

The hypothalamus controls adjustment processes that keep the organism in homeostasis and ensure its physical survival and its proliferation. It is viewed as the hierarchically foremost centre of the autonomic nervous system. Via the **Fasciculus longitudinalis dorsalis** it is reciprocally and anatomically connected to all hierarchically 'inferior' autonomic centres in the brainstem and spinal cord. Key features of the hypothalamus include:

- temperature regulation
- regulation of fluid balance
- regulation of food intake and metabolism
- sleep and circadian rhythms
- influence of sexual and social attachment behaviour

In order to fulfil these tasks, coordinated changes are required at several levels of control, i.e. changes to organ functions, hormonal changes and behavioural changes. The hypothalamus can fulfil this overarching coordination function because it has connections to the rest of the autonomic nervous system, to the endocrine, the neuroendocrine and the limbic system and it also has 'programmes' for their coordinated activity in the form of neuronal circuits.

NOTE

The hypothalamus is the most important central coordination centre of homeostasis.

An example of the activity of the hypothalamus is the regulation of fluid balance: with osmoreceptors the hypothalamus registers the inner state of the body (e.g., hypovolemia). It then adjusts the peripheral organ functions via the autonomic nervous system to the current situation (e.g., increase in heart rate, vasoconstriction). Via the endocrine system, it increases ADH secretion and induces an intake of fluid (perception of 'thirst', fluid intake or search for a source of fluid) at the behavioural level. With the intake of fluid and the restoration of homeostasis this 'pattern of activity' can be ended.

Nuclei

The nuclei of the hypothalamus are described elsewhere (➤ Chap. 12.2.4). At this point – with the exception of the Nucleus paraventricularis which plays a particular role in the autonomic control – only the most important areas and nuclei for the control of the homeostasis will be summarised (➤ Table 13.11).

Nucleus paraventricularis

This nucleus is a particularly good example of the close interlocking of the control systems. Although it is regarded as 'a' nucleus, it contains different cell groups that have endocrine and autonomic control functions:

- magnocellular parts – projection to the neurohypophysis: oxytocin and ADH secretion
- parvocellular parts – releasing hormones for the adenohypophysis: CRH, dopamine
- parvocellular parts – projection to autonomic centres and preganglionic autonomic neurons in the brainstem and spinal cord

In this way, the nucleus controls the effectors of the endocrine and the autonomic system. The proximity of the various cells in one nucleus underlines the biological necessity of harmonising the autonomic nervous system and the endocrine system of the body with each other.

Connections

Afferents initially reach the lateral hypothalamus. From there, there are connections to the other hypothalamic nuclei which, in turn, are closely configured with each other. This enables the hypo-

Table 13.11 Nuclei of the hypothalamus and their homeostatic functions.

Area	Nucleus	Function
Area hypothalamica anterior	Nucleus suprachiasmaticus	Circadian rhythm
	Nuclei preoptici	Management of gonadotropin release in the adenohypophysis
	Nucleus supraopticus	ADH, oxytocin secretion
	Nucleus paraventricularis	ADH, oxytocin secretion, food intake; regulation of stress hormone secretion via CRH
Area hypothalamica intermedia	• Nucleus infundibularis (arcuatus) • Periventricular nerve cells	Management of the adenohypophysis; food intake habits
	• Nucleus ventromedialis • Nucleus dorsomedialis	Regulation of food and fluid intake behaviour
Area hypothalamica posterior	Nucleus posterior hypothalami, Corpora mamillaria	Thermal regulation, autonomic management
Area hypothalamica lateralis		Food intake behaviour

thalamus to harmonise and coordinate the functions of the various nuclei with each other. The efferent connections consist functionally of 3 groups:

- Connections to the limbic system (e.g., via the Corpora mamillaria)
- Connections to cortical areas (link to consciousness, perception of 'needs', e.g., thirst, hunger, satiation)
- Connections to the autonomic brainstem and spinal cord areas

Fasciculus longitudinalis dorsalis

The thalamus is connected via this tract system to the autonomic centres located underneath. The Fasciculus longitudinalis dorsalis (bundle of SCHÜTZ) passes through the brainstem right up into the spinal cord and releases fibres along its course to all the autonomic nuclei.

Amygdala

The amygdala (➤ Chap. 12.1.8) is a central nucleus of the limbic system (➤ Chap. 1.10) and is crucial for emotional evaluation of sensory perceptions. It plays an important role in reaction to stress and conveys fear and anxiety behaviour. The autonomic symptoms that are associated with the feeling of fear (tachycardia, increase in blood pressure, sweating, gastrointestinal symptoms, dry mouth) are conveyed via efferent connections of the amygdala to the hypothalamus (lateral nucleus), the periaqueductal grey and the autonomic brainstem areas.

Cortical areas

Closely connected to the hypothalamus are 2 cortical areas, to which is assigned particular importance in linking the hypothalamus to the consciousness. Both, in turn, are closely interlinked with each other and with other cortical areas.

Anterior cingulate cortex

The anterior cingulate cortex (➤ Chap. 12.1.6) is an important hub in the limbic system (➤ Chap. 1.10) and links the system to the neocortex and the insula, on the one hand, and via the hypothalamus and the brainstem to the autonomic nervous system on the other hand. Via these connections, emotions can influence the function of internal organs.

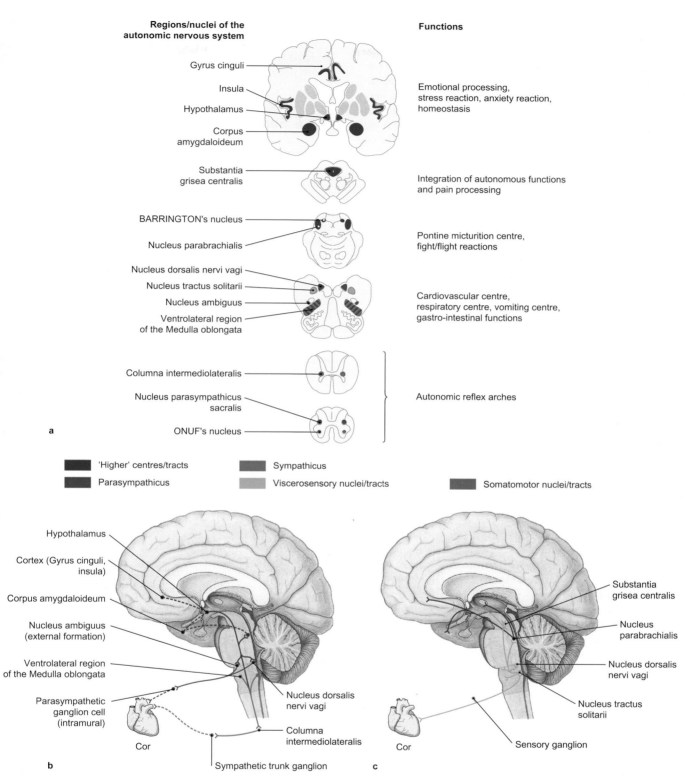

Regions/nuclei of the autonomic nervous system

- Gyrus cinguli
- Insula
- Hypothalamus
- Corpus amygdaloideum
- Substantia grisea centralis
- BARRINGTON's nucleus
- Nucleus parabrachialis
- Nucleus dorsalis nervi vagi
- Nucleus tractus solitarii
- Nucleus ambiguus
- Ventrolateral region of the Medulla oblongata
- Columna intermediolateralis
- Nucleus parasympathicus sacralis
- ONUF's nucleus

Functions

Emotional processing, stress reaction, anxiety reaction, homeostasis

Integration of autonomous functions and pain processing

Pontine micturition centre, fight/flight reactions

Cardiovascular centre, respiratory centre, vomiting centre, gastro-intestinal functions

Autonomic reflex arches

a

- 'Higher' centres/tracts
- Parasympathicus
- Sympathicus
- Viscerosensory nuclei/tracts
- Somatomotor nuclei/tracts

b
- Hypothalamus
- Cortex (Gyrus cinguli, insula)
- Corpus amygdaloideum
- Nucleus ambiguus (external formation)
- Ventrolateral region of the Medulla oblongata
- Parasympathetic ganglion cell (intramural)
- Cor
- Nucleus dorsalis nervi vagi
- Columna intermediolateralis
- Sympathetic trunk ganglion

c
- Substantia grisea centralis
- Nucleus parabrachialis
- Nucleus dorsalis nervi vagi
- Nucleus tractus solitarii
- Cor
- Sensory ganglion

Fig. 13.29 Central autonomous cerebral areas and nuclei. Lying on different levels of the CNS are nuclei and nerve cell groups, which are involved in the central control of the autonomic nervous system. These are closely connected to each other. **a** Autonomic nerve cells are located at the level of the spinal cord, brainstem, interbrain and forebrain. The subdivision into 'parasympathetic' and 'sympathetic' neurons exists up to the level of the lower brainstem. In the overlying levels, the two strands of the autonomic nervous system can no longer be sensibly distinguished. **b** Example for the interplay of visceral motorneurons with the regulation of internal organs. Neurons in the hypothalamus, the most important central nervous system autonomic conversion point, as well as neurons in the brainstem nuclei, reach the autonomic centres in the Medulla oblongata or in the spinal cord with their axons, either directly or via a neuronal chain. From there, preganglionic parasympathetic axons run via the cranial nerves – here via the N. vagus [X] – to their target organs. With their descending fibres, the same centres can also influence sympathetic neurons in the lateral horn of the spinal cord. In this way, the autonomic nervous system can be regulated in two directions. **c** Example for visceroafferents to the central nuclei. Viscerosensory information reaches the CNS via the Nucleus tractus solitarii, is converted there, and then either directly reaches the centres in the inferior brainstem (autonomic reflex arcs at the level of the brain) or reaches the more centrally located areas of the brain via ascending neural chains. [L127]

Insula

The insula is regarded by some authors as the 'primary interoceptive cortex' and thus contrasts functionally with the somatosensory cortex in the Gyrus postcentralis. It is – in the same way as in the gyrus – organised viscerotopically and receives, amongst others, afferents via the thalamus from the internal organs, skin and muscles. It integrates this information with emotions and cognitive information and is important for a conscious awareness of one's own body and the stimuli that emerge from this. It is, therefore, the cortical link between the 'unconscious' autonomic nervous system and the 'conscious' somatic nervous system.

Connections of the central autonomic areas of the brain and nuclei

The above described autonomic nuclei are, in multiple ways and means, often connected to each other via several switching points. This makes the central control of the autonomic nervous system complex. This complexity is a result of the many functions of the autonomic nervous system and the resulting required link to a wide range of brain areas, which, in turn, fulfil other functions. This highly simplified schematic diagram of the central connections (➤ Fig. 13.29) should facilitate an overview.

Visceroefferent tracts

The central collection point for descending visceroefferent information from the cortex and the limbic system is the **hypothalamus,** which is connected via the Fasciculus longitudinalis dorsalis to the visceral motor nuclei and centres in the brainstem and spinal cord (➤ Fig. 13.29). Below the control level of the hypothalamus there are still more efferents which reach the brainstem from the Substantia grisea centralis and the Nucleus parabrachialis. At the level of the brainstem the two visceral motor systems separate: parasympathetic efferents run from the visceral motor cranial nerve nuclei to the target organs and are converted in ganglia near the organs. Sympathetic efferents run from the autonomic centres of the brainstem to the lateral horn of the spinal cord and, after conversion, they run from there to the sympathetic ganglia (sympathetic trunk or prevertebrally) to the organs.

Visceroafferent tracts

The central collection point for afferent information from the periphery of the body is the **Nucleus tractus solitarii** (➤ Fig. 13.29). It receives visceroafferent information from the N. glossopharyngeus [IX] and the N. vagus [X]. It transmits the information and at the level of the Medulla oblongata it reaches the medullary control centres for heart, circulation and breathing as well as the visceral motor original nuclei of the N. vagus (Nucleus dorsalis nervi vagi; Nucleus ambiguus, external formation). The Nucleus tractus solitarii also conducts afferent information via the Fasciculus longitudinalis dorsalis to nuclei located further centrally, e.g., the Nucleus parabrachialis, the Substantia grisea centralis and the hypothalamus. With their projections, these areas, in turn, reach the limbic system (amygdala, Septum nuclei) and the cortical areas (anterior cingulate cortex, insula).

NOTE

Cortical control of the autonomic nervous system is – unlike cortical control in the somatic nervous system – a modulating factor as the basic functions of the autonomic nervous system necessary for survival are already ensured at the inferior reflex levels. If external stressors emerge ('danger'), cortical information can, via the hypothalamus and autonomic areas in the brainstem, influence visceromotor function and change the function of the organs. This influence on neocortical areas is not controlled consciously, but occurs by means of activation of phylogenetically old neuronal circuits. The effect of this influence is ultimately 'reported back' from the body via afferent information and, in this way, achieves perception ('I feel palpitations, if I am anxious').

13.9.6 Summary and outlook

The autonomic nervous system is of central importance for the **control of vital organ functions**. It maintains the homeostasis of the body and adjusts bodily functions to changing conditions. It does not act alone, but collectively with the endocrine system, the immune system and the somatic nervous system.

The autonomic nervous system is of particular importance for the **diagnosis and treatment of diseases.** Numerous medications act either directly or indirectly on autonomic reflex arcs or control mechanisms, in which the autonomic nervous system is also involved. The precise anatomical structures through which the autonomic nervous system exerts its effects are still partly unknown. The history of this is that the axons and ganglion cells are distributed in a more complex and more diffuse fashion and the effect is also not conveyed from one cell to another, but is directed via volume transmission to entire cell bonds. Neuromodulators play a decisive role in specifying the effect of the autonomic nervous system. Current research is attempting to decrypt the role of these neuromodulators and to find an 'autonomic code', which ultimately could lead to a deeper understanding of the control of organ functions.

13.10 Limbic system
Thomas Deller

┌─ **Skills** ────────────────────────────────────

After working through this chapter of the textbook, you should be able to:
• locate those areas of the brain that are usually grouped as the 'limbic system' on a specimen and name their most important connections (e.g., PAPEZ circuit)
• critically discuss the term 'limbic system'
• explain the most important functions of the limbic system (memory, emotions, reward learning, autonomic regulation)

└──

13.10.1 Overview

The term 'limbic system' implies a functional system – similar to the motor system or the somatosensory system. While the term 'system' in the motor or somatosensory systems is based on traceable anatomic and functional contexts, the term 'limbic system' developed historically (see below). It refers to a group of structures that are connected closely to each other anatomically, without immediately taking their functions into account. Thus, it is also understandable why both the term 'limbic system' as well as the components of this system are still debated very controversially to this day.

Functions

Important and medically relevant functions of the limbic system are:
• **Memory function:** it contains important nuclei (especially hippocampus formation) for declarative learning (knowledge of the world, biographical and episodic memory).

- **Emotional reactions:** nuclei in the limbic system (especially amygdala) 'evaluates' sensory impressions and memories and connect them to feelings; this is an important biological basis for anxiety and panic disorders.
- **Reward learning:** The limbic system is part of the motivational network of the brain and is thus involved in psychiatric illnesses with disorders of emotional experience and drive ('mood disorders'), which include, e.g., depression) or disorders of the reward system ('addiction diseases').
- **Autonomic regulation:** Connections between the limbic system and autonomic nervous system (especially the hypothalamus) form the biological basis for the influence of cognitive processes on the body. This is the biological basis for psychosomatic illnesses and autonomic symptoms in psychiatric conditions.

Historical background

Pierre Paul BROCA (French doctor, 1824–1880) was the first to describe significant limbic structures and to group them together. He noted that longitudinally running cortical structures are located around the Corpus callosum, which surround it like a fringe (Lat. limbus) (➤ Fig. 12.7). These structures, which are divided into an outer ring (including the Gyrus cinguli, Gyrus parahippocampalis) and an inner ring (including the hippocampus, fornix), were named by him as the '**Lobus limbicus**'.
James W. PAPEZ (American anatomist, 1883–1958) researched fibre connections in the brain and in 1937, on the basis of the strength of the anatomical connections between certain areas, which are partially located in the Lobus limbicus, he described a neuronal circuit, which to this day is called the 'PAPEZ circuit' (➤ Chap. 13.10.3). He suggested that this circuit controls the emotions of the brain. Even if this hypothesis is now outdated and important structures of the PAPEZ circuit can be associated with learning and memory, his proposal was of great scientific theoretical significance.
The first experimental indications of the structures in the temporal lobes being important for emotions were provided in 1939 by experiments performed by Heinrich Klüver (German and American psychologist, 1897–1979) and Paul Bucy (American neurosurgeon, 1904–1992), which proved that emotional and social behaviour in experimental animals significantly changed after removal of both temporal lobes.
Paul D. MCLEAN (American doctor and physiologist 1913–2007) ultimately introduced the term 'limbic system' into literature and expanded the limbic areas around the amygdala, in particular.

N O T E
Today, the term 'limbic system' is used to group areas of the brain that can influence autonomic and neuroendocrine reactions as well as emotions (fear, anger, euphoria, loathing). Therefore, the use of the term essentially has a didactic advantage in simplifying as far as possible the complex biological basis of emotions and psychological processes and, to a partial extent, representing them reproducibly.

13.10.2 Components of the limbic system

The limbic system can be divided into cortical parts and nuclei. In addition, there are a few further nuclei that are particularly closely connected to the limbic system:
- **cortical parts** of the limbic system:
  - cingulate cortex (including the Area retrosplenialis)
  - hippocampus formation (including the entorhinal cortex and the subiculum)

- **nuclei** of the limbic system:
  - Septal nuclei/diagonal band of BROCA
  - Amygdala
- **nuclei** closely connected to the limbic system (depending on the author, also components of the limbic system):
  - Nucleus anterior thalami
  - Nucleus accumbens
  - Corpora mamillaria
  - Nuclei ventromediales hypothalami
  - habenula nuclei
  - nuclei of the mesencephalon (including Area tegmentalis ventralis)

13.10.3 Neuronal circuits of the limbic system

The various nuclei can be assigned to different neuronal circuits. Due to the close anatomical connections with each other the same structures can also be involved in several circuits. Ultimately, there is no consensus in academic literature on *the* limbic circuits. At this point, the most clinically relevant and important connections for understanding the limbic system major will be presented.

Clinical remarks

'Can talking count as medical treatment?' The significance of **psychotherapy** in the treatment of illnesses is still under debate. The fact is that neuronal processes in the brain lead to behaviour and, vice versa, behaviour and cognitive processes can have an effect on the neuronal networks. The neuronal networks of the brain are plastic structures that are – depending on experiences in conjunction with the environment – constantly changing. This means that learning new forms of behaviour (behavioural therapy, sport and exercise therapy) and the conflict with one's own biography (deep psychological approaches, memory of past experiences) can, in principal, lead to biological changes, e.g., to neural changes of gene expression, protein composition, the number of newly formed nerve cells (neurogenesis), the structure of nerve cells (e g., number and form of synapses) and the function of neural networks. The limbic system is directly involved in many of these processes (biographical memories, emotions, learning of new behaviour). Psychotherapy can thus be considered as a form of therapeutic intervention that can change the brain in its function and structure.

PAPEZ circuit – 'declarative memory'
This circuit was described very early on due to the strong fibre connections between the participating areas (➤ Chap. 13.10.1). Its **switching stations** are:
- the hippocampus formation, and then via
- the fimbria/fornix to the
- Corpora mamillaria and further via the
- Tractus mamillothalamicus to the
- Nuclei anteriores thalami,
- to the Gyrus cinguli
and ultimately back to the hippocampus formation (➤ Fig. 12.11). The **importance of the circulation** of information within the 'PAPEZ circuit' is controversial. Indeed, key components of the PAPEZ circuit are involved in memory processes and their failure leads to disorders of episodic and biographical memory (hippocampus, Corpora mamillaria, Gyrus cinguli). A significant flow of information is with the transfer of information from the hippo-

campus formation to the Gyrus cinguli (➤ Chap. 12.1.6). This is connected to neocortical areas and is involved in the formation of memory tracks and the recall of memories. In this respect, the PAPEZ circuit can be regarded as an important element of the declarative memory system (➤ Chap. 12.1.6).

Amygdala circuit – 'emotional reactions'

The amygdala (➤ Chap. 12.1.8) is – just like the hippocampus formation – a central element of the limbic system. Cytoarchitecturally, 3 larger **core groups** can be differentiated (corticomedial, basolateral, centromedial core groups), of which the afferents and efferents differ in detail. For a general understanding of the amygdala circuit, only an overview of the connections of the amygdala and their functional relevance are given at this point.

Functionally, the amygdala is important for the control of **autonomic** (e.g., heart rate, blood pressure, respiratory rate) and **emotional reactions** (e.g., anxiety, aggression, sex drive, food intake behaviour). In addition, certain forms of learning (conditioning, fear conditioning) are dependent on the amygdala.

These functions are partly understandable due to the **anatomical connections** of the amygdala:

- In this way, the amygdala is closely connected to the **hypothalamus** (ventral amygdalofugal fibres; Stria terminalis), which explains their influence on the autonomic nervous system.
- The amygdala receives important input from the **hippocampus formation** and the **cingulate cortex.** Via this connection, for instance, biographical events are evaluated and connected to emotions. Via connections between the amygdala and the hippocampus formation, the result of this emotional evaluation is reported back to the hippocampus formation. This then decides about the transfer of a memory to the long-term memory.
- Ultimately, the amygdala is still connected to its numerous **brainstem nuclei** (e.g., Area tegmentalis ventralis), which can modulate its activity. Via these connections, e.g., the reward system (see below), emotional evaluation of experiences can be influenced.

> **N O T E**
> The **amygdala** plays a central role in emotions and emotionally-driven behaviour. Emotions are coupled with learning and memory via connections to the hippocampus. Emotions and autonomic reactions are linked through their connections to the hypothalamus.

Mesolimbic circuit – 'reward pathway'

Dopaminergic cells in the mesencephalon (Area tegmentalis ventralis) project to the **Nucleus accumbens.** This pathway is also known as the **'mesolimbic system'** (= mesencephalic-limbic tract) and forms the anatomical basis for success-dependent learning behaviour ('reward pathway'). The Nucleus accumbens is situated next to the anterior ventral striatum (some authors therefore also describe it as the 'ventral striatum') and receives afferents from the amygdala, the hippocampus and the prefrontal cortex. It projects to the pallidum.

It is known from deep brain stimulation that a stimulation of the Nucleus accumbens leads to euphoria and happy feelings. It can, however, also be activated physiologically via the mesolimbic sys-

tem, e.g., when a difficult task has been solved correctly. In this way, the 'correct' behaviour is valued and leads to **positive emotions** (the 'Aha! moment' or 'eureka effect', 'euphoria', 'happiness'). These reinforce the behaviour ('reward pathway'). Via connections to the basal motor system (projection to the pallidum), the Nucleus accumbens can 'practise what it preaches', i.e. a feeling of euphoria can lead to changes in behaviour.

Hypothalamic circuit – 'autonomic regulation'

This system connects the **limbic system** to the hypothalamus and via these to the **autonomic nervous system.** In this way, events, memories and emotions can trigger autonomic reactions such as an increase in heart rate. Essential components of this circuit are:

- the hippocampus formation (via fimbria/fornix),
- the amygdala (via the Stria terminalis; the ventral amygdalofugal fibres)
- the septal nuclei and
- the diagonal band of BROCA (via the Stria medullaris thalami) as well as
- various nuclei in the brainstem via the Tractus mamillotegmentalis; medial anterior horn bundle (see below),

all of which project to the hypothalamus.

Medial forebrain bundle – 'fibre bundle of the limbic system'

In academic literature, the term 'medial forebrain bundle' (**Fasciculus telencephalicus medialis**) is often found in connection with the limbic system. This includes a fibre bundle at the base of the brain, in which mainly axons of different nuclei of the limbic system run together:

- From rostral, these are **descending axons** from the basal prosencephalon, the amygdala and the olfactory medulla, which runs to the lateral hypothalamus and to the tegmentum of the brainstem. They connect limbic structures to the hypothalamus.
- **Ascending axons** originate caudally from brainstem structures that are connected to the limbic system. These include, amongst others, dopaminergic fibres from the Area tegmentalis ventralis to the Nucleus accumbens ('mesolimbic system'). An electrical stimulation of the medial anterior brain bundle can, therefore, lead to euphoria and happy feelings because the reward system of the brain is activated.

> ### Clinical remarks
>
> **Syndromes of the limbic system** are:
> - **hippocampus** – bilateral damage: disruption of the formation of new memory content (mainly anterograde amnesia); affected early on in ALZHEIMER's disease
> - **amygdala** – bilateral damage: KLÜVER-BUCY syndrome: uninhibited sex drive (hypersexuality), loss of sensation of fear, examination of all objects with the mouth (oral tendency), uninhibited exploration behaviour
> - **mesolimbic system** and **Nucleus accumbens** – addictive behaviour: 'reward pathways' is an important mechanism in the development of addiction
> - **Gyrus cinguli** – bilateral damage: akinetic mutism
> - **Corpora mamillaria** – bilateral damage: WERNICKE-KORSAKOW syndrome

Further reading

Books

Aumüller G, Aust G, Doll A. Duale Reihe – Anatomie. 4. A. Stuttgart: Thieme, 2017.

Benninghoff A, Drenckhahn D. Anatomie. Makroskopische Anatomie, Embryologie und Histologie des Menschen, Bd. 1. 17. A. München – Jena: Elsevier, 2008.

Benninghoff A, Drenckhahn D. Anatomie. Makroskopische Anatomie, Embryologie und Histologie des Menschen, Bd. 2. 16. A. München – Jena: Elsevier, 2004.

Blumenfeld H. Neuroanatomy Through Clinical Cases. Sunderland: Sinauer Ass., Inc., Publishers, 2002.

Büttner-Ennever JA, Horn AKE. Olszewski and Baxter's Cytoarchitecture of the Human Brainstem. 3rd ed. Basel: Karger, 2014.

Deller T, Sebesteny T. Fotoatlas Neuroanatomie, München: Elsevier, 2013.

Drake RL, Vogl W, Mitchell AWM. Gray's Anatomie für Studenten. München: Elsevier, 2007.

Drenckhahn D, Waschke J. Benninghoff/Drenckhahn – Taschenbuch Anatomie. 2. A. München: Elsevier, 2014.

Duvernoy HM, Cattin F, Risold P-Y. The Human Hippocampus: Functional Anatomy, Vascularization and Serial Sections. 4th ed. Heidelberg: Springer, 2013.

Feneis H. Anatomisches Bildwörterbuch der internationalen Nomenklatur. 10. A. Stuttgart: Thieme, 2008.

Förderreuther S. Kapitel Kopfschmerzen und andere Schmerzen, Trigeminusneuralgie. In: Diener H-C, Weimar C (Hrsg.). Leitlinien für Diagnostik und Therapie in der Neurologie. Herausgegeben von der Kommission „Leitlinien" der Deutschen Gesellschaft für Neurologie (AWMF-Leitlinie 030/016). Stuttgart: Thieme, 2012.

Grifka J, Kuster M. Orthopädie und Unfallchirurgie. Heidelberg: Springer, 2011.

Hacke W. Neurologie, 14. A. Heidelberg: Springer, 2015.

Hudspith MJ, Siddall PJ, Munglani R. Physiology of Pain in Foundations of Anesthesia by Hemmings and Hopkins. 2nd ed. St. Louis: Elsevier – Mosby, 2006.

Kahle W, Frotscher M. Taschenatlas Anatomie: Bd. 3, Nervensystem und Sinnesorgane. 12. A. Stuttgart: Thieme, 2018.

Kandel ER et al. Principles of Neural Science. 5th ed. New York: McGraw-Hill Professional, 2012.

Kretschmann H-J, Weinrich W. Klinische Neuroanatomie und kranielle Bilddiagnostik. 3. A. Stuttgart: Thieme, 2007.

Krstić RV. Human Microscopic Anatomy. Heidelberg: Springer, 1991.

Kummer B. Biomechanik. Köln: Deutscher Ärzte-Verlag, 2005.

Lang J, Wachsmuth W. Lanz-Wachsmuth – Praktische Anatomie – Bein und Statik. 2. A. Heidelberg: Springer, 2004.

Lang J. Klinische Anatomie der Nase, Nasenhöhle und Nebenhöhlen. Stuttgart: Thieme, 1988.

Lang KG. Augenheilkunde. 5. A. Stuttgart: Thieme, 2014.

Leonhardt H, Tillmann B. Rauber/Kopsch – Innere Organe, Bd. 2, Stuttgart: Thieme, 1987.

Lippert H, Pabst R. Arterial Variations in Man. München: J.F. Bergmann, 1985.

Lippert H. Lehrbuch Anatomie. 8. A. München: Elsevier, 2017.

Loeweneck H, Feifel G, Wachsmuth W. Lanz-Wachsmuth – Praktische Anatomie – Bauch, 2. A. Heidelberg: Springer, 2004.

Lüllmann-Rauch R. Taschenlehrbuch Histologie. 5. A. Stuttgart: Thieme, 2015.

Mai JK, Paxinos G. The Human Nervous System. 3rd ed. San Diego, London: Academic Press, 2012.

Moore KL, Dalley AF, Agur AMR. Clinically Oriented Anatomy. 7th ed. Wolters Kluwer Health, 2011.

Moore KL, Persaud TVN, Torchia MG, Viebahn C. Embryologie. 6. A. München: Elsevier, 2013.

Müller-Vahl H, Mumenthaler M, Stöhr M, Tegenhoff M. Läsionen peripherer Nerven und radikuläre Syndrome. 10. A. Stuttgart: Thieme, 2014.

Netter FH. Atlas der Anatomie, 6. A. München: Elsevier, 2015.

Nieuwenhuys R, Voogd J, van Huijzen Chr. Das Zentralnervensystem des Menschen. 2. A. Springer, Heidelberg, 1991.

Pape H.-Ch. et al. Physiologie. 8. A. Stuttgart: Thieme, 2018.

Paulsen F, Waschke J. Sobotta Atlas der Anatomie – Band 2: Innere Organe. 24. A. München: Elsevier, 2017.

Paulsen F. Anatomy and physiology of the nasolacrimal ducts. In: Weber R, Keerl R, Schaefer SD, Della Rocca RC (eds). Atlas of Lacrimal Surgery. Berlin, Heidelberg, New York: Springer, 2007:1-13.

Paulsen K. Einführung in die Hals-, Nasen-, Ohrenheilkunde. Stuttgart: Schattauer, 1978.

Purves D et al. Neuroscience, 3rd ed. Sunderland: Sinauer Ass., Inc., Publishers, 2004.

Robertson D et al. Primer on the Autonomic Nervous System. 3rd ed. San Diego, London: Academic Press, 2012.

Rohen J, Lütjen-Drecoll E. Funktionelle Anatomie des Menschen. Stuttgart: Schattauer, 2006.

Rohen J, Lütjen-Drecoll E. Funktionelle Embryologie. 5. A. Stuttgart: Schattauer, 2016.

Schiebler TH, Korf H-W. Anatomie. 10. A. Heidelberg: Steinkopff, 2007.

Schünke M, Schulte E, Schumacher U. Prometheus Lernatlas der Anatomie – Allgemeine Anatomie und Bewegungssystem. 4. A. Stuttgart: Thieme, 2014.

Schünke M. Funktionelle Anatomie – Topografie und Funktion des Bewegungssystems. 2. A. Stuttgart: Thieme 2014.

Speckmann E-J, Hescheler J, Köhling R. Physiologie. 6. A. München: Elsevier, 2013.

Squire LR et al. (eds.). Fundamental Neuroscience. 4th ed. San Diego, London: Academic Press, 2012.

Standring S. Gray's Anatomy. 41st ed. Edinburgh: Churchill Livingstone – Elsevier, 2015.

Steward O. Functional Neuroscience. New York: Springer, 2000.

Strutz J, Mann W. Praxis der HNO-Heilkunde. Kopf- und Halschirurgie. 3. A. Stuttgart: Thieme, 2017.

Szabo K, Hennerici MG (Hrsg.). The Hippocampus in Clinical Neuroscience. Front Neurol Neurosci. Basel: Karger, 2014.

Tillmann B, Schünke M. Taschenatlas zum Präparierkurs. Eine klinisch orientierte Anleitung. Stuttgart: Thieme, 1993.

Tillmann B, Töndury G, Zilles K. Rauber/Kopsch – Bewegungsapparat, Bd. 1. 3. A. Stuttgart: Thieme 2003.

Tillmann B, Töndury G, Zilles K. Rauber/Kopsch – Topographie der Organsysteme, Systematik der peripheren Leitungsbahnen, Bd. 4. Stuttgart: Thieme, 1988.

Tillmann B, Wustrow F. Kehlkopf. In: Berendes J, Link R, Zöllner F. (Hrsg.) Hals-Nasen-Ohren-Heilkunde in Praxis und Klinik. Bd. IV/1. Stuttgart, New York: Thieme, 1982:1-101.

Tillmann B. Farbatlas der Anatomie Zahnmedizin – Humanmedizin. Stuttgart: Thieme, 1997.

Von Lanz T, Wachsmuth W. Lanz-Wachsmuth – Praktische Anatomie – Arm. 2. A. Heidelberg: Springer, 2004.

Welsch U, Kummer W. (Hrsg.). Lehrbuch Histologie, 4. A. München: Elsevier, 2014.

Zilles K, Tillmann B. Anatomie. 1. A. Heidelberg: Springer, 2010.

Articles and essays

Abdul-Khaliq H, Berger F. Die Diagnose wird häufig zu spät gestellt. Dtsch Arztebl Int 2011;108(31-32):1433 ff.

Antoniadis G et al. Iatrogene Nervenläsionen. Dtsch Arztebl Int 2014;111 (16):273 ff.

Assmus H, Antoniadis G, Bischoff C. Karpaltunnel-, Kubitaltunnel- und seltene Nervenkompressionssyndrome. Dtsch Arztebl Int 2015;112 (1-2):14 ff.

Bajo VM, King AJ. Cortical modulation of auditory processing in the midbrain. Frontiers in Neural Circuits 2013;6:114.

Benarroch EE. Circumventricular organs, receptive and homeostatic functions and clinical implications. Neurology 2011;77(12):1198–204.

Bigioli P et al. Upper and lower spinal cord blood supply: The continuity of the anterior spinal artery and the relevance of the lumbar arteries. J Thorac Cardiovasc Surg 2004;127:1188–92.

Bosco G, Poppele RE. Proprioception from a spinocerebellar perspective. Physiological Reviews 2001;81:539–68.

Bouthillier A, van Loveren HR, Keller JT. Segments of the internal carotid artery: a new classification. Neurosurgery 1996;38:425–32.

Cascio CJ. Somatosensory processing in neurodevelopmental disorders. J Neurodevelop Disorder 2010;2:62–9.

Chiappedi M, Bejor M. Corpus callosum agenesis and rehabilitative treatment. Italian Journal of Pediatrics 2010;36:64–70.

Claes S et al. Anatomy of the anterolateral ligament of the knee. Journal of Anatomy 2013;223:321–8.

Deluca J, Diamond BJ. Aneurysm of the anterior communicating artery: A review of neuroanatomical and neuropsychological sequelae. J Clin Exp Neuropsych 1995;17:100–21.

Eftekhar B et al. Are the distributions of variations of circle of Willis different in different populations? Results of an anatomical study and review of literature. BMC Neurology 2006;6:22

Elbert T et al. Alteration of digital representations in somatosensory cortex in focal hand dystonia. Neuro Report 1998;9(16):3571–5.

Eliot L. The trouble with sex differences. Neuron 2011;72(6):895–8.

Esaki T et al. Surgical management for glossopharyngeal neuralgia associated with cardiac syncope: two case reports. Br J Neurosurg 2007;21(6):599–602.

Etkin A, Egner T, Kalisch R. Emotional processing in anterior cingulate and medial prefrontal cortex. Trends Cognitive Sci 2011;15:85–93.

Fowler CJ, Griffiths D, de Groat WC. The neural control of micturition. Nat Rev Neurosci 2008;9:453–66.

Gates P. Work out where the problem is in the brainstem using "the rule of 4". Pract Neurol 2011;11:167–72.

Goost H et al. Frakturen des oberen Sprunggelenks. Dtsch Arztebl Int 2014;111 (21):377 ff.

Goto F, Ban Y, Tsutumi T. Bilateral acute audiovestibular deficit with complete ocular tilt reaction and absent VEMPs. Eur Arch Otorhinolaryngol 2011;268:1093–6.

Griffiths TD et al. Sound movement detection deficit due to a brainstem lesion. J Neurol Neurosurg Psychiatry 1997;62:522–6.

Günther P, Rübben I. Akutes Skrotum im Kinder- und Jugendalter. Dtsch Arztebl Int 2012;109(25):449 ff.

Hamon M et al. Consensus document on the radial approach in percutaneous cardiovascular interventions: position paper by the European Association of Percutaneous Cardiovascular Interventions and Working Groups on Acute Cardiac Care and Thrombosis of the European Society of Cardiology. EuroIntervention 2013;8:1242–51.

Handley TPB et al. Collet-Sicard syndrome from thrombosis of the sigmoid-jugular complex: A case report and review of the literature. Int J Otolaryngol. 2010;2010:1–5.

Hendrikse J et al. Distribution of cerebral blood flow in the circle of Willis. Radiology 2005;235:184–9.

Hoksbergen AW et al. Absent collateral function of the circle of Willis as risk factor for ischemic stroke. Cerebrovasc Dis 2003;16:191–8.

Janni W et al. Sentinel-Node-Biopsie und Axilladissektion beim Mammakarzinom. Dtsch Arztebl Int 2014;111 (14):244 ff.

Jelev L. Some unusual types of formation of the Ansa cervicalis in humans and proposal of a new morphological classification. Clin Anat 2013;26(8):961–5.

Johanson CE et al. Multiplicity of cerebrospinal fluid functions: New challenges in health and disease. Cerebrospinal Fluid Res 2008;5:10.

Kapoor K, Singh B, Dewan LI. Variations in the configuration of the circle of Willis. Anat Sci Int 2008;83:96–106.

Kawashima T, Sasaki H. Gross anatomy of the human cardiac conduction system with comparative morphological and developmental implications for human application. Ann Anat 2011;193:1–12.

Kutta H, Knipping S, Claassen H, Paulsen F. Update Larynx: funktionelle Anatomie unter klinischen Gesichtspunkten. Teil 1: Entwicklung, Kehlkopfskelett, Gelenke, Stimmlippenansatz, Muskulatur. HNO 2007;55:583–98.

Kutta H, Knipping S, Claassen H, Paulsen F. Update Larynx: Funktionelle Anatomie unter klinischen Gesichtspunkten. Teil 2: Kehlkopfschleimhaut, Blutgefäßversorgung, Innervation, Lymphabfluss, Altersveränderungen. HNO 2007;55:661–75.

Kutta H, Steven P, Paulsen F. Anatomical definition of the subglottic region. Cells Tissues Organs 2006;184:205–14.

Labenz J et al. 2015. Epidemiologie, Diagnostik und Therapie des Barrett-Karzinoms. Dtsch Arztebl Int 2015;112 (13):224 ff.

Labib S et al. Congenital insensitivity to pain with anhydrosis: a report of a family case. Pan Afr Med J 2011;9:33–8.

Lanz U, Engelhardt TO, Giunta R. Neues aus der Handchirurgie. Bayerisches Ärzteblatt 2012;9:432 ff.

Lavezzi AM, Matturri L. Functional neuroanatomy of the human pre-Bötzinger complex with particular reference to sudden unexplained perinatal and infant death. Neuropathology 2008;28:10–6.

Lloyd S. Accessory nerve: anatomy and surgical identification. J Laryngol Otol 2007;121(12):1118–25.

Lopez C, Blanke O. The thalamocortical vestibular system in animals and humans. Brain Research Reviews 2011;67:119-46.

Mai H-X, Cheng L, Chen Q-C. Neural interactions in unilateral colliculus and between bilateral colliculi modulate auditory signal processing. Frontiers in Neural Circuits 2013;7:68.

Marinkovic S, Milisavljevic M, Puskas L. Microvascular anatomy of the hippocampal formation. Surg Neurol 1992;37:339–49.

Melzack R, Wall PD. Pain mechanism: A new theory. Science 1965;150(3699):971–9.

Meyer K. Primary sensory cortices, top-down projections and conscious experience. Prog Neurobiol 2011;94(4):408–17.

Ossipov MH, Dussor GO, Porecca F. Central modulation of pain. J Clin Invest 2010;120(11):3779–87.

Palacek J. The role of dorsal columns pathway in visceral pain. Physiol Res 2004;53:125–30.

Paulsen F et al. Arching and looping of the internal carotid artery with relation to the pharynx – frequency, embryology, and clinical implications. J Anat 2000;197:373–81.

Paulsen F, Tillmann B. Functional anatomy of the posterior insertion of the human vocal ligament. Eur Arch Otorhinolaryngol 1997;254:442–8.

Paulsen F, Tillmann B. Struktur und Funktion des ventralen Stimmbandansatzes. Laryngo-Rhino-Otol 1996;75:590–6.

Paulsen F. Anatomie und Physiologie der ableitenden Tränenwege. Ophthalmologe 2008;105:339–45.

Paulsen F. The human nasolacrimal ducts. Adv Anat Embryol Cell Biol 2003;170:1–106.

Raptis D et al. Differentialdiagnose und interdisziplinäre Therapie des Analkarzinoms. Dtsch Arztebl Int 2015;112(14):243 ff.

Rogers RC, McTigue DM, Hermann GE. Vagovagal reflex control of digestion: afferent modulation by neural and "endoendocrine" factors. Am J Physiol 1995;268(1 Pt 1):G1–10.

Rüb U et al. Anatomically based guidelines for systematic investigation of the central somatosensory system and their application to a spinocerebellar ataxia type 2 (SCA2) patient. Neuropathol Appl Neurobiol 2003;29:418–33.

Safari A, Khaledi AA, Vojdani M. Congenital insensitivity to pain with anhidrosis (CI-PA): A case report. Iran Red Crescent Med J 2011;13(2):134–8.

Schaller B, Lyrer Ph. A. spinalis-anterior-Syndrom: Eine wichtige Differentialdiagnose zu den akuten nicht-traumatischen Rückenmarksquerschnittssyndromen. Praxis 2001;90:1420–7.

Schild HH. Therapieoptionen beim Chylothorax. Dtsch Arztebl Int 2013;110(48);819 ff.

Szabo K et al. Hippocampal lesion patterns in acute posterior cerebral artery stroke. Stroke 2009;40:2042–5.

Tascioglu AO, Tascioglu AB. Ventricular anatomy: illustrations and concepts from antiquity to renaissance. Neuroanatomy 2005;4:57–83.

Thakar A, Deepak KK, Kumar SS. Auricular syncope. J Laryngol Otol 2008;122(10):1115–7.

Thömke F et al. Cerebrovascular brainstem diseases with isolated cranial nerve palsy. Cerebrovasc Dis 2001;13:147–55.

Thompson D. Hydrocephalus. Neurosurgery 2009;27:130–4.

Tsivgoulis G et al. Bilateral ageusia caused by a unilateral midbrain and thalamic infarction. J. Neuroimaging 2011;21:263–5.

Tubbs RS et al. Cranial roots of the accessory nerve exist in the majority of adult humans. Clin Anat 2014;27(1):102–7.

Wengen DF et al. Diagnostik der Liquorrhoe bei Schädelbasisläsionen. Schweiz Med Wochensch 2000;130:1715–25.

Wiesmann M et al. Identification and anatomic description of the anterior choroidal artery by use of 3D-TOF source and 3D-CISS MR imaging. AJNR 2001;22:305–10.

Wilson MH et al. Cerebral venous system and anatomical predisposition to high-altitude headache. Ann Neurol 2013;73:381–9.

Wise E, Malik O, Husain M. Lesson of the month. Is that your arm or mine? Clin Med 2010;10:633–4.

Wittkowski W, Bockmann J, Kreutz MR, Böckers TM. Cell and molecular biology of the pars tuberalis of the pituitary. Int Rev Cytol 1999;185:157–94.

Wright BL, Lai JT, Sinclair AJ. Cerebrospinal fluid and lumbar puncture: a practical review. J Neurol 2012;258 (8):1530–45.

Wülker N, Mittag F. Therapie des Hallux valgus. Dtsch Arztebl Int 2012;109(49):857 ff.

Zylka-Menhorn V. A. radialis ist Zugang erster Wahl. Dtsch Arztebl Int 2013:110(10):398 ff.

Further reading

Index

Index

G

O

W

X

Y

Z